DIAGNOSTIC MEDICAL SONOGRAPHY

Abdomen and Superficial Structures

DIAGNOSTIC MEDICAL SONOGRAPHY

Abdomen and Superficial Structures

FIFTH EDITION

Diane M. Kawamura, PhD, RT(R), RDMS, FSDMS, FAIUM
Professor Emeritus, School of Radiologic Sciences
Brady Presidential Distinguished Professor Emeritus
Weber State University
Ogden, Utah

Tanya D. Nolan, EdD, RT(R), RDMS
Professor
School of Radiologic Sciences
Weber State University
Ogden, Utah

. Wolters Kluwer

Philadelphia • Baltimore • New York • London
Buenos Aires • Hong Kong • Sydney • Tokyo

Acquisitions Editor: Nicole Dernoski
Development Editor: Eric McDermott
Editorial Coordinator: Oliver Raj
Editorial Assistant: Kristen Kardoley
Marketing Manager: Kirsten Watrud
Production Project Manager: Kirstin Johnson
Manager, Graphic Arts & Design: Stephen Druding
Manufacturing Coordinator: Beth Welsh
Prepress Vendor: S4Carlisle Publishing Services

Fifth Edition

9 8 7 6 5 4 3 2 1

Printed in Singapore

Library of Congress Cataloging-in-Publication Data

Names: Kawamura, Diane M., editor. | Nolan, Tanya D., editor.
Title: Diagnostic medical sonography. Abdomen and superficial structures /
  [edited by] Diane M Kawamura, Tanya D. Nolan.
Other titles: Abdomen and superficial structures
Description: Fifth edition. | Philadelphia: Lippincott Williams & Wilkins,
  [2023] | Includes bibliographical references and index. | Summary:
  "Kawamura and Nolan's Diagnostic Medical Sonography: Abdomen and
  Superficial Structures, 5th Edition provides an up-to-date,
  comprehensive, and consistent treatment of abdominal sonography. And is
  an integral part of the updated Diagnostic Medical Sonography Series"—
  Provided by publisher.
Identifiers: LCCN 2022016361 (print) | LCCN 2022016362 (ebook) | ISBN
  9781975174972 (hardcover) | ISBN 9781975174989 (ebook)
Subjects: MESH: Abdomen—diagnostic imaging | Ultrasonography—methods |
  Digestive System—diagnostic imaging | Urogenital System—diagnostic
  imaging
Classification: LCC RC944 (print) | LCC RC944 (ebook) | NLM WI 141 | DDC
  617.5/507543—dc23/eng/20220608
LC record available at https://lccn.loc.gov/2022016361
LC ebook record available at https://lccn.loc.gov/2022016362

shop.lww.com

To Mimi Berman (Volume I) and Marveen Craig (Volume II), who invited me to join their team and to oversee and develop Volume III Abdomen. As the fifth edition is nearing closure, my appreciation is elevated for Mimi and Marveen's first edition help as they were insightful, encouraging, role models, mentors, etc.

To my late husband, Bryan, who provided me with confidence and who always supported my professional endeavors. I miss my favorite companion and best friend. To our wonderful children, Stephanie and Nathan, who continue to inspire me to appreciate how important it is to learn new things and to enjoy learning. To all my colleagues on campus and in the profession who provide encouragement, support, and stimulating new challenges.
—DIANE M. KAWAMURA

To my husband and best friend, Trent, whose unconditional love and encouragement has sustained me through every challenge and enriched my life's journey. To my amazing children, Joseph, Ethan, and Spencer, for inspiring me to become a better person and for filling my dreams with hope and joy. To my many colleagues, for giving me the strength and motivation to aim high, learn more, and be determined to the end.
—TANYA D. NOLAN

And to students and professionals who will use this book:
"Any piece of knowledge I acquire today has a value at this moment exactly proportioned to my skill to deal with it. Tomorrow, when I know more, I recall that piece of knowledge and use it better."—Mark Van Doren, Liberal Education (1960)
—DIANE M. KAWAMURA, TANYA D. NOLAN

CONTRIBUTORS

Sharlette Anderson, MHS, RDMS, RVT, RDCS
Sonography Educator
Clinical Sonographer
Foulton, Missouri

Anjum N. Bandarkar, MD
Pediatric Radiologist, Section Chief–Ultrasound
Department of Imaging
Mid-Atlantic Permanente Medical Group
Tysons Corner, Virginia

Teresa M. Bieker, MBA-H, RT(R), RDMS, RDCS, RVT, CRA
Radiology Manager
Division of Ultrasound
UCHealth, University of Colorado Hospital
Aurora, Colorado

Joie Burns, MS, RT(R)(S), RDMS, RVT
Emeritus Professor, Radiologic Sciences
Boise State University
Boise, Idaho

Catherine Carr-Hoefer, CRA, RT(R), RDMS, RDCS, RVT, FSDMS
Sound Imaging Consulting, LLC
Corvallis, Oregon

Aaron M. Chandler, BA, RDMS, RVT
Lead Sonographer
Alta Bates Summit Medicare Center
Oakland, California

Tara K. Cielma, BS, RT(S), RDMS, RDCS, RVT
Lead Sonographer, Clinical Education
Department of Diagnostic Imaging and Radiology
Children's National Hospital
Washington, District of Columbia

M. Robert DeJong, RDMS, RDCS, RVT, FAIUM, FSDMS
Bob DeJong, LLC
Ultrasound Education Company
Rosedale, Maryland

Kevin D. Evans, PhD, RT(R)(M)(BD), RDMS, RVS, FSDMS, FAIUM
Professor, Division Director, Radiologic Sciences & Respiratory Therapy
Director, Laboratory for Investigatory Imping
The Ohio State University College of Medicine
Columbus, Ohio

Tim S. Gibbs, BS, RT(R), RDMS, RVT, CTNM
Adjunct Faculty
Orange Coase College
Anaheim, California

Barbara Hall-Terracciano, BS, RT(R)(M), RDMS
Clinical Sonography
Author/Editor
St. George, Utah

Charlotte Henningsen, MS, RT(R), RDMS, RVT, FSDMS, FAIUM
Director for Faculty Development in Teaching and Learning
Director and Professor Center for Advanced Ultrasound Education
AdventHealth University
Orlando, Florida

Diane M. Kawamura, PhD, RT(R), RDMS, FSDMS, FAIUM
Professor Emeritus, School of Radiologic Sciences
Brady Presidential Distinguished Professor Emeritus
Weber State University
Ogden, Utah

George M. Kennedy-Antillon, AS, RDMS, RDCS, RVT
Instructor/Sonographer
School of Medicine
University of Colorado Anschutz Medical Campus
Denver, Colorado

Wayne C. Leonhardt, BA, RDMS, RVT
Ultrasound Education Consultant
Master Scanning Laboratory Clinical Vascular Instructor
Medical Arts, DMS Program, Gurnick Academy
San Mateo, California
Staff Sonographer
Mission Imaging and Mission Hospital
Asheville, North Carolina

Tanya D. Nolan, EdD, RT(R), RDMS
Professor
School of Radiologic Sciences
Weber State University
Ogden, Utah

Ambree Penrod, MEd, RT(R), RDMS
Assistant Professor
School of Radiologic Sciences
Weber State University
Ogden, Utah

Javier Rosario, MD, FACEP
Division Director, Emergency Ultrasound
UCF/HCA Emergency Medicine Residency Program of
  Greater Orlando
Orlando, Florida

Aubrey J. Rybyinski, BS, RDMS, RVT
Senior Clinical Manager
NAVIX Diagnostix
Taunton, Massachusetts

Jeanine Rybyinski, AAS, RDMS, RVT
Staff Sonographer
Inspira Health Network
Turnersville, New Jersey

Kellie A. Schmidt, BS, RDMS, RVT, RDCS
Lead Diagnostic Medical Sonographer
Division of Ultrasound
University of Colorado Hospital
Aurora, Colorado

Cathie Scholl, DHSc, RDMS, RVT
Associate Professor
Cardiovascular Sonography Program
Nova Southeastern University
Clearwater, Florida

Susan Raatz Stephenson, MS, MAEd, RDMS, RVT, RT(CT)(ARRT)
Global Education Manager–General Imaging
Siemens Healthineers
Pagosa Springs, Colorado

Amber Wooten, MSHS, RT(R), RDMS, RVT
Program Director/Assistant Professor
Diagnostic Medical Sonography
Arkansas State University
Jonesboro, Arkansas

PREFACE

The fifth edition of *Diagnostic Medical Sonography: Abdomen and Superficial Structures* is updated to reflect the major developments that have occurred since the last edition. Educators and colleagues encouraged us to produce a fifth edition to incorporate new advances used to image, to refresh the foundational content, and to continue to provide information that recognizes readers have diverse backgrounds and experiences. The result is a textbook that can be used as either an introduction to the profession or a reference for the profession. The content lays the foundation for a better understanding of anatomy, physiology, and pathophysiology to enhance the caregiving role of the sonographer practitioner, sonographer, sonologist, or student when securing the imaging information on a patient.

The first section is focused on Sonography Fundamentals. Readers are introduced to pertinent professional terminology, ergonomics, anatomy, scanning planes, and patient positions. Adopting universal terminology permits every sonographer to communicate consistent information about the profession, how he or she scans the patient, and the anatomy and pathology that are sonographically represented.

The following four sections are divided into specific content areas including abdominal sonography, superficial structure sonography, neonatal and pediatric sonography, and special study sonography. Doing this allowed the contributors to focus their attention on a specific organ or system. This simulates application in that while scanning, the sonographer investigates the organ or system, moves systematically to the next organ or system, and completes the examination by synthesizing all the information to obtain the total picture.

We made every attempt to produce an up-to-date and factual textbook while presenting the material in an interesting and enjoyable format to capture the reader's attention. To do this, we provided detailed descriptions of anatomy, physiology, pathology, and the normal and abnormal sonographic representation of these anatomic and pathologic entities with illustrations, summary tables, and images, many of which include valuable case study information.

Our goal is to present as complete and current of a text as possible, while recognizing that by tomorrow, the textbook must be supplemented with new information reflecting the dynamic sonography profession. With every technologic advance made in equipment, the sonographer's imagination must stretch to create new applications. With the comprehensive foundation available in this book, the sonographer can meet that challenge.

Diane M. Kawamura
Tanya D. Nolan

We appreciate the continued support, ideas, and collaboration of Anne Marie Kupinski, Susan Stephenson, and Julia Dmitrieva who have worked on the volumes of *Diagnostic Medical Sonography*. We also acknowledge Ambree Penrod for her contributions to the accompanying workbook. Their input and ideas were a significant contribution to the project.

Our thanks and gratitude go to all the authors and contributors of the fifth edition who gave of their expertise, time, and energy, updating the content with current information to use in obtaining a more accurate imaging examination for our patients.

We thank the many sonographers and physicians for their assistance in obtaining images. A continued recognition for the support and images acquired by Taco Geertsma, MD, Ede, the Netherlands, at Ultrasoundcases.info, Copyright ownership: SonoSkills, the Netherlands, and Siemens Medical Solutions USA, Inc.; Philips Medical Systems, Bothell, Washington; GE Healthcare, Wauwatosa, Wisconsin; Joe Anton, MD, Cochin, India; Dr. Nakul Jerath, Falls Church, Virginia; Monica Bacani and Rechelle Nguyen at Nationwide Children's Hospital in Columbus, Ohio; and Ted Whitten, ultrasound practitioner, Elliot Hospital, Manchester, New Hampshire.

Many thanks to the production team at Wolters Kluwer, who helped edit, produce, promote, and deliver this textbook. We especially thank in the development of this edition, and the previous edition, Sharon Zinner, Eric McDermott (development editor), Heidi Grauel (freelance editor), Oliver Raj (editorial coordinator), and Jennifer Clements (art director) for their patience, follow-through, support, and encouragement.

To our colleagues, students, friends, and family, who provide continued sources of encouragement, enthusiasm, and inspiration—thank you.

Diane M. Kawamura
Tanya D. Nolan

USING THIS SERIES

The books in the *Diagnostic Medical Sonography* series will help you develop an understanding of specialty sonography topics. Key learning resources and tools throughout the textbook aim to increase your understanding of the topics provided and better prepare you for your professional career. This user's guide will help you familiarize yourself with these exciting features designed to enhance your learning experience.

Chapter Objectives

Measurable objectives listed at the beginning of each chapter help you understand the intended outcomes for the chapter, as well as recognize and study important concepts within each chapter.

Glossary

Key terms are listed at the beginning of each chapter and clearly defined, then highlighted in bold type throughout the chapter to help you to learn and recall important terminology.

Pathology Boxes

Each chapter includes tables of relevant pathologies, which you can use as a quick reference for reviewing the material.

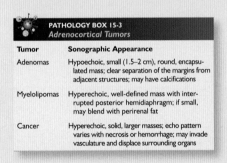

PATHOLOGY BOX 15-3
Adrenocortical Tumors

Tumor	Sonographic Appearance
Adenomas	Hypoechoic, small (1.5–2 cm), round, encapsulated mass; clear separation of the margins from adjacent structures; may have calcifications
Myelolipomas	Hyperechoic, well-defined mass with interrupted posterior hemidiaphragm; if small, may blend with perirenal fat
Cancer	Hyperechoic, solid, larger masses; echo pattern varies with necrosis or hemorrhage; may invade vasculature and displace surrounding organs

Resources

You will also find additional resources and exercises on thePoint, including a glossary with pronunciations, quiz bank, sonographic video clips, and weblinks. Use these interactive resources to test your knowledge, assess your progress, and review for quizzes and tests.

INTRODUCTION TO SONOGRAPHY

PART ONE

CHAPTER 1

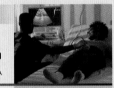

The Sonography Profession

DIANE M. KAWAMURA

OBJECTIVES

- Define the meaning of profession, professional, and professionalism.
- Identify the sonography legacy, the evolution of the profession, and the creation of an occupation.
- Compare the member benefits obtained for each sonography professional organization.
- Provide the rationale and function for each type of accreditation.
- Differentiate the different meaning of credential, certification, and licensure.
- State the importance of maintaining the credential.
- Analyze the essentials incorporated in the Scope of Practice and Clinical Standards.
- Discuss why the role of the sonographer is vital in health care.

KEY TERMS

accreditation
certification
credential
licensure
profession
professional
professionalism
scope of practice

GLOSSARY

sonogram pictorial (graphic) record of a sonography examination

sonographer highly skilled professional qualified by academic and clinical education who uses diagnostic ultrasound equipment to provide patient services that assist physicians in gathering sonographic data necessary to reach a diagnostic decision or a list of differential diagnostic findings

sonography imaging technique using ultrasound to produce a two-dimensional, three-dimensional, cross-sectional, or vascular flow imaging to create a graphical representation of the tissue; it is more of an inclusive term than ultrasonography

sonologist a physician who interprets sonograms

ultrasound acoustic oscillations (sound) having a frequency above the highest frequency limit of audible sound humans can hear (which is about 20 kHz)

This chapter introduces the sonography profession, which includes sonographers and sonologists. Sonographers are health care professionals who are educated to use imaging equipment, sound waves, and echoes to acquire and to evaluate sonograms in order to determine when sufficient imaging data have been recorded. Sonologists are physicians who interpret sonograms. Sonograms are the recorded images of a sonography examination.

IMPORTANT DEFINITIONS

Profession

A profession can be described as a group of disciplined individuals who adhere to ethical standards.[1,2] When sonography is defined as an occupation, its definition is limited and refers only to the activity the sonographer renders for

CONTENTS

PART THREE | SUPERFICIAL STRUCTURE SONOGRAPHY

PART FOUR | NEONATAL AND PEDIATRIC SONOGRAPHY

PART FIVE | SPECIAL STUDY SONOGRAPHY

CHAPTER 1

The Sonography Profession

DIANE M. KAWAMURA

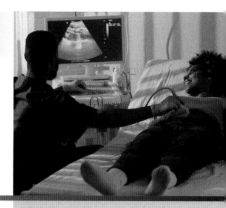

OBJECTIVES

- Define the meaning of profession, professional, and professionalism.
- Identify the sonography legacy, the evolution of the profession, and the creation of an occupation.
- Compare the member benefits obtained for each sonography professional organization.
- Provide the rationale and function for each type of accreditation.
- Differentiate the different meaning of credential, certification, and licensure.
- State the importance of maintaining the credential.
- Analyze the essentials incorporated in the Scope of Practice and Clinical Standards.
- Discuss why the role of the sonographer is vital in health care.

KEY TERMS

accreditation

certification

credential

licensure

profession

professional

professionalism

scope of practice

GLOSSARY

sonogram pictorial (graphic) record of a sonography examination

sonographer highly skilled professional qualified by academic and clinical education who uses diagnostic ultrasound equipment to provide patient services that assist physicians in gathering sonographic data necessary to reach a diagnostic decision or a list of differential diagnostic findings

sonography imaging technique using ultrasound to produce a two-dimensional, three-dimensional, cross-sectional, or vascular flow imaging to create a graphical representation of the tissue; it is more of an inclusive term than ultrasonography

sonologist a physician who interprets sonograms

ultrasound acoustic oscillations (sound) having a frequency above the highest frequency limit of audible sound humans can hear (which is about 20 kHz)

This chapter introduces the sonography profession, which includes sonographers and sonologists. Sonographers are health care professionals who are educated to use imaging equipment, sound waves, and echoes to acquire and to evaluate sonograms in order to determine when sufficient imaging data have been recorded. Sonologists are physicians who interpret sonograms. Sonograms are the recorded images of a sonography examination.

IMPORTANT DEFINITIONS

Profession

A profession can be described as a group of disciplined individuals who adhere to ethical standards.[1,2] When sonography is defined as an occupation, its definition is limited and refers only to the activity the sonographer renders for the salary the sonographer receives.[2] Although members of any profession can be linked to monetary compensation, the definition for an occupation and the definition for a profession are not synonymous. The sonography profession is made up of those individuals who have completed specialized academic courses and acquired clinical scanning competencies in an educational, a clinical, and/or a research environment. To ensure uniformity of each individual in the profession, a graduate sonographer must be competent to meet the profession's criteria.[1-3]

Professional

A professional is a member of a profession and adheres to the required codes of conduct, ethics, standards, and guidelines and is accountable to those they serve and to society.[1,2] Normally, professionals are perceived as competent, are known and respected for their specialized knowledge, and for keeping this knowledge current.[4] A sonographer should understand that professional behavior is determined from one's aptitudes, attributes, and attitudes.[5] Table 1-1 presents a summary of definitions and a positive example of professional aptitudes, attributes, attitude, and behavior.[5-9] Sonographers can determine if their professional standards

need to be enhanced by routine and thorough evaluation of how their aptitude, attributes, and attitude affect their professional behavior and their professional competency. Figure 1-1 illustrates the relationship of aptitude, attributes, and attitude to behavior.[10] One can judge someone's behavior but not their aptitude, attributes, and attitude.

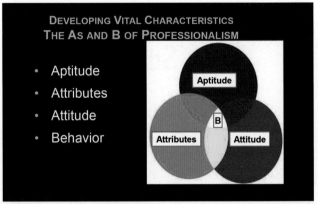

FIGURE 1-1 The three As and the B join to develop the vital characteristics of professionalism.

TABLE 1-1	Professional Aptitudes, Attributes, Attitude, and Behavior[5-9]	
	Definition	**Positive Characteristics**
Aptitudes	• Inherent/natural abilities for learning and performance • Competence to perform a specific type of work at a certain level • Capacity for learning • Skill matches position descriptions	• Ability to produce a diagnostic-quality sonographic image • Credentialed in one or more sonography specialty/specialties • Problem-solving skills • Emotional stability
Attributes	• Everything that makes up a person • Quality or characteristic owned by someone • Comprise a person's building block • Innate and come from within	• Self-confidence • Willingness to help others • Ability to follow directions • Empathy • Honesty, integrity • Conscientiousness • Emotional intelligence
Attitude	• What one thinks (one cannot judge attitude) • Set of feelings, memories, emotions, and beliefs • Internal and individual mindsets • Difficult to change attitude • Unlike attributes, attitudes are created	• Altruism—selflessness • Honor (integrity, honesty) • Respect • Caring, empathetic • Responsibility, accountability • Self-improvement • Scholarship • Leadership • Professional demeanor
Behavior	• What one does • Behavior can be judged • Behavior is how one responds to attitude	• Excellent communication skills • Patient treated as individual rather than an exam • Patients' best interest, rights, dignity, and confidentiality first • Accepts and incorporates supervisors' feedback • Makes deliberate choices • Takes responsibility for one's actions • Teaches and helps sonographers who are busy • Contributes to the profession and/or professional organization • Avoids making excuses, accepts responsibility, admits to mistakes and errors • Adheres to professional codes of conduct • Committed to lifelong learning and stays up to date on knowledge and skills • Dress, appearance, and behavior follow demeanor • Articulates gratitude and says thank you

Professionalism

The roof of professionalism is the profession. The profession is where disciplined individuals adhere to professional standards.[8] The word *professionalism* is based on the word *professional*, which describes a member of a profession. Professionalism does not refer to the task of completing a sonography examination but to how the sonographer completed the sonography examination. As illustrated in Table 1-1, promoting professionalism includes aligning one's aptitudes, attributes, and attitudes to enhance professional behavior.[5-7] When viewed as a competency or proficiency, professionalism uses practice methods recognized as being professional. These practice methods include upholding the profession's principles and standards.[1,2,4,5,8,11]

THE SONOGRAPHY LEGACY

Many historians believe that to know where we are going, we need to know where we have been. This belief provides the rationale to review a brief history to appreciate the sonography profession and its leadership.

Evolution of a Professional

In 1969, Joan Baker, Marilyn Ball, Margaret Byme, James Dennon, Raylene Husak, and L. E. Schnitzer gathered and initiated a proposal to create the American Society of Ultrasound Technical Specialists (ASUTS).[12] Baker and Schnitzer presented the proposal to the American Institute of Ultrasound in Medicine (AIUM) board of directors (BODs) explaining that the goal was to reach out to those individuals performing ultrasound procedures.[12,13] The AIUM board members did not oppose the request to establish a technical society, but many expressed a belief it would be a waste of time. ASUTS made its debut in 1970, at the AIUM's annual conference in Cleveland, Ohio. The conference had 187 registrants, which included 12 exhibitors and 13 technical specialists. Following the constitution and bylaws, the members proceeded to electing an ASUTS (BOD) comprised of 11 members to serve two-year terms and meeting the criteria of being an active member in the society and employed in sonographic technology.[12] Joan Baker became the first ASUTS president along with the remaining officers and six regional directors, each representing one of the six geographical regions in the North American continent.[13] In a short time period between 1969 and 1974, members of this group used their time, energy, and talent to create the goals and pathways of collaborating with other organizations. The ASUTS leadership identified the need to establish professional standards and was aware that the term "technical specialist" was not well received in the medical community.[12,13] Coming from Great Britain where radiography was used to describe x-ray technicians, Baker suggested the term "sonography" as a logical choice to incorporate sonar for those making an image with sound. History documents that the formation of ASUTS was initiated in 1969 and that it was created in 1970 and incorporated in 1972. The organization's name was officially changed to the Society of Diagnostic Medical Sonographers (SDMS) on September 16, 1980. With the advancements in equipment, diagnostic imaging, and membership, the name was again changed in 2016 to the Society of Diagnostic Medical Sonography. Changing "sonographers" to "sonography" made the name more inclusive to better represent the changes in the profession between 1980 and 2016 while maintaining the same acronym.

Creating the Occupation[12-14]

The ASUTS leaders determined that if the society was going to be successful, it was essential to create a new and separate occupation. The rationale for creating an occupation was to avoid the loss of diagnostic ultrasound to any other occupation that would require students to complete academic and clinical prerequisite education in a different field before gaining access to ultrasound education.

Establishing the new occupation had many challenges. The American Medical Association's (AMA's) Manpower Division was preparing to disband, which would create an unknown or a delayed procedure for creating a new occupation. The Manpower Division did not want to be involved with a new occupation. The United States Office of Education (USOE) released a statement discouraging the proliferation of allied health occupations and promoted new occupations such as ultrasound to be incorporated under the existing occupations. Joan Baker sought the assistance of Dr. Gil Baum, the current AIUM president. Dr. Baum successfully convinced the Manpower Division to respond to ASUTS' request. In 1973, the occupation of Diagnostic Medical Sonography (DMS) was created.[14] The ASUTS was very appreciative of Dr. Baum for his timely influence.[13,14]

The next challenge in the process was to work with the AMA's Department of Allied Health to compose a Document of Essentials that would have to be approved by all the collaborating organizations. Joan Baker, Jackie Ellis, and Betty Phillips met with the director of Allied Medical Professions and Services and two representative members with the Allied Medical Emerging Health Power of the AMA. Baker, Ellis, and Phillips presented the intentions of ASUTS. The outcome of the meeting required the ASUTS leadership team to develop and complete specific tasks. The outcome was the development of nine tasks, which included the foundation to develop the essentials for programmatic accreditation and the foundation to develop written and practice examinations to earn credentials.

PROFESSIONAL ORGANIZATIONS

A professional organization can also be referred to as a professional association. The word *association* can be ambiguous and can refer to different types of organizations.[15] One must review the infrastructure of an association to determine if it is synonymous with an organization.

When used as a verb, an association is a type of organization for individuals who share common interests and focus attention on promoting an area of interest such as art, history, science, alumni, etc. When used as a noun, the term *association* has a very broad meaning, one that can include different types of alliances, leagues, cooperatives, conventions, clubs, fellowships, unions, etc. An association can also be a collection of people forming an alliance to provide a particular service for a particular occupation or profession such as lawyers, accountants, or engineers. There may be an association of health care professionals having members of a specific imaging profession such as sonologists and sonographers.

The primary rationale why professional organizations were created was to provide continuing education (CE), to support the advancement of the specific profession, to support the interests of members employed in that profession, and to serve the public good.[15-17] Professional organizations can be at the state, regional, national, and/or international level.[18] In most cases, the members and the environment oversee the legitimate practice of any professional organization.[17] Different types of professional organizations can dramatically influence the required student education, student clinical experience, credential or certification, program accreditation, scope of practice, and requirements and evidence for completing continuing medical education (CME).

The main purpose of a member benefit organization is to create value for its membership.[15] Reflecting on history, a group of six sonographers saw a need to form an organization with the goal to reach out to those individuals performing sonography examinations.[12,13] The historical member benefits' value was the creation of a professional organization for sonographers performing examinations in all the specialty areas of sonography. This led to the formation of several sonography organizations composed of students, sonographers, physicians, researchers, and other sonography-associated practitioners.[16] The benefits provided for individual members include numerous resources such as a professional journal, educational conferences, virtual seminars or webinars, practice parameters, research grants, and codes of ethics.[18-20] Several organizations provide both CME credits and a CME tracking system.

In addition to providing current educational resources, numerous professional organizations provide members with opportunities to author, edit, and present current educational information. Student members often have discounted membership fees, education scholarships, and research grants.[18]

Professional member benefit organizations frequently recognize individual members who have shown outstanding achievements, such as outstanding educators, outstanding sonographers, memorial lecturers, fellow members, life members, and pioneer members. Sonography students may also be recognized for posters, essays, research, etc. Table 1-2 lists several member benefit sonography organizations and the acronyms for those primarily located in the United States.[18,21] The organizations' members may include students, sonographers, practitioners, physicians/sonologists,

researchers, educators, etc.[18] These professions usually provide its members with current information, employment opportunities, published professional journals, opportunities to submit peer-reviewed manuscripts, national annual conference, scholarships, professional liability insurance, personal medical insurance, virtual webinar courses, and CME.[19,20]

POSTSECONDARY ACCREDITATION

Accreditation is a voluntary evaluation process in order to maintain standards and educational quality. Although accreditation agencies may vary in the category of accreditation, there are similarities. One similarity is the agencies' goal to foster excellence by developing standards and guidelines. Another similarity in earning accreditation is the usual required periodic review process, which includes both self-review and peer review for continual analysis and documentation of academic quality and public accountability.[22,23] When accreditation is granted, it should symbolize the following: (1) There is recognition for performance, integrity, and quality. (2) The standards and guidelines were clearly met. (3) Appropriate methods were employed to evaluate the criteria. (4) Accreditation standards are being applied consistently and equitably.[22,24,25] The two basic types of educational accreditation are institutional and programmatic.[22,26]

Institutional Accreditation

Accreditation for higher education in most countries around the world is conducted by a government organization. In the United States, the institutional accreditation process is voluntary, and a nongovernmental process is employed to use the standards for measuring quality when evaluating institutions and its programs.[22,26] The U.S. Department of Education (USDE) does not perform accreditation but does oversee the postsecondary accreditation system by reviewing all of the federally recognized accrediting agencies.[26,27] The Council for Higher Education Accreditation (CHEA) is like the government USDE, except that it is a nongovernmental organization that oversees the accreditation process by reviewing the federally recognized agencies that set the accreditation standards.[28]

The accrediting agencies are accountable for enforcing their accreditation standards effectively.[27] The USDE also oversees that the Secretary of Education fulfills the legal requirement to publish a list of nationally recognized accrediting agencies.[27] The USDE's Office of Postsecondary Education (OPE) provides a database of postsecondary institutions and programs that have been accredited by accrediting agencies and the state approval agencies recognized by the U.S. Secretary of Education.[26,27] Accreditation by a recognized accrediting agency is one of the requirements for institutions to participate in federal student aid programs.[27] A student who wants federal and sometimes state grants and loans will need to attend a university, college, or program that is accredited by an approved agency.[28,29]

Institutional accreditation normally applies to an entire institution, indicating that each institutional part contributes to the achievement of the institution's objectives while recognizing that not every part is necessarily at the same level of quality.[26] The accreditation applies to the institution

TABLE 1-2 **Sonography Professional Organizations**[16,21]	
American Institute of Ultrasound in Medicine	AIUM
American Society of Echocardiography	ASE
American Society of Radiologic Technologists	ASRT
Society for Vascular Ultrasound	SVU
Society of Diagnostic Medical Sonography	SDMS
Society of Pediatric Echocardiography	SOPE
Sonography Canada	—
World Federation for Ultrasound in Medicine and Biology	WFUMB

as a whole and not to individual programs or units within the institution.[22] Two of the institutional accreditation types in the United States are national and regional. National accreditation agencies accredit approximately 85% of the colleges and universities focusing on accrediting trade and vocational schools as well as career programs that offer certifications and degrees.[28] Regional accreditation agencies accredit approximately 15% of the colleges and universities overseeing institutions that place a focus on academics and are state-owned or nonprofit colleges and universities. In the United States, there are six regional accrediting agencies that oversee higher education institutions within their particular geographic cluster of states.[28]

Programmatic Accreditation

There are a number of programmatic accrediting organizations where each represents a professional area such as sonography.[22] Most programmatic accrediting organizations have distinctive definitions of eligibility, criteria for accreditation, and operating procedures.[22,26] Programmatic accreditation by a specialized accrediting agency is an acceptable and recognized means of assuring a quality program.[22,26]

In the history of sonography, after creating the DMS occupation, the next challenge for ASUTS was to continue working with the AMA on the task of developing essentials for sonography program accreditation.[14] A primary education concern of the ASUTS was related to providing education and training opportunities for individuals interested in learning to be sonographers. Initially, when sonography was first introduced to the health care community, commercial ultrasound companies were the primary supporters of educational opportunities.[14] The four major equipment manufacturers continuously offered seminars nationwide to introduce the physical principles and techniques of sonography. These short-term courses ranged from 1 to 2 days.[14] Although the number of these short-term courses escalated and the participants emerged as trained and ready for employment, the ASUTS realized that the short-term programs could lower the quality of diagnostic examination results, which would contribute to lowering the credibility of the valuable diagnostic imaging tool. The ASUTS assumed responsibility for protecting the high standards of education required to produce competent practitioners and pushed even harder to establish educational programs.[13] Sonography programs were beginning to form but the graduating sonographers were insufficient to meet the critical workforce shortages.

The ASUTS agenda items were to stimulate the birth of sonography programs, to decrease the number of short-term courses, and to begin to work with the AMA's Department of Allied Medical Professions and Services—which later became known as the Committee on Allied Health Education and Accreditation (CAHEA). This committee worked with a diverse array of representatives, reflecting the multidisciplinary nature of DMS.[12,14]

Many interested medical and allied health organizations also collaborated in drafting the "Essentials of an Accredited Educational Program for the Diagnostic Medical Sonographer" between 1974 and 1979,[12,14] which were adopted in 1979 by eight organizations. That a 5-year span was required to complete the process can be attributed to the sheer number of organizations involved and the ongoing turf battles. The turf battle disputes included determining who should perform ultrasound procedures, where should the equipment and ultrasound procedures be performed within a hospital setting, who should or should not interpret the sonography examination, etc.[13] The collaborating organization's representatives and the organizations activated the formation of a Joint Review Committee on Education in Diagnostic Medical Sonography (JRC-DMS).[13,14] The JRC-DMS's first accreditation of educational programs occurred in January 1982.[13,14]

In 1992, the AMA presented a proposal for a new freestanding agency to replace CAHEA and its review committees and sponsoring organizations, educational institutions, and communities of interest to examine the current accreditation system. The proposal prompted the design of an independent allied health education accrediting body to respond to the needs of the allied health professions, educational institutions, students enrolled in allied health education programs, and the public. As a result of a task force and input from many communities of interest, CAHEA's proposed successor agency—the Commission on Accreditation of Allied Health Education Programs (CAAHEP)—became operational in mid-1994 to provide accreditation and related coordinating services. CAAHEP was committed to simplifying the existing accrediting process; to be more inclusive of allied health professions that provide entry-level education; and to serve as a stepping stone for future, more far-reaching developments.[30]

The Joint Review Committee on Education in Cardiovascular Technology (JRC-CVT) and the JRC-DMS have similar functions, and both are members of CAAHEP and these programmatic organizations are presented in Table 1-3. CAAHEP currently is the largest programmatic accreditor in the field of health sciences.[23] CAAHEP ensures oversight and due process to all programs that participate in its system of accreditation.[24]

The role of the JRC-CVT or JRC-DMS is to ensure quality sonography education that serves the public by completing a program evaluation to determine if the essentials have been met.[24] The evaluation is extensive and includes onsite program evaluation of course materials, academic courses, and clinical facilities. The JRC report is forwarded to the CAAHEP, which has established educational standards and guidelines to provide or deny accreditation based upon the evidence and recommendation of the JRC.[25] The CAAHEP BOD acts upon the recommendations of the JRC-DMS, confirming that appropriate procedures have been followed and that accreditation standards are being applied consistently and equitably when assessing applicant educational programs.[24]

TABLE 1-3 Programmatic Accreditation Organizations[18,30]	
Commission on Accreditation of Allied Health Education Programs	CAAHEP
Joint Review Committee on Education in Cardiovascular Technology	JRC-CVT
Joint Review Committee on Education in Diagnostic Medical Sonography	JRC-DMS

Laboratory Accreditation

The voluntary laboratory accreditation process provides standards of practice that help to ensure a high level of uniformity and enhance the quality of patient care.[18] Accreditation of DMS services helps sonographers and physicians to evaluate the strengths and weaknesses to determine the essentials needed to improve imaging outcomes (Table 1-4). Although laboratory accreditation is voluntary, accreditation does help the facility meet the criteria issued by governmental agencies and third-party payers.[31]

American College of Radiology

Since 1987, the American College of Radiology (ACR) has accredited a multitude of modalities.

The ACR Ultrasound Accreditation Program includes the evaluation of clinical images, relevant physician reports corresponding to the clinical images, and documentation of quality control.[32]

American Institute of Ultrasound in Medicine

The AIUM began developing the Ultrasound Practice Accreditation in 1995. The goals were to develop a method for evaluating proper education and training, proper experience, and proper understanding of the technology. The ultrasound practice for accreditation is to appraise evaluating the personnel education, training, and experience, document storage and record keeping, policies and procures safeguarding patients, personnel, and equipment, instrumentation, quality assurance, and case studies.[31]

Intersocietal Accreditation Commission

In 1991, the Intersocietal Commission for the Accreditation of Vascular Laboratories (ICAVL) became known as the Intersocietal Accreditation Commission (IAC). Its first accreditation division was the IAC Vascular Testing. In 1996, a division was created for the accreditation of echocardiography. In 2008, the organization incorporated vascular testing, echocardiography, and multiple diagnostic imaging and intervention-based procedures. The IAC Standards and Guidelines publication describes how to document the minimum standards for accreditation and the procedure for the accreditation application. The three divisions specific to ultrasound IAC Standards and Guidelines are Vascular Testing, Echocardiography, and Pediatric Echocardiography.[33,34]

CREDENTIALS, CERTIFICATION, LICENSURE

Credentials and Certification

Understanding and using the correct terminology, policies, and procedures for credential, certification, and licensure

TABLE 1-4 Laboratory Accreditation Organizations[18,31–34]	
American College of Radiology	ACR
American Institute of Ultrasound in Medicine	AIUM

Intersocietal Accreditation Commission
  IAC Vascular Testing
  IAC Echocardiography
  IAC Pediatric Echocardiography
	IAC

TABLE 1-5 Credentialing Organizations and Their Web Links[21,35–37]	
Credentialing Organization	**Web Links**
American Registry for Diagnostic Medical Sonography (ARDMS)[21]	https://www.ardms.org
American Registry of Radiologic Technologists (ARRT)[35]	https://www.arrt.org/
Cardiovascular Credentialing International (CCI)[36]	https://cci-online.org/
Sonography Canada[37]	https://sonographycanada.ca/

has relevance affecting the profession. Earning a credential verifies that a professional has achieved a baseline knowledge, skills, and the minimum level of competence. There are acceptable areas for health care providers to achieve a certification status that was earned after completing a specified level of education and clinical practice skills. For these levels, certification remains a formal process used to recognize and to validate an individual's qualifications.

The simplified definitions are as follows: A credential is awarded following an advanced level certification examination. The certification examination is typically created by following rigorous and precise protocols, has been psychometrically validated, and is usually delivered through a third-party testing service. Table 1-5 presents four credentialing organizations and their web links.

American Registry for Diagnostic Medical Sonography

Another ASUTS legacy was laying the foundation for sonographers to complete a certification examination and to earn a credential. After the creation of the DMS occupation, the ASUTS leadership continued collaborating with representatives from other organizations to develop the essentials for programmatic accreditation. Simultaneously, the ASUTS leadership developed the written and practice examinations to earn credentials.[13] Because of the issues encountered with the term "technical specialist" and the inability to prevent the terms "technician" and "technologist," the ASUTS leadership used the opportunity to adopt a new title for the profession.[13] The name chosen for the first examinations to earn credentials was the American Registry for Diagnostic Medical Sonography (ARDMS).[12,13] The ASUTS members on or before midnight, October 6, 1974, were "grandfathered," which means they were not required to take the written examination but would be required to take a proficiency test—which could have been a practical examination.[12]

From its creation in the 1970s, the ARDMS was the original credentialing organization offering certification examinations for all sonography specialties. The expansion of ARDMS certification examinations and credentials evolved to accommodate new developments in equipment and greater diversity in sonography examinations. The ARDMS expansion has created the opportunity for sonographers to earn credentials, for midwives to earn a certificate, and for physicians to earn certifications.[12]

Information from the ARDMS website is presented in Table 1-6 and serves as a guide to learn how to earn an ARDMS credential.[21] An applicant must have completed eligible requirements in education and clinical experience

TABLE 1-6 Earn an American Registry for Diagnostic Medical Sonography (ARDMS) Credential[18,21]

Credential: RDCS—Registered Diagnostic Cardiac Sonographer

Select the prerequisite meeting one's eligibility

Sonography Principles and Instrumentation (SPI)

Adult Echocardiography (AE) Examination	Pediatric Echocardiography (PE) Examination	Fetal Echocardiography (FE) Examination

Credential: RDMS—Registered Diagnostic Medical Sonographer

Select the prerequisite meeting one's eligibility:

Sonography Principles and Instrumentation (SPI)

Abdomen (AB) Examination	Breast (BR) Examination	Fetal Echocardiography (FE) Examination	Obstetrics and Genecology (OB/GYN) Examination	Pediatric Sonography (PS) Examination

Credential: RVT—Registered Vascular Technologist

Select the prerequisite meeting one's eligibility:

Sonography Principles and Instrumentation (SPI)

Vascular Technology (VT) Examination

Credential: RMSKS—Registered Musculoskeletal Sonographer

Select the prerequisite meeting one's eligibility:

Sonography Principles and Instrumentation (SPI)

Musculoskeletal Sonographer (MSKS) Examination

matching one of the specific prerequisites.[21] The next step is to pass an ARDMS specialty examination and the Sonography Principles and Instrumentation (SPI) examination. The SPI examination can be taken after completing a physics course and only needs to be passed once within 5 years of passing the specialty examination.[21]

American Registry of Radiologic Technologists

The American Registry of Radiologic Technologists (ARRT) offers credentialing examinations for sonographers. The primary and the postprimary are the two eligibility pathway requirements for an ARRT examination. Both pathways share the same ethics and examination requirements but have different education requirements. The primary eligibility pathway requires completion of an ARRT-approved educational program.[35]

The primary pathway is used by the majority of applicants to earn their first ARRT credential. There are two credentials that can be earned using the primary pathway and by passing either the sonography or the vascular sonography examination. When passing the sonography examination, the credential earned is RT(S). When passing the vascular sonography examination, the credential earned is RT(VS).[35]

The postprimary pathway is for the professional currently certified and registered with ARRT and would like to pursue an additional credential. The postprimary pathway may also be used by those who hold a credential from ARDMS. The breast sonography credential is RT(BS) and can be earned using the secondary pathway and by passing the breast sonography examination. The vascular sonography credential [RT(VS)] can be earned using either the primary pathway or the postprimary pathway. Table 1-5 and the ARRT website serve as reference guides to learn how to earn an ARRT credential.[35]

Cardiovascular Credentialing International

The Cardiovascular Credentialing International (CCI) offers credentialing examinations for cardiac and vascular specialists. At the time of preparing this chapter, CCI offered nine examinations designed to validate knowledge and competence and to help professionals leverage their credential to move their career to the next higher level.[36]

The Advanced Cardiac Sonographer (ACS) credential is designed to be a career track for sonographers practicing at an advanced level. The ACS credentialed sonographer should be committed to improving quality and efficiency, to performing advanced echocardiogram examinations, to preparing preliminary echocardiogram assessments, in order to develop and to implement educational plans, to facilitate continuous quality improvements, and to coordinate cardiac sonography research.[36]

The website provides detailed information on each of the nine examinations regarding qualification requirements, application process, information to assist the candidate to prepare for the examination, how to maintain the credential, and a strict code of ethics with high standards for candidates. Unlike the ARDMS, the CCI provides one examination for each cardiac and vascular specialty and that examination includes both specialty information and physics. Refer to Table 1-5 and the CCI website as a reference guide to learn how to earn a CCI credential.[36]

Sonography Canada

On January 1, 2014, Sonography Canada was launched with the merger of the national professional organization (Canadian Society of Diagnostic Medical Sonographers [CSDMS]) and the national credentialing organization (Canadian Association of Registered Diagnostic Ultrasound Professionals

[CARDUP]).[37] The launching of Sonography Canada provides a single voice to help promote the profession, education, credential, employment, and continuous education. Other benefits include increased and focused professional support, offering professional liability insurance, and providing continuing education such as through a national conference, and publishing a professional medical journal with current research and literature reviews.

It is common for clinics and hospitals to stipulate employment that requires the sonographer to have earned the Sonography Canada credentials. Earning a Sonography Canada credential signifies that the sonographer has met the national educational and competency requirements of the profession. The employment stipulation requiring a credential is of national importance in increasing awareness of the sonography professional. Knowing the important role a sonographer plays in health care has also increased public awareness.

After earning certification and gaining a credential, the sonographer has a professional responsibility to adhere to the Sonography Canada Professional Practice Guidelines and Member Policies.[37]

At the time of this writing, Sonography Canada grants a credential in three specialty areas: (1) the Canadian Registered Generalist Sonographer (CRGS)—an examination of the abdomen, male and female pelvis, obstetrics, peripheral veins for DVT, and superficial structures including (but not limited to) thyroid and scrotum[37]; (2) the Canadian Registered Cardiac Sonographer (CRCS)—an examination of the adult cardiac anatomy, function, physiology, pathology, and adult congenital assessment[37]; and (3) the Canadian Registered Vascular Sonographer (CRVS)—an examination dedicated to vascular ultrasound imaging including (but not limited to) the abdominal vessels, arterial and venous studies of the upper and lower limbs, head and neck, and physiologic arterial assessment.[37]

Maintaining Credentials

After earning a credential, one should maintain the credential. The most common methods credentialing organizations use to maintain a credential include a specified time period to earn a specified number of CE hours and a specified financial payment for the credential renewal fee.[17] The rationale for requiring CE (i.e., CME, continuing professional development [CPD], etc.) is to have some evidence in a rapidly changing health care environment that the professional has maintained documented learning experiences that serve to maintain, develop, or increase the knowledge skills and professional performance.

Sonographers have multiple resources to earn CE. Some of these include medical journal articles and completion of a short quiz, national conferences, virtual courses, and webinars.

Licensure

Licensure involves obtaining the legal right to practice or serve in a specific sonography role as approved by government legislation. Currently, in the United States, New Hampshire, New Mexico, North Dakota, and Oregon are the four states that have approved legislation requiring licensure of sonographers. Mandatory state licensure requirements vary in each state. It is recommended that sonographers evaluate state licensure requirements prior to accepting employment opportunities in a state requiring state licensure.

PREPARING FOR THE PROFESSION

Scope of Practice and Clinical Standards[38]

In December 1993, the first edition of the Scope of Practice for the Diagnostic Sonographer was endorsed by the ACR, the American Society of Echocardiography (ASE), and the SDMS. In May 2013, representatives of 16 organizations began the process of revising, developing, and updating a new document. On April 15, 2015, the Scope of Practice and Clinical Standards for the Diagnostic Medical Sonographer was endorsed by seven organizations: ASE, CCI, JRC-DMS, Society of Diagnostic Medical Sonography (SDMS), Society for Maternal-Fetal Medicine (SMFM), Society of Vascular Surgery (SVS), and Society for Vascular Ultrasound (SVU).

The document endorsed by these organizations is the only document for the scope of practice and clinical standards for DMS.[38] Because the information is of vital importance, sonographers and sonography students should review it on a periodic basis. This document may be found at: Scope of Practice (sdms.org).

The purpose of the document matches the title, which is to describe the scope of practice and clinical standards for DMS. This helps delineate the role of sonographers as members of the health care team who must always act in the best interest of the patient.

The section focused on the scope of practice includes the following: (1) limitation and scope; (2) definition of the profession; and (3) DMS certification/credentialing. The scope of practice is limited to what the law allows for specific education, experience, and demonstrated competency. The sonographers function as delegated agents of the physician and do not practice independently but with autonomy and responsibilities for their service and to make decision within the scope of their practice. The sonographer must understand that everything matters in patient care, must be committed to enhancing patient care, must focus on continuous quality improvement that increases knowledge, and must gain technical competency skills. To safely perform diagnostic sonographic procedures, the sonographer must use independent, professional, and ethical judgment and critical thinking.[38]

The section focuses on clinical standards including the following: (1) patient information assessment and evaluation; (2) patient education and communication; (3) analysis and determination of protocol for the diagnostic examination; (4) implementation of the protocol; (5) evaluation of the diagnostic examination results; (6) documentation; (7) implementation of quality improvement programs; (8) quality of care; (9) self-assessment; (10) education; (11) collaboration; and (12) ethics. The clinical standards in this section are designed to reflect the sonographer's behavior and performance levels expected in clinical practice. The standards reflect the principles common to all of the specialties within the sonography professions. The individual specialties or clinical areas may extend or enhance, but not limit, these general principles according to their specific practice requirements.[38]

Recommended Professional Terminology

Consistently using professional terminology increases accurate oral and written communication. In the earliest stages of the profession, ultrasound was used to identify the imaging modality, the equipment, the imaging examination or procedure, the acquired images, and the technical specialist who completed the examination.

In the Steven M. McLaughlin Memorial Lecture in 2007, Terry DuBose presented "The Profession's Identity—Words and Actions Matter." DuBose presented why the noun sonography was grammatically more correct than ultrasound for describing an image made using ultrasound energy. DuBose clarified that to refer to an image as an ultrasound is analogous to calling a photograph a light because it is made using reflected light, describing an image made using ultrasonic energy.[39]

Tables in this chapter represent the professional terminology. The sonographer is placed in a position to determine the best terminology needed to communicate to the patient. There may be patients who better understand being scheduled for an echo tech versus being scheduled for an echocardiography. The pregnant patient will request seeing images of the baby versus a fetus.

Entering the Profession

To enter the sonography profession, an essential prerequisite is to successfully complete a sonography program with specialized academic courses and supervised clinical experience. The graduating sonography student must be educationally prepared and clinically competent.[38] As students learn the anatomy and gain clinical experience, psychomotor skills are developed. Students stop looking at their hand and begin to focus their total attention on the monitor in order to analyze the anatomy and mentally direct their scanning hand.

Sonographers may often find themselves in an independent position and so must understand their important role in health care. It is extremely important to be able to recognize and differentiate normal and abnormal anatomy and to reject an image that is suboptimal. Correlating the patient's clinical history helps the sonographer perform a more targeted investigative imaging.[18] The sonologists' interpretation correlates the sonographic findings with the clinical findings, which results in a diagnosis and/or a list of differential diagnoses.

Following the academic preparation, the next step is to earn one or more of the credentials listed in Table 1-5.

SUMMARY

- The sonography profession includes sonographers and sonologists.
- Sonographers are educated to use imaging equipment.
- Sonologists interpret sonograms.
- Sonograms are recorded images of sonography examination.
- Sonographers are a professional group of disciplined individuals adhering to ethical standards.
- Professionals are members of a profession adhering to codes of conduct, ethics, standards, and guidelines.
- Professionalism is based on the word professional which describes a member of the profession; professional members are disciplined individuals who adhere to professional standards.
- In 1969, six sonographers initiated a proposal to create the ASUTS.
- ASUTS made its debut in 1970 at the AIUM's annual conference.
- Sonography is the logical name chosen for a profession using sonar to make an image or a graphic representation of anatomy.
- The AMA's Manpower Division created the occupation of DMS.
- ASUTS was officially changed to SDMS in September 1980 and renamed as the Society of Diagnostic Medial Sonography in 2016.
- In 1973, the occupation of DMS was created.
- ASUTS leadership develops the foundation criteria for programmatic accreditation and the written and practice examinations to earn credentials.
- Methods have been developed to earn CE credits to maintain credentials.
- Four states in the United States have approved legislation requiring licensure of sonographers.
- In 2015, the Scope of Practice and Clinical Standards for the Diagnostic Medical Sonographer document was endorsed by seven organizations.
- It is recommend to use consistent professional terminology to increase accurate oral and written communication and appropriate level of terminology to communicate with the patient.
- Determine the essential prerequisite required to qualify to enter the sonography profession.

REFERENCES

1. Australian Council of Professions. What is a profession? 2003. Accessed October 30, 2021. https://www.professions.org.au/what-is-a-professional/
2. Professional Standards Council. What is a profession? Accessed November 1, 2021. www.psc.gov.au/what-is-a-profession
3. Surbhi S. Difference between occupation and profession. 2018. Accessed October 30, 2021. https://keydifferences.com/difference-between-occupation-and-profession.html
4. Porcupile DW. What is professionalism? What does professionalism mean to you? September 9, 2015. Accessed January 5, 2022. http://graduate.auburn.edu/wp-content/uploads/2016/08/What-is-PROFESSIONALISM.pdf
5. Hammer DP. Professional attitudes and behaviors: the "A's and B's" of professionalism. *Am J Pharm Educ.* 2000;53:455–464.
6. Paans W, Wijkamp I, Wiltens E, Wolfensberger MV. What constitutes an excellent allied health care professional? A multidisciplinary focus group study. *J Multidiscip Healthc.* 2013;6:347-356. Assessed April 22, 2022. https://doi.org/10.2147/JMDH.S46784
7. Piccirilli G. 10 Characteristics of Professionalism in the Workplace. Published January 2, 2018. https://www.aapc.com/blog/40477-10-characteristics-of-professionalism-in-the-workplace/
8. Kirk LM. Professionalism in medicine: definitions and considerations for teaching. *Proc (Bayl Univ Med Cent).* 2007;20(1):13–16. doi:10.1080/08998280.2007.11928225
9. Indeed Editorial Team. Guide to professionalism in the workplace. August 30, 2021. Accessed November 4, 2021. https://www.indeed

.com/career-advice/career-development/the-ultimate-guide-to-professionalism

10. Kawamura DM. Behaving professionally: role model wanted. Stephen M. McLaughlin Memorial Lecture; 2016 SDMS Annual Conference, Orlando, Florida.

11. Cruess SR, Johnston S, Cruess RL. Professionalism for medicine: opportunities and obligations. August 10, 2007. Accessed November 11, 2021. https://www.mja.com.au/system/files/issues/177_04_190802/cru10332_fm.pdf

12. Hagen-Ansert AL. Society of Diagnostic Medical Sonographers: a timeline of historical events in sonography and the development of the SDMS: in the beginning. *J Diagn Med Sonogr.* 2006;22(4):272–278. doi:10.1177/8756479306291456

13. Baker J. *Society of Diagnostic Medical Sonographers: Focus on the Future.* Lippincott-Raven Publishers; 1975.

14. Hagen-Ansert AL, Barker JP. Society of Diagnostic Medical Sonographers: a history of the SDMS. Part II 1970-1980: development of the society and early educational efforts for sonographers. *J Diagn Med Sonogr.* 2007;23(4):218–223. doi:10.1177/8756479307304229

15. Balthazard C. #1 The four types of professional organizations. April 4, 2017. Accessed November 8, 2021. https://www.linkedin.com/pulse/four-types-professional-organizations-claude/

16. Indeed Editorial Team. Q&A: what is a professional organization? December 27, 2020. Accessed November 8, 2011. https://www.indeed.com/career-advice/career-development/what-is-a-professional-organization

17. Bhasin H. Professional organization—definition, meaning, types. March 5, 2020. Accessed November 4, 2021. https://www.marketing91.com/professional-organization/

18. Penny SM. *Introduction to Sonography and Patient Care.* 2nd ed. Wolters Kluwer; 2021.

19. American Institute of Ultrasound in Medicine. Practice parameters. Accessed November 11, 2021. https://www.aium.org/resources/guidelines.aspx

20. Society of Diagnostic Medical Sonography. Codes of ethics for the professional diagnostic medical sonography. Accessed November 11, 2021. https://www.sdms.org/about/who-we-are/code-of-ethics

21. American Registry of Diagnostic Medical Sonography (ARDMS). Accessed April 22, 2022. https://www.ardms.org/

22. Northwest Commission on Colleges and Universities. Accreditation? Accessed November 19, 2021. https://nwccu.org/accreditation/.

23. Council for Higher Education Accreditation. About CHEA. Accessed December 1, 2021. https://www.chea.org/about-chea

24. Joint Review Committee on Education in Diagnostic Medical Sonography. About us. Accessed November 26, 2021. https://www.jrcdms.org/

25. Commission on Accreditation of Allied Health Education Programs. Standards and guidelines for the accreditation of educational programs in diagnostic medical sonography. Accessed November 28, 2021. https://www.jrcdms.org/pdf/DMSStandards9-2021.pdf

26. Graduate Guide. Accreditation of postsecondary education in the United States. Accessed November 26, 2021. https://graduateguide.com/accreditation-of-postsecondary-education-in-the-united-states/

27. Database of Accredited Postsecondary Institutions and Programs. Accessed December 2, 2021. https://ope.ed.gov/dapip/#/home

28. Drexel University. Regional vs. national accreditation: why does it matter? Accessed December 5, 2021. https://www.online.drexel.edu/news/national-vs-regional-accreditation.aspx

29. Council for Higher Education Accreditation. Accreditation & recognition. Accessed December 1, 2021. https://www.chea.org/about-accreditation

30. Weithaus B. New directions for allied health education accreditation. *J Allied Health.* 1993;22(3):239–247.

31. American Institute of Ultrasound in Medicine. AIUM ultrasound practice accreditation. Accessed December 9, 2021. https://www.aium.org/accreditation/accreditation.aspx

32. American College of Radiology ACR ultrasound accreditation program. Accessed December 9, 2021. https://www.acraccreditation.org/modalities/ultrasound

33. Intersocietal Accreditation Commission. IAC standards and guidelines for echocardiography accreditation. Accessed December 9, 2021. https://intersocietal.org/programs/echocardiography/standards/

34. Intersocietal Accreditation Commission. IAC standards and guidelines for vascular testing accreditation. Accessed December 9, 2021. https://intersocietal.org/programs/vascular-testing/standards/

35. American Registry of Radiologic Technologists. Accessed December 14, 2021. https://www.arrt.org/

36. Cardiovascular Credentialing International. Accessed December 14, 2021. https://cci-online.org/

37. Sonography Canada. The national voice for diagnostic medical sonographers in Canada. Accessed January 12, 2022. https://sonographycanada.ca/

38. Society of Diagnostic Medical Sonography. *Scope of Practice and Clinical Standards for the Diagnostic Medical Sonographer.* Society of Diagnostic Medical Sonography; 2013. Accessed November 11, 2021. https://www.sdms.org/about/who-we-are/scope-of-practice

39. DuBose TJ. The profession's identity—words and actions matter. Paper presented at: SDMS 24th Annual Conference Proceedings; October 2007; Las Vegas, NV.

CHAPTER 2

Orientation to Scanning

DIANE M. KAWAMURA

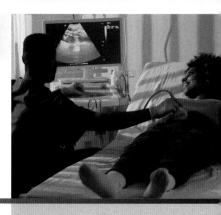

OBJECTIVES

- Identify anatomic definitions for directional terms, anatomic position, and anatomic planes.
- Demonstrate the sonography examination to include patient position, transducer orientation, image presentation, and image labeling.
- Define the terms used to describe image quality.
- Describe the echo patterns demonstrating how normal and pathologic conditions can be defined using image quality definitions.
- List and recognize the sonography criteria for cystic, solid, and complex conditions.
- Describe the appropriate patient preparation for a sonography evaluation.
- State what should and what should not be included in the sonographer's documentation of the sonography examination.
- Calculate sensitivity, specificity, and accuracy using the four outcomes of true positive, false positive, true negative, and/or false negative.

GLOSSARY

anechoic describes the portion of an image that appears echo-free

echogenic describes an organ or tissue that is capable of producing echoes by reflecting the acoustic beam

echopenic describes a structure that is less echogenic or has few internal echoes

heterogeneous describes tissue or organ structures that have several different echo characteristics

homogeneous refers to imaged echoes of equal intensity

hyperechoic describes image echoes brighter than surrounding tissues or brighter than is normal for that tissue or organ

hypoechoic describes portions of an image that are not as bright as surrounding tissues or are less bright than normal

isoechoic describes structures of equal echo density

KEY TERMS

accuracy

anechoic

coronal plane

echogenic

echopenic

heterogeneous

homogeneous

hyperechoic

hypoechoic

isoechoic

sagittal plane

sensitivity

specificity

transverse plane

This chapter focuses on the sonography examination of the abdomen and superficial structures. It was written to assist sonographers in acquiring, using, and understanding the sonographic imaging terminology used in the remainder of this textbook. Accurate and precise terminology allows effective communication among professionals.

The textbook is divided into five sections: introduction to sonography, abdominal sonography, superficial structure sonography, neonatal and pediatric sonography, and special study sonography.

ANATOMIC DEFINITIONS

The profession adopted standard nomenclature from the anatomists' terminology to communicate anatomic direction. Table 2-1 and Figure 2-1 illustrate how these simple terms help avoid confusion and provide specific information. A person in the conventional anatomic position stands erect, with feet together, the arms by the sides, and the palms and face directed forward, facing the observer. When sonographers use directional terms or describe regions or anatomic planes, it is assumed that the body is in the anatomic position.

There are three standard anatomic planes (sections), which are imaginary flat surfaces passing through a body in the standard anatomic position. The sagittal plane and coronal plane follow the long axis of the body and the transverse plane follows the short axis of the body[1] (Fig. 2-2).

The word *sagittal* literally means "flight of an arrow" and refers to the plane that courses vertically through the body and separates it into right and left portions. The plane that divides the body into equal right and left halves is referred to as the median sagittal or midsagittal plane. Any vertical plane on either side of the midsagittal plane is a parasagittal plane (para means "alongside of"). In most sonography cases, the term sagittal usually implies a parasagittal plane unless the term is specified as median sagittal or midsagittal. The coronal plane courses vertically through the body from right to left or left to right, and it divides the body into anterior and posterior portions. The transverse plane passes through the body from anterior to posterior and divides the body into superior and inferior portions and courses parallel to the surface of the ground.

SCANNING DEFINITIONS

Patient Position

Positional terms refer to the patient's position relative to the surrounding space. For sonographic examinations, the patient position is described relative to the scanning table or bed (Table 2-2 and Fig. 2-3). In clinical practice, patients are scanned in a recumbent, semierect (reverse Trendelenburg or Fowler), or sitting position. On occasion, patients may be placed in other positions, such as the Trendelenburg (head lowered) or standing position, to obtain unobscured images of the area of interest. Sonographers frequently convey information on patient position and transducer placement simultaneously. This terminology most likely was adopted from radiography, where it describes the path of the X-ray beam through the patient's body (*projection*), which results in a radiographic image (*view*). There is no evidence in the literature that this nomenclature has been adopted as a professional standard for sonographic imaging. Describing sonograms using the terms *projection* or *view* should be avoided. It is more accurate to describe the sonography image by stating the anatomic plane visualized, owing to the

TABLE 2-1	**Directional Terms**	
Term	**Definition**	**Example**
Superior (cranial)	Toward the head, closer to the head, the upper portion of the body, the upper part of a structure, or a structure higher than another structure	The left adrenal gland is superior to the left kidney.
Inferior (caudal)	Toward the feet, away from the head, the lower portion of the body, toward the lower part of a structure, or a structure lower than another structure	The lower pole of each kidney is inferior to the upper pole.
Anterior (ventral)	Toward the front or at the front of the body or a structure in front of another structure	The main portal vein is anterior to the inferior vena cava.
Posterior (dorsal)	Toward the back or the back of the body or a structure behind another structure	The main portal vein is posterior to the common hepatic artery.
Medial	Toward the middle or midline of the body or the middle of a structure	The middle vein is medial to the right hepatic vein.
Lateral	Away from the middle or the midline of the body or pertaining to the side	The right kidney is lateral to the inferior vena cava.
Ipsilateral	Located on the same side of the body or affecting the same side of the body	The gallbladder and right kidney are ipsilateral.
Contralateral	Located on the opposite side of the body or affecting the opposite side of the body	The pancreatic tail and pancreatic head are contralateral.
Proximal	Closer to the attachment of an extremity to the trunk or the origin of a body part	The abdominal aorta is proximal to the bifurcation of the iliac arteries.
Distal	Farther from the attachment of an extremity to the trunk or the origin of a body part	The iliac arteries are distal to the abdominal aorta.
Superficial	Toward or on the body surface or external	The thyroid and breast are considered superficial structures.
Deep	Away from the body surface or internal	The peritoneal organs and great vessels are deep structures.

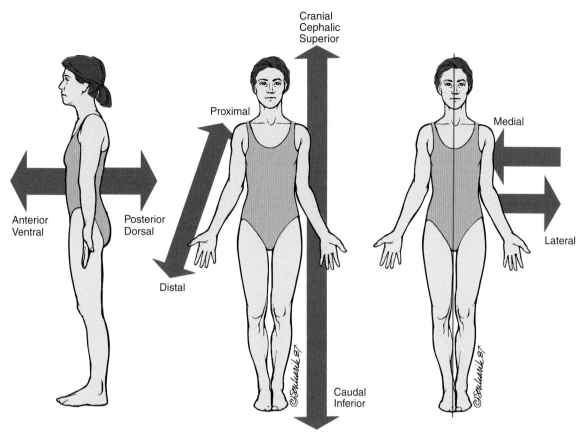

FIGURE 2-1 Directional terms. The drawing depicts a body in the anatomic position (standing erect, arms by the side, face and palms directed forward) with the directional terms. The directional terms correlate with the terms in Table 2-1.

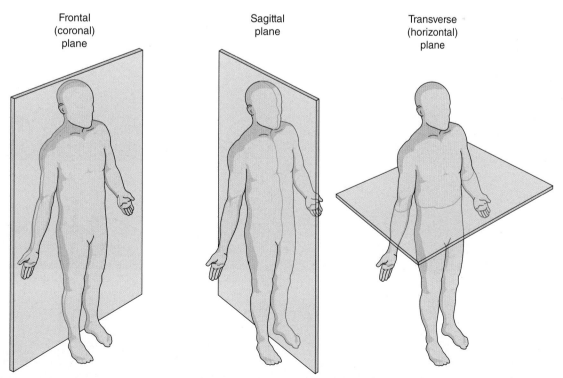

FIGURE 2-2 Anatomic planes. The standard anatomic position is used to depict the three imaginary anatomic flat surface planes. Both the sagittal and coronal planes pass through the long axis and the transverse plane passes through the short axis. (Reprinted with permission from Stephenson SR, Dmitrieva J. *Obstetrics and Gynecology*. 4th ed. Wolters Kluwer; 2018.)

TABLE 2-2	**Patient Positions**
Term	**Description**
Decubitus or Recumbent	The act of lying down. The adjective before the word describes the most dependent body surface.
Supine or dorsal	Lying on the back
Prone or ventral	Lying face down
RLD	Lying on the right side
LLD	Lying on the left side
Oblique	Named for the body side closest to the scanning table.
RPO	Lying on the right posterior surface, the left posterior surface is elevated
LPO	Lying on the left posterior surface, the right posterior surface is elevated
RAO	Lying on the right anterior surface, the left anterior surface is elevated
LAO	Lying on the left anterior surface, the right anterior surface is elevated

LAO, left anterior oblique; LLD, left lateral decubitus; LPO, left posterior oblique; RAO, right anterior oblique; RLD, right lateral decubitus; RPO, right posterior oblique.

transducer's orientation (i.e., transverse). A more specific description of the image would include both the anatomic plane and the patient position (i.e., transverse, oblique).

Transducer Orientation

The transducer's orientation as viewed on the monitor is the path of the insonating sound beam and the path of the returning echoes. Transducers are manufactured with an indicator (notch, groove, light) that is displayed on the monitor as a dot, arrow, letter of the manufacturer's insignia, or other delineation. *Scanning plane* is the term used to describe the transducer's orientation to the anatomic plane or to a specific organ or structure. The *sonographic image* is a representation of sectional anatomy. The term *plane* combined with the adjectives sagittal, parasagittal, coronal, and transverse describes the section of anatomy represented on the image (e.g., transverse plane).

Because many organs and structures lie oblique to the imaginary body surface planes, sonographers must identify sectional anatomy accurately to utilize a specific organ and structure orientation for scanning surfaces. The sonography imaging equipment provides a lot of flexibility to rock, slide, and angle the transducer to obtain sectional images of organs oriented obliquely in the body. For example, to obtain the long axis of an organ, such as the kidney, the transducer is placed obliquely and is angled off of the standard anatomic positions: sagittal, parasagittal, coronal, or transverse plane. Sonographers frequently use the terms *sagittal* or *parasagittal* to mean longitudinal in depicting the anatomy in a long-axis section. Although some images in this text are labeled sagittal or parasagittal, they are, in fact, longitudinal planes because the image is organ specific. For

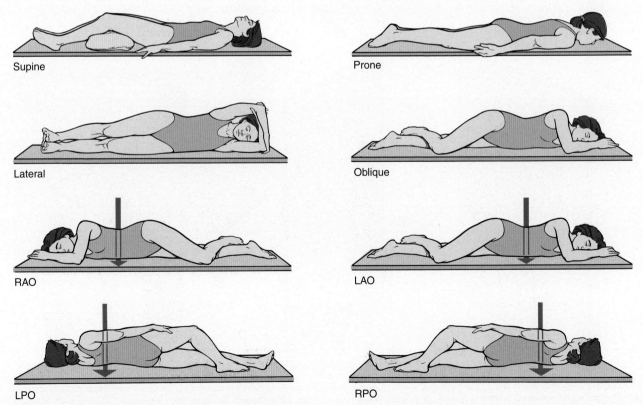

FIGURE 2-3 Patient positions. The various patient positions depicted in the illustration correlate with the descriptions in Table 2-2. LAO, left anterior oblique; LPO, left posterior oblique; RAO, right anterior oblique; RPO, right posterior oblique.

organ imaging, transverse planes are perpendicular to the long axis of the organ, and longitudinal and coronal planes are referenced to a surface. All three planes are based on the patient position and the scanning surface (Fig. 2-4A–C).

Image Presentation

When describing image presentation on the display monitor, the body, organ, or structure plane terminology, coupled with transducer placement, provides a very descriptive portrayal of the sectional anatomy being depicted. Current flexible, freehand scanning techniques may lack automatic labeling of the scanning plane. With the freehand scanning technique, quantitative labeling may be limited, which means reduced image reproducibility from one sonographer to another. Sonographers can usually select from a wide array of protocols for image annotation or employ postprocessing annotation. This is extremely important when the image of an isolated area does not provide other anatomic structures for a reference location. To ensure consistent practice, sonographers must correctly label all sonograms. With today's equipment, standard presentation and labeling are easily achieved along with additional labeling of specific structures and added comments.

The anterior, posterior, right, or left body surface is usually scanned in the sagittal (parasagittal), coronal, and transverse scanning planes. For organ or structure imaging, these same body surfaces are scanned with different angulations and obliqueness of the transducer to obtain longitudinal, coronal, or transverse scanning planes. With few exceptions, the transducer at the scanning surface is presented at the top of the image.[1,2] Images obtained using

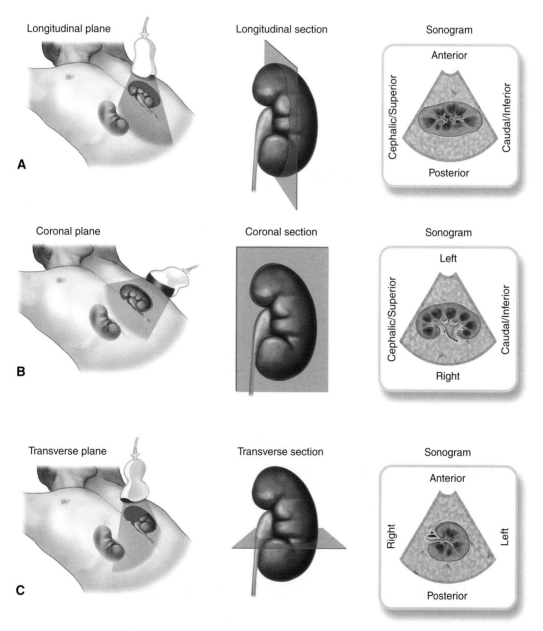

FIGURE 2-4 Transducer orientation. **A:** A parasagittal plane provides a longitudinal section of the kidney on the sonogram. **B:** The coronal plane provides a coronal section on the sonogram. **C:** The transverse plane provides a transverse section on the sonogram. The sonogram is the image the sonographer observes and evaluates on the monitor.

an endovaginal probe are usually flipped so that they are presented in the more traditional transabdominal transducer orientation, whereas images obtained using an endorectal probe are presented in the transducer–organ orientation. With neurosonography (neurosonology), the superior scanning surface is presented at the top of the image when the transducer is placed on the head.

These six scanning surfaces, anterior or posterior, right or left, endocavitary (vaginal or rectal), and the cranial fontanelle coupled with three anatomic planes (sagittal, coronal, and transverse) produce a combination of 14 different image presentations.

Longitudinal: Sagittal Planes

When scanning in the longitudinal, sagittal plane, the transducer orientation sends and receives the sound from either an anterior or posterior scanning surface. For a longitudinal plane, the transducer indicator is at the 12-o'clock position to the organ or to the area of interest. This always places the superior (cephalic) location on the image. From either the anterior or posterior body surface, the patient can be scanned in either erect, supine, prone, or an oblique position. The image presentation includes either the anterior or posterior, the superior (cephalic), and the inferior (caudal) anatomic area being examined[1,2] (Fig. 2-5A). Because the

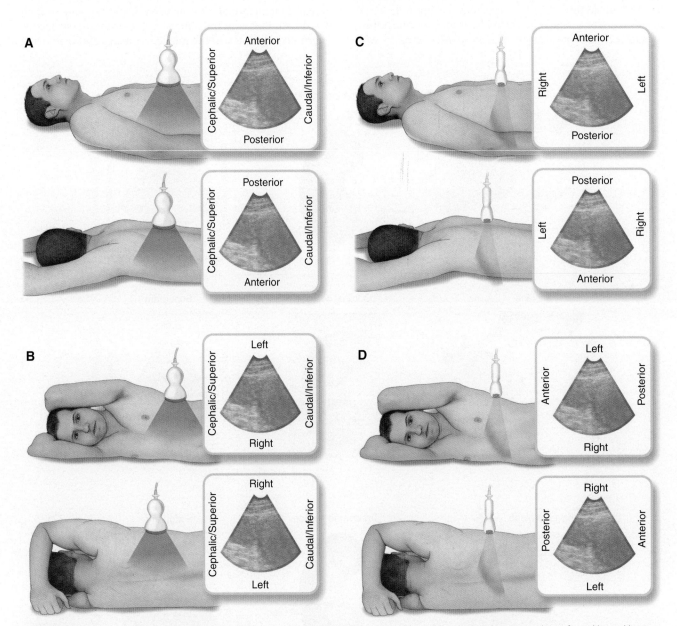

FIGURE 2-5 Image presentations. **A:** Longitudinal, sagittal plane. With the patient being scanned from either the anterior or posterior surface with or without obliquity, the image seen on the monitor demonstrates the scanning surface (anterior or posterior) and the superior (cephalic) and inferior (caudal) areas being examined. **B:** Longitudinal, coronal plane. With the patient being scanned from either the right or left surface with or without obliquity, the image seen on the monitor demonstrates the scanning surface (right or left) and the superior (cephalic) and inferior (caudal) areas being examined. **C:** Transverse plane, anterior or posterior surface. With the patient being scanned from either the anterior or posterior surface with or without obliquity, the image seen on the monitor demonstrates the scanning surface (anterior or posterior) and the right and left areas being examined. **D:** Transverse plane, right or left surface. With the patient being scanned from either the right or left surface with or without obliquity, the image seen on the monitor demonstrates the scanning surface (right or left) and the anterior and posterior areas being examined.

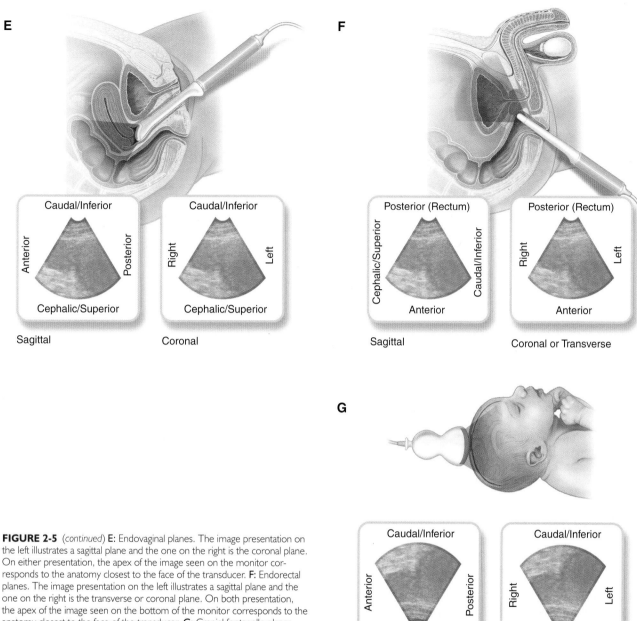

FIGURE 2-5 *(continued)* **E:** Endovaginal planes. The image presentation on the left illustrates a sagittal plane and the one on the right is the coronal plane. On either presentation, the apex of the image seen on the monitor corresponds to the anatomy closest to the face of the transducer. **F:** Endorectal planes. The image presentation on the left illustrates a sagittal plane and the one on the right is the transverse or coronal plane. On both presentation, the apex of the image seen on the bottom of the monitor corresponds to the anatomy closest to the face of the transducer. **G:** Cranial fontanelle planes. With the patient being scanned from either the anterior or posterior surface with or without obliquity, the image seen on the monitor demonstrates the scanning surface (anterior or posterior) and the superior (cephalic) and inferior (caudal) areas being examined.

longitudinal, sagittal image presentation does not demonstrate the right and left lateral areas, the adjacent areas can be evaluated and documented with transducer manipulation, by changing the transducer orientation or by changing the patient position.[2]

Longitudinal: Coronal Planes

When scanning in the longitudinal, coronal plane, the transducer orientation sends and receives the sound from either the right or left scanning surface. Because the transducer indicator is at the 12-o'clock position with respect to the organ or to the area of interest, the superior (cephalic) location is always imaged. From either the right or left body surface, the patient can be scanned in an erect, decubitus,

or an oblique position and the image presentation includes either the left or right, the superior (cephalic), and the inferior (caudal) anatomic areas being examined[1,2] (Fig. 2-5B). Because the longitudinal, coronal image presentation does not demonstrate the anterior or posterior areas, the adjacent areas can be evaluated and documented with transducer manipulation, by changing the transducer orientation or by changing the patient position.[2]

Transverse Plane: Anterior or Posterior Surface

Using the anterior or posterior surface, the transducer orientation for a transverse plane places the transducer indicator at the 9-o'clock position on either the anterior or posterior surface to the organ or to the area of interest. The right and left locations are always imaged. From either the anterior or posterior surfaces, the patient can be scanned in an erect, decubitus, or an oblique position. The image presentation includes either the anterior or posterior as well as the right and left anatomic areas being examined[1,2] (Fig. 2-5C).

Transverse Plane: Right or Left Surface

Using the right or left surface, the transducer orientation for a transverse plane places the transducer indicator at the 9-o'clock position on either the right or left surface to the organ or to the area of interest. From either the right or left surfaces, the patient can be scanned in an erect, decubitus, or an oblique position. The image presentation includes either the right or left and the anterior and posterior anatomic areas being examined[1,2] (Fig. 2-5D).

Endovaginal Planes

The patient is in the supine position for endovaginal imaging. The image presentation does not change if the system employs either an end-firing or an angle-firing endovaginal transducer. For the sagittal (longitudinal) plane, the transducer is placed at the caudal end of the body with the indicator at the 12-o'clock position. Both the endovaginal sagittal and translabial transducer orientations produce the same image presentation. The inferior (caudal) anatomy is presented at the top of the monitor with visualization of the anterior and posterior anatomic areas.

The coronal plane is obtained with the transducer at the caudal end of the body and the indicator at the 9-o'clock position. The top (apex) of the image is the inferior (caudal) area and the right and left anatomic areas can be visualized on the display monitor. The coronal plane is sometimes described using an older description reference to transverse plane[1] (Fig. 2-5E).

Endorectal Planes

The patient is most often in a left lateral decubitus position for the placement of either the end-firing transducer or the biplane endorectal transducer. When used for biopsy, both end-firing and biplane endorectal transducers place the biopsy guide anterior toward the prostate. For either the sagittal plane or the transverse or coronal plane, the anterior rectal wall is the scanning surface and is assigned to the bottom of the display monitor (Fig. 2-5F).

Cranial Fontanelle Planes

For neonatal brain examinations, the sagittal and coronal planes are most commonly accessed using the anterior fontanelle. For the sagittal plane, the transducer indicator is at the 6-o'clock position and indicates the anterior side of the brain. For the coronal plane, the transducer indicator is at the 9-o'clock position and indicates the right side of the brain (Fig. 2-5G).

UNDERSTANDING IMAGE QUALITY DEFINITIONS

The evaluation of sonographic image quality is learned and communicated using specific definitions. Normal tissue and organ structures have a characteristic echographic appearance relative to surrounding structures. An understanding of the normal appearance provides the baseline against which to recognize variations and abnormalities. These definitions describe and characterize the sonographic image.

An *echo* is the recorded acoustic signal. It is the reflection of the pulse of sound emitted by the transducer. Prefixes or suffixes modify the quality of the echo and are used to describe characteristics and patterns on the image.

Echogenic describes an organ or tissue that is capable of producing echoes by reflecting the acoustic beam. This term does not describe the quality of the image; it is often used to describe relative tissue texture (e.g., more or less echogenic than another tissue) (Fig. 2-6A, B). An aberration from normal echogenicity patterns may signify a pathologic condition or poor examination technique such as incorrect gain settings.

Anechoic describes the portion of an image that appears echo-free. A urine-filled bladder, a bile-filled gallbladder, and a clear cyst all appear anechoic (Fig. 2-6C). *Sonolucent* is the property of a medium allowing easy passage of sound (i.e., low attenuation). Sonolucent and transonic are misnomers that are often substituted for anechoic.[3] When the sonographic appearance is anechoic, sonographers frequently use the term *cystic*. When describing the appearance of the echo, the term anechoic is preferred. When describing the histopathologic nature of an anechoic structure, the term cystic or cyst-like is preferred (see "Clarifying Sonographic Characteristics").

If the scattering amplitude changes from one tissue to another, it results in brightness changes on an image. These brightness changes require terminology to describe normal and abnormal sonographic appearances. *Hyperechoic* describes image echoes brighter than surrounding tissues or brighter than normal for a specific tissue or organ. Hyperechoic regions result from an increased amount of sound scatter relative to the surrounding tissue. *Hypoechoic* describes portions of an image that are not as bright as surrounding tissues or less bright than normal. The hypoechoic regions result from reduced sound scatter relative to the surrounding tissue. *Echopenic* describes a structure that is less echogenic than others or has few internal echoes. *Isoechoic* describes structures of equal echo density. These terms can be used to compare echo textures (Fig. 2-6D).

Homogeneous refers to imaged echoes of equal intensity. A homogeneous portion of the image may be anechoic, hypoechoic, hyperechoic, or echopenic. *Heterogeneous* describes tissue or organ structures that have several different echo characteristics. A normal liver, spleen, or testicle has a homogeneous echo texture, whereas a normal kidney is heterogeneous, with several different echo textures.

Acoustic enhancement is the increased acoustic signal amplitude that returns from regions lying beyond an object that causes little or no attenuation of the sound beam such as fluid-filled structures. The opposite of acoustic enhancement is acoustic shadowing; both are types of sonographic artifacts. *Acoustic shadowing* describes reduced echo amplitude from regions lying beyond an attenuating object. An example is cholelithiasis, where there is a reduction in echo amplitudes distal to a strongly attenuating or reflecting structure (Fig. 2-6E). Air bubbles (bowel gas) do not allow transmission of the sound beam, and most of the sound is reflected. Often, sonographers refer to the shadowing caused by low reflectivity as soft or dirty shadowing.

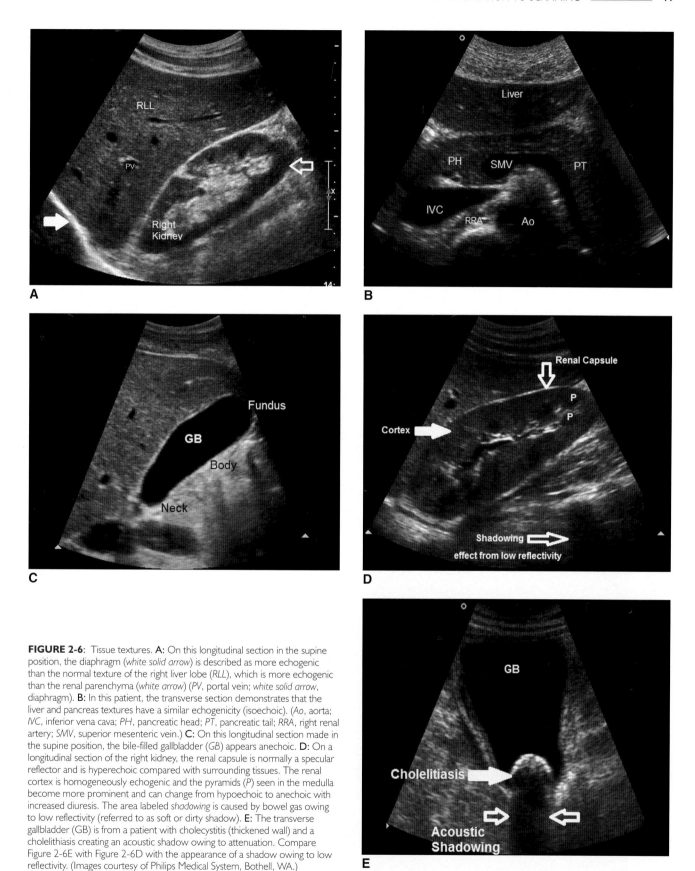

FIGURE 2-6: Tissue textures. **A:** On this longitudinal section in the supine position, the diaphragm (*white solid arrow*) is described as more echogenic than the normal texture of the right liver lobe (*RLL*), which is more echogenic than the renal parenchyma (*white arrow*) (*PV*, portal vein; *white solid arrow*, diaphragm). **B:** In this patient, the transverse section demonstrates that the liver and pancreas textures have a similar echogenicity (isoechoic). (*Ao*, aorta; *IVC*, inferior vena cava; *PH*, pancreatic head; *PT*, pancreatic tail; *RRA*, right renal artery; *SMV*, superior mesenteric vein.) **C:** On this longitudinal section made in the supine position, the bile-filled gallbladder (*GB*) appears anechoic. **D:** On a longitudinal section of the right kidney, the renal capsule is normally a specular reflector and is hyperechoic compared with surrounding tissues. The renal cortex is homogeneously echogenic and the pyramids (*P*) seen in the medulla become more prominent and can change from hypoechoic to anechoic with increased diuresis. The area labeled *shadowing* is caused by bowel gas owing to low reflectivity (referred to as soft or dirty shadow). **E:** The transverse gallbladder (GB) is from a patient with cholecystitis (thickened wall) and a cholelithiasis creating an acoustic shadow owing to attenuation. Compare Figure 2-6E with Figure 2-6D with the appearance of a shadow owing to low reflectivity. (Images courtesy of Philips Medical System, Bothell, WA.)

CLARIFYING SONOGRAPHIC CHARACTERISTICS

There are three other definitions frequently used to describe internal echo patterns: cystic, solid, and complex.

The diagnosis of a cyst is made on many asymptomatic patients based on specific sonographic characteristic appearances and only in certain situations, with a correlation to the patient's history. The sonographic criteria for cystic structures or masses are as follows: (1) Cysts retain an anechoic center, which indicates the lack of internal echoes even at high instrument gain settings. (2) The mass is well defined, with a sharply defined posterior wall indicative of a strong interface between cyst fluid and tissue or parenchyma. (3) There is an increased echo amplitude in the tissue beginning at the far wall and proceeding distally compared with surrounding tissue. This increased amplitude is better known as *through-transmission* or the *acoustic enhancement artifact*. It occurs because tissue located on either side of the cystic structure attenuates more sound than does the cystic structure. Reverberation artifacts can be identified at the near-wall if the cyst is located close to the transducer.[3] Edge shadowing artifacts may appear depending on the incident angle (refraction) and the thickness of the cystic wall at the periphery of the structure. The tadpole tail sign occurs with a combination of an edge shadow next to the echo enhancement (Fig. 2-7A).

A solid structure may have a hyperechoic, hypoechoic, echopenic, or anechoic homogeneous echo texture, or it may be heterogeneous because it contains many different types of interfaces. Usually, solid structures exhibit the following characteristics: (1) internal echoes that increase with an increase in instrument gain settings; (2) irregular, often poorly defined walls and margins; and

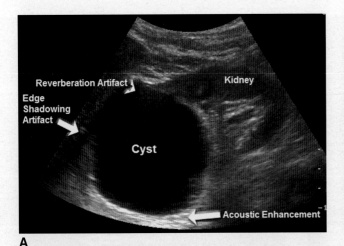

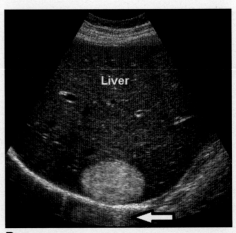

A

B

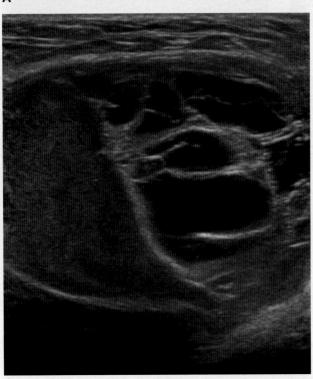

C

FIGURE 2-7 Interpretation. **A:** Cystic. A longitudinal section of the right kidney demonstrates a renal cyst. The sonographic criteria for a cyst are as follows: (1) anechoic center, (2) clear definition with a sharply defined posterior wall, (3) acoustic enhancement, (4) reverberation artifacts (*white arrowhead*), and (5) edge shadowing artifact. **B:** Solid. A transverse section through the right lobe of the liver demonstrates a hemangioma. The benign solid mass presents with the following sonographic criteria for a solid mass: (1) internal echoes that increase with increased gain settings and (2) low-amplitude echoes (*arrow*) or shadowing posterior to the mass. Irregular walls may be present when the solid mass is a calculus or a malignant tumor. **C:** Complex. The encapsulated mass is a complex structure exhibiting septa between echogenic and anechoic areas. (Images courtesy of Philips Medical System, Bothell, WA.)

(3) low-amplitude echoes or shadowing posterior to the mass owing to increased acoustic attenuation by soft tissue or calculi (Fig. 2-7B).

A complex structure usually exhibits both anechoic and echogenic areas on the image, originating from both fluid and soft tissue components within the mass. The relative echogenicity of a soft tissue mass is related to a variety of constituents, including collagen content, interstitial components, vascularity, and the degree and type of tissue degeneration (Fig. 2-7C).

The amplitude of echoes distal to a mass, structure, or organ can be used to evaluate the attenuation properties of that mass. *Transonic* or *sonolucent* refers to masses, organs, or tissues that attenuate little of the acoustic beam and result in images with distal high-intensity echoes.[3] An example is a cystic structure with the associated acoustic enhancement artifact. Masses that attenuate large amounts of sound show a marked decrease in the amplitude of distal echoes. An example is calculi, with the associated shadow artifact.

PREPARING FOR THE SONOGRAPHY EXAMINATION

Before the patient is scanned, it is important for the sonographer to obtain as much information as possible. The sonographer should be aware of the indications for the study and of any additional clinical information such as laboratory values, results of previous examinations, and related imaging examinations. The sonography examination should be tailored to answer the clinical questions posed by the overall clinical assessment.

Patient apprehension is reduced when the examination is explained. Apprehension may be lessened further by providing a clean, neat examination room, extending common courtesies and a smile, and letting the patient know that the sonographer enjoys providing this diagnostic service. It is important that patients know that they are the focus of the sonographer's attention.

The region of interest is visualized by planning the sonography examination to image in multiple planes, two of which are perpendicular to each other. Any abnormality is imaged with differing degrees of transducer and patient obliquity to collect more information. The patient is released only after sufficient information is documented, because being called back for a repeat examination will increase the patient's apprehension.

THE SONOGRAPHER'S DOCUMENTATION

The section on Scope of Practice and Clinical Standards introduced in Chapter 1 is relevant to the important role and the position of the sonographer related to the documentation required for a sonography examination.[4] The section entitled Scope of Practice and Clinical Standards states that the diagnostic medical sonographer functions as a delegated agent of the physician and does not practice independently.[4] In the Clinical Standards, Standard 1.6 Documentation and the AIUM practice parameter for documentation of a sonography examination clarifies the

sonographer is to be aware that the sonography examination is a legal document that becomes a permanent part of the patients' medical history.[4-6] The sonography examinations should be recorded for suitable diagnostic purposes and to allow subsequent review.[5] Table 2-3 provides a list of the minimum information to be documented with the examination.

Ideally, the sonographer has an opportunity to discuss these findings with the sonologist. As a team, the sonographer and sonologist determine when the documentation is sufficient to complete the sonography examination. When immediate action is indicated by the sonographic findings and the sonologist is unavailable to provide the official interpretive report, the sonographer should provide the referring physician with as much information as possible immediately following the examination.

The report should describe the sonographic findings only on what is documented, without offering a conclusion regarding pathology. The terminology presented earlier is very helpful. The report should include the scanning plane, normal tissue echogenicity, abnormal tissue texture (anechoic, hyperechoic, hypoechoic, isoechoic, cystic, solid or complex, focal or diffused, and shadowing or acoustic enhancement), measurements (vessels, ducts, organs, wall thickness, masses), location of measurements, and abnormal amounts of fluid collections. For example, a discussion of the sonographic findings would include a description of an echogenic mass that appears attached to the gallbladder wall that does not move as the patient changes position, whereas a diagnosis would include the statement that the patient has a polyp located in the gallbladder.

Sonographers should be competent, through education and experience, to provide images of adequate quality and written documentation of the sonographic findings. Sonographers should not provide any verbal or written sonographic findings to the patient or the patient's family.

While revealing their sonographic evaluation expertise, sonographers should always adhere to the scope of practice and the codes of medical ethics and/or professional conduct available from professional associations. A sonographer cannot act as a diagnostician.[5]

TABLE 2-3 Required Documentation for the Sonography Examination[4-6]

Patient's name and other identifying information (birthday, gender, etc.)

Identifying information of the facility where the examination was completed

Date, time, and length of the sonography examination

The output display standards to include both the thermal index and the mechanical index

Standard presentation and labeling of images to include anatomic location laterality (right, left, midline) when appropriate

Image orientation when appropriate

Completed oral or written summary of findings for the supervising interpreting provider or physician

SENSITIVITY, SPECIFICITY, AND ACCURACY[7]

Sonographers should be aware of a few statistical parameters developed to judge the efficacy of sonographic examinations. These statistics are frequently reported in the literature. A knowledge of these statistics allows the sonographer to provide a sound rationale for why a diagnostic procedure should or should not be performed.

There are four possible results for each sonographic examination correlated to an independent determination of disease, such as a biopsy or a surgical procedure. (1) A *true-positive result* means that the sonographic findings were positive and the patient does have the disease or pathology. (2) A *true-negative result* means that the sonographic findings were negative and the patient does not have the disease or pathology. (3) A *false-positive result* means that the sonographic findings were positive but the patient does not have the disease or pathology. (4) A *false-negative result* means that the sonographic findings were negative but the patient does have the disease or pathology. Sonographers should strive to increase both the true-positive and true-negative results.

The examination's sensitivity describes how well the sonographic examination documents whatever disease or pathology is present. Mathematically, it is determined by the equation [true positive ÷ (true positive + false negative) × 100]. If the number of false-negative examinations decreases, the sensitivity of the examination increases.

The examination's specificity describes how well the sonographic examination documents normal findings or excludes patients without disease or pathology. Mathematically, it is determined by the equation [true negative ÷ (true negative + false positive) × 100]. If the number of false-positive examinations decreases, the specificity of the examination increases.

The accuracy of the sonographic examination is its ability to find disease or pathology if present and to not find disease or pathology if not present. Mathematically, it is determined by the equation [true positive + true negative ÷ (all patients receiving the sonographic examination) × 100].

There are two other statistics that sonographers should be aware of. The positive predictive value indicates the likelihood of disease or pathology if the test is positive. Mathematically, it is determined by the equation [true positive ÷ (true positives + false positives) × 100]. The negative predictive value indicates the likelihood of the patient being free of disease or pathology if the test is negative. Mathematically, it is determined by the equation [true negatives ÷ (true negatives + false positives) × 100].

The mathematical formulas presented provide a percentage. If sensitivity, specificity, accuracy, and positive and negative predictive values are expressed by fractions between 0 and 1 rather than by a percentage, then the parameters are not multiplied by 100.

SUMMARY

- Learning and understanding accurate and precise terminology allow better communication among professionals.

- Developing standard protocols based on understanding patient positions, transducer orientations, and image presentations increases the accuracy of the sonography examinations.

- Sonographers describe sonographic findings with terminology that defines echo amplitude, echo texture, structural borders, characteristics of organs and anatomic relationships, sound transmission, and acoustic artifacts and identifies cystic, solid, and complex masses.

- The sonography examination relies on the skill, knowledge, and accuracy of the sonographer who must pay attention to the texture, outline, size, and shape of both normal and abnormal structures.

- The patient will benefit most when the sonographic appearance is correlated with patient history, clinical presentation, laboratory function tests, and other imaging modalities to compose a clinically helpful picture.

- True positive, true negative, false positive, false negative, sensitivity, specificity, and accuracy are statistical parameters used to judge the efficacy of sonography examinations.

REFERENCES

1. American Institute of Ultrasound in Medicine. *Standard Presentation and Labeling of Ultrasound Images*. 6th ed. American Institute of Ultrasound in Medicine; 2020. Accessed January 20, 2022. http://aium.s3.amazonaws.com/resourceLibrary/splv6.pdf
2. Tempkin BB. Scanning planes and scanning methods. In: Tempkin BB, ed. *Ultrasound Scanning: Principles and Protocols*. 4th ed. Elsevier Saunders; 2015:15–28.
3. American Institute of Ultrasound in Medicine. *Recommended Ultrasound Terminology*. 4th ed. American Institute of Ultrasound in Medicine; 2019. Accessed January 20, 2022. http://aium.s3.amazonaws.com/resourceLibrary/rut.pdf
4. Society of Diagnostic Medical Sonography. Scope of practice and clinical standards for the diagnostic medical sonographer. 2015. Accessed January 20, 2022. https://www.sdms.org/about/who-we-are/scope-of-practice
5. American Institute of Ultrasound in Medicine. AIUM practice parameter for documentation of an ultrasound examination. 2019. Accessed January 20, 2022. https://onlinelibrary.wiley.com/doi/epdf/10.1002/jum.15187
6. Penny SM. *Introduction to Sonography and Patient Care*. 2nd ed. Wolters Kluwer; 2021.
7. Kremkau FW. *Sonography: Principles and Instruments*. 10th ed. Elsevier; 2021.

CHAPTER 3

Ergonomic Practices for Abdominal Imaging

SUSAN RAATZ STEPHENSON

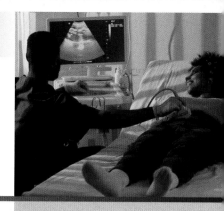

OBJECTIVES

- Recognize factors, both professional and personal, that increase the risk of developing musculoskeletal disorders (MSKDs).
- Classify symptoms of MSKD into three categories.
- Adapt the environment to reduce MSKD.
- Discuss correct and incorrect postures.
- Demonstrate exercises and stretches that aid in reducing repetitive stress injuries.

GLOSSARY

abduction moving away from the center of the body

ergonomics the creation of a safe workplace that involves the sonographer and ultrasound system positioning

extension a position that increases the angle of a joint (e.g., the unbending of the elbow, straightening of the spine)

flexion the decrease of an angle of a joint (i.e., bending of the elbow, curling of the spine)

hyperextension movement beyond the normal range of a joint

neutral position body position without flexion or extension

posture the position of the body

repetition repeated movements. When coupled with force and awkward body positions, repetition increases the risk of musculoskeletal disorders

repetitive stress injury cumulative injury because of repeated movement of a musculoskeletal structure

risk factor any behavior that increases the chances of developing musculoskeletal disorders

static posture fixed or unchanging position

workstation work area encompassing the equipment (i.e., ultrasound system, patient bed)

KEY TERMS

abduction

ergonomics

extension

flexion

hyperextension

musculoskeletal
disorders (MSKDs)

neutral position

repetitive stress injury

workstation

Musculoskeletal disorders (MSKDs)—injury to the muscles, nerves, ligaments, and tendons—result in a decrease in the ability to participate in both daily and work activities. Though often thought to be the result of work tasks, personal habits and life events change the risk. These include life changes such as pregnancy,[1] results of aging and disease treatment (i.e., use of statins),[2] and injury because of life activities (i.e., softball).

Work-related musculoskeletal disorders (WRMSKDs) occur in over half of working adults over 18 years, with the costs increasing with medical care, lost wages, and legal fees. A reduction in the accompanying symptoms can be anticipated upon retirement (>65 years); however, 40% of the time, problems continue.[3] Most medical professionals report working in pain because of the varied risk factors, resulting in the development of WRMSKDs.[3-10] Sonographers seldom anticipate that helping diagnose and ease patient suffering could lead to their own. Clinicians using an ultrasound system have indicated that the shoulder is the most common location for pain, closely followed by the lower back and wrist.[11,12] Table 3-1 provides a comparison of MSKDs for various medical professions, and Table 3-2 summarizes the days of work lost by sonographers because of varied symptoms.

PHYSICAL RISK FACTORS FOR WORK-RELATED MUSCULOSKELETAL DISORDERS

The reasons for the development of WRMSKDs are as varied as the person with complaints. Any movement or task creating an imbalance between a person and their environment describes a risk factor.[13] Usually associated with the work environment, many activities outside of work also contribute to MSKDs, thus adding to the cumulative injuries.

WRMSKD development depends on multiple factors, but there are key factors contributing to musculoskeletal problems. In this chapter, the focus is on work tasks that increase the risk of developing WRMSKD in sonographers. To begin, attention is paid to activities that increase risks:

- **Force** is the work needed to grasp, lift, or move an item. Examples include the tightness of grasp on the transducer or effort needed to hold and use a biopsy needle.
- **Vibration** refers to repeated, fast movement in any direction. Imaging systems vibrate while being pushed (force) during portable exams and some mechanical 3D transducers also vibrate.
- Sustained **body positions** are those that move out of a neutral position, thus fatiguing muscles and joints. When scanning a patient with the arm behind the body or with a head moved away from the central axis, the body placement is in a non-neutral position.
- **Contact pressure** of a body part against hard or sharp edges—for example, when the ventral wrist is placed on the desk while completing patient exams, the risk for developing carpal tunnel syndrome increases.
- Frequent **repetitive movements** using the same muscle groups or joints describe a repeated movement. This often occurs when a mouse is used to complete the tasks.
- **Temperature** is a final consideration because muscles that are cold have the potential to fail sooner than those used after a warm-up session.

The focus on WRMSKDs often falls on the physical risk factors, the interaction of stressors, and social setting. In the work environment, the inability to change task demands also increases the risks. These include the following:

- Lack of control over job tasks
- Increased production demands
- Communication failures
- Missing task variety resulting in boredom
- Lack of management support
- Job insecurity

CUMULATIVE MUSCULOSKELETAL DISORDER SIGNS AND SYMPTOMS

MSKDs are the result of accumulated **trauma** over a prolonged time; however, human bodies provide warning signs related to the severity of the injuries. Repeated exposure to a task reduces the body's ability to recover and repair itself. As a result, an injury is often not recognized or the cause of the symptoms is unable to be identified. The duration, signs, and symptoms provide clues to whether the pain is due to early-, intermediate-, or late-stage injuries.

An **early-stage injury** presents with aching, fatigue, stiffness, or discomfort in a muscle or joint. For example, the back or hand may ache; however, stretching and rest will resolve the symptoms. There will be no reduction in the ability to complete work or personal tasks. In essence,

TABLE 3-1 Percentage of Medical Professionals Working with Pain

Profession	Percentage (%)
Nurses	88
Sonographers	86
Obstetricians and midwives	85
Pregnant without history of pain	70
Other medical imaging professionals	45

TABLE 3-2 Nonfatal Occupational Injuries and Illnesses Resulting in Days Away from Work, by Nature of Injury, Private Industry, 2011

Nature of Injury	Number	Percent of Total	Typical Parts of Body Affected
Total	908,310	100.0	—
Sprains, strains, and tears	340,870	37.5	—
Sprains	84,560	9.3	Ankle, knee
Strains	209,740	23.1	Back, shoulder
Major tears to muscles, tendons, and ligaments	17,150	1.9	Shoulder, knee
Multiple strains, sprains, and tears	7,130	0.8	—
Sprains, strains, and tears, unspecified	22,290	2.5	—

From U.S. Bureau of Labor Statistics. Using workplace safety and health data for injury prevention. Accessed August 6, 2016. http://www.bls.gov/opub/mlr/2013/article/using-workplace-safety-data-for-prevention.htm

the work a body does is being balanced with contracting stretches, exercises, and rest.

As an injury progresses to the **intermediate stage**, pain is accompanied by the early-stage symptoms of aching and fatigue. In the event of a work injury, symptoms continue outside of the working environment and the advantages of structured stretching decrease. At this stage, the MSK injury begins to restrict activities, bringing lives out of "balance" even with stretching and rest. Commonly, pain disturbs sleep, and repetitive tasks—such as sewing, typing, and playing an instrument—become difficult.

Chronic injury adds another symptom, weakness or dropping of objects. At this stage, sleeping becomes difficult because of persistent pain. The work–life balance has become weighted toward the symptoms of pain, tiredness, aching, and weakness, with stretching, rest, and exercise having little effect. At this stage, work and personal life are restricted, with the possibility of surgery, physical therapy,

and medication as the only methods of relief. Failure of treatment methods to help may result in disability.[14] MSKD may progress through these stages, and everyone has a different development of symptoms—highlighting the importance of reporting symptoms.

UNDERSTANDING NEUTRAL BODY ALIGNMENT

Maintaining awkward body positions is one of the greatest risk factors encountered by scanning clinicians. The requirement for repeated, static contraction of muscles results in early fatigue, muscle integrity changes, circulation reductions, and buildup of metabolic waste. In preparing for exams, a neutral spine and arm position, decreased reach, and organization of work tools should be ensured (i.e., gel bottle and ultrasound system) (Figs. 3-1 and 3-2).

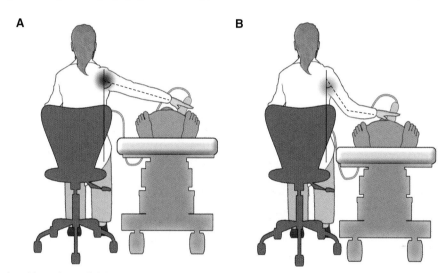

FIGURE 3-1 **A:** Positioning of the patient and chair at a distance increases the arm angle, thus increasing the risk of developing shoulder pain. This positioning also encourages leaning to the right as the arm becomes fatigued, placing stress on the right side of the body. **B:** Moving the patient toward the sonographer allows a decrease in the arm angle to less than 30 degrees, ensuring maintenance of a neutral, balanced spine.

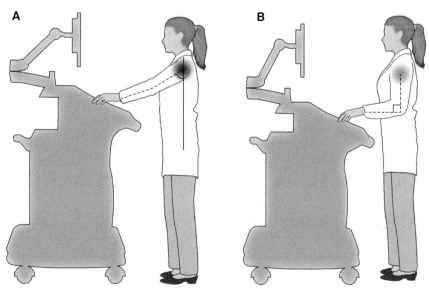

FIGURE 3-2 **A:** Placement of the ultrasound system and patient places the spine and the shoulder in a non-neutral position. **B:** Standing while scanning also requires placement of the spine in a neutral ventral to dorsal position. The arm is close to the side, parallel to the body, with a 90-degree elbow flexion. Note: Move the system control panel up or down to allow for proper body position.

The Neutral Wrist

The wrist joint is also one body part that is often ignored while scanning. It is a common occurrence to feel the need to ventrally flex, dorsally extend, or use radial and ulnar deviation of the wrist to obtain images (Figs. 3-3 and 3-4).[12,15]

No Pinch Zone

One of the tools used during ultrasound exams is the transducer that is transmits and receives the ultrasound signals. Used during each exam, awareness should be on the grip because the amount of force used may determine the development of MSK injuries to the upper extremity.[11,16] The global increase in patient obesity has led to the use of increasing axial force to acquire images.[11,16] Repetitive stress injuries any time similar muscle groups are used repeatedly, with wrist stress increasing the risk of developing carpal tunnel syndrome and de Quervain syndrome (Fig. 3-5).[17] Table 3-3 lists WRMSKDs of the upper body.

FITTING THE WORKSTATION

The evolution of the ultrasound system has allowed for a decrease in the size and weight of not only the system but also the transducers. Even with lighter equipment, a suboptimal room setup decreases the benefits of the workstation. It is well worth the extra time to set up the tools before beginning the exam.

Neutral Reach Zones

A neutral body position links directly with maintaining a balanced spine; an ergonomic shoulder, arm, and wrist position; and helping to reduce WRMSKDs. The two reach zones, horizontal and vertical, allow movement of the arm without extension. The **horizontal neutral zone** is close to the body, allowing for approximately a 45-degree medial and lateral rotation of the arm.[18] During the ultrasound exam, this area encompasses the transducer and control panel (Figs. 3-6 and 3-7).[18]

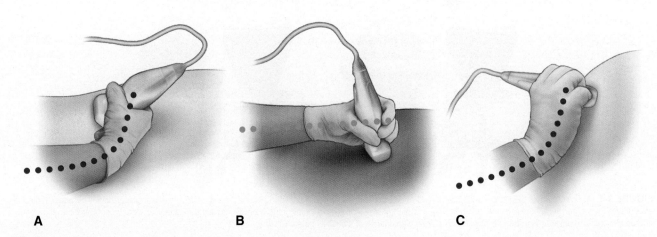

FIGURE 3-3 **A:** Dorsal flexion of the wrist. **B:** Neutral position. **C:** Dorsal extension of the wrist.

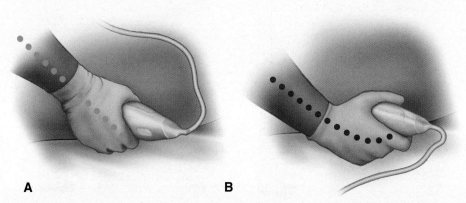

FIGURE 3-4 **A:** Neutral position of the wrist with a relaxed hand grip. The lateral fingers in contact with the patient help stabilize the transducer. **B:** Radial deviation of the wrist with a pinch grip using the thumb, index, and middle finger while imaging the dependent side of a patient. This type of grip increases the force needed to hold the transducer, resulting in hand and forearm fatigue.

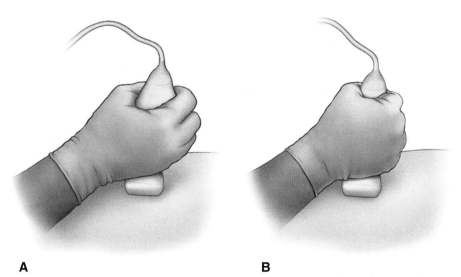

A **B**

FIGURE 3-5 A: A relaxed grip on the transducer allows for stability and decreased hand fatigue. **B:** A tight grip on the transducer accompanied with axial pressure on the patient increases the force on the joints and muscles. If it is difficult to release the transducer, the fingers or thumb locks after an exam, the grip is too tight.

TABLE 3-3	**Common WRMSKDs of the Upper Body**	
Disorders	**Occupational Risk Factors**	**Symptoms**
Tendonitis/tenosynovitis	Repetitive wrist motions Repetitive shoulder motions Sustained hyperextension of arms Prolonged load on shoulders	Pain, weakness, swelling, burning sensation, or dull ache over affected area
Epicondylitis (tendonitis or the medial or lateral elbow tendons)	Repeated or forceful rotation of the forearm and bending of the wrist at the same time	Same symptoms as tendonitis
Carpal tunnel syndrome	Repetitive wrist motions	Pain, numbness, tingling, burning sensations, wasting of muscles at base of thumb, dry palm
De Quervain disease	Repetitive hand twisting and forceful gripping	Pain at the base of thumb
Thoracic outlet syndrome	Prolonged shoulder flexion Extending arms above shoulder height Carrying loads on the shoulder	Pain, numbness, swelling of the hands
Tension neck syndrome	Prolonged restricted posture	Pain

WRMSKDs, work-related musculoskeletal disorders.
Canadian Centre for Occupational Health and Safety. Work-related musculoskeletal disorders (WMSDs). OSH Answers Fact Sheets. September 12, 2019. https://www.ccohs.ca/oshanswers/diseases/rmirsi.html. Reproduced with the permission of CCOHS, 2022.

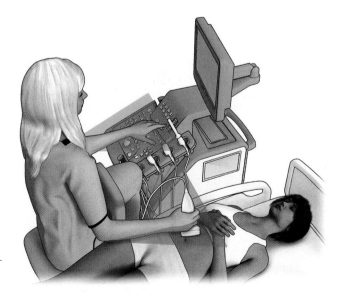

FIGURE 3-6 To decrease arm extension, place frequently used functions within the horizontal neutral zone. These include moving not only the patient but also controls such as the trackball, freeze, and mode activation keys. Rotate the control panel slightly away from the center within the horizontal zone to ensure a straight wrist and forearm. Regardless of the position (sitting vs. standing), ensure the elbow flexion remains at approximately 90 degrees.

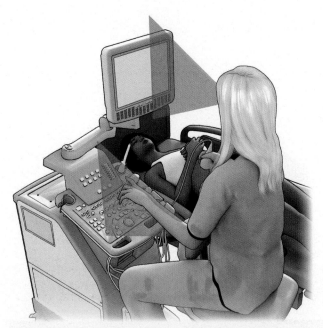

FIGURE 3-7 The vertical neutral zone includes system features above or below the control panel. The touchscreen or digital keyboard lies in this area as does the monitor. Proper placement of the monitor slightly toward the patient allows maintenance of a neutral spine and head position while decreasing shoulder use.

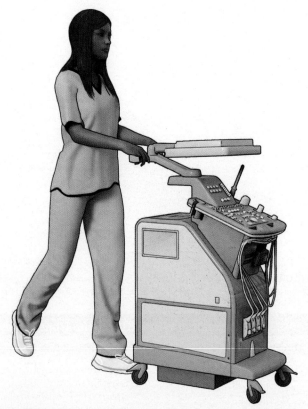

FIGURE 3-8 This sonographer has placed the transducer in the holders with the cables in the provided hooks below the control panel. The folded monitor provides an unobstructed view. The control panel is adjusted to a height at low chest, allowing for the maintenance of an appropriate elbow angle. Pushing the system requires less force than pulling the system.

The **vertical neutral zone**, located between 80 and 100 degrees of elbow flexion, includes the touch screen, digital keyboard, and the monitor. Temporary conditions, such as an injury or pregnancy, require adjustments to remain within the horizontal and vertical zones.[19]

Ultrasound System Ergonomics

Modern ultrasound systems allow for multiple adjustments to help maintain a **neutral body position**. One of the first adjustments is to raise or lower the control panel—remember to match the height to the chair and exam table. Another useful modification is to rotate the control panel to the right or left and change the front-to-back position.[20] Around the control panel, systems provide hooks to place transducer cables, thus supporting the weight and decreasing the twisting or torque on the wrist.

Most systems allow for independent monitor positioning, tilt, angle, and rotation, providing a method to decrease neck flexion and extension.[18] The system monitor is adjusted with the top at eye level and directly in front of the sonographer at a distance of approximately 40 inches (50 to 100 cm).[18] In the department that allows the patient to view the exam or in the event of multiple ultrasound-guided procedures, an auxiliary monitor should be considered. Other adjustments include changing the brightness to match the room lighting, expanding the ultrasound image size, and taking visual breaks by periodically looking at a distant object for 20 seconds every 20 minutes.[18]

Patients within an intensive care unit—whether adult, pediatric, or neonates—often require a portable exam. When transporting the system, pushing or pulling results in the use of increased force to move across varied floor surfaces

and thresholds. A smaller portable or laptop-style system requires less work and force to move to the patient's bedside. When moving a system, ensure the monitor is folded down, positioning of handles is at the lower chest, and there is proper storage of the transducer cables (Fig. 3-8). Remain diligent in the maintenance of a neutral body position for both the trunk and arms.

ERGONOMIC TOOLS

The design of modern ultrasound systems provides the ability to create an ergonomic work space. The adjustment of monitors and control panels and the use of lighter transducer cables help reduce risk factors when combined with additional tools such as adjustable exam tables and chairs, along with arm and cable supports. Table 3-4 provides information on additional adjustments to help reduce risk factors for developing WRMSKDs.

EXAM-SPECIFIC SETUP

Depending on the exam type (i.e., abdominal, thyroid), various adjustments of the ultrasound system and room are required to increase ergonomics. Adjustments of the environment include the following:

- Scheduling varied exam types to alter muscle groups used during the day

TABLE 3-4	**More About Using Ergonomic Tools**		
Tool	**Features**	**Aids In**	**Example**

Chair	Height adjustable
	Lumbar support
	Swivel chair and back
		Maintenance of
		  90-degree elbow flexion and
		  30-degree arm abduction
		Allows maintenance of the feet on
		  the floor or on the foot support	

Table	Narrow and height adjustable Removable components to aid in transducer placement	Reduces arm abduction	
Rolled-up towels Block and angle sponges[a,b]	Lumbar support with chair Upper limb support	Reduces fatigue	

Anti-fatigue floor mat	Provides cushion for lower
	  extremity
		Reduction of stress and force on
		  lower extremity joints	

Cable support[b,c]	Attaches to either the proximal or distal elbow	Reduces torque on the wrist Supports the cable weight	

(continued)

TABLE 3-4	**More About Using Ergonomic Tools** (*continued*)		
Tool	**Features**	**Aids In**	**Example**
Ergonomic transducer grip	Fits over the transducer	Decreases force required to hold transducer	
Properly fitting gloves	Helps maintain grip	Reduces grip force needed to grasp the transducer	

*a*Sports equipment, such as yoga blocks, provides a cost-effective solution.
*b*Clean between patient use or cover with a nonporous cover, such as a plastic bag, to reduce infection transmission.
*c*A commercially viable tennis elbow strap can be used as a substitute for ultrasound-specific supports.

From Industry standards for the prevention of work related musculoskeletal disorders in sonography. *J Diagn Med Sonogr.* 2017;33(5):370–391; OSHA. Positioning patients and equipment. Sonography 2008. Accessed February 6, 2020. https://www.osha.gov/SLTC/etools/hospital/sonography/access_patient.html; Harrison G, Harris A. Work-related musculoskeletal disorders in ultrasound: can you reduce risk? *Ultrasound.* 2015;23(4):224–230; Gonçalves JS, Shinohara Moriguchi C, Takekawa KS, Coury HJCG, Sato TO. The effects of forearm support and shoulder posture on upper trapezius and anterior deltoid activity. *J Phys Ther Sci.* 2017;29(5):793–798.

- Changing scanning position: sitting for some exams and standing for others
- Alternating scanning hands to vary the grip used
- Limiting portable exams that require static or awkward positions and forceful transducer handling

Abdominal

The upper and lower abdominal exam begins by **moving the patient** as close to the edge of the bed as possible to **reduce adduction** of the arm. A rolled towel or block is used for arm support. Raising the chair height also helps keep the arm abducted.

During imaging of either kidney, roll the patient onto their side. Imaging from the flank in the left lateral or right lateral decubitus prevents the need to press the transducer into the exam table, thus reducing the force needed to obtain renal images. If changing the patient position into a decubitus position still requires adduction of the arm, consider sitting or standing to obtain the required views. In the case of gallbladder imaging in the left lateral decubitus position, stand to place the arm in the optimal angle. Adjust the monitor and control panel when moving from sitting to standing.

Obese patients create a different set of challenges. Many systems have a penetration setting and all systems allow the use of a lower-frequency transducer. Both methods can help **decrease** the need for excessive **axial compression (force)** to obtain optimal images. In the presence of a pannus, ask the patient to support the area out of the scan area, change their position (i.e., Trendelenburg for lower abdomen), or use commercially available retraction devices.

Neck Structures

Many sonographers image the neck structures (i.e., carotid, thyroid, and salivary glands) with the patient positioned the same way as in abdomen exams. This provides a quasi-ergonomic imaging position for the left neck; however, there are several problems with this method. First, though the forearm rests on the patient's chest, shoulder abduction is often greater than suggested. Second, many female patients object to having the sonographer's arm across their breasts. Moving to the right side using this head-away position often requires arm abduction, support of the hand and forearm, and twisting of the wrist.

Imaging from the head of the patient alleviates many of these ergonomic problems. This permits patient positioning closer to the sonographer, **reduces arm abduction**, and helps with maintenance of a **neutral spine**.[21] When using this method to image neck structures, a support is used for the arm and hand. A parallel forearm and pronated hand is maintained to help decrease compression on the ulnar nerve and carpal

A   B   C

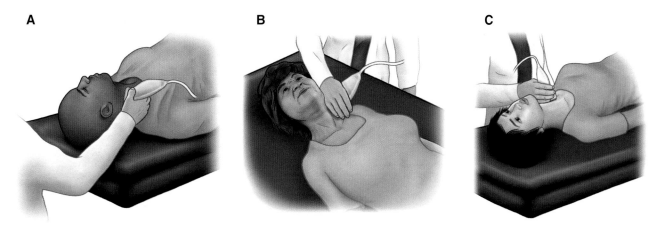

FIGURE 3-9 **A:** While imaging the right side of the neck, positioning of the patient head toward the sonographer allows for support of the arm. **B:** Left side neck imaging requires movement of the patient away from the sonographer at an angle. **C:** Consider standing to obtain central and left neck images.

tunnel structures (Fig. 3-9). The patient unable to lie supine on the exam table because of injury or breathing problems may require imaging while in a seated position. In this instance, ask the patient which position is best for the exam.

COUNTERACTING WORK-RELATED STRESS

WRMSKDs are a cumulative process involving personal and work behaviors. Both rest and stretching aid in reducing risk factors not only to decrease tension but also to increase joint and muscle flow.[14,15] Daily exercise contract and relax the muscles if simple movements are performed throughout the workday. As with any activity, warm up muscles before an exam and stretch afterward.[15] During a long exam, a 30- to 60-second **minibreak** every 20 minutes should be taken.

The remainder of this chapter provides simple exercises of the spine and upper extremity to help during the workday. Exercises are completed with both limbs for a set number of repetitions. This is a small set of available movements; as with all exercise, consult physicians before beginning.

Hand and Forearm Exercises

Each sonographic exam requires grasping of the transducer and reaching during use of the keyboard or touch panel. In the case of a biopsy procedure, the transducer should be held in a static position to follow the needle into the targeted anatomy. The result can be seen in hand fatigue, thumb and finger locking plus pain in both the hand and forearm. Many of the muscles and tendons of the hand originate in the forearm, thus exercising the hand also uses structures originating on the radius and ulna.[22] One method to counteract movements and force used during the exam involves completing simple yet effective hand exercises.[23–26] For examples of hand and forearm stretches, see Table 3-5.

Wrist and Forearm Exercises

The wrist, located between the digits and forearm, is the location for multiple nerves, tendons, and muscles. A wide superficial tendon sheath holds anatomy adjacent to the carpal bones. In the event of overuse, swelling occurs, compressing nerves and tendons, thus increasing the risk

TABLE 3-5	**Hand and Forearm Exercises**	
Exercise	**Movement**	**Example**
Thumb stretch	Place the hand flat on a counter, desk, or wall and flatten the palm keeping the wrist straight. Keep the digits and thumb close together. Move the thumb away from the index finger as far as possible without moving the fingers. To increase difficulty, place a rubber band around the index finger and thumb.	

(continued)

TABLE 3-5   Hand and Forearm Exercises (*continued*)

Exercise	Movement	Example
Thumb abduction	Place hand in a flat position with the thumb extended. Touch the end of the thumb to the base of the small finger, hold for 10–15 seconds, release and repeat. A rubber band around the base of the little finger and thumb increases the difficulty of this exercise.	
Digit (finger) stretch	Hold open hand in front with the palm inward. Touch the index finger and thumb, holding for 10 seconds. Open the hand, touching the second finger and thumb together, holding for 10 seconds. Perform the movement touching each digit to the thumb.	
Digit flexion/squeeze	The digits can be strengthened and exercised either with or without an object. These activities help improve grip strength and the flexion/squeeze and release sequence relaxes the hand and forearm muscles. The first movement, digit flexion, begins with the hand flat, digits together, and thumb extended. Slowly bend the fingers, starting at the distal joint, until a fist is created. Fold the thumb over the fingers, squeeze gently for 5–10 seconds, and release. If there is an object such as a tennis ball, therapy putty, or even a rolled wash cloth, the fist-sized object can be placed in the palm to complete the squeeze–release cycle.	
Wrist flexor stretch	Flexors of the wrist, located on the anterior side of the joint, allow to curl the wrist toward the forearm. To start this stretch, hold the arm in front of the body at a 90-degree angle, rotating the palm toward the floor. Point the fingers toward the ceiling while using the opposite hand; keeping the elbow straight, gently move the fingers toward the core. The stretch can be felt in the *anterior* forearm. Hold for 10–15 seconds, repeating two or three times.	

TABLE 3-5	**Hand and Forearm Exercises (*continued*)**	
Exercise	**Movement**	**Example**
Wrist extensor stretch	Stretching the extensors begins with the same body position as the flexor stretch. Point the fingers toward the floor, using the opposite hand; keeping the elbow straight, gently pull the fingers toward the core. The stretch will be felt in the *posterior* forearm. Hold for 10–15 seconds, repeating two or three times.	

From Christenssen W. Stretch exercises reducing the musculoskeletal pain and discomfort in the arms and upper body of echocardiographers. *J Diagn Med Sonogr.* 2001;17:123–140; Cursaro M, Rich J, Bradley J, Shirazim M, Edwards S. Ergonomics 2014: taking care of yourself. *J Am Soc Echocardiogr.* 2014;27(3):A36–A37; Gasibat Q, Simbak N, Abd Aziz A. Stretching exercises to prevent work-related musculoskeletal disorders—a review article. *Am J Sports Sci Med.* 2017;5:27–37; Stoffer-Marx M, Klinger M, Luschin S, et al. Functional consultation and exercises improve grip strength in osteoarthritis of the hand—a randomised controlled trial. *Arthritis Res Ther.* 2018;20(1):253.

of developing carpal tunnel syndrome and de Quervain syndrome.

Shoulder and Upper Trunk Exercises

Shoulder and back pain are common complaints for sonographers.[12] Even when using ergonomic practices, the shoulder and supporting musculature need to be released because of the static postures needed to complete the exam. As these muscles are worked, they metabolize nutrients, creating "waste" in the form of lactic acid, which is felt as fatigue, stiffness, and soreness. Stretching muscles helps move lactic acid from the muscles and move glycogen, muscle fuel, into the cells, thus aiding in decreasing the symptoms of overuse.[14,23] For examples of shoulder and upper trunk exercises, see Table 3-6.

TABLE 3-6	**Shoulder and Upper Trunk Exercises**	
Exercise	**Movement**	**Example**
Posterior shoulder	To complete this cross-chest stretch, place the arm across the chest with the palm up or down. Hook the opposite arm under the elbow. Gently pull the arm toward the body and shoulder toward the floor. Hold for 10–20 seconds, repeating with the contralateral side. This also stretches the trapezius muscle, which originates along the spine from the occipital bone to the upper lumbar spine. The insertion site is at the lateral clavicle, acromion, and scapular spine of the scapula.	
Anterior shoulder and pectoralis stretch	These movements stretch the anterior shoulder structures and pectoralis muscles. Maintain shoulder positions because this movement reduces the effectiveness of the stretch.	

(*continued*)

TABLE 3-6 Shoulder and Upper Trunk Exercises (*continued*)

Exercise	Movement	Example
	Stretch 1: Place the interlaced fingers on the base of the skull at the level of the occipital bone. Straighten the spine, move the elbows back, and inhale deeply to expand the chest. While holding the breath for 5–10 seconds, remember to relax the shoulders. Interlace the fingers behind the head at the occipital level. Move the elbows posterior, straighten the spine, and expand the chest.	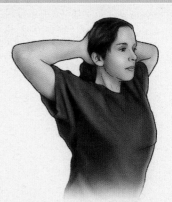
	Stretch 2: This stretch can also be done using a doorway. Place both arms, with both the elbows bent at 90 degrees and the upper arms parallel to the floor. Gently apply anterior pressure through leaning or pressing against the door.	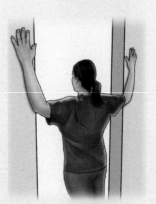
	Stretch 3: Grasp the hands behind the back, straighten the arms slowly raising the hands toward the ceiling. This can be done in either a standing or sitting position. Avoid leaning forward to increase the arm height, the goal is a slow gentle stretch.	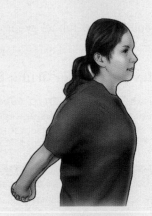
Overhead triceps stretch	The triceps muscle, located on the posterior upper arm, helps shoulder stabilization and extension of the elbow. To stretch the triceps, raise the arm above the head perpendicular to the floor. Bend the arm posterior, rotating the palm toward the body. Gently press the elbow posterior and toward the center.	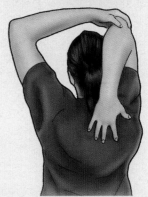

From Christenssen W. Stretch exercises reducing the musculoskeletal pain and discomfort in the arms and upper body of echocardiographers. *J Diagn Med Sonogr*. 2001;17:123–140; Cursaro M, Rich J, Bradley J, Shirazim M, Edwards S. Ergonomics 2014: taking care of yourself. *J Am Soc Echocardiogr*. 2014;27(3):A36–A37; Gasibat Q, Simbak N, Abd Aziz A. Stretching exercises to prevent work-related musculoskeletal disorders—a review article. *Am J Sports Sci Med*. 2017;5:27–37.

Neck, Sides, and Back

Daily tasks, such as lifting, bending, and twisting, increase the chance of back pain developing during the day. Sonographers report neck pain as often as shoulder pain,[12] underscoring the importance of performing a countermovement to job demands. When supporting muscles become strained and fatigued, they weaken, and thus decrease spinal stability, increasing the risk of injury. To decrease the chance of developing back pain, neutral spine alignment should be maintained while working, rest breaks need to be taken, and stretching should be added to the daily routine. Many of the suggested stretches benefit multiple areas of the body such as the upper trunk and shoulders. For examples of neck, side, and back stretches, see Table 3-7.

TABLE 3-7	**Neck, Side, and Back Exercises**	
Exercise	**Movement**	**Example**
Side stretch[a,b]	Stand with the feet at shoulder-width apart and grasp the hands above the head with the palms forward. Lean to one side, holding for 15 seconds. Repeat with the other side. This movement can also be done with the arm perpendicular to the floor on the dependent side or with the hand on the hip.	
Oblique stretch[b]	Begin in a neutral position, cross the arms across the upper torso. Keeping the back straight, rotate the shoulders side to side. Repeat multiple times. While in the fully rotated and neutral position, inhale deeply to add an upper back stretch.	
Low back extension[a]	Stand in a neutral position with feet at shoulder-width aprart. Place the fists lateral to the lower lumbar and superior to the posterior pelvis. Gently press the hips forward, arching the back. The stretch occurs in the lower back, abdomen, upper trunk, and anterior shoulders.	

(continued)

TABLE 3-7   Neck, Side, and Back Exercises (continued)

Exercise	Movement	Example
Low back flexion[c]	To maintain muscular balance while stretching, bend anterior keeping the knees slightly bent, grasping the thighs, calves, touch the toes or grasp the elbows. Allow the upper body to provide the weight for this stretch.	
Posterior neck[d]	Tilt the head forward, rotating the chin halfway to one shoulder. Hold for 10–15 seconds. Repeat with contralateral side.	
Lateral neck stretch[d]	Sit or stand with a neutral spine. Tilt the head to one side, pulling the chin into the chest. Return to the neutral position and repeat with the opposite side.	
	To add a shoulder stretch, pull the shoulder toward the floor opposite to the direction of the head.	

[a]This stretch also works the shoulders and abdominal muscles.
[b]Can be done while sitting.
[c]This movement also uses the shoulders, triceps, and upper back muscles.
[d]To increase the stretch, gently pull the head to the dependent side.

From Christenssen W. Stretch exercises reducing the musculoskeletal pain and discomfort in the arms and upper body of echocardiographers. *J Diagn Med Sonogr.* 2001;17:123–140; Cursaro M, Rich J, Bradley J, Shirazim M, Edwards S. Ergonomics 2014: taking care of yourself. *J Am Soc Echocardiogr.* 2014;27(3):A36–A37; Gasibat Q, Simbak N, Abd Aziz A. Stretching exercises to prevent work-related musculoskeletal disorders—a review article. *Am J Sports Sci Med.* 2017;5:27–37.

SUMMARY

- Align the body in a neutral scan position to avoid spinal rotation, flexion, or extension.
- Position the arms at midline or in front of the body.
- Keep the forearms, and thighs when sitting, parallel to the floor.
- Adjust the chair height to keep the feet flat on the floor.
- Arrange the work area (i.e., ultrasound system and patient) within the vertical and horizontal zones.
- Ask for help when moving patients.
- Continue learning stretches and preventative measures to reduce the risk factors for WRMSKDs.
- Report and document ergonomic concerns, continued pain or injury, and seek medical advice and care when appropriate.

REFERENCES

1. Thabah M, Ravindran V. Musculoskeletal problems in pregnancy. *Rheumatol Int*. 2015;35(4):581–587.
2. Auer J, Sinzinger H, Franklin B, Berent R. Muscle- and skeletal-related side-effects of statins: tip of the iceberg? *Eur J Prev Cardiol*. 2016;23(1):88–110.
3. Malik KM, Beckerly R, Imani F. Musculoskeletal disorders a universal source of pain and disability misunderstood and mismanaged: a critical analysis based on the U.S. model of care. *Anesth Pain Med*. 2018;8(6):e85532.
4. Kesikburun S, Güzelküçük Ü, Fidan U, Demir Y, Ergün A, Tan AK. Musculoskeletal pain and symptoms in pregnancy: a descriptive study. *Ther Adv Musculoskelet Dis*. 2018;10(12):229–234.
5. Wang J, Cui Y, He L, et al. Work-related musculoskeletal disorders and risk factors among Chinese medical staff of obstetrics and gynecology. *Int J Environ Res Public Health*. 2017;14(6):562.
6. Yan P, Li F, Zhang L, et al. Prevalence of work-related musculoskeletal disorders in the nurses working in hospitals of Xinjiang Uygur autonomous region. *Pain Res Manag*. 2017;2017:5757108.
7. United States Department of Labor, Occupational Safety and Health Administration. Ergonomics for the Prevention of Musculoskeletal Disorders. Publication No. 3182. OSHA; 2009.
8. United States Department of Labor, Occupational Safety and Health Administration. Clinical services: radiology. 2020. https://www.osha.gov/etools/hospitals/clinical-services/radiology
9. Barros-Gomes S, Orme N, Nhola LF, et al. Characteristics and consequences of work-related musculoskeletal pain among cardiac sonographers compared with peer employees: a multisite cross-sectional study. *J Am Soc Echocardiogr*. 2019;32(9):1138–1146.
10. Orme NM, Geske JB, Pislaru SV, et al. Occupational musculoskeletal pain in cardiac sonographers compared to peer employees: a multisite cross-sectional study. *Echocardiography*. 2016;33(11):1642–1647.
11. Murphey S. Work related musculoskeletal disorders in sonography. *J Diagn Med Sonogr*. 2017;33(5):354–369.
12. Evans K, Roll S, Baker J. Work-related musculoskeletal disorders (WRMSD) among registered diagnostic medical sonographers and vascular technologists: a representative sample. *J Diagn Med Sonogr*. 2009;25(6):287–299.
13. Occupational Health Clinics for Ontario Workers. Ergonomics & Pregnancy. Occupational Health Clinics for Ontario Workers Inc.; 2020.
14. Canadian Centre for Occupational Health and Safety. *Work-related Musculoskeletal Disorders (WMSDs)*. 2019. Accessed November 13, 2019. https://www.ccohs.ca/oshanswers/diseases/rmirsi.html
15. Harrison G, Harris A. Work-related musculoskeletal disorders in ultrasound: can you reduce risk? *Ultrasound*. 2015;23(4):224–230.
16. Dhyani M, Roll SC, Gilbertson MW, et al. A pilot study to precisely quantify forces applied by sonographers while scanning: a step toward reducing ergonomic injury. *Work*. 2017;58(2):241–247.
17. Gemark Simonsen J, Gard G. Swedish sonographers' perceptions of ergonomic problems at work and their suggestions for improvement. *BMC Musculoskelet Disord*. 2016;17:391.
18. OSHA. Positioning patients and equipment. Sonography 2008. Accessed February 6, 2020. https://www.osha.gov/etools/hospitals/clinical-services/sonography
19. Almeida HA. Pregnancy and ergonomics. In: Jorge RN, Mascarenhas T, Durante JA, et al, eds. BioMed Women: Clincial and Bioengineering for Women's Health. Taylor & Francis Group; 2016:11–18.
20. Industry standards for the prevention of work related musculoskeletal disorders in sonography. *J Diagn Med Sonogr*. 2017;33(5):370–391.
21. Baker JP, Coffin CT. The importance of an ergonomic workstation to practicing sonographers. *J Ultrasound Med*. 2013;32(8):1363–1375.
22. Moore KL, Dalley AF, Agur AMR. Arteries of Forearm. In: Moore KL, Dalley AF, Agur AMR, eds. Clinically Oriented Anatomy. Wolters Kluwer Health. Lippincott Williams & Wilkins; 2010:757-761.
23. Christenssen W. Stretch exercises reducing the musculoskeletal pain and discomfort in the arms and upper body of echocardiographers. *J Diagn Med Sonogr*. 2001;17:123–140.
24. Cursaro M, Rich J, Bradley J, Shirazim M, Edwards S. Ergonomics 2014: taking care of yourself. *J Am Soc Echocardiogr*. 2014; 27(3):A36–A37.
25. Stoffer-Marx M, Klinger M, Luschin S, et al. Functional consultation and exercises improve grip strength in osteoarthritis of the hand—a randomised controlled trial. *Arthritis Res Ther*. 2018;20(1):253.
26. Gasibat Q, Simbak N, Abd Aziz A. Stretching exercises to prevent work-related musculoskeletal disorders—a review article. *Am J Sports Sci Med*. 2017;5:27–37.

CHAPTER 4

The Abdominal Wall and Diaphragm

SHARLETTE ANDERSON

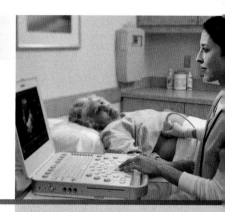

OBJECTIVES

- Describe the embryonic development of the abdominal wall.
- Locate the four quadrants of the abdominopelvic cavity and the nine regions of the abdomen.
- Describe the muscles, attachments, and connective tissue layers of the abdominal wall and diaphragm.
- Discuss the role of sonography, sonographic protocols, and scanning technique and the normal sonographic appearance of the abdominal wall and diaphragm.
- Describe the etiology and sonographic appearance of inflammatory processes involving the abdominal wall.
- Describe the etiology and sonographic appearance of abdominal wall trauma and hematoma formation.
- Discuss the different types of abdominal wall hernias and their sonographic appearance.
- Describe neoplasms of the abdominal wall and their sonographic appearance.
- Discuss the role of sonography and scanning techniques for evaluating diaphragmatic pathology.
- Distinguish sonographic image characteristics of technically adequate sonographic examinations of the abdominal wall and diaphragm.

GLOSSARY

abscess a cavity containing dead tissue and pus that forms owing to an infectious process
ascites an accumulation of serous fluid in the peritoneal cavity
erythema redness of the skin owing to inflammation
linea alba fibrous structure that runs down the midline of the abdomen from the xyphoid process to the symphysis pubis separating the right and left rectus abdominis muscles
peristalsis rhythmic wavelike contraction of the gastrointestinal tract that forces food through it
pneumothorax collapsed lung that occurs when air leaks into the space between the chest wall and lung

KEY TERMS

abdominopelvic cavity

abscess

aponeurosis

desmoid tumor

diaphragm

diaphragmatic hernia

diaphragmatic inversion

diaphragmatic paralysis

endometrioma

eventration

fascia

hematoma

inguinal canal

inguinal hernia

lipoma

neuroma

pleural effusion

rectus abdominis

rhabdomyolysis

sarcoma

seroma

The body is divided into two major cavities: the dorsal cavity and the ventral cavity. The dorsal, or posterior, cavity is completely encased in bone and is subdivided into the cranial cavity, which houses the brain, and the spinal cavity, which houses the spinal cord. The ventral cavity is divided by the diaphragm into the thoracic cavity superiorly and the abdominopelvic cavity inferiorly. The abdominopelvic cavity is subdivided into the abdomen and the pelvis though no physical barrier separates them. The abdominopelvic cavity is enclosed by the abdominal wall. This chapter focuses on the abdominal wall and diaphragm.

Sonography of the abdominal wall is an efficient and effective way of evaluating the integrity, structure, and function of the abdominal wall and diaphragm. Real-time imaging facilitates the evaluation of muscle contraction and relaxation as well as the motion of contents of the abdominal cavity. The ability to document motion helps sonographers demonstrate the motion of hernias through the layers of the abdominal wall, the changes in muscle fiber motion secondary to trauma or mass, and the changes in diaphragm motion related to paralysis or inflammation.

Sonography is a safe, cost-effective, and widely available method of imaging for most patients. Its portability and lack of radiation exposure support serial evaluation to monitor the progression of pathology and response to therapeutic measures. Although the transmission of any type of energy into the body has the potential to cause bioeffects, the benefits of sonographic evaluation of the abdominal wall and diaphragm by a competent sonographer far outweigh the risks, which, according to current literature, are negligible.[1,2]

EMBRYOLOGY

In the fourth week of development, the embryo folds from a flat disk into a tubular structure. The caudal end of the embryo folds cranially, moving the connecting stalk from the tail region of the embryo to the ventral surface, forming the site of the future umbilical cord insertion. At the same time, the sides of the disk fold ventrally, folding in part of the yolk sac to form the gut tube. This process also forms the ventral body cavity and the body walls (Fig. 4-1).

Diaphragmatic development is a complicated coordination of muscle, connective tissue, vessels, and nerves. Initially, the septum transversum develops to form a separation between the thoracic and abdominal cavities. It becomes anchored to the anterior wall of the embryo between the

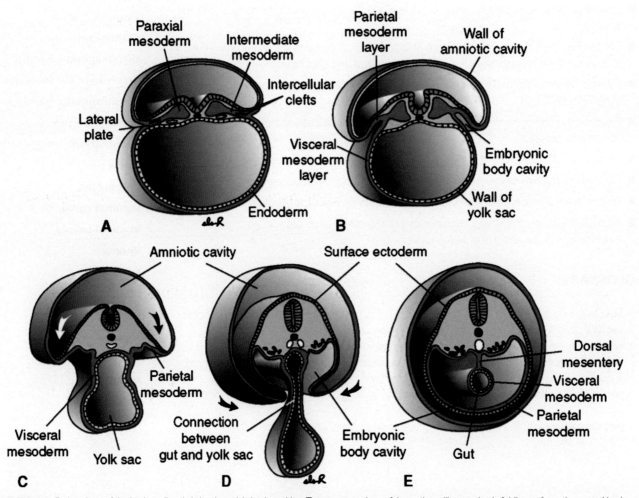

FIGURE 4-1 Embryology of the body wall and abdominopelvic body cavities. Transverse sections of the embryo illustrate body folding to form the ventral body wall, embryonic body cavities, and gut tube during the fourth week of development. As the embryo folds from a flat disk (**A,B,C,D**) into a tubular structure (**E**), the amnion is pulled ventrally to encircle the embryo and lateral plate mesoderm forms the visceral and parietal layers of the pleura and peritoneum (**C**). Mesoderm also forms the skeletal muscles of the abdominal wall. (Reprinted with permission from Sadler TW. *Langman's Medical Embryology*. 13th ed. Wolters Kluwer; 2015.)

heart and the liver. Paired pleuroperitoneal folds then extend medially from the lateral portions of mesoderm (the middle germ layer of the embryo) toward the septum transversum to form a scaffold for muscle fibers and connective tissue to form the diaphragm and its central tendon[3] (Fig. 4-2).

REGIONS AND QUADRANTS

To provide a more standardized way of describing the location of organs, pain, or pathology, the abdominopelvic cavity is divided into four quadrants by a midline vertical line extending from the xyphoid process to the symphysis pubis and a horizontal line through the umbilicus. The four quadrants are as follows: (1) right upper quadrant (RUQ), (2) left upper quadrant (LUQ), (3) left lower quadrant (LLQ), and (4) right lower quadrant (RLQ). For more specific descriptions, the abdomen is further divided into nine regions by dividing it with two vertical lines at the right and left midclavicular planes and two horizontal lines at the inferior costal margin and the level of the fifth lumbar vertebra and iliac tubercles. The nine regions are as follows: (1) right hypochondrium, (2) epigastrium, (3) left hypochondrium, (4) right lumbar, (5) umbilical, (6) left lumbar, (7) right iliac fossa, (8) hypogastrium, and (9) left iliac fossa[4,5] (Fig. 4-3).

ANATOMY

There are no physical divisions of the abdominal wall; it is a continuous structure. However, for descriptive purposes, it is divided into the anterior, right and left lateral, and posterior walls. The boundary between the anterior and lateral walls is indefinite, so clinicians often discuss the anterolateral abdominal wall as a single unit[4,5] (Fig. 4-4).

Anterolateral Abdominal Wall

The anterolateral wall extends from the thoracic cage to the pelvis. Superiorly, it is bounded by the cartilages of the 7th to 10th ribs and the xiphoid process. Inferiorly, it is bounded by the inguinal ligament and iliac crests, pubic crests, and pubic symphysis of the pelvic bones.[6,7]

Layers

When describing abdominal wall anatomy, it is important to distinguish between fascia and aponeuroses. A fascia is a fibrous tissue network located between the skin and the underlying structures. It is richly supplied with both blood vessels and nerves. The fascia is composed of two layers: a superficial layer and a deep layer. The superficial fascia is attached to the skin and is composed of connective tissue containing varying quantities of fat. The deep fascia is loosely connected to the superficial fascia by fibrous strands. The deep fascia covers the muscles and partitions them into groups. Although the deep fascia is thin, it is more densely packed and is stronger than the superficial fascia; however, neither the superficial fascia nor the deep fascia possesses any notable internal strength because they are a condensation of connective tissue organized into definable homogeneous layers within the body.[7,8]

Aponeuroses are layers of flat tendinous fibrous sheets fused with strong connective tissue that attach muscles to fixed points, functioning like a tendon, so they are quite strong. Aponeuroses have minimal vascularity and innervation. The abdominal wall aponeuroses are primarily located in the ventral abdominal regions with a primary function to join muscles to the body parts that the muscles act upon. The most readily known abdominal aponeurosis is the rectus sheath.[7,8]

The abdominal wall appears as a laminated structure when viewed in cross section.[7] From superficial to deep, the layers include the following: (1) skin, (2) subcutaneous tissue (superficial fascia), (3) muscles and their aponeuroses, (4) deep fascia, (5) extraperitoneal fat, and (6) the parietal peritoneum.[4,6,7] The skin attaches loosely to most of the subcutaneous tissue except at the umbilicus where the attachment is firm.[4,8]

The subcutaneous tissue anterior to the muscle layers makes up the superficial fascia. Superior to the umbilicus,

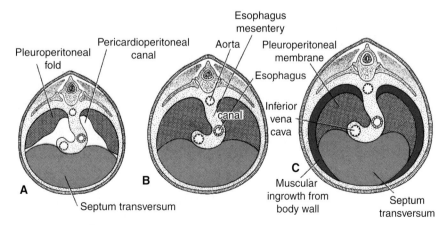

FIGURE 4-2 Embryology of the diaphragm. Transverse sections of the embryo illustrate the septum transversum and pleuroperitoneal membranes that provide scaffolding for the muscular development of the diaphragm separating the thoracic and abdominal cavities. **A:** The septum transversum separates the developing liver and heart on the ventral body wall. **B:** Pleuroperitoneal membranes grow from the dorsolateral body wall toward the septum transversum to form a scaffolding for muscle tissue as the diaphragm develops. **C:** Muscular tissue (mesoderm) grows over the scaffolding formed by the pleuroperitoneal membranes and septum transversum to form the diaphragm separating the thoracic and abdominopelvic cavities. (Reprinted with permission from Sadler TW. *Langman's Medical Embryology*. 13th ed. Wolters Kluwer; 2015.)

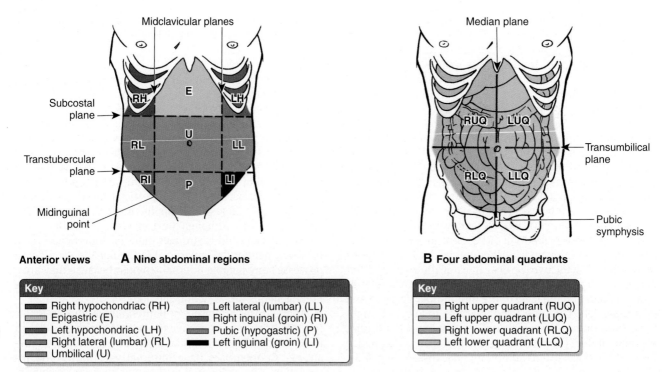

Midclavicular planes

Subcostal plane

Transtubercular plane

Midinguinal point

Anterior views **A Nine abdominal regions**

Median plane

Transumbilical plane

Pubic symphysis

B Four abdominal quadrants

Key	
▬ Right hypochondriac (RH)	▭ Left lateral (lumbar) (LL)
▭ Epigastric (E)	▬ Right inguinal (groin) (RI)
▬ Left hypochondriac (LH)	▬ Pubic (hypogastric) (P)
▬ Right lateral (lumbar) (RL)	▬ Left inguinal (groin) (LI)
▭ Umbilical (U)	

Key	
▭ Right upper quadrant (RUQ)	
▭ Left upper quadrant (LUQ)	
▭ Right lower quadrant (RLQ)	
▭ Left lower quadrant (LLQ)	

FIGURE 4-3 Abdominopelvic cavity subdivisions. **A:** The regions are formed by two sagittal (vertical) and two transverse (horizontal) planes. **B:** The quadrants are formed by the midsagittal plane and a transverse plane passing through the umbilicus at the iliac crest or the disk level between the L3-4 vertebrae. (Reprinted with permission from Moore KL, Agur AM. *Essential Clinical Anatomy.* 3rd ed. Lippincott Williams & Wilkins; 2007:119.)

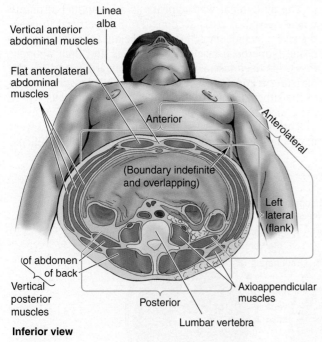

Linea alba

Vertical anterior abdominal muscles

Flat anterolateral abdominal muscles

Anterior

Anterolateral

(Boundary indefinite and overlapping)

Left lateral (flank)

of abdomen

of back

Vertical posterior muscles

Posterior

Axioappendicular muscles

Lumbar vertebra

Inferior view

FIGURE 4-4 Abdominal wall subdivisions. The transverse section illustrates the structural relationships of the abdominal wall. (Reprinted with permission from Moore K, Dalley A, Agur A. *Clinically Oriented Anatomy.* 6th ed. Lippincott Williams & Wilkins; 2010:186.)

it is consistent with that found in most regions. In contrast, inferior to the umbilicus, the deepest part of the subcutaneous tissue is reinforced with elastic and collagen fibers and is divided into two layers. The first is a superficial fatty layer (Camper fascia) containing small vessels and nerves.

Camper fascia gives the body wall its rounded appearance. The second layer is a deep membranous layer (Scarpa fascia) and it consists of a combination of fat and fibrous tissue that blends with the deep fascia.[4,8] The membranous layer continues into the perineal region as the superficial perineal fascia (Colles fascia)[4] (Fig. 4-5).

The three anterolateral abdominal muscle layers and their aponeuroses are covered by superficial, intermediate, and deep layers of extremely thin investing fascia.[4,8] The investing layer of fascia is located on the external aspects of the three muscle layers and is not easily separated from the external muscle layer, the epimysium. Varying thicknesses of membranous and areolar sheets of endoabdominal fascia line the internal aspects of the wall. Although the endoabdominal fascia is continuous, different regions are named based on the muscle or aponeurosis it lines. For example, the portion lining the deep surface of the transversus abdominis muscle and its aponeurosis is the transversalis fascia. Internal to the endoabdominal fascia is the parietal peritoneum. The distance separating the parietal peritoneum from the endoabdominal fascia is determined by the variable amounts of extraperitoneal fat in the fascia.[4] The parietal peritoneum is the outer layer of the serous membrane lining the abdominopelvic cavity formed by a single layer of epithelial cells and supporting connective tissue[4] (see Fig. 4-5).

Muscles

There are five bilaterally paired muscles in the anterolateral abdominal wall and one unpaired muscle (Table 4-1). Located bilaterally on the anterior abdominal wall are the rectus abdominis muscles (see Fig. 4-4). The rectus abdominis is a long, broad, vertical, strap-like muscle that is mostly enclosed in the rectus sheath. Also located on the

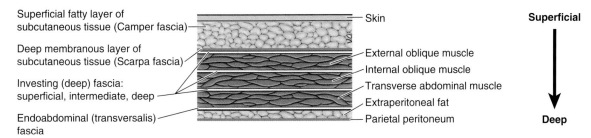

Superficial fatty layer of subcutaneous tissue (Camper fascia)

Deep membranous layer of subcutaneous tissue (Scarpa fascia)

Investing (deep) fascia: superficial, intermediate, deep

Endoabdominal (transversalis) fascia

Skin

External oblique muscle

Internal oblique muscle

Transverse abdominal muscle

Extraperitoneal fat

Parietal peritoneum

Superficial

Deep

FIGURE 4-5 Anterolateral abdominal wall. The section of the anterolateral abdominal wall inferior to the umbilicus illustrates the multilayered, laminar-appearing tissue and muscles located anterior to the peritoneal cavity.

TABLE 4-1 **Muscles of the Abdominolateral Wall**[1,2]	
Rectus abdominis (Figs. 4-4 and 4-6A)	Bilaterally paired, vertical muscle Origin: arises from the front of the pubic bone and pubic symphysis Insertion: inserts into the fifth, sixth, and seventh costal cartilages and the xiphoid process Action: acts to flex the trunk, to compress abdominal viscera, and to stabilize and control pelvic tilt
Pyramidalis (Fig. 4-6A)	Small, insignificant triangular muscle Origin: arises from the anterior surface of the pubis Insertion: inserts into the linea alba; lies anterior to the lower part of the rectus abdominis Action: acts to draw the linea alba inferiorly
External oblique (Figs. 4-4 and 4-6B, C)	Bilaterally paired, flat muscle Origin: arises from the external surface of the lower eight ribs Insertion: inserts in linea alba via an aponeurosis and into the iliac crest and pubis via the inguinal ligament Action: acts to compress and support abdominal viscera, flexes and rotate trunk
Internal oblique (Figs. 4-4 and 4-6B, C)	Bilaterally paired, flat muscle Origin: arises from the thoracolumbar fascia and the anterior two-thirds of the iliac crest Insertion: inserts into the inferior borders of the lower three ribs, linea alba, and pubis via a conjoint tendon Action: acts as a postural function of all abdominal muscles
Transversus abdominis (transverse abdominal; Figs. 4-4 and 4-6B, C)	Bilaterally paired, flat muscle Origin: arises from the internal surfaces of the lower eight costal cartilages (7–12), the thoracolumbar fascia, the anterior two-thirds of the iliac crest, and the lateral third of the inguinal ligament Insertion: inserts into the xiphoid process, linea alba with aponeurosis of internal oblique, pubic crest, and pectin pubis via a conjoint tendon Action: same as external oblique; acts to compress and support abdominal viscera

anterior abdominal wall in the rectus sheath is the pyramidalis muscle. The pyramidalis, a small triangular muscle, extends from its base, originating on the pubic bone to its apex inserting into the midline linea alba approximately halfway between the pubic symphysis and the umbilicus. This muscle lies deep to the anterior rectus fascia and superficial to the rectus abdominus muscle. The pyramidalis muscle is present in about 80% to 90% of people and can be easily harvested for use in reconstructive surgery when needed. Its function is poorly understood, but it helps to maintain tension on the linea alba, supporting the tone of the anterior abdominal wall[4,6,9] (Fig. 4-6).

There are three flat, bilaterally paired muscles of the anterolateral group. From superficial to deep, they include the following layers: (1) the external oblique, (2) the internal oblique, and (3) the transversus abdominis[4,6] (see Fig. 4-4 and Table 4-1). Coupled with the vertical orientation of the fibers of the rectus abdominis, the fibers in the three flat muscles are arranged to provide maximum strength by forming a supportive muscle girdle that covers and supports the abdominopelvic cavity. In the external oblique, the muscle

fibers have a diagonal inferior and medial orientation. The fibers of the internal oblique, the middle muscle layer, have a perpendicular orientation at right angles to those of the external oblique, running from lateral-inferior to superior-medial. The fibers of the innermost muscle layer, the transversus abdominis, are oriented transversely or horizontally, like a belt encircling the abdomen.[4,6]

Structures

The other structures within the anterolateral abdominal wall include the rectus sheath, linea alba, umbilical ring, and the inguinal canal.

The rectus sheath is a strong, dense connective tissue fascia that encases the rectus abdominis and pyramidalis muscles as well as some arteries, veins, lymphatic vessels, and nerves. The anterior and posterior layers of the rectus sheath are formed by the intercrossing and interweaving of the aponeuroses of the flat abdominal muscles. Additionally, each belly of the rectus abdominus muscle is divided into four sections by intersecting fascia, forming the "six-pack" that is visible on some people with highly toned abdominal

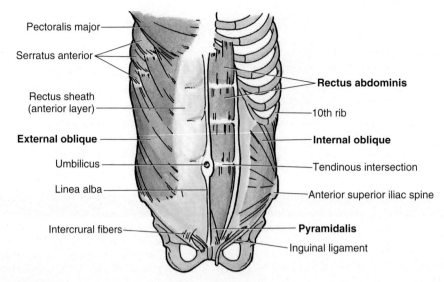

A Anterior view

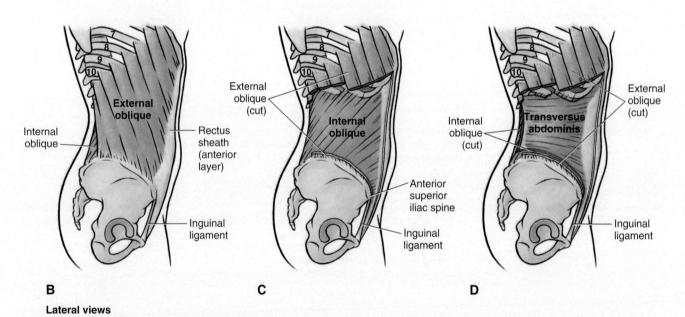

B

C

D

Lateral views

FIGURE 4-6 Abdominolateral wall muscles. **A:** The bilaterally paired, vertically oriented rectus abdominis muscles and the small triangular pyramidalis muscle are located on the anterior wall. **B–D:** The three flat, bilaterally paired muscles comprising the anterolateral group include the external oblique, the internal oblique, and the transverse abdominal. The strength of the muscles can be contributed to the collaborative relationship of the orientation of the fiber of each muscle. (Reprinted with permission from Moore KL, Agur AM. *Essential Clinical Anatomy*. 3rd ed. Lippincott Williams & Wilkins; 2007:122.)

muscles. At the lateral aspect of the rectus sheath, the aponeuroses fuse to form the linea semilunaris, which demarcates the interface of the rectus abdominus with the internal and external oblique and transversus abdominus muscles.[4,8] The posterior rectus sheath ends at the arcuate line, located halfway between the umbilicus and the pubis symphysis. The inferior, or distal, quarter of the rectus abdominus muscle is covered posteriorly by the transversalis fascia, which is all that separates the rectus muscles from the parietal peritoneum in the pelvic region[10] (Fig. 4-7A, B).

The linea alba (or white line) is a midline, dense connective tissue structure that separates the right and left bellies of the rectus abdominus muscle. It is a fusion of the aponeuroses that form the rectus sheath.[4,10] The linea alba extends from the xyphoid process to the pubic symphysis. Superiorly, the linea alba is wider and it narrows inferior to the umbilicus to the width of the pubic symphysis. The

linea alba transmits small vessels and nerves to the skin (Figs. 4-4, 4-6A, and 4-7A, B). In thin, muscular people, a groove is visible in the skin overlying the linea alba.

The umbilicus is the area where all layers of the anterolateral abdominal wall fuse.[4] The umbilical ring is a defect in the linea alba located deep to the umbilicus.[4] This is the area through which the fetal umbilical vessels passed into the umbilical cord to connect with the placenta. The umbilicus and umbilical ring are the remnants of that fetal connection.

The inferior border of the external oblique aponeurosis extends between the anterior superior iliac spine and the pubic tubercle forming the inguinal ligament.[10] Located in the inguinal region superior and parallel to the medial half of the inguinal ligament is the inguinal canal, a passageway through the abdominal wall that is formed during fetal development. It is an important canal where structures exit and enter the abdominal cavity, and the exit and entry pathways

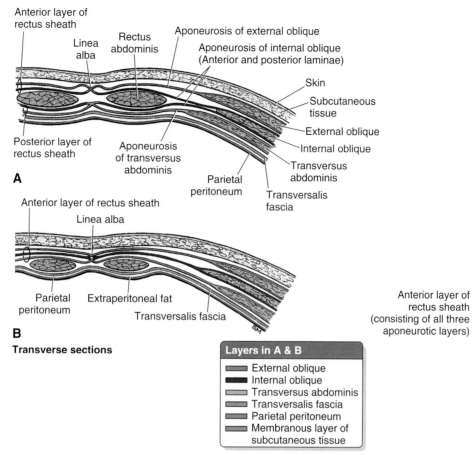

FIGURE 4-7 Abdominal wall structures. Transverse sections of the anterior abdominal wall (**A**) superior to the umbilicus with the posterior layer of the rectus sheath. **B:** Inferior to the umbilicus, the rectus sheath is separated from the parietal peritoneum only by the transversalis fascia. (Reprinted with permission from Moore KL, Agur AM. *Essential Clinical Anatomy*. 3rd ed. Lippincott Williams & Wilkins; 2007:123.)

are potential sites of herniation.[4,10,11] In adults, the inguinal canal is an oblique passage approximately 4 to 6 cm long. Functionally and developmentally distinct structures located within the canal are the spermatic cord in males and the round uterine ligament in females. Other structures included in the canal in both sexes are blood and lymphatic vessels and the ilioinguinal and genital nerves.[10] The entrance of the inguinal canal is formed by the deep inguinal ring at the superior end. The superficial (external) inguinal ring forms the exit at the inferior end. Normally, the inguinal canal is collapsed anteroposteriorly against the spermatic cord or round ligament. Between the two openings (rings), the inguinal canal has two walls (anterior and posterior), a roof, and a floor[10,11] (Table 4-2 and Fig. 4-8A, B).

Posterior Abdominal Wall

The posterior abdominal wall is composed of the lumbar vertebra, posterior abdominal wall muscles, diaphragm, fascia, lumbar plexus, fat, nerves, blood vessels, and lymphatic vessels. On the posterior abdominal wall, the thoracolumbar fascia is an extensive complex. Medially, it attaches to the vertebral column. In the lumbar region, the thoracolumbar fascia has posterior, middle, and anterior layers with enclosed muscles between them. The fascia is thin and transparent in the thoracic region, whereas it is thick and strong in the lumbar region. The posterior (the most superficial) and middle layers of the thoracolumbar fascia enclose the bilateral erector spinae muscles or the vertical deep back muscles in

the same manner that the rectus sheath encloses the rectus abdominus muscles.[4] The thoracolumbar fascia is stronger than the rectus sheath because it is thicker and has a central attachment to the lumbar vertebrae. The rectus sheath has no bony attachment and fuses with the linea alba. The lumbar part of the posterior sheath, extending between the 12th rib and the iliac crest, attaches laterally to the internal oblique and transversus abdominis muscles. The thoracic portion attaches to the latissimus dorsi[4] (see Fig. 4-9).

The anterior layer (which is the deepest layer) of the thoracolumbar fascia is the quadratus lumborum fascia, covering the anterior surface of the quadratus lumborum muscle.[4] It is thinner than the middle and posterior layers of the thoracolumbar fascia. The anterior layer attaches to the anterior surfaces of the lumbar transverse processes, to the iliac crest, and to the 12th rib. Laterally, the anterior layer is continuous with the aponeurotic origin of the transversus abdominis muscle. Superiorly, it thickens to form the lateral arcuate ligament, and inferiorly, it is adherent to the iliolumbar ligaments[4] (see Fig. 4-9).

Muscles

The muscles of the posterior abdomen are categorized as the superficial and intermediate extrinsic back muscles and the superficial layer, intermediate layer, and deep layer of intrinsic back muscles[4] (Table 4-3). The three main, bilaterally paired, muscles comprising the posterior abdominal wall are the psoas major, iliacus, and quadratus lumborum (Fig. 4-10).

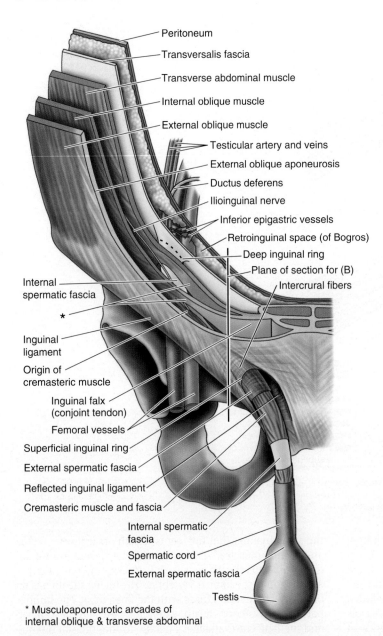

Peritoneum
Transversalis fascia
Transverse abdominal muscle
Internal oblique muscle
External oblique muscle
Testicular artery and veins
External oblique aponeurosis
Ductus deferens
Ilioinguinal nerve
Inferior epigastric vessels
Retroinguinal space (of Bogros)
Deep inguinal ring
Plane of section for (B)
Intercrural fibers

Internal spermatic fascia
*
Inguinal ligament
Origin of cremasteric muscle
Inguinal falx (conjoint tendon)
Femoral vessels
Superficial inguinal ring
External spermatic fascia
Reflected inguinal ligament
Cremasteric muscle and fascia
Internal spermatic fascia
Spermatic cord
External spermatic fascia
Testis

* Musculoaponeurotic arcades of internal oblique & transverse abdominal

A Anterior view

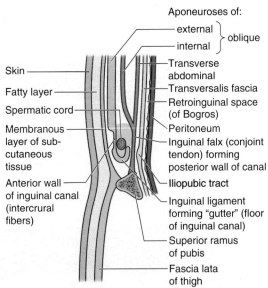

Aponeuroses of:
external ⎱ oblique
internal ⎰
Skin
Fatty layer
Spermatic cord
Membranous layer of sub-cutaneous tissue
Anterior wall of inguinal canal (intercrural fibers)
Transverse abdominal
Transversalis fascia
Retroinguinal space (of Bogros)
Peritoneum
Inguinal falx (conjoint tendon) forming posterior wall of canal
Iliopubic tract
Inguinal ligament forming "gutter" (floor of inguinal canal)
Superior ramus of pubis
Fascia lata of thigh

B Schematic sagittal section of inguinal canal

FIGURE 4-8 Inguinal canal. The anterior and posterior walls, the roof, and the floor of the inguinal canal are illustrated. **A:** The abdominal wall layers and the coverings of the spermatic cord and testis are seen in the anterior view. In females, the canal serves as the passageway for the round ligament. **B:** At the plane shown in (**A**), the sagittal section illustrates the composition of the canal. (Reprinted with permission from Moore K, Dalley A, Agur A. *Clinically Oriented Anatomy*. 6th ed. Lippincott Williams & Wilkins; 2010:204.)

TABLE 4-2	**Boundaries of the Inguinal Canal**[a]		
Boundary	**Deep Ring/Lateral Third**	**Middle Third**	**Lateral Third/Superficial Ring**
Posterior wall	Transversalis fascia	Transversalis fascia	Inguinal falx (conjoint tendon) plus reflected inguinal ligament
Anterior wall	Internal oblique plus lateral crus of aponeurosis of external oblique	Aponeurosis of external oblique (lateral crus and intercrural fibers)	Aponeurosis of external oblique (intercrural fibers), with fascia of external oblique continuing onto cord as external spermatic fascia
Roof	Transversalis fascia	Musculoaponeurotic arches of internal oblique and transverse abdominal	Medial crus of aponeurosis of external oblique
Floor	Iliopubic tract	Inguinal ligament	Lacunar ligament

[a]See Figure 4-8.

Reprinted with permission from Moore K, Dalley A, Agur A. *Clinically Oriented Anatomy*. 6th ed. Lippincott Williams & Wilkins; 2010:204.

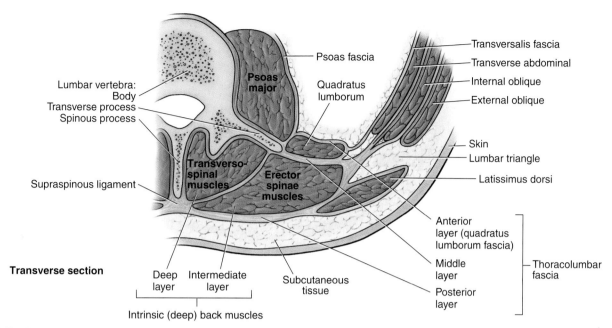

FIGURE 4-9 Posterior abdominal wall fascia. The relationship of the psoas fascia, the three layers of the thoracolumbar fascia, and quadratus lumborum fascia with the muscles and vertebrae are illustrated on this transverse section of the posterior abdominal wall. (Reprinted with permission from Moore KL, Agur AM. *Essential Clinical Anatomy.* 3rd ed. Lippincott Williams & Wilkins; 2007:300.)

TABLE 4-3 Muscles of the Posterior Abdomen Wall[1,2]

Psoas major (Figs. 4-8 and 4-9)	Bilaterally paired, long, thick, fusiform muscle Origin: arises from the bodies and transverse processes of lumbar vertebrae Insertion: inserts into the lesser trochanter of femur with iliacus via iliopsoas tendon Action: acts to flex the thigh; flexes and laterally bends the lumbar vertebral column
Iliacus (Fig. 4-9)	Bilaterally paired, triangular muscle Origin: arises from the iliac fossa and iliac crest and ala of the sacrum Insertion: inserts into the lesser trochanter of the femur Action: Acts to flex the thigh; if thigh is fixed, it flexes the pelvis on the thigh
Quadratus lumborum (Figs. 4-8 and 4-9)	Bilaterally paired, thick muscular sheet Origin: arises from the iliolumbar ligament and iliac crest Insertion: inserts into the 12th rib and transverse process of first four lumbar vertebrae Action: acts to flex vertebral column laterally and depress the last rib
Psoas minor (Fig. 4-9)	Bilaterally paired, long, slender muscle anterior to psoas major Origin: arises from the bodies of the 12th thoracic and first lumbar vertebrae Insertion: inserts into the iliopubic eminence at the line of junction of the ilium and the superior pubic ramus Action: acts to flex and laterally bends the lumbar vertebral column
Iliopsoas	Formed by the psoas and iliacus muscles Origin: arises from the iliac fossa, bodies and transverse processes of lumbar vertebrae Insertion: inserts into the lesser trochanter of the femur Action: acts to flex the thigh, flexes and laterally bends the lumbar vertebral column
Latissimus dorsi (Fig. 4-8)	Bilaterally paired, broadest back muscle Origin: arises from the lower six thoracic vertebrae, lumbar vertebrae, iliac crest via thoracolumbar fascia, sacrum, lower three or four ribs, and inferior angle of scapula Insertion: inserts into the intertubercular (bicipital) groove on the medial side of the humerus Action: acts to abduct, medially rotate, and extend arm at shoulder
Erector spinae (Fig. 4-8)	Location: a group of three columns of muscle located on each side of the vertebral column Action: acts as the chief extensor of the vertebral column
Transversospinal (Fig. 4-8)	Location: an oblique group of three muscles deep to the erector spinae Action: in the abdominal area, they act to stabilize vertebrae and assist with extension and rotation movements

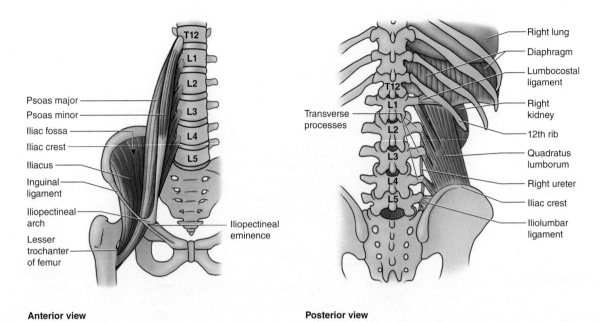

Anterior view

Posterior view

FIGURE 4-10 Posterior abdominal wall muscles. The anterior and posterior sections illustrate the musculoskeletal relationship of the major posterior abdominal wall muscles. (Reprinted with permission from Moore K, Dalley A, Agur A. *Clinically Oriented Anatomy.* 6th ed. Lippincott Williams & Wilkins; 2010:311.)

Layers

The posterior abdominal wall is covered with a continuous layer of endoabdominal fascia, which is continuous with the transversalis fascia.[4] The posterior wall fascia is located between the parietal peritoneum and the muscles. The psoas fascia (sheath) is attached medially to the lumbar vertebrae and pelvic brim. Superiorly, the psoas fascia is thickened and forms the medial arcuate ligament. Laterally, the psoas fascia fuses with both the quadratus lumborum fascia and the thoracolumbar fascia. Inferior to the iliac crest, the psoas fascia is continuous with that part of the iliac fascia that covers the iliacus[4] (see Fig. 4-9).

Diaphragm

The diaphragm is a fibromuscular domed structure separating the thoracic cavity from the abdominal cavity.[4,12] The convex superior surface forms the floor of the thoracic cavity, and the concave inferior surface forms the roof of the abdominal cavity. The concave surfaces form the right and left domes with the right dome slightly higher because of the presence of the liver and the central part slightly depressed by the pericardium.[4,12] The origin of the diaphragm is located at its periphery, which attaches to the inferior margin of the thoracic cage and the superior lumbar vertebrae.[4,12] The diaphragm is the primary muscle inspiration. The central part descends during inspiration to enlarge the thoracic cavity and ascends during expiration to increase thoracic pressure. The diaphragm varies in postural position (supine or standing) and varies in height based on the size and degree of abdominal visceral distention.[4,12]

The muscular part of the diaphragm is located peripherally with fibers that converge radially on the central tendon. The central tendon has no bony attachments and appears incompletely divided into what resembles the three leaves of a wide cloverleaf. Although it lies near the center of the diaphragm, the central tendon is closer to the anterior part of the thorax[4,12] (Fig. 4-11).

The area around the caval opening in the central tendon of the diaphragm is surrounded by a muscular part that forms a continuous sheet. The continuous sheet is divided into three parts based on its area of attachment: the sternal part, the costal part, and the lumbar part[4,12] (Table 4-4).

The diaphragmatic crura are musculotendinous bands that arise from the anterior surfaces of the bodies of the superior three lumbar vertebrae, the anterior longitudinal ligament, and the intervertebral disks. The right crus is larger and longer than the left crus and appears as a triangular mass anterior to the aorta.[4] It arises from the first three lumbar vertebrae and appears posterior to the caudate lobe of the liver. Fibers from the right crus extend anteriorly to form the esophageal hiatus.[4,12] The left crus arises from the first two lumbar vertebrae.[4]

Diaphragmatic Apertures

The diaphragmatic apertures (openings, hiatus) permit several structures (esophagus, blood vessels, nerves, and lymphatic vessels) to pass between the thorax and the abdomen.[4,12] The three larger apertures are the caval, esophageal, and aortic, and there are a number of small openings.[12,13] The caval hiatus is primarily for the inferior vena cava (IVC) as it ascends into the thoracic cavity.[4,13] The IVC shares the caval opening with the terminal branches of the right phrenic nerve and a few lymphatic vessels passing from the liver to the middle phrenic and mediastinal lymph nodes.[4,13] Located to the right of midline, at the junction of the right and middle leaves of the central tendon, the caval opening is the most superior and anterior of the three large diaphragmatic apertures. Because the IVC is adherent into the margin of the caval opening, diaphragmatic contraction during inspiration widens the opening, which allows the IVC to dilate and helps facilitate blood flow through this large vein to the heart.[4,12,13]

The esophageal hiatus is an oval opening located in the muscle of the right crus anterior and superior to the aortic

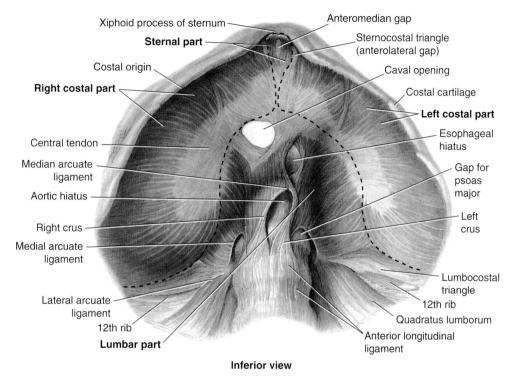

Xiphoid process of sternum
Anteromedian gap
Sternal part
Sternocostal triangle
(anterolateral gap)
Costal origin
Caval opening
Right costal part
Costal cartilage
Left costal part
Central tendon
Esophageal
hiatus
Median arcuate
ligament
Gap for
psoas
major
Aortic hiatus
Left
crus
Right crus
Medial arcuate
ligament
Lumbocostal
triangle
12th rib
Lateral arcuate
ligament
Quadratus lumborum
12th rib
Anterior longitudinal
ligament
Lumbar part

Inferior view

FIGURE 4-11 Diaphragm. The view of the concave inner surface forming the roof of the abdominopelvic cavity illustrates the fleshy sternal, costal, and lumbar parts of the diaphragm (outlined with *broken lines*). Identify the relationship of how each part attaches centrally to the trefoil-shaped central tendon, the aponeurotic insertion of the diaphragmatic muscle fibers. (Reprinted with permission from Moore K, Dalley A, Agur A. *Clinically Oriented Anatomy*. 6th ed. Lippincott Williams & Wilkins; 2010:306.)

TABLE 4-4	**Diaphragmatic Peripheral Attachments**[1,2]
Sternal part	Two muscular slips attach the diaphragm to the posterior aspect of xiphoid process. This part is not always present.
Costal part	Wide muscular slips bilaterally attach the diaphragm to the internal surfaces of the inferior six costal cartilages and their adjoining ribs. The costal parts form the right and left domes.
Lumbar part	The medial and lateral arcuate ligaments (two aponeurotic arches) and the three superior lumbar vertebrae form the right and left muscular crura that ascend and insert into the central tendon.

hiatus.[4,12] In 70% of individuals, both margins of the hiatus are formed by muscular bundles of the right crus. In 30% of individuals, a superficial muscular bundle from the left crus contributes to the formation of the right margin of the hiatus. The hiatus allows the esophagus to course from the thorax into the abdominal cavity and also serves as the passageway for the right and left trunks of the vagus nerve, esophageal branches of the left gastric vessels, and a few lymphatic vessels.[4,12,13]

The aortic hiatus passes between the crura posterior to the median arcuate ligaments at the inferior border of the T12 vertebra.[4,12] This opening in the posterior diaphragm allows the descending aorta to course from the thoracic cavity to the abdominal cavity. The thoracic duct; azygos vein; and, sometimes, hemiazygos veins are also transmitted through the aortic hiatus. The aorta does not pierce the diaphragm or adhere to the hiatus, which means diaphragmatic movements during respiration do not affect aortic blood flow.[4,12] The sternocostal triangle (foramen of Morgagni) is a small opening in the loose connective tissue between the sternal and costal attachments of the diaphragm. This triangle transmits lymphatic vessels from the hepatic diaphragmatic surface and the superior epigastric branch of the internal thoracic artery. The sympathetic trunk passes deep to the medial arcuate ligament and is accompanied by the least splanchnic nerves. In each crus, there are two small apertures: The right lesser aperture transmits the right greater and lesser splanchnic nerves and the left lesser aperture transmits the hemizygous vein (usually) and the left greater and lesser splanchnic nerves.[12]

Variants

Anatomic variants are composed of individual variations in fat and muscle content. In more muscular individuals, each lateral muscle layer tends to be identifiable, whereas in less well-developed individuals, muscle groups tend to be indistinct. Furthermore, some muscular components, like the psoas minor and pyramidalis muscles, are partially or completely absent in a significant portion of the population. It is important to note that in obese patients, the fatty layer variation can be significant.

SONOGRAPHIC APPEARANCES AND TECHNIQUES

Abdominal Wall

Sonography should be the first modality of choice for imaging abdominal wall structures because it is fast; widely available; and provides a valuable, inexpensive, and noninvasive method of imaging.[7,14,15] The ability to perform real-time imaging that demonstrates changes in anatomy with changes in patient position and other maneuvers makes sonography ideal for evaluating structures in motion. Imaging the normal abdominal wall and detecting pathologic processes such as inflammatory lesions, hemorrhage, hernia, or masses makes sonography of the abdominal wall an excellent modality for diagnosing pathology. Many clinical questions can be answered with the use of sonography in evaluating posttrauma or postsurgical patients. It is extremely important to understand the normal sonographic appearance of the abdominal wall and the appropriate instrumentation and scanning techniques necessary to achieve that appearance.

The superficial nature of the abdominal wall and its lesions demands excellent near-field imaging. Newer, high-frequency, short–focal zone transducers (7.5 MHz or higher linear array transducers) are the optimum tools for scanning this area.[7,14,15] Focal zone placement at the area of interest is especially important. Sonography enables the viewer to see the superficial layers of the abdomen.[7] In morbidly obese patients, a linear probe may not provide sufficient penetration, requiring the sacrifice of image resolution with a lower-frequency curvilinear probe in order to visualize the desired anatomy.

In some instances, a standoff device or other scanning technique may be indicated when scanning the superficial cutaneous layers to avoid a "main-bang" transducer artifact. Excellent standoff devices exist in the form of flotation pads constructed of liquid-filled microcell sponges, synthetic polymer blocks, and silicone elastomer blocks. Each of these substances is dense enough to stand alone and offers uniform consistency to minimize artifacts. In a pinch, a thick mound of ultrasound gel can be utilized, but air bubbles can create artifacts. When it is necessary to scan over a surgical wound, any protective dressing is removed, and a commercially available adhesive plastic membrane can be applied directly to the wound to provide a smooth, safe scanning surface. The use of sterile gel and a sterile probe cover aids in protecting the patient from any bacterial contamination.[16] The sonographer should use light transducer pressure while scanning to eliminate distortion of the superficial layers.

Demonstration of various layers of the normal abdominal wall and a contiguous diaphragm should not be limited to patients with superficial lesions. It should be an integral part of every high-quality sonographic abdominal study (Fig. 4-12).

Diaphragm

Sonographically, the diaphragm appears as a thin, curvilinear, hyperechoic band on children and adults. Conversely, the fetal diaphragm has a hypoechoic appearance. The abdominal side of the diaphragm produces a thin, curved line representing the diaphragm–liver interface. An additional thin, hyperechoic line, an artifactual mirror image of the diaphragm–liver interface, may sometimes be seen on the thoracic side (Fig. 4-13). Another thick, hyperechoic line can be seen on the diaphragm–lung interface. Occasionally, reverberation artifacts from air in the lung originate from this area. The diaphragmatic crura lie anterior to the upper abdominal aorta and appear as thin, hypoechoic bands that thicken during deep inspiration. The crus of the right hemidiaphragm contains medium-density echoes. In some patients, diaphragmatic slips appear as round, focal, hyperechoic masses when seen in a transverse section. They should not be mistaken for focal liver or peritoneal masses. They can be clarified by rotating the transducer from its transverse orientation and scanning along their long axis, noting their change to an elongated appearance.

The diaphragm should be closely evaluated for symmetric motion on real-time scanning. Absence of normal motion with respiration should prompt further, targeted evaluation. The left and right hemidiaphragm and pleural space should be documented on every abdominal sonogram.[17]

ABDOMINAL WALL PATHOLOGY

A thorough understanding of the anatomy and sonographic appearance of the superficial layers of the abdominal wall,

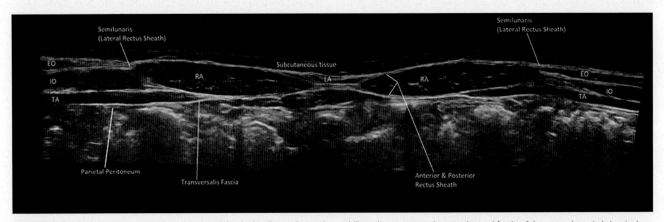

FIGURE 4-12 A panoramic image of the anterior abdominal wall superior to the umbilicus demonstrates the muscles and fascia of the anterolateral abdominal wall. *EO,* external oblique muscle; *IO,* internal oblique muscle; *LA,* linea alba; *RA,* rectus abdominus muscle; *TA,* transversus abdominus muscle.

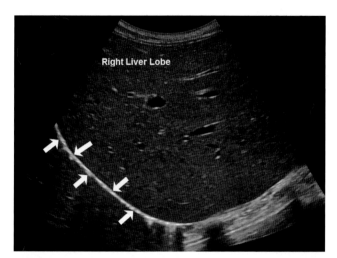

FIGURE 4-13 Diaphragm. A longitudinal section through the right liver lobe shows the normal sonographic appearance of the thin, curvilinear, hyperechoic diaphragm (*arrows*). On the chest-side of the diaphragm, the mirror image artifact of the liver can be identified in the pleural cavity.

and the tissues and organs directly beneath it, is essential before pathologic changes can be fully appreciated. Three major categories of disease affect the abdominal wall, the peritoneum, and the abdominal spaces. Both the tissues of the abdominal wall and the membranes lining its spaces are affected by inflammatory, traumatic, and neoplastic changes.

Inflammatory Response: Abscess

It is vitally important that sonographers understand the medical aspects of inflammation, as well as its sonographic appearance. Inflammation can be acute or chronic. Acute inflammation frequently results from cuts, scrapes, crushing injuries, or surgical trauma that produces tissue damage such as mesh for hernia repair.[7] Deep abdominal organs can also be the source of infection spreading to the abdominal wall.[7,15,18,19] Consequently, an inflammatory response can occur whenever bacterial infection damages the skin and underlying tissues. The four main indications of inflammatory response are heat, redness, pain, and swelling.[20–22]

In most patients with acute inflammation, the body will return to normal. This process of resolution can be hastened by using anti-inflammatory drugs. Such drugs block the body's natural inflammatory reactions, allowing removal of debris and fluid exudates associated with the inflammation via the circulatory and lymphatic systems.

If resolution occurs slowly, other consequences may result. Fibrous tissue growth invades areas of long-standing cellular and fluid exudates to form scar tissue. This process, called organization, is responsible for the development of adhesions following surgery. If sufficient necrosis of the involved tissues occurs, resolution does not take place and a cavity containing dead tissue and pus forms. The liquid pus in such a cavity consists of living and dead microorganisms, necrotic tissue, exudate, and granulocytes. The cavity is called an abscess.[21,22]

Abscesses are space-occupying lesions that can assume a variety of shapes owing to their fluid content. They are typically round or ovoid with irregular borders (Fig. 4-14A, B).

Because of their internal pressure, however, they can exert a mass effect, causing compression and/or displacement of surrounding structures. Abdominal wall abscesses frequently occur as a result of postsurgical incisional infections or exist as extensions of a superficial intraperitoneal abscess. Less frequently, tuberculous paraspinal abscesses may also track along the musculofascial plane into the lateral and posterior abdominal walls.[18–22]

Wherever abscesses occur, the usual treatment involves antibiotic therapy and sometimes drainage to facilitate resolution. Failure of an abscess to resolve can lead to thickening of its contents as a result of the reabsorption of water (inspissation), and eventually, calcifications develop. If the cause of the acute inflammation is not eliminated, the processes of tissue injury and repair will continue simultaneously, producing chronic inflammation.[21,22]

Chronic suppurative inflammation or pyogenic inflammation occurs when persistent infection results in abscess formation. Suppurative inflammation describes a condition in which a purulent exudate is accompanied by significant liquefactive necrosis; it is the equivalent of pus. The term suppurative refers to this formation of pus. Body defenses may be poor because the blood supply to the area is limited. If so, chronic suppurative inflammation can easily occur, requiring surgical drainage and the use of specific antibiotics to affect a cure.[21,22]

Superficial abdominal wall abscesses can be associated with surgical or external trauma, and, much less frequently with deep organ rupture, neoplasms, tuberculous, or bacterial abscesses.[7,15] In evaluating superficial abscesses, precise scanning is required to display the superficial layers of the skin, subcutaneous fat, muscle planes, and the peritoneum. The most clinically important aspect of treating abscesses is to determine whether the abscess is intraperitoneal or extraperitoneal. This is done by demonstrating the peritoneal line.

Superficial wound abscesses commonly result from intraoperative contamination. In such cases, sonography may have limited diagnostic value because the diagnosis can usually be made easily on physical examination. However, sonographic guidance is often used to drain or place a drainage tube into these types of abscesses to aid resolution. Most incisional abscesses are superficially located and display clinical signs of erythema, tenderness, purulence, and induration of the wound.[22] There have been several reported cases of abdominal wall abscesses forming around laparoscopic cholecystectomy gallstones that have fallen out of the gallbladder during perforation or removal. During imaging, there may be calcific shadowing if the patient has had a cholecystectomy via laparoscopy.[18] If the abscess develops below the fascial plane, detection by physical examination alone can be difficult. There have been many cases where abscesses have formed from cancer that had perforated bowel or other structures. The sonographer should look for fluid collections in the prehepatic space and thickening of the bowel wall.[23] Aspiration of a soft tissue abscess under sonographic guidance may be indicated so that the specimen can be sent to the laboratory for culture and sensitivity testing.[22]

The differential diagnosis of superficial abscesses includes rectus sheath hematomas and hernias, in addition to noninfected fluid collections.[7,23] Clinical history and patient symptoms are critically important when seeking to narrow

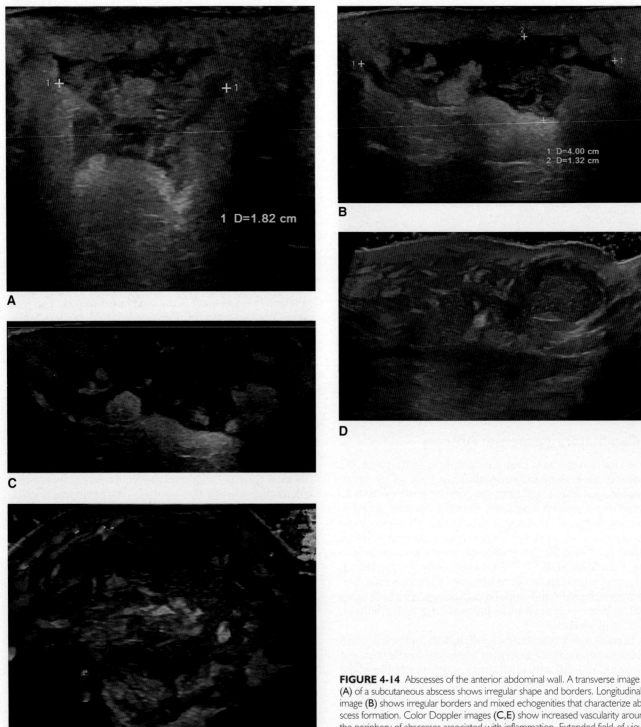

FIGURE 4-14 Abscesses of the anterior abdominal wall. A transverse image (**A**) of a subcutaneous abscess shows irregular shape and borders. Longitudinal image (**B**) shows irregular borders and mixed echogenities that characterize abscess formation. Color Doppler images (**C,E**) show increased vascularity around the periphery of abscesses associated with inflammation. Extended field-of-view image (**D**) shows abscess extension to the peritoneum. (Images courtesy of Ted Whitten, Ultrasound Practitioner, Elliot Hospital, Manchester, NH.)

the differential diagnosis because the sonographic appearance can be quite similar for various conditions.

Sonographically, most abscesses appear as hypoechoic fluid masses, with irregular borders and may have internal patterns ranging from uniformly echo-free to mildly or even highly echogenic.[7,15] The presence of particulate debris or microbubbles floating within an abscess cavity is generally the cause of its increased echogenicity. If the particulate matter is uniformly distributed throughout the abscess,

it may create a fluid-debris level within the abscess or it may be difficult to recognize and differentiate the abscess from surrounding structures. Despite their variable internal textures, however, most abscesses demonstrate posterior enhancement, revealing their fluid nature[7,15,22] (Fig. 4-14C–E).

Abscesses vary in contour from flat to oval or bonnet shaped. Occasionally, large abscesses may compress adjacent structures and cause confusion in the differentiation of extraperitoneal versus intraperitoneal locations.[7]

Table 4-5 describes the common types of tissue changes associated with abscesses and their corresponding sonographic patterns. Because sonographic diagnosis is very technique- and operator-dependent, it is critical to understand how instrumentation and scan technique can alter the echo image from within an abscess. Occasionally, septations may be seen within abscesses.[15] Such findings require documentation because their presence contraindicates percutaneous drainage. Fortunately, septated abscesses occur infrequently within the peritoneal cavity.

To permit contact scanning, postoperative patients' surgical dressings must be removed. Current guidelines recommend the use of sterile probe covers and sterile gel to prevent contamination.[16] Commercially available sterile plastic pads can be used to cover the wound rather than a probe cover. The point is to have a sterile barrier between the patient's wound and the transducer. Following scans of wounds or interventional procedures, the transducer should undergo high-level disinfection according to site policy and manufacturer guidelines.[16,24]

The search for an abscess must be conducted in a systematic fashion, with special attention and care given to areas of swelling or tenderness. If there is any open wound, incision, drain site, or enterostomy, it is important to use sterile gel and a sterile transducer cover as a precaution against infectious contamination.[16,24] When possible, the regions around such sites should be scanned by angling the transducer to view the area beneath.

As the sonographer scans to evaluate for abscess, special techniques may be necessary to enhance the appearance of any suspicious lesions. Because the gain setting may affect the overall appearance of lesions, it is important to vary the gain. When gain settings are excessively high, small fluid collections may be overlooked because they are artifactually filled with echoes, making them have a solid appearance. In contrast, when extremely low gain settings are used, there is a risk of making a homogeneously solid mass appear cystic or overlooking solid components in a mixed (complex) lesion. Moderate gain settings are useful in demonstrating the far wall of an abscess, but low gain may also be required to avoid the strong reverberation artifacts frequently seen at, or obscuring, the near walls. A standoff pad can also be used to better visualize the near wall of a superficial abscess. Maximum information about an abscess is best obtained by creating multiple images at different gain settings and machine parameters.

The shape of an abscess and its relationship to surrounding structures are valuable information if the clinician is planning percutaneous needle aspiration. Sonography aids in planning a safe aspiration route and monitoring the procedure, and it also provides a means of evaluating the effectiveness of therapy.

Trauma/Tear

Abdominal muscles may be injured by penetrating wounds, blows to the abdomen, or by hyperextension strain. Subcutaneous edema or muscle contusions are commonly seen with blunt trauma. Traumatic hernias, which go unnoticed because of more apparent injury, may be missed.[14,25] A contused muscle will appear thicker and very hypoechoic if edema is present. In cases of extravasated blood and inflammatory reactions, a disorganized, coarse echo pattern is common. A similar appearance may be seen with rhabdomyolysis (the breakdown of muscle caused by injury).

With violent hyperextension strain, it is possible for the rectus muscle to rupture, causing tearing of the inferior epigastric artery. Such patients present with a tender mass, sonographically resembling the appearance of a superficial hematoma.[7,15]

Hematomas

Hematomas are generally associated with muscular trauma that results in hemorrhage. They can also result from

TABLE 4-5	**Sonographic Appearances**		
Collection	**Location**	**Sonographic Characteristics**	**Acoustic Transmission**
Abscess	Near surgical site or painful area, subphrenic, subhepatic, paracolic gutters, and left perihepatic, perisplenic, and pelvis	Shape: lenticular or shape of space. Anechoic, with irregular or smooth borders; may have internal echoes, septations, fluid-fluid level; abscesses that contain gas are echogenic and may shadow.	Usually good
Hematoma	Near wound or surgical site	Shape: lenticular or shape of space. Change with stage of resolution; fresh blood is hypoechoic, as is clotted blood; fragmentation of clot creates internal echoes and anechoic areas with some scattered echoes; fluid–fluid level may be caused by cholesterol in breakdown of red blood cells; longstanding hematoma may have thick contours.	Coincides with stage; good-to-slow or decreased; may increase owing to fluid portion
Ascites	Most dependent areas of body, cul-de-sac, Morrison pouch, paracolic gutter, pararenal areas, perihepatic, midabdominal	Anechoic if benign, ascites if exudative, internal echoes if malignant; bowel and implants in anechoic ascitic fluid	Increased
Urinoma	Adjacent to kidneys	Usually anechoic unless infected	Increased
Lymphocele	Adjacent to renal transplant	Usually anechoic but may have septations	Increased

Courtesy Mimi Berman, PhD, RDMS.

infection, debilitating disease, collagen disorders, pregnancy, and childbirth. Straining, coughing, anticoagulant therapy, and surgery can also be precipitating factors.[7,14,15,25] Among the most common superficial abdominal wall hematomas are those occurring within the rectus sheath.

Sonography is valuable during the conservative management of even large hematomas because of its ability to monitor their size and resolution as they resorb (hypoechoic phase) and liquefy (anechoic phase). An important reality is that hematomas are not limited to the anterior abdominal wall but can also involve the lateral or retroperitoneal muscles.[7]

Sonographic patterns closely follow the pathologic evolution of the hematoma. Recent blood collections tend to appear echo-free, becoming more hyperechoic as they organize, although the reverse may also occur (see Table 4-5). Hematomas and thrombi behave differently, depending on their size and location. Generally, wound hematomas that occur within the body resolve over time. The sonographic characteristics of the borders of such masses differ from their centers. In contrast, abdominal wall hematomas or those surrounded by a capsule gradually change to an anechoic state.[4,15]

A seroma is a collection of serum in the tissue resulting from a surgical incision or from the liquefaction of a hematoma. The normal small seroma formation during the incisional healing process usually resolves. Without resolution, the seroma may require aspiration drainage to alleviate pain and/or visible swelling. The sonographic appearance of a seroma ranges from anechoic to hypoechoic[7] (Fig. 4-15A–C).

When bleeding is secondary to anticoagulant therapy, a wide range of sonographic appearances is possible (Fig. 4-15C). Although it is uncommon to scan such patients during active bleeding, the relative lack of coagulation would likely produce an echo-free or an unusual, layered appearance. The layered appearance is caused by the settling of moderately hyperechoic red blood cells to the bottom of the lesion. The fibrin content of the clot makes it hypoechoic compared with the red blood cells. Movement of blood can sometimes be produced in such patients by changing their positions. Serial examination with high-resolution sonography, which clearly delineates the muscular layers of the abdominal wall, is a valuable way to study the response of such lesions to treatment.[26]

Hernias

There are two main categories of abdominal wall hernias: (1) ventral (anterior or anterolateral abdominal wall) and (2) groin (indirect inguinal, direct inguinal, and femoral).[10,11,27] Diaphragmatic hernias occur with less frequency and are presented later in this chapter. If the abdominal wall muscles are excessively weak through an acquired or congenital wall defect, the viscera lying beneath may protrude, resulting in a hernia. It has been found that three major factors aid in a weak abdominal wall. These are abnormal collagen metabolism; pressure overload such as obesity, heavy lifting, coughing, smoking, familial tendency or straining that may contribute to either hernia formation or increased growth of an existing hernia; and insufficient protein intake.[28–30] Natural weak areas include where vessels penetrate the abdominal wall; where fetal migration of testis, spermatic cord, or round ligament occurred; and through aponeurosis.[10,30]

Ventral Hernias

Primary ventral hernias account for 75% of the repaired ventral hernias in the United States and are one of the most common surgical treatments worldwide.[31,32] Laparoscopic repair has become the preferred treatment method whenever possible because there is less tissue damage and the patient recovers faster.[31] Abdominal wall hernias consist of three parts: the sac, the contents of the sac, and the covering of the sac (Fig. 4-16). Hernia contents vary. Of the hernias diagnosed by sonography, most contain only fat, which may be intraperitoneal (mesenteric or omental) or peritoneal in origin.[15,30] If a hernia does contain intraperitoneal fat, it may contain bowel later in its course. When bowel is included in hernia contents, the risk of complications is increased compared with those containing only intraperitoneal fat owing to strangulation, which may result in ischemia caused by a compromised blood supply.[15,30] Some hernias contain free fluid of intraperitoneal origin.[30]

Epigastric and hypogastric hernias occur in the linea alba and are named for the abdominal regions where they occur. Epigastric hernias occur through the widest part of the linea alba anywhere from 3 cm below the xiphoid process and 3 cm above the umbilicus. Hypogastric hernias occur within the inferior portion of the linea alba where the deep fascia is absent. Usually, such hernias begin as a small defect of protruding extraperitoneal fat. Over a period of months or years, that fat is forced through the linea alba, pulling behind it a small peritoneal sac that often contains a small piece of the omentum or bowel.[33,34]

Although the clinical presentation of a Spigelian hernia is rare, sonographically detected spigelian hernias are more common.[30,35] A Spigelian hernia can occur anywhere along the course of the Spigelian fascia, which is the complex aponeurotic tendon located between the flat anterolateral muscles along the semilunar line.[30,35] Spigelian hernias are difficult to detect clinically because they lie beneath the external oblique fascia; the fascia forms a layer of the sac coverings.[36] Almost all Spigelian hernias are located at the inferior end of the semicircular line, inferior to the arcuate line where the posterior rectus sheath is absent.[30,35] The Spigelian hernia may be listed as an inguinal hernia because its location is within 2 cm of the internal inguinal rings and its symptoms are similar to indirect inguinal hernias.[30] Of note, if the hernia is on a pediatric patient, nearly 50% are associated with an undescended testis. When imaging a pediatric patient for cryptorchism, the sonographer may want to check for a hernia as well[37] (Fig. 4-17A–C).

Two complications that may occur in midline hernias are strangulation (compromised blood supply causing ischemia) and incarceration, which means the hernia is nonreducible (an irreducible sac where contents cannot be pushed back into the abdomen or through torn muscles).[34] An incarcerated hernia cannot be manually pushed back into the peritoneal cavity, but its vascular supply is generally intact. If the blood flow becomes compromised, the hernia is then classified as strangulated. This may be caused by extrinsic compression of vessels because of edema or by the vessels becoming twisted, impairing perfusion of the hernia contents. Surgery is generally indicated because these two conditions are vulnerable to serious complications. With an incarcerated or strangulated hernia, complicating factors may include edema of the protruding structure and constriction of the opening through

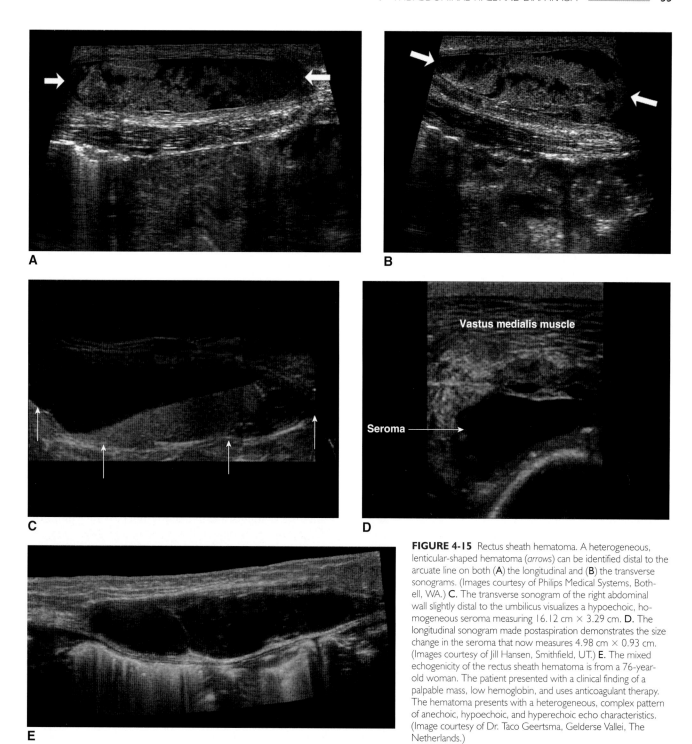

FIGURE 4-15 Rectus sheath hematoma. A heterogeneous, lenticular-shaped hematoma (*arrows*) can be identified distal to the arcuate line on both (**A**) the longitudinal and (**B**) the transverse sonograms. (Images courtesy of Philips Medical Systems, Bothell, WA.) **C.** The transverse sonogram of the right abdominal wall slightly distal to the umbilicus visualizes a hypoechoic, homogeneous seroma measuring 16.12 cm × 3.29 cm. **D.** The longitudinal sonogram made postaspiration demonstrates the size change in the seroma that now measures 4.98 cm × 0.93 cm. (Images courtesy of Jill Hansen, Smithfield, UT.) **E.** The mixed echogenicity of the rectus sheath hematoma is from a 76-year-old woman. The patient presented with a clinical finding of a palpable mass, low hemoglobin, and uses anticoagulant therapy. The hematoma presents with a heterogeneous, complex pattern of anechoic, hypoechoic, and hyperechoic echo characteristics. (Image courtesy of Dr. Taco Geertsma, Gelderse Vallei, The Netherlands.)

which intra-abdominal contents have emerged, leading to compromised blood flow, which progresses to necrosis and will require surgery[38] (Fig. 4-17D–F).

An incisional hernia occurs at the site of a surgical incision in the abdominal area where the surgical procedure created a weak point in the abdominal wall. This is considered a delayed surgical complication, which may be diagnosed months or even years after the surgical procedure. Incisional hernias are more commonly encountered with vertical rather than with transverse incisions. The occurrence rate may be as high as 28% after abdominal surgery.[39] A subtype of an incisional hernia is a parastomal hernia. A parastomal hernia is a common complication occurring adjacent to a stoma in about half of the patients who have an enterostomy.[40] Elderly, obese, or malnourished patients are more prone to develop incisional hernias. Infection, which impairs wound healing, is also a predisposing factor.

Groin Hernias

Groin hernias are fairly common with approximately 2% in the adult population and are comprised of three components—the neck, sac and contents. Groin hernias increase in frequency

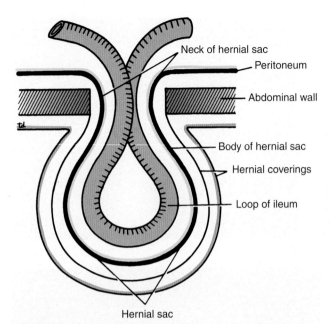

Neck of hernial sac

Peritoneum

Abdominal wall

Body of hernial sac

Hernial coverings

Loop of ileum

Hernial sac

FIGURE 4-16 Components of a hernia. Abdominal wall hernias consist of three parts: the sac, the contents of the sac, and the covering of the sac. (Reprinted with permission from Snell RS. *Clinical Anatomy*. 7th ed. Lippincott Williams & Wilkins; 2003.)

as people age, from 0.25% at age 18 to 4.2% at age 75, and are eight times more likely with a family history.[30,34] There is a 20% to 27% chance a male will develop an inguinal hernia in his lifetime and between 3% and 6% chance a female will develop an inguinal hernia in her lifetime.[41–43] These occur in the ilioinguinal crease at the junction of the abdomen and the thigh and the adjacent areas immediately above and below.[30] Although groin hernias are almost always inguinal or femoral, at times, Spigelian hernias are also included in this category.[30,37]

Inguinal hernias, which make up 75% of all hernias, can be either direct or indirect, depending on their route to the inguinal canal. Femoral hernias are outside the inguinal canal; but owing to their location, they are often considered with inguinal hernias.[40,41] Both direct and indirect inguinal hernias are above the inguinal ligament and are more common on the right side. Indirect inguinal hernias are one of the most common forms of hernia, occurring 10 times more often in males than in females. Indirect hernias are twice as common as direct hernias.[41] Indirect hernias pass through the deep inguinal ring and extend superficially and inferomedially down the inguinal canal (Fig. 4-18A–E). Indirect hernias protrude through a defect in the inguinal ring through enlargement of the vaginalis.[34,42] They can extend down into the scrotum in males and the labia majora in females. Nearly a third of inguinal hernias are bilateral, but unilateral hernias are located most often on the right side. Boys and young men are commonly seen with an indirect inguinal hernia, where bowel follows the pathway the testes descended during fetal development.

Direct inguinal hernias are caused by a weakness or tearing of the transversalis fascia, usually occurring in elderly men with weak abdominal muscles. Direct inguinal hernias are rarely found in women. Direct inguinal hernias enter through the floor of the inguinal canal, medial to the deep inguinal ring and the inferior epigastric arteries.[30,35,42]

Femoral hernias occur less frequently than inguinal hernias; in fact, only 5% to 15% of groin hernias are femoral. Femoral hernias are located medial to the femoral vein and inferior to the inguinal ligament, within the femoral canal, usually on the right side. The neck and sac extend inferior to the groin and pubic tubercle, appearing as a bulge in the upper thigh. Femoral hernias do not enter the scrotum.[34] There is a higher incidence of femoral hernias in females than in males.[34]

Other Hernias

There are multiple other hernias that occur, and these include sports hernia (groin and pubic area), lumbar hernia (defects in lumbar muscles or the posterior fascia below the 12th rib and above the iliac crest), pelvic hernias, traumatic hernias, recurring hernias, and multiple hernias.

Sonographic Evaluation

Because sonography is a quick, painless, inexpensive, and widely available imaging method, it should be widely used to image all abdominal wall hernias.[10,30,38] The use of power Doppler during imaging has made visualizing incarcerated hernias more easy to diagnose.[36] The use of 3D sonographic imaging provides high diagnostic accuracy as well as better visualization of lesions and surrounding tissues.[44] One-third of patients with groin hernias have no symptoms; when present, they are generally palpable masses and may cause burning or sharp pain. A diagnostic imaging referral is often required because of the limitations of clinical assessment alone for a significant proportion of patients with symptoms suggestive of a hernia but without a lump or bump.[41] In one study, sonography was found to be accurate and have a higher sensitivity compared with herniography, which at one time was the imaging procedure of choice for hernia evaluation. Patients are frequently referred for computed tomography (CT) or magnetic resonance (MR) imaging for hernia evaluation, especially with nonspecific clinical findings. The three major advantages of sonography over other imaging modalities are the ability to scan the patient in both upright and supine positions, the ability to include dynamic maneuvers such as Valsalva and compression, and the ability to document motion in real time. Dynamic abdominal scanning may be the new gold standard.[30,39,45]

Often, when the patient performs the Valsalva maneuver, the hernia content moves distally and the hernia neck widens. When the patient relaxes, the hernia content moves back toward the abdomen and the sac narrows, a lack thereof may indicate another type of mass[30,39,46] (Fig. 4-18D, E). Using the transducer for compression can reduce the hernia and push contents back toward the abdomen. When the compression is released, the hernia will return to the precompression position.[30,46] The third thing is to employ both supine and upright patient positions. In an upright position, most hernias enlarge; others may only be visible in the upright position[30,39,45] (Fig. 4-19A–C). Color Doppler is also helpful to evaluate presence or absence of flow within the hernia (see Fig. 4-17B).

This scanning protocol allows for the documentation of a significant amount of information, including (1) demonstrating an abdominal wall or groin defect; (2) determining the presence of bowel loops within a lesion; (3) exaggeration of the lesion on straining of the abdominal musculature; (4) reducibility of the lesion with pressure; and (5) vascularity of the hernia contents.

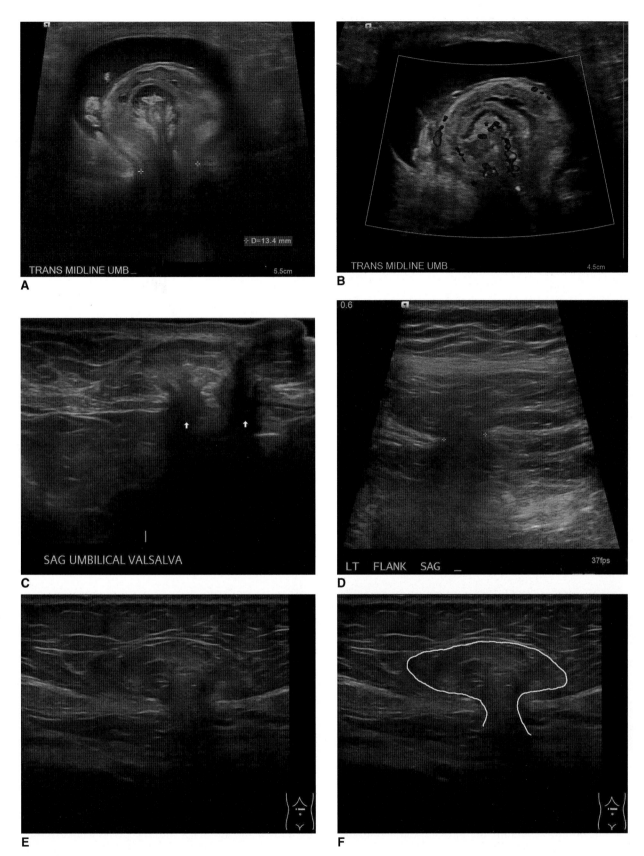

FIGURE 4-17 Ventral hernias: **A:** A transverse image at the level of the umbilicus shows bowel and fluid protruding through the umbilical ring. The neck of the hernia is located between the calipers. **B:** Color Doppler demonstrates vascular flow within the hernia contents, reducing concerns for strangulation and ischemia. **C:** This sagittal image of the umbilicus with Valsalva maneuver reveals two defects in the umbilical ring with two hernia necks (*arrows*). **D:** This sagittal image of the left lateral abdominal wall displays a lumbar hernia located at the lateral margin of the left abdomen. The neck is shown between the calipers. **E:** This transverse image shows a midline ventral wall hernia in the epigastric region. These occur at the medial attachment of the rectus abdominus muscle to the linea alba. **F:** The ventral wall hernia seen in image (**E**) is outlined. (Images courtesy of Ted Whitten, Ultrasound Practitioner, Elliot Hospital, Manchester, NH.)

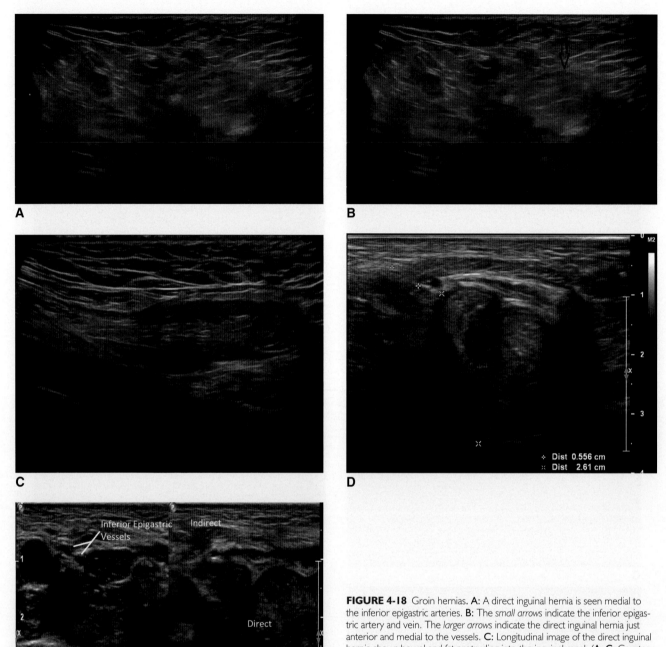

FIGURE 4-18 Groin hernias. **A:** A direct inguinal hernia is seen medial to the inferior epigastric arteries. **B:** The *small arrows* indicate the inferior epigastric artery and vein. The *larger arrows* indicate the direct inguinal hernia just anterior and medial to the vessels. **C:** Longitudinal image of the direct inguinal hernia shows bowel and fat protruding into the inguinal canal. (**A–C:** Courtesy of Ted Whitten, Ultrasound Practitioner, Elliot Hospital, Manchester, NH.) **D:** Longitudinal image of a patient with both direct and indirect inguinal hernias. The neck of the direct hernia, entering the inguinal canal through a tear in the transversalis fascia, is much larger than the neck of the indirect hernia, which enters through the deep inguinal ring. **E:** Transverse image of coexisting direct and indirect hernias with and without Valsalva. The relationship of each type of hernia to the inferior epigastric vessels is clearly shown along with the importance of the Valsalva maneuver to aid in the visualization of the hernias. (**D, E:** Courtesy of Amanda Auckland.)

Sonography can determine the location, size, and contents of a hernia. At the site of a hernia, interruption of the peritoneal line separating the muscles and abdominal contents is seen. Sonography can demonstrate the size of the defect and whether the hernia sac is fluid filled or contains peristaltic bowel or mesenteric fat. Besides peristaltic motion, gas in the bowel produces the typical shadowing artifact. Mesenteric fat, which also appears to be highly reflective, lacks both peristalsis and shadowing. Ascites can complicate the appearance of hernia by producing a fluid-filled sac. At times, the fluid can be evacuated out of the hernial sac and back into the peritoneal cavity when transducer pressure is applied to the area.

A high-frequency linear array transducer should be used to evaluate for a hernia, but a curved-array, lower-frequency transducer may be required on obese patients. The larger field of view provides good visualization of landmarks. It is important to capture dynamic events on video clips to document motion.

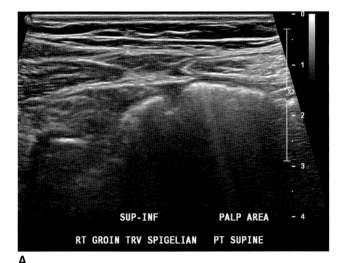

A

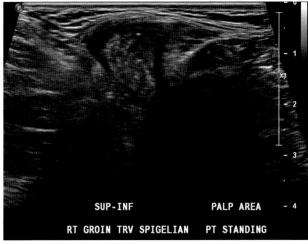

B

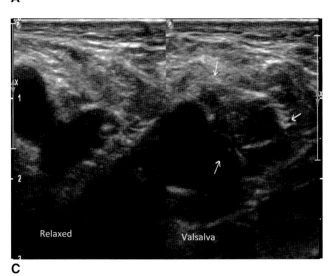

C

FIGURE 4-19 Images of a Spigelian hernia with the patient in supine (**A**) and standing (**B**) positions demonstrate the importance of utilizing multiple patient positions and maneuvers to optimize visualization of hernias. **C:** Transverse image of femoral hernia, indicated by the arrows in the Valsalva image. These images show the relationship of the femoral hernia to the common femoral vessels. The femoral canal is located inferior to the inguinal canal. They also demonstrate the importance of utilizing the Valsalva maneuver to optimize visualization of hernias. (Image courtesy of Amanda Auckland.)

A key landmark for distinguishing direct from indirect inguinal hernia sonographically is the inferior epigastric artery and vein. On a transverse sonographic image, the deep inguinal ring lies just lateral to the inferior epigastric vessels. If the hernia is seen lateral to these vessels, it is an indirect inguinal hernia. If the defect is seen medially to the inferior epigastric vessels, the hernia enters the inguinal canal through the transversalis fascia and is a direct inguinal hernia[47] (see Fig. 4-8).

Neoplasms

Abdominal wall tumors include (1) lipomas, (2) desmoid tumors, (3) soft tissue sarcomas, (4) metastatic carcinoma, (5) endometriomas, and (6) melanomas.[48] There are several reports of endometriomas undergoing malignant transformation, and this appears to be occurring with more frequency.[49,50] Malignant transformation of endometriomas most often results in serous cystadenocarcinoma, sarcoma, or clear cell carcinoma.[49–52] Cancers are now being found from long-term inflammation from mesh abscesses. Since the inception of the use of mesh to aid in replacing abdominal wall layers, complications have arisen in the form of abscesses and cancer.[7,15,53] Most lesions are readily diagnosed by physical examination and clinical history. Sonography, CT, MR, and fine-needle biopsy, however, are all valuable tools to help narrow the differential diagnosis of soft tissue masses of the abdominal wall.

Lipoma

Lipomas are benign fatty tumors and are among the most common benign masses of the abdominal wall and subcutaneous tissues. They can be found anywhere fat is present.[54] Lipomas are often surgically removed for cosmetic reasons, because they can grow to be very large. Lipomas are removed via surgical excision or liposuction, depending on their size.

Lipomas are usually hyperechoic to isoechoic to subcutaneous tissue and can be difficult to separate from adipose tissue if located superficially; most have a thin fibrous capsule defining the mass.[54] Unlike other solid masses, lipomas usually present with good through-transmission. They tend to be soft; compressible; and, in some cases, movable. Transducer pressure must be moderate and consistent to prevent displacement of the mass during scanning (Fig. 4-20). If a suspected lipoma presents with an atypical sonographic appearance, recommended follow-up includes further diagnostic testing and MR imaging. Lipomas are most often found in the subcutaneous tissues but sometimes are located in the peritoneal cavity, arising from the mesentery, omentum, or, rarely, the parietal peritoneum. Occasionally, a lipoma will torse around its pedicle, causing severe pain. The sonographer should be diligent in evaluating the superficial area as well as deeper structures in cases of acute-onset abdominal pain to be alert to the possible event of a torsed lipoma.[55,56]

Desmoid Tumors

Desmoid tumors may also be known as aggressive fibromatosis, desmoid-type fibromatosis, or deep musculoaponeurotic fibromatosis.[57] They are generally benign fibrous tissue neoplasms, which arise from muscle, fascia, or aponeuroses, and are commonly found in the anterior abdominal wall. They are also found in intra-abdominal and extra-abdominal (limbs, neck, thorax) locations; however, regardless of their location, the pathology is the same. The tumor is most frequently found in patients between the ages of 25 and 40 years.[57,58] Although these tumors can occur in either sex, they are more frequent in women and are often related to pregnancy. Childbirth, trauma, or hormonal changes during pregnancy are thought to be predisposing factors.[57] There is also a marked increase in desmoid tumors in patients with Gardner syndrome (familial polyposis syndrome). They are also often related to previous abdominal surgery. The vast majority of desmoid tumors are sporadic, with only 7.5% to 16% being hereditary related to Gardner syndrome; however, the hereditary type occurs more often in the abdomen and abdominal wall.[57,58]

Desmoid tumors often present as nontender, benign masses but can be infiltrating aggressive tumors that destroy adjacent structures.[58] Active surveillance with multiple imaging modalities has become the preferred first-line treatment over surgery owing to the incidence of spontaneous regression and a high recurrence after surgical intervention. Current guidelines advise surgery only when required to manage patient symptoms or when the tumor is aggressive.[57,59] Recurrence treatment includes radiation therapy, nonsteroidal anti-inflammatory drugs (NSAIDs), hormones, interferon, and chemotherapy, each of which has associated complications. Recently, high-intensity focused ultrasound (HIFU) has been utilized to ablate recurrent desmoid tumors with promising success and fewer side effects than systemic treatments.[57,60] Spontaneous regression of desmoid tumors has been recorded; the estimated recurrence rate is 20% to 60% depending on the location, size, and margin excision of the tumor.[54,58]

Sonographically, desmoid tumors are relatively homogeneous, hypoechoic-to-isoechoic masses with only occasional internal hyperechoic characteristics. Because they often

exhibit posterior enhancement, the sonographer must use strict criteria for a cystic mass so as not to mistake the tumor for a cyst. Size and margins are critical because of the capability for extension into other tissues. The tumor should be evaluated with color Doppler imaging as color flow may be seen within the tumor and is associated with the more aggressive forms of desmoid tumor.[57,58] Some desmoid tumors appear to be encapsulated sonographically, yet pathologic examination reveals no apparent capsule (Fig. 4-21A, B).

Neuromas

Neuromas are most commonly found postinjury, normally after surgery when a nerve gets damaged and swelling occurs. Neuromas occur at the end of a severed nerve and are found in 37% of posthernia repair patients. The most common symptom is pain in the region with or without palpable nodule.[54]

Sonographically, a neuroma is usually solitary, hypoechoic, and may or may not have enhancement. A neuroma does not demonstrate a specific blood flow pattern. It is important to assess patients with previous abdominal surgery for a neuroma when no other cause for pain can be found.[61,62]

Endometrioma

An endometrioma of the abdominal wall is typically found postoperatively and usually occurs after cesarean sections, laparotomies, or laparoscopies. Rarely, they are spontaneous and not associated with previous surgical procedure. The mass may be painful, and the pain may or may not be related to the patient's menstrual cycle. Subcutaneous endometriosis of the abdominal wall results in a palpable mass whereas lesions located within the muscles of the abdominal wall may not.[7,51,54,63,64]

Abdominal wall endometrioma most presents sonographically as a nodular hypoechoic or mixed (complex) mass that often displays vascularity with color or power Doppler imaging. Endometriomas may have a spiculated appearance, indicating infiltration of surrounding tissues.[64,65] It is imperative that the sonographer do a thorough evaluation of the endometrioma for evidence of infiltration into the abdominal fascia, document the lesion's depth from the skin surface, and measure it as accurately as possible.[63,64] Elastography of abdominal wall endometrioma has recently been shown to provide valuable information because there is a fibrotic component in endometrial tissue as well as the cells associated with the inflammatory response to functional endometrium in ectopic locations. This can be especially helpful when the endometrioma is isoechoic to surrounding tissues.[64]

The greatest risk for abdominal wall endometrioma is history of C-section.[64] The condition has been found in women with no previous history of endometriosis.[66] Approximately 7% to 10% of women in the general population have endometriosis.[64] The relationship between history of c-section and abdominal wall endometrioma has been postulated to be a combination of iatrogenic seeding of endometrial cells into the wound and the flow of endometrial cells into the peritoneal cavity with amniotic fluid during the procedure.[62,64,65]

Sarcoma

Sarcomas arising from the abdominal wall include liposarcoma, rhabdomyosarcoma, and fibrosarcoma; there is also

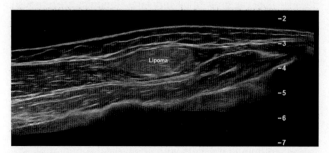

FIGURE 4-20 Lipoma. A longitudinal image presents a superficially located, well-defined, and hyperechoic area relative to the adjacent musculature lipoma. The intramuscular lipoma can be distinguished from the subcutaneous fat. (Image courtesy of Philips Medical Systems, Bothell, WA.)

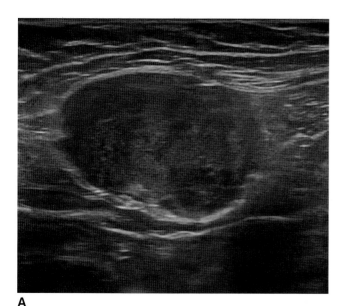

A

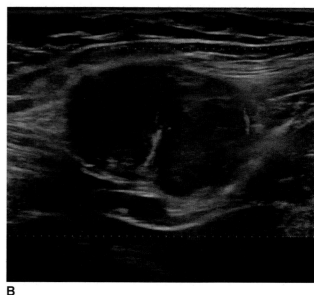

B

FIGURE 4-21 **A:** Desmoid fibromatosis located within the abdominal wall. **B:** Demonstration of color flow within the desmoid tumor that may suggest the tumor has an aggressive nature. (Images courtesy of Dr. Taco Geertsma, Hospital Gelderse Vallei, Ede, The Netherlands.)

an increasing incidence of endometriomas transforming into sarcomas.[67] These tumors can become quite large before producing symptoms. As a result, they often may be difficult to differentiate from large pancreatic tumors, renal tumors, or splenomegaly.[48,67] The sarcoma family of histiocytoma, osteosarcoma, angiosarcoma, fibrosarcoma, and a few rhabdomyosarcomas are seen in 0.03% to 8% of patients with history of receiving radiation therapy. There is a high incidence of recurrence with sarcomas. Postexcision radiation therapy is often required to aid in lowering the recurrence.[7,68]

Sonographically, soft tissue sarcomas are hypoechoic or isoechoic in comparison to the surrounding muscle. Sonography can be used to locate and identify the mass, but MR imaging is usually performed to determine its size, shape, and if there is involvement with surrounding tissues (Fig. 4-22A–C).

Metastatic Carcinoma

Metastatic carcinoma to the abdominal wall is frequently related to extension from a nearby primary carcinoma. For instance, in cases of primary ovarian carcinoma, there is a high incidence of clinically unsuspected metastases to the aortic and pelvic lymph nodes, diaphragm, peritoneum, and omentum. The abdominal wall may also be the site of distant metastases as a result of tracking during laparoscopic procedures. Endometrial sarcomas have been found in the abdominal wall, when this cancer is rare without a primary uterine cancer. It has been found in posthysterectomy patients; the cancer appears to be the result of malignant transformation of abdominal wall endometrioma.[67] Note that superficial cutaneous melanomas (occult or recurrent) and pigmented nevi, which are clearly demarcated from normal skin, rarely occur in the anterior abdominal wall. Quite often, they are found subcutaneously. Metastasis may occur as an isolated finding, but more often it is seen in patients with widespread metastatic disease elsewhere. All aggressive neoplasms should be resected with a clear margin to aid in lower recurrence rates.[69,70]

The broad spectrum of sonographic patterns seen in both primary and metastatic carcinomas makes it imperative that sonographers take time to observe the boundaries of the mass and whether it invades adjacent structures. The sonographer should add color or power Doppler imaging to evaluate for increased vascularity. Elastography can also be highly valuable when evaluating solid tumors. If at all possible, the sonographer should try to relate the abdominal wall mass to its primary source.

Some malignant masses are anechoic, with their deposits or extensions appearing very hyperechoic in contrast. Some are well circumscribed, whereas others are spiculated. When imaging a solid-appearing mass, the sonographer must use color Doppler, because malignant neoplasms will demonstrate increased vascularity at the wall periphery and internal vascularity of the mass.[71] Elastography can also help delineate the mass from normal, surrounding tissue. Melanomas typically appear to be hypoechoic and may demonstrate posterior enhancement. Other masses, particularly rhabdomyosarcomas, are hyperechoic. Tissue necrosis can produce echo-free areas within such masses, giving them a complex or mixed appearance. When scanning, the sonographer should vary the gain, make slight changes in the transducer angle, and be alert to the subtlest changes (Fig. 4-23A–C).

DIAPHRAGMATIC PATHOLOGY

The diaphragm is formed around the 4th to 12th week of gestation. It is formed by muscular fibers and is the division between the thoracic and abdominopelvic cavities. It is in these weeks that the diaphragm may not attach appropriately, causing pain, paralysis, herniation, eventration, and peridiaphragmatic abnormalities.[72] Often, pleural effusions are seen adjacent to the diaphragm. Sonography has replaced fluoroscopy as the method of choice for studying diaphragmatic motion because of its ability to examine patients without the need for radiation and can easily be performed at bedside.

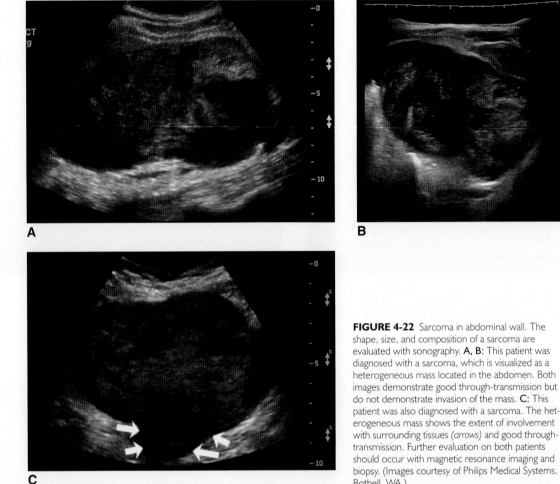

FIGURE 4-22 Sarcoma in abdominal wall. The shape, size, and composition of a sarcoma are evaluated with sonography. **A, B:** This patient was diagnosed with a sarcoma, which is visualized as a heterogeneous mass located in the abdomen. Both images demonstrate good through-transmission but do not demonstrate invasion of the mass. **C:** This patient was also diagnosed with a sarcoma. The heterogeneous mass shows the extent of involvement with surrounding tissues *(arrows)* and good through-transmission. Further evaluation on both patients should occur with magnetic resonance imaging and biopsy. (Images courtesy of Philips Medical Systems, Bothell, WA.)

M-mode is used to demonstrate diaphragmatic motion and can be performed serially to evaluate the status of diaphragmatic paralysis or dysfunction (Fig. 4-24A, B). One can also infer information about the duration of diaphragmatic paralysis by evaluating the thickness of the intercostal muscles on the affected side compared with the unaffected side. Although it was initially used primarily to evaluate pediatric patients with diaphragmatic dysfunction, sonographic evaluation of the diaphragm is gaining momentum as a valuable tool in the evaluation of diaphragmatic dysfunction in mechanically ventilated patients as well as in patients with prolonged shortness of breath following COVID-19 infection.[73,74] Evaluation of diaphragmatic excursion with M-mode and measurement of diaphragmatic thickness upon maximum expiration provide important information that can be used to predict the likelihood of successful weaning of patients from mechanical ventilation and can be used to help determine when to place COVID-19 patients on mechanical ventilation. It is also used to monitor patients who experience prolonged shortness of breath and fatigue as they recover from COVID-19 infection.[73,74]

The presence of fluid adjacent to the diaphragm (pleural effusion or ascites) prominently displays the central diaphragmatic tendon as a thin, linear echo covering the dome of the liver. Peripheral muscle insertions may also be seen posteriorly (sagittal scan) and posterolaterally (transverse scan) as thick, triangle-shaped, hypoechoic bands. The presence of gas in the stomach and bowel can make the left hemidiaphragm more difficult to scan than the right. However, patient exploration of multiple sonographic windows can usually provide access for images of diagnostic quality.

Pleural Effusions

Pleural effusion, also known as hydrothorax, is an accumulation of fluid within the pleural cavity. There are over a million people with pleural effusions each year, and there are many different causes. The most common causes are cancer, heart failure, pneumonia, and pulmonary embolism.[75]

Sonographic imaging for pleural effusions has increased detection from 47% to 93%. Sonography can visualize pleural fluid when there is only 5 to 20 mL of fluid compared with the 200 cc required for visualization with chest radiography. Sonographic guidance for thoracentesis has also decreased the pneumothorax rate to a low 3% as compared with 18% when performed with clinical guidance alone. Sonography can be performed at the bedside and in the emergency room without moving the patient to another department, saving time and money. Advocates for thoracic sonography feel that pathology is easily detected and that pleural effusions are better quantified if the patient is scanned in a sitting position.

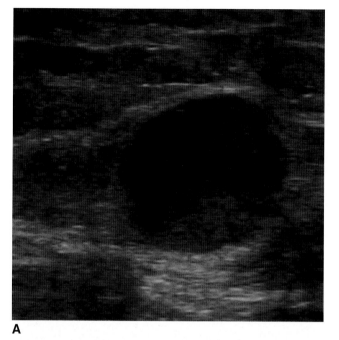

A

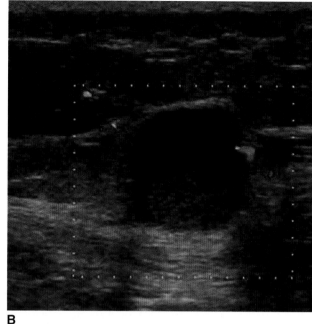

B

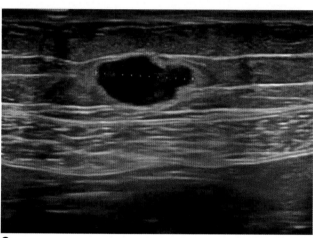

C

FIGURE 4-23 A: A cystic lesion containing a solid mass within the abdominal wall that biopsy proved to be metastasis of an endometrial carcinoma. B: Color Doppler demonstrating blood flow within the periphery of the mass. C: A hypoechoic mass within the abdominal wall that biopsy proved to be metastasis of a melanoma. (Images courtesy of Dr. Taco Geertsma, Hospital Gelderse Vallei, Ede, The Netherlands.)

Thoracic sonography has increased the detection of pleural effusion, greatly reducing the underestimation associated with chest radiography.[76-79] A high-frequency linear probe should be the first modality of choice to perform thoracic sonography so that detailed sonographic features can be better visualized to determine whether the effusion is simple or complex with/without septations.[79,80] In the critical care setting using sonography for thoracic pathology from trauma, sonography has been reported to have 92% to 100% sensitivity and specificity greater than chest radiography, which has a sensitivity and specificity of 39% to 81%. Sonography has been established as the best method for detecting pleural effusions.[77-80]

Sonographically, pleural effusion has four typical appearances: (1) of echo-free or anechoic areas on one or both sides of the chest superior to the diaphragm, (2) complex nonseptated fluid, (3) complex septations seen within fluid collection, and (4) hyperechoic.[77,80] The lung, compressed by the fluid, does not change shape and the diaphragm appears as a hyperechoic band. Depending on effusion extent, often part of the lung can be seen floating in the effusion (Fig. 4-25A–C). Thoracentesis is frequently done under sonographic guidance because of the ability to visualize the anatomy in real time; it also improves fluid collection and decreases the rate of complications like pneumothorax or hemothorax.[77,79,80] Sonography-guided thoracentesis has become the gold standard and is considered the best practice.[77]

Paralysis

Sonography is of particular investigative value when a chest radiograph demonstrates an elevated or obscured hemidiaphragm. Diaphragmatic paralysis can be unilateral or bilateral, is caused by a damaged phrenic nerve, and can be detected by showing absent or paradoxical motion on the affected side compared with a normal or exaggerated excursion on the opposite side.[30,81] It can occur in patients with arthritis of the neck owing to extrinsic compression of the phrenic nerve. Recovery from infectious or traumatic

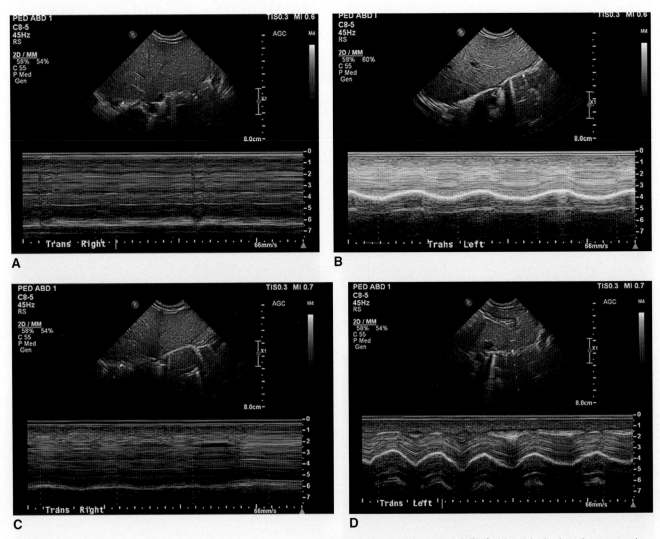

FIGURE 4-24 A–D: M-mode of the diaphragm depicting paralysis on the right (**A**) with normal motion on the left (**B**). Serial examination later demonstrates improved motion in the right hemidiaphragm (**C**). The appearance of the left diaphragm (**D**) shows an artifact resulting from the diaphragm moving in and out of the M-mode sample area with lung artifact obscuring part of the diaphragmatic motion. (Images courtesy of Madeline Soderstrom.)

paralysis takes an extended time and occurs in two out of three patients. Paralysis owing to surgical trauma may have a shorter recovery time. Diaphragmatic paralysis can be demonstrated by minimal or no thickening of the hemidiaphragm during inspiration, whereas thickening of the diaphragm demonstrates diaphragmatic shortening. The normal excursion of the diaphragm is easily visualized with sonography and documented with M-mode. Measuring the diaphragmatic thickness in the zone of apposition can show paralysis of one side of the diaphragm. This is an easy, noninvasive method of assessing diaphragmatic function.[81] Unlike fluoroscopy, sonography can easily demonstrate the diaphragm even in the presence of peridiaphragmatic masses or fluid collections, and can be used to monitor the recovery of the diaphragm.[72]

Eventration

Congenital eventration appears as an abnormal bulge or pouch in the diaphragmatic contour that moves normally with respiration. It is visualized as an abnormal elevation of the hemidiaphragm, typically on the right. The liver typically maintains its association with the diaphragmatic surface even when eventration is present unless ascites is present, in which case, fluid may be seen filling the pouch separating the liver from the diaphragm.

Eventration is the abnormal elevation of the diaphragm owing to focal thinning of the muscle fibers that fail to develop appropriately during gestation or is acquired in adulthood as a complication of other diaphragmatic issues such as paralysis or muscular atrophy.[81,82] In the presence of eventration, the diaphragm can give way, progressing to diaphragmatic hernia when abdominal organs protrude through a weakened section. Left diaphragmatic hernias are easier to image than right diaphragmatic hernias, owing to the echogenicity of the liver versus the fluid-filled stomach.[72,81] Congenital eventration results from incomplete muscularization of the membranous diaphragm. Acquired eventration is related to muscular weakness resulting most often from phrenic nerve injury but can also be caused by

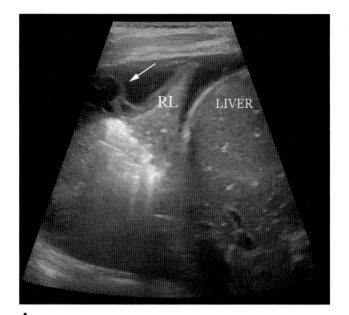

A

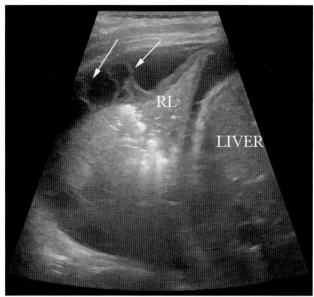

B

C

FIGURE 4-25 Complex pleural effusion. **A, B:** The sonographic chest evaluation from the right posterior surface is performed on a pediatric patient with a history of pneumonia. The sonogram reveals a loculated pleural effusion with thick adhesions *(arrows)* seen superior to the right lobe of the liver. The right lung *(RL)* is seen as well. The adhesions can make thoracentesis more difficult, but sonography can help guide the procedure. **C:** Sonographic evaluation from the coronal right chest in a different pediatric patient demonstrates a complex pleural effusion *(PE)* superior to the right lobe of the liver. The right lung *(RL)* is also visualized.

focal ischemia or infarct. This condition accounts for 5% of all diaphragmatic defects.[72,81,82]

Diaphragmatic eventration may be partial (segmental) or complete (total), unilateral or bilateral. With segmental eventration, the anterior portion of the right hemidiaphragm is most often affected. Congenital eventration is most often this type. Extensive eventration or hernias of the diaphragm are linked to neonatal morbidity and mortality because of impaired lung development owing to reduced space in the thoracic cavity.[72,81,82] Congenital eventration has been linked to many causes, including intrauterine infections and traumatic birth injuries. Acquired eventration can result from surgical intervention of the chest, thermal injuries, and syndromes such as Guillain–Barré.[81,82] Unilateral eventration may be associated with rib anomalies, whereas bilateral eventration is often associated with trisomy 13–15 and 18 and with Beckwith–Wiedemann syndrome. Diaphragmatic eventration has the same effect as diaphragmatic paralysis

in that it limits movement of the diaphragm and inhibits ventilation.[72,82]

Hernia

Diaphragmatic hernias may be either congenital or acquired. Congenital diaphragmatic hernia affects 1 in 2,500 to 5,000 live births and results from diaphragmatic fusion failure, maldevelopment, or localized weakness.[72,83,84] Approximately 40% of affected infants also have other genetic or structural abnormalities and with up to 30% mortality rate.[72,84,85] Acquired diaphragmatic hernias may also develop following surgery, other trauma, or increased intrathoracic or intra-abdominal pressure. Acquired diaphragmatic hernias are often small and difficult to detect sonographically.[86] Diaphragmatic hernias allow abdominal contents to enter the thorax, and approximately 85% of diaphragmatic hernias are through the left posterior lateral diaphragm. This allows stomach,

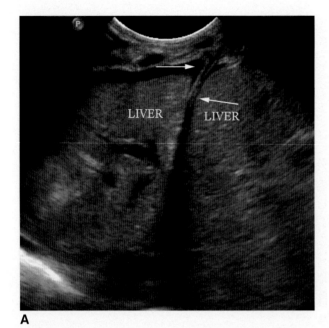

A

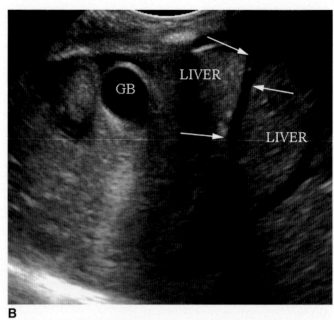

B

FIGURE 4-26 Diaphragmatic hernia. **A:** The sonographic evaluation on a prenatal patient reveals a diaphragmatic hernia. The liver is seen on both sides of the diaphragm (*arrows*). **B:** The gallbladder (*GB*) is also seen superior to the diaphragm. (Images courtesy of Dr. Nakul Jerath, Falls Church, VA.)

small bowel, and even spleen to enter the thorax, sometimes shifting the mediastinum and heart.[72,83,84]

The normal fetal diaphragm appears as a thin, hypoechoic band separating the thorax from the abdomen. With congenital diaphragmatic hernia of the left side, sonography may show the presence of a fluid-filled stomach or bowel in the lower thorax, displacing the fetal heart anteriorly or to the right.[72] When the hernia occurs on the right, the liver, or bowel, will be seen within the chest cavity, and the stomach will be below the diaphragm (Fig. 4-26A, B). In adults, the esophagus, and perhaps part of the stomach, may be seen within the chest cavity on the left.[86]

Sonographic imaging to determine fetal survival rate can use volumetric measurements of the lung-to-head ratio using 3D sonography. The lung measurements are obtained in cross-sectional images of the head and four-chamber view of the heart. Fetal lung vasculature has also been suggested as an assessment into the fetal outcome. Right fetal diaphragmatic hernias generally have a poorer outcome than left fetal diaphragmatic hernias. Up to 25% of congenital diaphragmatic hernias are not detected on prenatal sonography. Neonatal lung ultrasound is proving of great value in evaluation of congenital diaphragmatic hernia.[72,83,84]

Inversion

Diaphragmatic inversion, often associated with pleural effusion, presents as the diaphragm curving in a convex manner toward the abdomen, with the center of the diaphragm bulging inferiorly. It is often accompanied by asynchronous motion between the right and left hemidiaphragm. Inversion is a result of increased pressure in the pleural cavity which impairs diaphragmatic motion.[87,88]

Rupture

Penetrating injuries or blunt trauma may produce rupture of the diaphragm. With blunt thoracoabdominal trauma, 7% of patients have diaphragmatic rupture after a traumatic injury and up to 15% with a lower chest injury.[89] In rare instances, rupture may occur secondary to severe infection (e.g., amebiasis), vaginal childbirth, physical exercise, defecation, or violent coughing.[90]

Posttraumatic diaphragmatic rupture requires surgical closure. The preoperative diagnosis of diaphragmatic rupture is difficult to make when multiple injuries and other life-threatening conditions exist simultaneously. Its presence may first be suggested by imaging studies such as chest radiography, peritoneal lavage, sonography, scintigraphy, CT, and MR. Any delay in making the diagnosis increases the chances of intestinal strangulation and emergent surgery with added morbidity and mortality of up to 25%.[89,91]

The disruption of diaphragmatic echoes and visualization of herniated abdominal viscera are the sonographic signs of diaphragmatic rupture. Extensive (< 10 cm long) ruptures have also been reported.[91]

Neoplasms

The most common benign tumor of the diaphragm is the lipoma. Although an uncommon site for neoplastic disease, tumors of the diaphragm can be either primary or secondary. The most common malignant primary neoplasm is the fibrosarcoma or undifferentiated sarcoma.[72,92] Secondary involvement usually occurs with local invasion by adjacent pleural, peritoneal, or thoracic and abdominal wall malignancies.[92]

Disruption or interruption of the diaphragm at the site of metastatic implants can be visualized sonographically. The mass is usually heterogeneous, occasionally with cystic areas and possible extension into contiguous organs.[93,94]

SUMMARY

- Anterior abdominal wall extends from the xyphoid process to the symphysis pubis and is made up of the skin layer, the subcutaneous layer, and a musculofascial layer.
- Anterolateral abdominal wall is made up of the rectus abdominis, transverse, internal oblique, and external oblique muscles.
- Sonography should be the first modality of choice for imaging abdominal wall and diaphragm because it is a fast, widely available, inexpensive, and noninvasive method of imaging.
- The abdominal wall and membranous lining are affected by inflammatory, traumatic, and neoplastic changes.
- Inflammatory response can occur whenever bacterial infection damages the skin and underlying tissues.
- Four main indications of inflammatory response are heat, redness, pain, and swelling.
- Sonographically, an abscess can appear anechoic or have internal echoes; may be irregular or smooth bordered; and if the abscess contains gas, it may be echogenic with shadowing.
- Hematomas can be postsurgical or associated with trauma.
- Hematomas of the anterior abdominal wall can also involve the lateral or retroperitoneal muscles.
- The sonographic appearance of a hematoma varies with the stage of resolution, but it varies from hypoechoic to echogenic.
- A seroma is a collection of serum in the tissue resulting from a surgical incision or from the liquefaction of a hematoma and can range from anechoic to hypoechoic.

- A hernia occurs when the abdominal wall muscles are weak and the viscera lying beneath protrude.
- Strangulation (compromised blood supply causing ischemia) and incarceration, which means the hernia is nonreducible, are the two types of complications that may occur with midline hernias.
- Hernias are normally classified as ventral or groin and include umbilical, inguinal, femoral, epigastric, and spigelian hernia.
- Inguinal hernias make up 75% of all hernias and can be either direct or indirect, depending on route to the inguinal canal.
- Sonographic criteria for abdominal wall hernia include demonstration of an abdominal wall defect, presence of bowel in the lesion, exaggeration of the lesion on straining of the abdominal muscles, and reducibility of the lesion with pressure.
- Neoplasms of the abdominal wall include lipomas, desmoid tumors, sarcomas, and metastatic tumors.
- Metastatic carcinoma to the abdominal wall is frequently related to extension from a nearby primary carcinoma.
- Primary and metastatic carcinomas present a broad spectrum of sonographic patterns, meaning the sonographers should take care to (1) evaluate the boundaries of the mass and if it invades adjacent structures; (2) add color or power Doppler to evaluate vascularity; and (3) use elastography when evaluating solid tumors.
- Sonography can be used to visualize diaphragmatic paralysis, diaphragmatic hernia, inversion or rupture of the diaphragm, diaphragmatic neoplasms, and pleural effusion.

REFERENCES

1. Izadifar Z, Babyn P, Chapman D. Mechanical and biological effects of ultrasound: a review of present knowledge. *Ultrasound Med Biol.* 2017;43(6):1085–1104.
2. American Institute of Ultrasound in Medicine. Prudent clinical use and safety of diagnostic ultrasound. AIUM. AIUM Official Statements Web site. Published 2019. Accessed May 7, 2021.
3. Sefton EM, Gallardo M, Kardon G. Developmental origin and morphogenesis of the diaphragm, an essential mammalian muscle. *Dev Biol.* 2018;440(2):64–73.
4. Moore K, Dailey A, Agur A. *Clinically Oriented Anatomy.* 7th ed. Wolters Kluwer Health; 2014.
5. Cirocchi R, Boselli C, Renzi C, et al. The surface landmarks of the abdominal wall: a plea for standardization. *Arch Med Sci.* 2014;10(3):566–569.
6. Flynn W, Vickerton P. Anatomy, abdomen and pelvis, abdominal wall. In: *StatPearls.* StatPearls Publishing; 2021.
7. Mansoori B, Paspulati RM, Herrman KA. Mesentery, omentum, peritoneum: abdominal wall pathologies. In: Hamm B, Rose PR, eds. *Abdominal Imaging.* Springer-Verlag; 2013:1623–1635.
8. Kirchgesner T, Demondion X, Stoenoiu M, et al. Fasciae of the musculoskeletal system: normal anatomy and MR patterns of involvement in autoimmune diseases. *Insights Imaging.* 2018;9:761–771. doi:10.1007/s13244-018-0650-1
9. Cirocchi R, Cheruiyot I, Henry BM, et al. Anatomical variations of the pyramidalis muscle: a systematic review and meta-analysis. *Surg Radiol Anat.* 2021;43:595–605. doi:10.1007/s00276-020-02622-4
10. Mahadevan V. Anatomy of the anterior abdominal wall and groin. *Surgery.* 2012;30(6):257–260
11. Ellis H. Anatomy of the anterior abdominal wall and inguinal canal. *Anaesth Intens Care Med.* 2009;10(7):315–317.
12. Bains KNS, Kashyap S, Lappin SL. *Anatomy, Thorax, Diaphragm.* In: StatPearls, StatPearls Publishing; 2022. https://www.ncbi.nlm.nih.gov/books/NBK519558/
13. Kelley LL, Petersen CM. *Sectional Anatomy for Imaging Professionals.* 3rd ed. Elsevier; 2013.

14. Matalon S, Askari R, Gates JD, Patel K, Sodiskson AD, Khurana B. Don't forget the abdominal wall: imaging spectrum of abdominal wall injuries after nonpenetrating trauma. *Radiographics.* 2017;37:1218–1235. doi:10.1148/rg.2017160098
15. Jain N, Goyal N, Mukherjee K, Kamath S. Ultrasound of the abdominal wall: what lies beneath? *Clin Radiol.* 2013;68:85–93.
16. Nyhsen CM, Humphreys H, Koerner RJ, et al. Infection prevention and control in ultrasound—best practice recommendations from the European Society of Radiology Ultrasound Working Group. *Insights Imaging.* 2017;8(6):523–535. doi:10.1007/s13244-017-0580-3
17. The AIUM practice parameter for the performance of an ultrasound examination of the abdomen and/or retroperitoneum. *J Ultrasound Med.* 2022;41:E1–E8. doi:10.1002/jum.15874
18. Ray S, Kumar D, Garai D, Khamrui S. Dropped gallstone-related right subhepatic and parietal wall abscess: a rare complication after laparoscopic cholecystectomy. *ACG Case Rep J.* 2021;8(5):e00579. doi:10.14309/crj.0000000000000579
19. Sibomana I, Ishimwe M, Maniriho B, Nyampinga C, Ruhangaza D, Gahemba I. Actinomycetoma of the colon presenting as abdominal wall abscess. Case report and review of the literature. *Int J Surg Case Rep.* 2021;80:1–3. doi:10.1016/j.ijscr.2021.105679
20. Mahajan PS, Kolleri J, Farghaly H. Rare case of primary anterior abdominal wall abscess: ultrasound, CT, and MRI features. *Cureus.* 2021;13(12):e20618. doi:10.7759/cureus.20618
21. Rote NS. Innate immunity: inflammation and wound healing. In: Huether SE, McCance KL, eds. *Understanding Pathophysiology.* 6th ed. Elsevier; 2017:134–157.
22. Thorton J, Hellmich T. Current management of abscesses. AHC Media. 2016;3/19–14/19.
23. Vasileios R, Anna G, Christos L, et al. Abdominal wall abscess due to acute perforated sigmoid diverticulitis: a case report with MDCT and US findings. *Case Rep Radiol.* 2013;2013:565928. doi:10.1155/2013/565928
24. AIUM practice parameter for the performance of selected ultrasound-guided procedures. *J Ultrasound Med.* 2016;35:1–40. doi:10.7863/jum.2016.35.9.5

25. Chhikara A, Chawla S, Singh G, et al. Traumatic rectus sheath haematoma. *Int J Sci Res.* 2016;5:45–46.

26. Ferrier J, Kingston K. The role of ultrasound in the differential diagnosis of palpable abdominal wall lesions. Poster presented at: British Medical Ultrasound Society; September 2020.

27. Picasso R, Pistoia F, Zaottini F, et al. High-resolution ultrasound of spigelian and groin hernias: a closer look at fascial architecture and aponeurotic passageways. *J Ultrason.* 2021;21(84):53–62. doi:10.15557/JoU.2021.0008

28. Dessy LA, Mazzoccih M, Fallico N, Anniboletti T, Scuderi N. Associate between abdominal separation and inguinal or crural hernias: our experience and surgical indications. *J Plast Surg Hand Surg.* 2013;47:209–212.

29. Hernandez-Gascon B, Mena A, Pena E, Pascual G, Bellón JM, Calvo B. Understanding the passive mechanical behavior of the human abdominal wall. *Ann Biomed Eng.* 2013;41(2):433–444.

30. Stavros AT, Rapp CT. Dynamic ultrasound of hernias of the groin and anterior abdominal wall. In: Rumack CM, Wilson SR, Charbonneau JW, et al, eds. *Diagnostic Ultrasound.* Vol 1. 4th ed. Elsevier Mosby; 2011:486–523.

31. Pawlak M, Bury K, Smietanski M. The management of abdominal wall hernias—in search of consensus. *Videosurg Miniinv.* 2015;10(1):49–56.

32. Latifi R. Practical approaches to definitive reconstruction of complex abdominal wall defects. *World J Surg.* 2016;40:836–848.

33. Burcharth J, Pedersen MS, Pommergaard HC, Bisgaard T, Pedersen CB, Rosenberg J. The prevalence of umbilical and epigastric hernia repair: a nationwide epidemiologic study. *Hernia.* 2015;19:815–819.

34. Murphy KP, O'Connor OJ, Maher MM. Adult abdominal hernias. *AJR Am J Roentgenol.* 2014;202:506–511.

35. Rankin A, Kostusiak M, Sokker A. Spigelian hernia: case series and review of the literature. *Visc Med.* 2019;35:133–136. doi:10.1159/000494280

36. Srivastava KN, Agarwal A. Spigelian hernia: a diagnostic dilemma and laparoscopic management. *Indian J Surg.* 2015;77(suppl 1):35–37. doi:10.1007/s12262-014-1085-7

37. Balsara ZR, Martin AE, Wiener JS, Routh JC, Ross SS. Congenital spigelian hernia and ipsilateral cryptorchidism: raising awareness among urologists. *J Urol.* 2014;83:457–459.

38. Hamid YI, Khattab EM, Abdel A, Isamail A, Baioumy S. Evaluation high-resolution sonography and colour Doppler in assessment of complicated anterior abdominal wall hernia. *Eur J Mol Clin Med.* 2021;8(3):4087–4096.

39. Beck WC, Holzman MD, Sharp KW, Nealon WH, Dupont WD, Poulose BK. Comparative effectiveness of dynamic abdominal sonography for hernia vs computed tomography in the diagnosis of incisional hernia. *J Am Coll Surg.* 2013;216(3):447–453.

40. Khreiss W, Shah AA, Sarr MG. Prevascular hernias of the abdominal wall: a difficult problem, a difficult repair. *Hernia.* 2015;19:517–521.

41. Fitzgibbons RJ Jr, Forse RA. Groin hernias in adults. *N Engl J Med.* 2015;372(8):756–763.

42. Jorgenson E, Makki N, Shen L, et al. A genome-wide association study identifies four novel susceptibility loci underlying inguinal hernia. *Nat Commun.* 2015;6:10130.

43. Hammoud M, Gerken J. Inguinal hernia. In: *StatPearls* [Internet]. StatPearls Publishing; 2022. https://www.ncbi.nlm.nih.gov/books/NBK513332/

44. Wu J, Wang Y, Yu J, Chen Y, Pang Y. A fast detection and diagnosis algorithm for abdominal incisional hernia masses with automated 3D ultrasound images. Presented at: 2013 6th International Conference on Biomedical Engineering and Informatics; 2013:86–90.

45. Arend CF. Static and dynamic sonography for diagnosis of abdominal wall hernias. *J Ultrasound Med.* 2013;32:1251–1259.

46. Yildirim D, Ekci B, Gurses B, Sahin M, Gumus T. Dynamic power Doppler ultrasonography of anterior abdominal wall hernias: confirmation of incarceration. *J Med Ultrason.* 2013;40:33–38.

47. Jamadar DA, Jacobson JA, Morag Y, et al. Sonography of inguinal region hernias. *Am J Roentgenol.* 2006;187(1):185–190.

48. Ballard DH, Mazaheri P, Oppenheimer DC, et al. Imaging of abdominal wall masses, masslike lesions, and diffuse processes. *Radiographics.* 2020;40(3):684–706.

49. Wagner JM, Rebik K, Spicer PJ. Ultrasound of soft tissue masses and fluid collections. *Radiol Clin North Am.* 2019;57(3):657–669.

50. Lai YL, Hsu HC, Kuo KT, Chen YL, Chen CA, Cheng WF. Clear cell carcinoma of the abdominal wall as a rare complication of general obstetric and gynecologic surgeries: 15 years of experience at a large academic institution. *Int J Environ Res Public Health.* 2019;16(4):552. doi:10.3390/ijerph16040552

51. Usta TA, Sonmez SE, Oztarhan A, Karacan T. Endometrial stromal sarcoma in the abdominal wall arising from scar endometriosis. *J Obstet Gynaecol.* 2014;34(6):541–542.

52. Ijichi S, Mori T, Suganuma I, et al. Clear cell carcinoma arising from cesarean section scar endometriosis: case report and review of literature. *Case Rep Obstet Gynecol.* 2014;2014:642483. doi:10.1155/2014/642483

53. Duymus ME, Opci I. Squamous-cell carcinoma due to mesh infection after umbilical hernia operation: third case of the literature. *Scott Med J.* 2021;66(3):158–161.

54. Bashir U, Moskovic E, Strauss D, et al. Soft-tissue masses in the abdominal wall. *Clin Radiol.* 2014;69:e422–e431.

55. Choi H, Ryu D, Choi JW, et al. A giant lipoma of the parietal peritoneum: laparoscopic excision with the parietal peritoneum preserving procedure—a case report with literature review. *BMC Surg.* 2018;18:49. doi:10.1186/s12893-018-0382-7

56. Sathyakrishna BR, Boggaram SG, Jannu NR. Twisting lipoma presenting as appendicitis—a rare presentation. *J Clin Diagn Res.* 2014;8(8):7–8.

57. Mastoraki A, Schizas D, Vassiliu S, et al. Evaluation of diagnostic algorithm and therapeutic interventions for intra-abdominal desmoid tumors. *Surg Oncol.* 2022;41:101724.

58. Lou L, Teng J, Qi H, Ban Y. Sonographic appearances of desmoid tumors. *J Ultrasound Med.* 2014;33:1519–1525.

59. Kasper B, Baumgarten C, Garcia J, et al. An update on the management of sporadic desmoid-type fibromatosis: a European consensus initiative between sarcoma PAtients EuroNet (SPAEN) and European organization for research and treatment of cancer (EORTC)/Soft tissue and bone sarcoma group (STBSG). *Ann Oncol.* 2017;28:2399–2408.

60. Mo S, Chen J, Zhang R, et al. High-intensity focused ultrasound ablation for postoperative recurrent desmoid tumors: preliminary results. *Ultrasound Med Biol.* 2022;48(4):638–645.

61. O'Reilly MAR, O'Reilly PMR, Sheahan JN, Sullivan J, O'Reilly HM, O'Reilly MJ. Neuromas as the cause of pain in the residual limbs of amputees. An ultrasound study. *Clin Radiol.* 2016;71(10):1068.e1–1068.e6.

62. AlSharif S, Ferre R, Omeroglu A, El Khoury M, Mesurolle B. Imaging features associated with posttraumatic breast neuromas. *AJR Am J Roentgenol.* 2016;206:660–665.

63. Savelli L, Manuzzi L, DiDonato N, et al. Endometriosis of the abdominal wall: ultrasonographic and Doppler characteristics. *Ultrasound Obstet Gynecol.* 2012;39:336–340.

64. Cocco G, Delli Pizzi A, Scioscia M, et al. Ultrasound imaging of abdominal wall endometriosis: a pictorial review. *Diagnostics.* 2021;11(4):609. doi:10.3390/diagnostics11040609

65. Ecker AM, Donnellan NM, Shepherd JP, Lee TT. Abdominal wall endometriosis: 12 years of experience at a large academic institution. *Am J Obstet Gynecol.* 2014;210:1.e1–1.e5.

66. Ruiz MP, Wallace DL, Connell MT. Transformation of abdominal wall endometriosis to clear cell carcinoma. *Case Rep Obstet Gynecol.* 2015;2015:123740. doi:10.1155/2015/123740

67. Chen Z, Wu J, Liu X, et al. Low-grade endometrial stromal sarcoma in the abdominal wall: a metastatic or protopathic one? *Int J Clin Exp Path.* 2016;9:3593–3599.

68. Neuberg M, Mir O, Levy A, et al. Surgical management of soft tissue tumors of the abdominal wall: a retrospective study in a high-volume sarcoma center. *J Surg Oncol.* 2021;124:679–686. doi:10.1002/jso.26566

69. Yang F. Radical tumor excision and immediate abdominal wall reconstruction in patients with aggressive neoplasm compromised full-thickness lower abdominal wall. *Am J Surg.* 2013;205:15–21.

70. Gaopande VL, Joshi AR, Khandeparkar SGS, Deshmukh SD. Merkel cell carcinoma of the abdominal wall. *Indian Dermatol Online J.* 2015;6(4):269–273.

71. Chung EM, Biko DM, Arzamendi AM, Meldrum JT, Stocker JT. Solid tumors of the peritoneum, omentum, and mesentery in children: radiologic-pathologic correlation: from the radiologic pathology archives. *Radiographics.* 2015;35(3):1–25.

72. Alamo L, Gudinchet F, Meuli R. Imaging findings in fetal diaphragmatic abnormalities. *Pediatr Radiol.* 2015;45:1887–1900

73. Holtzhausen S, Unger M, Lupton-Smith A, Hanekom S. An investigation into the use of ultrasound as a surrogate measure of diaphragm function. *Heart Lung.* 2018;47(4):418–424.

74. Guarracino F, Vetrugno L, Forfori F, et al. Lung, heart, vascular, and diaphragm ultrasound examination of COVID-19 patients: a comprehensive approach. *J Cardiothorac Vasc Anesth.* 2021;35(6):1866–1874. doi:10.1053/j.jvca.2020.06.013

75. Jany B, Welte T. Pleural effusion in adults-etiology, diagnosis, and treatment. *Dtsch Arztebl Int.* 2019;116(21):377–386. doi:10.3238/arztebl.2019.0377

76. Ledwidge M. Rule out pleural effusion and chest mass. In: Sanders RC, Hall-Terracciano B, eds. *Clinical Sonography: A Practical Guide.* 5th ed. Lippincott Williams & Wilkins; 2016:704–712.

77. Sikora K, Perea P, Mailhot T, et al. Ultrasound for the detection of pleural effusions and guidance of the thoracentesis procedure. *ISRN Emerg Med.* 2012;2012:676524. doi:10.5402/2012/676524.

78. Schleder S, Dornia C, Poschenrieder F, et al. Bedside diagnosis of pleural effusion with a latest generation hand-carried ultrasound device in intensive care patients. *Acta Radiol.* 2012;53:556–560.

79. Prina E, Torres A, Carvalho CRR. Lung ultrasound in the evaluation of pleural effusion. *J Bras Pneumol.* 2014;40(1):1–5.

80. Heffner JE, Klein JS, Hampson C. Diagnostic utility and clinical application of imaging for pleural space infections. *Chest.* 2010;137(2):467–479.

81. Laghi FA, Saad M, Shaikh H. Ultrasound and non-ultrasound imaging techniques in the assessment of diaphragmatic dysfunction. *BMC Pulm Med.* 2021;21:85. doi:10.1186/s12890-021-01441-6

82. Hu J, Wu Y, Wang J, Zhang C, Pan W, Zhou Y. Thorascopic and laparoscopic plication of the hemidiaphragm is effective in the management of diaphragmatic eventration. *Pediatr Surg Int.* 2014;30:19–24.

83. Corsini I, Parri N, Coviello C, Leonardi V, Dani C. Lung ultrasound findings in congenital diaphragmatic hernia. *Eur J Pediatr.* 2019;178:491–495. doi:10.1007/s00431-019-03321-y

84. Nawapun K, Sandaite I, Dekonninck P, et al. Comparison of matching by body volume or gestational age for calculation of observed to expected total lung volume in fetuses with isolated congenital diaphragmatic hernia. *Ultrasound Obstet Gynecol.* 2014;44:655–660.

85. Zalla JM, Stoddard GJ, Yoder B. Improved mortality rate for congenital diaphragmatic hernia in the modern era of management: 15 year experience in a single institution. *J Pediatr Surg.* 2014;50:524–527. doi:10.1016/j.jpedsurg.2014.11.002

86. Revin RA, Shrikrishna U. Post-traumatic diaphragmatic hernia-delayed presentation with complications. *J Evol Med Dent Sci.* 2020;9(9):692–696. link.gale.com/apps/doc/A620338036/HRCA?u=anon~546ab849&sid=googleScholar&xid=4c5dc8b1

87. Patel K, Cheema TK, Singh A. Inverted diaphragm: more than just pleural effusion. *Am J Respir Crit Care Med.* 2018;197:A3228.

88. Hassan M, Mercer RM, Rahman NM. Thoracic ultrasound in the modern management of pleural disease. *Eur Respir Rev.* 2020;29:190136. doi:10.1183/16000617.0136-2019

89. Bhatia S, Kaushik R, Singh R, Sharma R. Traumatic diaphragmatic hernia. *Indian J Surg.* 2008;70:56–61.

90. Goyal VK, Solanki SL. Anesthetic management of a case of spontaneous rupture of diaphragm. *Saudi J Anaesth.* 2014;8(suppl 1):128–129.

91. Dwari AK, Mandal A, Das SK, et al. Delayed presentation of traumatic diaphragmatic rupture with herniation of the left kidney and bowel loops. *Case Rep Pulmonol.* 2013;2013:814632. doi:10.1155/2013/814632

92. Melis M, Rosen G, Hajdu CH, Pachter HL, Raccuia JS. Primary rhabdomyosarcoma of the diaphragm: case report and review of the literature. *J Gastrointest.* 2013;17:799–804.

93. Bothale KA, Mahore SD, Patrikar AD, Mitra K. A rare case of inflammatory myofibroblastoma of diaphragm. *Indian J Surg.* 2013;75(1):S243–S246.

94. Kumar VKDP, Shetty S, Saxena R. Primary hydatid cyst of the diaphragm mimicking diaphragmatic tumour: a case report. *J Clin Diagn Res.* 2015;9(8):1–5.

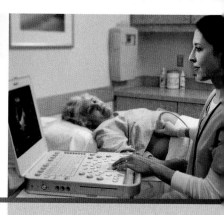

CHAPTER 5

The Peritoneal Cavity

JOIE BURNS

OBJECTIVES

- Identify the potential spaces of the peritoneum and the organs and/or ligaments that divide them on diagrams.
- Identify the potential spaces of the peritoneum on sonograms.
- State the organs located in the peritoneum.
- Describe the scanning techniques used to image the potential spaces and diseases of the peritoneum.
- Explain the role the greater omentum and mesentery play in limiting the extent of pathology.
- Recognize the sonographic appearance of benign and malignant changes seen in the peritoneum.
- Analyze sonographic images of the peritoneum for pathology.

GLOSSARY

abscess a pocket of infection typically containing pus, blood, and degenerating tissue

bare area surface area of a peritoneal organ devoid of peritoneum

biloma a collection of extravasated bile that can occur with trauma or rupture of the biliary tract

diverticulum a small pocket communicating with a larger cavity or tube

free fluid fluid outside of vessels, bowel, and organs, seen in the potential spaces

hematoma an extravasated collection of blood localized within a potential space or tissue

hemoperitoneum extravasated blood within the peritoneal cavity

hilum area of the organ where blood vessels, lymph, and nerves enter and exit

iatrogenic treatment induced; may be intentional or unintentional

lymphocele an extravasated collection of lymph

mesentery two layers of fused peritoneum that conduct nerves, lymph, and blood vessels between the small bowel/colon and the posterior peritoneal cavity wall

parietal peritoneum peritoneum lining the walls of the peritoneal cavity

peritoneal organs solid organs and some portions of the bowel within the peritoneal cavity that are covered by visceral peritoneum

potential space an empty fold where the peritoneal layer reflects between two organs or an organ and peritoneal wall, which may contain fluid and other materials when disease is present

KEY TERMS

abscess

ascites

biloma

diverticulum

hematoma

hemoperitoneum

iatrogenic

lymphocele

mesothelioma

omental caking

peritoneal implants

potential space

pseudomyxoma peritonei

seroma

urinoma

(continued)

> **retroperitoneal organs** organs posterior to the parietal peritoneum that are typically covered on their anterior surface or fatty capsule by parietal peritoneum
>
> **seroma** fluid collection composed of blood products located adjacent to or surrounding transplanted organs in the early transplantation period
>
> **visceral peritoneum** peritoneum encasing peritoneal organs

Sonography plays a significant role in the identification of disease processes within the peritoneal cavity; therefore, the peritoneal cavity is an important area of the body for sonographers to be familiar with. There are many disease processes of peritoneal organs that may result in pathology of the peritoneal cavity, including metastasis and a variety of fluid collections. Because of its ability to differentiate between cystic and solid lesions and collections, sonography excels at imaging the potential spaces within the abdominopelvic cavity. Sonography's real-time capabilities and use of sound waves instead of ionizing radiation make it an excellent technology for imaging as well as biopsy or aspiration guidance. A thorough understanding of the anatomy of the peritoneal cavity, especially its divisions, will assist sonographers in determining the presence and extent of disease processes.

ABDOMINOPELVIC CAVITY

The abdominopelvic cavity can be described by two commonly accepted methods using superficial landmarks. The first, Addison lines, divides the abdominopelvic cavity into nine regions by drawing two parasagittal (vertical) lines and two axial (horizontal) lines. The first of the axial lines is called the *transpyloric line* and is determined by drawing an imaginary line halfway between the manubrial notch and the superior pubic symphysis. Instead of using the transpyloric line, some choose to use the subcostal line, a line drawn at the inferior border of the last rib, for its ease of visualization. The second of the axial lines is called the *transtubercular line* and is determined by drawing an imaginary line halfway between the transpyloric line and the superior pubic symphysis. This line also intersects the anterior superior iliac spines of the pelvis. The parasagittal lines are drawn halfway between the manubrial notch and the acromioclavicular joint, called the *midclavicular line* or *mammary line*. These lines divide the abdomen into right and left hypochondriac regions; right and left lumbar and iliac regions bilaterally; and epigastric, umbilical, and hypogastric regions centrally[1] (Fig. 5-1).

The abdominopelvic cavity may also be described in quadrants. One imaginary line is drawn vertically from the tip of the xiphoid process to the superior pubic symphysis along the sagittal midline plane, and a horizontal line is drawn at the level of the umbilicus. This divides the abdominopelvic cavity into the right upper quadrant (RUQ), right lower quadrant (RLQ), left upper quadrant (LUQ), and left lower quadrant (LLQ). This simpler method is the one most commonly employed in the clinical setting[1] (Fig. 5-2). The sonographer must be well versed in the anatomy that is found in each of these regions in order to correlate clinical findings with the sonographic examination.

ANATOMY OF THE PERITONEAL CAVITY

A thin sheet of tissues, called the *peritoneal membrane*, divides the abdominal cavity into peritoneal and retroperitoneal compartments. The largest of the body cavities is the peritoneal cavity, encompassing the abdomen and pelvis.

The peritoneal cavity is formed by the fourth embryonic week and is derived from the mesoderm.[2] The abdominopelvic cavity is lined with a thin continuous layer of peritoneum. The cavity is completely sealed in males but communicates with the external environment via the fallopian tubes in females. Peritoneum that envelops the organs is referred to as *visceral peritoneum*, and the peritoneal layer that lines the walls of the abdominopelvic cavity is referred to as *parietal peritoneum*. This thin layer coating all surfaces of the peritoneal cavity and its organs secretes a small amount of serous fluid, approximately 50 mL, which acts to lubricate visceral surfaces, allowing them to move without friction.[1]

As organs develop along the posterior abdominal wall and protrude into the peritoneal cavity, they are covered by visceral peritoneum except at their hilum, where blood vessels, nerves, and lymph enter and exit the organ. The hila of peritoneal organs are considered bare areas because they lack a peritoneal covering. These bare areas are part of the retroperitoneum.

Divisions of the Peritoneal Cavity

The peritoneal cavity is generally divided into two compartments: the greater sac and the lesser sac. The *greater sac* is the largest, housing the liver, spleen, stomach, first portion of the duodenum, jejunum, ileum, cecum, transverse colon, sigmoid colon, and the upper two-thirds of the rectum.[1] This large sac contains several potential spaces that must be evaluated for free fluid.

The *lesser sac* may be thought of as a diverticulum of the greater sac and is also referred to as the omental bursa by some. The lesser sac does not contain any organs. This potential space lies immediately posterior to the stomach, extending superiorly to the left suprahepatic recess between the posterior left lobe of the liver and the left hemidiaphragm.

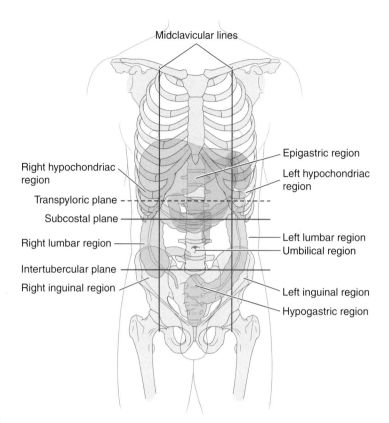

FIGURE 5-1 Addison lines. Nine regions of the abdominopelvic cavity based on Addison lines. The abdominal cavity is divided into nine regions by two sagittal midclavicular lines and two axial lines, the transpyloric line, and the transtubercular line.

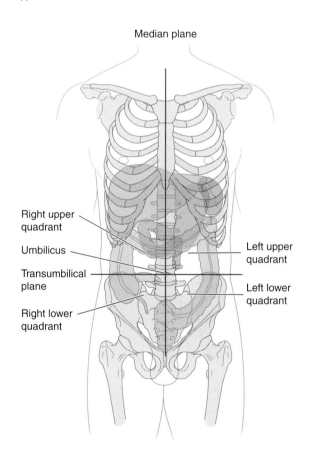

FIGURE 5-2 Quadrants of the abdominopelvic cavity. The abdominal cavity can be divided into four quadrants: right upper quadrant, right lower quadrant, left upper quadrant, and left lower quadrant.

The lesser sac extends inferiorly into the fold of the greater omentum. This may also be referred to as the *inferior recess of the lesser sac* or *omental bursa*. Note that this fold is patent in infants and small children but generally fuses in adults, thereby significantly limiting the caudal extent of the lesser sac (Fig. 5-3A, B). The lesser sac's anterior wall is formed by the posterior stomach, whereas superiorly it is enclosed by the lesser omentum, also called *hepatogastric ligament*. The splenorenal and gastrosplenic ligaments create the left lateral wall of this pocket (Fig. 5-4). The omental foramen, also called the *foramen of Winslow*, is located at the right lateral aspect of the lesser sac and is the only opening communicating with the greater sac. This opening is found posterior to the *hepatoduodenal ligament*, the thickened right border of the lesser omentum that guides the portal triad into the liver (Fig. 5-4).

The lesser omentum—also called the *small omentum*, *gastrohepatic omentum*, and *gastrohepatic ligament*—is a fused double layer of peritoneum stretching between the lesser curvature of the stomach and the left sagittal fissure for the ligamentum venosum (transverse fissure). This ligament creates the anterior superior border of the lesser sac, separating it from the supracolic compartment of the greater sac (Fig. 5-5).

Within the greater sac is a large apron-like double-layered sheet of peritoneum called the *greater omentum* that extends inferiorly from the greater curvature of the stomach and transverse colon. The greater omentum extends inferiorly, anterior to the bowel, folds inward, and travels superiorly to attach on the transverse colon. The anterior and posterior adjacent layers are separate in infants but typically fused

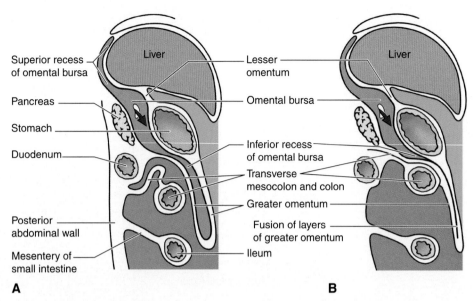

FIGURE 5-3 Lesser sac—schematic sagittal sections, lateral view. Note the patent inferior recess of the lesser sac in the infant (**A**) and the fused nature of the same space in the adult (**B**). The *red arrow* indicates the omental foramen.

in adults and contain a variable amount of fat[3] (Fig. 5-3). The greater omentum functions to prevent the parietal peritoneum of the anterior abdominal wall from adhering to the visceral peritoneum. This mesenteric drape is very mobile and moves to areas of inflammation, surrounding the inflamed area by creating adhesions to wall off infection (Fig. 5-6A, B). It also acts to cushion the abdominal organs to prevent trauma and acts to prevent the loss of body heat from abdominal organs.

The greater omentum subdivides the greater sac into a supracolic (above the colon) compartment and an infracolic (below the colon) compartment. The supracolic compartment is located anterior to the greater omentum and stomach and inferior to the liver. The infracolic compartment is located posterior to the greater omentum, surrounding the small bowel and colon within the remainder of the greater sac (Fig. 5-7). This division is important because it limits the spread of infected materials, pus, ascitic fluid, and malignant

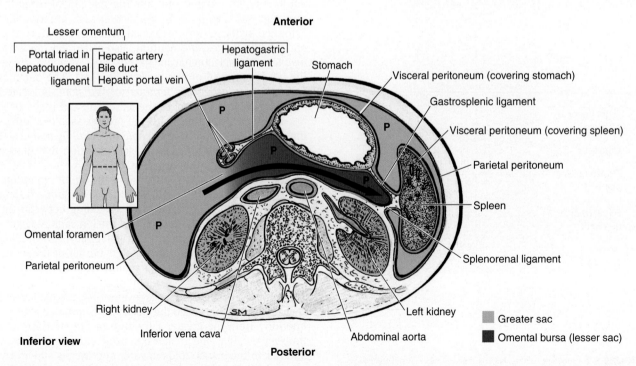

FIGURE 5-4 Omental foramen. The *black arrow* extends through the omental foramen through the width of the lesser sac. The opening is posterior to the hepatoduodenal ligament. The lesser space is seen immediately posterior to the stomach. *P,* peritoneal cavity.

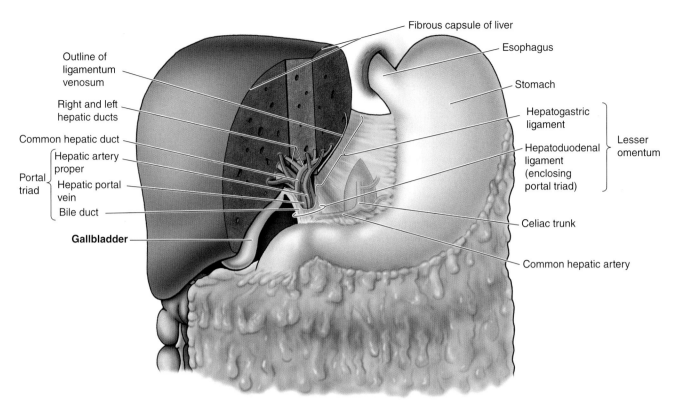

FIGURE 5-5 Lesser omentum. The lesser omentum is a double layer of peritoneum that stretches between the lesser curvature of the stomach and the left sagittal fissure for the ligamentum venosum.

cells within the peritoneal cavity. Communication between these two compartments is via the paracolic gutters, the lateral borders of the ascending and descending colon.

Potential Spaces of the Peritoneum

As organs grow into the peritoneal cavity, several pockets and recesses are formed by the organs, their vascular connections, and suspensory ligaments, thereby creating a complex landscape for sonographers to examine when performing abdominal and pelvic examinations. Ligaments divide portions of the peritoneal cavity. Sonographers require a working knowledge of these ligaments to understand where to look for fluid within the peritoneal sac and how to image and describe its location. See Table 5-1 for a description of the ligaments of the peritoneal cavity.

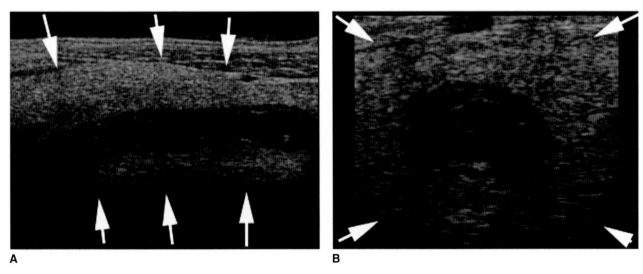

A   **B**

FIGURE 5-6 Greater omentum. **A:** Longitudinal image in a patient with appendicitis demonstrates hyperechoic omental fat (*arrows*) surrounding the inflamed appendix. **B:** Transverse image again demonstrates the hyperechoic omental fat (*arrows*) seen surrounding the inflamed appendix. (Images courtesy of Ultrasound-Cases.info, owner SonoSkills.)

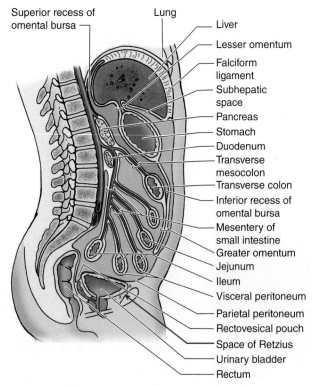

Superior recess of omental bursa
Lung
Liver
Lesser omentum
Falciform ligament
Subhepatic space
Pancreas
Stomach
Duodenum
Transverse mesocolon
Transverse colon
Inferior recess of omental bursa
Mesentery of small intestine
Greater omentum
Jejunum
Ileum
Visceral peritoneum
Parietal peritoneum
Rectovesical pouch
Space of Retzius
Urinary bladder
Rectum

FIGURE 5-7 Divisions of the peritoneal cavity. *Green* represents the supracolic compartment of the greater sac; *pink* represents the infracolic compartment of the greater sac; and *blue* represents the lesser sac.

Potential spaces are areas created by the peritoneal layer, reflecting between two organs or an organ and the peritoneal wall (typically posterior). A potential space is an empty fold; however, when disease is present, fluid or other materials may collect in this space. Because many pathologies present with excretions (ascitic fluid, blood, pus) into the peritoneal cavity, sonographers must examine these potential spaces and characterize the fluid as part of the abdominal and pelvic examinations. The following text includes anatomic descriptions of each major potential space of the peritoneal cavity.

Left Anterior Subphrenic Space

The left anterior subphrenic or suprahepatic space is an extension of the greater sac between the diaphragm and the anterior superior liver leftward of the falciform ligament.

Left Posterior Suprahepatic Space

The left posterior suprahepatic space is also called the *superior recess of the lesser sac*; this space is an extension of the lesser sac between the diaphragm and the posterior superior liver. See Figures 5-3 and 5-7.

Right Subphrenic Space

The right subphrenic or suprahepatic space is an extension of the greater sac between the right hemidiaphragm and the anterior superior liver rightward of the falciform ligament (Fig. 5-8).

TABLE 5-1	**Ligaments of the Peritoneal Cavity**
Gastrohepatic ligament	Also called the lesser omentum, smaller omentum, and gastrohepatic omentum, it connects the lesser curvature of the stomach and the left sagittal fissure for the ligamentum venosum (transverse fissure) of the liver.
Hepatoduodenal ligament	Thickened free edge of the lesser omentum through which courses the portal triad; it connects the liver to the duodenum.
Falciform ligament	Double-layered fold of peritoneum that ascends from the umbilicus to the liver; contained within it is the ligamentum teres. The falciform ligament passes onto the anterior and then the superior surface of the liver before splitting into two layers. The right layer forms the upper layer of the coronary ligament; the left layer forms the upper layer of the left triangular ligament.
Coronary ligament	Bifurcation of the falciform ligament layers that fuse with the parietal peritoneum to form borders of the bare area of the liver, suspending the liver from the diaphragm. The right branch becomes the coronary ligament and the left branch becomes the left triangular ligament, limiting the greater sac at its cephalad extent into anterior and posterior compartments in the right subphrenic area.
Left triangular ligament	Formed by the left branch of the falciform ligament and the parietal peritoneum, it forms the left extremity of the bare area of the liver.
Splenorenal ligament	Also called the lienorenal ligament, it connects the splenic hilum to the posterior abdominal wall, through which the splenic vein and artery travel.
Gastrosplenic ligament	It connects the stomach to the spleen and inferior diaphragm.
Broad ligament	A suspensory ligament that extends from the lateral uterine sidewalls to the pelvic sidewalls, dividing the pelvis into anterior and posterior compartments in the female
Ligamentum teres	Remnant of the fetal umbilical vein, which is contained within the falciform ligament; it passes into a fissure on the visceral liver surface to join the left branch of the portal vein in the porta hepatis.
Ligamentum venosum	It exhibits as a fibrous band (remnant of the ductus venosus) attached to the left branch of the portal vein. It ascends in a fissure on the visceral liver surface to attach above the inferior vena cava. In fetal circulation, oxygenated blood flows to the liver via the umbilical vein (ligamentum teres). Most of the blood bypasses the liver via the ductus venosus (ligamentum venosum) and enters the inferior vena cava.

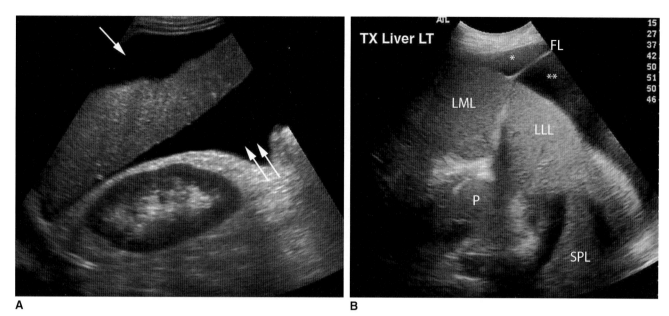

FIGURE 5-8 Subphrenic spaces. **A:** Right anterior subphrenic space and hepatorenal space. Longitudinal image of the right upper quadrant demonstrates fluid within the right anterior subphrenic space (*single arrow*); ascites is also seen within the hepatorenal space (*double arrows*). **B:** Right anterior subphrenic space and left anterior subphrenic space. Transverse image of the epigastrium demonstrates fluid within the right (*) and left (**) anterior subphrenic spaces separated by the falciform ligament. *LLL,* left lateral lobe of liver; *LML,* left medial lobe of liver; *P,* pancreas; *SPL,* spleen. (Image **A:** Courtesy of Philips Medical Systems, Bothel, WA.)

Hepatorenal Space

The hepatorenal space is also referred to as *Morrison pouch.* This peritoneal potential space is created by the peritoneum, reflecting from the liver over the right kidney and right posterior peritoneal wall. When the patient is in a supine position, this space is the most gravity-dependent potential space of the abdominal cavity, collecting fluid from the supracolic area and the lesser sac. See Figure 5-8.

Omental Bursa

The omental bursa, or lesser sac, is sandwiched between the posterior stomach and parietal peritoneum covering the anterior pancreas (front to back) and the splenorenal and gastrosplenic ligaments and epiploic foramen (side to side). In cases of posterior gastric wall perforation or inflammation

or trauma to the pancreas, fluid or a pseudocyst may be identified in this space (Fig. 5-9).

Right and Left Paracolic Gutters

The right and left paracolic gutters are potential spaces or grooves found along the lateral ascending and descending colons that conduct fluids between the supracolic compartment of the abdomen and the infracolic compartment of the inferior abdomen and pelvis. They are important in determining the extension of disease[1] (Fig. 5-10).

Vesicorectal Space

The vesicorectal space or cul-de-sac in the male is the potential space created by the peritoneal reflection over the rectum and posterior bladder wall. When the male is in the

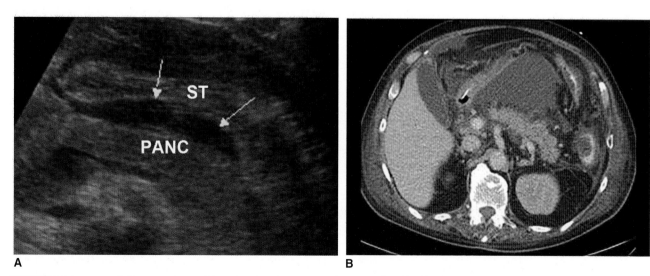

FIGURE 5-9 Lesser sac. **A:** Transverse image of the epigastrium demonstrates a hematoma (*arrows*) within the lesser sac in a patient with acute pancreatitis. The posterior wall of the stomach (*ST*) borders the hematoma anteriorly. The pancreas (*PANC*) forms the posterior border. **B:** The computed tomography scan shows the large fluid collection with debris in the omental bursa in a patient with pancreatitis. (Images courtesy of UltrasoundCases.info, owner SonoSkills.)

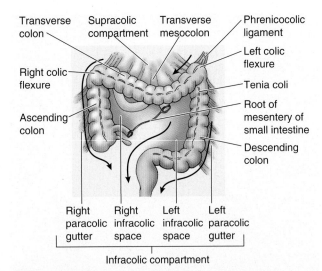

FIGURE 5-10 Paracolic gutters. This diagram demonstrates the flow of fluid and other materials between the infracolic and supracolic compartments.

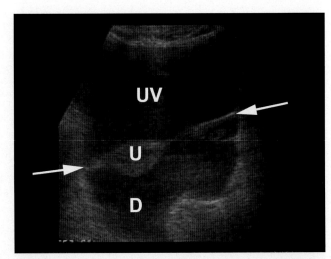

FIGURE 5-12 Female pelvis. Transverse image of the female pelvis demonstrates hemoperitoneum in the pouch of Douglas (*D*) and uterovesical pouch (*UV*) outlining the uterus (*U*) and broad ligaments (*arrows*) bilaterally. (Image courtesy of UltrasoundCases.info, owner SonoSkills.)

supine position, this space is the most gravity-dependent potential space of the pelvic cavity draining fluid from the infracolic area. See Figures 5-7 and 5-11.

Rectouterine Space

The rectouterine space is also called the *rectovaginal pouch*, *pouch of Douglas*, or *posterior cul-de-sac* in the female. This potential space is created by the parietal peritoneum draping over the anterior rectum, posterior vaginal wall, and posterior uterus. When the female is in a supine position, this space is the most gravity-dependent potential space of the pelvic cavity draining fluid from the infracolic area. See Figures 5-11B and 5-12.

Uterovesical Space

The uterovesical space is also called the *uterovesical pouch* or *anterior cul-de-sac* in the female and is the potential space created by the peritoneal reflection over the uterine fundus,

anterior uterus, broad ligament, and posterior urinary bladder. See Figures 5-11B and 5-12.

Space of Retzius

The space of Retzius is also called the *prevesical* or *retropubic space* and is an extraperitoneal potential space located between the anterior wall of the urinary bladder and the pubic symphysis. See Figures 5-7 and 5-11A, B.

SONOGRAPHIC EVALUATION OF THE PERITONEAL CAVITY

The parietal peritoneum lining the inner anterior abdominal wall may be visualized using a high-frequency 5- to 12-MHz linear transducer. The peritoneum appears as a thin hyperechoic continuous line posterior to the moderately hypoechoic

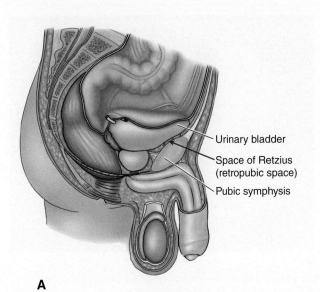

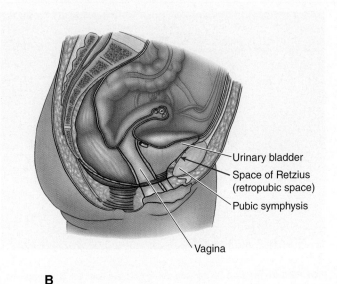

FIGURE 5-11 Male and female pelvic anatomy. **A:** Right lateral view of male. **B:** Right lateral view of female.

internal oblique and rectus abdominis abdominal wall muscles. Bowel filled with gas, fluid, and fecal material will be identified deep to this anterior parietal peritoneum and can be observed in peristalsis. Sonographers may examine the anterior abdominal wall parietal peritoneum when evaluating for an abdominal wall hernia or delineating the position of an abscess or hematoma.

The visceral peritoneum and parietal peritoneum of the posterior peritoneal wall are typically not appreciated because of their depth. A lower-frequency 2- to 5-MHz curvilinear or sector transducer is required to adequately visualize these deeper structures.

Generally, the peritoneal cavity is not evaluated as the primary focus of a diagnostic examination. Typically, the peritoneal organs are the focus of the examination, with the potential spaces of the peritoneal cavity viewed secondarily. A scanning technique that focuses specifically on the peritoneal cavity called focused assessment with sonography in trauma (FAST) or extended focused assessment with sonography in trauma (E-FAST) may be used to assess the peritoneal potential spaces for free fluid in trauma situations.[4]

The FAST examination is performed by acquiring longitudinal and transvers images to include the Morrison pouch (Fig. 5-13), the posterior right hemidiaphragm/liver interface (Fig. 5-14), the spleen/left kidney interface in the left upper quadrant (LUQ) (Fig. 5-15), and the pouch of Douglas[4] (Fig. 5-16A, B). The triage scanning technique has proven to be sensitive to detecting as little as 200 mL of pleural fluid. Additionally, the paracolic gutter and solid intraperitoneal organs may be imaged, depending on institutional protocol (Fig. 5-17). FAST has proven to be very effective in hemodynamically unstable patients suffering blunt abdominal trauma. Computed tomography remains the gold standard for imaging hemodynamically stable patients with possible abdominal trauma whenever possible.[5,6]

More detailed scanning techniques related to these the FAST and E-FAST approaches are discussed in detail in Chapter 25, Point-of-Care Ultrasonography, of this textbook.

When free fluid is observed within the peritoneal cavity, the sonographer should assess it for specific characteristics,

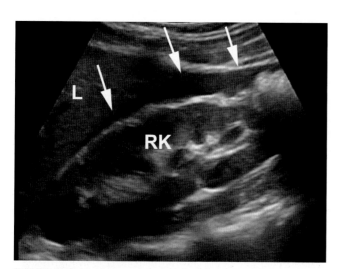

FIGURE 5-13 Morrison pouch. Longitudinal image of the right upper quadrant demonstrates a small amount of free fluid (*arrows*) in the Morrison pouch. *L*, liver; *RK*, right kidney. (Image courtesy of UltrasoundCases.info, owner SonoSkills.)

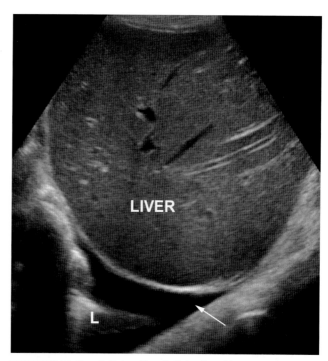

FIGURE 5-14 Pleural effusion. Pleural effusion (*arrow*) is seen superior to the right hemidiaphragm within the chest cavity. Lung tissue (*L*) is seen suspended within the fluid. No fluid is seen inferior to the diaphragm in the subphrenic space. (Image courtesy of Philips Medical Systems, Bothel, WA.)

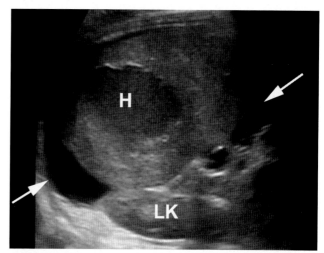

FIGURE 5-15 Left upper quadrant (LUQ). Transverse image of the LUQ demonstrates free fluid (*arrows*) and a splenic hematoma (*H*) following abdominal trauma and splenic rupture. *LK*, left kidney. (Image courtesy of UltrasoundCases.info, owner SonoSkills.)

taking images that demonstrate whether the fluid is simple or complex and to determine whether it is loculated or freely mobile (Figs. 5-18 and 5-19). This may require using a higher-frequency transducer, increasing the scanning gain above that optimally used during scanning, and imaging from multiple angles of incidence to detect fine septa or particles within the fluid. The patient's position may also be changed, rolling the patient into a lateral decubitus or Trendelenburg position, to demonstrate fluid movement.

Free fluid must be differentiated from cystic masses of the peritoneum. Ascites will demonstrate bowel moving freely

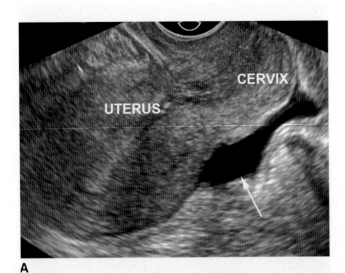

A

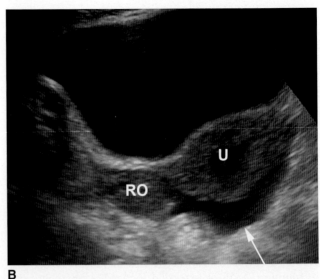

B

FIGURE 5-16 Posterior cul-de-sac (pouch of Douglas). **A:** Sagittal transvaginal image of the midline pelvis demonstrates free fluid in the posterior cul-de-sac (*arrow*). **B:** Transverse transabdominal image of the female pelvis demonstrates free fluid in the posterior cul-de-sac (*arrow*). *RO*, right ovary; *U*, uterus.

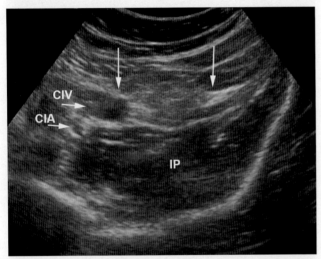

FIGURE 5-17 Paracolic gutters. Transverse image of the left paracolic gutter demonstrates normal musculature and vasculature. The *arrows* demonstrate where free fluid could collect. *CIA*, common iliac artery; *CIV*, common iliac vein; *IP*, iliopsoas muscle.

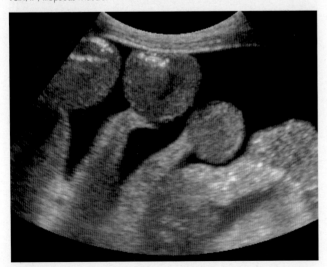

FIGURE 5-18 Simple ascites. Sagittal view demonstrates simple ascites outlining the small bowel and mesentery floating freely within the fluid. (Image courtesy of Philips Medical Systems, Bothel, WA.)

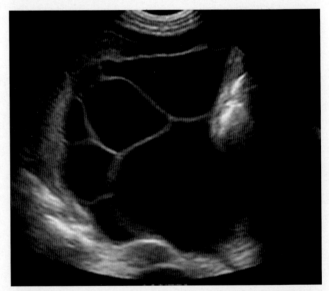

FIGURE 5-19 Loculated ascites. Complex loculated ascites demonstrates multiple septa with apparent sequestered pockets of fluid. (Image courtesy of Philips Medical Systems, Bothel, WA.)

within it. Free fluid will follow the contour of peritoneal organs, filling sharp corners and interfaces of recesses and potential spaces. Cystic masses may demonstrate a mass effect on surrounding tissues, tending to have a circular or oval shape without sharp corners or angles (Figs. 5-20 and 5-21).

When assessing the paracolic gutters and posterior rectouterine/rectovesical space for fluid, it may be necessary to decrease the gain settings to identify small amounts of fluid adjacent to hyperechoic gas-filled bowel and to accommodate for enhancement posterior to a urine-filled bladder. Additionally, color and/or power Doppler imaging should be employed at the most sensitive settings possible to evaluate septa and other solid-appearing masses within the peritoneal cavity for blood flow. When blood flow is identified with color or power Doppler imaging, it may be helpful to include spectral Doppler tracings with resistive indices.

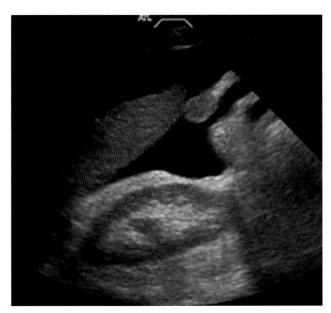

FIGURE 5-20 Ascites. Longitudinal image of the right upper quadrant demonstrates simple ascites in Morrison pouch and the right subphrenic space. Note the sharp fluid-filled corners created at organ interfaces and how organs project into the fluid that fills the available spaces. (Image courtesy of Philips Medical Systems, Bothel, WA.)

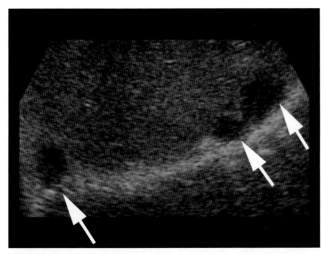

FIGURE 5-21 Tuberculomas. Fluid-filled structures (*arrows*) seen around the periphery of the liver represent tuberculomas. Note that these fluid collections are spherical and do not conform to the periphery of the organ or available space. (Image courtesy of UltrasoundCases.info, owner SonoSkills.)

PATHOLOGIES OF THE PERITONEAL CAVITY

Although the peritoneum does normally secrete a small amount of serous fluid to lubricate the surfaces of the peritoneal organs, it is typically not appreciated during a sonographic examination. A small amount of fluid, up to 20 mL, is commonly seen in the pouch of Douglas following ovulation in menstruating females. Fluid and solid or semisolid materials identified in other potential spaces may indicate a pathologic process and should be investigated further. The rest of this section discusses common peritoneal abnormalities.

Ascites

Ascites is ascitic or free fluid found within the peritoneal cavity that may be associated with a variety of causes, including liver failure, abdominal trauma, or malignancy.[7,8] Ascitic fluid typically collects in the Morrison pouch, the paracolic gutters, and the pouch of Douglas when the patient is in the supine position. There are two types of ascites: transudative and exudative. *Transudative ascites* is characterized by a lack of protein and cellular materials in the fluid.[5] Transudative ascites typically has a simple appearance and is often associated with portal hypertension and congestive cardiac disease[9] (Fig. 5-20). *Exudative ascites* is fluid that seeps out from blood vessels and contains a large amount of protein and cellular material.[8] Exudative ascites typically results in a more complex and echogenic appearance to the fluid and is associated with renal failure, inflammatory or ischemic bowel disease, peritonitis, and malignancy[9] (Fig. 5-22).

Peritoneal Abscess

A peritoneal abscess may be identified in a potential space or adjacent to an inflamed or perforated organ—the right subphrenic space being the most common because of the high frequency of appendicitis and duodenal ulcers.[10] Sonographically, the abscess typically appears as a thick-walled fluid collection that may contain ischemic tissue, pus, and blood components. The sonographic appearance is variable and may be anechoic, solid appearing, or multiseptated or contain a debris or fluid–fluid level (Fig. 5-23). No blood flow should be visualized within the abscess pocket, but hyperemia may be demonstrated surrounding the thick, shaggy wall. Air may be present within the abscess demonstrating a hyperechoic anterior interface that is gravity dependent with a "dirty" shadow posterior. Scanning from a coronal horizontal approach to avoid bubbles may allow improved imaging of an air-containing abscess. Primary abscesses may occur adjacent to an inflamed organ, such as the bowel with diverticulitis or appendicitis, or as a surgical complication. Additionally, parasitic abscesses may occur in peritoneal organs. These are often ingested and

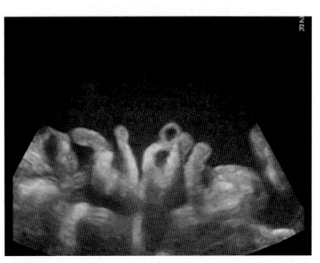

FIGURE 5-22 Exudative ascites. Exudative ascites associated with peritoneal metastases is seen. Note the particulate appearance of the fluid and the bowel matted to the posterior wall. (Image courtesy of UltrasoundCases.info, owner SonoSkills.)

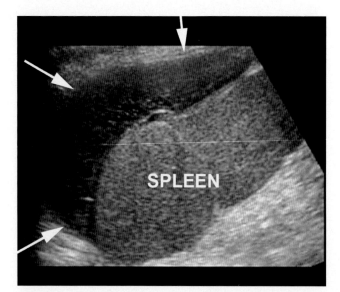

FIGURE 5-23 Peritoneal abscess. Perisplenic abscess (*arrows*) is seen in the left upper quadrant. Note the complex echogenicity and the rounded edges that demonstrate this is not free fluid. (Image courtesy of UltrasoundCases. info, owner SonoSkills.)

transported through the portal system into the liver and spleen. The most common is *Echinococcus granulosus*. An existing fluid collection such as a hematoma or cyst may become an abscess when it becomes infected secondarily.

Hemoperitoneum

Hemoperitoneum may be seen with blunt abdominal trauma resulting in abdominal viscera or vasculature bleeding into the peritoneal cavity. The trauma may also be iatrogenically induced, such as following a biopsy, angioplasty, or other surgical intervention. Once the blood organizes, it is typically referred to as a *hematoma*.

Hematoma

A hematoma is a blood clot or focal area of coagulated blood occurring as a postsurgical complication, following trauma such as an automobile accident, or occurring spontaneously in patients with hemophilia or other coagulation diseases, or those taking anticoagulant medications.[11] Large hematomas may be associated with a drop in hematocrit. Hematomas are typically found immediately adjacent to the tissue or vessel that has been disrupted, deep to a surgical incision, or in a dependent potential space of the peritoneal cavity (Morrison pouch, paracolic gutters, or posterior cul-de-sac).

Hematomas have a variable appearance depending on their age (Fig. 5-24A, B). The evolution of clotting blood is relatively predictable when the patient is not taking blood thinning or thrombolytic medications. Initial bleeding is anechoic; however, within a few hours, the collection will become somewhat larger, more echogenic, and complex in appearance as fibrin is deposited. Over a few days, the hematoma will become completely solid, appearing with an echogenicity similar to that of the parenchyma of the normal spleen or liver. Color or power Doppler imaging may assist the sonographer in identifying the hematoma because it will be devoid of blood flow and may demonstrate a mass effect on surrounding tissues. Eventually, the clot will progress into the lytic phase, retracting to become smaller in size with an increasingly complex appearance, and ending with complete or partial resorption by the body. Residual hematoma may be replaced by scar tissue, resulting in a hyperechoic fibrotic retracted area. Long-standing hematomas may develop a thin eggshell calcification around the periphery. A thorough patient history will assist the sonographer in recognizing potential scar tissue in a patient with a history of trauma.

Pseudomyxoma Peritonei

Pseudomyxoma peritonei (PMP) is a rare borderline malignant process that results when a benign appendiceal or

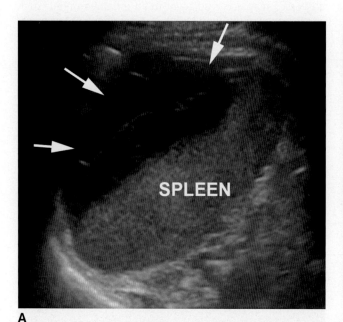

A

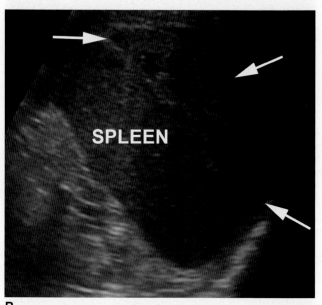

B

FIGURE 5-24 Hematoma. **A:** Sagittal image demonstrates a hypoechoic fluid collection (*arrows*) consistent with an acute splenic hematoma in a patient with recent abdominal trauma. **B:** Transverse image in the same patient a few weeks later demonstrates a nearly solid appearance (*arrows*). (Images courtesy of UltrasoundCases.info, owner SonoSkills.)

ovarian adenoma ruptures, spilling epithelial cells into the peritoneum.[12-14] These cells develop into noninvasive peritoneal implants that secrete a gelatinous mucus into the peritoneal cavity.[13,14] The cells spread from the appendix in the right paracolic gutter into the right subdiaphragmatic space and into the intraperitoneal potential spaces of the pelvis. As the mucus accumulates within the abdominopelvic cavity, it takes up space around the bowel and causes fibrosis of the peritoneal membranes, creating adhesions.[15] The 10-year survival rate of PMP patients is 30% because of the complications associated with recurrence and treatment.[13] Symptoms and imaging findings include abdominal pain and distension, omental caking, posterior fixation of bowel loops and mesentery, bowel obstruction, and small bowel fistula.[14] Treatments include palliative surgical debulking to remove visible implants, chemotherapy, cytoreductive surgery, and perioperative/postoperative chemotherapy.[13,14] This final treatment is the most aggressive therapy and involves stripping parietal peritoneum from the abdominopelvic cavity and surgical removal of the right colon, greater and lesser omentum, spleen, gallbladder, and uterus and ovaries in females. Unfortunately, therapy is relatively ineffective in completely eradicating all of the cells, resulting in periodic recurrence over time.[16]

Sonographically, PMP most commonly appears as simple or multiloculated ascites. It may also present as several thin-walled cysts of varying sizes scattered throughout the peritoneum[14] (Fig. 5-25A, B). PMP may rarely appear as a hypoechoic solid mass.[14] Identifying the primary adenoma as well as the complexity of the concomitant ascites is important.

Fluid Collections

Seroma

A seroma is a fluid collection composed of blood products located adjacent to or surrounding transplanted organs in the early postsurgical period. They are typically anechoic but may contain septa.[5]

Lymphocele

Lymphoceles are collections of lymphatic fluid outside of the lymph system owing to disruption of the lymphatic vessels or lymph node resection. These collections are generally simple but may contain septations. Lymphoceles are slower to develop following surgery and typically present 4 to 8 weeks after surgery.[17] The delayed onset can help establish the diagnosis of lymphocele. In the peritoneal cavity, a lymphocele may be seen following prostatectomy and lymph node dissection. The body may spontaneously resorb smaller collections, whereas larger collections may require more aggressive interventions ranging from percutaneous aspiration to surgery or sclerosis.[5,17]

Biloma

A biloma is an anechoic collection of bile located within the peritoneal cavity outside of the biliary tree.[11] It is typically associated with hepatic transplant because of a biliary leak or biliary tree ischemia, but it may also be the sequela of trauma, biopsy, or cholecystectomy (Fig. 5-26).

Urinoma

A urinoma is associated with a rupture of the urinary tract. It is typically found adjacent to the kidney in the perirenal space of the retroperitoneum. When urine is free within the peritoneal cavity, it is more appropriately called *urine ascites*. Urine will appear as simple anechoic fluid. The bladder wall should be evaluated for discontinuity in cases of urine ascites.

Peritoneal Masses

Mesenteric Cysts

Mesenteric cysts may occur anywhere along the mesentery, but the majority originate from the small bowel mesentery.

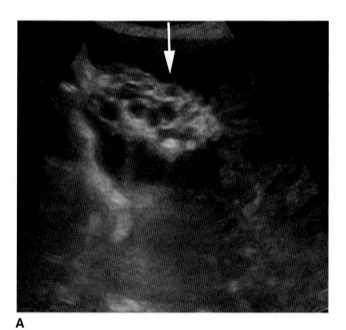

A

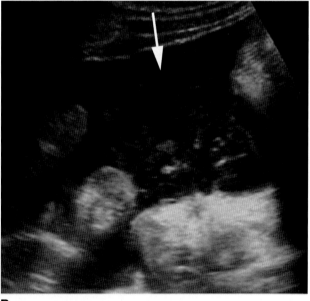

B

FIGURE 5-25 Pseudomyxoma peritonei. **A:** A multicystic appearance of pseudomyxoma peritonei (*PMP*) (*arrow*) is seen within the peritoneal cavity secondary to a mucinous carcinoma of the appendix. **B:** Complex mucinous *ascites* (*arrow*) is seen in the same patient. (Images courtesy of UltrasoundCases.info, owner SonoSkills.)

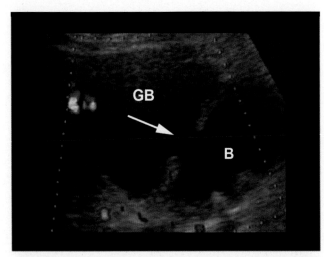

FIGURE 5-26 Biloma. Gallbladder (*GB*) wall perforation (*arrow*) with adjacent biloma (*B*). (Image courtesy of UltrasoundCases.info, owner SonoSkills.)

Variable in size, these benign cysts grow slowly over time with peritoneal serous secretions. These unilocular cysts may be pedunculated and may torse, hemorrhage, or cause bowel obstruction because of a mass effect[16] (Fig. 5-27A, B).

Mesenteric Adenopathy

Mesenteric adenopathy, also called lymphadenopathy, describes the enlargement of the lymph nodes along the mesentery or on the bowel. Adenopathy may be associated with inflammatory diseases of the bowel such as colitis and appendicitis and with viral infections. Adenopathy may also be associated with primary malignancy, such as lymphoma, or metastatic malignancy, such as colon cancer. Multiple lymph nodes become visible along the mesentery adjacent to the inflamed bowel. The lymph nodes lose their oval shape and become more rounded as they increase in size (Fig. 5-28A, B).

Peritoneal Mesothelioma

Peritoneal mesothelioma is a relatively rare primary malignant tumor of the peritoneum and is associated with asbestos exposure. Masses occur most frequently along the pleura and peritoneum, metastasizing by direct invasion into adjacent organs. The tumor may appear as a generalized thickening of the peritoneum, mesentery, omentum, and bowel or as a discrete nodule (Fig. 5-29). It is frequently associated with a small amount of ascites and may demonstrate areas of calcification.[16]

Peritoneal Implants and Omental Caking

Peritoneal implants are associated with peritoneal metastasis, appearing as multiple small polypoid masses projecting from the parietal peritoneum. Concomitant findings of complex ascites and omental caking are commonly seen.[18] Peritoneal implants are most commonly associated with primary cancers of the ovary, stomach, and colon[12,16,18] (Fig. 5-30A, B).

Omental caking is a thickening of the greater omentum because of malignant infiltration.[3] Omental caking is indicative of peritoneal metastasis, also called peritoneal carcinomatosis, and is commonly associated with primary cancers of the ovary, stomach, and colon.[12,16,18] It is frequently associated with a significant amount of complex ascites and peritoneal implants of nodular metastatic masses along the parietal peritoneum.[18] Sonographically, an omental cake appears as a moderately echogenic, homogeneous, thick, soft tissue layer deep to the anterior wall (Fig. 5-31A, B).

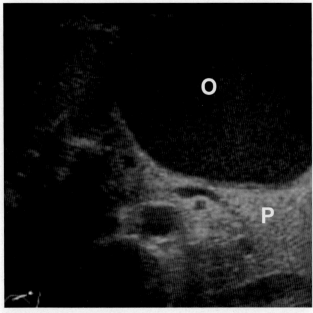

A

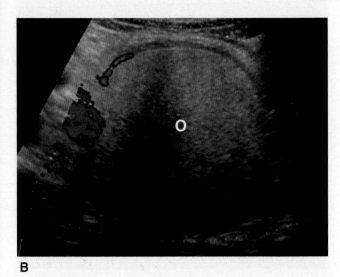

B

FIGURE 5-27 Omental cyst. **A:** Transverse epigastric image demonstrates an omental cyst (*O*) anterior to the pancreas (*P*). **B:** Sonogram demonstrates an omental cyst nearly filled with clot. Color Doppler image demonstrates flow around the periphery of the cyst. (Images courtesy of UltrasoundCases.info, owner SonoSkills.)

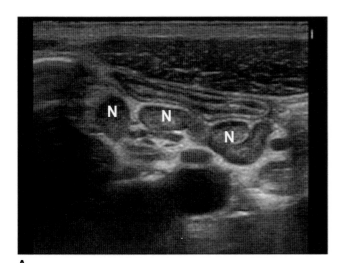

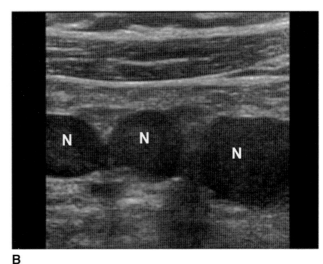

A **B**

FIGURE 5-28 Mesenteric lymphadenopathy. **A, B:** Mesenteric lymph node (*N*) enlargement in two patients with colitis. (Images courtesy of UltrasoundCases. info, owner SonoSkills.)

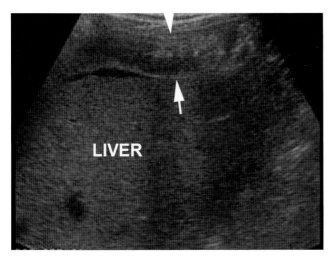

FIGURE 5-29 Peritoneal mesothelioma. Peritoneal mesothelioma seen as a solid mass (*arrows*) of the peritoneum at the anterior aspect of the liver. (Image courtesy of UltrasoundCases.info, owner SonoSkills.)

INTERVENTIONAL APPLICATIONS

Because of its real-time capability and ability to demonstrate vasculature, sonography-guided biopsy and aspiration of the peritoneal cavity and its contents are frequently performed.

Paracentesis

Paracentesis is the aspiration of ascitic fluid from the peritoneal cavity and may be done for diagnostic or therapeutic purposes.[7,8,17] This sterile procedure is typically performed by percutaneous placement of a Yueh catheter or other needle into the peritoneal cavity, typically in the area of the right paracolic gutter. In a diagnostic paracentesis, a small amount of fluid may be drawn into a syringe to be sent to the laboratory for testing. When greater amounts of ascitic fluid are present, a therapeutic paracentesis may be performed. Up to 6 L of fluid may be withdrawn for palliative purposes when the patient is experiencing respiratory

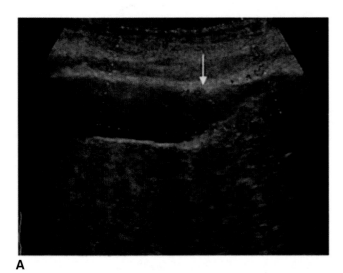

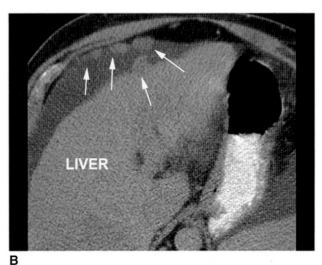

A **B**

FIGURE 5-30 Peritoneal implants. **A:** Lobulated solid masses (*arrow*) are seen projecting from the peritoneum anterior to the liver. A small amount of ascites is also seen. **B:** Computed tomography demonstrates solid polypoid masses (*arrows*) seen extending from the peritoneum consistent with peritoneal implants. (Images courtesy of UltrasoundCases.info, owner SonoSkills.)

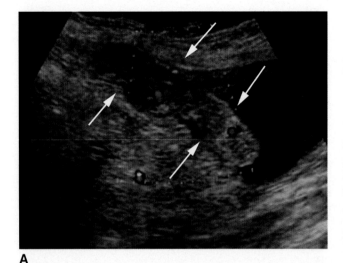

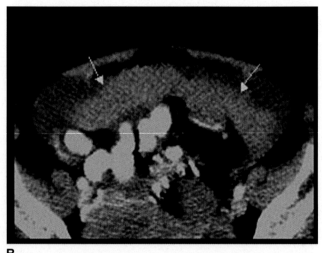

A   **B**

FIGURE 5-31 Omental caking. **A, B:** Sonogram and computed tomography images demonstrate an omental cake (*arrows*) with some vascularity seen on color Doppler imaging in a patient with ovarian cancer. (Images courtesy of UltrasoundCases.info, owner SonoSkills.)

difficulty and/or extreme abdominal pressure because of a large quantity of ascites. Large quantities of ascitic fluid are commonly associated with portal hypertension, requiring frequent drainage in the later stages of the disease.

Percutaneous Abscess Drainage

Percutaneous abscess drainage (PAD) is another sterile procedure that may be performed using sonographic guidance.[17] A small flexible catheter is inserted into the abscess pocket, and abscess contents are aspirated into a syringe to be sent to the laboratory for analysis.[19] The physician may choose to leave a drainage catheter in the abscess to allow for gravitational drainage and antibiotic instillation.

SUMMARY

- Many disease processes and fluid collections may occur within the peritoneal cavity.
- The abdominopelvic cavity can be divided into nine regions using Addison lines: right and left hypochondriac, right and left lumbar, right and left iliac, epigastric, umbilical, and hypogastric regions.
- The abdominopelvic cavity can also be divided into four quadrants: right upper quadrant, right lower quadrant, left upper quadrant, and left lower quadrant.
- The quadrants and regions are used to describe the location of fluid collections and disease processes.
- The abdominopelvic cavity is lined with a thin continuous layer of peritoneum.
- The peritoneum that surrounds the organs is referred to as visceral peritoneum.
- The peritoneum that lines the walls of the abdominopelvic cavity is referred to as parietal peritoneum.
- The peritoneum secretes a small amount of serous fluid that acts as a lubricant, allowing the organs to move without friction.
- The peritoneal cavity is divided into the larger greater sac, which contains the peritoneal organs, and the smaller lesser sac, which does not contain any organ.
- The greater omentum helps prevent the parietal peritoneum from adhering to the visceral peritoneum and also

functions to move to areas of inflammation, surrounding the area and walling off infection.
- The greater omentum subdivides the greater sac into a supracolic and an infracolic compartment; this separation helps limit the spread of infection and malignancy.
- Ligaments also divide the peritoneal cavity and form boundaries for potential spaces.
- A potential space is normally an empty fold except in the case of disease, when fluid and other materials may collect.
- When free fluid is visualized in the peritoneal cavity, it is important to determine whether the fluid is simple or complex and freely mobile or loculated.
- Ascites is free fluid within the peritoneal cavity and may occur with liver disease, portal hypertension, cardiac disease, malignancy, or abdominal trauma.
- The Morrison pouch, the paracolic gutters, and the pouch of Douglas are the most common locations for ascites to collect when the patient is supine.
- Transudative ascites is a simple ascites that lacks protein and cellular materials and is frequently associated with portal hypertension and congestive cardiac disease.
- Exudative ascites is fluid that seeps out of blood vessels, contains large amounts of protein and cellular material, and has a more echogenic or complex appearance. It is typically associated with renal failure, peritonitis, inflammatory bowel disease, and malignancy.

- A peritoneal abscess is a walled-off collection of pus, ischemic tissue, and blood products. The sonographic appearance is variable.
- Hemoperitoneum refers to free blood within the peritoneal cavity.
- A hematoma is a blood clot or focal area of congested blood frequently occurring following trauma or surgical procedures or occurring spontaneously in patients with clotting disorders.
- PMP occurs following the rupture of a benign appendiceal or ovarian adenoma. Epithelial cells are released into the peritoneum and secrete a gelatinous mucous into the peritoneal cavity.
- Sonographically, PMP appears as simple or multiloculated ascites or as several thin-walled cysts of various sizes.

- Seromas, lymphoceles, or bilomas may also occur in the peritoneal cavity following surgery or trauma.
- Mesenteric lymphadenopathy refers to enlargement of the lymph nodes along the mesentery or bowel and may be associated with inflammatory bowel disease.
- Peritoneal implants, complex ascites, and omental caking are seen with metastatic cancers of the ovary, stomach, and colon.
- Paracentesis is a diagnostic or therapeutic procedure performed to remove ascites from the peritoneal cavity.
- Percutaneous abscess drainage may be performed under sonographic guidance to better define the infection and to reduce the infectious load.

REFERENCES

1. Moore KL, Dalley AF, Agur AM. *Clinically Oriented Anatomy.* 7th ed. Wolters Kluwer Health; 2013.
2. Moore KL, Persaud TVN, Torchia MG. *Before We Are Born: Essentials of Embryology and Birth Defects.* 9th ed. Elsevier Health Science; 2015.
3. Que Y, Wang X, Liu Y, et al. Ultrasound-guided biopsy of greater omentum: an effective method to trace the origin of unclear ascites. *Eur J Radiol.* 2009;70(2):331–335.
4. Ollerton JE, Sugrue M, Balogh Z, D'Amours SK, Giles A, Wyllie P. Prospective study to evaluate the influence of FAST on trauma patient management. *J Trauma.* 2006;60(4):785–91.
5. Beck-Razi N, Gaitini D. Focused assessment with sonography for trauma. *Ultrasound Clin.* 2008;3:23–31.
6. Sanders RC, Winter TC. *Clinical Sonography: A Practical Guide.* 4th ed. Lippincott Williams & Wilkins; 2006.
7. Hou W, Sanyal AJ. Ascites: diagnosis and management. *Med Clin North Am.* 2009;93:801–817.
8. Gines P, Cardenas A, Arroyo V, et al. Management of cirrhosis and ascites. *N Engl J Med.* 2004;350:1646–1654.
9. Malde HM, Gandhi RD. Exudative v/s transudative ascites: differentiation based on fluid echogenicity on high resolution sonography. *J Postgrad Med.* 1993;39:132–133.
10. Pick TP, Howden R, eds. *Gray's Anatomy: Anatomy, Descriptive and Surgical.* Random House; 1995.
11. Chen CJ, Chang WH, Shih SC, et al. Clinical presentation and outcome of hepatic subcapsular fluid collections. *J Formos Med Assoc.* 2009;108:61–68.
12. Joshi M. Sonography of adnexal masses. *Ultrasound Clin.* 2008;3:369–389.
13. Jarvinen P, Lepisto A. Clinical presentation of pseudomyxoma peritonei. *Scand J Surg.* 2010;99:213–216.
14. Teo M. Peritoneal-based malignancies and their treatment. *Ann Acad Med Singapore.* 2010;39:54–57.
15. Nagarajan P, Renehan A, Saunders MP, et al. Sugarbaker procedure for pseudomyxoma peritonei (Intervention Protocol). *Cochrane Database Syst Rev.* 2006;1:CD005659.
16. Dähnert W. *Radiology Review Manual.* 5th ed. Lippincott Williams & Wilkins; 2003.
17. Childs DD, Tchelepi H. Ultrasound and abdominal intervention: new luster on an old gem. *Ultrasound Clin.* 2009;4:25–43.
18. Mironov S, Akin O, Pandit-Taskar N, et al. Ovarian cancer. *Radiol Clin North Am.* 2007;45:149–166.
19. Phillips CL, Williams PL, Watkinson AF. Pelvic drainage: image guidance and technique. *Ultrasound Clin.* 2009;4:73–81.

CHAPTER 6

Vascular Structures

AUBREY J. RYBYINSKI

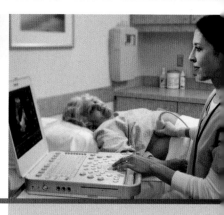

OBJECTIVES

- Identify the role of diagnostic medical sonography in the assessment of abdominal vascular structures.

- Perform sonographic evaluation of the abdominal vascular system.

- Describe the patient preparation, equipment considerations, and scanning techniques and Doppler protocols for normal and abnormal abdominal vascular structures.

- Identify circulatory anatomy, name the layers of blood vessels, and distinguish the difference between arteries and veins.

- Recognize the sonographic appearance and relational anatomy of the abdominal vascular system.

- Describe the pathology, etiology, clinical signs and symptoms, and sonographic appearance or aortic pathology to include atherosclerosis, aneurysms, dissection, rupture, inflammatory aneurysms, stenosis, and vascular insufficiency.

- Discuss the complications of an aortic graft, including pseudoaneurysms, graft aneurysms, hematomas, abscesses, and occlusions.

- Describe the pathology, etiology, clinical signs and symptoms, and the sonographic appearance for venous abnormalities, including vena caval obstruction, tumors, venous enlargement, thrombosis, aneurysm, hepatic venous abnormalities (Budd–Chiari syndrome), and portal venous abnormalities (portal thrombosis and portal venous hypertension).

- Formulate a list of differential diagnosis based on correlating the patient's clinical history, laboratory values, results of related diagnostic procedures, and the sonographic tissue characteristics.

- Identify technically satisfactory and unsatisfactory sonographic examinations of the vascular system.

KEY TERMS

anastomosis

aneurysm, pseudoaneurysm

Budd–Chiari syndrome

ectasia

Marfan syndrome

nutcracker phenomenon

parvus, pulsus tardus

postprandial, preprandial

splanchnic arteries

TIPS

GLOSSARY

anastomosis a connection between two vessels

arteriovenous fistula connection allowing communication between an artery and a vein

ectasia dilatation, expansion, or distention

endograft a metallic stent covered with fabric and placed inside an aneurysm to prevent rupture

graft any tissue or organ for implantation or transplantation

prosthesis an artificial substitute for a body part

pseudoaneurysm caused by a hematoma that forms as a result of a leaking hole in an artery; this pulsating, false (pseudo)aneurysm forms outside the arterial wall

thrombosis the formation of a thrombus (clot) in a blood vessel

This chapter stresses the importance of learning how to identify normal and abnormal abdominal vessels and how to assess normal and abnormal blood flow. The many branches of arterial flow and the confluences of venous return provide a comprehensive road map for identifying normal and abnormal anatomy and anatomic relationships. Current sonography equipment makes it possible to accurately image smaller vessels and to detect intraluminal abnormalities such as thrombi and tumors.[1] Current instrumentation provides the ability to assess blood flow, to obtain hemodynamic information regarding the many factors that influence the dynamics of blood flow, and the hemodynamic consequences of vascular disease.

SONOGRAPHY EXAMINATION

Patient Preparation

It is recommended that all patients fast for at least 4 hours prior to vascular scanning and refrain from chewing gum or smoking. Fasting tends to reduce the amount of air in the abdomen, which has the potential to obscure the anatomy of interest. In emergency situations, however, scanning can be accomplished without any patient preparation.[2] If Doppler interrogation is desired, studies should be performed in a consistent manner to reduce result variability. Many factors affect blood flow hemodynamics including ingestion of a meal, respiratory changes, and postural changes. In some instances, it may be helpful to perform preprandial and postprandial studies to aid in the diagnosis of abnormal blood flow states.

Equipment Considerations

With an understanding of the relationship between resolution and beam penetration, the sonographer may select either a sector or linear transducer operating at the highest clinically appropriate frequency. For adults, the common grayscale scanning frequency is 5 MHz and lower. Doppler is essential for investigating blood flow hemodynamics. The Doppler frequency may vary from the imaging frequency. Color-flow instrumentation provides rapid evaluation and visualization of blood flow and can reduce examination time.

Scanning Techniques

Most of the abdominal vasculature can be identified with the patient lying in the supine position. Standard scanning of the aorta and inferior vena cava (IVC) commences with the transducer placed in the subxiphoid position and oriented to the transverse plane. Because of their proximity, the aorta and IVC can be demonstrated in the transverse plane simultaneously, and once they are identified, gain settings should be adjusted to reveal their characteristic echo-free lumen. Some reverberation artifact may be present along the anterior aspect of each vessel. This is considered normal because of the strong reflective interface of each of the vessels' walls. Scanning continues inferiorly until the aortic bifurcation is reached. Images are recorded at 1- to 2-cm intervals along the course of the aorta and IVC, and additional sections are recorded in any area of disease. Once transverse scanning is completed, the aorta and IVC should be imaged in longitudinal sections. Images are recorded in segments to demonstrate the entire length of each vessel.

If specific arterial branches or venous tributaries are being investigated, the examination should begin with the transducer positioned near the vessel's origin. Transducer manipulations are then carried out in an attempt to follow the course of the vessel. Images are recorded to demonstrate vessel length as clearly as possible and any disease that may be present.

A sonographer examining the many vascular branches and pathways in the abdomen must have a working knowledge of the general course throughout. Once each vessel's site of origin is known and the general course of the abdominal vasculature is learned, sonographic examination is made easier. Diligent Doppler sampling is the most reliable and accurate method for confirming arteries versus veins.

VASCULAR ANATOMY

Blood is distributed throughout the body by a vast network of arteries and veins. In the systemic circulation, arteries transport blood from the heart to the muscles and organs, and veins transport blood from the muscles and organs back to the heart. Typically, blood vessels are composed of three distinct layers: (1) the tunica intima, (2) the tunica media, and (3) the tunica adventitia. The tunica intima, the innermost section of a vessel wall, consists of an endothelial lining and elastic tissue. Elastic fibers and smooth muscle constitute the second layer, the tunica media. The outer portion of the vessel wall, the tunica adventitia, is composed of elastic and collagen fibers.[3]

Although arteries and veins are histologically similar, there are differences in the distribution of each tissue within the walls that reflect pressure differences between the two systems. For example, arterial walls are thicker and contain more elastic and smooth muscle fibers than veins. This is true especially in the tunica media, which is the thickest layer of an artery and is largely responsible for its very elastic and contractile characteristics. Because of the thickness of arterial walls, they tend to maintain a constant shape and do not readily collapse in conjunction with low blood pressure.[3,4]

Because veins have less smooth muscle and elastic tissue, they are unable to contract to force through blood. Venous return to the heart is, therefore, accomplished through the pressure gradient difference between the arterial and venous network, breathing, and skeletal muscle contractions. Valves are also an important part of the veins located in the extremities. The circulatory network of blood vessels, the vasa vasorum, is located within their walls.[5]

Abdominal Aorta and Aortic Branches

Anatomy

The aorta is the main artery of the chest and abdomen from which all other branch vessels are derived. For reference purposes, the aorta is divided into segments along its path (Fig. 6-1).

The aorta originates from the left ventricle. As it leaves the heart, systemic circulation begins. The aorta arises from the left ventricular outflow tract and then courses slightly

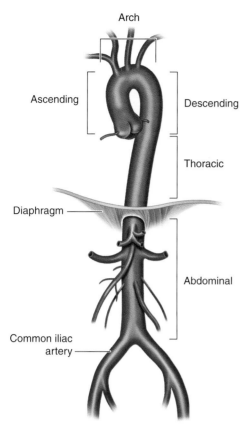

FIGURE 6-1 Segments of the aorta. The common reference segments, ascending, arch, descending, thoracic, and abdominal aorta can be identified on the illustration.

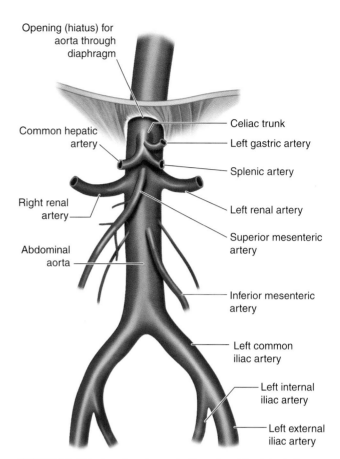

FIGURE 6-2 Major branches. An anterior illustration of the abdominal aorta showing the anatomic location of its major branches.

posterior, a short distance medial, and then superior to form the ascending aorta. It then curves lateral and posterior to form the aortic arch. As the aorta completes its curve at the arch, it begins to descend inferiorly into the chest. This portion, the descending aorta, soon gives rise to the thoracic aorta. Once the aorta penetrates the diaphragm, it is termed the *abdominal aorta* until it bifurcates into the common iliac arteries prior to entering the pelvic cavity. It is the abdominal aorta that is most accessible to sonographic examination (Fig. 6-2).

As it courses through the abdomen, several major vessels branch off of the abdominal aorta. The first branch is the celiac axis (CA; also known as the celiac trunk). It originates from the anterior aspect of the aorta and is usually found within the first 2 cm. The CA is a short vessel, approximately 1 cm long. It divides into three branches: (1) the hepatic artery, (2) the left gastric artery, and (3) the splenic artery.[3,4] The vessel may present with anatomic variations on the number of branches (Fig. 6-3A–C).

The hepatic artery leaves the CA at approximately a 90-degree angle, and it crosses the midline and courses toward the right side of the abdomen, following the upper border of the pancreatic head. At the duodenum, the hepatic artery turns anteriorly to enter the liver hilum, following the course of the main portal vein. Intrahepatically, the artery then divides into left and right branches at the portal fissure to supply the left and right hepatic lobes, respectively.[3,4,6,7] The left gastric artery initially has an anterior and a superior course from the CA. It then turns lateral to the left side of the abdomen to supply the stomach and esophagus with

blood.[3,4,6,7] The splenic artery takes a horizontal course from the CA and follows the upper margin of the pancreatic body posteriorly. Along its route to the spleen, it generates arterial branches to the stomach and pancreas.[3,4,6,7]

The second major branch vessel, the superior mesenteric artery (SMA), also originates from the anterior surface of the aorta approximately 1 to 2.5 cm distal to the CA (although this distance varies), and occasionally it may branch off of the CA. As it begins to course inferiorly, it travels posterior to the pancreatic body and anterior to the uncinate process. It then continues inferiorly, paralleling the aorta. The left renal vein, duodenum, and uncinate process pass between the SMA anteriorly and the aorta posteriorly. The *nutcracker phenomenon* refers to the compression of the left renal vein between the aorta and the SMA (like a nut in a nutcracker) (Fig. 6-4A). Several branches arise along the length of the SMA and are responsible for supplying the small and large bowel with blood (Fig. 6-3A–C).

The renal arteries are located just inferior to the SMA. The right renal artery tends to arise from the right lateral aspect of the aorta, whereas the left renal artery tends to arise from the left lateral or posterolateral aspect of the aorta. Both then course posterolaterally to enter the respective kidneys.[3,4,6,7]

The inferior mesenteric artery (IMA) is the last major branch to arise from the abdominal aorta before it bifurcates. It originates from the anterior aspect of the aorta and runs slightly inferiorly and to the left side of the abdomen. It is responsible for supplying the distal portion of the colon with blood.

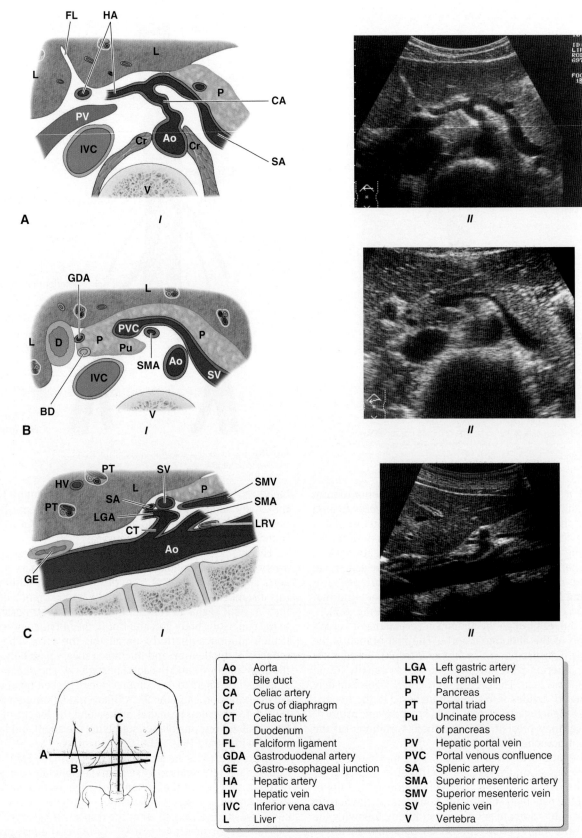

Ao	Aorta	LGA	Left gastric artery
BD	Bile duct	LRV	Left renal vein
CA	Celiac artery	P	Pancreas
Cr	Crus of diaphragm	PT	Portal triad
CT	Celiac trunk	Pu	Uncinate process
D	Duodenum		of pancreas
FL	Falciform ligament	PV	Hepatic portal vein
GDA	Gastroduodenal artery	PVC	Portal venous confluence
GE	Gastro-esophageal junction	SA	Splenic artery
HA	Hepatic artery	SMA	Superior mesenteric artery
HV	Hepatic vein	SMV	Superior mesenteric vein
IVC	Inferior vena cava	SV	Splenic vein
L	Liver	V	Vertebra

FIGURE 6-3 Relationships. The abdominal aorta and its branches are illustrated along with representative sonograms. **A:** The level of the transverse section is made through the celiac trunk. **B:** The level of the transverse section is made through the pancreas. **C:** The level of a longitudinal section is made through the upper aorta. (Reprinted with permission from Moore KL, Agur AMR, Dalley AF II. *Essential Clinical Anatomy.* 5th ed. Wolters Kluwer Health; 2015:191. See page 191 of resource book.)

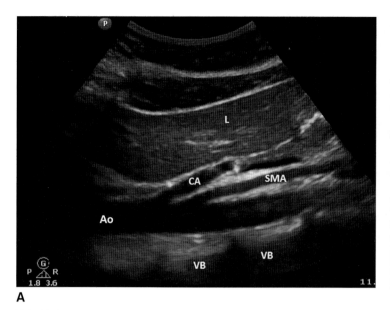

A

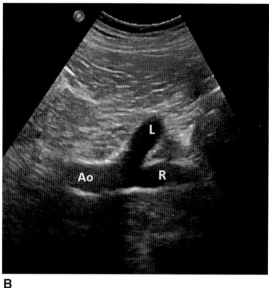

B

FIGURE 6-4 Longitudinal aorta. **A:** The longitudinal plane through the proximal abdominal aorta *(Ao)* demonstrating the celiac axis *(CA)* and superior mesenteric artery *(SMA)*. The liver *(L)* is anterior to the aorta, and the vertebral bodies *(VB)* are posterior to the aorta. **B:** With the patient positioned in a right lateral decubitus, the longitudinal plane demonstrates the bifurcation of the aorta into the right common *(R)* and left common *(L)* iliac artery at the level of the umbilicus.

At about the level of the umbilicus, the aorta bifurcates into the left and right common iliac arteries. The common iliac arteries are about 5 cm in length (right somewhat longer than the left) and course inferiorly and posteriorly until they branch into the external and internal (hypogastric) iliac arteries. As a result of their fairly deep location in the pelvis, the iliac arteries can be very difficult to image. Full bladder techniques as well as left and right lateral decubitus position may be necessary to visualize them (Fig. 6-4B).[3,4,6,7]

Sonographic Appearance

Sonographically, the lumen of the aorta and other vascular structures appear anechoic. It is important that the sonographer optimizes gain settings to demonstrate normal vessels as anechoic structures. In the longitudinal plane, slightly to the left of midline, the proximal aorta can be seen as an anechoic tubular structure following a somewhat anterior and inferior course within the abdomen. The spine lies immediately posterior to it, providing a highly reflective echo boundary. As the aorta courses inferiorly, it tapers and becomes smaller in caliber. In the proximal aspect of the aorta, both the CA and the SMA can be seen as they arise anteriorly. A longitudinal section provides the best scanning plane to image the proximity of the CA and SMA (see Figs. 6-3C and 6-4).

In transverse scan planes, the aorta takes on a more rounded appearance and again can be seen lying anterior to the spine. Because the transducer is moved inferiorly from the xiphoid process, the first aortic branch to be encountered is the CA. It appears as an anechoic tubular structure that divides into the hepatic artery and the splenic artery. If viewed in the appropriate plane, the image may resemble the spread wings of a seagull (see Fig. 6-3A). The hepatic artery branches off of the right side of the CA and can be followed transversely and superiorly as it travels to enter the liver hilum. The splenic artery branches off of the left side of the CA and courses to the left side of the abdomen to enter the splenic hilum (Fig. 6-5A). The splenic artery can be quite tortuous and is difficult to image in its entirety, especially in elderly patients.

The left gastric artery can occasionally be seen in its proximal aspect. This vessel, however, is usually smaller in caliber than the neighboring hepatic and splenic arteries and is more difficult to image consistently.

After moving the transducer inferiorly, the SMA can be seen. It appears rounded and is surrounded by an echodense collar consisting of mesentery and fat (see Fig. 6-3B).

Immediately inferior to the level of origin of the SMA are the origins of the renal arteries. They are best appreciated in the transverse plane because of their relationship to the acoustic beam. The renal arteries arise from the lateral aspect of the aorta and continue their course, respectively, to the right and left to enter the kidneys. From the right flank, a coronal plane shows the aorta and bilateral renal arteries and gives the appearance of a peeled banana (Fig. 6-5B, C). A transverse plane at this level can demonstrate the nutcracker phenomenon, with the left renal vein being compressed between the aorta and SMA (Fig. 6-5D).

The IMA can be seen approximately midway between the renal arteries and the aortic bifurcation arising antero-laterally from the aorta, sometimes having the appearance of pumpkin stem (Fig. 6-5E). Soon after its origin, the IMA makes an abrupt turn in the posteroinferior direction. High-frequency probes and compression of overlying bowel loops greatly facilitate visualization of this artery, as does color-flow Doppler.

At the level of the umbilicus, the right and left common iliac arteries can be seen as they arise from the aortic terminus as rounded and anechoic vessels emerging from a common source (distal aorta). In the longitudinal plane, the common iliac artery can be seen bifurcating into the external and internal (hypogastric) iliac arteries. Further,

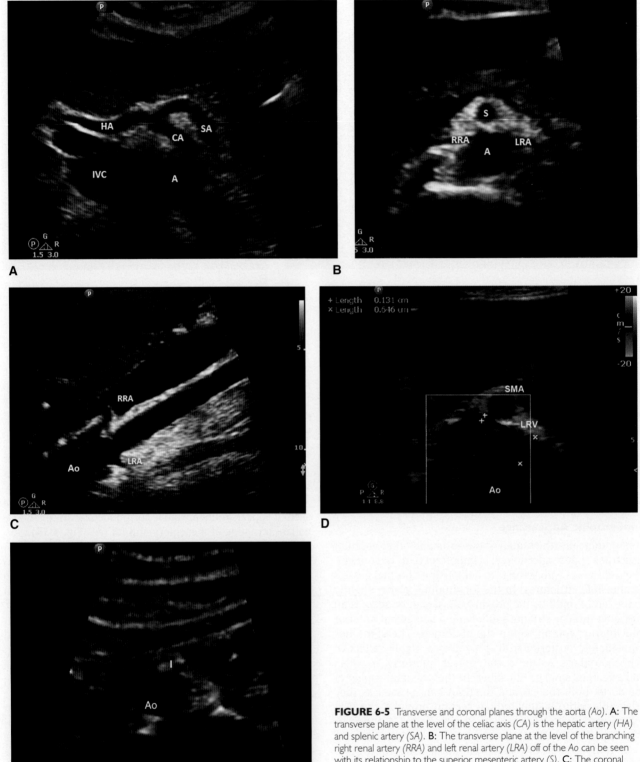

FIGURE 6-5 Transverse and coronal planes through the aorta *(Ao)*. **A:** The transverse plane at the level of the celiac axis *(CA)* is the hepatic artery *(HA)* and splenic artery *(SA)*. **B:** The transverse plane at the level of the branching right renal artery *(RRA)* and left renal artery *(LRA)* off of the *Ao* can be seen with its relationship to the superior mesenteric artery *(S)*. **C:** The coronal plane demonstrating the renal artery origins. This sonographic appearance is referred to as the "banana peel." **D:** The transverse image demonstrating the left renal vein *(LRV)* being compressed *(cursors)* between the *A* and superior mesenteric artery *(SMA)*, which is known as the "nutcracker phenomenon." **E:** Transverse image of the *Ao* and inferior mesenteric artery *(I)*. *IVC*, inferior vena cava.

more comprehensive imaging of the iliac arteries is accomplished by placing the transducer in the iliac fossa and angling medially with the scan plane oriented approximately 45 degrees from midline. Demonstration of the length of the iliac arteries is thus achieved. At times, successful imaging of the iliac arteries requires a distended urinary bladder. In this case, the transducer is placed in the midline of the pelvis and oriented 45 degrees from midline. Lateral angulation will result in visualization of the iliac vessels.

Abdominal Veins

Anatomy

The IVC is the large vessel that returns blood to the right atrium from the lower limbs, pelvis, and abdomen. It is formed by the junction of the paired common iliac veins slightly anterior and to the right of the fifth lumbar (L5) vertebral body. The IVC travels superiorly in the abdomen, enters the thoracic cavity and then the right atrium at the level of the eighth thoracic (T8) vertebral body. As the vena cava nears the heart, it courses somewhat anteriorly to form a hockey stick–like configuration before it terminates in the right atrium (Fig. 6-6A, B).

There are many tributaries to the IVC, but most cannot be seen because of their small size. The veins most consistently seen entering the IVC are the common iliac veins at its formation, the renal veins, and the hepatic veins. The right renal vein is generally shorter than the left renal vein because of the right kidney's proximity to the IVC. The left renal vein traverses the abdomen, coursing anterior to the aorta and posterior to the SMA to finally enter the lateral aspect of the IVC.

The hepatic veins also drain directly into the IVC or right atrium. Normally, there are three hepatic veins: (1) the left, (2) the right, and (3) the middle (Fig. 6-7).

Sonographic Appearance

Sonographically, the IVC is an anechoic structure slightly to the right of midline. Unlike the aorta, which has a relatively consistent diameter and a rounded appearance in the

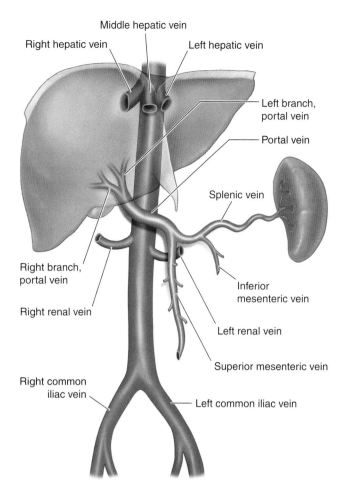

FIGURE 6-7 Abdominal veins. The most often sonographically visualized veins and their relationships are depicted on the illustration of the inferior vena cava, its tributaries, and the formation of the portal venous system.

transverse plane, the IVC tends to have a more oval shape. It also responds to respiratory variations. During inspiration, the IVC collapses, owing to the decreased pressure within the thoracic cavity, allowing prompt blood flow from the IVC into the right atrium. The opposite is true for expiration

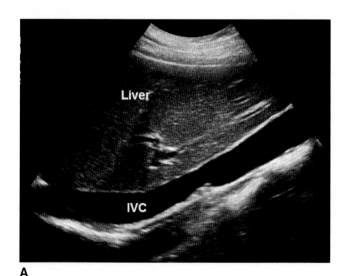

A

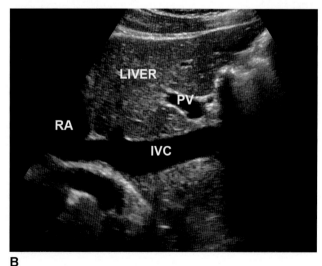

B

FIGURE 6-6 Normal inferior vena cava *(IVC)*. **A:** A longitudinal sonogram through the IVC demonstrating the hockey stick configuration as the vessel as it nears the right atrium *(RA)*. **B:** Image displaying the relationship of the IVC draining into the RA. *PV*, portal vein. (**A:** Courtesy of Philips Medical System, Bothell, WA.)

in which the IVC expands during this maneuver. With suspended inspiration, the IVC expands because of increased intrathoracic pressure and decreased blood flow into the heart. During the Valsalva maneuver, the IVC collapses because of the increased abdominal pressure associated with this technique.[8,9]

The hepatic veins are best demonstrated in a transverse plane with the transducer just inferior to the xiphoid process and angled cephalic. Identification of the right, middle, and left hepatic veins is relatively easy because they converge to empty into the IVC (Fig. 6-8A). Partial imaging of the right hepatic vein with simultaneous imaging of the middle and left hepatic veins will result in a rabbit ear appearance (Playboy Bunny sign).

Optimal imaging of the renal veins is also accomplished using a transverse scanning approach. The renal veins should be visualized at about the same level as the renal arteries (just inferior to the origin of the SMA) (Fig. 6-8B). The right renal vein is best imaged with the transducer placed in the right lateral abdomen over the right kidney and angled medially. The renal vein is identified as an echo-free tube exiting the renal hilum. When attempting to visualize the left renal vein, the transducer is placed (in a transverse orientation) in the midline of the abdomen just inferior to the SMA origin. The left renal vein is seen as an anechoic tubular structure coursing between the SMA and the aorta to enter the lateral aspect of the IVC.

Portal Venous System Anatomy

The portal venous system is composed of the veins that drain blood from the bowel and spleen and is separated from the IVC.

The main portal vein is formed at the junction of the splenic vein and the superior mesenteric vein, which can be identified with sonography in most patients (see Fig. 6-7).

To image the portal venous system, it is easiest to begin by placing the transducer in the midline of the abdomen substernally with a transverse orientation. The splenic vein can be used as an initial reference point because it is easily seen in this plane. The splenic vein emerges from the splenic hilum and courses medially and superiorly within the abdomen, bordering the posterior surface of the pancreatic body and tail. It is identified sonographically as a tubular structure with a superomedial course within the abdomen coursing anterior to the SMA as it nears the midline. At its termination, the splenic vein can be seen to increase in diameter. This is the point at which the splenic vein merges with the superior mesenteric vein to form the main portal vein (Fig. 6-9A). The junction of the superior mesenteric vein and the splenic vein is known as the *portal confluence*, and this confluence is immediately posterior to the neck of the pancreas. Visualization of the superior mesenteric vein is accomplished by placing the transducer over the portal confluence (transverse orientation) and rotating the transducer 90 degrees. The length of the superior mesenteric vein will be displayed having a longitudinal course within the abdomen that parallels that of the IVC posteriorly (Fig. 6-9B).

The main portal vein travels somewhat obliquely and anteriorly within the abdomen before it enters the liver hilum (Fig. 6-9C). Placement of the transducer over the portal confluence and subsequent clockwise rotation eventually demonstrates the portal vein in its long axis. It can then be followed into the liver where it soon divides into left and right branches.

Other vessels contributing to portal venous circulation include the inferior mesenteric vein, coronary vein, pyloric vein, cystic vein, and paraumbilical veins. These generally are not seen on routine abdominal examinations but may be identified in abnormal states and are discussed later in this chapter.

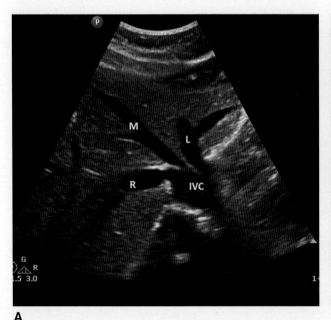

A

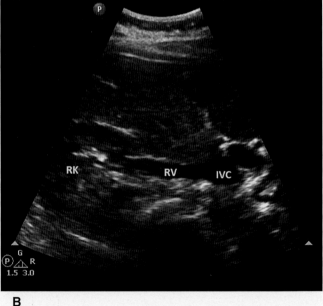

B

FIGURE 6-8 Transverse sections. **A:** A transverse plane through the liver showing the right hepatic vein *(R)*, middle hepatic vein *(M)*, and left hepatic vein *(L)*, and they drain into the inferior vena cava *(IVC)*. **B:** A transverse plane through the right kidney *(RK)* demonstrating the right renal vein *(RV)* as it drains into the IVC.

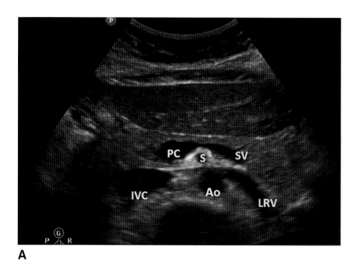

A

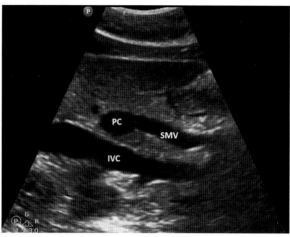

B

C

FIGURE 6-9 Portal system. **A:** Transverse sonogram through the upper abdomen showing the splenic vein *(SV)* as it converges with the superior mesenteric vein to form the portal confluence *(PC)*, the beginning of the portal vein. **B:** The longitudinal sonogram demonstrating the superior mesenteric vein *(SMV)* as it courses parallel to the inferior vena cava *(IVC)* which is seen posterior. **C:** An oblique plane through the right upper quadrant visualizes the portal vein *(PV)* as it enters the liver and branches into the right portal vein *(RPV)* and the left portal vein *(LPV)*. Ao, aorta; *LRV*, left renal vein. (**C:** Courtesy of Philips Medical System, Bothell, WA.)

Relational Anatomy of the Arteries and Veins

To perform sonography, it is clinically useful to know the relationship of abdominal arteries and veins to each other as well as to the ducts and organs.[10] Figure 6-10 illustrates the information summarized in Table 6-1.

ARTERIAL ABNORMALITIES

Atherosclerosis

Description

Atherosclerosis is a form of arteriosclerosis in which the intimal lining of the arteries is altered by the presence of any combination of focal accumulation of lipids, complex carbohydrates, blood and blood products, fibrous tissue, and/or calcium deposits. The media of the arterial wall is also changed (Fig. 6-11).[11]

Etiology

The cause is not known, but several factors have been linked to the progression of atherosclerosis and they include hyperlipidemia, hypertension, cigarette smoking, and diabetes mellitus.[12]

Clinical Signs and Symptoms

Generally, there are no symptoms of atherosclerosis until a significant stenosis develops. Then, symptoms vary and are related to the particular stenotic vessel. These are discussed later. Atherosclerotic disease also disposes to the development of aneurysms. There are generally no symptoms unless complications arise because they are often diagnosed as a result of screening or other imaging studies.

Sonographic Appearance

The sonographic findings of atherosclerosis include luminal irregularities (representative of the various changes of the intimal lining of the artery), tortuosity, and vessel wall calcification.

The wall irregularities detected by sonography can be seen as low-level echoes along the internal walls of the aorta with a propensity for development at the areas of bifurcation or the branch vessels.[1,13] In and of themselves, these areas of plaque formation are not terribly important unless they produce hemodynamically significant stenosis of a particular

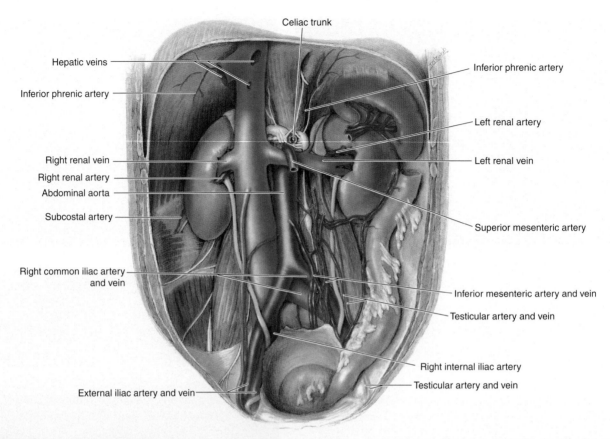

FIGURE 6-10 Relationships. Collective illustration of the major branches of the aorta, inferior vena cava, and the portal system helps visualize the abdominal vascular and organ relationships.

TABLE 6-1	**Relational Anatomy**
Vessels	**Relational Anatomy**[a]
Aorta	Anterior to the spine Left of the inferior vena cava More posterior proximally than distally
Inferior vena cava	Anterior to the spine Right of the aorta Courses anteriorly to enter right atrium
Hepatic artery	Anterior to the portal vein Left of the common bile duct Superior to the head of the pancreas
Splenic artery	Superior to the body and tail of the pancreas
Superior mesenteric artery	Posterior to the body of the pancreas and the splenic vein Anterior to the aorta
Right renal artery	Posterior to the inferior vena cava
Splenic vein	Posterior to the body and tail of the pancreas Inferior to the splenic artery
Superior mesenteric vein	Right of and parallel to the superior mesenteric artery
Left renal vein	Anterior to the aorta Posterior to the superior mesenteric artery Anterior to the right renal artery
Portal vein	Anterior to the inferior vena cava
Common bile duct	Anterior to the portal vein Right of the hepatic artery

[a]The left and right directional terms refer to the patient's anatomy.

branch artery. Detection of a hemodynamically significant stenosis is discussed in detail later in this chapter.

In elderly persons, tortuosity of the aorta is often seen leftward in the patient but occasionally can be right sided.[6] Imaging of the vessel is best carried out in the transverse plane because this affords a clearer picture of the course of a tortuous aorta.

Aortic wall calcification is easily detected as an echogenic focus in the arterial wall, which at times may produce acoustic shadows.

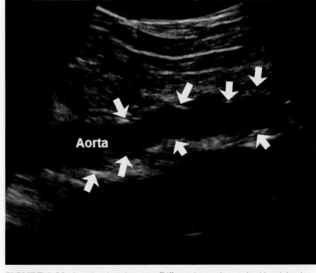

FIGURE 6-11 Arteriosclerotic aorta. Diffuse plaque (*arrows*) with minimal acoustic shadowing can be seen in the longitudinal sonogram through the distal portion of an aorta. (Image courtesy of Philips Medical System, Bothell, WA.)

Aneurysms of the Abdominal Aorta

Description

An aneurysm is a focal abnormal dilatation of a blood vessel caused by a structural weakness in its wall. True aneurysms involve all three layers of the arterial wall. A false aneurysm (also called a pseudoaneurysm) is an extravascular hematoma communicating with the intravascular space. A saccular aneurysm is a saclike protrusion of the aorta toward one side or the other, is usually larger than a circumferential, and is connected to the aorta by a channel or an opening that varies in size. Most true aneurysms are fusiform and circumferential. A fusiform aneurysm is a gradual and progressive dilatation of the complete circumference of the vessel, which varies in diameter and length. A dissecting aneurysm is when a longitudinal tear in the arterial wall allows bleeding to occur into the wall. Saccular and circumferential aneurysms occur more often in the abdominal aorta, whereas dissecting aneurysms are less common and occur more often in the thoracic aorta (Fig. 6-12). Most abdominal aortic aneurysms occur below the level of the renal arteries.[12]

Etiology

Smoking is a risk factor for aneurysm as well as atherosclerosis. Syphilis and other diseases can cause aneurysms, although these are not very common causes.[2,12]

Clinical Signs and Symptoms

Generally, patients with aneurysms are asymptomatic, and the presence of an aneurysm is suspected during palpation of a pulsating mass in the region of the umbilicus, or by calcification seen on an abdominal radiograph. Patients with an expanding aneurysm may have vague lower back or abdominal pain.[2]

Sonographic Appearance

At the diaphragm, normal aortic diameters have been cited at approximately 2.5 cm.[6] During its course, inferiorly the aorta tapers, reaching a diameter of about 1.5 to 2.0 cm at the level of the iliac arteries.[6] Ectasia of the aorta, as seen with atherosclerosis, is manifested by a slight widening of the normal aortic diameter up to 3.0 cm. There are also aortic wall irregularities, owing to the atherosclerotic changes that take place in this disease process. A true aneurysm is identified sonographically as a dilatation of the aorta ≥3.0 cm near its bifurcation point, a focal dilatation along the course of the aorta, or lack of normal tapering of the aorta.[14-17]

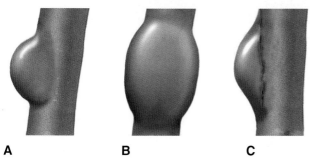

FIGURE 6-12 Aneurysms. The illustration presents three types of true aneurysms: **(A)** saccular, **(B)** fusiform, circumferential, and **(C)** dissecting.

Aneurysms vary in size and can range from 3 to 20 cm as a result of the abnormal blood flow patterns within an aneurysm. If thrombus is formed, it can usually be detected by sonographic techniques and is a common finding. Sonographically, thrombus typically produces a low-level echo pattern and tends to accumulate along the anterior and lateral walls of the aortic lumen (Fig. 6-13A–H).[14,15] Adequate demonstration of the thrombus may require that gain settings be increased from initial settings to display the low-level echoes associated with thrombus. It may also be necessary to scan coronally or obliquely through the aorta to demonstrate thrombus. These maneuvers may help reduce confusion between reverberation artifacts and actual thrombus. Occasionally, there may be calcification within the thrombus. An interesting phenomenon that has been reported in association with aortic aneurysm thrombus is that of an anechoic crescent sign (Fig. 6-13C). In these instances, the anechoic area within the lumen of the aneurysm was found at surgery to be serosanguineous fluid or liquefying clot. When evaluating the aorta for aneurysm formation, it is important to distinguish this finding from aortic dissection because the surgical treatments are different.

Thrombus within the aorta may be difficult at times to visualize, especially in an obese or a gassy patient. Anterior reverberation artifacts from a calcific anterior aortic wall may obscure the clot as well. Instances have been reported in which an obstruction clot of the aorta was not detected sonographically.[18] If an obstructing clot is suspected on clinical grounds, Doppler examination of the aorta can confirm the presence or absence of flow within it, thereby solving the problem (Fig. 6-13D).

If an aneurysm is detected during sonographic examination, it is prudent to attempt to identify the origins of the renal arteries as well as to extend the examination to the iliac arteries to look for aneurysmal involvement in these areas.

Associated renal artery aneurysm in conjunction with abdominal aortic aneurysm has been reported to be 1% or less.[19] Nonetheless, it is important for the surgeon to know of this coexistence because of the difference in treatment procedures. When the renal arteries are involved in an aneurysm, renal artery enlargement generally coexists with aortic dilatation. Demonstration of this complication, however, can be quite difficult because large aneurysms tend to displace surrounding bowel superiorly and subsequently cover the renal artery origins.[19] Consequently, diligent scanning techniques involving multiple patient positions and numerous transducer angulations may be necessary before adequate visualization of the renal artery origins is achieved. Color-flow Doppler may also aid visualization of the renal arteries in such patients. If efforts to identify the renal arteries are unsuccessful, an attempt should be made to visualize the SMA. Because of the proximity of the renal arteries to the SMA, any aneurysm shown to involve the SMA also involves the renal arteries.

Abdominal aneurysms may also extend into the iliac arteries. When this occurs, the iliac arteries will be abnormally dilated, and the thrombus may or may not be present in the dilated areas. Isolated iliac artery aneurysms are an occasional finding.[2] On occasion, aneurysm thrombosis may lead to peripheral thromboembolism or acute limb ischemia.

The accuracy rate for the sonographic detection of aortic aneurysms approaches 100% in most reports.[5,20-22] Because of this, sonography is a very good screening tool as the first step

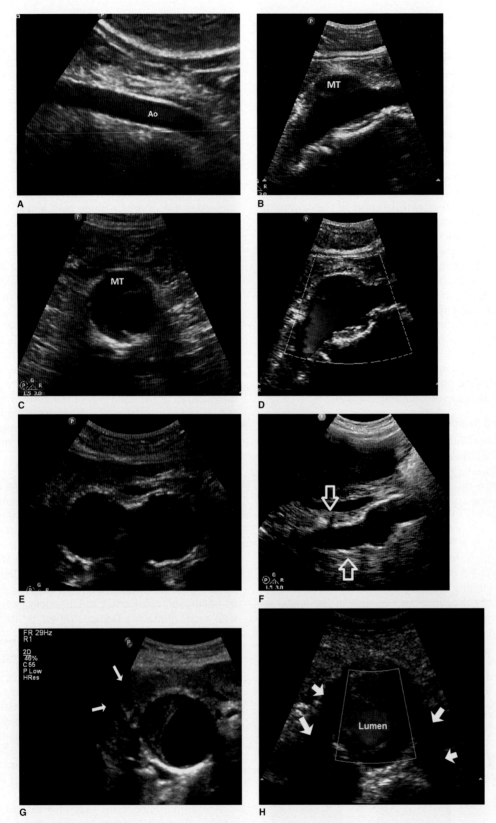

FIGURE 6-13 Aneurysms. **A:** The longitudinal plane sonogram demonstrating a normal caliber aorta (*Ao*). **B:** The longitudinal section demonstrating an abdominal aortic aneurysm with mural thrombus (*MT*). **C:** On the same patient, the transducer is turned 90 degrees from the longitudinal plane for a transverse image of the aneurysm. The mural thrombus has the appearance of a crescent sign because the thrombus has begun to liquefy. **D:** Doppler instrumentation aids in proving blood flow as well as visualizing subtle mural thrombus compared to the total size of the aneurysm. **E:** Longitudinal image demonstrating juxtarenal and infrarenal aortic aneurysms. **F:** The sonogram obtained with a coronal plane demonstrating the renal artery origins (*arrows*) proving infrarenal aneurysm. **G, H:** These transverse sonograms display an abdominal aortic aneurysm. **G:** A transverse sonogram demonstrates the anechoic crescent sign (*arrows*) due to the area within the thrombus that has liquefied. **H:** A transverse sonogram with color Doppler provides evidence of blood flow as well as the residual lumen compared to the total size of the aneurysm. On both sides of the vessel, refraction creates shadowing artifacts (*arrows*). (**G** and **H:** Courtesy of Philips Medical System, Bothell, WA.)

in the evaluation of suspected aortic aneurysm and can be used to monitor the growth of aneurysms over time.[23] However, there are some important considerations to keep in mind to avoid misdiagnosis of an aneurysm. Tortuosity may make the aortic diameter appear larger than it is. This occurs when the plane of imaging is not truly perpendicular to the aortic walls. Therefore, careful observations should be made of the aortic curvature in these instances to avoid misrepresentation of a tortuous aortic segment as an aortic aneurysm. Excessive air in the abdomen or obesity may obscure the distal aorta and iliac vessels and render some aneurysms invisible. Lymphadenopathy may also confound the picture.[21,22]

Normally, the abundant lymph nodes that are linked together chainlike along the anterior and lateral aspects of the aorta are invisible sonographically. When enlarged, however, their appearance can be dramatic—and initially confusing. Sonographically, enlarged lymph nodes are echo poor, but with increased gain settings, fine internal echoes may be appreciated. Several patterns of lymph node enlargement have been described: isolated large masses, which tend to develop along the aortic chain; mantle-like distributions of enlarged nodes draped atop the aorta and IVC; symmetric nodal enlargement along the aortic chain bilaterally; multiple spindle-shaped nodes dispersed in the mesentery; and large, confluent masses surrounding the aorta and IVC.[14] It is conceivable that the mantle-like configurations and the confluent mass effects may be confused with aortic aneurysm with thrombus. Close inspection of the area should reveal linear separations between lymph node masses. In addition, the general appearance of extensive lymph node enlargement seems to be slightly more irregular, or "lumpy," than an aortic aneurysm. The most reliable and accurate tool to use to determine artery versus vein versus lymph node is to Doppler sample for the presence or absence of arterial or venous flow patterns.

The rates with which sonography can accurately detect renal artery involvement and other abnormalities (ruptured aneurysm) are unfortunately not as high as those for aneurysm detection. Therefore, other diagnostic imaging tests may be necessary to further evaluate these complications if they are suspected.[24]

Although other imaging procedures may be the primary tool used to evaluate the extent of various aortic pathologies, sonographic evaluation is a sensitive and specific imaging technique of choice for screening patients suspected of having aortic aneurysms. The sonographic measurements are accurate, repeatable, and noninvasive and do not involve ionizing radiation.[20,25]

Aortic Dissection

Description

In aortic dissection, there is a separation of the layers of the arterial wall by blood or hemorrhage, which generally begins in the proximal portion of the aorta. According to the DeBakey model, there are three types of dissections (Fig. 6-14). Type I and type II involve the ascending aorta and the aortic arch, and type III involves the descending aorta at a level below the left subclavian artery. There is a high incidence of mortality with type I and type II dissections because of the propensity of the dissection to extend into

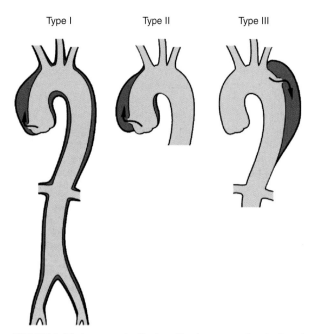

Type I   Type II   Type III

FIGURE 6-14 Aneurysm classifications. The three types of aortic dissections illustrated were categorized by DeBakey.

the pericardium. Once dissection has begun, it may extend for varying distances along the length of the aorta.[26] The Stanford classification is used to separate aortic dissections into those that need surgical repair and those that usually require only medical management. The Stanford classification divides dissections by the most proximal involvement. Type A "**a**ffects **a**scending **a**orta" and requires surgical management. Type B "**b**egins **b**eyond the **b**rachiocephalic vessels" and is treated with medical management with blood pressure control. Dissections that involve the aortic arch but not the ascending aorta have been addressed in the American surgical consensus 2020.[27]

Etiology

The etiology of aortic dissection is not clear. Presumably, the dissection results from a tear of the intimal lining of the aorta. It has been demonstrated, however, that this is not always the case, and postulation has been made that rupture of the vasa vasorum can initiate a dissection.[12,27] Hypertension is strongly associated with dissections, and cystic medial necrosis of the vessel is also well recognized as an underlying cause. Other entities that contribute to aortic dissection include Marfan syndrome, pregnancy, aortic valve disease, congenital cardiac anomalies (coarctation, aortic hypoplasia, bicuspid aortic valve, persistent patent ductus arteriosus, atrial septal defect, and tricuspid valve abnormalities), Cushing syndrome, pheochromocytoma, and catheter-induced needle wounds.[12,27–29]

Clinical Signs and Symptoms

Intense chest pain is the most common symptom of aortic dissection. Abdominal, as well as lower back, arm, or leg, pain may occur, depending on the extent of the dissection. There may also be vomiting, paralysis, transient blindness, coma, confusion, syncope, headache, and dyspnea, and extremity pulses may be absent.[26,27,29]

Sonographic Appearance

Sonographically, aortic dissection appears as a thin, linear echo flap within the arterial lumen (Fig. 6-15).[30] Because of the presence of blood flow along both sides of the dissection, there is usually motion of the flap with each cardiac cycle. Doppler interrogation is an additional diagnostic aid, providing demonstration of arterial blood flow on both sides of the flap. When evaluating a patient for aortic dissection, it is important to utilize both longitudinal and transverse imaging planes to carefully examine the aorta because an intimal flap can be overlooked if it is located laterally in the artery.[26]

Aortic Rupture

Description

Abdominal aortic aneurysms of any size may rupture, but the risk increases with aneurysms larger than 7 cm in diameter.[21,31,32] Most aneurysms rupture into the peritoneal space, with no predilection for a specific site. They may also rupture into the duodenum, left renal vein, IVC, or urinary tract. An aortic rupture is a medical emergency because the mortality rate for untreated aortic rupture is virtually 100%; with surgery, the mortality rate ranges between 40% and 60%.[33]

Clinical Signs and Symptoms

Typically, aortic rupture presents clinically as central back pain and hypotension.[6,12]

Sonographic Appearance

Because of the leakage of blood outside the vessel, aortic rupture may be diagnosed by identification of a hematoma in the abdomen in association with aneurysmal dilatation of the aorta. These hematomas may be located close to the aorta or may extend to varying degrees through the retroperitoneum. Aortic rupture may appear in a variety of stages, from a completely cystic mass to a complex mass. If large enough, the hematomas may also displace surrounding

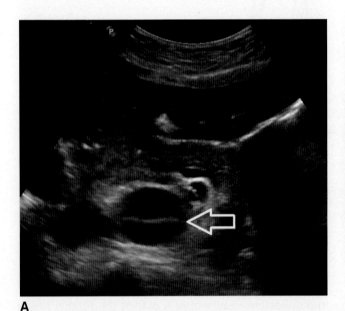

A

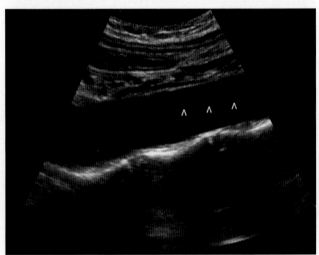

B

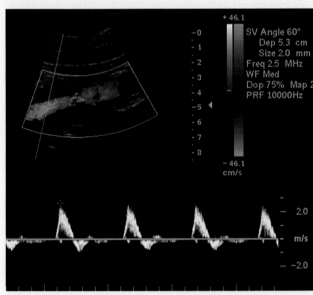

C

FIGURE 6-15 Dissecting aneurysm. **A:** A transverse sonogram of the aorta demonstrating a linear flap (arrow) with the arterial lumen consistent with dissection. **B:** On a longitudinal sonogram through an abdominal aorta, a thin linear echo flap (carets) is noted paralleling the anterior wall. **C:** The Doppler interrogation showing narrowing of an aorta flow with increased speed. (**A:** Courtesy of Jill Langer, MD, Hospital of University of Pennsylvania, Philadelphia, PA. **B** and **C:** Courtesy of Philips Medical System, Bothell, WA.)

organs and structures.[12] Other findings suggestive of aortic aneurysm rupture include irregular intra-abdominal fluid collections in association with aortic aneurysm and diffuse irregular hypoechoic areas near an aortic aneurysm.

It is difficult to identify the actual rupture site by sonographic examination, although they may be inferred by hematoma "geography." Computed tomography (CT), on the other hand, is well suited for the detection of aortic rupture and is the diagnostic test of choice because it allows for clear depiction of the extent and density of the hematoma as well as the site of rupture.[34] For high-risk patients, contrast-enhanced three-dimensional magnetic resonance angiography (MRA) is a preferred and accurate examination with iodinated contrast material or carbon dioxide contrast agents.[35]

Inflammatory Aneurysms

Description

Inflammatory aneurysms are enveloped by a dense, fibrotic reaction, generally including many inflammatory cell infiltrates and fatty tissue. This fibrotic reaction is also vascular in nature and involves the retroperitoneum to different degrees. The inflammatory reaction around the aneurysm may become adherent to the duodenum, sigmoid colon, small bowel, ureter, iliac vein, and IVC.[36–39]

Inflammatory aneurysms are an uncommon entity, reportedly between 5% and 20% of all aortic aneurysms.[37] They tend to occur in relatively younger persons than arteriosclerotic aneurysms. Even though the risk of rupture is less than that of a "normal" aneurysm, rupture is still a possible scenario.

Etiology

The cause of inflammatory aneurysms is uncertain, but because they are always seen in the presence of aneurysm, it has been postulated that the aneurysm itself may be the cause of the inflammatory reaction.[36,38]

Clinical Signs and Symptoms

Clinically, the symptoms of inflammatory aneurysms are similar to those of aortic aneurysm. Other symptoms may develop in accordance with the extent of inflammatory involvement to the neighboring areas. These may include leg edema, bothersome pulsations in the epigastrium, and constipation. Hydronephrosis with concomitant flank pain may develop in the presence of ureteral obstruction, and there may be anorexia, early satiety, and dyspnea if bowel adheres to the aneurysmal inflammation.[38,40]

Sonographic Appearance

Typically, the sonographic features of an inflammatory aneurysm include aneurysmal dilatation of the aorta with a hypoechoic mantle, usually seen anterior and lateral to a thickened aortic wall.[36–38] CT can also demonstrate this phenomenon, and it is actually better able to depict the extension of the inflammatory process to the surrounding structures in the retroperitoneum.[37]

It is important to distinguish inflammatory aneurysms from a condition known as retroperitoneal fibrosis.[36] Whereas inflammatory aneurysms are always associated with an aortic aneurysm, retroperitoneal fibrosis is not. In addition, the makeup of the two fibrotic reactions is somewhat different. The symptoms of retroperitoneal fibrosis generally do not occur until there is vascular or ureteral compromise. Sonographically, it appears as an echo-free area around the anterior and lateral aspects of the aorta, similar to that seen in association with inflammatory aneurysms, although no aneurysm is present.[41]

AORTIC BRANCH VESSEL ANEURYSMS

Splanchnic Artery Aneurysms

Splenic Artery Aneurysms

Description

Splenic artery aneurysms are the most common type of splanchnic artery aneurysm. These usually occur in the middle to distal aspect of the splenic artery. There is apparently a female preponderance. Splenic artery aneurysms, although not very common, are life threatening (Fig. 6-16A–C).[40,42]

Etiology

The causes of splenic artery aneurysm encompass fibromuscular disease of the renal arteries, pancreatic inflammation, peptic ulcer disease, primary arterial injury, and mycotic lesions. There is also a greater potential for patients with portal hypertension and multigravidas to develop splenic artery aneurysms.[32,40,42,43]

Clinical Signs and Symptoms

The symptoms vary and may range from none to nonspecific left side upper quadrant pain, nausea, vomiting, and a palpable mass if the aneurysm is large enough. There is about a 10% risk of rupture of a splenic artery aneurysm into the peritoneal cavity, with a lesser incidence of rupture into the gastrointestinal tract, spleen, or pancreas.[40]

Hepatic Artery Aneurysms

Description

Hepatic artery aneurysms are the second most common type of splanchnic vessel aneurysms encountered. About 75% of all hepatic aneurysms are extrahepatic in origin. The remaining 25% occur intrahepatically, the right hepatic arterial branch being more often affected than the left.[44,45] Hepatic artery aneurysms are rare and tend to male preponderance (Fig. 6-17).[40,42]

Etiology

The most common causes of reported hepatic arterial aneurysms are systemic infection, arteriosclerosis, and blunt abdominal trauma. Other less common causes include iatrogenic trauma, vasculitis as a result of pancreatitis, chronic cholecystitis, polyarteritis, and congenital abnormalities.[45–49]

Clinical Signs and Symptoms

Generally, hepatic artery aneurysms are silent or asymptomatic until the aneurysm attains a large size or tapers. When symptoms do occur, they are often vague and unclear and may include epigastric pain (two-thirds of patients), gastrointestinal bleeding because of rupture of the aneurysm into the biliary tract and resulting hemobilia, or obstructive jaundice.[45,46] Because of the propensity of hepatic artery

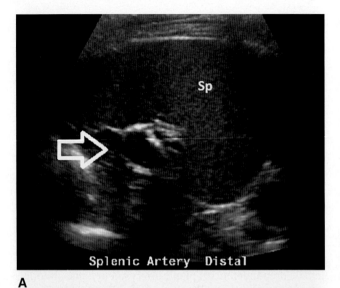

A

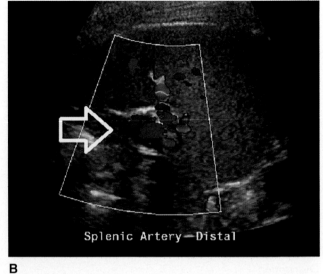

B

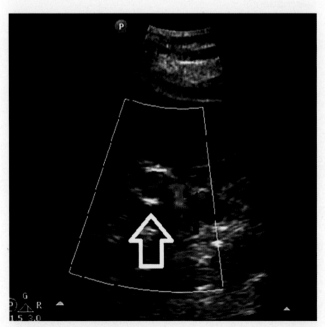

C

FIGURE 6-16 Splenic artery aneurysm. **A:** The sonogram demonstrating the spleen *(Sp)* and a splenic artery aneurysm *(arrow)* near the hilum. **B:** The color Doppler image demonstrating flow within the splenic artery aneurysm *(arrow)*. **C:** A calcified splenic artery aneurysm *(cursors)* with measurements can be identified on the two sonograms.

FIGURE 6-17 Hepatic artery aneurysm. The color Doppler sonogram demonstrates a hepatic artery aneurysm *(arrow)*.

aneurysms to rupture, early detection is important so that prompt treatment can be obtained.

Superior Mesenteric Artery Aneurysms

Description

SMA aneurysms are the rarest of the splanchnic arterial aneurysms (reported incidence approximately 1 in 12,000). Branch SMA aneurysms are also quite rare.[40,42]

Etiology

The most common cause that has been cited in the pathogenesis of SMA aneurysms is cystic medial necrosis (mycotic aneurysm), which accounts for approximately 58% of the aneurysms detected. Arteriosclerosis, medial degeneration, and trauma have also been associated with SMA aneurysms.[42]

Clinical Signs and Symptoms

There may be intestinal angina and postprandial abdominal pain in association with an SMA aneurysm. General abdominal pain and fever (in association with mycotic aneurysms) may also be present.[40,42] Again, as with the other splanchnic vessel aneurysms, the symptoms are generally vague and nonspecific.

Sonographic Appearance of Splanchnic Artery Aneurysms

Sonographically, splanchnic artery aneurysms appear similar to one another. The distinguishing feature is location in the abdomen. All splanchnic aneurysms may appear as an anechoic or a complex abdominal mass. Arterial pulsations or thrombus may or may not be discernable.[50] By demonstrating continuity of the mass with one of the splanchnic arteries, splanchnic artery aneurysms can be identified with a higher degree of confidence, but this is a difficult task to accomplish. Therefore, in order to confirm or refute the vascular nature of the lesion, Doppler sonography should always be used to further investigate an anechoic or a complex mass in the upper abdomen. In the case of a splanchnic artery aneurysm, the Doppler signal demonstrates arterial pulsations. Color-flow Doppler technology is also of benefit in this type of setting because the characteristic swirling blood flow patterns in these aneurysms are easily recognized.

Renal Artery Aneurysms

Description

Renal artery aneurysms have been encountered with increasing frequency, although the overall incidence remains relatively low.[51] Most renal artery aneurysms tend to be extrarenal, but there are reports of intrarenal aneurysms. Generally, surgical intervention is required in the presence of aneurysms greater than 1.5 cm and if there is associated pain, bleeding, or hypertension. The prevalence of renal artery aneurysm rupture is about 20%.[2]

Etiology

Renal artery aneurysms are most commonly a result of atherosclerosis and polyarteritis, and represent true aneurysms; congenital abnormalities account for a relatively smaller portion of them. Aneurysms resulting from iatrogenic trauma, blunt trauma, or penetrating trauma are considered false aneurysms and tend to be among the least common types.[2]

Clinical Signs and Symptoms

The symptoms encountered with renal artery aneurysm may include a palpable mass, hypertension, and blood in the urine along with flank pain.[2]

Sonographic Appearance

A renal artery aneurysm appears as an anechoic mass along the extent of the renal artery, or occasionally intrarenally. Calcification of the wall may be present, and other findings may or may not include thrombus formation along the periphery of the mass and pulsations. Demonstrating continuity of the mass with the renal artery is a useful indicator of renal artery aneurysm. Doppler interrogations are an excellent method of distinguishing the vascular nature of a suspicious mass in this area because renal artery aneurysms will demonstrate arterial blood flow signals. Color-flow Doppler can also rapidly demonstrate blood flow within an aneurysm (Fig. 6-18A, B).

Care must be taken in the evaluation of renal artery aneurysms because it is possible to mistake a normal left renal vein for a left renal artery aneurysm, especially in thin patients.[2] This is because of the fact that the left renal vein is prominent as it exits the renal hilum, but as it passes over the aorta to enter the IVC, it narrows. At this point, part of the aortic wall may not be visualized owing to the angle of incident sound beam, and subsequently, the renal vein may appear to arise from the aorta. In order to clarify this situation, it may be helpful to study the area in question during suspended inspiration. If the structure is truly venous, the entire venous path should dilate, affording better visualization. If the vessel is arterial, inspiration techniques will not affect its size. Doppler investigation is probably the method of choice to determine the nature of the area in question. If the "mass" is found to have characteristic continuous low-velocity flow, it is most likely the renal vein. If arterial pulsations can be detected, the vessel is most likely the renal artery.

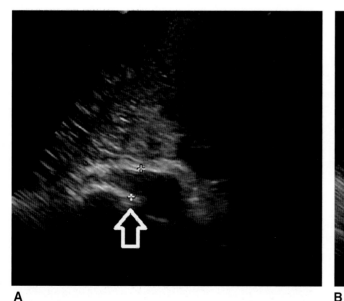

A

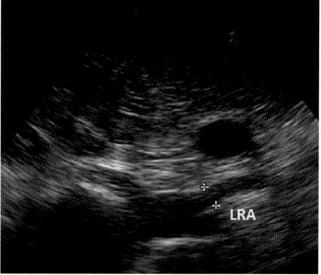

B

FIGURE 6-18 Renal artery aneurysm. **A:** A right renal artery aneurysm *(calipers)* at the vessel origin *(arrow)*. **B:** On the same patient, the left renal artery *(LRA)* origin is normal.

Iliac Artery Aneurysms

Description

Iliac artery aneurysms are most often associated with (continuations of) abdominal aortic aneurysms. Isolated iliac aneurysms are possible, however, and when they occur, they tend to be bilateral. Isolated internal iliac aneurysms are rare. Half of all untreated iliac aneurysms rupture, making this the most common complication of iliac aneurysms.[2,52]

Etiology

Most iliac aneurysms are arteriosclerotic in origin. Other less common causes include external or surgical trauma, pregnancy, congenital abnormality, syphilis, and bacterial infection.[2,52]

Clinical Signs and Symptoms

Iliac artery aneurysms typically go unrecognized clinically and are often discovered unexpectedly. Because of compression on surrounding structures, large iliac aneurysms may produce urologic, gastrointestinal, or neurologic symptoms. Pain may also be present, and a mass may be palpable on physical examination.[2]

Sonographic Appearance

An iliac artery aneurysm appears as a primarily anechoic mass in the pelvis. Smaller aneurysm may be difficult to identify in the presence of profuse bowel gas. Pulsations may be present. Thrombus may also be present along the periphery of the mass, and calcific changes may be visualized within the wall. Continuity with the iliac artery is a strong indicator for iliac artery aneurysm, and Doppler interrogation reveals a turbulent arterial signal. Because of the strong tendency toward bilaterality, the contralateral iliac artery should also be examined carefully (Fig. 6-19A, B).[2]

AORTIC GRAFTS AND ASSOCIATED COMPLICATIONS

Diagnostic medical sonography is useful not only for the detection of arterial abnormalities such as aneurysms but also for the assessment of aortic grafts and their related complications.

Description

An aortic graft, endograft, or prosthesis is usually a man-made structure used to repair an aortic aneurysm. Grafts can be made of various materials, including Teflon (DuPont, Wilmington, DE) and Dacron (INVISTA, Wichita, KS). The name of the graft is usually in reference to the vessel they are attached to, and the attachment may be anastomosed in an end-to-end anastomosis to the normal portion of the vessel after the aneurysm is removed.[53] In some instances, the original aneurysm may be retained and actually sewn around the prosthesis as a stabilizer.[13] In aortofemoral bypass surgery, the diseased segment of the aorta is left intact and end-to-side anastomotic technique is used, resulting in graft placement anterior and adjacent to the native vessel.[53] An endovascular repair of abdominal aortic aneurysms (EVAR) is a minimally invasive surgical procedure that involves deploying a stent graft into the aorta with subsequent exclusion of the aneurysm. In essence, an aortic stent graft is designed to prevent recurrent flow into the aneurysm sac by diverting the arterial flow through the graft material. Over time, because of the loss of dynamic arterial flow, the aneurysm sac is expected to contract and thereby is not likely to rupture.[54]

Sonographic Appearance

Sonographically, graft replacements are easily detected by their characteristic wall brightness and, at times, it may also be possible to see their ribbing. The graft walls are also straighter than native vessel walls. At the level of the

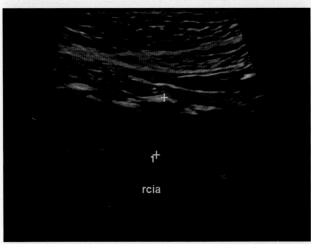

A

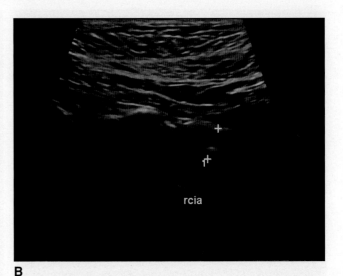

B

FIGURE 6-19 Iliac artery aneurysms. **A** and **B**: A fusiform infrarenal abdominal aortic aneurysm extending into both the right and left common iliac arteries was diagnosed in a 65-year-old man. **A**: The 1.6 cm diameter was measured in the right common iliac artery *(rcia)*. **B**: A large calcification is noted within the rcia. The sonographer should note the size of the residual lumen compared to the total size of the aneurysm. The calipers in these images demonstrate the increased width of the right common iliac artery (rcia) due to aneurysm.

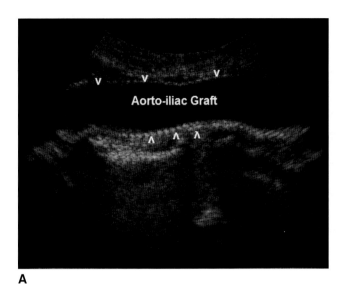

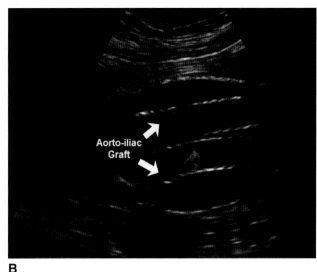

A

B

FIGURE 6-20 Aortic graft. **A** and **B**: The longitudinal images made through end-to-end anastomoses of an aortoiliac graft can be seen with its characteristic ribbing *(carets)*. **A**: Sonogram demonstrating the characteristic ribbing seen on synthetic aortobifemoral bypass grafts *(carets)*. **B**: Two limbs within the aneurysm sac seen with endovascular repairs.

proximal anastomosis, the graft is usually seen to dive posteriorly and continue its course inferiorly with a slight angulation toward the anterior abdominal wall.[2] The graft then bifurcates, and a connection should be demonstrated at the iliac artery level or the common femoral artery level, depending on the extent of the prosthesis. The sonographic appearance of EVAR grafts is characterized by wall brightness within the aneurysm sac and, like prosthetic grafts, endografts are straighter than the native vessel walls (Fig. 6-20A, B). Oftentimes, the endografts are of a bifurcated design where the bifurcated iliac limbs are visualized considerably more proximally in the aorta rather than at the aortoiliac bifurcation itself.

Complications

Pseudoaneurysms

Of all aortic graft complications, pseudoaneurysms are perhaps the most common.[2,53,55] They occur at the site of anastomosis and result from bleeding at this site or from trauma. In essence, there is a pulsating hematoma connected to the lumen of the graft–native vessel interface. The presence of a pulsating mass is usually the first clinical evidence that a pseudoaneurysm may be forming. It may be demonstrated as a graft ending abruptly in an anechoic mass, but is more often seen as a pulsating fluid collection near the site of anastomosis. Doppler interrogation of the mass reveals turbulent arterial signals, and color-flow Doppler affords a dramatic representation of the swirling blood flow patterns within pseudoaneurysms as well as their leakage site.

Graft Aneurysms

Graft aneurysms result from degeneration of the graft material and appear sonographically as focal dilatations of the actual graft material. These are not common complications of aortic grafts.

Hematomas

Hematomas are a normal part of the healing process of graft replacement surgery. Sonographically, they may present as an anechoic or a complex mass in the area of the graft.

Abscess

Abscesses may also have a sonographic appearance consistent with an anechoic or a complex mass in the area of a graft. Consequently, it may be impossible to differentiate between abscesses and hematomas by sonographic appearance alone. In these instances, clinical signs such as tenderness in the area, history of fever, leukocytosis, and local erythema may be useful in differentiating an infectious process from a hematoma. If there is any question, aspiration of the fluid under sonographic guidance will be diagnostic.

Occlusion

Graft occlusion was an elusive complication for sonographers until the advent of Doppler technology. Now, it is relatively simple to verify flow through a graft. Once the graft is located by real-time scanning, the Doppler sample volume cursor is moved into the graft lumen. If flow is present, it registers as arterial pulsations. The absence of flow denotes occlusion of the graft. Often, even though there is a compete occlusion, real-time B-mode imaging cannot demonstrate the occluding clot.[53] Therefore, duplex Doppler is essential in this diagnosis. Color-flow Doppler dramatically represents flow within a graft and can be used in conjunction with conventional Doppler to confirm graft patency.

Endoleaks

Endografts have been associated with device-related complications called *endoleaks* and are graded type I through V. Endoleaks occur as a result of an incomplete seal between the endograft and the native wall of the aorta (type I) or because the IMA or lumbar artery have not been excluded

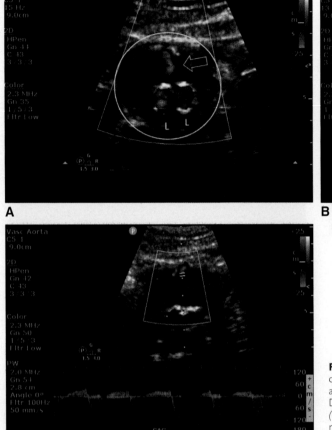

FIGURE 6-21 Endoleaks. **A:** Transverse image taken during an aortic duplex sonography examination on a patient that is status post endovascular aortic aneurysm repair *(EVAR)*. The sac *(circle)* and limbs are identified *(L)*. Doppler flow is demonstrated within the aneurysm and outside of the graft *(arrow)*. **B:** Optimized Doppler settings demonstrating flow within the aneurysm sac *(arrow)* consistent with endoleak. **C:** The spectral Doppler sampling of the area suspected of flow within aneurysm sac demonstrating the characteristic to-and-fro pattern.

by the device and continue to provide a source of arterial flow into the aneurysm sac (type II). Type II is the most common. There are also rare instances where an endoleak occurs as a result of endograft failure because of stump disconnection, fabric disruption (type III), or graft porosity (type IV). Enlargement of the residual sac without visualized endoleak is referred to as endotension (type V). It is a poorly understood phenomenon and is thought to occur when increased graft permeability allows pressure to be transmitted through the aneurysm sac, affecting the native aortic wall, but this is only a theory. A consequence of an endoleak is that there is continued blood flow around the graft within the aneurysm, which, in turn, may result in fatal consequences stemming from aneurysm expansion and eventual rupture.[56] It can sometimes be difficult to determine the type of endoleak, in which case additional imaging such as a CT scan can be performed.

Endoleaks are identified on duplex by meticulous Doppler sampling and attention to the presence or absence of color outside the endograft. Attention to the endograft in grayscale is critical to determine the presence of graft compression, luminal defects, and separation of modular junctions. Color-flow Doppler is used to determine extrastent flow. Use of the most sensitive color Doppler scale settings is required to determine low-velocity leaks. Flow that is associated with an endoleak is relatively uniform, persists into diastole,

and is reproducible in all scanning planes (Fig. 6-21A–C). Spectral Doppler should be used to determine the speed and flow direction for any suspected extrastent flow. The endograft should be closely inspected at the proximal and distal fixation sites to document the presence or absence of endoleaks. The sonographer should also obtain velocity waveforms from each iliac limb extension to evaluate for any potential stenosis from graft compression.[57]

VASCULAR STENOSIS

The discussion of arterial abnormalities would not be complete if the subject of stenosis was not mentioned. Until recently, angiography, and no other method of medical imaging, was very successful in the actual investigation of abdominal visceral artery stenosis. With continued improvement and refinements in duplex and color-flow Doppler technology, much interest has been generated in developing criteria for evaluating suspected visceral artery stenoses.[58]

Several studies have shown that blood flow volumes through the visceral arteries can be assessed by Doppler techniques with a relative degree of accuracy when compared to more invasive methods.[59–65] Doppler blood flow volume studies are time consuming, and their accuracy is limited by several inherent problems of the technique such as underestimation of vessel diameter and overestimation

TABLE 6-2   Doppler Findings with Vascular Stenosis

1. Vessel lumen narrowed by atheromatous plaque or arteriosclerotic changes
2. Poststenotic dilatation
3. Increased velocities in the area of stenosis
4. Downstream changes: turbulence (increases as the percentage of stenosis increases), decreased velocities, slowed acceleration during systole, and relative elevation of diastolic velocities

of average blood flow velocity. Even if Doppler techniques could precisely estimate flow volumes, its routine use in the clinical setting would seem to be limited, as evidenced by prior investigations of significant peripheral occlusive arterial disease. It has been established that volume flows are not particularly helpful in the assessment of stenotic lesions because collateral pathways "normalize" flow volume beyond areas of stenosis. Sonographers identify significant stenosis by recognizing the physiologic blood flow changes associated with significantly compromised arteries. Doppler findings in association with vascular stenosis are identified in Table 6-2. Because it may be difficult to visualize occlusive plaque in the visceral arteries with grayscale sonography, Doppler interrogation becomes very important in the assessment of visceral arteries. Before abnormal Doppler signals can be appreciated, it is essential to be familiar with normal Doppler waveform patterns of the major abdominal visceral arteries (Fig. 6-22A–E).

Although there is some variability between different investigators' data, there are accepted and established guidelines to follow when evaluating for potential renal artery and mesenteric artery stenoses.[66,67]

Renal Artery Stenosis

Description

Renal artery stenosis is a significant medical problem because of its association with uncontrollable hypertension. Other consequences of renal artery stenosis include decreased glomerular filtration rate and ischemic renal damage.[68,69] It is estimated that up to 6% of all hypertensive patients have significant renal artery stenosis as the underlying cause of their hypertension. Identification of these individuals allows corrective intervention that will reduce or minimize the progressive negative sequelae associated with renovascular hypertension.

Etiology

Renal artery stenosis is caused by atherosclerotic plaque, generally located at its origin from the aorta or within its first 2 cm. It may also be caused by fibromuscular dysplasia. These lesions are usually located in the distal two-thirds of the renal artery.

Patient Selection

Of all hypertensive individuals, it has been determined that those with a greater than 10% prevalence of having a significant renal artery stenosis include children, onset age younger than 30 years (especially females), onset age older than 50 years (mostly male smokers), poorly controlled hypertension, rapidly worsening hypertension, severe hypertension (diastolic pressure >115 mm Hg), peripheral vascular disease, cerebrovascular disease, coronary artery disease, abdominal aortic aneurysm, aortic dissection, renal artery stenosis, renal insufficiency of unknown cause, renal function deterioration on angiotensin-converting enzyme, blood pressure that responds well to angiotensin-converting enzyme, elevated renin plasma, abdominal bruit, grades 3 to 4 hypertensive retinopathy, and unilateral small kidney.[67,70,71]

Diagnostic Technique and Criteria

Sonography equipment provides color-flow imaging to identify flow abnormalities and spectral Doppler measurements to provide the quantitative data to determine the severity of stenosis.[71] Two methods are used in sonography evaluation of renal artery stenosis, and a combination of these two methods will enhance the examination results. The direct method relies on detection of blood flow changes that occur at a hemodynamically significant stenosis, whereas the indirect method relies on identification of blood flow changes that occur distal to a significant stenosis. Both methods require attention to Doppler technique being crucial to the examination.

Direct Method

The direct method involves direct visualization and Doppler interrogation of the aorta and renal arteries along their entire length. The examination begins with longitudinal images of the abdominal aorta. A central stream Doppler trace is obtained at or slightly above the renal artery origins (near the level of SMA), and an angle-corrected peak systolic velocity measurement is recorded. All velocity measurements should be made with a Doppler angle of less than 60 degrees. The renal arteries are then imaged, and the Doppler sample volume walked through their length. Doppler spectral and angle-corrected peak systolic velocities are recorded at the vessel origins and at their proximal, middle, and distal segments. The maximum peak systolic velocity from each side is noted and used to calculate the renal artery to aortic ratio (RAR).[58,59,72–75] Stenosis is diagnosed if there is a 50% to 60% reduction in the lumen diameter, which is considered hemodynamically significant (Table 6-3).[59,76–79]

Direct imaging and Doppler interrogation may be technically more difficult on obese individuals, as well as those with excessive bowel gas. Right lateral and left lateral decubitus patient positions may help in delineation of the renal arteries as well as multiple transducer positions and varying degrees of probe pressure. The major limitations of this method include incomplete visualization of the renal arteries, potential overestimation of blood flow velocities because of suboptimal Doppler angles (those >60%) and vessel tortuosity, and the inability to detect accessory renal arteries (Fig. 6-23).

There may be instances in which a Doppler angle of 60 degrees or less will not be obtainable despite the best efforts of the sonographer. Using a Doppler angle of greater than 60 degrees will lead to falsely elevated velocities. Abnormal velocities obtained with suboptimal Doppler angles should be viewed with suspicion. In these instances, poststenotic turbulence should be identified before significant stenosis is suggested.

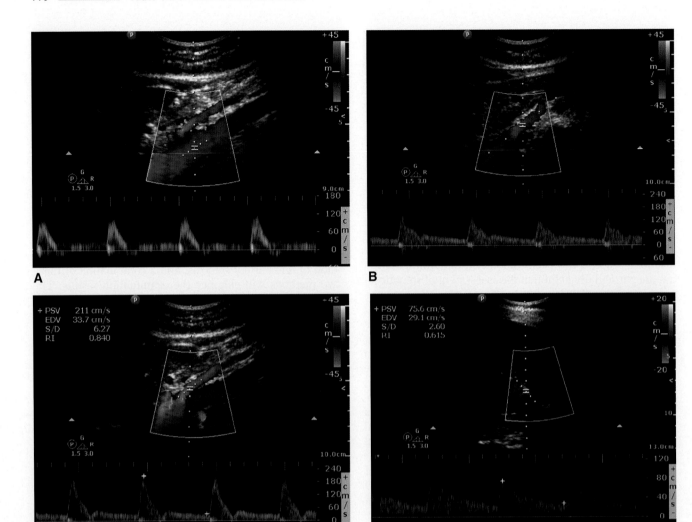

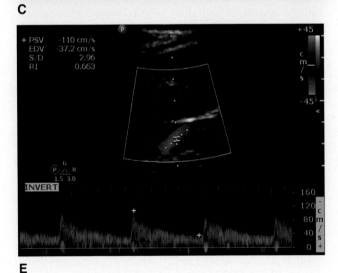

FIGURE 6-22 Normal Doppler waveforms. **A:** The normal Doppler wave-form for the aorta varies with location. The flow state superior to the renal arteries has a narrow, well-defined systolic complex with forward flow during diastole. The blood in diastole is represented as that part of the waveform closest to the zero baseline. **B:** The major branches of the celiac artery supply the liver and spleen organs that both have low-resistance arterial beds. The arterial waveform is affected by prandial states and caloric food composition. **C:** The superior mesenteric artery supplies the small bowel and proximal colon that also have low-resistance arterial beds. The arterial waveform is affected by prandial states. **D:** The hepatic arterial system has low-resistance flow characteristics with large amounts of continuous forward flow through-out diastole. When the hepatic artery and portal vein velocities are obtained in a fasting patient and compared, it is considered normal if the hepatic artery is equal to or slightly less than portal vein velocity. **E:** In this patient, the examination shows the normal low-pulsatility right renal artery. Doppler spectrum is seen with a PSV of 110 cm/second. The forward flow present in diastole is because of the low resistance in the renal vascular bed. *PSV*, peak systolic velocity.

TABLE 6-3 Criteria for Detection of at Least 50%–60% Renal Artery Stenosis[70,76,79,80]

DIRECT EVALUATION OF THE MAIN RENAL ARTERY

PSV > 180–200 cm/sec
RAR > 3.3–3.5
Poststenotic turbulence

INTERNAL (INTRARENAL) EVALUATION OF THE SEGMENTAL/INTERLOBAR ARTERIES

Absence of ESP
AT > 0.07 sec (increasing the time to 0.10 increases specificity)
Tardus–parvus waveform
RI difference between kidneys exceeding −0.5

IN-STENT STENOSIS

PSV > 250 cm/sec
Poststenotic turbulence

OTHER HEMODYNAMIC PARAMETERS

AI = measured from the slope of the initial acceleration point over the transmitted frequency

AI, acceleration index; AT, acceleration time; ESP, end-systolic peak; PSV, peak systolic velocity; RAR, renal-to-aorta ratio; RI, resistive index.

A significant number of individuals have accessory renal arteries. Duplex Doppler and even color-flow Doppler have not proven to be very helpful in identifying accessory renal arteries. A stenosis in an unrecognized accessory renal artery will result in a falsely negative examination.

Indirect (Intrarenal) Method

The indirect method involves Doppler evaluation of the segmental or interlobar arteries in the upper, middle, and lower poles within the kidney. The rationale for evaluating each pole is to document if a stenotic accessory artery is feeding one of the renal poles. An abnormal waveform detected with Doppler in that segment compensates and adds information to the direct method where it is possible to miss accessory renal arteries.

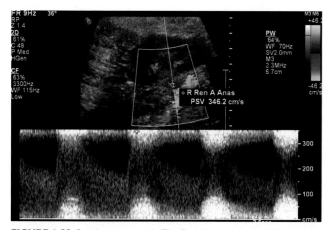

FIGURE 6-23 Renal artery stenosis. The Doppler examination demonstrates elevated velocities, spectral broadening, and aliasing present at the site of stenosis. The velocity is calculated to be 346 cm/second. (Image courtesy of Jill Langer, MD, Hospital of the University of Pennsylvania, Philadelphia, PA.)

Using color and/or power Doppler is essential and is helpful in identifying the intrarenal vessels and in determining an optimal angle of incidence. If a feeding artery has a high-grade stenosis, it can cause the pulsus parvus et tardus changes in intrarenal arterial flow signals (*pulsus* is beat; *tardus* is slow; *parvus* is small). A tardus–parvus waveform demonstrates a delay in the time to maximum systole and a increase in the acceleration index. If the intrarenal segmental and interlobar arteries are normal, the waveform will display an early systolic peak (ESP) or notch at the beginning of systole. With renal artery stenosis greater than 60%, the ESP is absent.

The systolic acceleration time (AT) is measured from the start of systolic upstroke to the first peak or ESP. Systolic ATs greater than 0.07 seconds are consistent with a main renal artery stenosis exceeding 60%.[69,70,77,81] If 0.10 to 0.12 seconds is used as the cutoff for significant stenosis, then specificity increases.[70] The resistive index (RI) is obtained from both the kidneys. An RI difference more than −5 increases the probability of a stenosis in the kidney with the lower RI value (Fig. 6-24A–D).[70]

It cannot be understated that either direct or indirect methods of obtaining accurate hemodynamic Doppler parameters require experience. The sonographer must pay attention to technique. With the patient in either a decubitus or an oblique position, the scan plane through the posterior axillary line will result in a shorter Doppler distance and a better Doppler angle to interrogate the intrarenal vessels. Color Doppler should be used to visualize the vessel path to assist with the incident Doppler angle. Maintaining a Doppler incident angle between 0 and 30 degrees helps define the ESP. An angle greater than 30 degrees may not allow demonstration of the ESP.[82] To spread out the cardiac cycle to better visualize and measure each component, set the Doppler sweep speed to display only 2 to 3 seconds at a time. The pulse repetition frequency is adjusted so that the waveform fills the entire spectral window and the transducer frequency selected provides a large frequency shift and larger waveform. This enhances the definition of the ESP and improves caliper placement for measurements.

The limitations associated with indirect evaluation include obese body habitus, excessive bowel gas, inability to differentiate between severe stenosis and occlusion of the main renal artery, and inability to detect stenosis less than 60%.

Postrenal Artery Stent Imaging

Postrenal artery duplex stent imaging is performed using the same protocol as nonstented renal arteries. The difference is that the stent is well visualized and brightly echogenic. After renal artery stents are placed, the diameter of the stented vessel may be slightly increased when compared to the diameter of the native artery distal to the stent. Because of this, a flow gradient may be present at the distal end of the stent because of diameter mismatch between the stented segment and the native renal artery. If so, the peak systolic velocity may increase slightly and disordered flow will be apparent as the flow moves from the slightly larger diameter stented segment to the smaller diameter native arterial segment. Careful attention must be given to these flow patterns to make the distinction of whether the flow shift is because of size mismatch or the flow shift is because of a flow-reducing stenosis either in the stent or

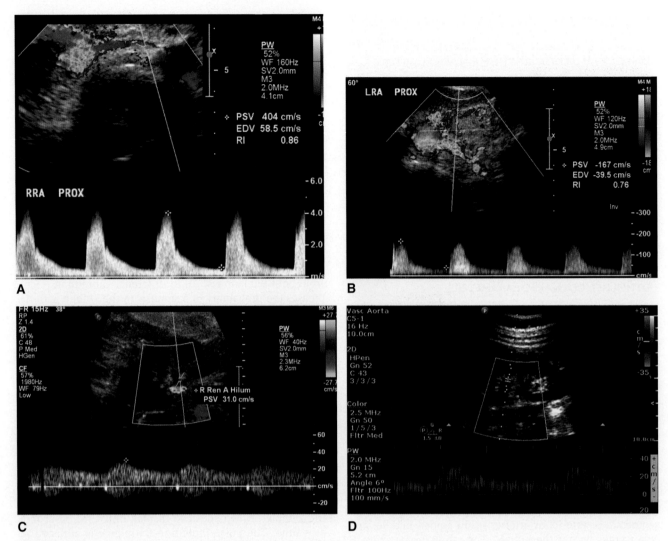

FIGURE 6-24 Resistive index difference. **A** and **B**: A 76-year-old woman with history of uncontrolled hypertension, hyperlipidemia, coronary artery disease, and renovascular disease has had coronary artery bypass surgery and carotid endarterectomy presented for renal artery follow-up evaluation. **A**: The transverse image of the right renal artery displays peak systolic velocity (PSV) of 404 cm/second, end-diastolic volume (EDV) of 58.5 cm/second, and a resistive index (RI) of 0.86. **B**: The left renal artery displays PSV of 167 cm/second, EDV of 39.5 cm/second, and an RI of 0.76. There is a 0.10 cm/second RI difference between the right renal arterial stenosis and the left renal artery. **C**: On a different patient, there is delayed systolic upstroke seen distal to a significant stenosis. **D**: This examination of a normal intrarenal flow pattern demonstrates a sharp systolic upstroke. (**C**: Courtesy of Jill Langer, MD, Hospital of the University of Pennsylvania, Philadelphia, PA.)

just distal to the stent docking site.[83] Velocity criteria for classification in stent stenosis of renal arteries include a peak systolic velocity of greater than 250 cm/second and the presence of poststenotic turbulence (Fig. 6-25).[83]

Mesenteric Artery Stenosis (Mesenteric Insufficiency)

Description

Chronic mesenteric insufficiency is a complex problem that has been difficult to recognize clinically because presenting symptoms are vague and closely related to other abdominal disease processes. One vascular surgeon reports that the average time from initial patient complaint to actual diagnosis is 18 months.[84]

Mesenteric insufficiency results from lack of adequate blood supply to the intestinal tract because of underlying vascular compromise: either acute occlusion of the mesenteric

vessels via embolic phenomenon or atherosclerotic disease with associated significant stenosis and/or occlusion of the mesenteric vessels.

Individuals at increased risk of developing mesenteric arterial disease include those with a history of smoking, hypertension, coronary artery disease, peripheral atherosclerotic disease, chronic renal insufficiency, and diabetes mellitus.

Classical symptoms of chronic mesenteric ischemia include progressive postprandial pain, weight loss, change in bowel habits, and an epigastric bruit.[85] Other symptoms that may be encountered include diarrhea, fear of eating, nausea/vomiting, and constipation.[86]

Acute mesenteric insufficiency is a catastrophic event necessitating immediate diagnosis and surgical intervention. Thus, angiography is still considered the primary diagnostic tool to demonstrate suspected acute mesenteric insufficiency.

Chronic mesenteric insufficiency results from hemodynamically significant stenosis and/or occlusion in two of the three arteries, which comprise the mesenteric circulation.[85,87]

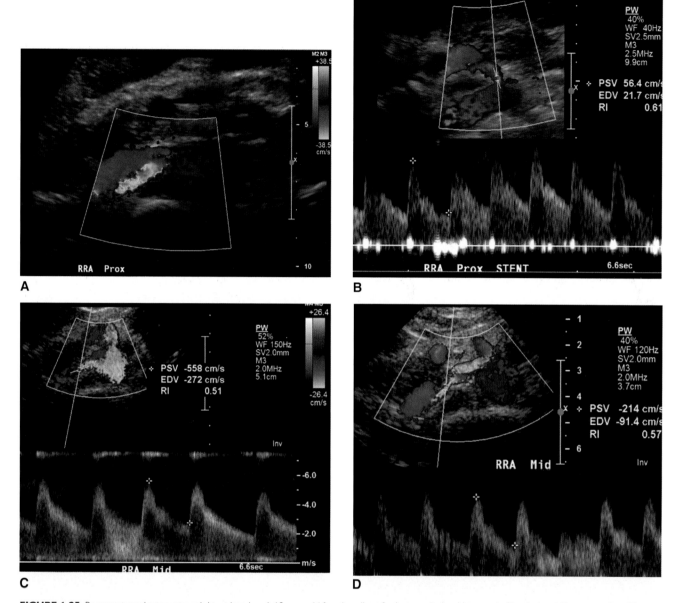

FIGURE 6-25 Recurrent renal artery stenosis/stent imaging. A 19-year-old female college freshman noted sudden onset of headaches ×5 or more days. The college health center found her blood pressure to be 220/130 mm Hg. There were no associated neurologic symptoms with her headache. A computerized tomography angiography of the abdomen demonstrated a right renal artery *(RRA)* stenosis. Following a percutaneous balloon angioplasty and stenting of her RRA, this postintervention renal artery duplex was performed. **A:** The transverse color Doppler displays a wide, patent RRA. **B:** The longitudinal image displays a wide, patent RRA with normal velocity peak systolic velocity *(PSV)* of 56.4 cm/second and end-diastolic volume *(EDV)* of 21.7 cm/second. **C:** Six months post-RRA stenting, the duplex RRA stent surveillance shows significantly elevated velocity of PSV of 558 cm/second and EDV of 272 cm/second. **D:** The patient had a repeat endovascular balloon dilatation and RRA stent. The postoperative RRA velocities returned to PSV of 214 cm/second and EDV of 91.4 cm/second. Note the resistive index *(RI)* on each image.

It is a much less ominous disease and can be corrected with minimally invasive methods or with bypass surgical techniques.[88] Because of the vague symptoms exhibited by a majority of patients and the reported uncommonness of chronic mesenteric insufficiency, physicians have been reluctant to pursue angiography, with its inherent risks, for many of these patients. Duplex and color-flow Doppler sonography appears to be a more acceptable noninvasive technique to initially evaluate patients suspected of having chronic mesenteric ischemia.

Examination

Because the diagnosis of chronic mesenteric ischemia depends on identifying significant stenosis and/or occlusion in two of the three mesenteric arteries, the examination protocol should include sonography and Doppler evaluation of the CA, SMA, and IMA. The common hepatic and splenic artery should also be evaluated because abnormal flow patterns in these vessels can confirm suspected CA occlusion.

Patients are evaluated after an overnight fast. Each vessel should be scanned throughout its length in search of focal velocity increases and associated poststenotic turbulence, paying particular attention to their proximal portions because this is where the majority of stenotic lesions are found. The SMA is usually best evaluated from a longitudinal imaging plane, whereas the CA should be evaluated from a variety of planes to best outline its course. Many times, axial scanning more clearly reveals the sometimes tortuous course of this artery. Velocity measurements are made with Doppler angles between 40 and 60 degrees. Color-flow Doppler may be used as an aid in visualizing the mesenteric vessels in difficult patients and is also helpful in placing the Doppler sample volume and Doppler angle cursor. Occasionally, a color bruit may be seen and is a helpful finding in suggesting significant stenosis; however, duplex Doppler spectral tracings should always be used to confirm abnormal blood flow patterns demonstrated by color-flow examination and common anomalies such as the SMA and CA sharing a common trunk.

Some institutions also perform postprandial scanning to help determine normal responses of SMA flow. Ensure an over-the-counter energy drink has been used effectively as the "stress meal" for postprandial studies.

Doppler Findings in Superior Mesenteric Artery

In a prepandial (fasting) state, Doppler spectral analysis of the normal SMA reveals a characteristic pattern that is associated with a highly resistant vascular bed. There is a sharp rise in flow during systole and a rapid falloff during diastole, with reversal of flow below the baseline (see Fig. 6-22C). In the postprandial state (after ingestion of a meal), the blood flow characteristics change and exhibit reduced or absent reversal of flow during the diastolic phase of the cardiac cycle concomitant with increased peak forward diastolic flow.[89] Velocity changes begin to occur within 15 minutes of meal ingestion, with near doubling of baseline peak systolic velocities occurring at about 45 minutes. After 90 minutes, blood flow velocity returns to baseline levels.[85] The diastolic flow goes through similar changes, with the maximum diastolic flow reaching approximately three times the baseline values at approximately 45 minutes postmeal.[85]

With a significant stenosis of the SMA, a loss of the reversed flow component, even in the preprandial state, occurs. Abnormally high velocities with associated poststenotic turbulence are also detected in the narrowed region of the vessel. Visually, poststenotic dilatation and arteriosclerotic plaque may be seen. A splanchnic peak velocity >275 cm/second is considered highly indicative of a severely compromised blood flow, and CA peak systolic velocities >200 cm/second have been associated with greater than 70% stenosis.[89] Because breathing may exert periodic effects on splanchnic arterial hemodynamics, which may affect an underestimation of arterial stenosis, it is recommended that mesenteric Doppler examinations be performed during expiration[89] (Fig. 6-26). Occlusion of the SMA is diagnosed when there is no Doppler signal detected in a reliably visualized vessel.

Doppler Findings in the Celiac Artery

In a prepandial state, CA flow resembles that of other vessels supplying a low-resistant vascular bed with a rapid systolic upstroke followed by gradually decreasing velocities during diastole. Flow never reaches zero. During the postprandial state, some increase in CA velocities is noted, but not to the same extreme as those seen in the SMA.

Doppler findings suggesting significant celiac artery stenosis include a localized area of high velocity, a peak systolic velocity of >200 cm/second, poststenotic turbulence, and blunted flow downstream from a high-grade stenosis. Visually, poststenotic dilatation may also be recognized (Fig. 6-27A, B).

Doppler Findings in the Inferior Mesenteric Artery

Even though the IMA is a relatively important vessel, especially in regard to collateral flow in the presence of significant stenosis and/or occlusion of both the SMA and CA, it has not been studied much. Although sonographic examination

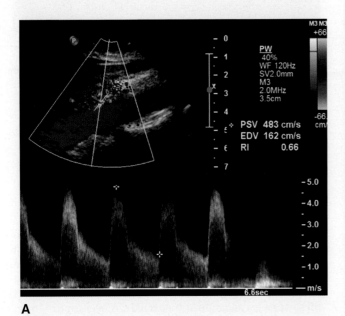

A

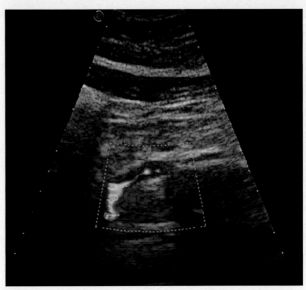

B

FIGURE 6-26 Superior mesenteric artery (SMA) stenosis. **A:** Doppler evaluation of an SMA stenosis was made on this patient with a peak systolic velocity (PSV) of approximately 483 cm/second and end-diastolic volume (EDV) of approximately 162 cm/second. **B:** Intraluminal narrowing of the color Doppler signal in this stenotic SMA. RI, resistive index.

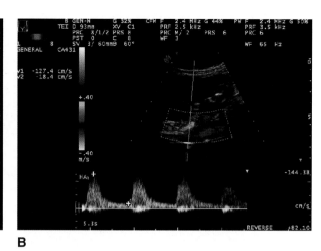

A   **B**

FIGURE 6-27 Doppler analysis. **A:** Spectral Doppler tracing of the celiac artery with a calculated velocity of 250 cm/second. **B:** In the presence of significant celiac artery disease flow pattern, changes will be present in branch vessels such as the hepatic and splenic arteries. This image demonstrates turbulent flow patterns within the hepatic artery.

is difficult because of its size and overlying small bowel, in the majority of patients referred for mesenteric arterial evaluation, it is feasible to demonstrate the IMA using high-frequency probes, bowel compression techniques, and color-flow imaging.

Preprandial flow in the IMA resembles that of the SMA. There is, however, higher resistivity associated with the IMA. When the IMA provides collateral flow to the intestinal tract, it will enlarge, making it easier to identify.

Postprandial Scanning

Postprandial scanning protocol begins with initial fasting evaluation of the mesenteric arteries for identification of stenosis. Afterward, the stress meal is given, and peak systolic velocities in the SMA are recorded at 5- to 10-minute intervals. A positive scan for chronic mesenteric ischemia consists of identification of significant stenosis of two of the three mesenteric arteries and no significant change in the SMA postprandial velocities.

Pitfalls and Limitations

There are several pitfalls and limitations to be aware of when performing mesenteric insufficiency evaluation. Compression of the CA can occur from the median arcuate ligament. This median arcuate ligament syndrome causes celiac artery compression by causing narrowing of the celiac artery at the end of deep expiration or at rest and in some patients at the end of inspiration. Median arcuate ligament compression syndrome can become the pathogenesis of hepatic and splenic artery disease (Table 6-4; Fig. 6-28).

Although much has been learned regarding mesenteric blood flow in normal and abnormal states, much still needs to be learned to help improve the accuracy and reliability of duplex and color-flow Doppler in the evaluation of chronic mesenteric ischemia.

Hepatic Artery with a Hepatic Transplant

Description

The area of hepatic artery Doppler examination is important in the investigation of liver transplant recipients. The portable nature of the technique makes it a very good tool for the

TABLE 6-4 Pitfalls and Limitations When Performing Mesenteric Insufficiency Evaluation

1. Owing to body habitus, and overlying bowel gas, it may be impossible to interrogate the mesenteric arteries.
2. Incomplete interrogation of the vessel. Although most stenosis occurs at the vessel origins or within their first 2–3 cm, distal disease would be overlooked if the length of the vessel was not entirely examined.
3. Collateral flow may lessen the accuracy of Doppler parameters. There is speculation that adequate collateral perfusion through a normally patent mesenteric vessel may cause a decrease in the velocities detectable through a stenotic one. It has also been demonstrated that in isolated, single-vessel disease, compensatory flow increases occur in the nondiseased vessel, and this phenomenon, too, has the potential to negatively affect the accuracy of Doppler criteria.
4. Vessel tortuosity can cause confusing Doppler information. It may be difficult to differentiate between actual stenosis and vessel tortuosity.
5. The celiac compression syndrome may be mistaken for a celiac axis stenosis. Elevated celiac axis velocities and poststenotic turbulence can be detected in the celiac axis resulting from compression of the median arcuate ligament of the diaphragm. During inspiration, and subsequent Doppler evaluation, the high velocities and poststenotic turbulence disappear.

detection of postsurgical complications such as occlusion of the hepatic artery or occlusion of the portal system (which are discussed in "Venous Abnormalities" section).

Technique

Initially, the transducer is placed intercostally to identify the portal vein. After the portal vein is visualized, the transducer is maneuvered to identify the hepatic artery, usually located anterior to the portal vein. The Doppler sample volume is electronically moved into the area of interest to identify blood flow. Color-flow Doppler instrumentation is very helpful for hepatic artery localization and subsequent placement of the sample volume. In a normal examination, the Doppler flow pattern is pulsatile and has a high diastolic flow component owing to the low resistance of the blood bed

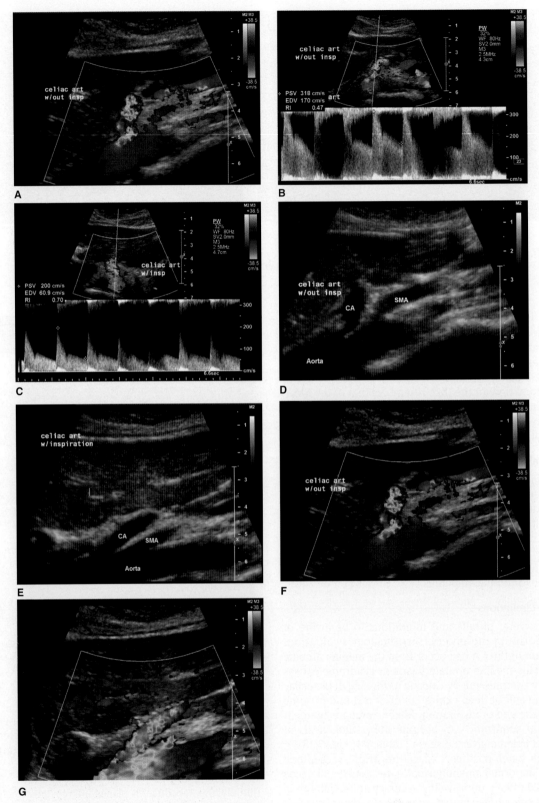

FIGURE 6-28 Median arcuate ligament compression. A 32-year-old woman has an asymptomatic abdominal bruit during routine physical examination. Four months prior, her most recent pregnancy was complicated by a coronary artery dissection of the left anterior descending artery and myocardial infarction at approximately 3 weeks postdelivery. Initial treatment was an intra-aortic balloon pump and she did not require percutaneous coronary intervention. Postdischarge, the patient was managed medically and successfully completed cardiac rehabilitation. The aorta, celiac artery, and superior mesenteric artery *(SMA)* were obtained using Doppler angle correction with the cursors parallel to flow. **A:** A color bruit was present in the celiac artery on this longitudinal image. Using respiratory maneuvers, Doppler images were obtained of the celiac artery **(B)** with suspended respiration and **(C)** with deep inspiration. Grayscale images were also obtained of the celiac axis *(CA)* with suspended respiration **(D)** and with deep inspiration **(E)**. The celiac artery peak systolic flow/diastolic flow at rest during suspended respiration was peak systolic velocity *(PSV)* of 318 cm/second and end-diastolic volume *(EDV)* of 170 cm/second. With deep inspiration, the celiac artery flow decreased significantly to PSV of 200 cm/second and EDV of 70 cm/second. **F:** Color-flow changes of the celiac artery demonstrated the presence of significant mosaic turbulence at rest **(G)** that returned to laminar flow pattern with inspiration. Furthermore, on grayscale interrogation, the celiac artery trunk demonstrated evidence of luminal narrowing that resolved with deep inspiration.

in the liver. Absent or very blunted flow is almost always indicative of hepatic arterial obstruction and is most critical in the immediate postoperative period. If hepatic arterial occlusion occurs in the later period of transplant recovery, its significance is not as profound because of the collateral circulation that has had a chance to develop.[59]

Although it is a less common complication of liver transplant, hepatic artery stenosis can be identified by Doppler and is recognized as a focal elevation of hepatic artery velocity with associated poststenotic turbulence.[90]

Originally, it was hoped that liver transplant rejection could be reliably detected using hepatic artery duplex scanning techniques as well. In these instances, the hepatic arterial Doppler signal was expected to show evidence of increased vascular resistance, depicted as a decreased diastolic flow component in the spectral tracing, but these findings turned out to be inconsistent.[59,90,91]

VENOUS ABNORMALITIES

Vena Caval Obstruction

In order to assess the IVC for the presence of obstruction, it is important to remember the effects of normal respiration on the IVC. These effects include (1) the IVC caliber decreases during initial inspiration; (2) after suspended respiration, the IVC enlarges to its maximum diameter; (3) the IVC caliber enlarges during expiration; and (4) during the Valsalva maneuver, the IVC caliber diminishes, nearly obliterating the lumen owing to the increased abdominal pressure created by this technique. Because of the variations in the caliber of the IVC during respiration, it is imperative that IVC examinations be done in a consistent manner. This is usually best accomplished by examining while the patient suspends inspiration.[8]

Description

When blood flow in the IVC is obstructed, the normal response of the vessel is to increase in caliber below the point of obstruction. Because of the elastic capacity of the veins, the expansion of the IVC can be quite dramatic.

Etiology

The most common cause of IVC obstruction is right-sided heart failure, which itself has many causes. IVC obstruction may also have its origins with an enlarged liver, para-aortic lymph node enlargement, retroperitoneal masses or tumors, and pancreatic tumors. A congenital IVC valve may also obstruct the lumen of the IVC.[12]

Clinical Signs and Symptoms

The signs and symptoms may include abdominal pain, ascites, or tender hepatomegaly. Lower extremity edema may also be present in the more severe forms of IVC blockage.[12]

Sonographic Appearance

In the presence of obstruction, the IVC tends to dilate below the level of obstruction. Respiratory changes are decreased or absent below the obstructed segment.[92]

In right-sided heart failure, the proximal IVC and hepatic veins become congested, resulting in a concurrent increase in diameter. Respiratory changes are markedly decreased or absent.

Solid, complex, or echo-poor tumors in the retroperitoneum or pancreas may be seen to impinge on the IVC. If large enough, they can obstruct the vessel, and dilatation below the impingement would be recognized. Intravenous tumors, primary or metastatic, also obstruct flow within the IVC.[13,93] Again, dilatation of the vein below the tumor mass will be identified. Severe obstruction or compression of the IVC may result in enlargement of the ascending lumbar vein, which is recognized as an anechoic structure posterior to and midway between the aorta and IVC in transverse imaging planes.

In the superior vena cava obstruction syndrome, collateral vein formation and enlargement may develop involving the epigastric veins, the ligamentum teres, and the caudate lobe veins.[90]

Tumors of the Inferior Vena Cava

Tumors of the IVC may be primary, metastatic, or an extension from a tumor.

Primary Tumors

Primary tumors of the IVC, most of which are leiomyomas or leiomyosarcomas, tend to be uncommon (vascular incidence of only 2%). These types of tumors tend to develop in women, and the median age of detection is 61 years. With leiomyosarcomas, metastasis to the liver and lung has been reported in 40% to 50% of cases. A 36% recurrence rate is also reported, and prognosis is poor.[94,95]

Metastasis or Extension of Tumors

Malignant invasion of the IVC may occur from renal carcinoma (the most commonly reported incidence at 9% to 33%), secreting and nonsecreting adrenal tumors, retroperitoneal sarcomas, hepatocellular carcinomas, teratomas, and lymphomas.[96]

Clinical Signs and Symptoms

The symptoms are generally unremarkable, but this depends on tumor size and the degree of obstruction they present to the IVC. With tumors of large proportions, leg edema as well as ascites and abdominal pain may develop.[92] This is true for the primary tumors of the IVC as well as those that are metastatic.

Sonographic Appearance

Tumors within the IVC tend to appear as echogenic foci. Occasionally, they may be isodense with the blood in the lumen, in which case they are more difficult to visualize. Tumors, especially the larger primary types, may be heterogeneous, with areas of necrosis.

Depending on tumor size and degree of obstruction, there may be normal or increased IVC caliber as well as loss of respiratory changes. Because of the similarity in echographic appearance of vascular tumor masses, the differential diagnosis is large and includes primary vascular neoplasm, malignant IVC mass, thrombus (chronic), and large primary tumors outside the vessel.[96] The latter differential is important because large tumors distort their surroundings, thereby making normal anatomy difficult to identify.

Doppler and color-flow instrumentation can aid in the diagnosis of vena caval obstruction by tumors. Normally, blood flow in the middle and distal IVC is of low velocity and varies with respiration. Flow velocities decrease with inspiration and increase with exhalation. Near the heart, the effects of right atrial hemodynamics become evident in the Doppler spectra, revealing complex triphasic waveforms. When the cava is partially obstructed, distinct blood flow patterns may be recognized, but these will depend on the degree of obstruction present. Milder forms of obstruction do not produce appreciable blood flow changes; however, with more severe forms of impingement and obstructive lesions, blood flow changes can be quite dramatic. Respiratory changes distal to a significant obstruction will be severely diminished or absent, whereas blood flow velocities within the narrowed segment caused by the obstruction lesion will elevate. With duplex Doppler technique, it is necessary to move the sample volume along the length of the IVC to look for increased flow velocity. Abnormal flow velocity findings may be useful in suggesting vena cava obstruction when the obstructing lesion is echopenic. Color-flow Doppler may be of greatest asset in these cases because the blood flow path is more easily seen than with conventional grayscale sonography (Fig. 6-29). Complete occlusion of the IVC results in absence of detectable blood flow by Doppler interrogation.

When an IVC mass is identified during sonography, it is important to attempt to identify (1) the presence of a primary tumor and its site; (2) the cranial extent of the tumor mass (does it involve the hepatic veins or the right atrium?); and (3) possible tumor involvement or invasion of the wall of the vessel (CT is better able to show this type of involvement than sonography).[96] To localize a lesion in the IVC, it should be placed into one of the three (or a combination) designated segments because surgical management depends on its cranial extent. The upper IVC is that part of the vessel that is seen between the right atrium and the hepatic veins. The middle IVC includes the part between the hepatic veins and the renal veins, and the lower IVC is the portion that lies below the renal veins.[95]

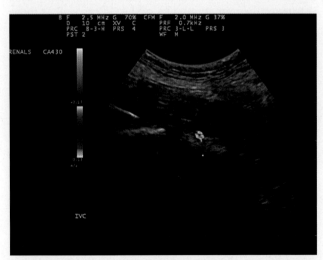

FIGURE 6-29 Vena cava obstruction. The sagittal image of the inferior vena cava *(IVC)* demonstrates that it is distended with intraluminal echoes and absent color Doppler signal consistent with thrombus. (Image used with permission from Navix Diagnostix, Taunton, MA.)

Renal Vein Enlargement

Discussion and Etiology

There are several reasons why renal veins enlarge, including increased flow because of a splenorenal or gastrorenal shunt in patients with portal hypertension or portal thrombosis, tumor involvement from a renal cell carcinoma, and increased flow from an arteriovenous malformation in the kidney.[97-99]

In portal hypertension, several collateral pathways are apt to develop as the pressure in the portal system increases. Consequently, blood flow is diverted to the collaterals, which may in turn fistulize to the left renal vein as a means of relieving the increased pressure.[1] The same mechanism can take place in a patient with portal venous thrombosis.

It has been determined that the prevalence of renal vein involvement in renal cell carcinoma is approximately 21% to 55%.[100] When invasion occurs, obstruction to the renal vein results in dilatation. Expansion may also be the direct result of tumor growth.

In arteriovenous malformation, there is an abnormal connection between the arterial and venous vessels. Because of the higher pressure in the arterial system, blood is routed directly from the artery into the vein, thus increasing blood flow through the veins. A natural response for the vein under increased blood volume is to dilate. Arteriovenous fistulas may occur for a number of reasons, including blunt or penetrating trauma, biopsy complications, tumor involvement, nephrectomy, and idiopathic causes.[99]

Clinical Signs and Symptoms

The symptoms in the presence of an enlarged renal vein are generally associated with the underlying disease process and are not the result of the venous enlargement. With portal venous hypertension and gastrorenal or splenorenal shunting, there may be no obvious distinguishing clinical features.

Tumor involvement of the renal veins usually produces no specific symptoms that would lead to suspicion of tumor extension. Such findings are generally made during the routine workup of patients with known renal cell carcinoma.

In patients with small arteriovenous malformations, generally no clinically significant symptoms are recognized. With larger malformations, however, there may be hematuria, abdominal pain, abdominal bruit, congestive heart failure, and cardiomegaly with possible systolic hypertension, diastolic hypertension, and renal ischemia.[2,99]

Sonographic Appearance

Evaluation of symmetry between the renal veins is useful in differentiating the types of disease processes that may cause venous enlargement.[98] If enlargement of the renal veins is bilateral or symmetric, the disease process most likely involves the IVC at a level above the insertion of the renal veins. Such may include congestive heart failure and tumor involvement or thrombosis of the IVC.

Unilateral renal vein enlargement may indicate tumor involvement, portal venous hypertension with renal vein collateral anastomosis, or arteriovenous fistula. In portal venous hypertension, there is isolated left renal vein involvement, whereas either the left or the right renal vein may be involved by tumor invasion or arteriovenous fistula.

Sonographically, an enlarged renal vein is defined as one with a diameter in excess of 1.5 cm. Another sonographic

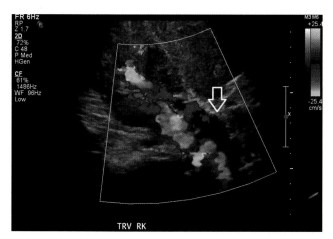

FIGURE 6-30 Renal vein thrombus. The examination demonstrates absent color Doppler in the main renal vein with intraluminal echoes that are present consistent with thrombus (arrow). This thrombus was a result of renal mass tumor.

finding suggestive of increased flow volume into the renal vein is an abrupt IVC dilatation at the level of the renal insertion point.[98]

Blood flow patterns can be determined with Doppler techniques and may be useful in differentiating the various types of renal vein enlargement. For instance, in the presence of a gastrorenal or splenorenal shunt associated with portal hypertension or in the presence of an arteriovenous malformation, disturbed or turbulent venous flow signals are evident in the enlarged renal vein. Velocities may also be abnormally rapid.

With tumor involvement, an echogenic focus is usually present in the vessel lumen (Fig. 6-30). If this is a finding during sonography examination, the IVC should be searched carefully to identify the extension of the tumor beyond the renal veins.

Pitfalls

In a tumor-free vessel, reverberation artifact may mimic a tumor or possibly a thrombus. It is also possible that some metastatic tumors may appear isoechoic with the surrounding blood, making them very difficult to identify.

The left renal vein may appear enlarged at the point where it crosses over the aorta before entering the IVC. It should be noted that this is a normal finding in many persons. Dilatation should be suspected only if the entire length of the renal vein is enlarged, especially in conjunction with any of the other findings associated with renal vein enlargement.

Although duplication of the IVC is not common, it is possible that a duplicated IVC could be misinterpreted as left renal vein enlargement. To avoid this confusion, it is wise to follow the vessel in question to its origin if possible.[98]

Renal Vein Thrombosis

Etiology

Renal vein thrombosis may occur in disorders such as nephrotic syndrome, renal tumors, renal transplantation, trauma, infant dehydration, and/or compression of the renal vein secondary to extrinsic tumor.[97]

Clinical Signs and Symptoms

The symptoms of acute renal venous thrombosis may include loin or flank pain, leg swelling, proteinuria, and hematuria.[97]

Sonographic Appearance

With renal vein thrombosis, the renal vein is dilated at a point proximal to the occlusion. In many cases, the thrombus is visible in the vessel lumen. Thrombus generally appears as an echogenic focus, especially in long-standing cases. In the more acute phase, however, thrombus may not appear echogenic, but isoechoic to the surrounding blood. In these instances, Doppler interrogation may be helpful (no venous signal is heard in the presence of renal vein occlusion). The acute phase of renal vein thrombosis causes enlargement of the kidney and loss of normal renal architecture.[97]

Venous Aneurysms

Description

Venous aneurysms are rare vascular abnormalities that may be incidentally discovered. They tend to occur principally in the neck or lower extremity veins. They have, however, been reported to occur in most major veins.[64] Portal vein aneurysm is the most common type of visceral venous aneurysm and has been reported in the main portal vein, the confluence of the splenic and superior mesenteric veins, and intrahepatic portal vein branches at bifurcation sites.[101] In recent years, there has been an increase in the number of venous aneurysm cases reported in the portal venous system.[102]

Etiology

Several theories have been developed to explain the cause of venous aneurysms. They include weakening of the vessel wall by pancreatitis, portal hypertension, and embryonic malformations (congenital anomalies). There is a greater presence of aneurysms in patients who have chronic liver disease, portal hypertension, pancreatitis, trauma, and postsurgical complication.[101]

Clinical Signs and Symptoms

Usually, no symptoms are associated with small aneurysms of the portal venous system. When an aneurysm enlarges, it may cause the commonly reported symptoms such as duodenal compression, common bile duct obstruction, chronic portal hypertension, jaundice, recurrent crampy abdominal pain, upper gastrointestinal bleeding, obstruction of the portal vein as a result of thrombus, and rupture of the aneurysm.[12]

Sonographic Appearance

Sonographically, portal venous aneurysms can be recognized as anechoic distended vessels that may or may not contain thrombus. Doppler techniques can be used to verify the venous nature of the echo-free structure by detecting a turbulent venous signal in the lesion. Included in the differential diagnosis (especially in the absence of Doppler data) are neoplastic cysts and visceral arterial aneurysms.

Once detected, pulsed and color Doppler examination can be used in follow-up of most patients. CT and MRA are more costly and invasive examinations that are used to determine location and relationship to adjacent organs, and angiography is used for surgical planning.[103] Employing Doppler helps define the pathology by being able to detect portal vein to hepatic vein fistulas by showing their connections and noting turbulent venous flow within the aneurysm. Doppler spectra in nonfistulated aneurysms do not show turbulent flow.

Other venous aneurysms are rare, but it stands to reason that they would resemble a portal vein aneurysm, except for their location within the abdomen. Doppler investigation should be used to help define the vascular nature of any suspicious anechoic lesion within the abdomen.

Hepatic Venous Abnormalities

Budd–Chiari Syndrome

Description and Etiology

Budd–Chiari syndrome is defined as the occlusion of some or all of the hepatic veins and/or occlusion of the IVC. Two types are recognized: primary Budd–Chiari syndrome is the resultant occlusion of the hepatic veins or IVC by a congenital web or fibrous cord. In secondary Budd–Chiari syndrome, occlusion of the hepatic veins and/or IVC occurs by tumor or thrombus formation.

Sonographic Appearance

Color-flow Doppler is superior to grayscale sonography in the evaluation of suspected Budd–Chiari syndrome because of its ability to detect flow in otherwise unseen veins.[71,104,105] Recognized sonographic and Doppler findings of Budd–Chiari syndrome include absent or sluggish flow in the IVC (oftentimes, in the primary type), visualization of the obstructing membrane, absent flow in some or all of the hepatic veins, reversed flow in portions of the obstructed hepatic veins, damped Doppler spectra with loss of normal triphasic flow pattern of obstructed hepatic veins, identification of intrahepatic venovenous collaterals, and identification of extrahepatic collaterals. The intrahepatic collaterals appear as either a curved configuration resembling a hockey stick or a spider web pattern.[104]

Evaluation of suspected Budd–Chiari should also include examination of the portal vein because a 20% incidence of portal venous occlusion has been reported in these patients.[71,106]

Portal Venous Abnormalities

Portal Venous Thrombosis

Description and Etiology

Portal venous thrombosis can be caused by a variety of pathologic states, including portal hypertension, inflammatory abdominal processes (appendicitis, peritonitis, pancreatitis, and colon diverticulum), trauma, postsurgical complications, hypercoagulability states (oral contraceptives, pregnancy, migratory thrombophlebitis, antithrombin III deficiency, polycythemia vera, and thrombocytosis), abdominal neoplasms (hepatocellular, colonic, and pancreatic), renal transplant, and benign ulcer disease.[1,44,107–110] It can also be idiopathic. A potential complication of portal vein thrombosis is bowel ischemia and perforation.

Clinical Signs and Symptoms

A patient with portal vein thrombosis may exhibit symptoms such as abdominal pain, low-grade fever, leukocytosis, hypovolemia, and shock. Shock is unlikely unless there is an associated bowel infarction. Abdominal rigidity, elevated liver function test results, nausea, and vomiting may also be present. Changes in bowel habit, hematemesis, and melena can occur.[4,111]

Sonographic Appearance

Portal venous thrombosis goes through several stages, and its sonographic appearance varies at different stages of the disease process.[108] In the first stage, there is echogenic thrombus in the vessel lumen, and then thrombus and smaller collaterals are visible in the immediate area. Finally, larger collaterals (cavernomatous transformation of the portal vein) are observed in the absence of an identifiable portal vein. The latter two stages are usually seen in benign processes and are because of chronic disease.

Direct signs of portal venous thrombosis include visualization of a clot in the lumen of the portal vein (Fig. 6-31A–C). Clot often appears more echogenic than the surrounding blood; however, in an acute process when thrombus is fresh, the clot may appear hypoechoic and be difficult to identify. A localized bulge of the vein at the clot level may also be recognized. Because improper gain settings and reverberation artifact may appear as clot within the lumen of the portal vein, careful attention to technique is critical to avoid misdiagnosis of portal vein thrombosis.

The normal caliber of the portal vein has been established to be smaller than 13 mm.[110] In the event of an acute thrombotic episode, the caliber is likely to exceed 13 mm, but in a more chronic process, it may indeed be less than 13 mm.[109]

Indirect evidence of portal vein thrombus includes lack of normal portal vein landmarks, collateral vessel formation in the area of the portal vein, and increased caliber of the superior mesenteric and splenic veins.[108] It has been demonstrated that in some cases of complete obliteration of the portal vein by thrombus, the thrombus actually appeared isodense with the liver parenchyma. The only indication of portal involvement was echoic margins surrounding the clot, which were generated from the portal vein walls.[1]

In cavernous transformation of the portal vein, multiple wormlike, serpiginous vessels can be seen in the region of the portal vein. This particular process is the result of long-standing thrombus and subsequent collateral vessel formation.[112]

Duplex and color-flow Doppler prove to be more useful than conventional grayscale sonography in the detection of portal vein thrombosis.[100,113] With Doppler, the diagnosis of portal venous thrombosis is suggested by demonstration of absent flow within the vein. Several investigators have shown that the negative predictive value of portal vein thrombus is higher than its positive predictive value.[113] The reasons for false-positive Doppler scans include undetectable slow flow within the portal vein and technical factors. Some have proposed rescanning the portal vein in equivocal cases postprandially to confirm the absence of flow.[90] Recently, it has been suggested that a hepatic artery RI of ≤0.50 may be useful in corroborating suspected portal venous thrombus.[113] This finding was determined more useful in acute portal vein thrombus because it was generally not seen in chronic portal venous thrombus with collateral formation.[113]

Sonography can also be used to detect rare superior mesenteric vein and splenic vein thromboses.[107,108] Sonographically, the signs of thrombosis appear similar to those

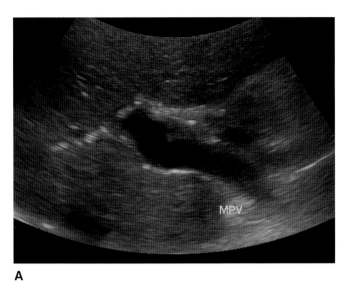

A

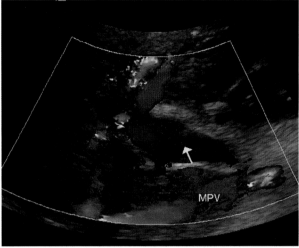

B

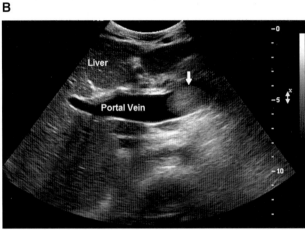

C

FIGURE 6-31 Portal venous thrombosis. **A:** The grayscale image demonstrating echoes within the main portal vein *(MPV)* as it enters the liver. **B:** The color Doppler image shows a filling defect consistent with portal vein thrombosis *(arrow)*. **C:** On a different patient, the transverse sonogram displays an echogenic clot in the portal vein lumen *(arrow)*. (**A** and **B:** Courtesy of Shana Huber, RDMS, RVT, Hospital of the University of Pennsylvania, Philadelphia, PA; **C** courtesy of Philips Medical Systems, Bothell, WA.)

seen in portal vein thrombosis. Echogenic material may be visualized directly inside the vessel lumen, and the caliber of the superior mesenteric and splenic veins may be increased, especially in the acute phase. The absence of flow is detectable by Doppler techniques in the presence of total obstruction of the vein, whereas flow characteristics may be normal or diminished when thrombus is partially occlusive.

Color-flow Doppler provides for easier demonstration of porta-hepatic collaterals associated with cavernous transformation of the portal vein. Color-flow Doppler may also be better suited to detect partial portal vein thrombosis. In such instances, color-flow voids within the portal vein may be apparent in areas of thrombus formation.[91]

It is difficult to differentiate between thrombus and tumor with sonography alone. Other findings, such as primary tumor or lymphadenopathy, may be useful in pinpointing the correct diagnosis. Some recent studies, however, have illustrated the potential utility of duplex and color-flow Doppler in the differentiation of tumor thrombus from clot thrombus.[84,114,115] In all of the studies, the majority of tumor thrombi showed evidence of tumor vascularity. It was generally identified by color flow as a patchy or spotty pattern of color within the clot.[114,115] Doppler spectra revealed pulsatile arterial flow in two of the studies[84,114] and continuous venous flow with nearly constant amplitude in

the other.[115] Optimization of Doppler parameters is essential to document this flow.

Portal Venous Hypertension

Description

Portal hypertension is an increase in the portal venous pressure. Normally, pressure in the portal venous system is sustained between 0 and 5 mm Hg. In the pathologic state of portal hypertension, it increases to 10 to 12 mm Hg or more.[12]

Etiology

Portal hypertension may be induced by an increase in the splanchnic blood flow or by increased hepatic vascular resistance.[12] Conditions associated with increased splanchnic blood flow include splenic, hepatic, and mesenteric arteriovenous fistulas resulting from either trauma or rupture of an aneurysm into the splanchnic vessel circulation. These particular mechanisms are not common causes in the United States.[12]

Conditions associated with increased resistance to hepatic vascular flow include extrahepatic obstruction of the portal vein, such as thrombosis, and presinusoidal obstruction of portal vein radicles in which there is fibrosis of the portal triads. These can be idiopathic or associated with schistosomiasis, chronic arsenic or vinyl chloride toxicity, congenital hepatic fibrosis, granulomatous disease, or neoplastic infiltration. Perhaps, the most common cause of portal hypertension in the United States is sinusoidal and postsinusoidal obstruction, as is seen with fatty infiltration and inflammation of the liver in patients with acute alcoholic hepatitis and cirrhosis. Budd–Chiari syndrome or hepatic venous obstruction may also be a mechanism of portal hypertension. In these instances, hepatic venous occlusion results from congenital webs or thrombosis or neoplasia.[12]

Clinical Signs and Symptoms

In more advanced cases of portal hypertension, there may be ascites and gastrointestinal bleeding. Other complications include poor renal function and impaired coagulation,[68,98,116] but these symptoms are nonspecific, and the total clinical picture must be correlated with physical and sonographic findings to arrive at the correct diagnosis.

Sonographic Appearance

In healthy persons, the portal vein diameter is usually less than 13 mm. It has been proposed that the presence of a larger portal vein is suggestive of portal venous hypertension, but this is not a consistent finding. Interestingly, in persons with known portal hypertension, portal vein caliber was frequently reported to be normal or small compared to that of normal persons. This is probably because of the development of collateral circulation pathways in patients with more severe portal hypertension. Increased portal vein caliber is not regarded as a reliable indicator of portal venous hypertension.[117] Measurements and diagnosis of portal venous hypertension should consider physiologic factors affecting portal vein measurements (meal, respiration, and posture). Goyal et al.[118] attempted to define discriminating measurement criteria of the portal veins keeping the physiologic factors constant. All measurements were taken in patients with an overnight fast, in a supine position, and at deep inspiration. The largest diameters of the portal vein, splenic vein, and superior mesenteric vein were recorded and analyzed. Their results indicate that the upper limits of normal for the portal vein, splenic vein, and superior mesenteric vein are 16 mm, 12 mm, and 11 mm, respectively. Measurements above these discriminating values were 72% sensitive, 91% accurate, and 100% specific for the diagnosis of portal vein hypertension. It remains to be seen whether these criteria hold up in larger study populations.

In order to diagnose portal venous hypertension, it is important to look for the secondary effects of increased pressure within the portal system, including collateral channel development and abnormal respiratory responses. More recently, Doppler techniques have been investigated in the hope they might allow the physician to more confidently diagnose portal venous hypertension, especially in the absence of visible collateral pathways or other changes associated with portal hypertension.

The collateral network associated with portal hypertension can be extensive and can involve many areas such as coronary vein, gastroesophageal veins, umbilical vein, pancreatic duodenal veins, gastrorenal, and splenorenal veins.

It has been noted that a dilated coronary vein (vein of the stomach located in the midepigastric area and visualized as a tortuous anechoic structure measuring more than 5 mm and following the lesser omentum) was detected in the majority of patients with portal hypertension. This, along with the identification of esophageal varices, is a good indicator of portal hypertension. Because esophageal varices and coronary vein enlargement seem to be involved quite frequently in association with portal hypertension (80% to 90%),[119] it would be prudent to search the midepigastric region thoroughly to identify any of these collateral pathways. Of course, visualization of the collaterals depends on their size—larger ones being much more readily visible than smaller ones. Esophageal varices are also the most clinically significant of the collateral pathways because of their propensity to bleed, and a positive correlation between increasing size of the coronary vein and risk of variceal bleeding has been established.[120] Other collaterals are seen but not to the extent of the coronary vein and esophageal varices.

About 10% to 20% of patients with portal hypertension may also have a patent umbilical vein. This structure is seen in the falciform ligament as a tubular area of 3 mm or greater.[121]

Pancreatic and duodenal collaterals may also be present. They would be located in the region of the descending duodenum, lateral to the pancreatic head. Depending on the amount of air in the duodenum at the time of study, as well as the size of the collateral vessels, they may be easy or difficult to identify.[116]

Splenorenal and gastrorenal venous involvement is detected in the area of the splenic hilum, renal hilum, and the greater curvature of the stomach, respectively. Their proximity may make it difficult to distinguish them from one another.[106] With this particular type of collateral, blood may also be spontaneously shunted to the left renal vein to relieve the high pressure in the system, in which case the caliber of the left renal vein also increases. If unilateral left renal vein enlargement is present, portal venous hypertension with gastrorenal or splenorenal shunting may be a cause.[119] Other causes would include arteriovenous fistula of the kidney or tumor involvement.

Retroperitoneal and paravertebral collateral vessels as well as omental collaterals may be detected, although their position in the abdomen makes it difficult to do so.[119] Investigators have reported imaging dilated cystic veins of the gallbladder in patients with portal hypertension. The technique utilizes a high-frequency transducer and pulsed-wave Doppler.[122]

Other related sonographic findings in the presence of portal hypertension may include a comma-shaped portal trunk, increased periportal echogenicity, increased caliber of the splenic and superior mesenteric veins, ascites, and an enlarged spleen.[28]

Respiratory effects on the portal system have been studied in an attempt to diagnose portal hypertension by abnormal findings. It has been stated that portal venous caliber does not change much with respiration[28]; therefore, respiratory dynamics of the superior mesenteric vein and the splenic vein have been investigated for usefulness in detecting portal venous hypertension.

In normal subjects, the caliber of both the superior mesenteric and splenic veins is less than 1 cm. During suspended inspiration, the diameters increased by 14% to 100% in the majority of normal subjects. In persons who developed portal hypertension as a result of cirrhosis, vessel diameters were usually 1 cm or greater, and the inspiration-induced caliber changes were less than 10%.[123,124]

The role of Doppler sonography in the detection of portal venous hypertension is continually undergoing investigation.[125] One of the most useful aspects of color Doppler in the evaluation of portal venous hypertension is its superior ability to identify collateral vessels that are otherwise "invisible" with conventional grayscale sonography.[64,71]

Although current research has led to the conclusion that Doppler sonography can reliably measure portal flow, there is much variability between normal and abnormal flow, and specific criteria have not been established to diagnose portal vein hypertension.[61,65,126,127] However, more recent studies indicate a more proactive role for duplex Doppler-derived flow estimates in determining the effectiveness of medical treatments by comparing individual patient baseline flows to postinterventional flows.[128]

Because of the inherent inaccuracies of Doppler-derived estimates and wider variability of portal flow, qualitative Doppler signs of portal vein hypertension are being sought to aid in its diagnosis.

The qualitative Doppler examination begins with visualization of the portal vein and its branches, by placing the transducer at the right intercostal spaces overlying the liver. This intercostal approach generally affords better detection of Doppler signals by virtue of better Doppler angles. Doppler interrogation is then carried out in the right, left, and main portal veins.[129] Once accomplished, flow is assessed in the superior mesenteric vein and along the splenic vein. Transducer positions for the latter examination are determined by the position of the vessels and the angle necessary to obtain Doppler data.

In normal subjects, portal vein blood flow velocity is 16.0 ± 0.5 cm/second. In fasting adults, portal vein blood flow velocity ranged from 8 to 18 cm/second. After ingestion of a meal, velocities increased by 50% to 100%. The flow characteristics in the majority of the normal subjects were a wavy continuous pattern (70%) and traveled toward the liver (hepatopetally). Flow in the superior mesenteric and splenic veins was also antegrade.[120]

Several blood flow abnormalities may be detected in patients with portal hypertension, including flow reversal (hepatofugal) in the portal veins—in some cases, this reversal of flow was detected only when the patient was asked to suspend inspiration. Reversed flow in the superior mesenteric vein suggested mesentericocaval shunting and prompted the examiner to look for collaterals in the pelvis. Reversed flow in the splenic vein and associated increase in left renal vein caliber along with high-velocity, turbulent blood flow suggested splenorenal shunting. This prompted the examiner to look closely for collateral flow in the splenic and renal hilar areas. Hepatofugal flow was also detected in the left gastric (coronary), paraduodenal, and paraumbilical veins. The flow observed using Doppler techniques in collateral vessels tended to be fast and turbulent.[120]

It was also noted that the venous flow pattern in the portal system was continuous in approximately 72% of persons who had portal hypertension and associated cirrhosis. Blood flow velocity tended to be slower than in normal control subjects.[130] Because blood flow velocity in the portal vein is widely variable and consistent, useful criteria for the diagnosis of portal venous hypertension have not been forthcoming.[71]

There is still no clearly established role for Doppler sonography in the assessment of portal venous hypertension.[71,90]

This is probably due in part to the complex nature of portal venous flow and resultant wide variations reported of normal and abnormal blood flow patterns.

PORTOSYSTEMIC SHUNT EVALUATION

Major clinical complications of portal hypertension include variceal hemorrhage and ascites.[71] Sclerotherapy can be used to control variceal bleeding in some patients, but if it is not successful, other treatments are necessary to control the bleeding. The creation of surgical portosystemic shunts can be used to decompress the portal vein pressure, thus reducing the risk of variceal hemorrhage. Four types of shunts can be created, namely, portocaval, mesocaval, splenorenal, and, more recently, transjugular intrahepatic portosystemic.

Portocaval Shunts

Portocaval shunts have been the most commonly used. These shunts are made by end-to-side or side-to-side anastomosis of the portal vein to the IVC. Portocaval shunts are generally amenable to sonography examination. Patency in these shunts can easily be confirmed with duplex and color-flow Doppler by showing venous flow across the shunt from the portal vein into the IVC. The absence of flow would suggest shunt failure. Indirect signs of shunt patency in instances of nonvisualization of the shunt would include hepatopetal flow proximal to shunt anastomosis and hepatofugal flow distal to shunt anastomosis. Persistent hepatopetal flow distal to shunt anastomosis would suggest shunt occlusion or severe stenosis.

Mesocaval Shunts

Mesocaval shunts are created with an H configured synthetic graft connecting the midsuperior mesenteric vein with the IVC. These shunts are more difficult to evaluate because of their deep position within the abdomen and overlying bowel gas. Persistent scanning with the aid of color-flow Doppler, however, generally results in adequate assessment of shunt patency. If the graft is visualized, duplex and color-flow Doppler can be used to demonstrate flow across the shunt. If the graft cannot be visualized, graft patency can be inferred by demonstration of flow entering the IVC at a level below the renal veins.[71,90]

Splenorenal Shunts

Splenorenal or Warren shunts are made by connecting the distal splenic vein to the renal vein, and these are the most difficult types of shunts to assess with sonography. Color-flow Doppler seems essential for assessment of graft patency, which can be inferred by demonstration of well-defined splenic and renal limbs of the graft with appropriately directed flow.[71,90,91,131] The splenic limb of the shunt is usually best identified from an anterior approach, whereas the renal limb is best visualized from a coronal or flank approach. Graft occlusion or compromise is suggested by identification of collateral vessels in the left upper quadrant in lieu of well-defined limbs of the shunt, or occlusion of the distal splenic vein at the splenic hilum.[71,90]

Transjugular Intrahepatic Portosystemic Shunts

Transjugular intrahepatic portosystemic shunts (TIPSs) have been developed to avoid the surgical risks associated with the creation of portocaval, mesocaval, and splenorenal shunts. TIPS procedures involve placement of a metal stent between a hepatic vein and an intrahepatic portal vein via transcatheter route through the jugular vein. On sonography, the TIPSs are usually easily seen as a bright tubular structure within the hepatic parenchyma connecting the portal vein with one of the hepatic veins (Fig. 6-32). Complications of these shunts include stenosis at either the portal or hepatic vein anastomosis, or occlusion of the shunt. Because identification of shunt dysfunction relies on the demonstration of relative changes in portal blood flow, it is important to perform both pre-TIPS and baseline post-TIPS examinations.[132]

Suggested protocol for evaluation of TIPS includes that all scans be performed after the patient fasts and velocity measurements are taken with Doppler angles between 40 and 60 degrees (Table 6-5).[133-136]

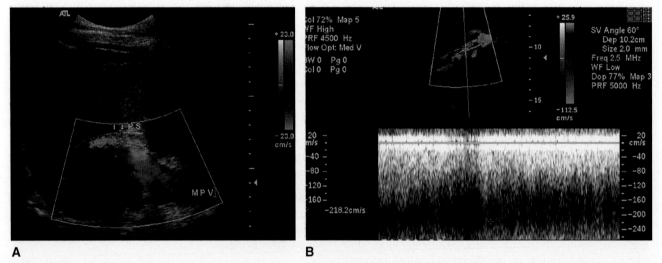

A　　　　　　　　　　　　　　　　**B**

FIGURE 6-32 Transjugular intrahepatic portosystemic shunt *(TIPS)*. **A:** The normal color Doppler image demonstrating a TIPS. **B:** Significantly elevated velocity of 218 cm/second was obtained within the shunt. *MPV,* main portal vein. (Images courtesy of M. Robert DeJong RDMS, RDCS, RVT, The Johns Hopkins Medical Institutions, Baltimore, MD.)

TABLE 6-5　Protocol and Criteria for Evaluation of TIPS

PRE-TIPS EXAMINATION INCLUDES

1. Measurement of maximum blood flow velocity and determination of blood flow direction within the extrahepatic portal vein, superior mesenteric vein, splenic vein at the confluence of the superior mesenteric vein, and the three hepatic veins
2. Identification of collaterals and blood flow direction within post-TIPS examination

PRE-TIPS EXAMINATION INCLUDES

1. Repeat of pre-TIPS examination
2. Evaluation of the shunt at three places: portal anastomosis, midportion, and hepatic vein anastomosis

REPORTED SIGNS OF TIPS STENOSIS INCLUDE

1. Drop in portal vein velocities to pre-TIPS levels
2. Focal, high-velocity blood flow within the shunt and associated poststenotic turbulence
3. Reversal of flow in the hepatic vein draining the TIPS (may also occur in TIPS occlusion)
4. More than 20% reduction of flow through the stent as measured at midstent from baseline studies
5. Detection of either an increase or a decrease of midsegment shunt blood flow velocity in excess of 50 cm/sec

REPORTED SIGNS OF TIPS OCCLUSION INCLUDE

1. Return of hepatopetal blood flow in the portal vein (may also occur in severe shunt stenosis)
2. Absence of blood flow within the TIPS stent

TIPS, transjugular intrahepatic portosystemic shunt.

SUMMARY

- Current equipment provides the ability to assess blood flow, to obtain hemodynamic information regarding the many factors that influence the dynamics of blood flow, and the hemodynamic consequences of vascular disease.
- Blood vessels are composed of three distinct layers: (1) the tunica intima (innermost), (2) the tunica media (middle), and (3) the tunica adventitia (outermost).
- The aorta is the main artery of the chest and abdomen from which all other branch vessels are derived.
- The first branch is the celiac artery (also known as the CA or trunk) and originates from the anterior aspect usually within the first 2 cm of the abdominal aorta.
- The CA is approximately 1 cm long before it divides into the (1) hepatic artery, (2) left gastric artery, and (3) splenic artery.
- The second major abdominal aorta branch vessel is the SMA, which also originates from the anterior surface of the aorta approximately 1 to 2.5 cm distal to the celiac artery.
- Inferior to the SMA, the right renal artery arises from the right lateral aspect of the aorta, whereas the left renal artery arises from the left lateral or posterolateral aspect of the aorta. Both then course posterolaterally to enter the respective kidneys.
- The IMA is the last major branch to arise from the abdominal aorta before it bifurcates.
- At the umbilicus, the aorta bifurcates into the left and right common iliac arteries that course inferiorly and posteriorly.
- The IVC is the large vessel that returns blood to the right atrium from the lower limbs, pelvis, and abdomen.
- The IVC is formed by the junction of the paired common iliac veins slightly anterior and to the right of the L5 vertebral body and courses superiorly in the abdomen, enters the thoracic cavity, and enters the right atrium at the level of the T8 vertebral body.
- The veins most consistently seen entering the IVC are the common iliac veins at its formation, the renal veins, and the hepatic veins.
- The right renal vein is generally shorter than the left renal vein because of the right kidney's proximity to the IVC.
- The left renal vein traverses the abdomen, coursing anterior to the aorta and posterior to the SMA to finally enter the lateral aspect of the IVC.
- The three hepatic veins—(1) the left, (2) the right, and (3) the middle—drain directly into the IVC or right atrium.
- The effects of normal respiration on the IVC include (1) IVC caliber decreases during initial inspiration; (2) IVC enlarges during expiration and is its maximum diameter after suspended respiration; and (3) during the Valsalva maneuver, the IVC caliber diminishes, nearly obliterating the lumen owing to the increased abdominal pressure created by this technique.
- The main portal vein is formed at the junction of the splenic vein and the superior mesenteric vein, which can be identified with sonography in most patients.
- The sonographic findings of atherosclerosis include luminal irregularities (representative of the various changes of the intimal lining of the artery), tortuosity, and vessel wall calcification.

- A true aneurysm is identified sonographically as a dilatation of the aorta ≥3.0 cm near its bifurcation point, a focal dilatation along the course of the aorta, or lack of normal tapering of the aorta.
- Thrombus typically produces a low-level echo pattern and tends to accumulate along the anterior and lateral walls of the aortic lumen.
- Aortic dissection appears as a thin, linear echo flap within the arterial lumen.
- Aortic rupture with leakage of blood outside the vessels may be diagnosed by identification of a hematoma in the abdomen in association with aneurysmal dilatation of the aorta.
- Inflammatory aneurysms manifest with dilatation of the aorta with a hypoechoic mantle, usually seen anterior and lateral to a thickened aortic wall.
- The most common splanchnic artery aneurysms are splenic aneurysms followed by hepatic aneurysms with SMA aneurysms being the rarest.
- Renal artery aneurysms have been encountered with increasing frequency, although the overall incidence remains relatively low.
- Iliac artery aneurysms are most often associated with (continuations of) abdominal aortic aneurysms.
- An aortic graft, endograft, or prosthesis is usually a manmade structure used to repair an aortic aneurysm and is easily detected by their characteristic wall brightness, and at times their ribbing.
- Complications of aortic grafts include pseudoaneurysm, graft aneurysms, hematomas, abscesses, occlusions, and endoleaks.
- Renal artery stenosis, a significant medical problem associated with uncontrollable hypertension, can be evaluated using two methods that can be combined to enhance examination results.
- Both evaluation methods require attention to Doppler technique being crucial to the accuracy of the examination.
- The direct method involves direct visualization and Doppler interrogation of the aorta and renal arteries along their entire length relying on blood flow changes that occur at a hemodynamically significant stenosis.
- The indirect or intrarenal method involves Doppler evaluation of the segmental or interlobar arteries in the upper, middle, and lower renal poles and relies on identification of blood flow changes that occur distal to a significant stenosis.
- Postrenal artery duplex stent imaging is performed using the same protocol because nonstented renal arteries with the difference being the stent will be well visualized and brightly echogenic.
- Mesenteric insufficiency results from lack of adequate blood supply to the intestinal tract because of underlying vascular compromise as a result of acute occlusion of the mesenteric vessels or atherosclerotic disease.
- In a preprandial (fasting) state, Doppler spectral analysis of the normal SMA reveals a characteristic pattern associated with a highly resistant vascular bed.
- In the postprandial state (after ingestion of a meal), the SMA blood flow characteristics change and exhibit reduced or absent reversal of flow during the diastolic phase of the cardiac cycle concomitant with increased peak forward diastolic flow.

- With obstruction, the IVC tends to dilate below the level of obstruction, and respiratory changes are decreased or absent below obstructed segment.
- Tumors of the IVC may be primary, metastatic, or an extension from a tumor.
- Tumors within the IVC tend to appear as echogenic foci and occasionally isodense with the blood in the lumen.
- In arteriovenous malformation, there is an abnormal connection between the arterial and venous vessels.
- Doppler evaluation of symmetry and blood flow patterns between the renal veins is useful in differentiating the types of disease processes that may cause renal vein enlargement.
- An enlarged renal vein has a diameter in excess of 1.5 cm.
- With renal vein thrombosis, the renal vein is dilated at a point proximal to the occlusion.
- Venous aneurysms are rare vascular abnormalities that may be incidentally discovered.
- Portal venous aneurysms can be recognized as anechoic distended vessels that may or may not contain thrombus.
- Doppler evaluation of portal venous aneurysms can be used to verify the venous nature of the echo-free structure by detecting a turbulent venous signal in the lesion.
- Primary Budd–Chiari syndrome is the occlusion of the hepatic veins or IVC by a congenital web or fibrous cord, and secondary Budd–Chiari syndrome is occlusion of the hepatic veins and/or IVC by tumor or thrombus formation.

- Portal venous thrombosis can be idiopathic or it can be caused by a variety of pathologic states, and its sonographic appearance varies at different stages of the disease process.
- Direct signs of portal venous thrombosis include visualization of a clot in the lumen of the portal vein.
- Portal hypertension is an increase in the portal venous pressure.
- The collateral network associated with portal hypertension can be extensive and can involve many areas such as coronary vein, gastroesophageal veins, umbilical vein, pancreatic duodenal veins, gastrorenal, and splenorenal veins.
- The creation of surgical portosystemic shunts can be used to decompress the portal vein pressure that reduces the risk of variceal hemorrhage.
- Four types of shunts can be created, namely, portocaval, mesocaval, splenorenal, and, more recently, transjugular intrahepatic portosystemic.
- Optimize instrumentation settings to demonstrate normal arterial and venous lumen as anechoic structures.
- The sonography examination of the vascular system relies on the skill, knowledge, and accuracy of the sonographer who must pay attention to the texture, outline, size, and shape of both normal and abnormal structures.
- The patient will benefit most when the sonographic findings are correlated with patient history, clinical presentation, laboratory function tests, and other imaging modalities to compose a clinically helpful picture.

REFERENCES

1. Boozari B, Bahr MJ, Kubicka S, et al. Ultrasonography in patients with Budd–Chiari syndrome: diagnostic signs and prognostic implications. *J Hepatol.* 2008;49(4):572–580.
2. Sutherland T. Demystifying abdominal ultrasound. *Aust Fam Physician.* 2009;38(10):797–800.
3. Moore K, Dalley A, Agur A. *Essential Clinical Anatomy.* 6th ed. Wolters Kluwer; 2019.
4. Woolgar JD, Ray R, Maharaj K, et al. Colour Doppler and grey scale ultrasound features of HIV-related vascular aneurysms. *Br J Radiol.* 2002;75(899):919–929.
5. Size GP. *Inside Ultrasound Vascular Reference Guide.* Inside Ultrasound, Inc; 2013.
6. Valeriani E, Riva N, Di Nisio M, Ageno W. Splanchnic vein thrombosis: current perspectives. *Vasc Health Risk Manag.* 2019;15:449–461. doi:10.2147/VHRM.S197732
7. Hagen-Ansert SL. The vascular system. In: Hagen-Ansert SL, ed. *Textbook of Diagnostic Ultrasonography.* 8th ed. Mosby; 2017:141–189.
8. Owen C, Meyers P. Sonographic evaluation of the portal and hepatic systems. *J Diagn Med Sonogr.* 2006;22(5):317–328.
9. Polak J. Hemodynamic considerations in peripheral vascular and cerebrovascular disease. In: Pellerito JS, Polak J, eds. *Introduction to Vascular Ultrasonography.* 6th ed. Elsevier Saunders; 2012:3–19.
10. Kim JM, Kim KW, Kim SY, et al. Technical essentials of hepatic Doppler sonography. *Curr Probl Diagn Radiol.* 2009;38(2):53–56.
11. Gotlieb AI, Liu A. Blood vessels. In: Rubin E, Strayer D, Rubin R, et al., eds. *Rubin's Pathology: Clinicopathologic Foundations of Medicine.* 6th ed. Lippincott Williams & Wilkins; 2005:435–478.
12. Blumberg SN, Maldonado TS. Mesenteric venous thrombosis. *J Vasc Surg Venous Lymphat Disord.* 2016 Oct;4(4):501–507. doi:10.1016/j.jvsv.2016.04.002
13. Pellerito J. Anatomy and normal Doppler signatures of abdominal vessels. In: Pellerito JS, Polak J, eds. *Introduction to Vascular Ultrasonography.* 6th ed. Elsevier Saunders; 2012:439–449.
14. Saeyeldin AA, Velasquez CA, Mahmood SUB, et al. Thoracic aortic aneurysm: unlocking the "silent killer" secrets. *Gen Thorac Cardiovasc Surg.* 2019;67(1):1–11. doi:10.1007/s11748-017-0874-x
15. Benson RA, Meecham L, Fisher O, Loftus IM. Ultrasound screening for abdominal aortic aneurysm: current practice, challenges and controversies. *Br J Radiol.* 2018;91(1090):20170306. doi:10.1259/bjr.20170306
16. Gerhard HM, Gardin JM, Jaff MR, et al. Guidelines for noninvasive vascular laboratory testing: a report from the American Society of Echocardiography and the Society for Vascular Medicine and Biology. *Vasc Med.* 2006;11:183–200.
17. American Institute of Ultrasound in Medicine. AIUM practice guidelines for the performance of diagnostic and screening ultrasound examinations of the abdominal aorta in adults. 2015. Accessed March 9, 2021. http://www.aium.org/resources/guidelines/abdominalAorta.pdf
18. Mohler ER. Abdominal aorta imaging. In: Mohler ER, Gerhard-Herman M, Jaff MR, eds. *Essentials of Vascular Laboratory Diagnosis.* Blackwell Publishing; 2005:68–71.
19. Di Candio G, Lencioni R, Ferrari M, et al. Abdominal aortic aneurysms: efficacy of sonography for preoperative assessment. *Eur J Ultrasound.* 1996;4(1):5–20.
20. Sprouse LR, Meier GH, Lesar CJ, et al. Comparison of abdominal aortic aneurysm diameter measurements obtained with ultrasound and computed tomography: is there a difference? *J Vasc Surg.* 2003;38(3):466–471.
21. Hudson P, Englund R, Hanel KC. What is the most important dimension of an abdominal aortic aneurysm? *J Vasc Technol.* 1996;20(4):213–216.
22. Chun KC, Anderson RC, Smothers HC, et al. Risk of developing an abdominal aortic aneurysm after ectatic aorta detection from initial screening. *J Vasc Surg.* 2020;71(6):1913–1919. doi:10.1016/j.jvs.2019.08.252
23. Lal B, Cerveira J, Seidman C, et al. Observer variability of iliac artery measurements in endovascular repair of abdominal aortic aneurysms. *Ann Vasc Surg.* 2004;18(6):644–652.

24. Clancy K, Wong J, Spicher A. Abdominal aortic aneurysm: a case report and literature review. *Perm J.* 2019;23:18.218. doi:10.7812/TPP/18.218

25. Ali MU, Fitzpatrick-Lewis D, Miller J, et al. Screening for abdominal aortic aneurysm in asymptomatic adults. *J Vasc Surg.* 2016;64(6):1855–1868. doi: 10.1016/j.jvs.2016.05.101

26. Catalano O, Siani A. Ruptured abdominal aortic aneurysm: categorization of sonographic findings and report of 3 new signs. *J Ultrasound Med.* 2005;24:1077–1083.

27. Lombardi JV, Hughes GC, Appoo JJ, et al. Society for Vascular Surgery (SVS) and Society of Thoracic Surgeons (STS) reporting standards for type B aortic dissections. *J Vasc Surg.* 2020;71(3):723–747. doi:10.1016/j.jvs.2019.11.013

28. Rossi S, Rosa L, Ravetta V, et al. Contrast-enhanced versus conventional and color Doppler sonography for the detection of thrombosis of the portal and hepatic venous systems. *Am J Roentgenol.* 2006;186(3):763–773.

29. Clevert DA, Weckbach S, Kopp R, et al. Imaging of aortic lesions with color coded duplex sonography and contrast-enhanced ultrasound versus multislice computed tomography (MS-CT) angiography. *Clin Hemorheol Microcirc.* 2008;40(4):267–279.

30. Kaban J, Raio C. Emergency department diagnosis of aortic dissection by bedside transabdominal ultrasound. *Acad Emerg Med.* 2009;16(8):809–810.

31. Chaikof EL, Dalman RL, Eskandari MK, et al. The Society for Vascular Surgery practice guidelines on the care of patients with an abdominal aortic aneurysm. *J Vasc Surg.* 2018;67(1):2–77.e2. doi:10.1016/j.jvs.2017.10.044

32. Clevert DA, Schick K, Chen MH, et al. Role of contrast enhanced ultrasound in detection of abdominal aortic abnormalities in comparison with multislice computed tomography. *Chin Med J.* 2009;122(7):858–864.

33. Chaikof EL, Brewster DC, Dalman RL, et al. SVS practice guidelines for the care of patients with an abdominal aortic aneurysm: executive summary. *J Vasc Surg.* 2009;51(13):799–800.

34. Galesić K, Brkljacić B, Sabljar-Matovinović M, et al. Renal vascular resistance in essential hypertension: duplex-Doppler ultrasonographic evaluation. *Angiology.* 2000;51(8):667–675.

35. Adriaans BP, Wildberger JE, Westenberg JJM, Lamb HJ, Schalla S. Predictive imaging for thoracic aortic dissection and rupture: moving beyond diameters. *Eur Radiol.* 2019;29(12):6396–6404. doi:10.1007/s00330-019-06320-7

36. Lee WK, Mossop PJ, Little AF, et al. Infected (mycotic) aneurysms: spectrum of imaging appearances and management. *Radiographics.* 2008;28(7):1853–1868.

37. Rogers S. Sonographic evaluation of arteritis. *J Diagn Med Sonogr.* 2005;21:128–134.

38. Paravastu S, Murray D, Ghosh J, et al. Inflammatory abdominal aortic aneurysms (IAAA): past and present. *Vasc Endovascular Surg.* 2009;43(4):360–363.

39. Willing SJ, Fanizza-Orphanos A, Thomas HA. Mycotic aneurysm of the abdominal aorta. Diagnosis by duplex sonography. *J Ultrasound Med.* 1989;8(9):527–529.

40. Wang TKM, Desai MY. Optimal surveillance and treatment of renal and splenic artery aneurysms. *Cleve Clin J Med.* 2020;87(12):755–758. doi:10.3949/ccjm.87a.19140-2

41. Wang J, Lee YZ, Cheng Y, et al. Sonographic characterization of arterial dissections in Takayasu arteritis. *J Ultrasound Med.* 2016;35(6):1177–1191. doi:10.7863/ultra.15.07042

42. Lorelli D, Cambria RA, Seabrook GA, et al. Diagnosis and management of aneurysms involving the superior mesenteric artery and its branches: a report of four cases. *Vasc Endovascular Surg.* 2003;37:59–66.

43. Ouchi T, Kato N, Nakajima K, et al. Splenic artery aneurysm treated with endovascular stent grafting: a case report and review of literature. *Vasc Endovascular Surg.* 2018;52(8):663–668. doi:10.1177/1538574418785252

44. Lee HK, Park SJ, Yi BH, et al. Portal vein thrombosis: CT features. *Abdom Imaging.* 2008;33(1):72–79.

45. Malkowski P, Pawlak J, Michalowicz B, et al. Thrombolytic treatment of portal thrombosis. *Hepatogastroenterology.* 2003;50(54):2098–2100.

46. Pasha FS, Gloviczki P, Stanson AW, et al. Splanchnic artery aneurysms. *Mayo Clin Proc.* 2007;82:472–479.

47. Schweiger ML, Redick EL, Siegel LA, et al. Hepatic arterial pseudoaneurysm after placement of transjugular intrahepatic portosystemic shunt. *J Ultrasound Med.* 1997;16:437–439.

48. Turkvatan A, Okten RS, Ersa K, et al. Hepatic artery aneurysm: imaging findings. *J Ank Univ Fac Med.* 2005;58:73–75.

49. Germanos S, Soonawalla Z, Stratopoulos C, et al. Pseudoaneurysm of the gastroduodenal artery in chronic pancreatitis. *J Am Coll Surg.* 2009;208(2):316.

50. Berek P, Kopolovets I, Dzsinich C, Bober J, Štefanič P, Sihotský V. Interdisciplinary management of visceral artery aneurysms and visceral artery pseudoaneurysms. *Acta Medica (Hradec Kralove).* 2020;63(1):43–48. doi:10.14712/18059694.2020.14

51. Zwiebel WJ, Mountford RA, Halliwell MJ, et al. Splanchnic blood flow in patients with cirrhosis and portal hypertension: investigation with duplex Doppler US. *Radiology.* 1995;194(3):807–812.

52. Richards T, Dharmadasa A, Davies R, et al. Natural history of the common iliac artery in the presence of an abdominal aortic aneurysm. *J Vasc Surg.* 2009;49(4):881–885.

53. Roth SM, Bandyk DF. Duplex imaging of lower extremity bypasses, angioplasties, and stents. *Semin Vasc Surg.* 1999;12(4):275–284.

54. Lee WA, Wolf YG, Fogarty TZ, et al. Does complete aneurysm exclusion ensure long term success following endovascular repair? *J Endovasc Ther.* 2000;7:494–500.

55. Bandyk DF. Surveillance after lower extremity arterial bypass. *Perspect Vasc Surg Endovasc Ther.* 2007;19:376–383.

56. Nerlekar R, Warrier R, de Ryke R, et al. A comparative study of ultrasound and computed tomography for the follow up of abdominal aortic aneurysms after endovascular repair. *J Vasc Ultrasound.* 2006;30(2):81–85.

57. Johnson BL, Arko FR, Wolf Y, et al. Update: quantitative duplex ultrasound assessment of aortic aneurysms after endovascular repair. *J Vasc Surg.* 2003;27(3):165–170.

58. Taylor DC, Kettler MD, Moneta GL, et al. Duplex ultrasound scanning in the diagnosis of renal artery stenosis: a prospective evaluation. *J Vasc Surg.* 1988;7:363–369.

59. Radermacher J, Chavan A, Bleck J, et al. Use of Doppler ultrasonography to predict the outcome of therapy for renal artery stenosis. *N Engl J Med.* 2001;344:410–417.

60. Manoharan A, Gill RW, Griffiths KA. Splenic blood flow measurements by Doppler ultrasound: a preliminary report. *Cardiovasc Res.* 1987;21:779–782.

61. Gaitini D, Thaler I, Kaftori JK. Duplex sonography in the diagnosis of portal vein thrombosis. *Rofo.* 1990;153(6):645–649.

62. Qamar MI, Read AE, Skidmore R, et al. Transcutaneous Doppler ultrasound measurement of celiac axis blood flow in man. *Br J Surg.* 1985;72:329–393.

63. Qamar MI, Read AE, Skidmore R, et al. Pulsatility index of superior mesenteric artery blood velocity waveforms. *Ultrasound Med Biol.* 1986;12:772–776.

64. Gillespie DL, Villavicencio JL, Gallagher C, et al. Presentation and management of venous aneurysms. *J Vasc Surg.* 1997;26(5):845–852.

65. Bombelli L, Genitoni V, Biasi S, et al. Liver hemodynamic flow balance by image-directed Doppler ultrasound evaluation in normal subjects. *J Clin Ultrasound.* 1991;19(5):257–262.

66. Mitchell EL, Moneta GL. Mesenteric duplex scanning. *Perspect Vasc Surg Endovasc Ther.* 2006;18(2):175–183.

67. American Institute of Ultrasound in Medicine. AIUM practice parameter for the performance of duplex sonography of native renal vessels. 2019. Accessed May 2, 2022. https://www.aium.org/resources/guidelines/renalVessels.pdf

68. Hoffman U, Edwards JM, Carter S, et al. Role of duplex scanning for the detection of atherosclerotic renal artery disease. *Kidney Int.* 1991;39:1232–1239.

69. Poe PA. Color duplex ultrasound evaluation of renal and mesenteric arteries. *J Vasc Ultrasound.* 2003;27(3):177–183.

70. Samadian F, Dalili N, Jamalian A. New insights into pathophysiology, diagnosis, and treatment of renovascular hypertension. *Iran J Kidney Dis.* 2017;11(2):79–89.

71. Pellerito JS, Revzin M. Ultrasound assessment of native renal vessels. In: Pellerito JS, Polak J, eds. *Introduction to Vascular Ultrasonography.* 6th ed. Elsevier Saunders; 2012:517–539.

72. Dubbins PA. The kidney. In: Allan P, Dubbins P, McDicken WN, et al., eds. *Clinical Doppler Ultrasound.* 2nd ed. Churchill Livingstone Elsevier; 2006:185–213.

73. Schoepe R, McQuillan S, Valsan D, Teehan G. Atherosclerotic renal artery stenosis. *Adv Exp Med Biol.* 2017;956:209–213. doi:10.1007/5584_2016_89

74. Martin T, Nanra R, Wlodarczyk J, et al. Renal hilar Doppler analysis in the detection of renal artery stenosis. *J Vasc Technol.* 1991;15:173–180.

75. Moneta G, Lee R, Yeager R, et al. Mesenteric duplex scanning: a blinded prospective study. *J Vasc Surg.* 1993;17:79–86.

76. Zierler RE. Natural history of atherosclerotic renal artery stenosis. *Perspect Vasc Surg Endovasc Ther.* 1999;11:55–67.

77. Soares GM, Murphy TP, Singha MS, et al. Renal artery duplex ultrasonography as a screening and surveillance tool to detect renal artery stenosis: a comparison with current reference standard imaging. *J Ultrasound Med.* 2006;25:293–298.

78. Coombs P. Color duplex of the renal arteries: diagnostic criteria and anatomical windows for visualization. *J Vasc Ultrasound.* 2004;28(2):89–95.

79. Raju S, Hollis K, Neglen P. Obstructive lesions of the inferior vena cava: clinical features and endovenous treatment. *J Vasc Surg.* 2006;44(4):820–827.

80. Pellerito JS, Revzin M. Evaluation of organ transplants. In: Pellerito JS, Polak J, eds. *Introduction to Vascular Ultrasonography.* 6th ed. Elsevier Saunders; 2012:579–613.

81. Motew SJ, Cherr GS, Craven TE, et al. Renal duplex sonography: main renal artery versus hilar analysis. *J Vasc Surg.* 2000;32(3):462–471.

82. Crutchley TA, Pearce JD, Craven TE, et al. Clinical utility of resistive index in atherosclerotic renovascular disease. *J Vasc Surg.* 2009;49(1):148–155.

83. Rocha-Singh K, Jaff MR, Lynne K. Renal artery stenting with noninvasive duplex ultrasound follow up: 3 year results from the renaissance renal stent trial. *Catheter Cardiovasc Interv.* 2008;72(6):853–862.

84. Lencioni R, Caramella D, Sanguinetti F, et al. Portal vein thrombosis after percutaneous ethanol injection for hepatocellular carcinoma: value of color Doppler sonography in distinguishing chemical and tumor thrombi. *Am J Roentgenol.* 1995;164:1125–1130.

85. Zwolak RM, Fillinger MF, Walsh DB, et al. Mesenteric and celiac duplex scanning: a validation study. *J Vasc Surg.* 1998;27(6):1078–1087.

86. Armstrong PA. Visceral duplex scanning: evaluation before and after artery intervention for chronic mesenteric ischemia. *Perspect Vasc Surg Endovasc Ther.* 2007;19(4):386–392.

87. Bowie J, Bernstein JR. Retroperitoneal fibrosis: ultrasound findings and case report. *J Clin Ultrasound.* 1976;4(6):435–437.

88. Oderich G, Bower T, Sullivan T, et al. Open versus endovascular revascularization for chronic mesenteric ischemia: risk stratified outcomes. *J Vasc Surg.* 2009;49(6):1472–1479.

89. Bertino RE, Saucier NA, Barth DJ. The retroperitoneum. In: Rumack CM, Wilson SR, Charbonneau JW, et al., eds. *Diagnostic Ultrasound.* Vol 1. 4th ed. Elsevier Mosby; 2011:447–485.

90. Luong S, Miller J. Calcification and narrowing of the inferior vena cava. *J Diagn Med Sonogr.* 1991;7:154–156.

91. Williams C, Benson CB, Rhodes A, et al. American Registry of Diagnostic Medical Sonographers: survey of practice abdominal and in superficial sonography. *J Diagn Med Sonogr.* 1996;12(1):18–21.

92. Jia YP, Lu Q, Gong S, et al. Postoperative complications in patients with portal vein thrombosis after liver transplantation: evaluation with Doppler ultrasonography. *World J Gastroenterol.* 2007;13(34):4636–4640.

93. England RA, Wells IP, Gutteridge CM. Benign external compression of the inferior vena cava associated with thrombus formation. *Br J Radiol.* 2005;78:553–557.

94. Singh-Panghaal S, Karcnik TJ, Wachsberg RH, et al. Inferior vena caval leiomyosarcoma: diagnosis and biopsy with color Doppler sonography. *J Clin Ultrasound.* 1997;25(5):275–278.

95. Sorrell K, Harris S, Hanna J, et al. Renal vein and inferior vena cava tumor thrombus: presentation and mapping of venous extension with color duplex ultrasound. *J Vasc Ultrasound.* 2006;30(1):9–15.

96. McGahan JP, Blake LC, deVere White R, et al. Color flow sonographic mapping of intravascular extension of malignant renal tumors. *J Ultrasound Med.* 1993;12:403–409.

97. Sidhu R, Lockhart ME. Imaging of renovascular disease. *Semin Ultrasound CT MR.* 2009;30(4):271–288.

98. Ferrante A, Di Stasi C, Pierconti F, et al. Incidental finding of right renal venous aneurysm in a patient with symptomatic ipsilateral renal carcinoma: a case report. *Cardiovasc Pathol.* 2005;14(6):327–330.

99. Yura T, Yuasa S, Ohkawa M, et al. Noninvasive detection and monitoring of renal arteriovenous fistula by color Doppler. *Am J Nephrol.* 1991;11(3):250–251.

100. Valla DC. The diagnosis and management of the Budd-Chiari syndrome: consensus and controversies. *Hepatology.* 2003;38(4):793–803.

101. Gaba RC, Hardman JD, Bobra SJ. Extrahepatic portal vein aneurysm. *Radiol Case Rep.* 2016;4(2):291. doi: 10.2484/rcr.v4i2.291.

102. Ozbek SS, Killi MR, Pourbagher MA, et al. Portal venous system aneurysms: report of five cases. *J Ultrasound Med.* 1999;18(6):417–422.

103. Jin B, Sun Y, Li Y-Q, et al. Extrahepatic portal vein aneurysm: two case reports of surgical interventions. *World J Gastroenterol.* 2005;11(14):2206–2209.

104. Chaubal N, Dighe M, Hanchate V, et al. Sonography in Budd-Chiari syndrome. *J Ultrasound Med.* 2006;25(3):373–379.

105. Indeck M, Puyau F, Kerstein MD. Balloon septostomy for membranous obstruction of the vena cava in Budd-Chiari Syndrome. *Vasc Endovascular Surg.* 1984;18:399–402.

106. Andrew A. Portal hypertension: a review. *J Diagn Med Sonogr.* 2001;17:193–200.

107. Condat B, Pessione F, Denninger MH, et al. Recent portal or mesenteric venous thrombosis: increased recognition and frequent recanalization on anticoagulant therapy. *Hepatology.* 2000;32(3):466–470.

108. Bradbury MS, Kavanagh PV, Bechtold RE, et al. Mesenteric venous thrombosis: diagnosis and noninvasive imaging. *Radiographics.* 2002;22(3):527–541.

109. Miller VE, Berland LL. Pulsed-Doppler duplex sonography and CT of portal vein thrombosis. *AJR Am J Roentgenol.* 1985;145(1):73–76.

110. Parmar HH, Shah JJ, Shah BB. Imaging findings in a giant hepatic artery aneurysm. *J Postgrad Med.* 2000;46:104–105.

111. Umpleby HC. Thrombosis of the superior mesenteric vein. *Br J Surg.* 1987;74(8):694–696.

112. Gibson PR, Gibson RN, Donlan JD, et al. Duplex Doppler ultrasound of the ligamentum teres and portal vein: a clinically useful adjunct in the evaluation of patients with known or suspected chronic liver disease or portal hypertension. *J Gastroenterol Hepatol.* 1991;6(1):61–65.

113. Colli A, Cocciolo M, Mumoli N, et al. Hepatic artery resistance in alcoholic liver disease. *Hepatology.* 1998;28(5):1182–1186.

114. Evans K, Schneider J. Tumor masquerading as a portal vein thrombosis. *J Diagn Med Sonogr.* 2004;20(3):188–193.

115. Ciancio G, Vaidya A, Savoie M, et al. Management of renal cell carcinoma with level III thrombus in the inferior vena cava. *J Urol.* 2002;168(4 pt 1):1374–1377.

116. Iwao T, Toyonaga A, Oho K, et al. Value of Doppler ultrasound parameters of portal vein and hepatic artery in the diagnosis of cirrhosis and portal hypertension. *Am J Gastroenterol.* 1997;92(6):1012–1017.

117. Tchelepi H, Ralls PW, Randall R, et al. Sonography of diffuse liver disease. *J Ultrasound Med.* 2002;21(9):1023–1032.

118. Goyal AK, Pokharna DS, Sharma SK. Ultrasonic measurements of portal vasculature in diagnosis of portal hypertension, a controversial subject reviewed. *J Ultrasound Med.* 1990;9:45–48.

119. von Herbay A, Frieling T, Häussinger D. Color Doppler sonographic evaluation of spontaneous portosystemic shunts and inversion of portal venous flow in patients with cirrhosis. *J Clin Ultrasound.* 2000;28(7):332–339.

120. Goyal N, Jain N, Rachapalli V, et al. Non-invasive evaluation of liver cirrhosis using ultrasound. *Clin Radiol.* 2009;64(11):1056–1066.

121. Moneta GL, Taylor DC, Yeager RA, et al. Duplex ultrasound: applications to intra-abdominal vessels. *Perspect Vasc Surg.* 1989;2(2):133–148.

122. Taourel P, Blanc P, Dauzat M, et al. Doppler study of mesenteric, hepatic, and portal circulation in alcoholic cirrhosis: relationship between quantitative Doppler measurements and the severity of portal hypertension and hepatic failure. *Hepatology.* 1998;28(4):932–936.

123. Perisić MD, Culafić DjM, Kerkez M. Specificity of splenic blood flow in liver cirrhosis. *Rom J Intern Med.* 2005;43(1–2):141–151.

124. Bolognesi M, Sacerdoti D, Mescoli C, et al. Different hemodynamic patterns of alcoholic and viral endstage cirrhosis: analysis of explanted liver weight, degree of fibrosis and splanchnic Doppler parameters. *Scand J Gastroenterol.* 2007;42(2):256–262.

125. Kutlu R, Karaman I, Akbulut A, et al. Quantitative Doppler evaluation of the splenoportal venous system in various stages of cirrhosis: differences between right and left portal veins. *J Clin Ultrasound.* 2002;30(9):537–543.

126. Matveyenko AV, Donovan CM. Metabolic sensors mediate hypoglycemic detection at the portal vein. *Diabetes.* 2006;55(5):1276–1282.

127. Leen E, Goldberg JA, Anderson JR, et al. Hepatic perfusion changes in patients with liver metastases: comparison with those patients with cirrhosis. *Gut.* 1993;34(4):554–557.

128. Orban Schiopu AM, Balas BI, Diculescu M. The effect of a combined treatment with propranolol and isosorbide-5-mononitrate on Doppler ultrasound parameters in patients with cirrhosis and portal hypertension. *Rom J Gastroenterol.* 2005;14(2):123–127.

129. Segawa M, Sakaida I. Diagnosis and treatment of portal hypertension. *Hepatol Res.* 2009;39(10):1039–1043.

130. Cosar S, Oktar SO, Cosar B, et al. Doppler and gray-scale ultrasound evaluation of morphological and hemodynamic changes in liver vasculature in alcoholic patients. *Eur J Radiol.* 2005;54(3):393–399.

131. Culafic D, Perisic M, Vojinovic-Culafic V, et al. Spontaneous splenorenal shunt in a patient with liver cirrhosis and hypertrophic caudal lobe. *J Gastrointestin Liver Dis.* 2006;15(3):289–292.

132. Abbitt PL. Ultrasonography. Update on liver technique. *Radiol Clin North Am.* 1998;36(2):299–307.

133. Hirooka K, Hirooka M, Kisaka Y, et al. Doppler waveform pattern changes in a patient with primary Budd-Chiari syndrome before and after angioplasty. *Intern Med.* 2008;47(2):91–95.

134. Kruskal JB, Newman PA, Sammons LG, et al. Optimizing Doppler and color flow US: application to hepatic sonography. *Radiographics.* 2004;24(3):657–675.

135. Manatsathit W, Samant H, Panjawatanan P, et al. Performance of ultrasound for detection of transjugular intrahepatic portosystemic shunt dysfunction: a meta-analysis. *Abdom Radiol (NY).* 2019;44(7):2392–2402. doi:10.1007/s00261-019-01981-w

136. Abraldes JG, Gilabert R, Turnes J, et al. Utility of color Doppler ultrasonography predicting tips dysfunction. *Am J Gastroenterol.* 2005;100(12):2696–2701.

CHAPTER 7

The Liver

M. ROBERT DEJONG AND JEANINE RYBYINSKI

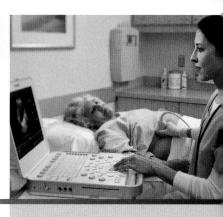

OBJECTIVES

- Identify the normal anatomy of the liver including the liver lobes, segments, fissures, ligaments, and hepatic vasculature.
- Describe the different lobar divisions of the liver including anatomic, functional, and Couinaud's segmental divisions.
- List some of the various functions of the liver.
- Discuss the laboratory values associated with liver function.
- Explain the patient preparation, scanning technique, and sonographic appearance of the normal liver.
- Discuss the pathophysiology and sonographic appearance of diffuse liver diseases including fatty infiltration, hepatitis, and cirrhosis.
- Describe the differential diagnoses, clinical signs, symptoms and sonographic appearance of cystic and solid liver lesions.
- Discuss ultrasound contrast enhancement of the liver, when to use it, and how it helps with diagnosing solid masses.
- Discuss the benefits of elastography of the liver.

GLOSSARY

AFP (alpha-fetoprotein) a tumor marker frequently elevated in cases of hepatocellular carcinoma and certain testicular cancers

ALP (alkaline phosphatase) an enzyme found in liver tissue that can be elevated with biliary obstruction

ALT (alanine aminotransferase) a liver enzyme most specific to hepatocellular damage

AST (aspartate aminotransferase) an enzyme found in all tissues, but in largest amounts in the liver; an increase can indicate hepatocellular damage

falciform ligament fold in the parietal peritoneum that extends from the umbilicus to the diaphragm and contains the ligamentum teres

Glisson capsule a fibroelastic, connective tissue layer that surrounds the liver and the portal triads

hepatofugal blood flow away from the liver; normal flow in the hepatic veins is hepatofugal

hepatomegaly enlarged liver

hepatopetal blood flow toward the liver; normal flow in the portal vein is hepatopetal

jaundice yellowish pigmentation of the skin and whites of the eyes caused by increased levels of bilirubin in the blood

KEY TERMS

adenoma

Budd–Chiari syndrome

candidiasis

cavernous hemangioma

cirrhosis

contrast-enhanced ultrasound

diffuse hepatocellular disease

echinococcal cyst

elastography

fatty infiltration

focal nodular hyperplasia

hepatitis

hepatocellular carcinoma

lipoma

liver abscess

hematoma

liver metastases

Pneumocystis infection

polycystic liver disease

(continued)

ligamentum teres remnant of the obliterated left umbilical vein seen as a triangular echogenic focus dividing the medial and lateral segments of the left lobe of the liver in the transverse plane

ligamentum venosum remnant of the ductus venosus seen as an echogenic line separating the caudate lobe from the left lobe

main lobar fissure divides the right and left lobes of the liver; seen in the sagittal plane as an echogenic line between the gallbladder neck and the main portal vein

porta hepatis known as the gateway to the liver, a fissure where the portal vein and hepatic artery enter the liver and the common hepatic duct exits

Riedel lobe anatomic variant in which the right lobe is enlarged and extends inferiorly as a tongue-like projection

The liver is an organ that is essential for life. It is the largest gland and solid organ in the body and is considered an accessory organ of digestion. It is important for the sonographer to understand the anatomy, physiology, and the various pathologies of the liver. The liver can be easily evaluated with ultrasound, and the use of new technologies—such as contrast and elastography—can help provide a lot of information about the liver for the physician. When a disease process of the liver is suspected, a sonography examination is commonly the first imaging test ordered because it can be quickly scheduled, has high patient acceptance, and does not use nephrotoxic contrast agents. Ultrasound can be used to measure the size of the liver, evaluate it for various masses and cysts, evaluate and stage parenchymal disease, and provide guidance for biopsies. This chapter will not cover biliary pathology because it is covered in another chapter. Liver transplants are covered in another chapter as well as in another book in this series.

ANATOMY

Embryology

Early in the fourth week of fetal development, the liver, gallbladder, and bile duct system develop from the endoderm. The hepatic diverticulum, also called the liver bud, develops from the ventral aspect of the foregut of the endoderm and gives rise to the parenchyma of the liver as well as the gallbladder and bile ducts. During week 5, the diverticulum differentiates into the origin of the cystic duct and the gallbladder in the caudal portion and the two endodermal cellular buds begin forming the right and the left hepatic lobes.[1-3] These solid cell buds grow into columns or cylinders that branch and form networks, which will envelope the vitelline and umbilical veins and become the liver sinusoids. The columns of endodermal cells in the liver parenchyma grow into the surrounding mesoderm. The mesoderm provides the hemopoietic tissue, which forms blood cells, until the bone marrow and spleen take over the process in late fetal life, and the connective tissue for the portal tracts and the fibrous liver capsule that becomes Glisson capsule.[1,3] As the terminal branches of the right and left hepatic lobes canalize, the bile duct system is formed. The development of the Kupffer cells starts in the yolk sac and they will eventually migrate to the fetal liver.

Both lobes are equal in size until the beginning of the sixth week, at which time the right lobe (RL) becomes larger, with the caudate and quadrate lobes developing from the RL. The left lobe actually undergoes some degeneration. At week 6, the liver fills most of the abdominal cavity and, relative to other organ development, the liver becomes less active.[1,2]

Hemopoiesis takes place in the liver at week 6, peaks at 12 to 24 weeks, and ceases at birth.[1,4] At week 10, lymphocyte formation occurs in the liver, which also ceases at birth. Coagulation factors are manufactured at 10 to 12 weeks and bile is produced by 13 to 16 weeks,[1] but the fetal liver does not take part in digestion until after birth.[5]

Oxygenated blood and nutrients are delivered to the fetus through the umbilical vein, which ascends and divides into two branches.[6,7] The left branch joins the portal vein and enters the liver and the right branch, the ductus venosus, flows directly into the inferior vena cava (IVC), bypassing the liver[5,8] (Fig. 7-1). Normally, both of these vessels deteriorate into fibrous cords sometime after birth. The left umbilical vein becomes the ligamentum teres, or round ligament, and the ductus venosus becomes the ligamentum venosum. Both the ligamentum teres and the ligamentum venosum can become recanalized as collateral vessels in patients with portal hypertension.[8]

Location and Size

The liver fills the right hypochondrium, epigastric region, and the left hypochondrium as far as the mammillary line. Most of the RL and usually the entire left lobe are protected by the ribs; therefore, intercostal scanning may be needed to visualize the entire liver. The liver can provide an acoustic window through which the upper abdomen and retroperitoneum may be imaged (Fig. 7-2A, B). The liver is wedge or triangular in shape with its base to the right and its apex to the left. Sonographically, the liver displays a medium-level homogeneous echo pattern owing to the nonspecular reflections from the hepatocytes. Interspersed within the parenchyma are tubular, fluid-filled structures representing the branches of the portal and hepatic veins. The liver is usually more echogenic, or it can also appear to be isoechoic, to the normal renal cortex (Fig. 7-3A, B). The liver is less echogenic than the normal pancreas and spleen. Disease processes can change these relationships. An example is when a normal right kidney appears to be

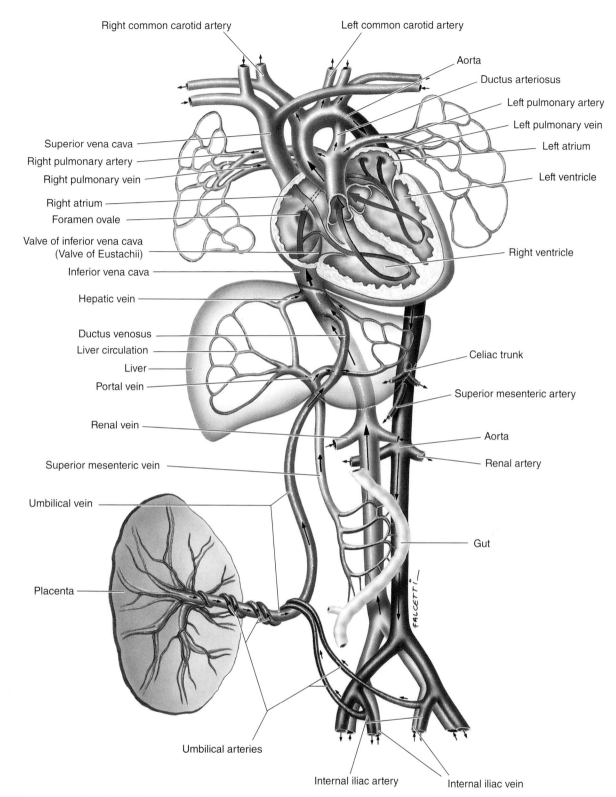

Right common carotid artery

Left common carotid artery

Aorta

Ductus arteriosus

Left pulmonary artery

Left pulmonary vein

Left atrium

Left ventricle

Superior vena cava

Right pulmonary artery

Right pulmonary vein

Right atrium

Foramen ovale

Valve of inferior vena cava
(Valve of Eustachii)

Right ventricle

Inferior vena cava

Hepatic vein

Ductus venosus

Liver circulation

Liver

Portal vein

Celiac trunk

Superior mesenteric artery

Aorta

Renal artery

Renal vein

Superior mesenteric vein

Umbilical vein

Gut

Placenta

Umbilical arteries

Internal iliac artery

Internal iliac vein

FALCETTI

FIGURE 7-1 Fetal circulation. The umbilical vein carries oxygenated blood from the placenta to the fetus, ascends the fetal abdomen, and courses toward the liver. A portion of blood flow is allowed to bypass the fetal liver via the ductus venosus. After birth, both veins close and exist as ligaments; the umbilical vein becomes the ligamentum teres and ductus venosus becomes the ligamentum venosum.

more echogenic than the liver in a patient with hepatitis, whose inflamed liver is abnormally hypoechoic.

The liver varies somewhat in shape and size, depending on the patient's body type, the size of the left lobe, and the length of the RL. The weight of a normal liver varies but usually ranges from about 1,200 g in an adult female to about 1,600 g in an adult male.[7] The weight of the liver is approximately 1/36th of the total body weight for an adult as compared to approximately 1/18th of the total body weight for an infant.[9] The normal transverse measurement of the liver can range from 20 to 22.5 cm, the anteroposterior (AP) measurement from 10 to 12.5 cm, and the length

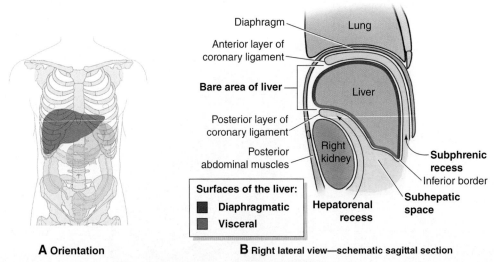

FIGURE 7-2 Liver location. **A:** The liver occupies the right hypochondrium, the greater part of the epigastric region, and extends in varying degrees into the left hypochondrium as far as the mammary line.[3] The lateral segment of the left lobe and the length of the right lobe determine the contour and shape of the liver. Overall, the liver can be described as irregular, hemispheric,[2] or wedge-shaped.[3] **B:** The relationship of the liver to surrounding anatomy is illustrated in a lateral, sagittal section.

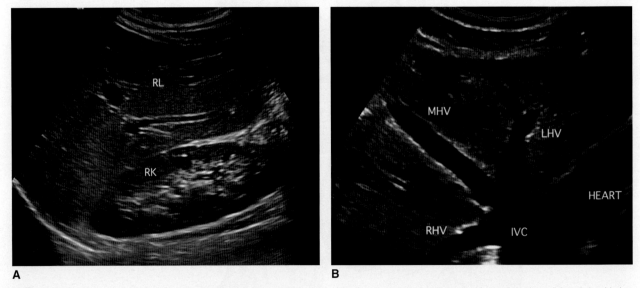

FIGURE 7-3 Normal sonographic anatomy. **A:** sagittal image of the right lobe (RL) of the liver demonstrating the normal increased echogenicity relationship between the normal liver and normal right kidney (RK). **B:** A transverse image demonstrating the normal homogeneous echo pattern of the liver and the three main hepatic veins, the right hepatic vein (RHV), the middle hepatic vein (MHV), the left hepatic vein (LHV), and the inferior vena cava (IVC).

from 13 to 15.5 cm, although some references go as high as 17 cm.[11] An AP measurement can be obtained on the same image as the length if needed. The length of the liver is obtained by measuring the liver from the diaphragm to the tip of the RL at the right midclavicular level, which is an imaginary vertical line that goes through the middle of the clavicle.[10,11] The liver's size can increase with increased height and body surface area and decrease with age.[10] Liver length is needed to determine if hepatomegaly is present.

Kratzer and coworkers did an extensive sonographic liver measurement study on 2,080 subjects. They found that the average liver length at the midclavicular line was 14.0 ± 1.7 cm. The average length for male subjects was 14.5 ± 1.6 cm and for female subjects 13.5 ± 1.7 cm.[12] Their technique allows for easy assessment and accurate follow-up

examinations. They also demonstrated that body mass index, height, sex, age, and frequent alcohol consumption in men influenced liver size.[12]

Perihepatic Relationships

The liver is an intraperitoneal organ that is covered by a capsule that is composed of two adherent layers. One layer is an outer serous layer that is derived from the visceral peritoneum and covers the liver except at the bare area near the diaphragm, the porta hepatis, and the area where the gallbladder is attached to the liver. The inner layer is a dense, fibroelastic connective tissue called Glisson capsule, which is named after the British physician and anatomist Francis Glisson, who was the first person to describe the layer of connective tissue that covers the entire liver and each lobule. Glisson capsule contains blood, lymphatic vessels, and nerves and is highly echogenic by sonography.[10,13,14] Distention of the capsule from liver disease or swelling can cause pain, and lymphatics may ooze fluid into the peritoneal space.[13] Glisson capsule also ensheaths the portal triad, which consists of a branch of the hepatic artery, portal vein, and bile duct, which explains why the portal triad has echogenic borders.

The external surfaces of the liver are described as the diaphragmatic and visceral surfaces. The diaphragmatic surface is the anterosuperior surface of the liver and is smooth and convex, fitting beneath the curvature of the diaphragm. The posterior aspect of the diaphragmatic surface

is not covered by the visceral peritoneum and is called the bare area. The bare area is a small triangular area where the liver connects to the diaphragm, and although it is not covered by the visceral peritoneum, it is covered by Glisson capsule. The bare area lies between the anterior and posterior folds of the coronary ligament and is clinically important because it represents an area where disease, such as an abscess or tumor, can spread from the abdominal cavity to the thoracic cavity because the barrier in the form of the visceral peritoneum is absent[9,15] (Fig. 7-4 A–D).

The visceral surface of the liver faces inferiorly and posteriorly with its shape determined by the surrounding organs. It is uneven and concave and is covered by the peritoneum except in the fossa of the gallbladder, the

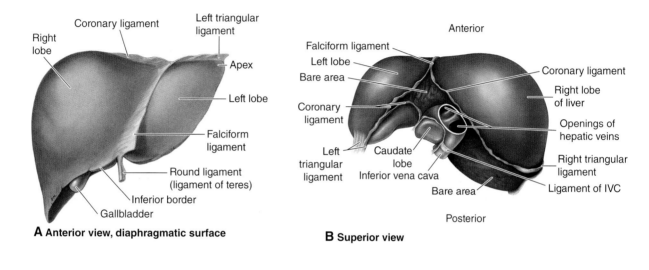

A Anterior view, diaphragmatic surface

B Superior view

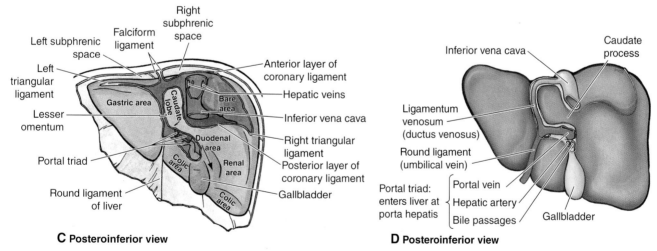

C Posteroinferior view

D Posteroinferior view

FIGURE 7-4 Normal anatomy. **A:** Anterior surface. The ligamentum teres begins at the umbilicus and courses within the falciform ligament to a deep notch called the umbilical notch, which is located on the anterior surface of the liver. The falciform ligament divides the liver into right and left anatomical lobes and will become the coronary ligaments. Opposite the cartilage of the ninth rib is the fossa for the gallbladder fundus.[9] **B:** Posterior surface. The posterior portion of the liver is round and broad on the right and narrow on the left.[3] The caudate lobe lies between the inferior vena cava (*IVC*) and the ligament venosum, which is not marked on this image.[3,9] The posterior surface is in direct contact with the diaphragm and is attached by loose connective tissue. Most of the liver is covered by peritoneum except for the bed of the gall bladder, the porta hepatis, and where the liver is in direct contact with the diaphragm called the bare area. The bare area is bounded by the superior and inferior reflections of the coronary ligament, which connect the liver to the diaphragm.[9] **C:** Posterior inferior view of visceral area: The right subphrenic space is seen between the right lobe of the liver and the inferior surface of the diaphragm. The left subphrenic space is seen between the diaphragm and the spleen. From lateral to medial, the right lobe has three impressions—the colic impression, which is a flattened or shallow area for the hepatic flexure; more posterior is the larger and deeper impression for the right kidney; and lying along the neck of the gallbladder, the duodenal impression is a narrow, poorly marked area.[3] On the left, the gastric impression for the ventral surface of the stomach is a large, hollow area extending to the liver margin. **D:** Visceral surface. The visceral surface is concave and faces posterior, caudal, and to the left.[3,9] The caudate process is just anterior to the *IVC* and connects the caudate lobe to the right lobe.[9] On this image, the ligamentum venosum is seen with the caudate lobe located between the ligamentum venosum and the *IVC*. The portal triad as it enters the liver via the porta hepatis is illustrated.

porta hepatis, and the IVC groove. It is in contact with the esophagus, the stomach including the pylorus, the first part of the duodenum, the right hepatic flexure, the transverse colon, the lesser omentum, the gallbladder, the right kidney, and the right adrenal gland.

Ligaments

The liver is tethered to the undersurface of the diaphragm, the anterior wall of the abdomen, the lesser curvature of the stomach, and the retroperitoneum by eight ligaments, seven of which are either parietal or visceral peritoneal folds and one of which is a round, fibrous cord. These ligaments are as follows: the coronary, falciform, ligamentum teres (round ligament), ligamentum venosum, right and left triangular, gastrohepatic, and hepatoduodenal ligaments.[15] The largest of these ligaments is the coronary ligament. They are described in Table 7-1 and can be identified on Figures 7-4 and 7-5. Understanding the location of these various ligaments can help in identifying the location of various pathologies and fluid collections.

Lobar Anatomy

The lobes of the liver can be described based on their anatomic or external landmarks or their functional anatomy,

which is based on the portal and hepatic veins. Because the author may not specify which method is being used, the literature can be confusing and may appear to be contradictory. The next section presents each method separately. The sonographic images are presented in the segmental division because sonographers evaluate and document the liver using internal landmarks.

Anatomic Division

The anatomic division of the liver is based on external markings that divide the liver into right, left, caudate, and quadrate lobes. This method uses the falciform ligament on the anterior surface to divide the liver into its left and right lobes and considers the caudate and quadrate lobes as part of the RL. A simulated "H" configuration on the visceral surface has the ligamentum venosum and the ligamentum teres separate the caudate and the quadrate lobes from the left lobe, the porta hepatis separates the caudate from the quadrate, and the main lobar fissure (MLF) separates the caudate and the quadrate from the RL (Fig. 7-6).

Right Lobe

The RL occupies the right hypochondrium and is six times larger than the left lobe with this method.[5] It is separated from the left lobe by the falciform ligament on its anterior surface and by the left intersegmental fissure on its visceral

TABLE 7-1	**Ligament Attachments to the Liver**
Ligament	**Description**
Coronary	The coronary ligament attaches the superior surface of the liver to the inferior surface of the diaphragm. The coronary ligament consists of an anterior and a posterior layer that create a triangular area that is devoid of peritoneum which is called the bare area of the liver. The anterior layer is formed by the reflection of the parietal peritoneum and is continuous with the right layer of the falciform ligament. The posterior layer is reflected from the caudal margin of the bare area onto the right adrenal gland and right kidney and is sometimes referred to as the hepatorenal ligament.[15] The anterior and posterior folds unite to form the triangular ligaments.[15,16]
Falciform	The term falciform ligament is derived from Latin, meaning sickle shaped. It is a broad and thin fold of peritoneum that anchors the anterior surface of the liver to the anterior abdominal wall. It is used to separate the anatomic right and left liver lobes. It extends from the liver to the abdominal wall between the diaphragm and umbilicus.[9,15,16] At its base or free edge, the ligamentum teres is released from between its layers.[15]
Ligamentum teres	The ligamentum teres, or round ligament, is a fibrous cord that is the remnant of the left umbilical vein.[9,15] The round ligament divides the left lobe into medial and lateral sections. It ascends from the umbilicus in the free margin of the falciform ligament into the umbilical fissure where it is in continuity with the ligamentum venosum and joins the left branch of the portal vein.[9]
Ligamentum venosum	The ligamentum venosum is the obliterated ductus venosus and is usually attached to the left branch of the portal vein and can be in continuance with the ligamentum teres within the left intersegmental fissure. The ligamentum venosum is invested by the peritoneal folds of the lesser omentum within a fissure between the caudate and left lobe.
Triangular	The right and left triangular ligaments are named because of their triangular shape. They are formed by the apposition of the upper and lower ends of the coronary ligament and extend from the diaphragm of the liver.[9] The right triangular ligament attaches the right lobe of the liver to the diaphragm.[15] The left triangular ligament is the larger of the two. It lies anterior to the esophagus and connects the posterior part of the upper surface of the left lobe to the diaphragm.[9]
Gastrohepatic	The gastrohepatic ligament connects the liver to the lesser curvature of the stomach. It is composed of two folds of visceral peritoneum and originates on the undersurface of the liver. It extends from the fissure of the ligamentum venosum and porta hepatis; courses caudally to attach to the lesser curvature of the stomach and to the first portion of the duodenum; and, together with the hepatoduodenal ligament, forms the lesser omentum.[5,15]
Hepatoduodenal	The hepatoduodenal ligament is a thick anatomical structure wrapped in the peritoneum that constitutes part of the lesser omentum. It extends between the porta hepatis and the superior part of the duodenum. The opening behind the free edge of the hepatoduodenal ligament is the epiploic foramen or foramen of Winslow, which is the only communication between the lesser sac and the peritoneal cavity.[9] The hepatoduodenal ligament encloses the portal triad to protect it because it provides the blood supply to the liver and drains the bile into the duodenum.

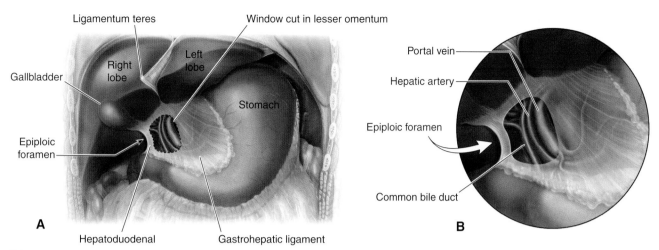

FIGURE 7-5 Ligaments. **A:** The gastrohepatic ligament originates on the undersurface of the liver and courses caudal to attach to the lesser curvature of the stomach and the first portion of the duodenum. The hepatoduodenal ligament is located on the right free edge of the gastrohepatic ligament, surrounds the portal triad, and forms the anterior boundary of the epiploic foramen or the foramen of Winslow. **B:** Enlarged cutaway view of the hepatoduodenal ligament showing the portal triad.

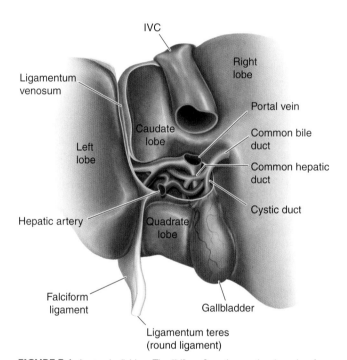

FIGURE 7-6 Anatomic division. The "H" configuration on the visceral surface of the liver is as follows: An imaginary line from the gallbladder fossa to the inferior vena cava (IVC) fossa makes the right vertical limb. This separates the right lobe from the caudate and quadrate lobes. The left vertical limb is a line created by the falciform ligament and the ligamentum venosum and separates the left lobe from the caudate and quadrate lobes.[9]. The transverse limb is the porta hepatitis and separates the caudate and quadrate lobes. The gallbladder fossa is shallow and oblong, extending from the inferior margin to the right border of the porta hepatis.[9] The IVC fossa is a short, deep depression between the caudate lobe and the right lobe.

surface.[16] It is somewhat quadrilateral. The posterior surface is marked by three fossae: the porta hepatis, the gallbladder, and the IVC.[17]

Caudate Lobe

The caudate lobe (CL) is anatomically distinct from the left and right lobes and is situated on the posterosuperior surface of the RL opposite the 10th and 11th thoracic vertebrae. It is located between the IVC posteriorly and the ligamentum venosum anteriorly.[18,19] The ligamentum venosum separates the caudate from the left lobe. The left margin of the caudate forms the hepatic boundary of the superior recess of the lesser sac. The caudate process is a small elevation of hepatic tissue that extends obliquely and laterally, from the lower aspect of the CL to the undersurface of the RL. It is situated behind the porta hepatis and separates the gallbladder fossa from the commencement of the fossa for the IVC. The papillary process is an anteromedial extension of the CL, which may appear separate from the CL and mimic lymph nodes.[10,15] Physiologically, the CL is considered independent from the liver vasculature because it has its own arterial supply and venous drainage. Blood drains from the CL directly into the vena cava via the small caudate veins.[9]

Quadrate Lobe

Anatomists describe the quadrate lobe as a distinct lobe, but it is physiologically and sonographically the same as the medial segment of the left lobe. The quadrate lobe is located on the undersurface of the liver between the middle and the left hepatic vein. Situated on the visceral surface, it is bounded posteriorly by the porta hepatis, anteriorly by the inferior margin of the liver, and laterally by the gallbladder fossa on the right and the fissure for the ligamentum teres on the left.[15]

Left Lobe

The left lobe is situated in the epigastric and left hypochondriac regions. Anatomically, it is separated from the RL by the falciform ligament on its anterior surface. On the visceral surface, the fissure for the ligamentum teres separates it from the quadrate lobe, and the fissure for the ligamentum venosum separates it from the CL.[15] The left lobe is flatter and smaller than the right and can vary in size. Its superior surface is slightly convex, is molded to the diaphragm, and tapers off to the left at about the left mammary line.[9,15]

Sonographic Segmental Division

Ultrasound can easily divide the liver into three lobes and four segments using the main lobar fissure, the hepatic veins, and the ligamentum venosum and ligamentum teres (Fig. 7-7A). The lobes and segments are the RL, with an anterior and a posterior segment, the left lobe, with a medial and a lateral segment, and the CL.[15] A combination of scanning planes that includes transverse, oblique, and parasagittal is needed to delineate the landmarks to identify the lobes and segments.

Right and Left Lobes

The MLF is a line that connects the gallbladder and the IVC and contains the middle hepatic vein (MHV). It is used to separate the liver into right and left lobes (Fig. 7-7B). It is seen sonographically as an echogenic line that runs obliquely between the neck of the gallbladder and right portal vein (RPV) (Fig. 7-7C).

The right intersegmental fissure divides the RL into its anterior and posterior segments. The sonographic landmark for the right intersegmental fissure is the right hepatic vein (RHV) (Fig. 7-7D–F).

The left intersegmental fissure divides the left lobe into medial and lateral segments. The sonographic landmarks used to define this fissure are the left hepatic vein (LHV); the ascending branch of the left portal vein (LPV); and more inferiorly, the hyperechoic ligamentum teres (Fig. 7-7G–J). In patients with ascites, the externally located falciform ligament may be a visible landmark for separation of the medial and lateral segments of the left lobe (Fig. 7-7K).

The sonographer should understand that the hepatic veins are intersegmental—that is, they run between the segments—and that the portal veins are intrasegmental, because they will travel within the segments, except for the ascending portion of the LPV, which runs in the left intersegmental fissure (Fig. 7-7L). The RPV divides into an anterior segmental branch and a posterior segmental branch, supplying blood to each respective segment (Fig. 7-7M). The LPV divides into medial and lateral segment branches supplying blood to their respected segments (Fig. 7-7N). Both portal veins and hepatic veins have distinguishing features by sonography that enable differentiation between them (Table 7-2).[10,17,26]

Caudate Lobe

The CL is located in the posterior aspect of the liver and corresponds to the anatomic CL. Sonographically, three anatomic landmarks identify the CL. The anterior border of the CL is the fissure for the ligament venosum, which appears as a hyperechoic line that separates the CL from the left lobe, the IVC runs along the posterior aspect of the CL and the main portal vein (MPV) is located at the inferior aspect of the CL, separating it from the head of the pancreas (Fig. 7-7O, P).[15,16,19]

The CL is functionally distinct from the right and left lobes because it has its own bile ducts and receives its blood supply from both right and left portal and hepatic arterial branches.[10,19] It is drained by short venous channels that extend from its posterior aspect and drain directly into the IVC (Fig. 7-7Q).[19] This independent blood supply has significant clinical implications that will produce changes in the size of the lobe with certain pathologies.[20,21] The portal veins and hepatic arteries of the CL have a short intrahepatic course, which is not as readily affected by hepatic fibrosis. CL enlargement and RL shrinkage are seen in patients with

cirrhosis and may be attributed to the discrepancy between blood perfusion of the two lobes.[22] CL enlargement is also seen in patients with Budd–Chiari syndrome, which is thrombosis of the hepatic veins, cavernous transformation of the portal vein, and end-stage primary sclerosing cholangitis, which is a long-term inflammation and scarring of the bile ducts.

Couinaud's Hepatic Segment Classification

In 1957, Claude Couinaud (pronounced kwee-NO), a French surgeon, described a detailed method of liver segmentation, which has become the universal nomenclature for hepatic lesion localization.[10] It is currently the most widely used system to describe functional liver anatomy. The Couinaud classification system creates eight functionally separate liver segments, counted in a clockwise fashion. Traditionally, the hepatic segments were numbered using Roman numerals I to VIII, but the Arabic numerals 1 to 8 are now preferred (Fig. 7-8A–F). The CL is segment 1, the left lobe makes up segments 2 to 4, and the RL makes up segments 5 to 8 (Table 7-3).[10,23,24] The division is based on the hepatic and portal vein branches. Each of the eight segments has its own branch of a portal vein, hepatic artery, hepatic vein, and bile duct. This allows the surgeon to resect a segment of a hepatic lobe, allowing the vascular supply to the remaining lobes to be left intact. The hepatic veins provide the boundaries of each segment. In Couinaud's segmental anatomy, the three planes of the right, middle, and left hepatic veins divide the liver vertically. The MHV lies in the MLF and divides the liver into right and left lobes. This vertical plane courses from the IVC to the gallbladder fossa and is also known as the Cantlie line. The portal plane is a horizontal plane where the portal vein bifurcates and further divides the liver into superior and inferior segments. These three vertical planes and one horizontal plane divide the liver into the eight segments as summarized in Table 7-3.[10,23,24] These segmental divisions do not coincide completely with the lobar anatomy divisions because the quadrate lobe is now the medial segment of the left lobe, the anatomic left lobe is now the lateral segment of the left lobe, and the CL is considered a separate lobe.

The Couinaud classification system of eight independent functional segments is important for the sonographer to understand because computed tomography (CT) and magnetic resonance imaging (MRI) will report the location of liver masses based on these eight segments. If the CT report states that the mass is in segment V, the sonographer will know to concentrate on the RL between the RHV and the MHV and posterior to the RPV. If the CT report states that the mass is in segment III, the sonographer will know to look in the left lobe lateral to the LHV. When a liver mass is initially discovered on an ultrasound examination, the sonographer should try and determine which segment contains the mass.[10,23] This can be difficult with ultrasound, and the sonographer may only be able to narrow the location down to the left medial or lateral lobe using the LHV or ligamentum teres, the right anterior or posterior segment using the RHV or the CL.

Anatomic Variations

Variations of the liver include variations in shape, variations in lobe size, thinning of the left lobe, congenital absence of the left lobe, diaphragmatic indentations called pseudofissures,

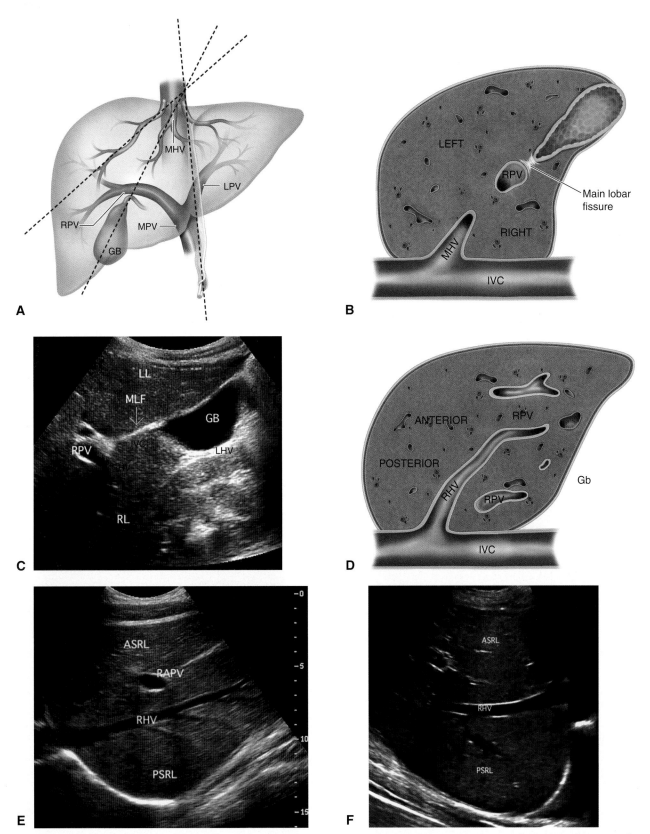

FIGURE 7-7 Segmental division. **A:** A "see-through" anterior to posterior profile. The dotted lines will be referenced in subsequent illustrations and sonograms. Segmental anatomy. **B:** An illustration through vertical plane B (Fig. 7-7A), which represents the main lobar fissure, which is seen sonographically between the gallbladder neck and the RPV and is used to divide the liver into its segmental right and left lobes. **C:** A parasagittal scan displays a portion of the *MLF*, seen as a linear echogenic line extending from the *RPV* to the *GB* separating the *RL* from the *LL*. **D:** An illustration through vertical plane C (Fig. 7-7A), the right intersegmental fissure, where the *RHV* courses between the right anterior and right posterior branches of the portal vein. **E:** A parasagittal scan through the *RHV*, which is the sonographic landmark dividing the right lobe of the liver into anterior and posterior segments. **F:** A transverse scan through the *RHV* dividing the liver into *ASRL* and *PSRL*.

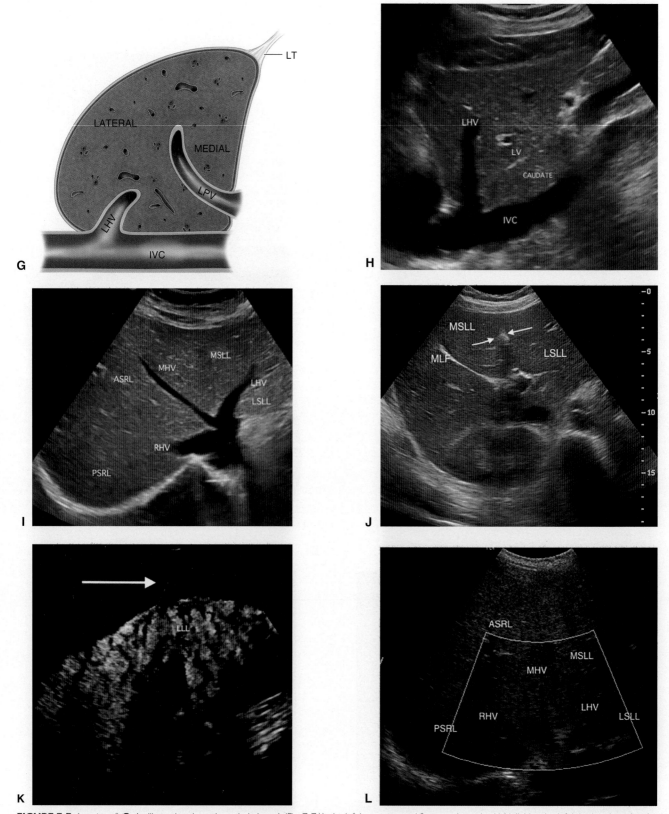

FIGURE 7-7 (*continued*) **G:** An illustration through vertical plane A (Fig. 7-7A), the left intersegmental fissure, where the *LHV* divides the left lobe into lateral and medial segments. **H:** A parasagittal scan through the *LHV* and *IVC*. The caudate lobe is seen between the *IVC* and the *LV*. **I:** A transverse scan through the *LHV* dividing the left lobe of the liver into medial and lateral segments. **J:** *LT* (*small arrows*) is seen in the left lobe of the liver in the transverse plane as a rounded echogenic structure with an acoustic shadow. It serves as a landmark separating the *MSLL* and the *LSLL* of the left lobe. The *LT* should not be mistaken for a liver lesion. **K:** On this transverse image of a patient with cirrhosis and ascites, the falciform ligament (*arrow*) can be identified coursing between the anterior abdominal wall and the *LLL* which is very nodular. **L:** A transverse scan demonstrates the hepatic veins and liver segments. The *MHV* separates the right and left liver lobes. The *LHV* separates the *MSLL* from the *LSLL*. The *RHV* divides the *ASRL* from the *PSRL*.

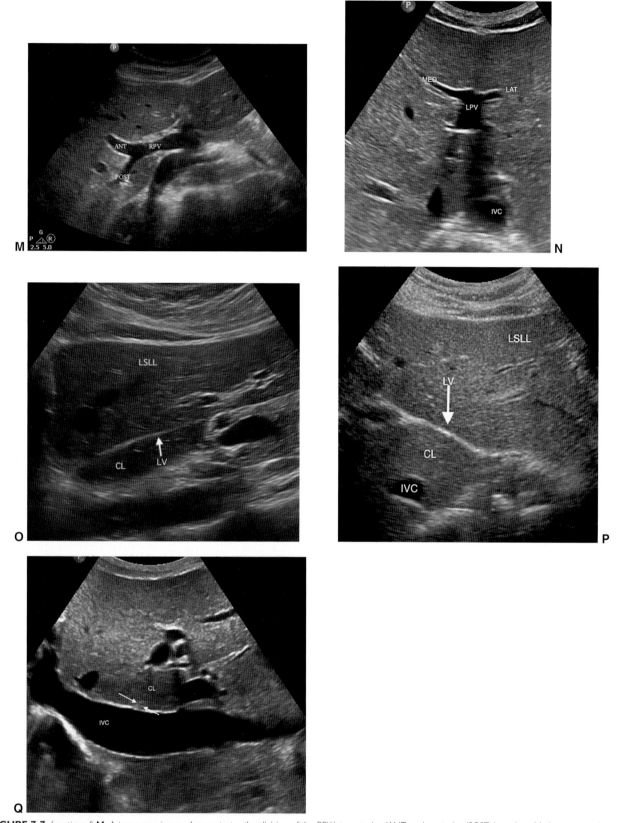

FIGURE 7-7 (continued) **M:** A transverse image demonstrates the division of the *RPV* into anterior (*ANT*) and posterior (*POST*) branches. **N:** A transverse image demonstrates the division of the *LPV* into medial and lateral branches. **O:** A sagittal scan demonstrates the *LSLL*, which is delineated from the *CL* by a linear echogenic line representing the *LV* (*arrow*). **P:** The anatomy identified on this transverse scan includes the *LSLL*, which is delineated from the *CL* by the *LV* (*arrow*). **Q:** A parasagittal image demonstrates a small vein (*arrows*) draining directly from the *CL* into the *IVC*. *ASRL*, anterior segment of the right lobe; *CL*, caudate lobe; *GB*, gallbladder; *IVC*, inferior vena cava; *LHV*, left hepatic vein; *LL*, left lobe; *LLL*, left lobe of the liver; *LPV*, left portal vein; *LSLL*, lateral segment of the left lobe; *LV*, ligamentum venosum; *LT*, ligamentum teres; *MHV*, middle hepatic vein; *MLF*, main lobar fissure; *MPV*, main portal vein; *MSLL*, medial segment left lobe; *PSRL*, posterior segment right lobe; *RAPV*, right anterior portal vein; *RL*, right lobe; *RHV*, right hepatic vein; *RPV*, right portal vein.

TABLE 7-2	**Sonographic Criteria for Differentiating the Portal Veins and Hepatic Veins**[10,17,26]
Origin and drainage	Observe the point of origin and drainage of the vessels. Portal vein branches can be traced back to the main portal vein, distinguishing them from the hepatic veins draining into the IVC.
Echogenic walls	The portal vein runs with branches of the hepatic artery and of a bile duct and is known as a portal triad. The portal triad is covered by Glisson capsule, which is highly reflective, making the walls of the portal vein appear to be hyperechoic in contrast to the liver parenchyma. By contrast, the hepatic veins are surrounded by parenchymal tissue and have rather imperceptible margins. Specular reflection may occur if the sound beam strikes a main hepatic vein wall perpendicularly, resulting in a high-amplitude, echogenic margin that will disappear when the insonation angle is <90 degrees.
Branching patterns	An angle is formed as vessels bifurcate. For the portal vein, its vessels branch such that the angle's apex point toward the porta hepatis. For the hepatic veins, branching occurs such that the angle's apex points toward the IVC and heart.
Caliber changes and Doppler signal	The direction of blood flow also dictates the caliber of the venous radicles. The caliber of the hepatic veins becomes greater as it courses toward the IVC and diaphragm. The caliber of the portal veins decreases further from its point of origin, the porta hepatis. The hepatic veins have a pulsatile waveform whereas the portal vein has a continuous waveform.
Segmental location	Hepatic veins are interlobar and intersegmental, coursing between lobes and segments. Portal veins are intrasegmental, coursing within lobar segments.

IVC, inferior vena cava.

high posterior hepatodiaphragmatic interposition of the colon, and situs inversus (Fig. 7-9A–C).[9,20,25] A common variant that can mimic hepatomegaly is called a Riedel lobe, which is a downward projection of the RL. (Note that the proper name is Riedel lobe and not Riedel lobe.) It is more common in women than in men. Sonographically, a Riedel lobe is identified as a finger-like or a tongue-like projection of the RL that extends past the ribs and may reach as far as the iliac crest[25] (Fig. 7-10A, B). A Riedel lobe can be felt clinically, and the patient may be referred for a liver ultrasound to rule out a liver mass or hepatomegaly. To differentiate it from a mass, the sonographer must observe consistency of the echotexture between the Riedel lobe and the rest of the RL. To differentiate it from hepatomegaly, the sonographer should note that the rest of the liver's size appears normal, and that the lobe comes to a point, whereas with hepatomegaly, the lobe has a more rounded edge (also see Fig. 7-16F, G). In hepatomegaly, the RL of the liver can displace the right kidney downward and up toward the diaphragm whereas a Riedel lobe "skims" across the top of the kidney.

Vascular System

The liver is a unique organ in that it receives a blood supply from two different sources. The hepatic artery supplies about 20% to 30% of the blood supply to the liver and 40% to 50% of oxygenated blood. The remaining 70% to 80% is supplied by the portal venous blood, which is nutrient rich and contains oxygenated blood, supplying 50% to 60% of the oxygenated blood owing to its greater volume. The portal vein and the hepatic artery mix their blood in the liver sinusoids, which are drained by the central hepatic vein (Fig. 7-11A–C).

Hepatic Arteries

The common hepatic artery supplies oxygenated blood to the liver, pylorus of the stomach, duodenum, pancreas, and gallbladder. It is the largest branch of the celiac axis or trunk and the only branch that courses to the right across the epigastric region of the abdomen. The common hepatic artery passes anterior to the pancreas, and then inferiorly

to the right toward the first part of the duodenum. It gives off the right gastric artery, which will anastomose with the left gastric artery. The common hepatic artery then travels upward, lying to the left of the common bile duct and anterior to the portal vein. As it courses toward the porta hepatis, it gives off the gastroduodenal artery and then becomes the proper hepatic artery, terminating into the right and left hepatic arteries that will supply blood to the right and left lobes, respectively. The cystic artery arises off of the right branch and the middle hepatic artery usually arises from the left branch (Fig. 7-11D–H).

Portal Veins

The MPV measures approximately 8 cm in length and has a maximum diameter of 13 mm. It originates just to the right of the midline at the junction of the splenic vein and superior mesenteric vein (SMV) anterior to the IVC and posterior to the neck of the pancreas. It carries blood containing nutrients and toxins from the gastrointestinal (GI) tract, except for the lower section of the rectum, the pancreas, gallbladder, and the spleen. The MPV courses upward and toward the porta hepatis within the hepatoduodenal ligament and is posterior to the hepatic artery and the common bile duct. Before entering the liver, the MPV divides into a smaller LPV and into a larger RPV with each branch entering the liver separately (Fig. 7-11I).[10,26] The LPV lies more anterior and superior to the RPV. The LPV can be divided into transverse and umbilical portions. The LPV, prior to its bifurcation, gives off a branch that supplies the medial segment of the left lobe[10] and a branch for the lateral segment of the left lobe (Fig. 7-11J). Both are intrasegmental in their course.[26] Prior to the bifurcation is the umbilical portion of the LPV, named because in utero, the umbilical vein is attached at this point.[9] The umbilical portion of the LPV provides blood to the CL through small branches that are not visualized sonographically. The size of the LPV and its angle of bifurcation with the MPV vary, depending largely on the size and configuration of the left lobe.[17] The main branches of the LPV originate from the umbilical portion and supply liver segments 2, 3, and 4. The RPV bifurcates at various distances from the MPV to

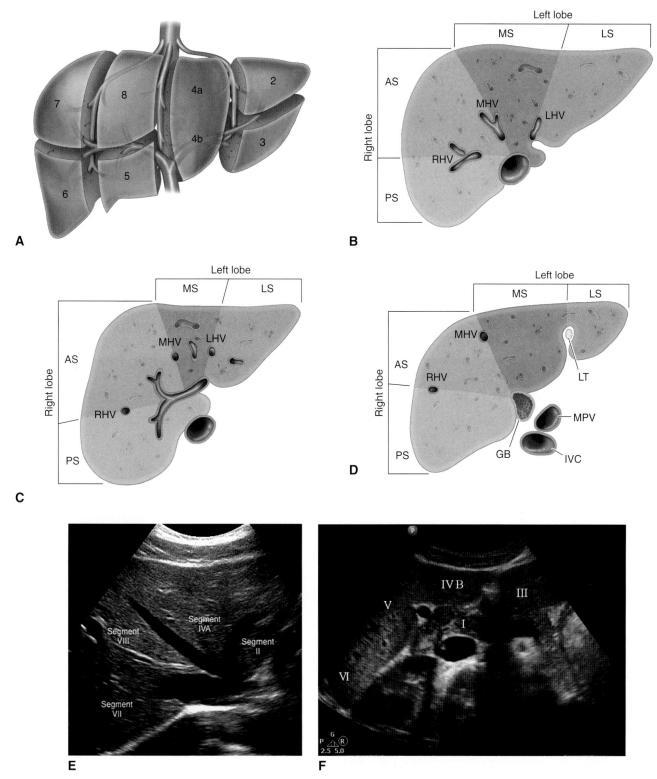

FIGURE 7-8 Couinaud's anatomy. **A:** An illustration of the eight segments and how they are identified in a clockwise fashion. The hepatic veins divide the liver vertically into four segments and the portal veins divide the liver horizontally creating eight segments. The caudate lobe is segment 1 and is seen on the posterior aspect of the liver, it is not seen in an anterior view. **B:** A cross-sectional illustration high in the liver at the level of the hepatic veins identifies the four superior segments in Couinaud's anatomy (*PS* = segment 7, *AS* = segment 8, *MS* = segment 4a, and *LS* = segment 2). **C:** A cross-sectional illustration at a midlevel through the liver identifies the right and left portal vein branches that correspond with the horizontal boundary. **D:** A cross-sectional illustration low in the liver at the level of the gallbladder and ligamentum teres identifies the four inferior segments in Couinaud's anatomy (*PS* = segment 6, *AS* = segment 5, *MS* = segment 4b, and *LS* = segment 3). **E:** A transverse scan at the level of the hepatic veins demonstrates the superior segments. **F:** A transverse scan through the gallbladder and ligamentum teres demonstrates the inferior segments.

TABLE 7-3	Couinaud's Segmental Anatomy[10,23,24]
Caudate Lobe	
Segment I	Caudate lobe is situated posteriorly and is anterior to the IVC and separated from the left lobe by the ligamentum venosum.
Left Lobe	
Segment II	Lateral segment of left lobe located above (superior) the portal plane and lateral to the LHV
Segment III	Lateral segment of left lobe located below (inferior) the portal plane and lateral to the LHV
Segment IVa	Medial segment of left lobe located above (superior) the portal plane and between the MHV and LHV
Segment IVb	Medial segment of left lobe located below (inferior) the portal plane and between the MHV and LHV; includes the quadrate lobe
Right Lobe	
Segment V	Anterior segment of right lobe located below (inferior) the portal plane and between the MHV and RHV
Segment VI	Posterior segment of right lobe located below (inferior) the portal plane and lateral to the RHV
Segment VII	Posterior segment of right lobe located above (superior) the portal plane and lateral to the RHV
Segment VIII	Anterior segment of RL located above (superior) the portal plane between the MHV and RHV

IVC, inferior vena cava; LHV, left hepatic vein; MHV, middle hepatic vein; RHV, right hepatic vein; RL, right lobe.

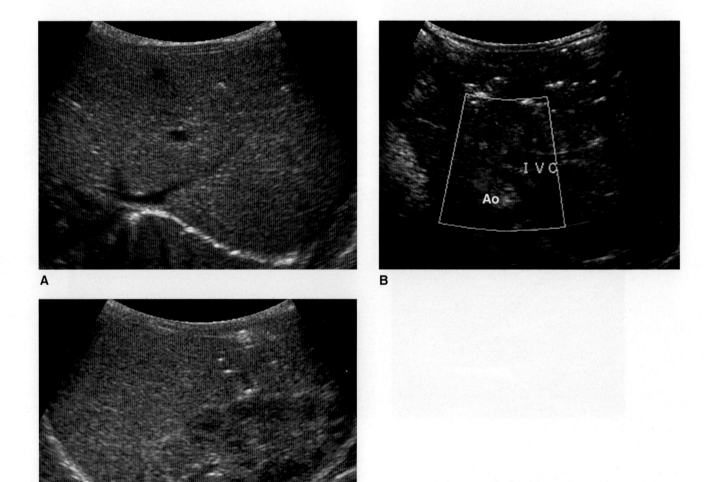

FIGURE 7-9 Situs inversus. **A:** Transverse scan on a newborn at midline demonstrating the liver in the left upper quadrant. **B:** Color Doppler image showing the inferior vena cava (*IVC*) on the left side of the abdomen and the aorta (*Ao*) on the right side. **C:** Parasagittal scan on the left side showing the right lobe of the liver and the right kidney.

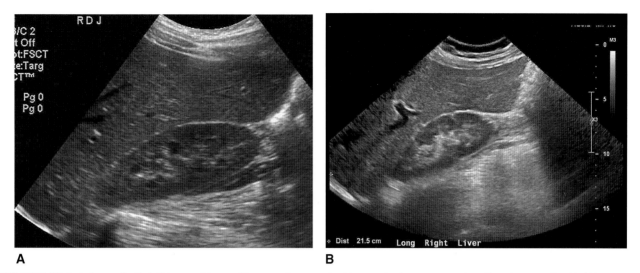

FIGURE 7-10 A: An image of a Riedel lobe on a 36-year-old woman demonstrating this normal variant as an extension of liver tissue past the right kidney. **B:** Another example of a patient with a Riedel lobe and the liver measured 21.5 cm.

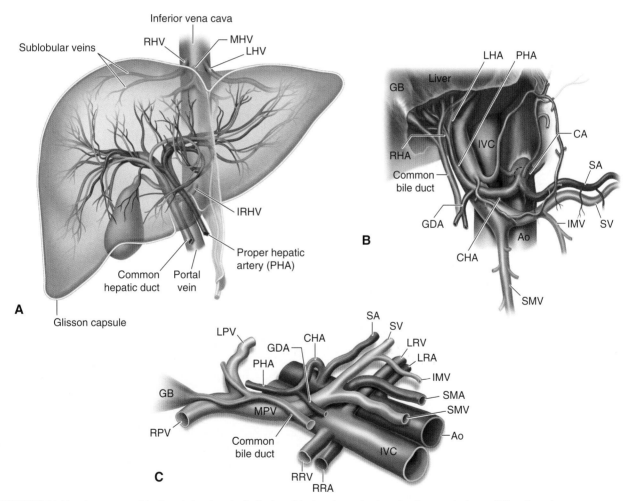

FIGURE 7-11 Vascular anatomy of the liver. **A:** Intrahepatic distribution of the hepatic arteries, hepatic veins, portal veins, and biliary ducts. An accessory or inferior right hepatic vein is illustrated draining directly into the *IVC* and is a variant identified in some patients. **B:** The vessels and ducts of the upper abdomen. **C:** A recumbent view of the relationship between the vessels and ducts of the upper abdomen.

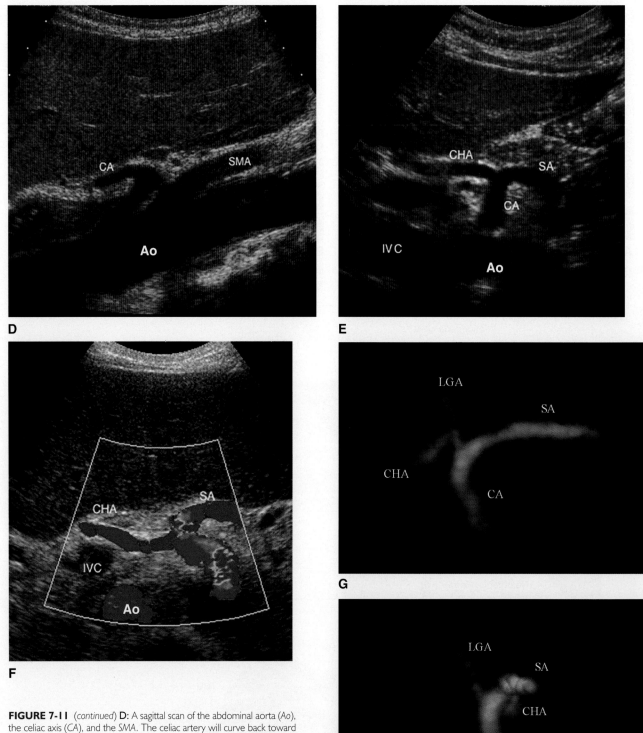

FIGURE 7-11 *(continued)* **D:** A sagittal scan of the abdominal aorta (*Ao*), the celiac axis (*CA*), and the *SMA*. The celiac artery will curve back toward the liver while the *SMA* will run parallel to the aorta. **E:** A transverse midline scan images the *CHA* and *SA* as they come off of the *CA*. This appearance of *CA*, *CHA*, and *SA* is called the tail of a whale sign. The third branch of the *CA*, the *LGA*, is not seen. **F:** Color Doppler image of the *CA* and the *CHA* and *SA*. Because of the curviness of the vessels at times flow is going away from the transducer, blue signals, and then toward the transducer, red signals. **G:** A three-dimensional power Doppler image with grayscale subtraction displays the *CA* branching into the *SA*, *CHA*, and the least often detected third branch, the *LGA*. **H:** A lateral view of the same 3D data set offering better visualization of the *LGA*.

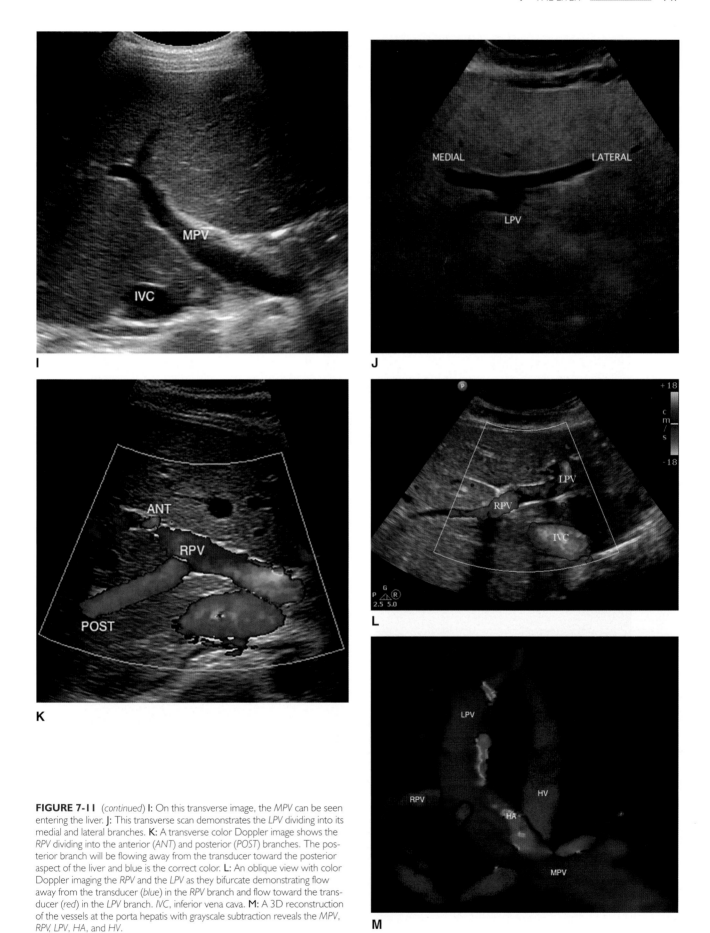

FIGURE 7-11 (*continued*) **I:** On this transverse image, the *MPV* can be seen entering the liver. **J:** This transverse scan demonstrates the *LPV* dividing into its medial and lateral branches. **K:** A transverse color Doppler image shows the *RPV* dividing into the anterior (*ANT*) and posterior (*POST*) branches. The posterior branch will be flowing away from the transducer toward the posterior aspect of the liver and blue is the correct color. **L:** An oblique view with color Doppler imaging the *RPV* and the *LPV* as they bifurcate demonstrating flow away from the transducer (*blue*) in the *RPV* branch and flow toward the transducer (*red*) in the *LPV* branch. *IVC*, inferior vena cava. **M:** A 3D reconstruction of the vessels at the porta hepatis with grayscale subtraction reveals the *MPV*, *RPV*, *LPV*, *HA*, and *HV*.

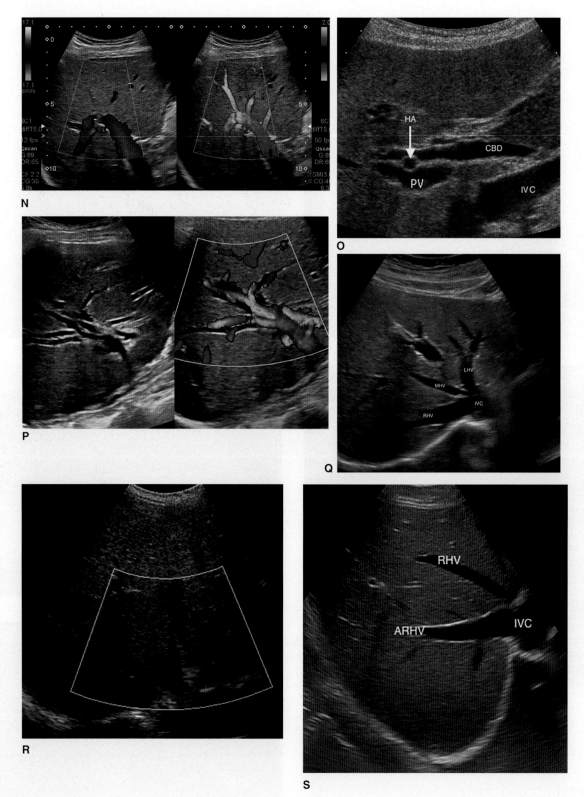

FIGURE 7-11 (*continued*) **N:** A side-by-side image of the portal vein with color Doppler image on the left and microflow imaging on the right demonstrating the branches coming off of the portal vein, which are not seen with conventional Doppler. With microflow imaging, slower flow and smaller vessels can be detected with better spatial resolution and improved sensitivity. **O:** An image showing the relationship of the *CBD* with the *PV* and *HA*. Both the *CBD* and *HA* should be anterior to the *PV*. **P:** The grayscale image on the left shows multiple tubular structures called the parallel-channel sign. The color Doppler image on the right shows that the parallel-channel sign represents dilated bile ducts, structures void of color, and normal portal veins, vessels with color. **Q:** The *RHV*, *MHV*, and *LHV* are seen in this transverse scan draining into the *IVC*. Transducer placement is at the sternum angling toward the patient's head. **R:** On this transverse color Doppler image, all three hepatic veins are seen with hepatofugal flow, which represents flow exiting the liver as they drain into the *IVC*. **S:** A transverse oblique image through the right lobe demonstrating an *ARHV* and the *RHV* draining into the *IVC*. The middle and left hepatic veins are not seen in this image. *Ao*, aorta; *ARHV*, accessory or inferior right hepatic vein; *CA*, celiac artery; *CBD*, common bile duct; *CHA*, common hepatic artery; *GB*, gallbladder; *GDA*, gastroduodenal artery; *HA*, hepatic artery; *HV*, hepatic vein; *IMV*, inferior mesenteric vein; *IRHV*, inferior right hepatic vein; *IVC*, inferior vena cava; *LGA*, left gastric artery; *LHV*, left hepatic vein; *LPV*, left portal vein; *LRA*, left renal artery; *LRV*, left renal vein; *MHV*, middle hepatic vein; *MPV*, main portal vein; *PHA*, proper hepatic artery; *PV*, portal vein; *RHV*, right hepatic vein; *RPV*, right portal vein; *RRA*, right renal artery; *RRV*, right renal vein; *SA*, splenic artery; *SMA*, superior mesenteric artery; *SMV*, superior mesenteric vein; *SV*, splenic vein.

supply the right anterior and right posterior intrahepatic lobar segments (Fig. 7-11K–N).[9] The RPV divides into an anterior branch that supplies blood to segments 5 and 8, and a posterior branch that supplies blood to segments 6 and 7. Segment 1, the CL, is not considered to be part of either the right or left lobe and receives blood from multiple branches from both the left and right portal veins. The hepatic artery, portal vein, and intrahepatic duct course parallel to each other with hepatic and portal blood flowing into the liver and bile flowing in the opposite direction out of the liver (Fig. 7-11O). Intrahepatic ducts are not visualized routinely. If biliary radicles and portal venous radicles are imaged simultaneously side by side, the appearance, referred to as the parallel-channel sign, is used to diagnose biliary obstruction (Fig. 7-11P). Color or power Doppler imaging can distinguish the vessel from the bile duct. The biliary system is discussed in more detail in a later chapter.

Hepatic Veins

The hepatic veins are best visualized on transverse scans by angling the transducer toward the patient's head from a subcostal approach. An intercostal approach from the right can also be helpful to evaluate them. The hepatic veins drain directly into the superior aspect of the IVC and all three veins, the right, middle, and left, should routinely be demonstrated emptying into the IVC (Fig. 7-11Q–S).[27]

The RHV is the largest of the three hepatic veins and is located in the right intersegmental fissure and is used to divide the right hepatic lobe into anterior segments 5 and 8 and posterior segments 6 and 7. The RHV drains segments 5, 6, 7, and 8. A common anatomical variant is an accessory inferior right hepatic vein (IRHV). There is controversy regarding the incidence based on autopsies ranging from 61.4% to 88%,[28] and based on sonography, color Doppler, and CT imaging; the incidence has been reported from 10% to 28.33%.[28] When identified, the IRHV is visualized on a transverse section below the RHV (Fig. 7-11A and S).[10,29] Attempting to identify an IRHV variant can be clinically important for several reasons: (1) The entire main RHV is resected during a hepatectomy, and the RL can be preserved along with the hypertrophic IRHV. (2) Thrombus has been identified in the IRHV in patients with hepatocellular carcinoma (HCC). (3) Finally, the RL's main drainage vein becomes the IRHV in patients with Budd–Chiari syndrome.[28,29] The MHV is located in the MLF, separates the right and left lobes, and drains segments 4 of the left lobe and segments 5 and 8 of the RL.[10] The smaller LHV is located in the cephalic portion of the left intersegmental fissure and divides the left lobe into lateral and medial segments[27] and drains segments 2, 3, and 4. A common variant is for the MHV and the LHV to join and become a common trunk before emptying into the IVC.

Sonographic Distinction between Portal and Hepatic Veins

It is important to be able to differentiate between the portal and hepatic veins sonographically. The five criteria used to distinguish hepatic veins and portal veins are described in

Table 7-2. The easiest way to differentiate between the two vessels is by spectral Doppler imaging because each vessel has its own distinct waveform.

Porta Hepatis

The porta (gate) hepatis (liver) is a fissure where the portal vein and hepatic artery enter the liver and the bile duct exits the liver.[9] In the normal relationship of these three structures within the hepatoduodenal ligament, the bile duct is ventral and lateral, the hepatic artery is ventral and medial, and the portal vein is dorsal (see Fig. 7-11B, C).[15]

It is important to evaluate these structures and measure the bile duct in either a transverse or longitudinal section. To do this, the splenic vein should be located on a transverse section and followed to the right, where it is joined by the SMV and becomes the portal–splenic confluence (Fig. 7-12A). From the confluence, the MPV will course toward the liver and appear round. The transducer should be positioned at an oblique angle, approximately 45 degrees (from right shoulder to left hip), until the long axis of the MPV, bile duct, and hepatic artery are identified. A measurement of the bile duct should be made by placing the calipers along the inner wall to the opposing inner wall of the duct. The published values for the normal internal diameter of the bile duct vary from 4 to 8 mm. A transverse section through the portal triad creates what is called the Mickey Mouse sign (Fig. 7-12B). This is just a quick overview, and in-depth knowledge of the biliary system can be acquired from Chapter 8.

The bile duct and hepatic artery may be confused because of their proximity, their similar internal diameter, and common anatomic variations of these structures. Color Doppler imaging can help in distinguishing the bile duct from the hepatic artery owing to the presence of flow in the artery and absence of flow in the bile duct (Fig. 7-12C). In addition, Berland and colleagues[29] found several reliable sonographic signs to differentiate the bile duct from the hepatic artery, including evaluating the porta hepatis with Doppler techniques:

- Only pulsations should be exhibited by an artery or a vein.
- An artery can indent the wall of a duct or a vein, but the reverse is not true. This is probably because of the lower venous and ductal pressures and the thicker, less easily deformed arterial wall.
- The duct can occasionally decrease several millimeters in caliber during an examination and can have various calibers along its course, whereas arteries are uniform in caliber.
- The artery may not parallel the portal vein or may do so only for a short distance, whereas the duct parallels the portal vein closely.
- Arteries may be tortuous and loop in and out of the scanning plane.
- Arteries produce pulsatile Doppler signals, veins produce continuous Doppler signals, and ducts produce no signal.

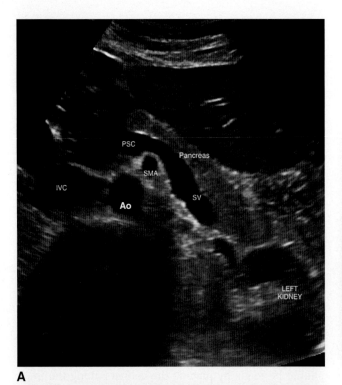

A

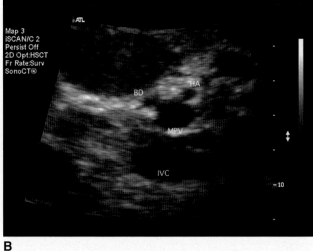

B

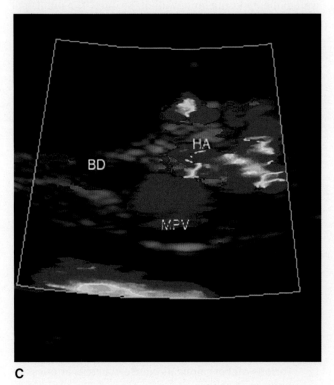

C

FIGURE 7-12 A: Transverse section demonstrating the splenic vein (*SV*) and portal–splenic confluence (*PSC*). Locating the confluence at the level of the pancreas helps identify the origin of the main portal vein (*MPV*). **B:** An image of a portal triad showing the hidden "Mickey Mouse" sign. The *MPV* represents the face; the bile duct (*BD*) the right ear; and the hepatic artery (*HA*) the left ear. **C:** A color Doppler image of the hidden "Mickey Mouse" sign showing flow in the *MPV* and *HA* and no flow in the *BD*. *Ao*, aorta; *SMA*, superior mesenteric artery.

Microscopic Structures

Hepatic lobes are made up of the basic functional unit of the liver, which is the liver lobule.[5,6] The liver parenchyma is made up of 50,000 to 100,000 individual lobules (Fig. 7-13A, B).[4] Within each lobule, small bile canaliculi lie adjacent to the cellular plates and receive the bile produced by the hepatocytes

to carry it toward the bile duct branches in the triad regions (Fig. 7-13C).[4,6,13] These branches open into the interlobular bile ducts accompanying the hepatic artery and portal vein, except that bile flows in the direction opposite to that of blood in these vessels.[4,6] Bile ducts join other bile ducts and eventually form two main trunks, the right and left hepatic ducts, which eventually join to become the common hepatic duct.[6,7]

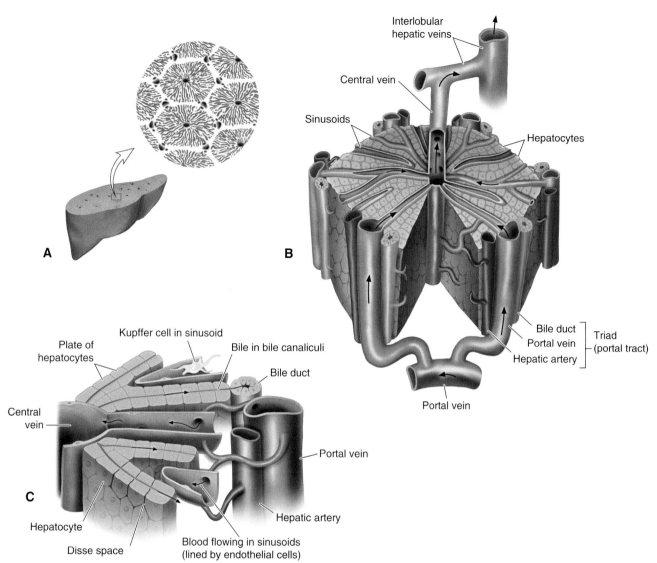

FIGURE 7-13 Microscopic anatomy. **A:** An enlarged sectional cut of the liver shows the hexagonal shape of its lobules. Each lobule measures several millimeters in length and 0.8 to 2 mm in diameter.[4,9] **B:** The *arrows* indicate the direction of blood flow on this representation of one liver lobule. Constructed around a central hepatic vein, each lobule is composed principally of many cellular plates, or hepatocytes, the functional cells of the liver. The cellular plates radiate centrifugally from the central hepatic vein like wheel spokes.[4] Hepatocytes are capable of regenerating, which allows damaged or resected liver tissue to regrow.[13] A lobule has six corners. At each corner is a portal triad, so named because three basic structures are always present: a branch of the hepatic artery, a branch of the portal vein, and a bile duct.[6,7] **C:** An enlarged schematic view of a small portion of one liver lobule illustrates the sinusoids and portal triad. Sinusoids are small capillaries that have a highly permeable endothelial lining located between the cellular plates. The sinusoids receive a mixture of portal venous and hepatic arterial blood.[4,13] The blood drains into the central hepatic vein in the middle of each lobule and flows into the interlobular hepatic veins.[4,13] Unlike other capillaries, sinusoids are also lined with phagocytic cells known as Kupffer cells.[5,6,13] Kupffer cells belong to the reticuloendothelial system and function to remove foreign substances, such as bacteria and depleted white and red blood cells, from the blood.[5,6] The Disse space, located between the endothelial lining and the hepatocyte, drains interstitial fluid into the hepatic lymph system.[4,13] Small bile canaliculi are adjacent to the cellular plates and receive the bile produced by the hepatocytes.[4,13]

PHYSIOLOGY

The liver is an organ essential to life and performs more than 500 separate functions.[4,13] A single liver cell is so diversified in its activities that it is analogous to a factory for many chemical compounds, a warehouse with short- and long-term storage capabilities, a power plant producing heat, a waste disposal plant excreting waste, and to a chemistry lab regenerating tissue that has not been too severely damaged. These functions are carried out by three types of cells in the parenchyma: the hepatocyte, which carries out most metabolic functions; the biliary epithelial cells, which line the biliary system, bile ducts, canaliculi, and gallbladder; and the Kupffer cells, which are phagocytic and belong to the reticuloendothelial system.[4]

It is not necessary to know these liver functions in great detail to obtain quality sonograms; however, because hepatic diseases alter these functions and produce identifiable clinical manifestations, it is important to have a basic understanding of some normal functions (Table 7-4).[2,4–9,13]

TABLE 7-4　Hepatic Function[2,4–9,13]

Bile formation and secretion	Bilirubin, or bile pigment, is a major end product resulting from the breakdown of hemoglobin by Kupffer cells and other reticuloendothelial cells. Bilirubin, bound to plasma protein, travels via the bloodstream to the liver, where it is conjugated (i.e., made water soluble) and excreted into bile. Bile is produced continuously by the hepatic cells at a rate of 700–1,200 mL a day. Bile salts are formed from cholesterol in the hepatic cells, and they emulsify fats and assist in the absorption of fatty acids from the intestinal tract. Calculus formation occurs if the bile salt content is abnormally high owing to cholesterol precipitation.
Carbohydrate metabolism	The liver acts as a glucose buffer. It removes excess glucose from the blood, stores it, and returns it to the blood when the glucose concentration begins to fall. Functions of carbohydrate metabolism include (1) glycogenesis, the conversion of glucose to glycogen for storage; (2) glycogenolysis, the reduction of glycogen to glucose; and (3) gluconeogenesis, formation of glycogen from noncarbohydrates such as protein, amino acids, and fatty acids, which maintains a relatively normal blood glucose concentration.
Fat metabolism	Fatty acids are a source of metabolic energy. Approximately 60% of all preliminary breakdown of fatty acids occurs in the liver. Functions of fat metabolism include (1) beta-oxidation of fatty acids and formation of acetoacetic acid, a soluble acid that passes from the liver cells into the extracellular fluid; (2) formation of lipoprotein by synthesis of fat from glucose and amino acids; (3) formation of cholesterol, which forms bile salts and phospholipids; and (4) conversion of proteins and carbohydrates to fat to be transported as a lipoprotein for storage in the adipose tissue.
Protein metabolism	Protein metabolism functions include (1) deamination of amino acids, which is necessary before they can be used for energy or converted into carbohydrates or fats; (2) formation of urea by the liver, removing ammonia from the body fluid; (3) formation of approximately 85% of the plasma proteins (except approximately 45% of the gamma-globulins) at a maximum rate of 50–100 g/day; and (4) interconversions or synthesizing of amino acids and other compounds vital to the metabolism of the body.
	The reticuloendothelial tissue performs an essential part in protein anabolism by synthesizing various blood proteins (prothrombin, bilinogen, albumins, accelerator globulin, factor VII) and other less important coagulation factors. Blood proteins are essential for normal circulation, because they maintain water balance, contributing to the blood's viscosity.
Reticuloendothelial tissue activity	The activity of the reticuloendothelial tissue in the liver starts before birth with the production of blood cells, a process called hemopoiesis. By birth, this function is carried out by the bone marrow. Plasma has three major types of protein: albumin, globulin, and fibrinogen. All of the albumin and fibrinogen and 50% or more of the globulins are formed in the liver. The rest of the globulins are formed by the lymphatic and other reticuloendothelial systems. The function of albumins is to provide colloid osmotic pressure, which prevents plasma loss from the capillaries. Fibrinogen polymerizes into long fibrin threads during blood coagulation, forming blood clots to help repair leaks in the circulatory system. Globulins perform a number of enzymatic functions in the plasma. The principal function of globulins is to provide natural and acquired immunity against invading organisms.
	After a circulation time of approximately 120 days, red blood cells die. It is assumed that these cells simply wear out with age and rupture during passage through a tight spot in the circulatory system. The reticuloendothelial tissue of the spleen and the liver digests the hemoglobin released from the ruptured red blood cells. In this process, the iron from destroyed red cells is released back into the blood, bone marrow, or to other tissues.
	Large numbers of bacteria invade the body through the intestinal tract, passing through the mucosa into the portal blood. The sinuses of the liver where the blood passes are lined with Kupffer cells, which are tissue macrophages. Kupffer cells form an effective particulate filtration system. Almost all of the bacteria from the GI tract undergo phagocytosis.
Storage depot	The liver has the capacity to store enough vitamin A to prevent a deficiency for as long as 1–2 years[4] and enough vitamin D and vitamin B$_{12}$ to prevent deficiency for 1–4 months. The liver also stores glycogen, fats, and amino acids and can metabolize them into glucose or vice versa, depending on the body's needs.
	Aside from iron in the hemoglobin, by far the greatest proportion of iron is stored in the liver in the form of ferritin. When the body becomes iron deficient, the ferritin releases iron. The liver is also the storage depot for copper and for some poisons that cannot be broken down or detoxified and excreted, such as dichlorodiphenyltrichloroethane.
Blood reservoir	Approximately 1,000–1,100 mL of blood flows from the portal vein through the liver sinusoids each minute, and another 350–400 mL flows through the hepatic artery. As a blood reservoir, the liver has the capacity to enlarge and store 200–400 mL of blood with a rise of only 4–8 mm Hg in hepatic venous pressure. If there is hemorrhage and large amounts of blood are being lost in the circulatory system, the liver releases its blood from that stored in the sinusoids to help compensate for this loss in blood volume.

TABLE 7-4	**Hepatic Function**[2,4-9,13] (*continued*)
Heat production	The liver, a significant metabolizer, produces heat as a result of its chemical reactions. On average, 55% of the energy of food ingested becomes heat during ATP formation. Even more heat is produced during the ATP cell formation process.
Detoxification	To a great degree, the liver is a detoxifier, converting chemicals, foreign molecules, and hormones to compounds that are not as toxic or biologically active. When amino acids are burned for energy, they leave behind toxic nitrogenous wastes that are converted to urea by the liver cells. These moderate amounts of urea are then easily removed by the kidney or sweat glands.
Lymph formation	Under resting conditions, the liver produces between one-third and one-half of all the body's lymph.

ATP, adenosine triphosphate; GI, gastrointestinal.

LIVER FUNCTION TESTS

Liver function tests, commonly referred to as LFTs, are a group of blood tests that can tell the physician how the liver is performing under normal and diseased conditions. This group of tests is also referred to as a liver panel and includes total bilirubin, alanine aminotransferase (ALT), aspartate aminotransferase (AST), AST/ALT ratio, alkaline phosphatase (ALP), gamma-glutamyl phosphatase (GGT), and albumin. AST may also be referred to as aspartate transaminase or the older serum glutamic-oxaloacetic transaminase (SGOT), which is no longer used. ALT may also be referred to as alanine transaminase or the older serum glutamic-pyruvic transaminase (SGPT), which is also no longer used. Patients undergoing certain invasive procedures or surgery will have their bleeding times evaluated, especially if they have liver disease because one of the functions of the liver is to make clotting factors. These tests include prothrombin time (PT) and partial thromboplastin time (PTT). To evaluate for dilated biliary ducts is the main reason an ultrasound is ordered on a patient with increased LFTs. The presence of dilated ducts will mean that the patient will need to be treated surgically to relieve the obstruction. If the ducts are normal, then the reason for the increased values will be a medical condition such as hepatitis, fatty liver disease, overuse of over-the-counter drugs such as acetaminophen, prescription drugs such as statin drugs, alcohol abuse, and primary or metastatic disease. (The most common cause of acute liver failure in the United States is an overdose of acetaminophen, usually as a suicide attempt.) The most common laboratory tests are listed in Table 7-5.[26,31-33] Normal reference ranges are not provided because they can vary by gender and age, and values can be updated periodically. The range of normal values used will be on the patient's report next to their current value, with abnormal values indicated and clearly marked as high or low.

TABLE 7-5	**Liver Function Tests**[26,31,33]		
Test	**Explanation**	**Result**	**Clinical Indication**
Bilirubin	It is formed in large part from heme of destroyed erythrocytes. Heme is converted to biliverdin and then another enzyme changes it into bilirubin (unconjugated). Unconjugated or indirect bilirubin is bound to albumin and transported to liver cells. The liver conjugates the bilirubin with glucuronic acid, making it soluble in water. Most of this conjugated bilirubin goes into the bile.	Indirect values are increased.	Body is making too much bilirubin, usually owing to an increase in red blood cell breakdown such as hemolytic anemia and hemolysis, or diseases that affect the liver's ability to conjugate, such as Gilbert syndrome or Crigler–Najjar syndrome. Typically, causes of increased indirect values cannot be diagnosed with ultrasound.
	Conjugated or direct bilirubin is not excreted but remains in the blood. Bilirubin is conjugated by liver enzymes, becomes water soluble, and is excreted in feces and urine.	Direct values are increased.	Clinical indications include hepatocellular jaundice from hepatitis or cirrhosis; obstructive liver disease; intrahepatic cholestasis, alcoholic hepatitis, primary biliary cirrhosis, or posthepatic jaundice from lower biliary tract obstruction, biliary stones, pancreatic head pathology, especially cancer. Typically, causes of increased direct values can be diagnosed with ultrasound.
			Most laboratories report the total value and the direct (conjugated) value. The indirect (unconjugated) value is calculated by subtracting the direct value from the total.

(*continued*)

TABLE 7-5   **Liver Function Tests**[26,31,33] (*continued*)

Test	Explanation	Result	Clinical Indication
ALT	It is a necessary enzyme in Krebs cycle for tissue energy production, with largest amounts in the liver, smaller amounts in the kidney, heart, and skeletal muscle. When damage to these tissues occurs, ALT increases. ALT is a rather specific indicator of hepatocellular damage. It is used in conjunction with AST to help distinguish between cardiac and hepatic damage. AST levels are very high and ALT levels are only mildly elevated with cardiac damage. ALT can differentiate between hemolytic jaundice when there is no rise in ALT and jaundice owing to liver disease with high ALT levels. Hepatitis, cirrhosis, Reye syndrome, and toxic drug treatment can be monitored with ALT.	Values are increased.	Clinical indications include liver cell damage owing to hepatitis, cirrhosis, or liver tumors; Reye syndrome, or biliary tract obstruction; other diseases involving the liver, heart failure, alcohol or drug abuse; its levels are elevated with some renal diseases, some musculoskeletal diseases, systemic lupus erythematosus, other conditions that cause trauma or hypoxia, and hemolysis. Ratio of AST to ALT can be meaningful. AST levels are higher in cirrhosis and metastatic carcinoma of the liver. ALT levels are usually higher in acute hepatitis, alcoholic liver disease, and nonmalignant hepatic obstruction.
AST	An enzyme found in all tissues, but largest amounts are present in in cells that use the most energy, such as liver, heart, and skeletal muscles. AST is released with injury to cells.	Values are increased.	In hepatitis, it is elevated before jaundice appears; cirrhosis, shock, or trauma may cause lesser elevation; other conditions include Reye syndrome and pulmonary infarction. Damaged cardiac cells have other correlating examinations. Ratio of AST to ALT is significant (see clinical indications for ALT).
ALP	This enzyme is found in the tissues of liver, bone, intestine, kidney, placenta; higher levels are normal with new bone formation in children and in pregnancy; it is normally excreted in bile.	Values are increased.	Clinical indications include biliary obstruction from tumors or space-occupying lesions, hepatitis, metastatic liver carcinoma, pancreatic head carcinoma, cholelithiasis, or biliary atresia; elevation may also occur from bone or kidney origin and from congestive heart failure owing to hepatic blood flow obstruction.
LDH	An enzyme in all tissues, LDH is normally not used for liver evaluation because other enzyme values are more specific. LDH_4 and LDH_5 are found in liver, skeletal, kidney, placenta, and striated muscle tissue.	Values are increased for LDH_4 and LDH_5.	Liver damage owing to cirrhosis, chronic viral hepatitis, etc.
GGTP or GGT	Responsible for the transport of amino acid and peptide across cell membranes, it is found chiefly in liver, kidney, and pancreas, with smaller amounts in other tissues. The test is the most sensitive indicator of alcoholism and is also sensitive to other liver diseases.	Values are increased.	Clinical indications include marked elevation in liver disease and posthepatic obstruction; moderate elevation with liver damage from alcohol, drugs, chemotherapy; elevation may also be owing to pancreatic, kidney, prostate, heart, lung, or spleen disease.
PT	Test used to determine pathologic deficiency of clotting factors due either to liver dysfunction or to absence of vitamin K.	Values are increased.	Bleeding disorder, correlated with obstructive disease, PT can be corrected with parenteral vitamin K; when correlated with parenchymal disease, scarred nonfunctioning liver tissue does not produce prothrombin.
Albumin	The smallest protein molecule, it makes up the largest proportion of total serum protein. It is almost totally synthesized by the liver. Albumin plays an important role in total water distribution or osmotic pressure because of its high molecular weight. With dehydration, albumin levels increase. A lack of albumin in the serum allows fluid to leak out into the interstitial spaces and into the peritoneal cavity causing ascites.	Values are decreased.	Chronic liver disease, especially cirrhosis; ascites from cirrhosis, right-sided heart failure, cancer, or peritonitis; other conditions related to the GI tract, inflammation, pregnancy, and aging.
		Values are increased.	Clinical indications include hemolysis, other conditions related to dehydration, exercise, anxiety, depression.

TABLE 7-5	**Liver Function Tests**[26,31,33] (*continued*)		
Test	**Explanation**	**Result**	**Clinical Indication**
A/G ratio	Albumin divided by globulins equals the ratio. When evaluating liver disease, serum globulin is produced by the Kupffer cells and albumin is synthesized in the liver. In chronic liver disease, the A/G ratio is reversed where albumin is decreased and globulin is elevated.	Decreased total protein with decreased albumin and elevated globulin (reversed A/G ratio)	Chronic liver disease, especially cirrhosis, ascites from cirrhosis; right-sided heart failure, cancers, or peritonitis and other conditions related to the GI tract; and inflammation, pregnancy, and aging
AFP	A globulin formed in yolk sac and fetal liver, it is normally present only in trace amounts after birth; produced with primary carcinoma of the liver and certain types of testicular cancer.	Values are increased.	In nonpregnant adults, carcinoma of the liver, as in hepatocellular carcinoma; in the pediatric patient, hepatoblastoma

AFP, alpha-fetoprotein; A/G, albumin/globulin; ALP, alkaline phosphatase; ALT, alanine aminotransferase; AST, aspartate aminotransferase; GGTP or GGT, gamma-glutamyl transpeptidase; GI, gastrointestinal; LDH, lactic dehydrogenase; PT, prothrombin time.

SONOGRAPHIC EXAMINATION TECHNIQUE

Indications for Examination

The two most common indications for a sonographic examination of the liver include right upper quadrant (RUQ) or abdominal pain and abnormal LFTs. Other reasons include jaundice, abnormal findings on a CT or MRI exam, concerns for metastatic disease to the liver, and evaluating the liver for an abscess or hematoma.[24] Ultrasound can also be used as guidance for invasive procedures on the liver and is discussed in another chapter.

Patient Preparation

The liver itself can be visualized without any patient preparation; however, because frequently the biliary system is evaluated at the same time, the patient is instructed to take nothing by mouth (NPO), after midnight or 6 to 8 hours before the study. Patients should take needed medications with sips of water and abstain from smoking or chewing gum as these activities will increase the amount of gas in the stomach and intestines. The sonographer should be aware of any patient that is an insulin-dependent diabetic and attempt to schedule them first thing in the morning or arrange an alternate preparation so that the patient does not have a hypoglycemic episode.

Patient Instructions

Breathing Instructions

Because the liver moves with respiration, the sonographer should determine how the patient should breathe during the exam, which is usually a combination of breath holding and normal breathing. Normal, also known as quiet, breathing may be used with intercostal scanning whereas deep suspended inspiration technique is generally used for subcostal images. Scanning the patient on deep inspiration will allow the liver to descend below the ribs, displace bowel gas inferiorly, and provide better visualization. Asking the patient to stop breathing at a certain point while scanning, called suspended respiration, or scanning on expiration is often best for intercostal scanning. A helpful maneuver is

called the belly-out technique, where the patient is asked to take in a breath and hold it while pushing out their belly.

Patient Positioning

A subcostal and/or intercostal imaging approach is common while scanning the liver, starting with the patient supine. Expansion of the rib spaces can be aided by having the patient raise their right arm and place their hand above or under their head. The study begins with the patient in a supine position for initial documentation of the liver size and parenchymal evaluation. Additional scanning planes include having the patient turn into a left posterior oblique (LPO) and/or a left lateral decubitus position (LLD) also known as right side up (RSU). As the patient gradually turns from the left LPO position to the LLD position, the RL of the liver typically descends inferiorly and rotates medially to expose more of the superior portion of the liver. With intercostal probe placement, the oblique or decubitus position may offer better visualization of the portal vein and common hepatic duct. If the IVC is compressed owing to an enlarged liver, turning the patient into either an RPO or LPO position may alleviate the pressure from the liver and allow better visualization of the IVC. The lower liver segment may be best visualized with the patient in the right posterior oblique (RPO) position because this allows the liver to displace the duodenum and transverse colon inferiorly.[17] The dome of the liver is best seen with the patient holding their breath in a deep inspiration, placing the transducer parallel to the ribs and angling it toward the diaphragm from a subcostal position. Owing to the effects of gravity, an erect or semi-erect position may expose even more liver tissue. A good sonographer will use a variety of patient positions and techniques to obtain a complete study of the liver.

Scanning Technique

The liver is systematically evaluated in both the sagittal and transverse planes with oblique scanning planes utilized as needed until the entire liver parenchyma is adequately evaluated. Attention is paid to the size and echotexture of the liver, the intrahepatic and extrahepatic biliary ducts, blood vessels, and any pathology of the liver or pathology that affects the hepatobiliary system. The highest-frequency transducer that allows good visualization of the deepest part of the liver should be used. The sonographers should use their critical thinking skills to decide the best patient and transducer positions in order to obtain the best image. Even in a patient that had a cholecystectomy, turning the patient to a LLD position may improve visualization of the liver.

Protocols

All imaging protocols must be based on the standards of the governing societies and their accreditation organizations. Current scanning protocols and guidelines can be found at the American College of Radiology (ACR), www.acr.org, or the American Institute of Ultrasound in Medicine (AIUM), www.aium.org, websites and are free. Note that the two organizations, along with other ultrasound organizations, have worked together so that all protocols are identical between the various organizations. Protocols may vary or may need to be altered depending on sonographic findings and the condition and cooperation of the patient. It is more important to answer the clinical question than to obtain a "complete" protocol when the patient has difficulty cooperating or has an urgent condition such as trauma from a car accident.

Sagittal Images

Sagittal scanning typically begins with the midsagittal plane, just inferior to the sternum and xiphoid process. Next, the sonographer will evaluate the left lobe and then the RL although the sonographer can start with either lobe. The diaphragm and dome of the liver are visualized by angling the transducer superiorly. To evaluate the inferior margin of the RL of the liver, the sonographer can either slide the transducer down toward the area or angle the transducer toward the patient's feet. Therefore, a complete sagittal assessment requires the sonographer to move the probe superiorly and inferiorly throughout the sagittal scanning process. In the average adult patient, the RL of the liver is typically larger than the imaging field of view. This may present a challenge to the sonographer for measuring the length of the liver because the entire lobe cannot fit the image. If available, the sonographer can employ the extended field of view to obtain an accurate measurement. Sonographers should be careful to image all aspects of the liver from the lateral margin of the left lobe to the lateral margin of the RL. Documented sagittal and parasagittal images should include the left lobe segments, the proximal aorta and IVC, the CL and ligamentum venosum, the porta hepatis, the gallbladder if present, the RL segments, and the right kidney (Fig. 7-14A–F). Some departments now require a video clip through each lobe. A Riedel lobe, if present, is best documented in the sagittal plane.

Transverse Images

In the transverse imaging plane, the transducer is swept superiorly from the dome of the liver to the inferior margin of the liver. Again, the size of the adult liver in the transverse dimension prohibits fitting the entire liver on each transverse image plane. Therefore, the sonographer usually begins the assessment at the midsagittal, subxiphoid location to image the left lobe in a transverse approach from superior to inferior and then moves to a subcostal and/or intercostal probe position in order to image the RL from superior to inferior. Portions of the heart may be seen just superior to

the diaphragm of the left lobe and may be mistaken for a fluid collection on a still image. Usually, taking a video clip or documenting the cardiac valves in another image will let the radiologist know that this fluid structure is the heart. Imaging the dome of the liver is accomplished by angling the transducer superiorly toward the patient's right ear. Documented transverse images should include the left lobe from superior to inferior including the LHV and LPV, the CL and ligamentum venosum, and the aorta. Images of the RL will be documented from the dome to the right kidney, the RHV, MHV and RPV, the gallbladder if present, and the right kidney (Fig. 7-15A–F).

Technical Considerations

Transducer frequencies ranging from 1 to 9 MHz are used in the sonographic evaluation of the adult liver, and higher frequencies may be used on pediatric patients, especially neonates. The highest-frequency transducer should be used in order to achieve the best possible resolution without compromising penetration. If there is a lot of noise in the far field, then the transducer frequency is too high. Curved linear array transducers, preferably with a wide sector image, are best for evaluating the liver. A linear array transducer is useful for evaluating the anterior liver capsule, especially in patients with cirrhosis. Sector or vector transducers may be used for intercostal approaches, especially if there are issues with rib artifacts.[22] The focal point should be placed at or below the area of interest or at the level of the diaphragm for evaluating the entire liver. Current ultrasound units have built-in focusing techniques; therefore, the focal zone is no longer displayed on the image nor does the sonographer have the ability to adjust the placement of the focal zone. The time gain compensation (TGC) and the overall gain settings should be adjusted to give a uniform appearance of the hepatic parenchyma from the anterior to posterior margins of the liver. The normal liver should display a relatively homogeneous texture of medium-level echoes that are isoechoic or slightly more echogenic than the normal renal cortex.

Harmonic imaging is helpful to improve resolution but may have penetration issues. Because harmonic imaging reduces the near-field artifact, the sonographer may need to adjust the near-TGC control to increase the echo brightness of the echoes right beneath the Glisson capsule. Attention should be given to the far field to ensure that the far-field parenchyma is appropriately seen (Fig. 7-16A). If there is a lot of noise in the far field or if penetration is an issue when using harmonics, the sonographer may need to turn harmonics off or use the harmonic penetration mode to obtain far-field images and then turn it back on for the rest of the study. In this scenario, turning up the gain to increase echoes in the far field will introduce noise into the image, which may obscure pathology. Another option is to scan at the lower-frequency bandwidth of the transducer, which can be adjusted on the ultrasound machine by decreasing the frequency or in other units by turning the control to penetration mode. If the far field is obscure owing to a fatty liver, the best option is to use a lower-frequency transducer because penetration mode may still not visualize the far field. Compound imaging is helpful in reducing artifacts, improving the visualization of borders, and improving image

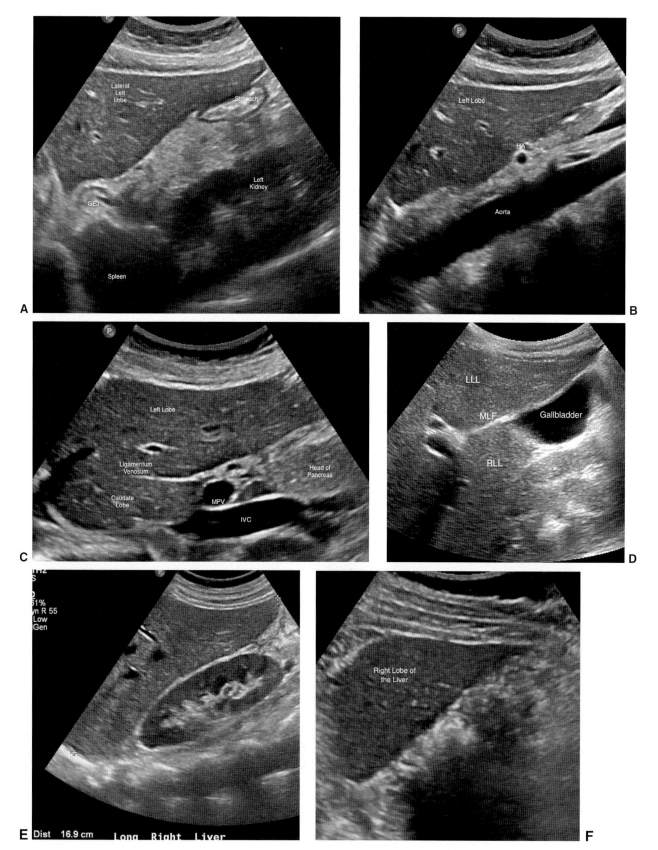

FIGURE 7-14 Sagittal protocol. **A:** A sagittal section through the lateral left lobe of the liver with the stomach and gastroesophageal junction (*GEJ*). On this patient, the spleen and left kidney are seen. **B:** A sagittal section through the left lobe at the level of the aorta. **C:** A sagittal section through the left lobe and caudate lobes of the liver at the level of the inferior vena cava (*IVC*) and ligamentum venosum. **D:** A sagittal section through the liver at the level of the main lobar fissure (*MLF*) and gallbladder. **E:** A sagittal section through the *RLL* and the right kidney demonstrating the normal echogenicity relationship between the two organs. In this image, the length of the liver is 16.9 cm. **F:** A sagittal section through the most lateral part of the right lobe of the liver. *HA*, hepatic artery; *LLL*, left lobe of liver; *MPV*, main portal vein; *RLL*, right lobe of liver.

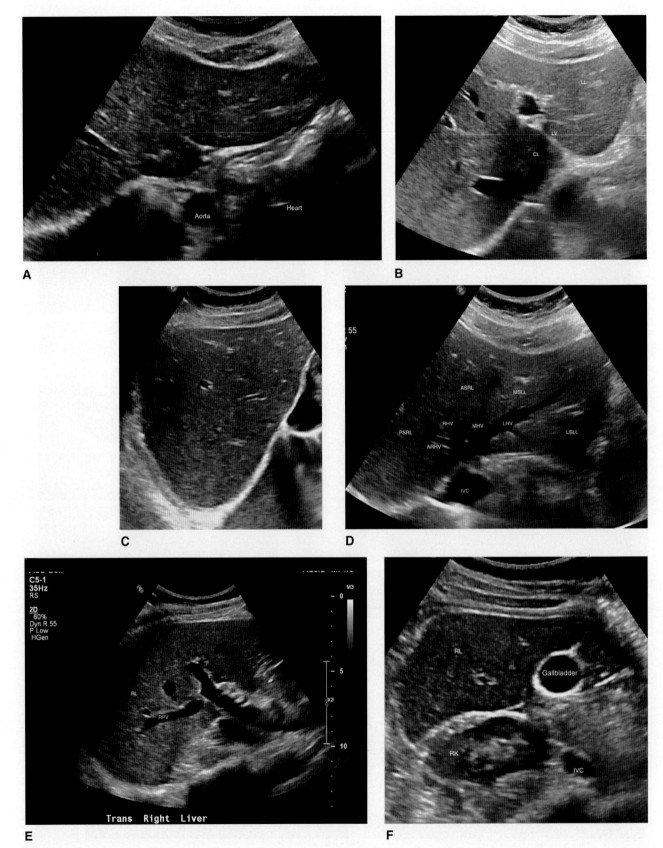

FIGURE 7-15 Transverse protocol. **A:** A transverse section through the superior aspect of the left lobe of the liver. **B:** A transverse section through the left lobe (*LL*), the caudate lobe (*CL*), and the ligamentum venosum (*LV*). **C:** A transverse section through the superior aspect of the right lobe of the liver at the dome. **D:** A transverse section through the liver at the level of the hepatic veins. **E:** A transverse section through the right lobe (*RL*) and the right portal vein (*RPV*). **F:** A transverse section through the inferior aspect of the right lobe of the liver (*RL*), the gall bladder, the right kidney (*RK*), and the inferior vena cava (*IVC*). *ARSV*, accessory right hepatic vein; *ASRL*, anterior segment of the right lobe; *LHV*, left hepatic vein; *LSLL*, lateral segment left lobe; *MSLL*, medial segment left lobe; *MHV*, middle hepatic vein; *PSRL*, posterior segment of the right lobe; *RHV*, right hepatic vein.

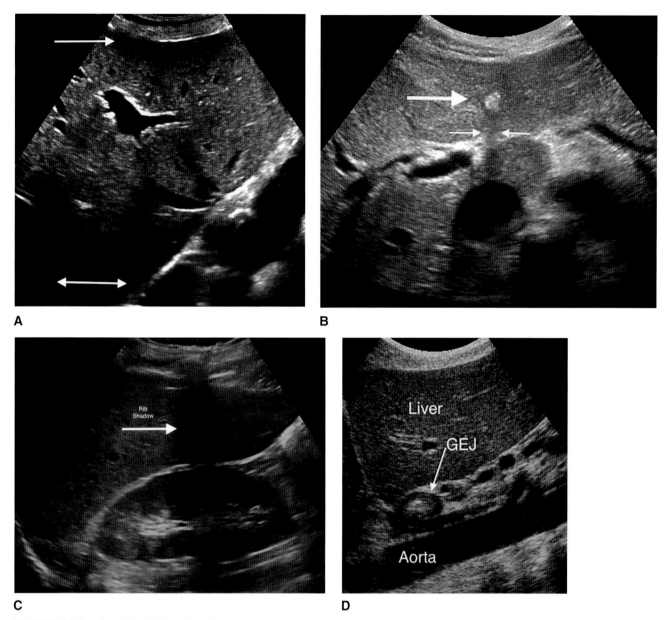

A   **B**

C   **D**

FIGURE 7-16 Scanning pitfalls. **A:** Although resolution is improved using harmonics, the sonographer needs to pay attention to the whole image. Harmonics help to reduce artifacts and the single *arrow* shows loss of echoes in the near field owing to elimination of the reverberation artifact. The double-headed *arrow* demonstrates penetration issues in the far field in this normal patient. **B:** The *arrow* points to the ligamentum teres that mimics a "bull's eye" lesion and casts a faint acoustic shadow as seen between the two *arrows*. One should recognize that this is not a mass owing to its location in the left lobe. **C:** When scanning intercostally with a curved linear array transducer, it is not uncommon to have an acoustic shadow from the rib. The sonographer should take an image showing the tissue under the acoustic shadow is normal so that this area is not mistaken for pathology or so that the small pathology under the rib is not missed. If needed, a sector type of transducer could be used because it can easily scan between the ribs owing to their small footprint. **D:** The gastroesophageal junction (*GEJ*) is located between the aorta and liver edge. The sonographer should not mistake this normal structure for a hepatic mass or lymph node.

quality. New transducer technologies, such as high-definition and matrix transducers, are also helping to improve image resolution. Abnormal areas should be evaluated by optimizing the area in question. Typically, the control settings at the beginning of the exam may not be appropriate for other parts of the liver. The sonographer should optimize each image before recording it or send it to picture archiving and communication systems (PACSs).

When using Doppler imaging, it is important to optimize the equipment settings for pulsed, color, and power Doppler imaging separately. Improper adjustment of velocity scale, wall filters, and Doppler gain controls can affect the quality of the Doppler image and cause errors in determining the flow direction, cause Doppler artifacts, and possibly cause a misdiagnosis. Wall filters for color and spectral Doppler imaging should be at their lowest setting to start and the be increased as needed. The color velocity scale will need to be adjusted for each artery and vein with a setting that provides good color fill-in with little to no aliasing. A setting to optimize the hepatic artery may cause little to no flow in the portal vein, giving the appearance of portal vein thrombosis. After the hepatic artery has been evaluated, the color velocity scale needs to be optimized for the portal vein, which may cause aliasing in the hepatic artery. On any vessel, setting

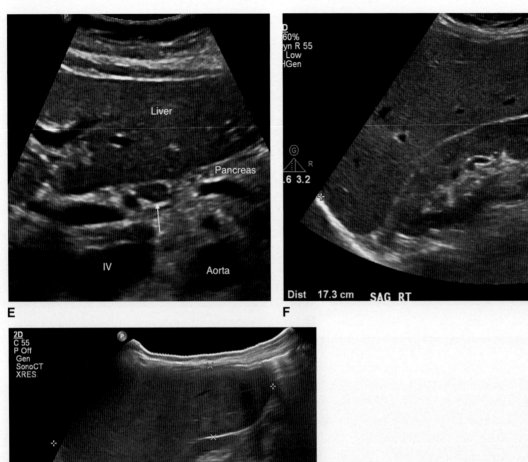

FIGURE 7-16 *(continued)* **E:** The *arrow* points to a small peri-portal lymph node in this patient with lymphoma. Notice the echogenic border between the liver and the node helping to confirm that the mass is not hepatic in origin. **F:** Sagittal image of a patient with a Riedel lobe. The liver measures 17.3 cm. **G:** Sagittal image of a patient with hepatomegaly using extended field of view to visualize the entire length of the liver, which measures 25.9 cm. Notice the rounded inferior edge of the liver, which is associated with hepatomegaly.

the color velocity to a very low value will cause aliasing, making it difficult to evaluate the flow direction inside the vessel. The color and spectral Doppler gains should be adjusted until echoes are seen in the background and then be turned down until the speckles disappear. This will ensure that the gain control is properly set. When a velocity needs to be measured, angle correction must be used and the cursor properly placed, which is usually parallel to the vessel walls with an angle less than 60 degrees. The incorrect use of angle correction will cause errors in velocity readings. Some vessels may be at angles between 0 and 30 degrees, such as the hepatic and portal veins, which is perfectly acceptable. Strict angles of 60 degrees are not needed in abdominal Doppler imaging and the angle of insonation must be properly set at an angle less than 60 degrees. Earlier, strict angles of 60 degrees were only required for the distal common carotid and proximal internal artery, but even that has changed. All of our ultrasound societies and accrediting bodies state that all Doppler angles must be less than 60 degrees. The sonographer should stay abreast of recommendations for angle correction.

Pitfalls

Normal anatomy can sometimes be mistaken for pathology because anatomic variants and artifacts can simulate pathologic conditions. The normal ligamentum teres, fat anterior to the liver or between the liver and right kidney, acoustic shadowing from vascular and biliary structures, and air in the biliary tree have all been cited as causes of pseudolesions or fluid collections. The normal ligamentum teres can be documented in the transverse plane in the left lobe of the liver. This fibrous structure is surrounded by fat and may appear as a hyperechoic or bulls eye lesion in the left lobe, mimicking a hemangioma or liver mass (Fig. 7-16B).[34] On a transverse section or with a right costal margin (RCM) view, the perinephric fat may appear echopenic, mimicking ascites. (The RCM view is obtained by placing the transducer parallel to the ribs in a subcostal approach and angling superiorly.) Careful evaluation in both sagittal and transverse planes and adjusting the gain or harmonic controls may help demonstrate that it is perinephric fat. Also, ascites is rarely limited to Morison pouch; so, noting lack of fluid around the liver or elsewhere in the body will confirm that this is not ascites. The ribs can cause shadowing throughout the examination, especially when using an intercostal scanning approach with a curved linear array transducer. This may require angling the transducer around the ribs so that the rib shadow does not obscure or mimic any pathology (Fig. 7-16C). When true acoustic shadowing is seen within the liver parenchyma, intraductal calculi should be considered. Other causes include a calcified hematoma, granulomatous deposits, or surgical metal clips. A common scanning pitfall is mistaking GI structures or bowel gas for pathology. Gas reflects sound and is always a problem because it interferes with the transmission of the sound beam. Thus, visualization of the liver parenchyma can be especially difficult if there is a lot of air in the stomach, the intestines are overdistended with gas or they are high in the abdomen, or there is air in the peritoneum called pneumoperitoneum. The gastroesophageal junction (GEJ) can mimic a bull's eye lesion in the liver (Fig. 7-16D). However, having the patient swallow will verify that it is the GEJ. Masses near the liver border can sometimes be confusing in determining their location, especially larger masses such as an upper pole renal mass. The sonographer needs to observe if there is a bright interface from Glisson capsule between the liver and the mass, confirming that it is extrahepatic. The sonographic features most often observed with an extrahepatic mass include displacement of the liver capsule inward and capsule discontinuity. Observed sonographic features of an intrahepatic mass are displaced hepatic vascular, external bulging of the liver capsule, and dilated ducts. A common pitfall is to mistake a Riedel lobe for hepatomegaly. The Riedel lobe will be long but will have normal AP dimensions. Hepatomegaly also tends to push the kidney posteriorly and superiorly toward the diaphragm and will enlarge in the AP dimension and extend below the anterior edge of the kidney (Fig. 7-16F, G).

HEPATOMEGALY

An enlarged liver is called hepatomegaly and is a nonspecific finding, which can be caused by a variety of diseases. It is defined as a liver that is enlarged beyond its normal size. Most ultrasound references state that a liver greater than 15.5 to 16 cm in size is considered enlarged. Some of the causes of hepatomegaly include hepatitis, hepatic tumors, alcoholic liver disease, nonalcoholic fatty liver disease (NAFLD), congestive heart failure, autoimmune disease, and obesity. Physicians will request an ultrasound when they suspect hepatomegaly and to make sure that the enlargement is not caused by a mass. Some common reasons that can be diagnosed by ultrasound include masses, cysts including polycystic liver disease, NAFLD, and the presence of a Riedel lobe.[17,21]

DIFFUSE HEPATOCELLULAR DISEASE

Hepatocellular disease causes dysfunction of the hepatocytes and interferes with normal liver function,[31] usually affecting the patient's LFTs,[32] which may be the indication for an ultrasound exam. Examples of diffuse hepatocellular disease include fatty infiltration, hepatitis, and cirrhosis. Parenchymal disease can affect the echogenicity of the liver, causing it to decrease with hepatitis or to increase in echogenicity with fatty infiltration and cirrhosis. The size of the liver is also affected; it can not only increase in size but also decrease in size. Sonography can detect these diffuse hepatocellular changes, and now using elastography, quantitative estimates of the severity of the parenchymal damage can be measured in certain pathologies. Elastography will be described later in this chapter.

Fatty Infiltration

Fatty infiltration, or steatosis, of the liver by itself usually does not significantly disrupt the liver's functions. Over time, however, the accumulation of fatty triglycerides within the liver cells may cause the liver lobules to separate and increase the organ's weight.[35] Alcohol abuse and obesity are the leading causes for the development of fatty infiltration.[25,35] Some other factors influencing fat deposition include diabetes, severe hepatitis, corticosteroid use, chemotherapy, parenteral hyperalimentation, protein malnutrition, metabolic disorders, pregnancy, cystic fibrosis, hyperlipidemia, and glycogen storage disease.[35,36] Two terms used to indicate that the patient's liver disease is not alcohol-related are NAFLD and nonalcoholic steatohepatitis (NASH). NASH is a progression of NAFLD with inflammation and liver cell damage that can progress to cirrhosis in up to 15% to 20% of patients.[37] Eliminating the cause of the fatty infiltration can reverse the process in patients with NAFLD and some patients with NASH.

Sonographic features depend on the severity of the disease. The key sonographic markers of fatty infiltration are diffuse increased echogenicity of the liver parenchyma and decreased acoustic penetration owing to the increased attenuation of the sound beam by the fat.[22] Hepatomegaly may be present. The normally bright portal triad walls diminish as the surrounding liver tissue becomes more hyperechoic, leading to poor delineation of the intrahepatic architecture. The cortex of the right kidney will appear unusually hypoechoic in contrast to the abnormally bright liver parenchyma. Increased sound attenuation makes penetration of the posterior liver and visualization of the diaphragm difficult (Fig. 7-17A, B). To see the posterior liver, the sonographer will need to decrease the frequency either by adjusting the control to a lower frequency or to penetration mode or by possibly turn off harmonics.

Although the process is usually diffuse, fatty infiltration may be focal, resembling a hyperechoic mass. Although this focal fatty pattern may mimic a mass, the margins are typically more angular and vessels are not displaced (Fig. 7-17C).[10,38] Another sonographic appearance is that of focal fatty sparing, making normal tissue appear as a hypoechoic area surrounded by the hyperechoic liver tissue. Focal fatty sparing is usually detected in the medial segment of the left lobe near the porta hepatis, anterior to the gallbladder or anterior to the portal vein. They may be solitary or multiple areas (Fig. 7-17D).[17]

Glycogen Storage Disease

An autosomal recessive disorder that can have detectable features on sonography is the glycogen storage disease. The most common type is classified as von Gierke disease type 1.

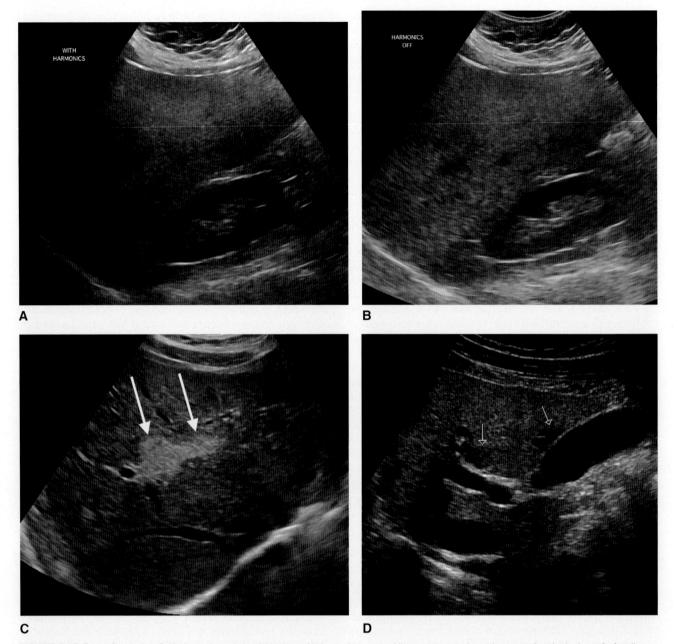

FIGURE 7-17 Fatty infiltration. **A:** Sagittal scan through the right lobe and kidney using a curved linear array transducer demonstrating classic signs of a fatty liver: heterogeneity, lack of visualization of internal vessels, marked difference in echogenicity between the liver and kidney, and decreased sound penetration limiting visualization of the diaphragm. This image was taken with harmonics turned on. **B:** The same patient as in figure **A** with harmonics turned off showing better penetration of the liver down to the diaphragm and with echoes that are better seen in the renal parenchyma. Using harmonics will improve resolution, but it may also affect penetration as demonstrated here. Sonographers need to evaluate the image and decide how they can improve it when needed. Leaving harmonics on constantly may not be the best for every image. **C:** A local increased echogenic area in the right lobe of the liver compatible with focal fatty infiltration (*arrows*). Note that it does not displace vessels, suggesting that this area is not a mass. **D:** Two areas of focal fatty sparing (*arrows*) are seen in classic locations as hypoechoic, irregularly shaped areas anterior to the gallbladder and portal vein. Because the liver is now hyperechoic from the fatty infiltration, normal liver tissue will appear as hypoechoic areas.

This disorder results from a defect in the enzyme glucose-6-phosphatase allowing excessive deposits of glycogen to be stored in the liver, intestinal tract, and kidneys.[10,39] Glycogen, normally broken down into glucose, is stored in the tissues, but the body is unable to synthesize it. This may cause severe hypoglycemia, abdominal distension, fatigue, and irritability.[36] von Gierke disease begins in infancy, but with early therapy, survival can continue into adulthood.[36,39,40]

Sonographic features of type 1 glycogen storage disease include a marked diffuse increase in parenchymal echogenicity and decreased penetration, indicating a fatty liver, hepatomegaly, and the possible presence of solid liver masses.[41] Typically, these masses are liver adenomas, which can occur in up to 40% of patients with von Gierke disease (Fig. 7-18).[10] Glycogen storage disease types 3 and 4 are more often associated with cirrhosis and potentially with HCC.[42]

Of note in the literature, patients with decreased glycogen stores have the opposite sonographic appearance of the liver compared to those with fatty infiltration. Cazier and Sponaugle[42] suggest there is a relationship between

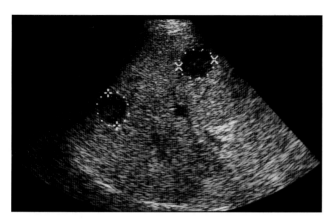

FIGURE 7-18 Glycogen storage disease with liver cell adenoma. A transverse image in a man with known glycogen storage disease demonstrates fatty infiltration of the liver and hypoechoic liver lesions consistent with liver cell adenomas (*cursors*).

glycogen phosphate and the attenuation properties of the liver. Malnourished individuals or those fasting for several days have depleted glycogen stores. The sonographic result is a noticeable decrease in the attenuation of the liver and a resultant apparent increase in the echogenicity or delineation of the periportal vascular markings. The liver pattern resembles that of a "starry sky."[42] In some cases, the normal renal cortex may appear more echogenic than

the liver. Normalization of the liver pattern relative to the kidney is achieved with adequate food intake if no other underlying process exists. Clinical correlation is necessary because decreased liver echogenicity can be seen with acute hepatitis, some diffuse infiltrative processes, leukemia, and some lymphomas.

Hepatitis

Hepatitis is an inflammation of the liver caused by reactions to viruses or toxins such as drugs or alcohol.[25,35] Types A, B, C, D, and E account for 95% of all acute hepatitis cases,[35] with the remaining caused by nonhepatotropic viruses such as cytomegalovirus (Table 7-6).[5,10,35] Common pathologic features of viral hepatitis are liver cell injury and swelling, varying cellular degeneration and possible necrosis, an immune system response, and regeneration.[35] Hepatitis A virus (HAV) is transmitted by a fecal–oral route, and symptoms typically resolve completely in less than 6 weeks.[10,35] Hepatitis B virus (HBV) occurs most frequently from sexual contact, blood transfusion, or sharing a contaminated needle and persists longer. Sonographers, as well as all health care workers, are encouraged to get the hepatitis B vaccine. Hepatitis C virus (HCV) is usually spread through direct contact with the blood or body fluid of a person who has the disease typically from sharing needles or unprotected sex. HCV can also be spread through blood transfusions and improperly disinfected medical

TABLE 7-6	Pathophysiology of Hepatitis[5,10,35]					
Hepatitis Type	Route of Transmission	Incubation Period (Days)	Fulminant Hepatitis	Chronic/ Carrier	Common Manifestations	Sonographic Appearance
HAV	Parenteral, fecal–oral, eating infected food or water, especially water and shellfish	15–50	Rare	No	Incubation period: headache, nausea, vomiting Prodromal phase (begins 2 wk after exposure, lasts 3–12 d, ends with jaundice): fatigue, anorexia, malaise, nausea with food odors; changes in taste suppress desire to smoke or drink alcohol; vomiting, headache, hyperalgesia, cough, and low-grade fever; elevations of AST, ALT, LDH₁, and LDH₂ Icteric phase (jaundice, lasts 2–6 weeks): abdominal pain and tenderness; elevated total bilirubin, dark urine, clay-colored stools; PT may be prolonged; may have pruritus if severe Recovery phase (resolution of jaundice 6–8 wk after exposure): Symptoms diminish but hepatomegaly may persist; LFTs return to normal within 2–12 wk.	Normal at first Acute phase: hyperechoic portal vein walls; hypoechoic parenchyma owing to swelling of liver Chronic phase: Increased amount of fibrous tissue and inflammatory cells surrounding hepatic lobules produces coarse echo pattern.
HBV	Sexual contact, mother to infant through breast milk, exposed to contaminated needles, blood, body fluids, or tattoo tools	14–180	Uncommon	Common (5%–10%)		
HCV	Sexual contact, exposed to contaminated needles, blood, body fluids, or tattoo tools	60–180	Uncommon	Common		
Hepatitis D virus	Contact with infected blood, unprotected sex, and infected needles with Hep B already	28–180	Common	Common		
Hepatitis E	Drinking contaminated water	14–56	Common in third trimester; uncommon otherwise	No		

ALT, alanine aminotransferase; AST, aspartate aminotransferase; HAV, hepatitis A virus; HBV, hepatitis B virus; HCV, hepatitis C virus; LDH, lactic dehydrogenase; LFT, liver function test; PT, prothrombin time.

equipment. If tattoo needles are not properly disinfected, there is a risk of being infected with HBV or HCV. Nearly half of all HCV cases develop into chronic hepatitis, and many chronic alcoholics with liver disease have antibodies to HCV.[35] Viral hepatitis accounts for 50% to 65% of all cases of fulminant hepatitis, although there are other causative agents such as viral infections and drug overdose.[35] With fulminant hepatitis, the onset of symptoms is more sudden and severe, leading to shock, coma, and, possibly, rapid death from marked liver necrosis. Liver transplantation may be lifesaving as massive hepatic necrosis is irreversible.[35]

The degree of hepatitis symptoms varies. These symptoms include fever, chills, nausea and vomiting, RUQ pain, hepatomegaly, and jaundice. Hepatitis is a nonobstructive, hepatocellular cause of jaundice and is the most common cause for a nontender gallbladder wall thickening.

Laboratory values usually include elevated ALT and AST. During the icteric phase, both the conjugated and unconjugated fractions of serum bilirubin are elevated, and PT increases with the severity of disease (Table 7-6). Health care workers should avoid exposure to viral hepatitis by wearing gloves and washing their hands after examining patients with hepatitis A.[35] Direct contact with blood and body fluids must be avoided in cases of hepatitis B and C.[35,36] Any accidental needle stick should follow these guidelines by the Centers for Disease Control (CDC)[43]:

- The needlesticks and cuts should be washed with soap and water.
- Splashes to the nose, mouth, or skin should be flushed with water.
- The eyes with should be irrigated with clean water, saline, or sterile irrigants.
- The incident should be reported to the supervisor.
- Immediate medical treatment should be sought.

The role of sonography in hepatitis is to evaluate for parenchymal changes, document liver size, and exclude biliary obstruction as the source of jaundice. In the acute phase, the parenchymal pattern ranges from normal to hypoechoic secondary to diffuse swelling of the liver cells caused by inflammation.[28] The portal vein walls appear much more hyperechoic against the hypoechoic background of the edematous parenchyma and is called the "starry sky" sign (Fig. 7-19A, B). Periportal collagenous markings are easily seen extending peripherally in the liver.[25] Gallbladder wall thickening may be noted (Fig. 7-19C).[10,25] By contrast, fibrosis resulting from chronic hepatitis along with secondary fatty change produces a coarser and more hyperechoic texture. The portal vein walls are less discrete compared to the more reflective parenchyma. Chronic active hepatitis has more serious consequences than chronic persistent hepatitis, because more patients progress to develop cirrhosis or liver failure.[10] Elastography can help monitor these patients.

Cirrhosis

In 2017, cirrhosis caused more than 1.32 million deaths worldwide, compared with 899,000 deaths in 1990.[44,45] In the United States, deaths from cirrhosis increased by 65% from about 20,600 people in 1999 to nearly 34,200 in 2016.[46] Cirrhosis is the ninth leading cause of death in the United States, with the leading causes being alcohol abuse, hepatitis B or C, and NASH.[44,45]

Cirrhosis is a general term for a diffuse process that destroys the normal architecture of the liver lobules. This process is the end result of chronic, severe damage to the liver cells, which leads to inflammation and subsequent necrosis.[10] Following inflammation, dense fibrous tissue septa form, which will separate the liver lobules and cause the parenchymal cells to degenerate, which may be followed by the formation of regenerative nodules.[10,35] The liver is the only organ in the body that can regenerate new healthy tissue. Initial changes cause liver enlargement, but continued insult results in atrophy of the liver. The parenchymal distortion may alter or compress biliary and vascular channels, leading to jaundice and portal hypertension.[8,21] The resulting jaundice develops more from impaired biliary excretion owing to primary liver cell injury than from biliary obstruction.[9] With portal hypertension, new vascular channels called collaterals can form, causing portal venous blood to bypass the liver (Fig. 7-20A).[21]

The incidence of NAFLD and NASH continues to rise, and they are rapidly growing causes of liver disease. Cirrhosis can develop from other disorders such as viral hepatitis, toxic drug and chemical reactions, biliary obstruction, and cardiac disease. Cirrhosis is also associated with metabolic defects such as glycogen storage disease, where glycogen is not released by the liver but builds up, and storage diseases that cause minerals to be deposited in the liver such as hemochromatosis (iron) and Wilson disease (copper).[35] Regardless of the etiology, cirrhosis can take one of four forms: alcoholic (Laennec, portal, or fatty), biliary (primary or secondary), postnecrotic owing to hepatitis, or metabolic (Table 7-7).[35,45,46]

LFT abnormalities depend on the stage and extent of disease. AST, ALT, lactic dehydrogenase (LDH4 and LDH5), and serum and urine conjugated bilirubin values are elevated. Serum ALP levels may also be elevated, whereas serum albumin level is decreased, and alpha-globulin protein levels are increased. No symptoms may appear for a long time. When clinical symptoms occur, patients may present with fatigue, weight loss, diarrhea, hepatomegaly, jaundice, and possible ascites. Hepatomegaly causes stretching of Glisson capsule, and patients may complain of a dull, aching pain in the epigastric region or RUQ. As the disease progresses, the liver returns to normal size and the RL begins to atrophy. The CL is usually spared or hypertrophies, probably because of its unique blood supply.[9] The chronic effects of cirrhosis, such as alterations in normal liver function, portal hypertension, and liver failure, are detailed in Table 7-8.[10,35,46]

The sonographic features of cirrhosis vary during disease progression. Early features include hepatomegaly and possible textural changes indicative of diffuse hepatocellular disease. These imaging features alone are nonspecific and unreliable in detecting the early histologic changes of cirrhosis. With superimposed fatty infiltration and fibrosis, the parenchymal pattern will display increased echogenicity compared to the normal renal cortex and decreased acoustic penetration. More specific sonographic features of cirrhosis are seen with late disease and can include liver atrophy, especially the RL, CL hypertrophy, surface nodularity, loss of delineation of intrahepatic vasculature, ascites, and findings related to portal hypertension (Fig. 7-20B–E). Parenchymal patterns can be heterogeneous owing to fibrosis, hypoechoic regenerative nodules, and superimposed fatty changes.[22,25,47] The

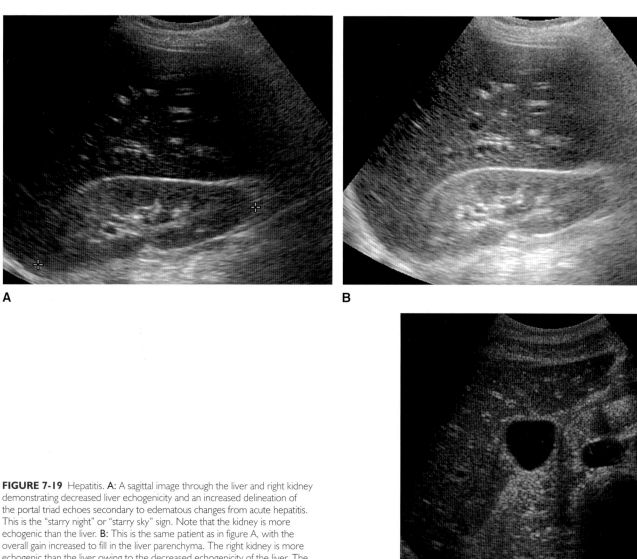

A

B

C

FIGURE 7-19 Hepatitis. **A:** A sagittal image through the liver and right kidney demonstrating decreased liver echogenicity and an increased delineation of the portal triad echoes secondary to edematous changes from acute hepatitis. This is the "starry night" or "starry sky" sign. Note that the kidney is more echogenic than the liver. **B:** This is the same patient as in figure A, with the overall gain increased to fill in the liver parenchyma. The right kidney is more echogenic than the liver owing to the decreased echogenicity of the liver. The kidney is normal, and the increased echogenicity of the kidney is not caused by medical renal disease. **C:** A transverse image of a patient with acute hepatitis demonstrating a thickened gallbladder wall. Hepatitis is the most common cause of a nontender, thickened gallbladder wall. Notice how bright the portal triad echoes appear owing to the decreased echogenicity of the liver.

incidence of HCC is significantly increased with macronodular cirrhosis, but hepatomas may be difficult to differentiate from regenerating nodules because both will appear as hypoechoic areas surrounded by the hyperechoic parenchyma. An elevated alpha-fetoprotein (AFP), biopsy of the lesion, or a contrast-enhanced ultrasound study (CEUS) can help to differentiate between the two (Fig. 7-20F–H).[47] Surface nodularity is diagnostic for cirrhosis, and the anterior liver capsule can be evaluated using a high-frequency linear array transducer or a higher-frequency curved linear array if a lot of ascites are present (Fig. 7-20I–K).[22] A lower-frequency transducer may be necessary to compensate for areas of increased attenuation. Some departments may determine the CL/RL ratio to establish the presence of caudate hypertrophy. This is accomplished by dividing the CL width by the RL width as measured on a transverse section using the MPV as a reference point. A C/RL ratio above 0.65 is considered indicative of cirrhosis.

Any secondary finding of cirrhosis should be documented and can include portal hypertension, splenomegaly, varices, collaterals, and ascites. The patency and flow direction of the portal vein should be documented with color and spectral Doppler imaging. Doppler signals should also be obtained from the hepatic artery, splenic vein, and any collaterals or varices. Common collaterals or varices include recanalization of the paraumbilical vein off of the LPV, esophageal varices, splenic varices, and a splenorenal shunt.[10,21] The portal vein velocities are often reduced and become hepatofugal, or directed away from the liver, and the hepatic artery will enlarge, also called hypertrophy, with elevated velocities to maintain hepatic perfusion (Fig. 7-20L–O).[8] The spleen can enlarge from portal congestion (Fig. 7-20P). It is not uncommon to find esophageal or splenic varices (Fig. 7-20Q). Another finding is a reconstituted umbilical vein arising from the LPV and flowing to the skin surface. The vessel can be followed just under the skin until it stops at the umbilicus.

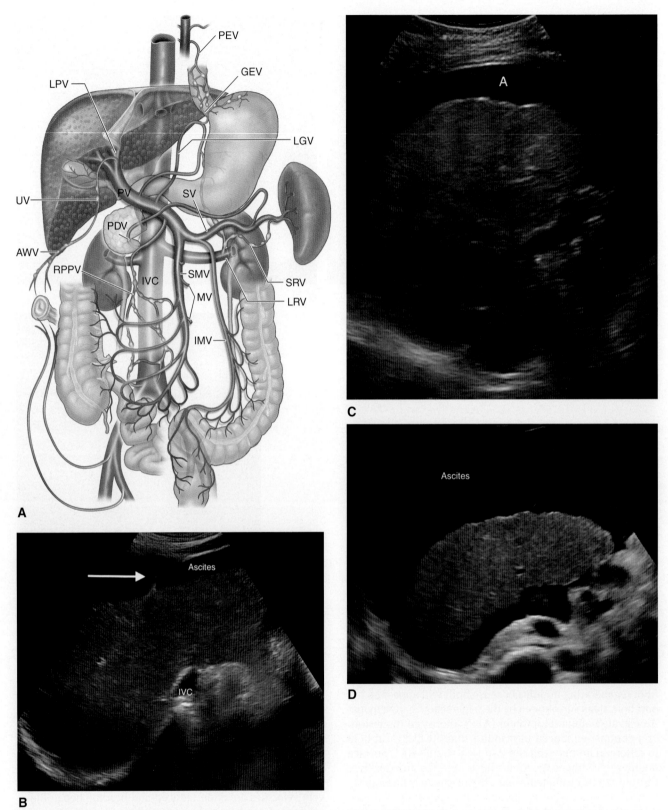

FIGURE 7-20 Cirrhosis. **A:** A drawing illustrating the various collateral vessels and pathways that may open up in patients with portal hypertension. **B:** A transverse scan demonstrates a cirrhotic liver with increased echogenicity. Ascites allows visualization of the falciform ligament *(arrow)*. **C:** On this patient with cirrhosis and ascites (A), the nodularity of the liver surface is seen. The nodularity can usually be better appreciated by scanning with a high-frequency linear array. **D:** A transverse scan on a patient with end-stage alcoholic liver disease. Ascites outlines the liver margins, which show considerable lobulation. The liver is also decreased in size.

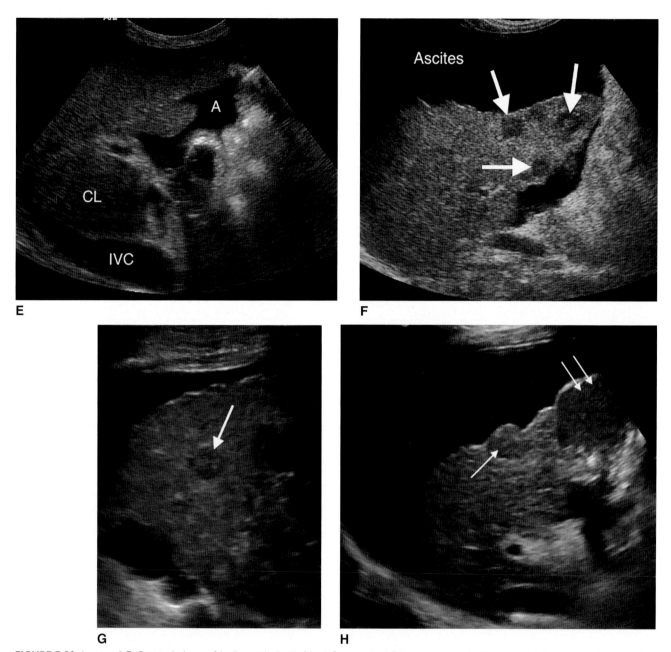

FIGURE 7-20 (continued) **E:** On a sagittal scan of the liver at the level of the *IVC*, an enlarged *CL* is seen associated with advanced cirrhosis. This enlargement is thought to be from alterations in the portal blood flow to the liver secondary to venous compression by fibrosis and regenerative nodules. Ascites (*A*). **F:** A sagittal image of a cirrhotic liver demonstrates multiple hypoechoic areas (*arrows*) that are compatible with regenerating nodules. Lab work, follow-up ultrasound, or CT or possibly a biopsy may be needed to prove that these nodules are not *HCCs* if clinically indicated. These were proven by biopsy to be regenerating nodules. **G:** This patient presented with elevated *AFP* and a history of cirrhosis. The *arrow* is pointing to a biopsy-proven *HCC*. Notice the similarity in appearance with the lesions in figure **F**. **H:** The sonogram on another patient with a biopsy-proven *HCC* (*double arrows*) also had a biopsy-proven regenerating nodule (*single arrow*).

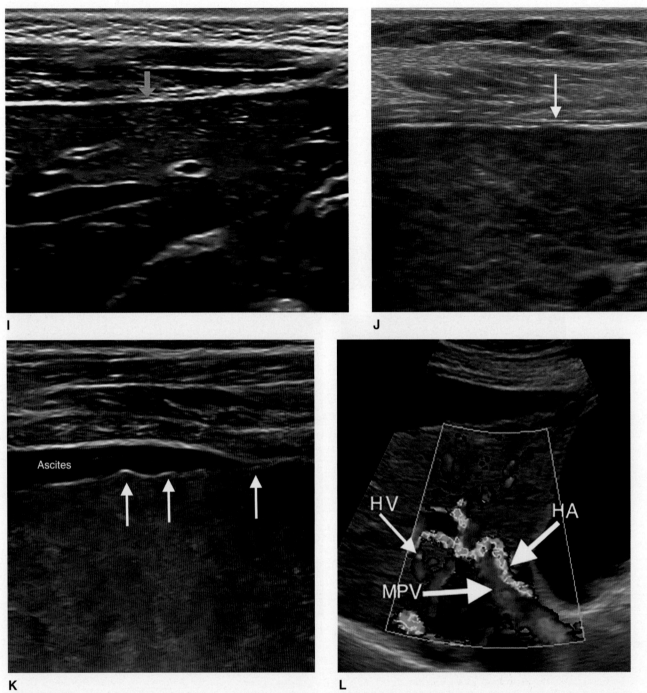

FIGURE 7-20 *(continued)* I: A high-frequency linear array image of a normal liver capsule (*arrow*). Notice how smooth it looks. J: A high-frequency linear array image of a patient with mild cirrhosis. Notice the nodularity of the parenchyma and the slight irregularity of the capsule (*arrow*). This patient did not have ascites. K: An image obtained with a high-frequency linear array transducer on a patient with cirrhosis and ascites. Notice the increased irregularity of the liver capsule (*arrows*) as opposed to the image in figure J, and the heterogeneity of the liver parenchyma. L: A color Doppler image demonstrates the corkscrew appearance of the *HA* that can occur because of decreased portal vein flow, which causes an increase in arterial flow. The hepatic and portal veins have nice color fill-in with no aliasing, whereas the *HA* is showing aliasing.

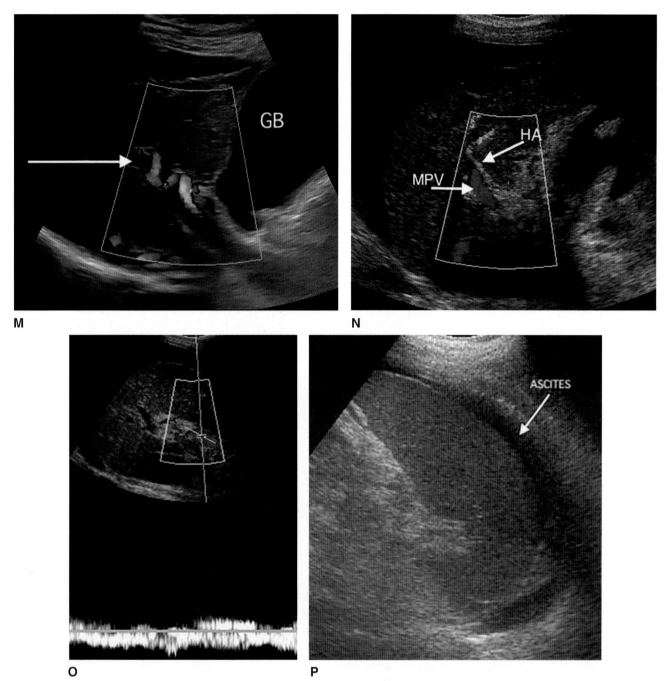

FIGURE 7-20 *(continued)* **M:** Increasing the color velocity scale reduces the aliasing inside the artery and causes the flow in the portal vein to not be displayed *(arrow)*, which could lead to a false impression of portal vein thrombosis. **N:** This color Doppler image demonstrates reversed flow, hepatofugal *(arrow)*, in the main portal vein and hepatopetal flow *(arrow)* of the hepatic artery on this patient with a cirrhotic liver. **O:** The spectral Doppler waveform from the main portal vein in figure **M** demonstrates hepatofugal flow. **P:** A transverse image of the spleen on the same patient as in figures **M** and **N** demonstrating splenomegaly from their portal hypertension. Some ascites *(arrow)* can be seen around the spleen.

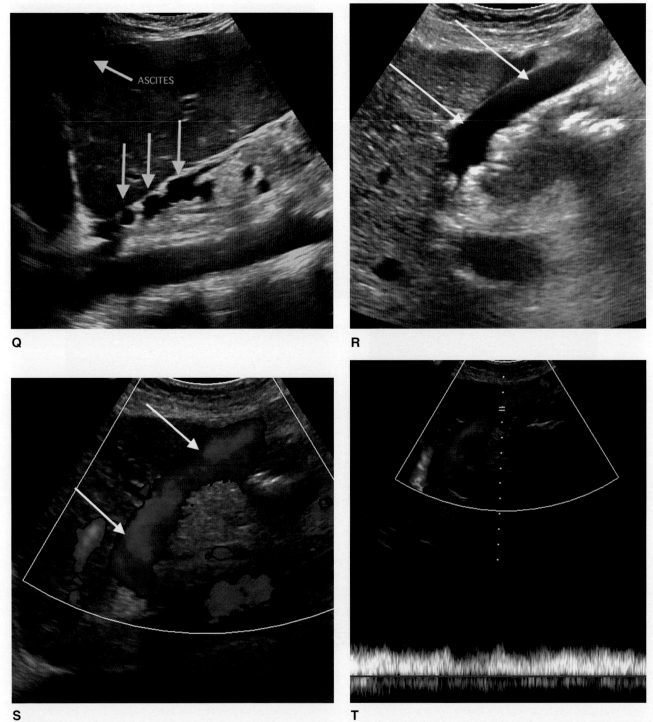

FIGURE 7-20 (*continued*) **Q:** A sagittal image demonstrating multiple cystic areas (*arrows*) superior to the aorta and posterior to the liver compatible with esophageal varices. Varices are filled and confirmed with color Doppler. Ascites is demonstrated superior to the liver (*arrow*). **R:** A sagittal image of the left upper quadrant showing a recanalized umbilical vein (*arrows*). **S:** A color Doppler image of the vessel in Figure **Q** (*arrows*) showing flow toward the skin surface. **T:** A spectral Doppler signal of the vessel in Figure **R** showing that the flow is venous.

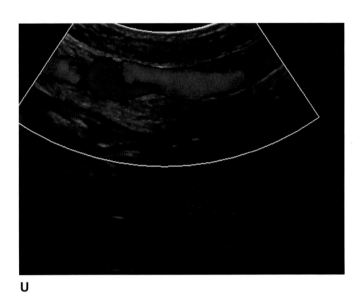

U

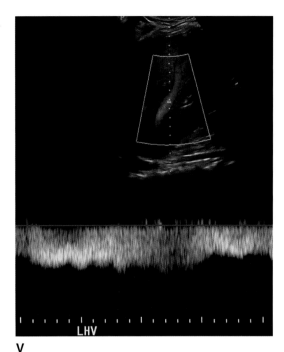

V

FIGURE 7-20 *(continued)* **U:** A color Doppler image following the recanalized umbilical vein from Figures **Q** to **S** showing continuation of the vessel under the skin, which would end at the area of the umbilicus. **V:** An example of a flattened hepatic vein signal that looks more like a portal vein, then a hepatic vein. *AFP*, alpha-fetoprotein; *AWV*, abdominal wall vein; *CL*, caudate lobe; *CT*, computed tomography; *GB*, gall bladder; *GEV*, gastroesophageal vein; *HA*, hepatic artery; *HCC*, hepatocellular carcinoma; *HV*, hepatic vein; *IMV*, inferior mesenteric vein; *IVC*, inferior vena cava; *LGV*, left gastric vein; *LPV*, left portal vein; *LRV*, left renal vein; *MPV*, main portal vein; *MV*, mesenteric veins; *PDV*, pancreaticoduodenal vein; *PEV*, paraesophageal vein; *PV*, portal vein; *RPPV*, retroperitoneal-paravertebral vein; *SMV*, superior mesenteric vein; *SRV*, splenorenal vein; *SV*, splenic vein; *UV*, umbilical vein.

TABLE 7-7	**Cirrhosis**[35,45]		
Type	**Etiology**	**Pathophysiology**	**Sonographic Appearance**
Alcoholic	Toxic effects of chronic, excessive alcohol intake (alcohol is a hepatotoxin that induces metabolic changes that damage hepatocytes)	Fat accumulation, inflammation (alcoholic hepatitis), and derangement of the lobular architecture by necrosis and fibrosis (cirrhosis)	In early stages, hepatomegaly; liver may appear hyperechoic compared to normal renal parenchyma; diffuse parenchymal changes lead to a diagnosis of hepatocellular disease. As cirrhosis progresses, hepatic tissue begins to atrophy and attenuates more sound; fibrosis appears more coarse; vascular structures are not as readily visualized and may present an irregular contour owing to nodular regeneration. With portal hypertension, splenomegaly and ascites may be seen.
Biliary	Primary: unknown, possible autoimmune mechanism; secondary: obstruction by cholelithiasis, stricture, or neoplasm	Primary: lobular bile ducts become inflamed and scarred; secondary: bile ducts become inflamed and scarred proximal to obstruction.	
Postnecrotic	Viral hepatitis, drugs, toxins, autoimmune destruction	Necrotic tissue is replaced with cirrhotic tissue, specifically fibrous, nodular scar tissue.	
Metabolic	Metabolic defects and storage disease (glycogen storage disease), Wilson disease, hemochromatosis, galactosemia	Morphologic changes resulting in inflammation and scarring	

TABLE 7-8	**Chronic Effects of Cirrhosis**[10,35,45]
Alteration in Function	**Symptoms and Signs**
PORTAL HYPERTENSION	
Collateral vessel development	Esophageal varices often lead to GI bleeding and possible hemorrhage, splenic varices, hemorrhoids, caput medusa (a radiating plexus of dilated periumbilical subcutaneous veins), spleno-renal shunt.
Increased portal vein pressure	Recanalization of the ligamentum teres (umbilical vein)
Increased portal vein pressure and decreased serum albumin level	Ascites, peripheral edema
Splenomegaly	Hematopoietic disorders: anemia, leukopenia, thrombocytopenia
Hepatorenal syndrome	Elevated serum creatinine, azotemia, oliguria; precursor of hepatic coma
Postsystemic shunting of blood	Hepatic systemic encephalopathy (precursor of confusion, coma, and convulsions)
HEPATOCELLULAR DYSFUNCTION	
Inability to remove conjugated bilirubin	Jaundice
Impaired bile synthesis	Malabsorption of fats and fat-soluble vitamins
Impaired plasma protein synthesis	Decreased level of albumin (precursor of edema and ascites)
Decreased synthesis of blood-clotting factors	Tendency to bleed
Impaired drug metabolism	Drug reactions and toxicity
Impaired gluconeogenesis	Glucose intolerance
Capillary congestion	Spider angiomas and palmar erythema
Decreased ability to convert ammonia to urea	Elevated blood ammonia level
Depressed metabolism of sex hormones	Women: menstrual disorders; men: testicular atrophy, gynecomastia, decrease in secondary sex characteristics

GI, gastrointestinal.

Because there is no fetus, there is nowhere else for the blood to go, and it enlarges the paraumbilical veins, creating what is called a caput medusae (head of Medusa) because the small, distended veins look like the snakes of Medusa's hair with the umbilicus being her head from Greek mythology (Fig. 7-20R–U). Doppler waveforms recorded from the hepatic veins may demonstrate continuous flow, described as "portalized" hepatic flow, as they lose their normal multiphasic appearance. This is caused by the noncompliance of the surrounding fibrous parenchyma that is causing the pressure in the liver to always exceed the pressure of the right atrium, causing the blood to continually flow out of the liver and into the heart (Fig. 7-20V).[8,21,22]

VASCULAR ABNORMALITIES

A variety of conditions can alter the blood flow pattern of the liver. Hemodynamic changes can range from simple vascular congestion to thrombosis and infarction with potential liver necrosis. Doppler imaging is a valuable tool for assessing changes within the hepatic artery, the portal system, and the hepatic veins. It is important to remember that both the hepatic artery and the portal vein bring flow into the liver, called hepatopetal, and both should be flowing in the same direction (Fig. 7-21A). Arterial inflow is characterized by a low-resistive Doppler waveform, indicating forward flow throughout the cardiac cycle (Fig. 7-21B). Normal portal venous inflow is characterized by a continuous monophasic flow with little pulsatility[8] and with a normal velocity between 15 and 18 cm/sec (Fig. 7-21C).[48] Portal vein flow velocity can increase after eating.[8] Hepatic vein flow is away from the liver, called hepatofugal, and toward the IVC and heart.[10] In healthy individuals, pulsed spectral tracings of the hepatic veins show pulsatility relative to right atrial filling, contraction, and relaxation.[8,49] This phasic hepatic venous pattern is sensitive to respiratory changes (Fig. 7-21D).[8]

A significant condition affecting liver hemodynamics is portal hypertension. The sonographic examination for portal venous hypertension and portal vein thrombosis is described in more detail in the the chapter on abdominal vasculature and the textbook on vascular structures in this series.

Hepatic Venous Outflow Obstruction

Budd–Chiari syndrome is an uncommon condition of hepatic venous outflow obstruction that can occur at any level from the small hepatic veins to the main hepatic veins, including the junction of the IVC and the right atrium. Budd–Chiari syndrome generally requires the occlusion of at least two hepatic veins to be clinically significant. Clinical features include abdominal pain, jaundice, ascites, hepatomegaly, and splenomegaly. The classic acute presentation is the clinical triad of ascites, hepatomegaly, and abdominal pain, although these findings are nonspecific. The possible causes

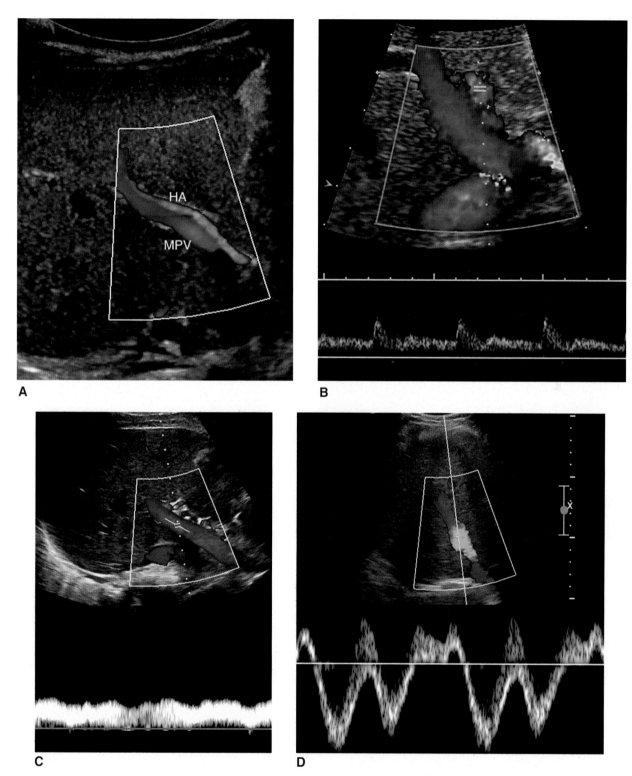

FIGURE 7-21 Normal hepatic vascular flow. **A:** Color Doppler image of a normal main portal vein (*MPV*), darker orange, and a normal hepatic artery (*HA*), brighter orange. The hepatic artery should be anterior to the portal vein. **B:** A spectral Doppler tracing demonstrating a normal, low-resistive waveform of the hepatic artery. Sometimes, using a write zoom of the area can aid in seeing the small hepatic artery better. **C:** Spectral Doppler waveform of the main portal vein showing continuous hepatopetal flow. **D:** Spectral Doppler tracing of the middle hepatic vein showing normal multiphasic flow. The flow in the hepatic veins reflects the changing pressures between the right side of the heart and the liver.

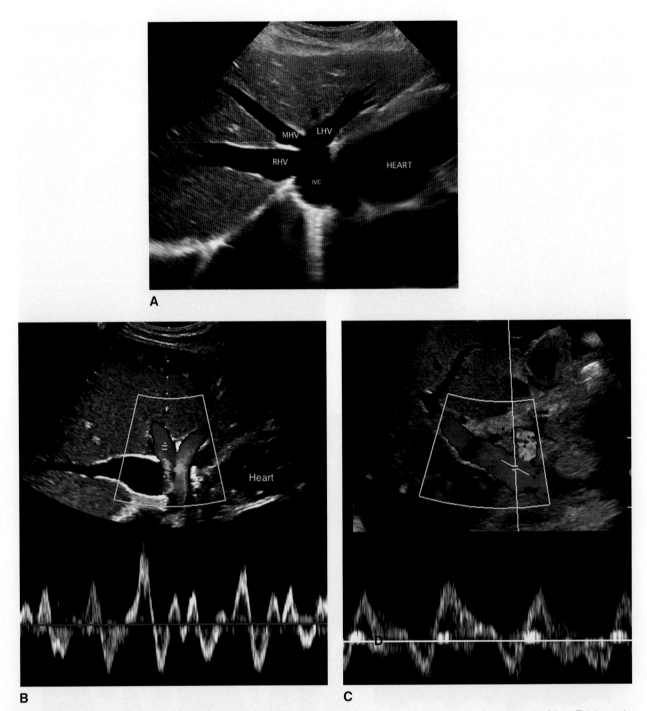

FIGURE 7-22 Liver congestion. **A:** A transverse scan of the inferior vena cava (*IVC*) and hepatic veins showing dilatation from right heart failure. This image demonstrates the Canadian Moose sign. **B:** Doppler tracing of the middle hepatic vein (*MHV*) waveform demonstrating the pulsatile W-type waveform pattern in this patient with congestive heart failure. When comparing with the waveform in Figure 21D, notice the increased flow above the baseline, which is flow back into the liver. **C:** The portal vein waveform from the same patient as in Figure **B**. The image was frozen with the color Doppler in the portal vein giving the appearance of hepatofugal flow. The pulsatile Doppler waveform shows that the flow is both above and below the baseline with the majority being hepatopetal. To avoid confusion, it would have been better to freeze the image when the portal vein flow was red. *LHV*, left hepatic vein; *RHV*, right hepatic vein.

are varied, although in a majority of cases, the etiology is never determined and is called idiopathic.[10] Thrombosis of the hepatic veins has been linked with several conditions such as oral contraceptive use, tumor invasion from HCC, renal or adrenal carcinoma, severe liver metastatic disease, Wilms tumor in pediatrics, and radiation to the liver with obliteration of small hepatic veins.[21]

The sonographic findings of Budd–Chiari syndrome depends on the degree of venous obstruction and the underlying cause. The hepatic veins may not be visible, may be narrow, or may have reversed flow. Grayscale imaging may show hypertrophy of the CL[50] owing to its direct venous drainage into the IVC,[10] as the blood from the other lobes is drained into the CL. Color Doppler imaging may occasionally demonstrate the enlarged caudate veins draining into the IVC. Other findings include portal hypertension, intrahepatic venous collaterals, ascites, splenomegaly, flow disturbances of the IVC, and extension of the thrombus into the IVC.[50] Because blood flows to unobstructed vessels, the flow may be to interlobular hepatic veins, subcapsular arcades, or it may be retrograde, hepatofugal, flow through branches of the portal veins. Doppler assessment is useful in demonstrating altered hemodynamics in the IVC, hepatic veins, and portal veins, as well as possibly identifying the site or level of obstruction.

Passive Liver Congestion

Passive edema of the liver, secondary to vascular congestion, is a complication related to heart failure.[49] The large volume of blood exiting the liver must pass through the hepatic veins to the IVC and enter the right side of the heart. Resistance to flow into the right side of the heart from cardiac or pulmonary disorders will cause secondary dilatation of these vessels. In the more acute phase, the liver enlarges, causing RUQ discomfort. Sonographically, the liver is easily evaluated, and dilated veins are readily visible. The IVC is dilated and may not change much in caliber with respiratory maneuvers (Fig. 7-22A). Pulsed Doppler waveforms of the hepatic vein may demonstrate a highly pulsatile W-type pattern[49] showing flow reversal during systole secondary to tricuspid regurgitation (Fig. 7-22B).[8] Sample volume tracings in the portal vein are also pulsatile with flow reversal away from the liver seen (Fig. 7-22C). In chronic disorders, the liver shrinks and becomes more fibrotic, but the hepatic veins will remain distended.[9] Of note is that all of the veins in the body will dilate and have pulsatile waveforms.

HEPATIC CYSTS

Hepatic cysts are commonly detected incidentally on an abdominal ultrasound or CT and usually have no clinical significance. They are uncommon, affecting about 5% of the population, and are usually reported in women. Hepatic cysts can vary in size, and most are less than 3 cm in size. Most patients are asymptomatic, although large cysts may cause pain or symptoms. Hepatic cysts are believed to be congenital in origin and thought to be the result of a malformation in the bile ducts, although the exact cause of this malformation is unknown. Cysts can be related to hereditary disorders such as polycystic liver disease (PLD). Other causes for cystic masses include hydatid disease, hematomas, abscesses, and necrotic tumors.

Congenital Cysts

Congenital cysts are often described as developmental because their prevalence increases with age.[25] They are discovered incidentally with imaging and are seen in fewer than 1% of patients less than 60 years of age but increases to 3% to 7% in older patients.[25] Solitary cysts are more common than multiple cysts, and the RL is affected twice as often as the left.[10,38] Cysts can be tiny or occupy large areas. In some patients, multiple or large cysts can cause hepatomegaly, palpable nodules, abdominal discomfort, or rarely localized bile duct compression causing jaundice.[38]

The imaging modality of choice for hepatic cysts is sonography. Lesions are typically round or oval (Fig. 7-23A, B). Sonographically, the imaging criteria for diagnosing a simple liver cyst are the same as any cyst and include the following:

1. A well-defined, thin-walled, cystic mass with a sharp posterior wall
2. No internal echoes (anechoic)
3. Distal acoustic enhancement
4. Lateral wall refractive edge shadowing

Sonographic diagnosis of a hepatic cyst is 95% to 100% accurate. Correlation with the patient's history, including the patient's age, can be helpful. Complex cysts may be caused by hemorrhage or infection. Differential diagnoses of complex cysts include bilomas, necrotic tumors, hepatic cystadenoma, parasitic masses, and intrahepatic hematoma or abscess.[10,38] CEUS may help with complicated cysts to help differentiate them from a malignant process.

There are two forms of PLD. PLD is caused by an autosomal dominant pattern and is characterized by the presence of differently sized cysts scattered throughout the liver with no cysts seen in the kidneys (Fig. 7-23C). The more common cause, representing 80% to 90% of all incidences of PLD, is a patient with autosomal dominant polycystic kidney disease (ADPKD), in which patients have cysts in both their liver and their kidneys (Fig. 7-23D). Most patients are asymptomatic, but occasionally, patients may have abdominal pain. Other symptoms are related to pressure from the enlarged liver and may include abdominal distention, early satiety, nausea, abdominal discomfort, back discomfort, and supine dyspnea. Histologically, the cysts are lined with cuboidal epithelium and are scattered randomly throughout the liver, causing disruption of the normal echo appearance. Cysts are numerous and can become detectable in the third or fourth decade of life, with women being affected more commonly than men. Differential diagnoses include Caroli disease, multiple abscesses, hepatic cysts with tuberous sclerosis, or degenerative metastasis. ADPKD will be discussed in detail in Chapter 12.

Acquired Cysts

Acquired cystic masses can be categorized as traumatic (hematoma, biloma), parasitic (echinococcal), or inflammatory (abscess).[38] They are often suspected prior to scanning because patients are usually symptomatic. The sonographic appearance ranges from classic cystic features to complex masses. In addition to localizing and measuring these lesions, it is important to characterize the appearance of acquired cysts and to correlate the sonographic presentation with clinical findings.

Hydatid Disease

The most common cause of hydatid disease in humans is *Echinococcus granulosus,* which is a parasitic tapeworm.[10] When a dog eats infested animal organs, the tapeworms mature in the dog's intestine and the ova are passed into their feces, which contaminates the ground. Cattle, sheep, and hogs serve as intermediate hosts. Humans become infected when they ingest parasite eggs by eating contaminated food or using water that was contaminated by the

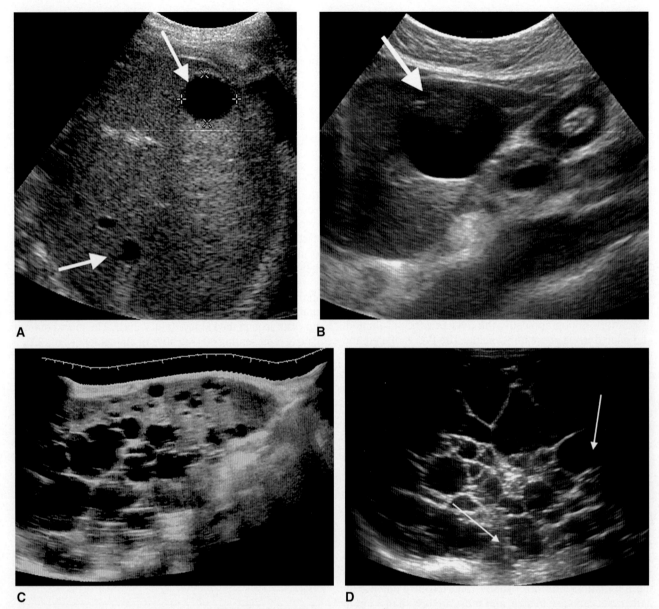

FIGURE 7-23 Congenital liver cysts. **A:** Congenital liver cysts (*arrows*) in an asymptomatic patient found incidentally on an exam to look for gallstones. The classic signs of a simple cyst are seen including thin walls, anechoic and acoustic enhancement. **B:** A simple cyst in the left lobe showing enhancement and a reverberation artifact (*arrow*). **C:** A sagittal extended field-of-view image demonstrating polycystic liver disease. The kidneys were normal in this patient. **D:** A sagittal image of the right lobe of the liver showing multiple cysts compatible with polycystic liver disease. This patient also had cysts in the kidneys, compatible with polycystic kidney disease, which is defined by the *arrows*. Sometimes, it can be difficult to know where the liver stops, and the kidney begins. Polycystic liver disease in isolation, in which patients have cysts only in the liver, is less common than autosomal dominant polycystic kidney disease with patients having cysts in both their liver and their kidneys.

stool from infected dogs. A person can also become infected from petting an infected animal.

The parasites were once confined to specific geographic areas, but international travel and markets for food products that have been fertilized with infected manure have increased their transmission. Sanitary measures can help reduce the incidence of this cyst.[9] Larvae ingested by a human hatch in the intestine and get into the bloodstream through the intestinal wall. Once in the blood, they can migrate and end up most often in the liver from portal flow. Although less frequently, they can also go to the lungs, the brain, or other organs.[9] The cysts may deform the organ, leading to unusual findings on palpation. Clinical symptoms range

from pain to anaphylactic shock if the cyst ruptures, which causes severe allergic reactions that can lead to death. Other symptoms include slight elevation of ALP, possibly jaundice if the cyst obstructs any bile ducts and portal hypertension.[9] If the larvae invaginate and develop, they become encysted and daughter cysts develop.[10] The original unilocular-looking cyst is eventually filled in by multiple cysts of varying size. The daughter cysts float in a protein-free, highly irritating hydatid fluid, which also contains hydatid sand.[9] It can take years after being infected for symptoms to occur. Patients with echinococcal cysts are rarely asymptomatic.

The sonographic appearance of echinococcal cysts depends on the course of larval maturation. The possibilities include a solitary cyst with possible mural or shell-like calcification, a mother cyst containing internal peripherally placed daughter cysts, fluid collections with septa yielding a honeycomb appearance, and solid-looking cysts, presenting with or without calcification (Fig. 7-24A–C).[17,26] Larger cysts may compress adjacent vessels or bile ducts.[39] During a stage of relative inactivity or parasite death, the germinal layer can fall away from the pericyst and infold within the cavity. This pattern has been referred to as the congealed water-lily sign.[26] As the lesion decreases in size, folds of the germinal layer become more tightly apposed and produce a more solid appearance.[10]

Schistosomiasis

Schistosomiasis is a common parasitic infection caused by *Schistosoma mansoni*, *S. japonicum*, *S. mekongi*, and *S. intercalatum*. It is prevalent in certain parts of the world such as Africa, Asia, Indonesia, China, Japan, South America, Egypt, and the Mediterranean.[9,39] In locations with contaminated water, immature worms can penetrate the skin from walking or swimming in affected water. It can enter the mesenteric veins via the lymphatics and bloodstream.[51] Eggs can travel to the intestine or migrate from the portal vein to the liver.[9,51] The ova will then penetrate the portal venous walls and lodge in the surrounding liver tissue. A granulomatous reaction occurs, inducing periportal fibrosis. The terminal portal vein branches can become occluded, causing portal hypertension and potentially cirrhosis.[51] Clinically, these patients will present with signs of portal hypertension, splenomegaly, gastroesophageal varices, hematemesis, and ascites. Hepatic function is commonly preserved until the late stages of the disease.

Sonographic features include hyperechoic thickened walls of the portal venules that display in a "clay-pipe stem" pattern (Fig. 7-25A, B) Periportal fibrosis is further characterized by the irregular hepatic surface and splenomegaly with portal and splenic vein dilatation. Early on, both portal and splenic veins maintain continuous hepatopetal flow with normal velocities; however. Portal hypertension will eventually develop.

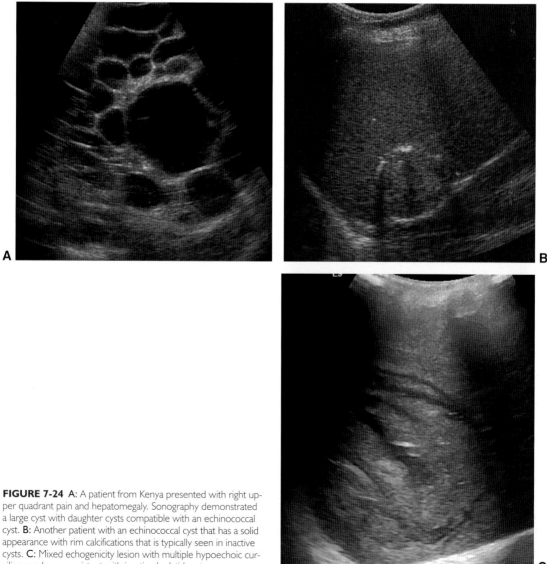

FIGURE 7-24 A: A patient from Kenya presented with right upper quadrant pain and hepatomegaly. Sonography demonstrated a large cyst with daughter cysts compatible with an echinococcal cyst. **B:** Another patient with an echinococcal cyst that has a solid appearance with rim calcifications that is typically seen in inactive cysts. **C:** Mixed echogenicity lesion with multiple hypoechoic curvilinear echoes consistent with inactive hydatid cyst.

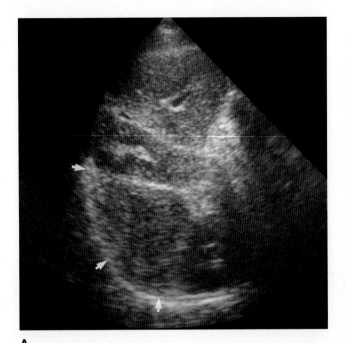

A

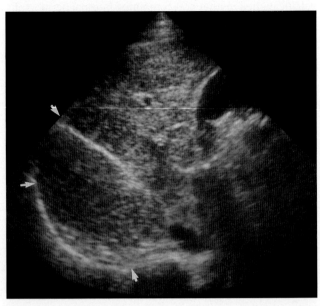

B

FIGURE 7-25 Schistosomiasis. **A:** This 30-year-old woman presented with right back pain. A calcification was noted on an abdominal radiograph, and the patient was referred for renal sonography evaluation. On both the sagittal (**A**) and transverse (**B**) sections of the liver, advanced periportal fibrosis provides the "turtle back" sonographic appearance (*arrows*). (Courtesy of Charlotte Henningsen, Florida Hospital College of Health Sciences, Orlando, FL.)

HEPATIC ABSCESSES

Because the liver receives blood from the portal circulation, it might seem that the liver would be more prone to infections with increased exposure to bacteria. However, the Kupffer cells remove the bacteria so efficiently that an infection rarely occurs. The cause of a hepatic abscess is usually a bacterial, amebic, or parasitic infection. The sonographic examination can noninvasively locate, measure, and characterize hepatic abscesses, which can be located in the intrahepatic, subhepatic, or subphrenic areas.[17] Patients with an abscess will present with pain, fever, and leukocytosis, which is elevated white blood cells. Ultrasound can also be used to guide an aspiration of the fluid for cultures so that the proper antibiotic or treatment can be determined.

Pyogenic Abscess

Pyogenic abscess is most often polymicrobial and accounts for almost 80% of all hepatic abscesses in the United States, with *Escherichia coli*, commonly referred to as *Escherichia coli* and Klebsiella pneumoniae being the two most frequently isolated pathogens. Recent studies suggest that Klebsiella pneumoniae is increasing as the most prominent bacteria causing an abscess. The abscess will develop when the reticuloendothelial system is compromised by altered immune function or when there is severe sepsis.

Biliary tract disease is now the most common source for a pyogenic abscess, replacing appendicitis as the main cause. Obstruction of bile flow allows for the bacteria to grow and proliferate and will usually produce multiple abscesses (Fig. 7-26A). Pyogenic bacteria enter the liver through direct extension (Fig. 7-26B) from adjacent organs or enter through the blood via the portal vein or hepatic artery. Common conditions that would lead to seeding from the portal vein include appendicitis, acute diverticulitis, and inflammatory bowel disease. Seeding from the hepatic artery can occur in systemic bacteremia from bacterial endocarditis, urinary sepsis, or from intravenous drug abuse. A pyogenic abscess in the subhepatic region may result from a cholecystectomy and is found in the gallbladder bed or in Morison pouch. In the subphrenic region, abscess formation results from bacteria spilling into the peritoneum from surgery, bowel rupture, a perforated peptic ulcer, or trauma.[17] The mortality rate can be 100% in untreated cases. Pyogenic abscesses produce varying symptoms, depending on the severity and extent of the process. Clinical symptoms may include fever, leukocytosis, elevated LFTs, RUQ pain, pleuritic pain, and hepatomegaly.

Several sonographic features have been described including the presence of single or multiple areas measuring 1 cm or larger, with 80% located in the RL. The shape of an abscess is variable, but a pyogenic abscess may be round or ovoid with walls that are usually irregular and poorly defined. Increased flow may be seen around the mass owing to peripheral hypervascularity (Fig. 7-26C). The internal echo pattern is usually heterogeneous and depends on the presence of debris, septations, or gas (Fig. 7-26D), but it is usually less echogenic than the hepatic parenchyma. Some abscesses will have a more homogenous pattern with acoustic enhancement owing to the fluid of the abscess.[10] The acoustic enhancement will help to differentiate them from a solid liver mass. The clinical features and echo enhancement are important considerations in the differential diagnosis, which includes cyst, hematoma, biloma, necrotic tumor, echinococcal cyst, and primary or metastatic cystadenocarcinoma.[38]

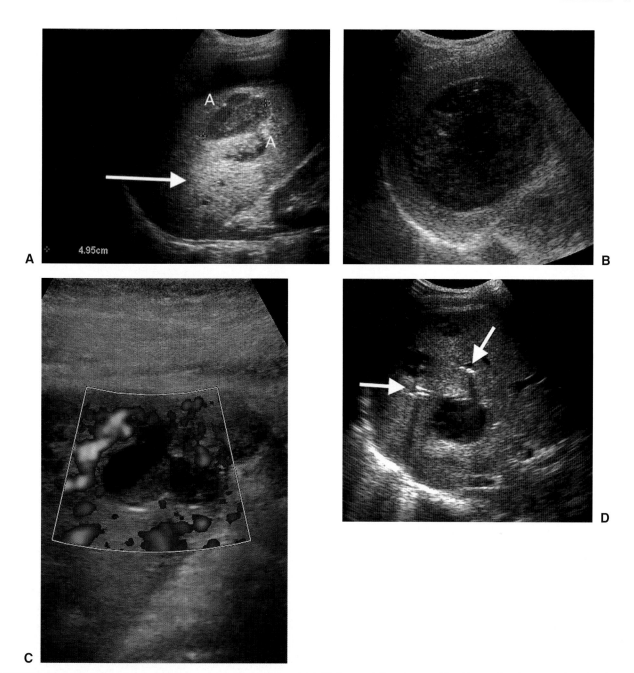

FIGURE 7-26 Pyogenic abscesses. **A:** A sagittal scan of a patient with two debris-filled pyogenic liver abscesses (*A*), with acoustic enhancement (*arrow*) demonstrated, that helped differentiate them from a solid mass. The cause of the abscesses was believed to be biliary in origin. **B:** A large liver abscess in a patient with cholecystitis. The abscess was present before surgery. **C:** Patient presented with pain and fever and a history of diverticulitis. Sonography shows a complex collection with acoustic enhancement in the left lobe of the liver compatible with an abscess. Power Doppler demonstrated increased flow around the abscess. **D:** Multiple gas-forming pyogenic liver abscesses in this patient with a history of diabetes and biliary obstruction. Notice the bright white reflectors (*arrows*) compatible with gas. Gas-producing abscesses are more common in diabetic patients and are associated with a high mortality rate.

Amebic Abscess

An amebic abscess occurs when the patient is infected with the parasite *Entamoeba histolytica* from eating food or drinking water that has been contaminated. This parasite causes amebiasis, which is an intestinal infection that can also be called amebic dysentery. After an infection has occurred in the GI tract, the blood from the intestines via the portal vein may carry the parasite to the liver. Once confined to tropical areas where crowded living conditions and poor sanitation exist, the amebic disease is now found in many developed countries. Humans serve as an intermediate host and are usually asymptomatic when the organism is confined to the GI tract.[10] When a liver abscess develops, patients will present with symptoms including RUQ pain, hepatomegaly, diarrhea, fever, chills, jaundice, and black tarry stool.[10] Reactive hepatomegaly is common. Laboratory tests can reveal moderate leukocytosis,[52] mild anemia, elevated LFTs, and positive serologic tests.[52] Fluid from the abscess can be aspirated and cultured. The fluid may be thick and chocolate colored and can become thinner with age.[9] The RL of the liver is more commonly affected than the left lobe, and this has been attributed to the fact that the RL portal blood flow is supplied predominantly by the SMV, whereas the left lobe portal blood flow is supplied primarily by the splenic vein. Before liquefaction, an echogenic mass may correlate with the presence of a new amebic abscess.[52] As the mass matures, it becomes more hypoechoic, contains fewer echoes, develops smoother walls, and demonstrates acoustic enhancement (Fig. 7-27). Color Doppler imaging will demonstrate the absence of internal blood flow. Without treatment, the abscess may rupture spreading into the abdominal cavity, the pleura, the lungs, the pericardium, and the brain. Untreated patients also have a high morbidity, approaching 100%. Patients that receive treatment have a high chance of being cured.

OTHER INFECTIOUS PROCESSES

HIV/AIDS

Opportunistic infections are illnesses that occur more frequently and are more severe in people with damaged immune systems, such as HIV and AIDS patients. With current effective HIV treatment, opportunistic infections of the past are less common in people with HIV, including what used to be the most common infection, *Pneumocystis* (Fig. 7-28). HIV/AIDS can affect the liver in different ways, but because of antiretroviral therapy, these complications have declined dramatically. Patients with HIV/AIDS may have coexisting diseases including HBV, HCV, NASH, and cirrhosis and their liver will have an ultrasound appearance of those conditions.

Fungal Infection

A possible liver complication in immunosuppressed patients, especially those receiving chemotherapy for blood

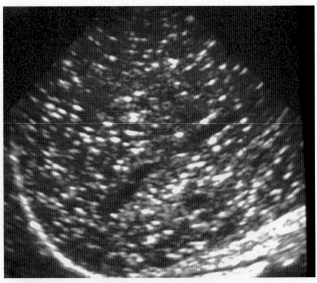

FIGURE 7-28 HIV/AIDS–related liver disease. A sagittal scan of the right lobe of the liver reveals multiple tiny focal calcifications (starry sky). This pattern is highly suggestive of, but not definitive for, disseminated *Pneumocystis* infection, which this patient did have.

malignancies is hepatic candidiasis. Spread of the fungus *Candida albicans* is through the bloodstream. Patients may experience some RUQ pain and fever. This mycotic infection can cause hepatomegaly that is detectable by sonography as well as have micro-abscesses. These abscesses display a "wheel within a wheel" imaging pattern (Fig. 7-29).[10] The outer hypoechoic wheel represents a fibrosis surrounding the inner echogenic wheel of inflammatory cells and a central hypoechoic area of necrosis.[10]

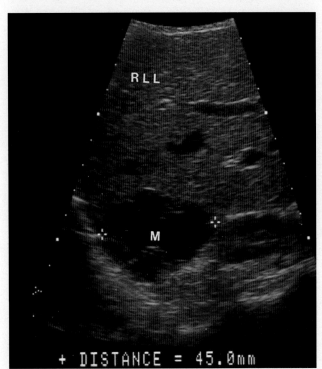

FIGURE 7-27 Amebic abscess. In the right lobe (*RLL*), a 4.5-cm complex cystic mass (*M*) is detected in a woman who lived for a time in Indonesia.

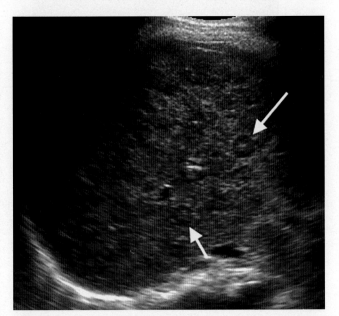

FIGURE 7-29 Candidiasis: microabscesses. Multiple small, hypoechoic masses, "wheels within wheels" (two are pointed out by *arrows*), are seen in an immunocompromised patient receiving high-dose chemotherapy. The patient presented for a sonography examination with fever. Although metastatic disease could have a similar appearance, the rapid appearance of multiple masses between short-term imaging sessions and the patient's clinical presentation was more indicative of a fungal infection.

HEMATOMA

The liver's abundant vascular supply makes it highly susceptible to hemorrhage when blunt force trauma to the abdomen ruptures or tears hepatic tissue. The liver and spleen are the most commonly injured organs in blunt abdominal trauma, with splenic trauma being the most common cause of internal bleeding or hemorrhage. In addition to trauma, hematomas can form secondary to interventional procedures, such as a liver biopsy, from rupture of a vascular neoplasm or aneurysm, or can be associated with pregnancy-induced hypertension.[9,53] Symptomatically, the liver is tender. With a significant bleed, the patient may physically collapse and show signs of shock as the blood pressure, pulse rate, and hematocrit levels drop.

Liver trauma is categorized based on severity and location. Classifications include contusion, subcapsular hematoma, central laceration, and transcapsular laceration with rupture through Glisson capsule.[53] With capsular disruption, both blood and bile can leak into the peritoneal cavity. Although CT is the imaging modality of choice, especially in blunt abdominal trauma, sonography is capable of detecting disruptions in the hepatic parenchyma associated with lacerations, localizing and measuring focal hematoma formation, and documenting hemoperitoneum. The sonographic appearance of a hematoma depends on the age of the bleed. Fresh hematomas are echogenic during the first day following injury as fibrin and erythrocytes are deposited to stop the bleeding and are echogenic (Fig. 7-30A).[53] Blood can be anechoic, but early in the evolution of a hematoma, acoustic enhancement may not be exhibited. Gradually, as a hematoma becomes organized and develops a clot, it appears as a complex fluid collection with both cystic and solid parts. Eventually, it undergoes complete liquefaction and becomes a seroma, which has an anechoic cystic pattern. A chronic hematoma may become calcified and produce an acoustic shadow. Frequently, the liver capsule will contain the hepatic hematoma, although disruption of the capsule may show free fluid in the abdomen and pelvis (Fig. 7-30B–D). A subcapsular hematoma produces a striking appearance as it displaces the liver medially and may have a crescent-shaped appearance (Fig. 7-30E).

BENIGN NEOPLASM

In neonates and infants, benign hepatic tumors are more common than malignant ones, whereas in older children and adults, they are less common than malignant ones.[50] Primary liver tumors may originate from the parenchymal cells or bile duct epithelium or may represent a mixture of the two. Sonography is an excellent imaging modality for liver tumors, and now with CEUS, the patient may be able to leave with a diagnosis instead of waiting to be scheduled for other imaging tests or a biopsy.

Cavernous Hemangioma

A cavernous hemangioma is the most common benign liver tumor occurring in up to 4% of the general population.[38,54,55] These lesions are not true neoplasms, because histologically they are composed of a large network of blood-filled vascular spaces lined with endothelium.[55] The spaces are separated by fibrous septa, which commonly proliferate centrally and extend peripherally. Hemangiomas are five times more common in women.[10] Lesions can occur at any age but increase in frequency with age.[55] Most hemangiomas are found incidentally because they cause no symptoms.[54,55] Most are solitary, but 10% to 20% of patients can have multiple hemangiomas. Typical hemangiomas measure less than 3 cm, but larger lesions are possible and are called giant hemangiomas.[10] Their location is typically in the posterior segment of the RL and in subcapsular locations, along the periphery of the liver.[10]

Sonography is reported to be more reliable than CT in detecting cavernous hemangiomas, especially those smaller than 1 cm.[51] The classic sonographic appearance is a homogeneous (58% to 73% of masses), hyperechoic (67% to 79% of masses) mass with sharp, well-defined margins and possible posterior acoustic enhancement (Table 7-9; Fig. 7-31A–C).[10,54] When hemangiomas are smaller than

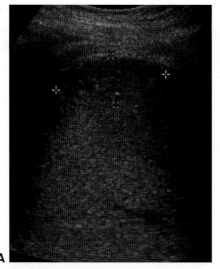
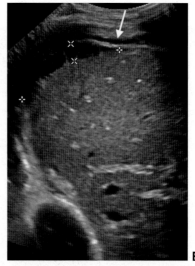

FIGURE 7-30 **A:** A transverse scan of the liver in a patient 1 hour post–liver core biopsy. The patient complained of abdominal pain, and sonography demonstrated a fresh hematoma at the biopsy site, which is seen between the calipers. Fresh hematomas are usually echogenic. **B:** A transverse scan of a patient in the left lateral decubitus position 4 hours post a blind liver biopsy through the ribs, who presented with very sudden swelling of his scrotum. The scan of the patient's liver revealed a subcapsular hematoma as seen between the calipers. The *arrow* is pointing to the bright white line of Glisson capsule, and fluid can be seen anterior to it.

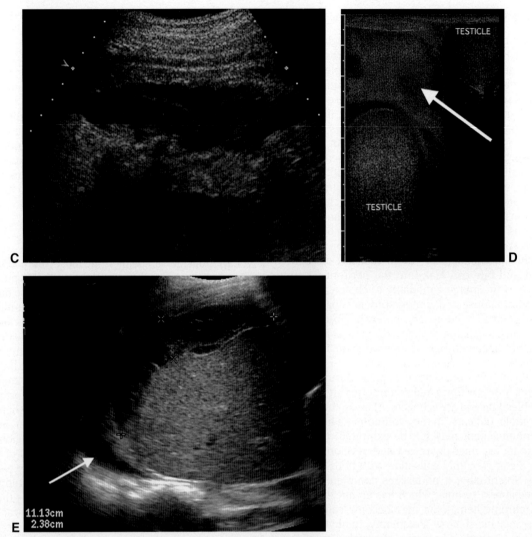

FIGURE 7-30 (*continued*) **C:** Same patient as in **B** scanning along their right flank demonstrates free fluid. **D:** Same patient as in **B** and **C**. A transverse scan of the patient's testicles shows echogenic fluid in the right side of the scrotum compatible with a hematocele. The left side of the scrotum and the left testicle were normal. This patient was leaking blood from his liver core biopsy, down his flank and into his scrotum. He was taken to interventional radiology to stop the bleeding from the liver. Follow-up exam in 2 weeks showed resolution of the hematocele. **E:** A transverse image of a subcapsular hematoma, which is outlined by the calipers on a patient who was in a motor vehicle accident. The *arrow* is pointing to a pleural effusion.

TABLE 7-9   Benign Liver Neoplasms

Neoplasm	Histologic Appearance	Clinical Signs	Sonographic Appearance
Cavernous hemangioma	Large network of vascular endothelial-lined spaces with red blood cells	No symptoms; 70%–95% occur in women; its frequency increases with age.	Usually homogeneous, hyperechoic mass with sharp, well-defined margins; may have posterior acoustic enhancement, usually in the posterior right segment
Focal nodular hyperplasia	Hepatocytes, Kupffer cells, bile duct elements, and fibrous connective tissue; central fibrous band with radiating septa separates mass into nodules; no known malignant potential	Usually asymptomatic, generally an incidental finding	May be hypoechoic, hyperechoic, or isoechoic with normal tissue; 0.5- to 20-cm well-circumscribed mass
Liver cell adenoma	Encapsulated, slightly atypical hepatocytes, often with areas of bile stasis, focal hemorrhage, and necrosis; malignant potential of a hepatoma; susceptible to hemorrhage	Usually symptomatic; incidence increases in women of childbearing age and is associated with oral contraceptive use	Usually hyperechoic relative to normal tissue; well-circumscribed mass; with hemorrhage, internal from anechoic to hyperechoic depending on age of bleed

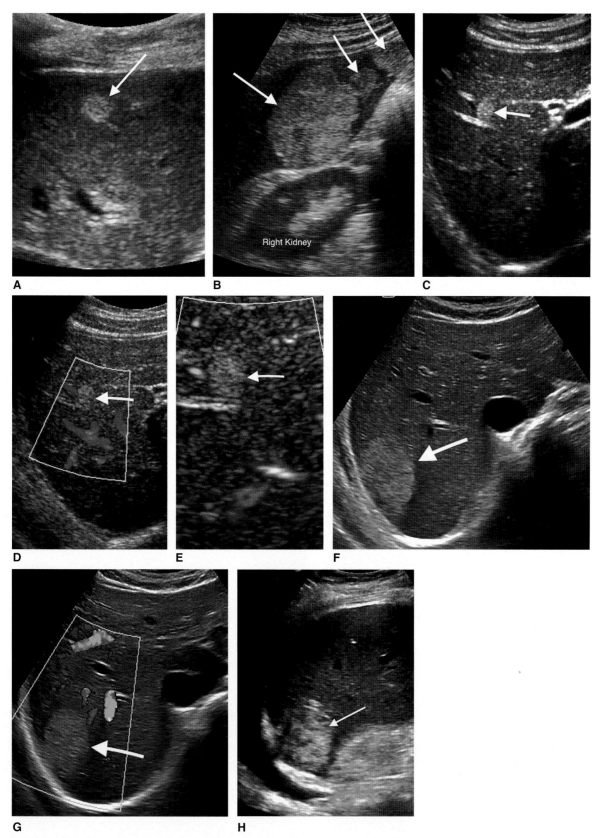

FIGURE 7-31 Cavernous hemangioma. **A:** Typical appearance and location of a hemangioma (*arrow*) in a liver seen under the capsule. This was found incidentally on a gallbladder ultrasound. Radiologists may use the term incidentaloma when they are found. **B:** Three hemangiomas (*arrows*) were found incidentally on
this patient, the larger one compatible with a giant hemangioma. **C:** A small hemangioma (*arrow*) is seen in this image. **D:** Same patient as in **C**; notice the lack
of flow seen with color Doppler image. **E:** A power Doppler image of the same patient as in **C** with the image zoomed still demonstrating lack of flow. **F:** Giant
hemangioma (*arrow*) found deep in the liver adjacent to the diaphragm. **G:** Same patient as in **F** using color Doppler imaging, which does not show any flow inside
the mass. **H:** A giant hemangioma (*arrow*) demonstrating a more heterogeneous echo texture. This appearance could be worrisome for a malignant mass, and
contrast-enhanced ultrasound could be used to help confirm that this is a hemangioma.

2.5 cm, acoustic enhancement may not be seen. Color Doppler and power Doppler imaging will not demonstrate any flow inside the hemangioma because the flow within them is too slow to be visualized with color Doppler imaging (Fig. 7-31D, E).[25] Larger lesions present with a more heterogeneous echo pattern[38] (Fig. 7-31F–H). If a cavernous hemangioma is suspected after sonography, a short-term follow-up ultrasound examination is accepted practice to monitor any change, or a CEUS can be performed. CEUS will show vascular enhancement along the periphery of the lesion and then completely fill in on delayed scans. Contrast applications will be discussed later in this chapter.

Focal Nodular Hyperplasia

Focal nodular hyperplasia (FNH) is the second most common benign liver mass.[10] An FNH nodule contains all the cellular elements of normal liver tissue, including hepatocytes, Kupffer cells, bile duct elements, and fibrous connective tissue, but it lacks the normal hepatic architecture.[50] It is more common in females, possibly owing to hormonal influence, with a male-to-female ratio of 1:8. About 80% of FNH are solitary, are usually less than 5 cm in diameter, and are often located in the RL or lateral segment of the left lobe. They are usually incidental findings with imaging. FNH liver lesions are typically asymptomatic, they rarely grow or bleed and will not become malignant. On nuclear medicine exams, because these masses contain Kupffer cells they will accumulate the injected technetium-99m (^{99m}Tc) sulfur and will appear as a hot spot on the scan.

Sonographically, the classic appearance of FNH is a subtle, isoechoic lesion that is difficult to identify within the normal liver parenchyma (Fig. 7-32A, B) and is referred to as a stealth lesion.[55] The lesion usually appears as a homogenous mass with variable echogenicity, including hypoechoic, isoechoic, or rarely hyperechoic.[39,54] Displacement of vascular structures may be seen, suggesting the possibility of the mass being an FNH. Even though the mass is not encapsulated, it is well circumscribed with a characteristic depressed central or eccentric stellate scar composed of dense fibrous connective tissue, proliferating bile ducts, and thin-walled blood vessels.[38,54] The echogenicity of both the FNH and its scar is variable, and they may be difficult to be seen with ultrasound. FNH masses characteristically demonstrate a central scar, and with color Doppler imaging, peripheral and central blood vessels are seen and blood flow may be seen in the center of the lesion from the feeding vessel. Ultrasound contrast may help to eliminate the need of further imaging with CT or MRI. CEUS demonstrates a typical spoke-wheel pattern followed by complete enhancement in the arterial phase, and the mass will remain hyper/isoechoic in the portal and late phases.

Hepatic Adenoma

With the increased usage of abdominal imaging, including ultrasound, benign liver tumors are being detected as incidental findings more frequently. It is important to be able to differentiate between an FNH and a hepatic adenoma (HCA). Both are benign masses that occur predominantly in women; however, it is important to differentiate an FNH from HCA because an HCA has potential for life-threatening complications, including the risk of spontaneous bleeding and the possibility of malignant transformation. HCA has

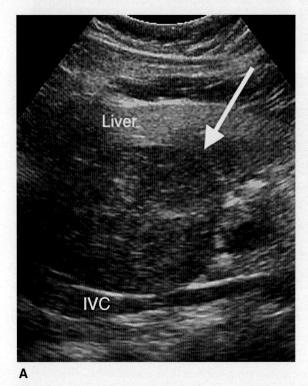

A

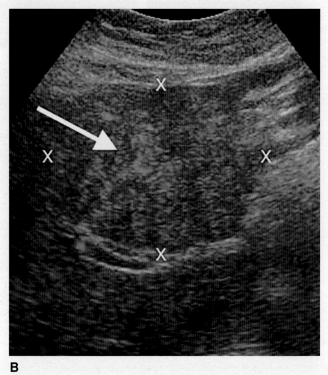

B

FIGURE 7-32 Focal nodular hyperplasia (*FNH*). **A:** Incidental finding on this female patient who was referred to sonography to evaluate for gallstones. The *FNH* mass (*arrow*) is slightly compressing the patient's inferior vena cava (*IVC*). Note the central scar in the middle of the mass. **B:** This patient was referred for a possible palpable mass. This *FNH* was more isoechoic and harder to delineate. The borders are marked by the Xs and the *arrow* points to the central scar.

a link to oral contraceptive use and is less common than an FNH.[56]

Unlike FNH masses, an HCA contains no bile duct or Kupffer cells and can be cold on technetium-99m (^{99m}Tc) sulfur imaging as a result of absent Kupffer cells. They are encapsulated masses consisting of atypical hepatocytes. They are usually solitary masses with defined margins and are more common in women, especially of childbearing age. Its association with long-term oral contraceptive use in women is well documented. Occasionally, these masses will occur in men taking anabolic steroids, and they can shrink or disappear after stopping the hormones. Patients with type I glycogen storage disease or von Gierke disease may have multiple adenomas. An HCA produces no significant laboratory value changes and is usually an incidental finding on imaging. Clinical symptoms of liver adenomas vary from the patient being asymptomatic to acute RUQ or epigastric pain. An HCA can rupture, causing severe abdominal pain and sudden intraperitoneal hemorrhage. Owing to the possibility of rupturing or becoming malignant, liver adenomas are usually surgically removed.

The sonographic appearance of an HCA is an encapsulated, well-circumscribed, hyperechoic mass with a hypoechoic halo. However, they may also appear as a hypoechoic or isoechoic mass relative to the normal liver parenchyma (Fig. 7-33A). An HCA is very vascular on color Doppler images, demonstrating flow in the center of the lesion as well as flow around the periphery (Fig. 7-33B). If the tumor

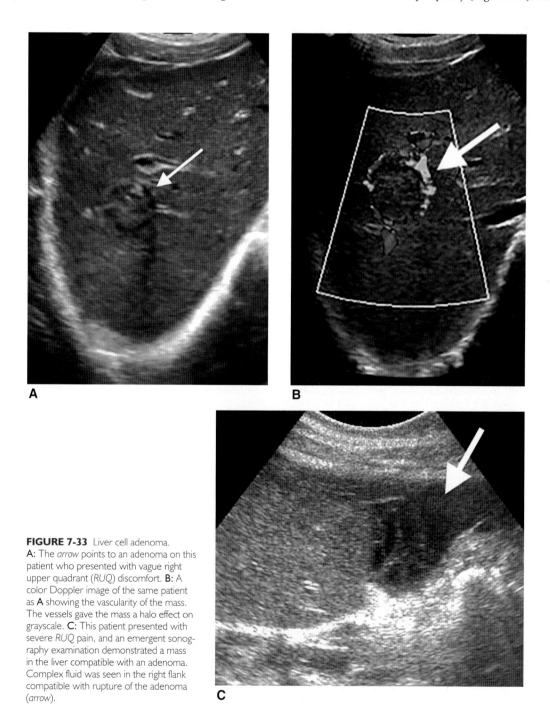

FIGURE 7-33 Liver cell adenoma. **A:** The *arrow* points to an adenoma on this patient who presented with vague right upper quadrant (*RUQ*) discomfort. **B:** A color Doppler image of the same patient as **A** showing the vascularity of the mass. The vessels gave the mass a halo effect on grayscale. **C:** This patient presented with severe *RUQ* pain, and an emergent sonography examination demonstrated a mass in the liver compatible with an adenoma. Complex fluid was seen in the right flank compatible with rupture of the adenoma (*arrow*).

hemorrhages, the sonographic appearance varies with the age and extent of bleeding from anechoic to hyperechoic (Fig. 7-33C). CEUS study can help to differentiate an HCA from other types of masses.

Table 7-9 summarizes the key features of these three benign liver neoplasms.

Lipoma

Intrahepatic lipomas are very rare and do not undergo malignant transformation.[39] Affected individuals are typically asymptomatic.[55] These masses may also be detected in children. The sonographic presentation of a lipoma is that of a highly echogenic lesion, which may be hard to distinguish from a hemangioma. Lipomas cause speed error artifacts because the speed of sound through fat is slower than that through normal liver tissue, causing the echoes distal to the mass to be displaced slightly deeper in the body, also causing a break in the solid line of the diaphragm.[39] A hemangioma does not cause a speed of sound artifact. CT can confirm the fatty nature of these lesions.

MALIGNANT NEOPLASMS

Primary Malignant Tumors

The most common malignant tumor of the liver is the hepatic cellular carcinoma, HCC, accounting for almost 90% of primary liver tumors. The second most common primary is the cholangiocarcinoma, which develops in the bile ducts, and will be discussed in detail in Chapter 8.

HEPATOCELLULAR CARCINOMA

HCC, also known as a hepatoma, is a cancer that starts in the hepatocytes. Liver cancer is more common in countries in sub-Saharan Africa and Southeast Asia than it is in the United States and is the fourth most common cancer worldwide,[57] accounting for more than 700,000 deaths each year.[35] HCC is more common in men than in women, with about a 3:1 ratio. In the United States, liver cancer is the most rapidly increasing cancer in both men and women. The American Cancer Society predicts that there will be over 42,000 new cases in 2021 with over 30,000 people dying from liver cancer.[58–60]

The major risk factors for developing an HCC include hepatitis, HBV or HCV, heavy alcohol consumption, aflatoxin ingestion, and NAFLD caused by obesity and insulin resistance.[35] The HCC incidence rate is found to increase in patients with NAFLD and nonalcoholic steatohepatitis (NASH). Patients with cirrhosis owing to HCV and heavy alcohol consumption are at a significantly higher risk of HCC than those with cirrhosis owing to alcohol consumption alone. Aflatoxin is a well-established hepatic carcinogen and is a fungus produced by molds of the *Aspergillus* species, which can contaminate corn, wheat, soybeans, groundnuts, tree nuts, and rice. Storing these foods in a moist, warm environment can lead to the growth of this fungus. The regions of the world with the highest levels of aflatoxin exposure are in sub-Saharan Africa, Southeast Asia, and China. In the United States, the majority of HCCs have been found to develop in patients with cirrhosis.[10,53,55] People

with hereditary hemochromatosis have a condition where the body takes up and stores more iron than it needs. As the iron builds up in the liver, it can lead to cirrhosis and eventually liver cancer.[33] Developing an HCC is unusual before the age of 40 and is more common in the sixth decade of life and beyond.[35] The 5-year survival rate is 3% to 34% depending on the stage of the cancer, according to the latest information from the American Cancer Society's website at the time of publication.[60]

HCC can be focal and limited to one area, multiple and occurring in numerous areas, or diffuse and infiltrating throughout the liver.[35,55] Physiologically, HCC interferes with normal hepatocyte function, causing biliary obstruction, jaundice, portal hypertension, ascites, portal vein thrombosis, and different metabolic disturbances. HCC commonly metastases to the lungs, portal vein, intra-abdominal lymph nodes, bone. and the mesentery and/or the omentum.[39]

Clinical symptoms of HCC include weight loss, nausea and vomiting, RUQ pain, pruritus, splenomegaly, a palpable mass, hepatomegaly, jaundice, and ascites. LFTs demonstrate increased levels of ALP, AST, and ALT. The most significant lab value is that of AFP, which will be elevated in about 70% of patients.[39] AFP is typically not detectable in a healthy person. The diagnosis of HCC is based on the patient's medical history, clinical symptoms, increased levels of AFP, imaging studies, and a biopsy of the mass. CEUS can help to make the diagnosis, possibly alleviating the need for a biopsy.

Sonographically, an HCC has a variety of appearances (Fig. 7-34A, B). In the cirrhotic liver, the masses are usually hypoechoic because the liver tissue is now very echogenic (Fig. 7-34C). A typical appearance of an HCC is a large dominant mass with smaller scattered satellite lesions. Masses may be hypoechoic or hyperechoic, homogeneous or heterogeneous, localized or diffuse. Color Doppler images will show chaotic internal vasculature (Fig. 7-34D). Cystic areas and calcifications inside the mass are uncommon. HCC tends to invade the portal vein in up to 60% of patients and the hepatic veins in 15% of patients. Tumor thrombus tends to dilate the vein more than bland thrombus and spectral Doppler images will show arterial signals inside the vein, which represents the arterial supply to the tumor (Fig. 7-34E).[49]

Sonography has the ability to localize and measure any mass and characterize the presentation of HCC, for example, when there are multiple masses or a diffuse presentation. Treatment and surgical resectability depend on the location of the masses and the extent of the liver affected, the presence of vascular invasion, and the degree of metastatic spread. Detected tumors should be classified as focal, multiple, or diffuse, and an effort should be made to define their location based on liver segments. Attention should be paid to displacement or tumor invasion of intrahepatic vessels, the IVC, and the extrahepatic portal venous system. Tumors can compress bile ducts, causing localized biliary dilatation. If HCC is discovered incidentally, the remainder of the abdomen should be scanned to evaluate and document any ascites or regional lymphadenopathy.

Treatment options for HCC include hepatic resection,[61] transarterial embolization or chemoembolization,[57,62] percutaneous ethanol injection,[57,62] radiofrequency ablation,[62] cryoablation,[62] chemotherapy, and targeted drug therapy.

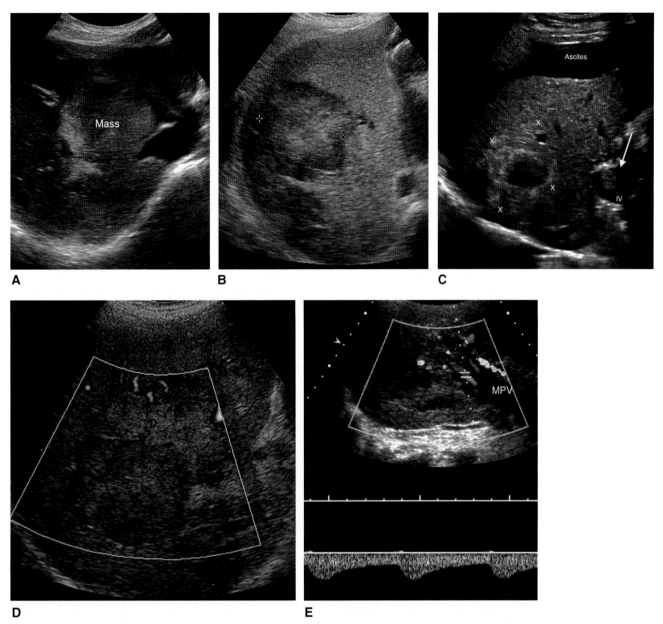

FIGURE 7-34 Hepatocellular carcinoma. **A:** A 61-year-old male presented with abnormal liver function tests (*LFTs*). The sonography examination found a hyperechoic mass that was later biopsied and an HCC was confirmed. This patient had a normal alpha-fetoprotein (*AFP*). **B:** This 62-year-old woman presented with abnormal LFTs. A hypoechoic mass (between the calipers) was seen by ultrasound. She then had her AFP drawn and it returned elevated. An ultrasound-guided biopsy confirmed that this was an HCC. **C:** This 48-year-old man with a history of alcohol abuse and cirrhosis was sent for a sonography examination to screen for HCC. A 6-cm heterogeneous mass (*calipers*) was seen in the right posterior lobe of the liver with another mass (*arrow*) pressing into the inferior vena cava (*IVC*) giving the appearance of a nonobstructive thrombus. His AFP was elevated. An ultrasound-guided biopsy confirmed that this was an HCC. **D:** The color box outlines a large infiltrative HCC. Power Doppler image shows small tortuous vessels inside the mass. **E:** Thrombus was noticed in the main portal vein on a patient with a biopsy-proven HCC. Color Doppler tracing showed flow and a spectral Doppler tracing demonstrated an arterial waveform inside the main portal vein (*MPV*). These findings are compatible with tumor thrombus from the HCC.

Ablation techniques are more successful on masses less than 3 cm in size. Embolization techniques block the branch of the hepatic artery feeding the tumor, which helps to kill off the cancer cells because their blood supply is solely from the hepatic artery. The healthy liver cells remain unharmed because they can get their blood supply from the portal vein. Embolization can be used on tumors larger than 5 cm in size. Liver transplant is an option, but unfortunately, donors are scarce and there is the possibility of tumor recurrence. Ultrasound can be used as a guidance technique for the

initial biopsy diagnosis and later for percutaneous treatments of HCC such as cryoablation and radiofrequency ablation.

Metastases

The liver is the second most common site of metastatic spread after lymph nodes. Metastatic liver disease is 18 to 20 times more common than a primary HCC.[10] Having metastatic disease will change the patient's prognosis and management. The majority of patients with metastatic disease will have multiple masses that will frequently involve both lobes. Almost any cancer can spread to the liver. The most common metastases come from colorectal cancers, followed by the pancreas and the breast. Other sites include the gallbladder, stomach, kidney, ovaries, and lung.[10] Cancer cells will break away from the primary cancer and travel through the bloodstream until they deposit in some tissue elsewhere in the body. The liver is very vulnerable to metastatic disease because of the large volume of blood it receives from both the hepatic artery and the portal vein. The portal vein will bring cancer cells from the colon and rectum whereas the hepatic artery will bring cancer cells from the rest of the body such as the breast, kidneys, and lung. Lymphatic spread of cancer can be from such sources as the pancreas and the ovary. Cancer of the gallbladder will spread to the liver by direct invasion.

Symptoms of liver metastatic disease may include hepatomegaly, jaundice, weight loss, abdominal swelling or bloating, and RUQ or abdominal pain; sometimes, the patient may even be asymptomatic. LFT values can be normal, although AST and ALT may be elevated, and ALP and bilirubin may be elevated if there is biliary obstruction. AFP is typically not elevated in liver metastatic disease. Multiple metastases give rise to multiple masses in the liver, suggesting that tumor seeding has occurred in episodes.[50] Hepatectomy is the recommended treatment option for patients with resectable liver metastasis. Intraoperative ultrasound can be used to verify the extent of the metastatic disease and to help plan the surgery. Unfortunately, at the time of surgery, the intraoperative ultrasound may show that the metastatic disease is more spread than what pre-op imaging showed, and the surgery may be canceled. It is hoped that CEUS may help identify these situations before surgery.

Sonographically, metastases have a wide variety of appearances, including hypoechoic, hyperechoic, isoechoic, anechoic, mixed areas of both hyperechoic and hypoechoic, as well as bull's eye or target appearance or diffuse (Fig. 7-35A–D).[10,50] Sonography examinations lack specificity for correlating the sonographic appearance of hepatic metastases to the primary cancer.[10,38] The literature reports that there may be some correlation between the ultrasound appearance of the metastatic lesion and its primary tumor. Hyperechoic masses are associated with a GI primary,[54] renal cell carcinomas,[10] neuroendocrine tumors, and choriocarcinoma. Hypoechoic masses can be seen with lymphoma[50] and breast, lung and pancreatic cancers. The target-like or "bull's eye" lesions are masses with an echogenic center surrounded by a hypoechoic ring and can be seen with lung cancer.[10] Some patients may display multiple patterns. Because there are typically more lesions in the liver than what is seen with ultrasound, using CEUS will help to define the extent of the disease because it will show lesions not appreciated on grayscale images.

Too often, the sonographer will be the one to discover that the patient has an unexpected cancer with the discovery of metastatic liver disease. When this happens, the sonographer should try to locate the primary tumor by including images of the pancreas, evaluating for upper abdominal lymph adenopathy, and including images of the pelvis in a female patient looking for large pelvic masses.

CONTRAST-ENHANCED ULTRASOUND

CEUS has proven useful in the evaluation of focal liver lesions. On April 1, 2016, the U.S. Food and Drug Administration (FDA) approved the use of Lumason (sulfur hexafluoride with a phospholipid shell) in both adult and pediatric liver applications. The kit contains everything needed to perform two injections (Fig. 7-36A). Lumason, internationally known as SonoVue, was first introduced in 2001.[63] Similar to contrast-enhanced CT or MRI, CEUS allows for an evaluation of lesions based on their vascular enhancement and flow characteristics.[55,64]

Grayscale sonography of liver lesions has limitations because lesions may be difficult to see in the setting of a fatty or cirrhotic liver and the sonographic appearances of many benign and malignant lesions overlap. Some lesions are isoechoic and cannot be appreciated on the grayscale image.[64,65] Studies have shown that without contrast, sonography is able to correctly characterize focal liver lesions 60% to 65% of the time but with contrast, the lesions are correctly characterized 86% to 95% of the time.[65] Conventional grayscale sonography was able to differentiate between benign and malignant lesions only 23% to 68% of the time, whereas CEUS was able to correctly make the distinction in 92% to 95% of patients.[65] CEUS is used to evaluate the vascularity and enhancement patterns of lesions found on grayscale sonography. Benign and malignant liver lesions each have different enhancement patterns on CEUS, frequently allowing for a more definitive diagnosis without further testing. Most masses have characteristic enhancing and flow patterns that can help distinguish between the different types of benign and malignant tumors, although there are some masses that remain undeterminable and will require a biopsy to determine their cell type.

Ultrasound contrast agents are microbubbles of gas stabilized by a lipid or protein shell. These shells are flexible, allowing the microbubbles to change size and shape easily as needed. The type of gas and the shell used will vary between the manufacturers of the different ultrasound contrast agents.[63,66,67] At the time of publication, there was only one FDA-cleared ultrasound contrast agent for liver ultrasound; however, there are other agents being used in cardiology as well as in other countries of the world. Each 1 mL of contrast contains 100 to 500 million microbubbles of gas that are smaller than red blood cells with a mean diameter of 1.5 to 2.5 μm.[63,66,68] These microbubbles can move within the capillaries and are large enough that they stay in the vascular system, making ultrasound contrast a true intravascular agent, unlike CT and MRI contrast agents that extravasate into the interstitial tissues. The gas of the microbubble is exhaled through the lungs and all microbubbles should clear the patient in 6 to 10 minutes. The body metabolizes the components of the shell.[66,67] CEUS has other advantages over contrast-enhanced CT or MRI, including real-time assessment of vascularity at higher frame rates, no exposure to ionizing radiation, portability of performance, and serial examination of patients without radiation or doses of contrast agents that may be nephrotoxic. Because ultrasound contrast is not nephrotoxic, it is not necessary to perform laboratory tests to assess renal function before administering the contrast agent. Another advantage is the narrow ultrasound beam that allows for

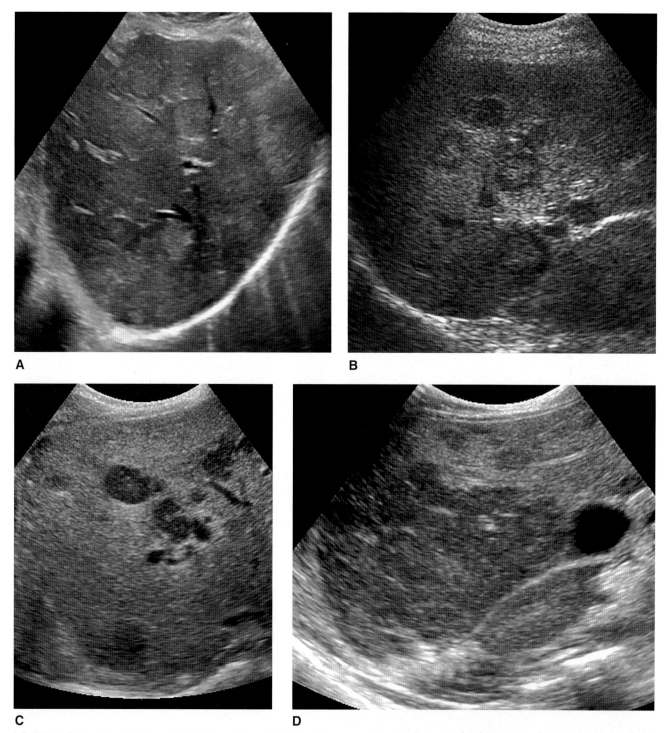

FIGURE 7-35 Hepatic metastasis. **A:** Multiple hyperechoic metastatic liver lesions are seen in this patient with a pancreatic primary. This 58-year-old man was referred to sonography for right upper quadrant (*RUQ*) pain. The diagnosis of pancreatic head cancer with liver metastases was unexpected. **B:** This patient also had unexpected finding of liver metastases. This sonogram shows the "bull's eye" lesions, an echogenic center with a hypoechoic rim. This patient had a primary lung cancer. **C:** Hypoechoic lesions are seen in this patient with lymphoma. **D:** This patient was jaundiced and was referred for a biliary ultrasound. The sonography examination showed unexpected findings of infiltrative liver metastases. This patient was discovered to have a left renal cell carcinoma.

improved visualization of vascularity in small structures such as septations or mural nodules in a cystic mass. CEUS can be used on patients who are allergic to CT and MRI contrast agents or have renal failure. It may be necessary to explain the difference between the contrast agents used in CT, MRI, and US because patients have been told that they cannot have contrast and will refuse the study. A potential advantage of CEUS is performing the study at the same time as the initial discovery of the liver lesion on the routine ultrasound. This will lead to great patient satisfaction and also help reduce health care costs because, potentially, an MRI or CT will not be needed. CEUS can also be used to assist with liver mass biopsies, especially with isoechoic lesions because the biopsy can be performed with contrast.[69,70]

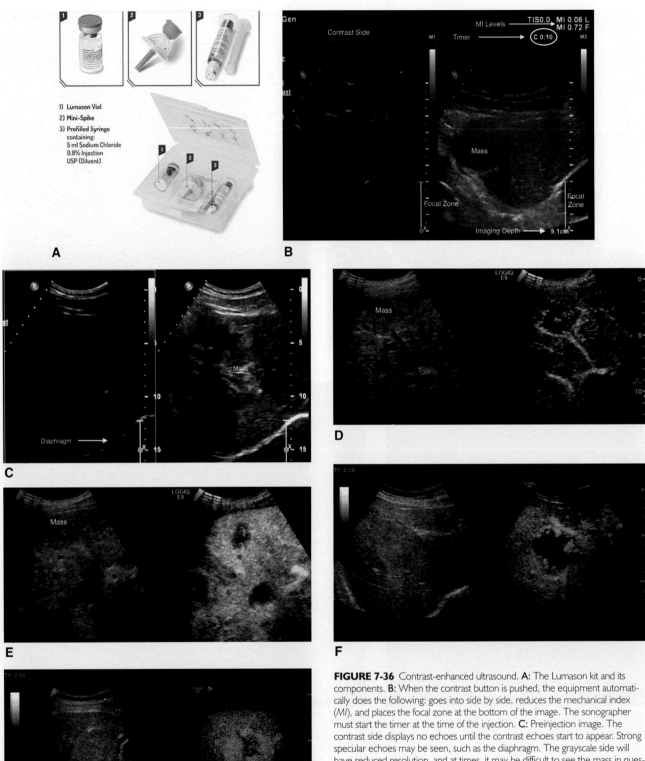

1) Lumason Vial
2) Mini-Spike
3) Prefilled Syringe
   containing:
   5 ml Sodium Chloride
   0.9% Injection
   USP (Diluent)

FIGURE 7-36 Contrast-enhanced ultrasound. **A:** The Lumason kit and its components. **B:** When the contrast button is pushed, the equipment automatically does the following: goes into side by side, reduces the mechanical index (*MI*), and places the focal zone at the bottom of the image. The sonographer must start the timer at the time of the injection. **C:** Preinjection image. The contrast side displays no echoes until the contrast echoes start to appear. Strong specular echoes may be seen, such as the diaphragm. The grayscale side will have reduced resolution, and at times, it may be difficult to see the mass in question. **D:** The contrast first starts to arrive in the liver from the hepatic artery. The brightest echoes represent arterial flow. Notice the feeding vessel that divides into branches around the mass. This is called the basket sign and is typical for *HCC*. **E:** Same patient as in D showing the portal venous phase. Now the *HCC* is only slightly brighter than the liver parenchyma. **F:** On a patient with an atypical hemangioma, a contrast-enhanced ultrasound (*CEUS*) demonstrates the typical appearance of peripheral nodular enhancement in the arterial phase. **G:** Same patient as in F demonstrating continued enhancement in the late phase.

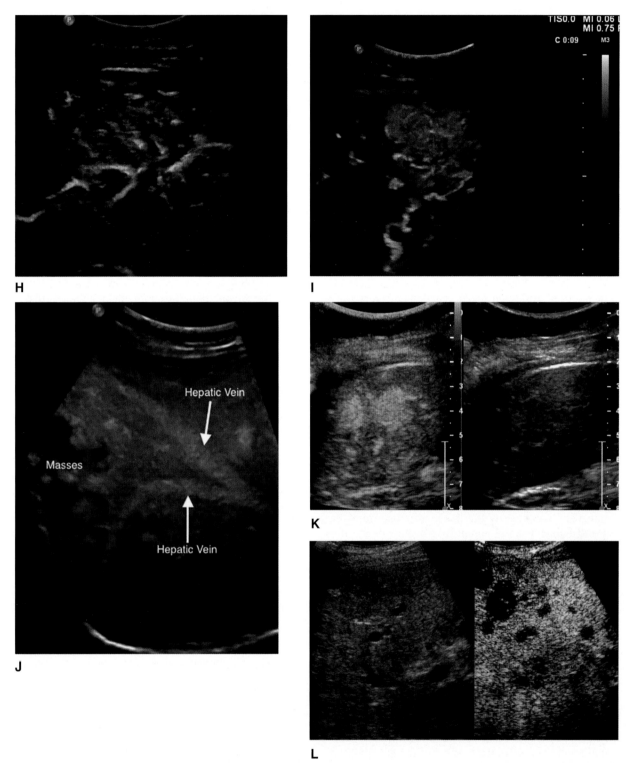

FIGURE 7-36 (*continued*) H: This *CEUS* of a patient with focal nodular hyperplasia (*FNH*) demonstrates the typical spoke-wheel vascular pattern. On real time, the characteristic rapid fill-in from the center outward was seen. I: This *HCC* demonstrates hyperenhancing 9 seconds after injection. A feeding artery is also seen. J: The portal venous phase in this patient with liver mets shows the lesions as hypoenhancing. Notice how the contrast outlines the hepatic veins. K: In the arterial phase on this patient with liver metastases, the lesions are seen as hyperenhancing. L: Lesions of a patient with liver metastases are hypoenhancing during the portal venous phase. (Image **A**: Courtesy of Bracco Imaging. Images **F** and **G**: Courtesy of GE Healthcare, Wauwatosa, WI. Images **I** and **J**: Courtesy of Philips Ultrasound, Bothell, Washington.)

An IV needs to be placed and the requirements for who can place an IV vary by state and institutions. Training may be needed just to have the legal rights to inject the contrast agent and remove the IV. Two people are required to perform the study because one person, the sonographer, needs to scan, whereas the other person, usually the radiologist, needs to perform the injection. A typical CEUS study requires at least 3 minutes of continuous documentation, leading to large video clips. Some PACSs may have a size limit on clips that can be stored or retrieved for viewing on the PACS workstation monitor. The sonographer should talk to the PACS administrator to warn them of these large clips and if there will be any issues storing or retrieving the clips. Current PACSs usually do not have storage and retrieving issues.

Adverse events to the contrast material are mild and transient, with the most common being headache and nausea. These typically resolve spontaneously. These reactions typically occur within the first 30 minutes after injection and the patient is kept in the area for 30 minutes, which includes the imaging time. Although severe reactions are very rare, it is recommended to have cardiopulmonary resuscitation equipment available. A large study from Europe with approximately 24,000 examinations had a serious adverse event rate of 0.0086%, which is lower than MRI and CT contrast reactions.[65,69] The requirements for requiring informed consent from the patient will vary among hospitals and clinics. For consistency, most ultrasound departments will follow the policy used for administering CT and MRI contrast.[66]

Normal scanning transducers are used to perform CEUS; however, the ultrasound unit must have contrast software installed. The contrast mode will cancel the linear US signals returned from the tissue and process and display the nonlinear responses from the microbubbles to form the contrast image. This allows for a vascular-only image to be obtained by suppressing the linear response from the tissues and enhancing the nonlinear response of the microbubbles. Manufacturers develop proprietary techniques for how they process and produce the contrast information. The contrast images are obtained at a low–acoustic output setting determined by the mechanical index (MI). A low MI is needed for continuous real-time imaging because it minimizes microbubble destruction and will allow dynamic evaluation of the three vascular phases, which are needed to classify the type of liver tumor. These vascular phases will be discussed later in the section. The focal zone will also be placed at the bottom of the image to help preserve the microbubbles because the acoustic pressure is highest in the focal zone. The contrast software will reduce the MI and place the focal zone at the bottom automatically (Fig. 7-36B). Once the lesion has been identified by conventional imaging, the contrast aspect of the examination can begin. The sonographer should image the lesion in the best imaging plane. The main requirement is to see normal liver parenchyma surrounding the mass. Lesions deeper than 8 cm may be difficult to assess, and the patient should be positioned to try to get the lesion closer to the transducer. The imaging plane does not matter and can be a sagittal, transverse, or even an oblique imaging plane. The contrast-specific setting will create a side-by-side image with one side for the contrast image and the other side for the grayscale image. The sonographer should not be alarmed with the contrast side of the screen because it will be black until

the contrast starts to appear and the contrast images are formed, although strong reflectors, such as the diaphragm, may remain barely visible. The grayscale side of the image may also appear degraded and not look like the precontrast images (Fig. 7-36C). As long as the lesion can be identified, the image is acceptable because the diagnosis is not made by using the grayscale image but by the contrast images. Most units will have the ability to adjust controls separately for each side. The sonographer will hold the transducer steady in one position for at least the first 3 minutes so that all phases can be accurately assessed. The arterial phase is an important aspect of a CEUS study, and good visualization of the lesion is needed during this phase. Usually, normal or quiet breathing will allow good visualization of the mass and the patient should be instructed to not take deep breaths during the examination. If the radiologist wants to see the arterial phase again, the sonographer can temporarily increase the MI by either turning on color Doppler or hitting the button that will quickly increase the MI. This is to destroy the microbubbles in the field of view at that time. Some units call this control "flash" because it generates a sound beam at a high MI and gives the appearance of a bright flash that flashes quickly on and off. Also unique to the contrast setting is a timer control. The timer should be started at the time of the injection and is displayed on the image. This is used for timing of the phases.[63,66,67] After the initial acquisition, the sonographer may scan other areas of the liver as needed, until no more contrast is seen. If there is a question on the first injection or if other lesions need to be evaluated, a second dose can be administered. Current recommendations are to limit contrast administration to a two-injection limit during a single examination. Usually, each vial contains enough contrast to allow for two injections. Prior to the injecting the second dose, there should be no contrast on the image. This is accomplished by increasing the MI temporarily to help destroy any remaining microbubble either by using color Doppler imaging for about 30 seconds or repeatedly hitting the flash button until no more contrast is seen on the image.

Because of the dual blood supply of the liver from the hepatic artery and the portal vein, there are three overlapping vascular phases in a CEUS study. Observing the patterns of the arterial, portal venous, and late phases will help to determine the nature of the liver lesion. The arterial phase provides the degree and pattern of the arterial vascular supply to the lesion (Fig. 7-36D). The appearance of a lesion in the liver should be described in terms of the degree and timing of enhancement. The degree of enhancement refers to the intensity of the signal relative to that of the adjacent normal parenchyma. It should be described as isoenhancing when it is equal to, hyperenhancing when it is greater than, and hypoenhancing when it is less than the normal liver parenchyma. The term sustained enhancement refers to the continuing enhancement of the lesion over time. A complete absence of enhancement is described as nonenhancing. The enhancement pattern should be described for each phase. The wash-in phase refers to the period of progressive enhancement from the arrival of the microbubbles to peak enhancement. The washout phase refers to the reduction in enhancement following the peak enhancement. For the liver, these phases are as follows: (1) The arterial phase begins about 10 to 20 seconds following injection and ends in 30 to 45 seconds. (2) The portal venous phase begins approximately 30 to 45 seconds after injection and ends in approximately 120 seconds (Fig. 7-36E). (3) The late phase starts approximately 120 seconds after injection and ends with microbubble disappearance in approximately 4 to 6 minutes.[63,66,68]

Benign Lesions

The typical CEUS features of a hemangioma include a peripheral nodular enhancement in the arterial phase that progresses in a centripetal direction with partial or complete fill-in of the lesion (Fig. 7-36F). In the late phase, the lesion remains hyperenhancing (Fig. 7-36G).[63,66,68,70]

An FNH appears as a hyperenhancing homogenous lesion in all phases. Hyperenhancement is usually marked in the arterial phase with a rapid fill-in from the center outward, centrifugal filling, toward the periphery. The presence of stellate vessels and a tortuous feeding artery are characteristics of an FNH (Fig. 7-36H). During the portal venous and late phases, it will remain hyperenhancing or may become isoenhancing. The centrally located scar may be seen as an unenhanced scar in both the arterial and portal phases.[66,71,72]

With CEUS, a liver adenoma will exhibit arterial hyperenhancement initially at the periphery with subsequent rapid centripetal filling. This is the opposite direction as seen with an FNH. There will be no washout or a weak washout in the portal venous phase.[66,71,72] This arterial enhancement pattern can also be seen in HCC and hyperenhancing metastases.

Malignant Lesions

HCC is the most common primary malignant mass of the liver and occurs in patients with a history of chronic liver disease. Ultrasound is often used as a screening modality; unfortunately, the ultrasound appearance of HCC is nonspecific, requiring further evaluation. In the past, this meant that the patient either had a biopsy or a CT or MRI with contrast, but with the advent of CEUS, these lesions can be further evaluated using ultrasound. An HCC will show hyperenhancement in the arterial phase and dysmorphic vessels and may have areas of unenhanced regions representing necrosis (Fig. 7-36I). A pattern of disorganized centripetal vessels, called a basket weave pattern, has been described with an HCC and is considered a specific characteristic of an HCC. In the portal venous and late phases, an HCC usually shows washout with hypoenhancement.[66,71,73]

Liver metastases can be characterized reliably as hypoenhancing lesions during the portal venous and late phases (Fig. 7-36J). In metastatic disease, the arterial phase is variable, and the lesions may show transient hyperenhancing (Fig. 7-36K) or will show contrast enhancement that is often chaotic with possible rim enhancement. This is followed by a rapid washout, which often begins within the arterial phase. In the portal venous phase, metastases will show washout that tends to be complete and rapid. Metastases will appear as black spots or holes against the background of the uniformly enhanced normal liver. These areas have been described as black punched-out areas (Fig. 7-36L). It is not surprising to see many more lesions with CEUS than what is seen on the normal grayscale image.[66,71–73] Hypoenhancement of lesions in the late phase characterizes malignancies, and almost all metastases show this feature regardless of their enhancement pattern in the arterial phase. Washout in the portal venous phase or the late phase is the most important feature distinguishing malignant lesions from benign lesions (Table 7-10).[62,65,70–72]

The reader is encouraged to read about the limitations of CEUS; how cirrhosis can affect the portal venous phase; and the CEUS appearance of nonmasses such as abscesses, hematomas and cysts.[62,69] The reader should keep current of new techniques, diagnostic criteria, and the different uses of CEUS outside the liver.

THE LIVER IMAGING REPORTING AND DATA SYSTEM

In 2014, the ACR created a work group to develop an algorithm to be used on the liver to grade liver masses called LI-RADS, the Liver Imaging Reporting and Data System, much like BI-RADS for the breast and TI-RADS for the

TABLE 7-10 CEUS Findings in Vascular Phases of Liver Masses[62,65,70–72]

Lesion	Arterial Phase	Portal Venous Phase	Late Phase
Hemangioma	Peripheral nodular enhancement; centripetal progression of enhancement	Complete or partial fill-in	Incomplete or complete enhancement; nonenhancing regions
FNH	Hyperenhancing spoke-wheel pattern of enhancement with inside-to-outside or centrifugal filling pattern; feeding artery	Hyperenhancing	Sustained enhancement; iso-hyperenhancing
		Nonenhancing central scar	Nonenhancing central scar
Adenoma	Diffuse or centripetal hypervascular enhancement; dysmorphic arteries	Isoenhancing, hyperenhancing, nonenhancing region	Sustained enhancement; isoenhancing; slightly hypoenhancing; nonenhancing regions
Metastasis	Rim enhancement; complete enhancement; diffuse hyperenhancement; nonenhancing regions	Fast washout	Washout
HCC	Hyperenhancing dysmorphic vessels	Iso to nonenhancing	Mild, delayed washout

CEUS, contrast-enhanced ultrasound; FNH, focal nodular hyperplasia; HCC, hepatocellular carcinoma.

thyroid. In June 2016, the algorithm was published. It is a classification system for liver masses to be used on patients with liver cirrhosis or chronic HBV without cirrhosis because these patients are at an increased risk to develop an HCC. In 2017, the ACR released an US LI-RADS to provide standardized terminology, technical recommendations, and a reporting framework for US examinations on patients at risk for developing HCC. The appropriate patient population for screening and surveillance are patients who are at risk for developing HCC but do not have a known mass. There are currently two LI-RADS for ultrasound. The first is for ultrasound, US LI-RADS, and the second is for CEUS, CEUS LI-RADS. The US LI-RADS is used to score liver masses in patients with cirrhosis or HBV to help determine the probability of any mass seen to be an HCC. The CEUS LI-RADS chart helps to determine if the mass is an HCC based on its ultrasound features and ultrasound contrast characteristics. There is also a CT/MRI LI-RADS. The reader is encouraged to visit the ACR website at www.acr.org to keep updated on changes to the LI-RADS recommendations and charts.

ELASTOGRAPHY

Elastography is a technique that uses ultrasound to assess the stiffness of the liver parenchyma and allows for a non-invasive assessment of diffuse liver fibrosis. Because the speed of sound will be faster through stiffer material, and because the liver tissue gets stiffer from the fibrosis, the speed of the sound beam will increase and be faster than that in normal liver tissue. The speed of the sound beam will correlate with the degree of liver fibrosis.

Chronic liver disease leads to the deposition of fibrous tissue within the liver. Liver fibrosis is an abnormal increase in collagen deposition and other components of the extracellular matrix in response to a chronic injury. As fibrosis progresses, there is increasing loss of liver function, increasing portal hypertension, and an increased risk for developing an HCC. Cirrhosis is a diffuse process that is characterized by fibrosis and the conversion of normal liver architecture into abnormal nodules. Staging of liver fibrosis is important to help determine prognosis and as a surveillance tool to evaluate for the progression or the regression of the disease. For patients with severe fibrosis or liver cirrhosis who are asymptomatic, the term "compensated advanced chronic liver disease" (cACLD) has been proposed.[76] For the clinician, the most important question in a patient with chronic liver disease is whether or not they have cirrhosis. Until the development of elastography, the only method for staging the degree of fibrosis was with a liver biopsy. However, a liver biopsy is invasive and has potential complications that can be severe in up to 1% of patients. The tissue obtained from a liver biopsy is prone to sampling errors, and there is also considerable interobserver variability with interpretation. One of the more common methods for staging liver fibrosis is using the METAVIR (Meta-analysis of Histological Data in Viral Hepatitis) scoring system, which is used to assess inflammation and fibrosis by the histopathologic evaluation of a liver biopsy. Although it was developed primarily to stage viral hepatitis, it has been adapted for other liver diseases. The stage of fibrosis is determined by evaluating the location and the degree of portal and peri-portal fibrosis, bridging fibrosis, which is fibrosis acting like

TABLE 7-11 **Staging of Fibrosis**[73,75]
• F0—No fibrosis
• F1—Portal fibrosis without septa
• F2—Portal fibrosis with few septa
• F3—Numerous septa without cirrhosis
• F4—Cirrhosis

a bridge between adjacent central veins, and the degree of nodularity. The fibrosis is graded on a 5-point scale from 0 to 4 and the stage represents the amount of fibrosis of the liver (Table 7-11).[73–75]

Diagnostic Criteria

The Society of Radiologists in Ultrasound (SRU) guidelines no longer recommends using METAVIR cutoff values and now recommends a low cutoff value below which there is a high probability of no or mild fibrosis and a high cutoff value above which there is a high probability of cACLD because these patients are at a risk for developing complications such as ascites, variceal hemorrhage, portal hypertension, and HCC.[76] Notice that the chart says recommendation as opposed to diagnosis. The SRU recommends that the report include the system vendor name, the technique used, shear wave elastography (pSWE) or 2D shear wave elastography (SWE), the probe used, the number of valid acquisitions, and the value of IQR/M.[76] Table 7-12 provides the liver stiffness values used for staging liver fibrosis at the time of publication.[76] This chart is universal, that is, it can be used for all vendors, unlike past charts that were vendor specific.

Clinical Indications

The main clinical indication for liver elastography is for staging the degree of fibrosis in patients with chronic liver disease. These patients may have chronic viral hepatitis or NAFLD, which is the number one underlying condition that leads to NASH. It should be noted that the stiffness of the liver and therefore the velocity through the liver can be affected by severe inflammation as indicated by ALT and AST with values that are five times higher than normal, biliary obstruction, acute hepatitis, and congestion from right-sided heart failure. These situations will cause the velocity to have falsely elevated values. Determining the presence of cirrhosis is important, because this will trigger the need to monitor the patient or begin treatment. Other indications for liver elastography include following patients with fibrosis, assessment of patients with known cirrhosis, the evaluation of patients with unexplained portal hypertension, and to follow the response to patients receiving therapy treatments that may help to treat their fibrosis.

Elastography Technologies

There are two main technologies for measuring the degree of fibrosis using ultrasound. Only the basic physics of these technologies will be discussed, and the reader is encouraged to read more about these technologies by reading journal articles or attending or watching seminars. Besides measuring liver stiffness, elastography is used on other organs such

TABLE 7-12 **Liver Stiffness Values Obtained with Acoustic Radiation Force Impulse Techniques in Patients with Viral Hepatitis and Nonalcoholic Fatty Liver Disease**[73,75]

Liver Stiffness Value	Recommendation
<1.3 m/sec or 5kPa	High probability of being normal
<1.7 m/sec or 9kPa	In the absence of other known clinical signs, rules out cACLD. If there are known clinical signs, further test may be needed for confirmation.
1.7–2.1 m/sec or 9–13 kPa	Suggestive of cACLD but need further test for confirmation
>2.1 m/sec or 13kPa	Rules in cACLD
>2.4 m/sec or 17kPa	Suggestive of CSPH

cACLD, compensated advanced chronic liver disease; CSPH, clinically significant portal hypertension.

as the breast, thyroid, and prostate. MRI also has a method to perform liver elastography, and the reader is encouraged to learn about this technique because this section will only discuss ultrasound methods. Transient elastography (TE) is a sonography-based technique that does not have any image guidance and has been reported to have accuracy issues with patients who have a body mass index greater than 30 to 35 kg/m^2, even using their XL probe.[75,77] The transducer emits an ultrasound pulse that vibrates the skin with a motor to create a passing distortion in the tissue to create shear waves. The transducer measures the velocity of the shear waves. The shear wave velocity can then be converted into liver stiffness and is expressed in kilopascals (kPa). TE cannot be used on patients with ascites because the fluid prevents propagation of the vibration wave and, therefore, frequently results in failure to obtain readings. The appropriate transducer is selected based on the size of the patient, and because there is no image guidance, the transducer is typically placed in the 9th to 11th intercostal space.[75,77] This is the type of unit that a nonsonography department will use for liver elastography, typically by hepatologists, and the results can only be expressed in kPa. The most common unit is the FibroScan, and patients or clinicians may ask if the department offers the FibroScan. At this point, the sonographer should educate the patient or clinician that the department offers shear wave liver elastography that also allows visualization of the liver to help determine the best location to obtain results, and that both technologies provide the same results.

SWE is imaging based and uses a standard ultrasound transducer on an ultrasound unit that has elastography software installed. Unlike TE, SWE also allows the evaluation of the liver parenchyma, diagnosis of any incidental pathology, and evaluation of any complications from cirrhosis. SWE uses a technique called acoustic radiation force impulse (ARFI) (pronounced arf-e). Remember that the term radiation does not always refer to ionizing radiation. In physics, radiation is the transmission of energy in the form of waves through a medium. With this technique, a push pulse is sent into the tissue that is of high intensity and has a short duration, approximately 0.3 seconds. The disturbance created travels perpendicular to the ARFI pulse through the tissue as a shear wave. The response of the tissue to the radiation force is determined by using conventional B-mode imaging pulses. Then, either the strain modulus is calculated, which

determines the quantitative shear wave velocity, expressed in m/s, or the Young modulus is calculated and expressed in kPa, thus allowing the results to be expressed in either kPa or m/sec. Because the velocity of the shear wave depends on tissue stiffness, stiffer areas have less displacement and softer regions move more. The best location for maximum shear wave generation is 4 to 4.5 cm from the transducer and is the optimal location for obtaining measurements. The ARFI push pulse is attenuated and reaches a point where adequate shear waves are not generated for accurate measurement. On most systems, this occurs between 6 and 8 cm in depth. The ARFI pulse is also attenuated in patients with more subcutaneous tissue.[77] Unlike TE, this technology is not limited by ascites because the ultrasound beam, which generates the shear waves, propagates through fluids. Some investigators suggest that ARFI techniques may be more accurate than TE. Because the FibroScan was initially used and only measured in kPa, many of the early papers use kPa so that comparisons between the two technologies can be made. Some authors have started to switch and have reported their findings in m/sec. There is a formula to convert between m/sec and kPa if needed. The initial approval of point SWE, pSWE, by the FDA only allowed units of m/sec. Currently, the measurements can be expressed in either unit.

SWE currently has two methods, which are pSWE, and 2D SWE. pSWE is analogous to pulsed Doppler because it uses a small sample volume–like box, called the region of interest (ROI), to obtain a single measurement. This method calculates the shear wave speed generated with ARFI within this ROI to provide a quantitative stiffness estimate, which can then be expressed in either m/s or kPa (Fig. 7-37A).[77] Owing to the energy needed to emit the ARFI beam, the transducer needs to "cool down" between measurements. During this time, which only lasts a few seconds, the machine will not allow another pulse to be sent out. Once the warning message goes away, the sonographer can take the next measurement. An average time to obtain the 10 measurements needed for a complete study is about 5 to 10 minutes.

The 2D SWE is analogous to a color Doppler box, where a larger-ROI box is used, and a color map shows areas of normal and increased stiffness (Fig. 7-37B, C). This method calculates the shear wave speed generated over the field of view, and each pixel is color coded based on the estimate of

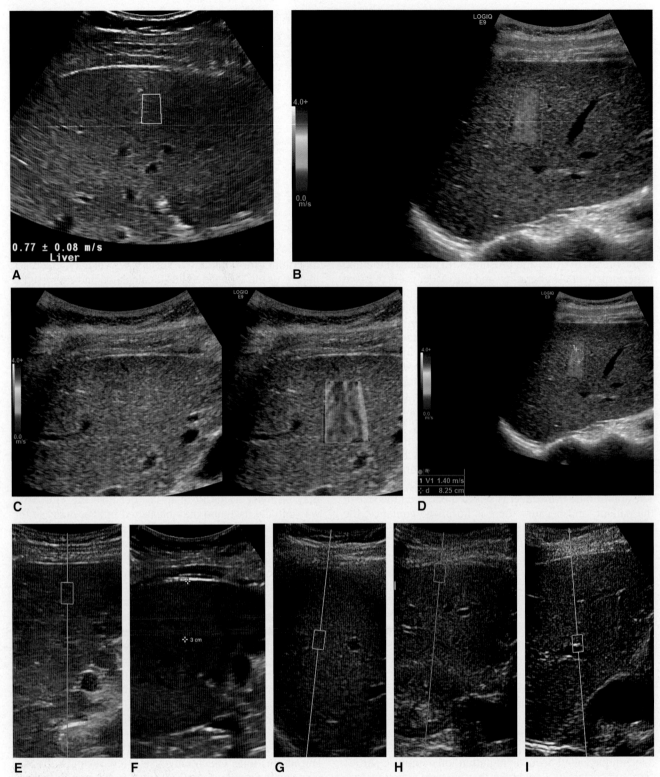

FIGURE 7-37 Elastography. **A:** Point shear wave elastography of a normal liver with proper placement of the *ROI*. **B:** The 2D *SWE* uses a larger box and a color map to show areas of normal or abnormal tissue. This is a normal patient because the only color seen is blue. **C:** This patient has areas of red in the *ROI*, which is compatible with stiff tissue. The *red* and *yellow* areas represent areas of stiff tissue. This patient had a cirrhotic liver. **D:** Same patient as in **B** obtaining a value in m/sec. **E:** The image demonstrates the proper placement of the *ROI* perpendicular to the liver capsule and at about 2.5 cm deep from Glisson capsule. **F:** Because this unit does not display the depth of the *ROI*, the sonographer measured 3 cm down to help with accurate placement of the *ROI* by placing the middle of the *ROI* box at 3 cm. **G:** This image shows an improper placement of the *ROI* because it is too deep and not perpendicular to the liver capsule. **H:** This image shows an improper placement of the *ROI* because it is too close to Glisson capsule and is not perpendicular to the liver capsule. **I:** This *ROI* is too deep and on a vessel.

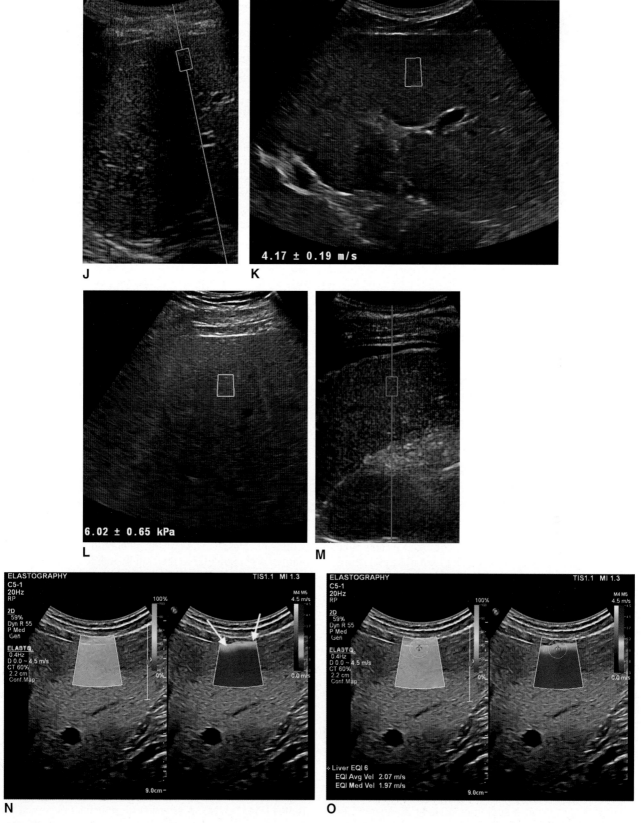

FIGURE 7-37 *(continued)* **J:** This *ROI* is on a rib and is not perpendicular to the liver capsule. **K:** This image is from a patient demonstrating proper *ROI* placement with a value of 4.17 m/sec suggestive of *CSPH*. **L:** This image shows proper *ROI* placement in a patient with the values expressed in kPa and has a measurement of 6.02 kPa. According to the chart: In the absence of other known clinical signs, *cACLD* is ruled out. If known clinical signs are present, the patient may need further test for confirmation. **M:** Proper *ROI* placement in a patient with ascites. **N:** An image of a 2D SWE with the top of the box placed in the reverberation artifact (*arrows*). The left side of the image is the quality map, which warns not to measure at the top of the box. **O:** Same patient as in N being measured in the reverberation artifact. The value is increased to 1.97 m/sec. This is suggestive of *cACLD*, but further testing is needed for confirmation.

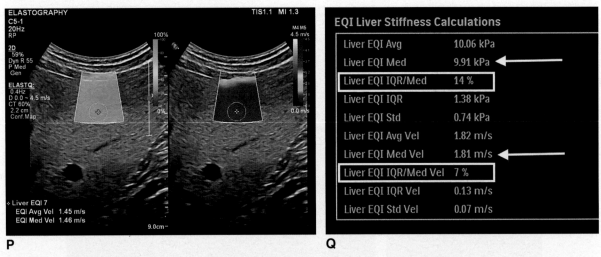

FIGURE 7-37 (continued) **P:** Same patient as in **N** and **O** measuring in the correct place with a measurement of 1.46 m/sec. Based on recommendations, the absence of other known clinical signs would rule out cACLD. **Q:** This is the summary page of the measurements, which contains the median, mean, standard deviation, and IQR values for both kPa and m/sec. The IQR/M ratio is normal at 14% for kPa and 7% for m/sec, indicating that this set of measurements is valid. The square indicates where the IQR/Med is located. EQI is vendor specific. The arrows point to the Med value both of which place this liver in the recommendation of "Suggestive of cACLD but need further test for confirmation." (Image courtesy of Amy Lex.) cACLD, compensated advanced chronic liver disease; CSPH, clinically significant portal hypertension; EQI, ElastQ Imaging (Elastography); EQI/Med, Quality assurance value that eliminates outliers; IQR/Med, interquartile range divided by the median value; Med, median; ROI, region of interest; SWE, shear wave elastography.

its shear wave velocity. A smaller ROI is placed within the field of view to display the mean stiffness estimate, which can then be expressed in either m/s or kPa (Fig. 7-37D).[77] The 2D SWE method can also be used to assess multiple areas of the liver inside the large ROI.

Performing a Liver Elastography Exam

At the time of publication, the following was the suggested protocol to perform a liver elastography examination and patient prep and is based on the 2020 update to the Society of Radiologists in Ultrasound Liver Elastography Consensus Panel from 2015.[76] The reader is encouraged to download this free article and read it; it can be found at https://pubs.rsna.org/doi/full/10.1148/radiol.2020192437 or by just searching for SRU 2020 elastography.

Patient Preparation

The patient should be fasting for 4 to 6 hours because eating will increase the blood flow to the liver, resulting in increasing the stiffness of the liver. Because eating can only cause an increase in liver stiffness, a patient with normal values after recently eating has no or mild fibrosis and there is no reason to reschedule the patient. The fibrotic liver in a nonfasting patient will have falsely increased elastography values, which could place their disease in a higher category. These patients should be rescheduled and reminded to be NPO after midnight.

Patient Position

Patients should be in a supine or a slight 30-degree LPO position with their right arm raised over their head as much as possible to open the rib space for the intercostal approach.

Transducer Position

The transducer is placed in an intercostal position and a location is determined that is free of blood vessels, rib shadow, the diaphragm, liver/kidney interface, the liver capsule, and any ligament. Although fibrosis of the liver is a heterogeneous process, the accuracy of the final value is best when it is made from multiple measurements from the same location.

Region of Interest Placement

The ROI will be placed in segment 7 or 8. The amount of displacement of the liver tissue is optimized when the ARFI pulse is perpendicular to the liver capsule so as to limit the amount of refraction of the pulse. As the box is placed in the liver, it should appear to be perpendicular, like a sample volume in a vessel. The transducer should not be angled but pointed perpendicular to the skin in an intercostal approach only. The top of the ROI box should be placed about 1.5 to 2 cm below Glisson capsule, not from the skin surface, but with the liver capsule parallel to the transducer face as well as the top of the ROI box (Fig. 7-37E). Current units do not measure the distance of the ROI, and the sonographer should measure it using calipers to determine the proper depth (Fig. 7-37F). Unfortunately, sonographers will need to fix that location in their mind because there is no method to mark the spot. The sonographer should ensure that the ROI is not too deep or too shallow and that does not include any vessel, ligament, or artifact (Fig. 73-7G–J). The sonographer should double check that the box is properly placed and that the top of the box is parallel to the liver capsule and transducer. Measurements can be obtained in either m/sec (Fig. 7-37K) or kPa (Fig. 7-37L) depending on the lab. Unlike TE, SWE can be used on patients with ascites (Fig. 7-37M). A reverberation artifact occurs at the liver capsule and the artifact should not be included in any measurements. This artifact is not seen with pSWE but is appreciated with 2D SWE.

The 2D SWE ROI is placed 1.5 to 2 cm from the capsule as long as any reverberation artifact is avoided when measuring. Using pSWE, the artifact is not seen; therefore, it is important to obtain measurements at least 1.5 cm below the liver capsule to avoid including this artifact in the measurement. With 2D SWE, the artifact appears as a stiff tissue right under the upper border of the ROI and should be avoided when obtaining measurements (Fig. 7-37N–P). The measurement ROI, which is usually a small circle, should be positioned 1.5 to 2 cm below the capsule and the measurement obtained where the quality map is green.

Patient Breathing

The measurement is performed on a neutral breath hold and lasts only for a few seconds. Before each measurement, patients should be asked to pause their breathing in a neutral, relaxed state. They should not take a deep breath in or completely exhale but just stop breathing. Taking a deep breath or using a Valsalva maneuver changes hepatic venous pressures, which can affect the stiffness measurements.

Measurements

Currently, using pSWE, it is recommended to obtain 10 measurements from 10 independent images from the same location, that is, to keep the ROI in the same place in the liver and not move it to different locations. Measurements that display as xxx or 000 should not be saved nor used to calculate the final value because these measurements have technical errors and the unit cannot not derive an accurate value. Five measurements may be appropriate for 2D SWE when a quality assessment parameter is used, usually called a quality map. Most systems will now report the interquartile ratio (IQR), which is used to assess the quality of the data. The IQR is a measurement of the statistical dispersion, being equal to the difference between the upper and lower quartiles of data. The recommended quality criteria include the number of acquisitions and the IQR-to-M ratio. The IQR/M should be lesser than 0.3 when values are expressed in kPa and lesser 0.15 for values expressed in m/sec, to prove that it is an accurate data set. If the IQR/M is greater than these values, each of the numbers should be evaluated and any outliers deleted. New measurements are then need to be obtained using the same area in the liver until the proper number of measurements has been achieved. It may appear that there is no consistency with the numbers and that they are "all over the place," which is why the IQR/M is so important (Fig. 7-37Q).

Liver elastography and its role in patient care continue to evolve and the sonographer should keep up to date on the advances in new scanning techniques, which includes comparing elastography measurement from the spleen and kidney to the liver, and new technologies that are currently being investigated such as dispersion.

With the advancements in CEUS and elastography, ultrasound will continue to play a major role in the evaluation of the liver. The sonographer who performs liver sonography needs to understand the anatomy, physiology, and the various diseases that can affect the liver and embrace these new ultrasound technologies and the technologies yet to come to help our patients obtain a diagnosis, hopefully sparing them from having a biopsy or other imaging tests.

SUMMARY

- The liver is an intraperitoneal organ and is the largest internal organ in the body, measuring 13 to 15 cm in a sagittal plane along the RL.
- The liver is divided into the right, left, and CLs and is covered by a connective tissue layer referred to as Glisson capsule.
- Lobular divisions of the liver are described as anatomic, based on external landmarks, such as fissures and ligaments, or segmental, based on hepatic function.
- The liver receives a unique double blood supply with the hepatic artery suppling oxygen-rich blood and the portal vein suppling nutrient-rich blood from the gastrointestinal tract. Both vessels can be seen entering the liver at the porta hepatis.
- The right, middle, and left hepatic veins drain directly into the IVC and are best visualized in a transverse plane with the transducer angled toward the cephalad portion of the liver.
- The liver performs over 500 functions, including bile formation and secretion; the metabolism of carbohydrates, fats, and proteins; production of clotting factors; vitamin storage; acting as a blood reservoir; detoxification of blood; and lymph formation.

- Liver function tests include ALT, which is most specific to hepatocellular disease, AST, ALP, lactic dehydrogenase, bilirubin, GGT, prothrombin time, and albumin.
- Diffuse hepatocellular disease, which affects the liver as a whole and can interfere with normal liver function, includes fatty infiltration, glycogen storage disease, hepatitis, and cirrhosis.
- Fatty infiltration of the liver can range from mild to severe and has many causes, but the most common causes are alcohol abuse and obesity. Sonographic features include a diffuse increase in the hepatic parenchymal echogenicity with a decrease in acoustic penetration.
- Hepatitis is an inflammation of the liver and can be caused by a virus or toxins such as drugs or alcohol. In the acute phase, the liver parenchyma may appear normal or hypoechoic owing to diffuse swelling of the liver cells, whereas the portal vein walls appear more hyperechoic in contrast to the hypoechoic parenchyma. In the chronic phase, the parenchyma may appear hyperechoic, similar to that of fatty infiltration.
- Cirrhosis is a chronic, progressive disease that destroys the normal architecture of the liver lobules and is caused most frequently by alcohol abuse. Other causes include biliary obstruction, metabolic disorders, and hepatitis.

- Sonographic features of cirrhosis vary with the stage of the disease and early on may include hepatomegaly and a diffuse increase in echogenicity. As the disease progresses, sonographic features can include a shrunken RL, hypertrophied CL, surface nodularity, hyperechoic parenchyma, loss of delineation of hepatic vasculature, possible portal hypertension, and ascites.
- Budd–Chiari syndrome is the obstruction of the hepatic venous outflow tract by tumor or thrombus in the hepatic veins.
- Hepatic cysts are more prevalent with increasing age, are usually asymptomatic, are discovered incidentally, and should meet the diagnostic criteria for a simple cyst.
- Polycystic liver disease becomes detectable in the third or fourth decade of life and is an inherited disorder usually associated with autosomal dominant polycystic kidney disease.
- Acquired liver cysts can be categorized as traumatic (hematoma, biloma), parasitic (echinococcal), or inflammatory (abscess) and range in sonographic appearance from cystic to complex masses.
- Candidiasis is a fungal infection spread via the blood in patients with HIV and other immunocompromised conditions that causes hepatomegaly, fatty infiltration, and focal liver masses that may demonstrate a "wheel within a wheel" or "bull's eye" appearance.
- Benign solid neoplasms of the liver include cavernous hemangiomas, FNH, lipomas, and liver cell adenomas.
- HCC is the most common primary malignant liver tumor in the United States, with the most common predisposing factor being cirrhosis.
- HCC or hepatoma interferes with normal hepatocyte function and may present as a focal nodule or multiple nodules or may diffusely infiltrate the liver. LFTs are abnormal and AFP is elevated in 70% of cases.
- Hepatomas range in sonographic appearance from hypoechoic to hyperechoic, portal vein invasion is common, and bile duct compression with subsequent dilatation is possible.
- Because of the large volume of blood the liver receives, metastatic liver tumors are 18 to 20 times more common than primary hepatic malignancies and may arise from many primary cancers, including GI, breast, pancreas, or pulmonary carcinoma.
- Sonographically, liver metastases may appear hypoechoic, hyperechoic, isoechoic, anechoic, complex, or have a bull's eye or target appearance.
- Contrast-enhanced ultrasound is used to characterize focal liver lesions when the grayscale findings are indeterminant.
- Liver elastography can evaluate the stiffness of the liver by measuring the speed of the shear wave produced by the liver. Increased stiffness of the liver will produce a faster sound wave through the liver.
- CT is useful in evaluating trauma and jaundiced patients, demonstrating liver masses, evaluating for metastasis, and displaying the global relationship of abdominal anatomy.
- PET/CT displays both anatomic and functional information and is used to evaluate for distant metastases.[77]
- MRI can characterize liver masses, evaluate for metastases, and evaluate the stiffness of the liver.[78]

REFERENCES

1. England MA. *Color Atlas of Life Before Birth: Normal Fetal Development*. 2nd ed. Elsevier Mosby; 1996.
2. Moore KL, Persaud TVN, Torchia MG. *Before We Are Born: Essentials of Embryology and Birth Defects*. 10th ed. Elsevier; 2020.
3. Moore KL, Persaud TVN, Torchia MG. *The Developing Human: Clinically Oriented Embryology*. 11th ed. Elsevier; 2019.
4. Guyton AC, Hall JE. *Textbook of Medical Physiology*. 14th ed. Saunders; 2020.
5. Tortora GJ, Derrickson B. *Principles of Anatomy and Physiology*. 16th ed. Wiley; 2020.
6. Marieb EN, Hoehn K. *Human Anatomy and Physiology*. 11th ed. Pearson-Benjamin Cummings; 2018.
7. FanPutte CN, Regan JL, Russo AF. *Seeley's Anatomy and Physiology*. 11th ed. McGraw-Hill; 2017.
8. Robinson KA, Middleton WD, AL-Sukaiti R, et al. Doppler sonography of portal hypertension. *Ultrasound Q*. 2009;25:3–13.
9. Netter FH. The CIBA collection of medical illustrations. In: Oppenheimer F, ed. *Digestive System*. 2nd ed. Vol. 3. Part III. CIBA Pharmaceutical; 1972.
10. Wilson SR, Withers CE. The liver. In: Rumack C, Wilson S, Charboneau J, eds. *Diagnostic Ultrasound*. 5th ed. Elsevier Mosby; 2017:74–138.
11. Parulekar SG, Balachandran A. Ultrasound measurements of the liver. In: Goldberg BB, McGahan JP, eds. *Atlas of Ultrasound Measurements*. 2nd ed. Elsevier Health Sciences; 2006:414–418.
12. Kratzer W, Fritz V, Mason R, et al. Factors affecting liver size. *J Ultrasound Med*. 2003;22:1155–1161.
13. Huether SE. Structure and function of the digestive system. In: Huether SE, McCance KL, eds. *Understanding Pathophysiology*. 6th ed. Elsevier; 2017:884–905.
14. Roan E. The effect of Glisson's capsule on the superficial elasticity measurements of the liver. *J Biomech Eng*. 2010;132(10):104504. doi:10.1115/1.4002369
15. Moore KL, Agur AM, Dalley AF. *Essential Clinical Anatomy*. 6th ed. Wolters Kluwer, 2019.
16. Hagen-Ansert S. Liver. In: Hagen-Ansert S, ed. *Textbook of Diagnostic Sonography*. 8th ed. Elsevier; 2017:190–247.
17. Abdel-Misih SRZ, Bloomston M. Liver anatomy. *Surg Clin N Am*. 2010;90:643–653.
18. Abdalla EK, Vauthey JN, Couinaud C. The caudate lobe of the liver: implications of embryology and anatomy for surgery. *Surg Oncol Clin N Am*. 2002;11:835–848.
19. DeJong MR. Liver scanning protocol. In: Tempkin BB, ed. *Sonography Scanning: Principles and Protocols*. 5th ed. Elsevier; 2020:71–100.
20. Cervone A, Sardi A, Conaway GL. Intraoperative ultrasound (IOUS) is essential in the management of metastatic colorectal liver lesions. *Am Surg*. 2000;66:611–615.
21. Swart J, Sheth S. Role of vascular ultrasound in the evaluation of liver disease. *Ultrasound Clin*. 2007;2:355–375.
22. Shin DS, Jeffrey RB, Desser TS. Pearls and pitfalls in hepatic ultrasonography. *Ultrasound Q*. 2010;26:17–25.
23. Ahuja AT, Griffith JF, Wong KT, et al. *Diagnostic Imaging Ultrasound*. Amirsys; 2007.
24. Chong WK, Shah MS. Sonography of right upper quadrant pain. *Ultrasound Clin*. 2008;3:121–138.
25. Ovel S. Liver. In: Ovel S, ed. *Sonography Exam Review*. 2nd ed. Elsevier; 2014:86–104.
26. Drose J. Sonographic abdominal anatomy. In: Sanders RC, Hall-Terracciano, eds. *Clinical Sonography: A Practical Guide*. 5th ed. Wolters Kluwer; 2015:381–393.
27. Li X, Xu X, Gong J. Clinical significance of inferior right hepatic vein. *Am J Med Case Rep*. 2016;4(1):26–30.
28. Makuuchi M, Hasegawa H, Yamazaki S, et al. The inferior right hepatic vein: ultrasonic demonstration. *Radiology*. 1983;148:213–217.
29. Berland LL, Lawson TL, Foley WD. Porta hepatis: sonographic discrimination of bile ducts from arteries with pulsed Doppler with new anatomic criteria. *AJR Am J Roentgenol*. 1982;138:833–840.

30. Drose J. Abnormal liver function tests: jaundice. In: Sanders RC, Hall-Terracciano, eds. *Clinical Sonography: A Practical Guide.* 5th ed. Wolters Kluwer; 2015:436–451.

31. Chernecky CC, Berger BJ. *Laboratory Tests and Diagnostic Procedures.* 6th ed. Elsevier Saunders; 2012.

32. Pagano KD, Pagano TJ. *Mosby's Diagnostic and Laboratory Test Reference.* 14th ed. Elsevier; 2018.

33. Joint Review Committee on Education in Diagnostic Medical Sonography. National Education Curriculum (NEC) for Sonography. 2016. Accessed April 11, 2021. www.jrcdms.org/nec.htm

34. Martin C, Hall-Terracciano B. Right upper quadrant mass: possible metastasis. In: Sanders RC, Hall-Terracciano, eds. *Clinical Sonography: A Practical Guide.* 5th ed. Wolters Kluwer; 2015:408–420.

35. Mann RE, Smart RG, Govoni R. The epidemiology of alcoholic liver disease. National Institute on Alcohol Abuse and Alcoholism. Accessed April 11, 2021. https://pubs.niaaa.nih.gov/publications/arh27-3/209-219.htm

36. Huether SE. Alterations of digestive function. In: Huether SE, McCance KL, eds. *Understanding Pathophysiology.* 7th ed. Elsevier; 2019:879–915.

37. Sables-Baus S. Fidanza SJ. Alterations of digestive function in children. In: Huether SE, McCance KL, eds. *Understanding Pathophysiology.* 7th ed. Elsevier; 2019:916–931.

38. Ramesh S, Sanyal AJ. Evaluation and management of non-alcoholic steatohepatitis. *J Hepatol.* 2005;42(suppl 1):S2–S12.

39. Li D, Hann LE. A practical approach to analyzing focal lesions in the liver. *Ultrasound Q.* 2005;21:187–200.

40. Dahnert W. *Radiology Review Manual.* 8th ed. Wolters Kluwer/Lippincott Williams & Wilkins; 2017.

41. Pozzato C, Botta A, Melgara C, et al. Sonographic findings in type I Glycogen Storage Disease. *J Clin Ultrasound.* 2001:29(8);456–461.

42. Cazier PR, Sponaugle DW. "Starry sky" liver with fasting: variations in glycogen stores? *J Ultrasound Med.* 1996;15(5):405–407.

43. The National Institute for Occupational Safety and Health; Centers for Disease Control and Prevention. Bloodborne infectious diseases: emergency needlestick information. Accessed April 11, 2021. https://www.cdc.gov/niosh/topics/bbp/emergnedl.html

44. Naghavi M, Bisignano C, Ikuta K, et al. The global, regional, and national burden of cirrhosis by cause in 195 countries and territories, 1990–2017: a systematic analysis for the Global Burden of Disease Study 2017. Accessed May 11, 2021. http://www.healthdata.org/research-article/global-regional-and-national-burden-cirrhosis-cause-195-countries-and-territories

45. Reinberg S. U.S. deaths from liver disease rising rapidly. HealthDay Reporter. Published July 19, 2018. https://www.webmd.com/digestive-disorders/news/20180719/us-deaths-from-liver-disease-rising-rapidly

46. Crawford JM. The liver. In: Cotran RS, Kumar V, Collins T, eds. *Robbins & Cotran Pathologic Basis of Disease.* 10th ed. Sanders; 2020:823–880.

47. Lefton HB, Rosa A, Cohen M. Diagnosis and epidemiology of cirrhosis. *Med Clin N Am.* 2009;93:787–799.

48. McGahan JP, Goldberg BB. *Diagnostic Ultrasound.* 2nd ed. Informa Healthcare; 2008.

49. Hertzberg BS, Middleton WD. Liver. In: Middleton, WD, Kurtz AB, Hertzberg BS, eds. *Ultrasound: The Requisites.* 3rd ed. Mosby; 2015:51–88.

50. Bissett RAL, Khan AN. *Differential Diagnosis in Abdominal Ultrasound.* 4th ed. WB Saunders; 2012.

51. Stone C. Schistosomiasis. *J Diagn Med Sonogr.* 2005;21(5):424–427.

52. Casillas VJ, Amendola MA, Gascue A, et al. Imaging of nontraumatic hemorrhagic hepatic lesions. *Radiographics.* 2000;20:367–378.

53. Friedman AC. *Radiology of the Liver, Biliary Tract, Pancreas and Spleen.* Williams & Wilkins; 1987.

54. Tchelepi H, Ralls PW. Ultrasound of focal liver masses. *Ultrasound Q.* 2004;20:155–169.

55. Kim TK, Jang HJ, Wilson SR. Hepatic neoplasms: features on gray scale and contrast enhanced ultrasound. *Ultrasound Clin.* 2007;2:333–354.

56. Weissleder R, Chen JW, Harisinghani MG, et al. *Primer of Diagnostic Imaging.* 6th ed. Elsevier Mosby; 2018.

57. Greten TF, Papendorf F, Bleck JS, et al. Survival rate in patients with hepatocellular carcinoma: a retrospective analysis of 389 patients. *Br J Cancer.* 2005;23:1862–1868.

58. Cancer.Net Editorial Board. Liver Cancer: Statistics. May 20, 2016. Accessed April 11, 2021. http://www.cancer.net/cancer-types/liver-cancer/statistics

59. National Cancer Institute. Cancer state facts: liver and intrahepatic bile duct cancer. Accessed April 11, 2021. https://seer.cancer.gov/statfacts/html/livibd.html

60. American Cancer Society. Early detection, diagnosis, and staging. Accessed April 11, 2021. https://www.cancer.org/cancer/liver-cancer/detection-diagnosis-staging.html

61. Zhou Y, Sui C, Li B, et al. Repeat hepatectomy for recurrent hepatocellular carcinoma: a local experience and a systematic review. *World J Surg Oncol.* 2010;8:55.

62. Minami Y, Kudo M. Radiofrequency ablation of hepatocellular carcinoma: current status. *World J Radiol.* 2010;28:417–424.

63. Claudon M, Dietrich CF, Choi BI, et al. Guidelines and good clinical practice recommendations for contrast enhanced ultrasound (CEUS) in the liver—Update 2020—WFUMB in cooperation with EFSUMB, AFSUMB, AIUM, and FLAUS. Accessed April 11, 2021. https://www.researchgate.net/publication/343196393_Guidelines_and_Good_Clinical_Practice_Recommendations_for_Contrast_Enhanced_Ultrasound_CEUS_in_the_Liver_-_Update_2020_WFUMB_in_Cooperation_with_EFSUMB_AFSUMB_AIUM_and_FLAUS

64. Tao F, Heiden RA, Bieuei F. Focal nodular hyperplasia. *Appl Radiol.* 2000;29:30–33.

65. Bertolotto M, Catalano O. Contrast-enhanced ultrasound: past, present, and future. *Ultrasound Clin.* 2009;4:339–367.

66. Barr RG. How to develop a contrast-enhanced ultrasound program. *J Ultrasound Med.* 2017;36(6):1225–1240. doi:10.7863/ultra.16.09045

67. Greis C. Technology overview: SonoVue (Bracco, Milan). *Eur Radiol Suppl.* 2004;14(suppl 8):P11–P15.

68. Burns PN, Wilson SR. Focal liver masses: enhancement patterns on contrast-enhanced images—concordance of US scans with CT. *Radiology.* 2007;242(1):162–174.

69. Nolsoe CP, Lorentzen T. International guidelines for contrast-enhanced ultrasonography: ultrasound imaging in the new millennium. *Ultrasonography.* 2016;35(2):89–103.

70. Castéra L, Foucher J, Bernard PH, et al. Pitfalls of liver stiffness measurement: a 5-year prospective study of 13,369 examinations. *Hepatology.* 2010;51(3):828–835.

71. Piscaglia F, Bolondi L. The safety of Sonovue® in abdominal applications: retrospective analysis of 23188 investigations. *Ultrasound Med Biol.* 2006;32(9):1369–1375.

72. Piscaglia F, Lencioni R, Sagrini E, et al. Characterization of focal liver lesions with contrast-enhanced ultrasound. *Ultrasound Med Biol.* 2010;36(4):531–550.

73. Rettenbacher T. Focal liver lesions: role of contrast-enhanced ultrasound. *Eur J Radiol.* 2007;64:173–182.

74. Konopke R, Bunk A, Kersting S. The role of contrast-enhanced ultrasound for focal liver lesion detection: an overview. *Ultrasound Med Biol.* 2007;33(10):1515–1526.

75. Chen S, Sanchez W, Callstrom MR, et al. Assessment of liver viscoelasticity by using shear waves induced by ultrasound radiation force. *Radiology.* 2013;266(3):964–970.

76. Barr RG, Ferraioli G, Levine D, et al. Elastography assessment of liver fibrosis: society of radiologists in ultrasound consensus conference statement. *Radiology.* 2015;276(3):845–861.

77. Barr RG, Wilson SR, Rubens D, Garcia-Tsao G, Ferraioli G. Update to the Society of Radiologists in ultrasound liver elastography consensus statement. *Radiology.* 2020;296:263–274.

78. Coenegrachts K. Magnetic resonance imaging of the liver: new imaging strategies for evaluating focal liver lesions. *World J Radiol.* 2009;1:72–85.

CHAPTER 8

The Gallbladder and Biliary System

TERESA M. BIEKER

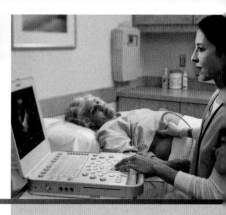

OBJECTIVES

- Illustrate surface, relational, and internal anatomy of the normal gallbladder and biliary system.

- Discuss the embryologic development, common anatomic variants, and congenital anomalies of the gallbladder and biliary tree.

- Describe the physiology of the gallbladder and biliary tree and include the laboratory values associated with normal and abnormal function.

- Explain the sonographic evaluation of the gallbladder and biliary tree to include patient preparation, protocol, and demonstrate completing the examination procedure.

- Describe the embryologic development, clinical signs and symptoms, and sonographic appearance for each of the following congenital anomalies: septate gallbladder, interposition of the gallbladder, biliary atresia, and choledochal cyst.

- Identify gallbladder pathology in terms of etiology, clinical signs and symptoms, and sonographic appearance for acquired diseases to include biliary sludge, cholelithiasis, acute cholecystitis, acute acalculous cholecystitis, complicated cholecystitis, chronic cholecystitis, wall thickening, cholestasis, neoplasms, hyperplastic cholecystoses, and miscellaneous pathology.

- Identify biliary system pathology in terms of etiology, clinical signs and symptoms, and sonographic appearance for acquired diseases to include postcholecystectomy, bile duct obstruction, cholangitis, other pathology, and AIDS cholecystopathy.

- Differentiate between the advantages and disadvantages of utilizing other gallbladder and biliary system imaging procedures to include radiography, nuclear medicine, computed tomography, and magnetic resonance.

KEY TERMS

acquired diseases

alanine aminotransferase (ALT)

aspartate aminotransferase (AST)

bilirubin

cholecystokinin (CCK)

congenital anomalies

extrahepatic biliary system

gallbladder

GLOSSARY

cholangitis inflammation of the bile ducts

cholecystectomy surgical removal of the gallbladder

cholecystitis acute or chronic inflammation of the gallbladder

cholecystokinin a hormone secreted into the blood by the small intestine that stimulates gallbladder contraction

choledocholithiasis calculi within the bile duct

cholelithiasis the formation or presence of calculi or bile stones within the gallbladder

common bile duct the duct that carries bile from the cystic and hepatic ducts to the duodenum

cystic duct the duct of the gallbladder that joins with hepatic duct to form the common bile duct

(continued)

gallbladder a pear-shaped sac that lies on the undersurface of the liver; the gallbladder holds bile from the liver until released through the cystic duct

junctional fold a fold within the gallbladder neck or body

phrygian cap a fold within the gallbladder fundus

pneumobilia air within the bile ducts

sludge solid, semisolid, or thickened bile within the gallbladder or bile ducts

sonographic Murphy sign pain over the gallbladder when the ultrasound transducer is used to compress the right upper quadrant

Sonography plays a key role in the evaluation of suspected gallbladder and biliary disease. Because the quality of sonographic examinations is strongly operator-dependent, it is crucial to understand the anatomy, physiology, pathology, techniques, and pitfalls of scanning these structures. The quality of education and the experience of a sonographer are directly related to accuracy of findings.[1] This is especially true of the gallbladder and biliary tree because scanning may require patience, skill, and appropriate technique. Sonography is considered the modality of choice to evaluate gallbladder and ductal pathology.

ANATOMY

The normal distended gallbladder is a pear- or teardrop-shaped sac measuring approximately 8 cm long and 4 to 5 cm in anteroposterior (AP) and transverse diameter. The normal wall measures less than 3 mm in thickness.[1,2] The gallbladder is located in the main lobar fissure between the right and left hepatic lobes (Fig. 8-1). It lies under the visceral surface of the liver, lateral to the second part of the duodenum, and anterior to the right kidney and transverse colon[3] (Fig. 8-2A, B).

The gallbladder is divided into a neck, body, and fundus (Figs. 8-2B and 8-3A, B). The narrowest portion is the neck, which lies to the right of the porta hepatis. The body is the central or main portion. The fundus varies considerably in position. Normally, the fundus is the most inferolateral portion of the gallbladder and it extends caudally and anteriorly below the inferior margin of the right hepatic lobe; however, it can extend as low as the right lower quadrant (RLQ) or as far left as the left anterior axillary line.[3]

Histologically, the gallbladder consists of an inner epithelial mucosa with folds, a muscular layer, a subserous layer, and an outer serosal surface. Mucous glands are found only in the gallbladder neck. Aberrant vestigial bile ducts of the liver may enter the adventitia (outermost covering) of the gallbladder and serve as a pathway for infection from the liver.[4]

The cystic duct arises from the superior aspect of the gallbladder neck and enters into the common bile duct (CBD) (Fig. 8-4).[2,3] It is 2 to 6 cm in length and its lumen contains a series of mucosal folds, the spiral valves of Heister, which prevent collapse or overdistention during sudden changes in position.[3]

The intrahepatic bile ducts run in juxtaposition to the portal veins and hepatic arteries. Together, these three structures form portal triads. The portal triads are surrounded by connective tissue and radiate through the lobes and segments of the liver. This fibrous connective tissue lines the portal vein walls, creating an echogenic appearance on sonography. The intrahepatic ducts join to form the right and left main hepatic ducts. The right and left main ducts unite at the porta hepatis to form the common hepatic duct (CHD). The cystic duct joins the CHD, forming the CBD. The CBD courses inferiorly within the hepatoduodenal ligament and anterior to the portal vein to the first portion of the duodenum and the head of the pancreas. In some cases, the CBD is surrounded by pancreatic tissue (Fig. 8-5A–D). The duct ends at the ampulla of Vater, which is difficult to visualize sonographically. Ducts can vary in their course, length, and site of anastomosis. For example, the CBD can be straight, curved, or angled.[2,3] There can also be accessory hepatic ducts.[3,4] Anatomically, the proximal duct is located at the liver, whereas the distal duct is located at the bowel. Central refers to the porta, and peripheral is the branching within the liver.[2]

On sonography, the duct is measured inner wall to inner wall. A normal intraluminal measurement for the intrahepatic duct is 2 mm, or no more than 40% of the portal vein.[2] Measurements for the CBD and CHD are controversial; however, the CHD typically does not exceed 6 mm, and the CBD should measure less than 7 to 8 mm (Fig. 8-6A–D).[5,6] There is also controversy over whether duct size increases with age or after a cholecystectomy. Normal diameters of up to 10 mm have been reported in asymptomatic populations.[2]

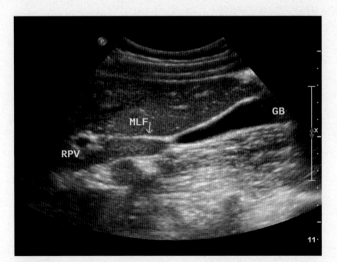

FIGURE 8-1 Longitudinal image of the normal gallbladder (GB). Note the anatomic landmarks: the main lobar fissure (arrow, MLF) and the right portal vein (RPV).

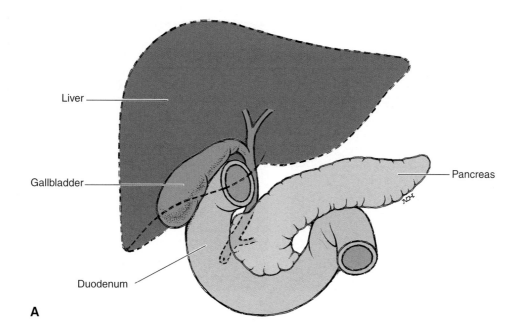

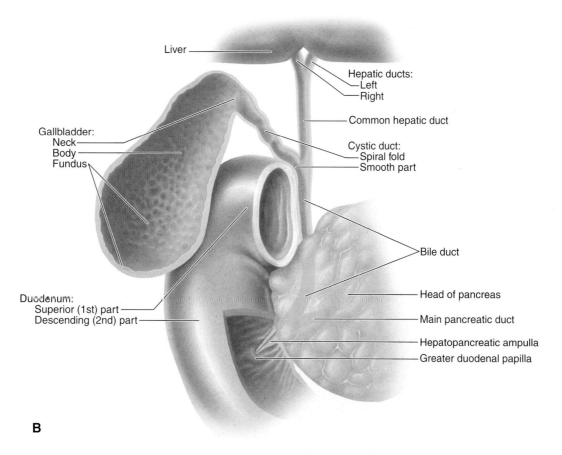

FIGURE 8-2 A: The illustration demonstrates the relationship of the normal gallbladder location to the liver, duodenum, and pancreas. **B:** The internal locations of the neck, body, and fundus and the ducts are labeled on this illustration. (**A:** Reprinted with permission from The Neil Hardy Collection 2008-05, Lippincott Williams & Wilkins; **B:** Reprinted with permission from Tank PW, Gest TR. *Lippincott Williams & Wilkins Atlas of Anatomy*. Wolters Kluwer Health/Lippincott Williams & Wilkins; 2009:236.)

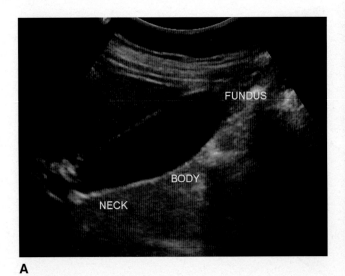

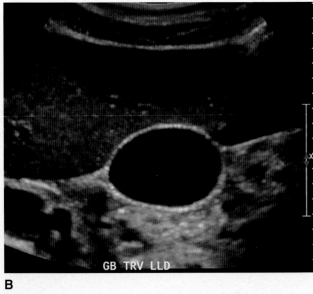

FIGURE 8-3 Sonographic images of the normal gallbladder. **A:** Longitudinal gallbladder. The distal fundus is more bulbous, whereas the neck is the narrowest portion. **B:** Transverse mid-gallbladder at the body with a normal appearing wall.

SECTIONAL VIEWS

Anatomic structures are sonographically identified by location and relationships with other structures. The schematic views with corresponding sonographic sectional images of the gallbladder and extrahepatic biliary tree demonstrate this relationship (Figs. 8-7A–C, 8-8A, B, 8-9A–C, and 8-10A, B).

PHYSIOLOGY

The biliary system transports bile, which is produced continually by hepatic parenchymal cells, to the duodenum, where it aids in digestion. Bile contains bile pigments (chiefly bilirubin), bile acids, cholesterol, lecithin, mucin, and other organic and inorganic substances. Bile helps to emulsify and promote the absorption of fats, and it also facilitates the actions of lipase, a pancreatic enzyme. The gallbladder concentrates and stores bile until needed and regulates biliary pressure.[3,4]

When food, especially fats, enters the small intestine, cholecystokinin (CCK) is secreted by the proximal small intestine, causing the gallbladder to contract and the sphincter of Oddi to relax. Bile is then released into the cystic duct, flows through the CBD, and enters the duodenum.[4] Gallbladder contraction can also be induced by commercially available "fatty meals" or by intravenous (IV) injections of CCK, although these methods are not commonly utilized. Gallbladder emptying may be diminished in some patients with gallstones. Residual gallbladder volume is known to increase during pregnancy. Sonography can monitor such gallbladder kinetics by measuring the gallbladder volume in various fasting and postprandial states.[7]

Several laboratory tests can be helpful in evaluating pathophysiology of the biliary tract. An increased WBC indicates infection. Aspartate aminotransferase (AST) and alanine aminotransferase (ALT) are enzymes produced by tissues of high metabolic activity, including the liver. Both values, but particularly the latter, can be mildly to moderately elevated in biliary obstruction. Lactic dehydrogenase (LDH), an enzyme, can be mildly elevated in obstructive jaundice. Alkaline phosphatase, another liver enzyme, markedly increases in obstructive jaundice. Bilirubin results from the breakdown of hemoglobin in red blood cells. Direct, or conjugated, bilirubin level tends to be elevated in obstructive (surgical) jaundice, whereas the indirect, or unconjugated, bilirubin level rises in hepatocellular disease and hemolytic anemias.[3,8] Although helpful, the results of liver function tests can be nonspecific and must be considered with the clinical presentation and the findings of diagnostic imaging. This can help identify trends; therefore, it is important to evaluate the laboratory results over time to determine if function is improving or deteriorating.

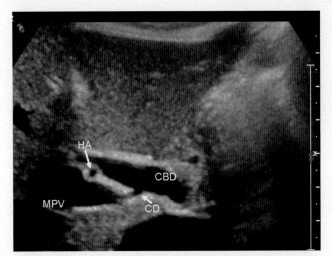

FIGURE 8-4 Sonographic image of the porta hepatis. The cystic duct is seen entering the dilated common bile duct (CBD) on the posterior margin. CD, cystic duct; HA, hepatic artery; MPV, main portal vein.

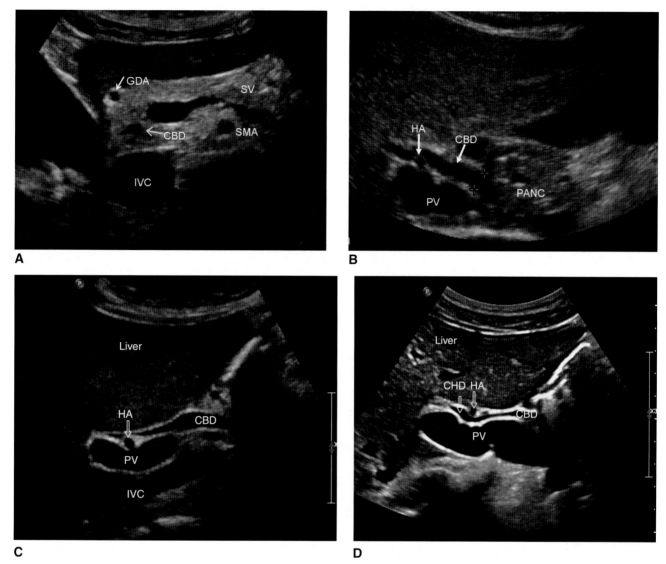

FIGURE 8-5 Sonographic images of the extrahepatic biliary tree. **A:** Short axis of the common bile duct (*CBD*) at the level of the pancreatic head. **B:** Long-axis view of the CBD coursing from the liver to the pancreatic head. **C:** Portal triad at the porta hepatis. **D:** Occasionally, a replaced hepatic artery is seen. The artery is located anterior to the duct, rather than between the duct and portal vein. *CHD*, common hepatic duct; *GDA*, gastroduodenal artery; *HA*, hepatic artery; *IVC*, inferior vena cava; *PANC*, pancreas; *PV*, portal vein; *SMA*, superior mesenteric artery; *SV*, splenic vein.

SONOGRAPHIC EXAMINATION, PREPARATION, PROTOCOL, AND PROCEDURE

Ideally, patients should not have anything by mouth for 6 to 8 hours prior to an examination of the gallbladder and biliary tree. Clear liquids are accepted. Fasting distends the gallbladder and reduces bowel gas for optimal visualization. The diagnosis of various gallbladder and ductal pathologies can be made with a partially contracted, nonfasting gallbladder in emergent situations, when the patient is not fasting.

The chief complaint and pertinent medical or surgical history should be verified with the patient. This includes the type, frequency, and duration of symptoms; location of pain; factors that aggravate or alleviate symptoms; prior similar episodes; and previous surgery or medical illnesses. Additional information, such as previous imaging studies, laboratory work, or clinic notes, is also helpful. The patient

should also be evaluated physically. Conditions such as jaundice and/or surgical scars should be noted.

The normal gallbladder has thin echogenic walls, an anechoic lumen, and posterior enhancement. The bile duct lumen should also appear anechoic; therefore, proper technique is important to avoid the presence of artifact filling these structures. The gallbladder is located in the main lobar fissure to the right of the ligamentum teres, anterior to the right kidney and lateral to the pancreatic head. Although its position can vary, the neck has a constant relationship to the region of the porta hepatis (Fig. 8-3A). The CBD is usually identified anterior to the portal vein and hepatic artery at the porta hepatis and should be followed throughout its course to the pancreatic head. The CHD and the right and left intraductal branches should also be evaluated. Dilated intrahepatic biliary ducts can be identified along the intrahepatic portal vein branches. The gallbladder and ducts are carefully evaluated for size, wall thickness, contents, course,

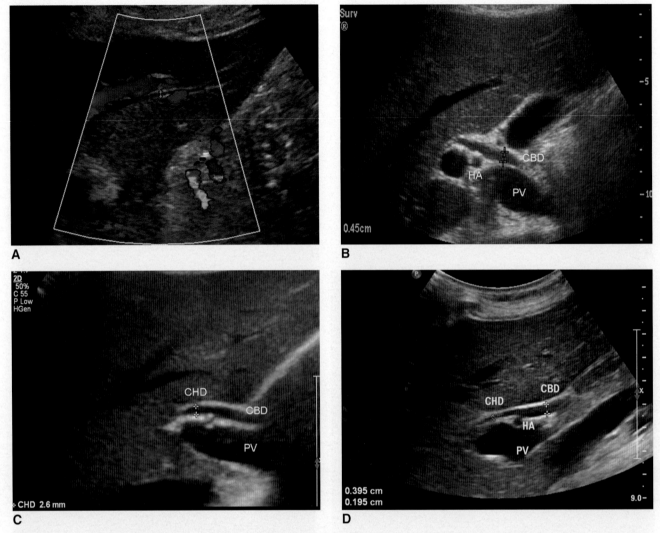

FIGURE 8-6 Normal measurements of the ductal system. **A:** Intrahepatic duct measuring less than 2 mm within the left lobe. **B:** Common bile duct *(CBD)*, less than 8 mm. **C:** Common hepatic duct *(CHD)*, less than 6 mm at the porta hepatis. The ducts are measured inner wall to inner wall. **D:** Another example of normal duct measurements at the porta. *HA*, hepatic artery; *PV*, portal vein.

and caliber. The presence or absence of pathology in the gallbladder, porta hepatis, and intrahepatic and extrahepatic biliary system should be documented.

Meticulous real-time examination of the gallbladder and bile ducts should be performed in all scan planes. A 3.5-MHz probe or higher-frequency probe should be utilized. In thinner patients, a 7.5-to-9-MHz probe can be used for optimal resolution. Proper setting of the overall gain, the time gain compensation, compression, spatial compounding, and dynamic range should be optimized for adequate and accurate visualization of the gallbladder. Using harmonics is also helpful in reducing artifacts within the gallbladder as well as identifying small stones (Fig. 8-11A, B).[5,9] The focal zone should be adjusted for each area of interest. The focal zone is the narrowest segment of the beam, and suspected calculi (or other pathology) should lie within this zone to demonstrate shadowing. Even then, many small calculi may not shadow. Changing the transducer frequency or angle may be necessary to bring the gallbladder into the focal zone. Also, removing compound imaging may help to visualize a shadow posterior to a small stone (Fig. 8-12).

The patient should be examined in two positions—typically supine and left lateral decubitus (LLD) or posterior oblique. A right lateral decubitus (RLD), erect (sitting or standing), or even prone positions may be necessary. While in the decubitus positions, small changes in the patient's angle, from 45 to 90 degrees, may improve visibility. The erect positions demonstrate gravity dependence. A prone position can show the mobility of stones and allows the liver to fall anteriorly, thereby providing an acoustic window and displacing bowel. Because the prone scanning position may be awkward, the technique may be varied by turning the patient prone for 10 to 15 seconds and then quickly returning the patient to an LLD position and rescanning the area.

Depending on the patient's body habitus and ability to cooperate, breathing techniques may also be beneficial. Suspended, full inspiration is often best, but sometimes, varying degrees of inspiration or expiration may also help. Breathing techniques are useful in moving organs inferiorly for improved subcostal access.

Another technique is to vary the scanning approaches. With the patient in an LLD position, scan should be performed subcostally with the transducer angled slightly toward the patient's right shoulder to elongate the portal vein and the bile duct at the porta hepatis. If this technique is not optimal, intercostal scanning may be necessary. Structures should be evaluated by scanning through many different windows to achieve the best angle and resolution. Gentle transducer pressure is useful often for pushing bowel away from the field of view.

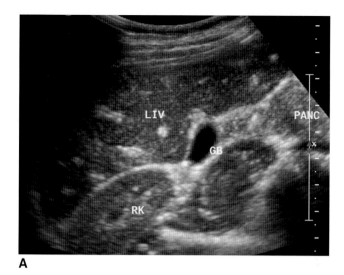

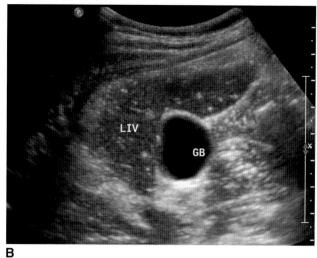

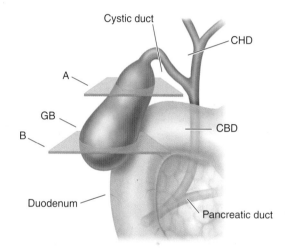

FIGURE 8-7 **A**: The sonogram of plane A demonstrates an axial plane near the gallbladder *(GB)* neck. **B**: A more distal transverse image through the gallbladder fundus *(GB)* is visualized at scanning plane B. **C**: The illustration demonstrates scanning planes A and B at different levels through the gallbladder. *CBD*, common bile duct; *CHD*, common hepatic duct; *LIV*, liver; *PANC*, pancreas; *RK*, right kidney.

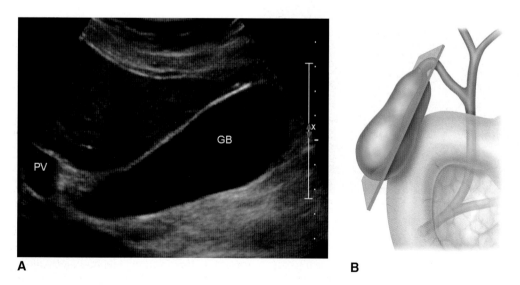

FIGURE 8-8 The sonogram (**A**) and illustration (**B**) demonstrate a longitudinal image through the gallbladder *(GB)* body and fundus. The portal vein is just posterior to the gallbladder.

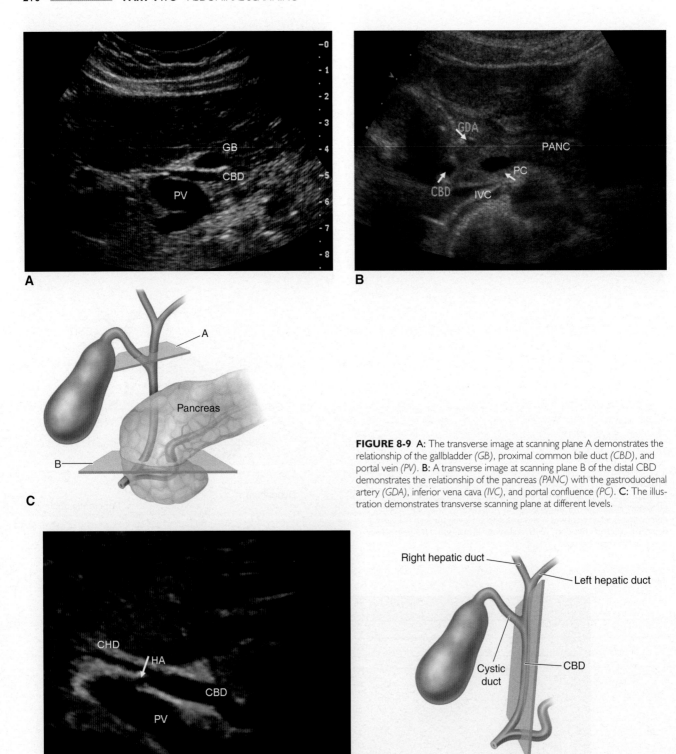

FIGURE 8-9 **A:** The transverse image at scanning plane A demonstrates the relationship of the gallbladder (GB), proximal common bile duct (CBD), and portal vein (PV). **B:** A transverse image at scanning plane B of the distal CBD demonstrates the relationship of the pancreas (PANC) with the gastroduodenal artery (GDA), inferior vena cava (IVC), and portal confluence (PC). **C:** The illustration demonstrates transverse scanning plane at different levels.

FIGURE 8-10 The sonogram (**A**) and illustration (**B**) demonstrate a longitudinal scanning plane through the common bile duct (CBD). CHD, common hepatic duct; HA, hepatic artery; PV, portal vein.

Owing to absorption, gallstones should produce a clean shadow. If echogenic foci are seen within the gallbladder and do not shadow, several techniques should be attempted. First, the gain distal to the foci should be reduced. Second, the frequency of the transducer should be increased. Third, the scanning angle should be changed to decrease the distance between the ultrasound beam and the stone. When a focal zone is used, the focus should be placed at or just below the stone. However, new technologies allow for and create multi focal images. Removing compound imaging may also be helpful to visualize a shadow posterior to a small stone.

While scanning, it is also important to determine if there is a sonographic Murphy sign. To evaluate, transducer pressure should be applied directly over the gallbladder. When positive, the patient will have focal pin-point tenderness. Care must be taken to ensure pressure is placed

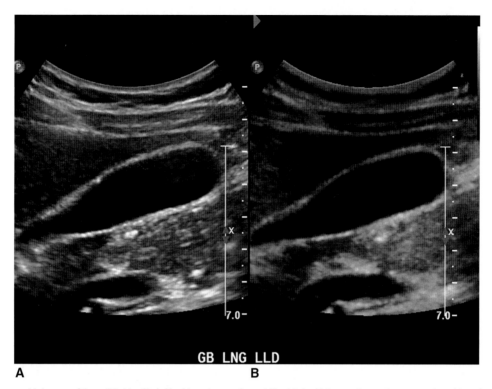

FIGURE 8-11 Sonographic images of the gallbladder (**A, left**) without harmonics and (**B, right**) with harmonics on the same patient. Note the decrease in artifact within the gallbladder lumen.

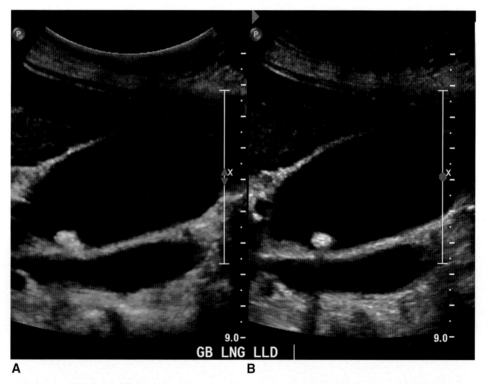

FIGURE 8-12 Sonographic images of the gallbladder (**A, left**) with compound imaging and (**B, right**) without compound imaging. Note the posterior shadow once compound imaging was renewed.

directly over the gallbladder and not the epigastrium or the liver. If the patient has received pain medication or is unresponsive, the sonographic Murphy sign will not be accurate.[5]

It is also valuable to interrogate the gallbladder and biliary structures with color Doppler imaging. This may be helpful in evaluating hyperemia in inflammatory conditions, in distinguishing solid masses from avascular pathology, and in differentiating intrahepatic and extrahepatic bile ducts from blood vessels.[2]

Meticulous scanning technique is crucial and can decrease or eliminate the need for other diagnostic tests.

CONGENITAL ANOMALIES AND NORMAL VARIANTS

There are many common gallbladder variations, including different shapes (e.g., hourglass), positions, folds, and/or septations (Fig. 8-13A, B). The gallbladder may occasionally contain a small infundibulum at the neck, Hartman pouch, where stones can collect. The phrygian cap is a common variant that forms when the fundus kinks or folds back on the body (Fig. 8-14). The gallbladder can be excessively mobile, ectopic (on the left, midline, and transversely), or low in the RLQ. It can also be located partially or totally embedded in the liver parenchyma, completely surrounded by peritoneum, in the abdominal wall or falciform ligament, contained in the retroperitoneum, or above the liver.[2-4]

Embryonic development of the liver, gallbladder, and biliary duct system arises from the hepatic diverticulum of the foregut in the fourth week of gestation. This diverticulum divides into two parts: a larger cranial part, which gives rise to the liver, and a smaller caudal part, which develops into the gallbladder and cystic duct. At the beginning of the fifth week, the hepatic ducts, extrahepatic duct system, gallbladder, cystic duct, and pancreatic duct are demarcated as a solid cord of cells. Ductal lumina begin development during the sixth week in the common duct and slowly progress distally. The lumen extends into the cystic duct by the 7th week, but the gallbladder remains solid until the 12th week. Therefore, most gallbladder anomalies probably occur between the 4th and 12th week.[10,11]

Agenesis of the gallbladder is rare. Often incidental, but dilated ducts and choledocholithiasis can be seen with agenesis of the gallbladder. Duplication of the gallbladder can be diagnosed prenatally and often involves duplication of the cystic duct.[2] Anomalies of the gallbladder alone do not generally give rise to any characteristic symptoms. Although some of the defects predispose to bile stasis and attacks of cholecystitis, the attacks themselves have usual aspects. The symptoms only call attention to the anomaly.[10]

Septate Gallbladder

A gallbladder septum may result from a congenital mucosal diaphragm, adenomyomatosis, or a combination of the two. Although a gallbladder septum may be an incidental finding during an otherwise normal examination, stasis of bile in the distal segment predisposes to calculus formation.[12] A single septum appears as a thin linear echo separating the gallbladder into compartments. Simple junctional folds may mimic a septum.

The multiseptated gallbladder is one of the rarest congenital gallbladder malformations. This anomaly may be associated with biliary colic or cholelithiasis or may be entirely asymptomatic without associated cholelithiasis.[13]

A multiseptated gallbladder can have variable sonographic appearances. There can be fine linear septa or a honeycomb pattern of clustered septations resulting in multiple communicating cyst-like compartments. Septa may cluster in the neck and body region of the gallbladder. Differential diagnoses include desquamated gallbladder mucosa (an unusual finding in acute cholecystitis) and hyperplastic cholecystoses (such as polypoid cholesterolosis or adenomyomatosis). Desquamated gallbladder mucosa appears as multiple, haphazardly arranged, linear, nonshadowing densities within the gallbladder lumen, which does not consistently arise from the gallbladder wall because they do in multiseptated gallbladder. Polypoid cholesterolosis may more often resemble multiseptated gallbladder, although the nonshadowing polypoid densities are more bulbous, and there is no bridging of the lumen by septa as in the multiseptated gallbladder. In adenomyomatosis, Rokitansky–Aschoff sinuses could be confused with the honeycomb pattern, but cyst-like Rokitansky–Aschoff sinuses are smaller and are actually within the thickened gallbladder wall; there is no bridging of the lumen itself to form cyst-like compartments.[13,14]

Interposition of the Gallbladder

Childhood jaundice is usual. Although interposition of the gallbladder (the absence of the CHD and cystic duct) is a rare anomaly, its diagnosis is important because it is surgically correctable. Normally, the right and left main hepatic ducts join to form the CHD, which are entered by the cystic duct to form the CBD. In interposition, the main hepatic ducts drain, separately or together, directly into the gallbladder. The gallbladder then drains directly into the CBD, although variants can also occur (Fig. 8-15). The cause of interposition of the gallbladder is unknown.[11]

A patient with interposition of the gallbladder presents with jaundice, which may be intermittent, abdominal

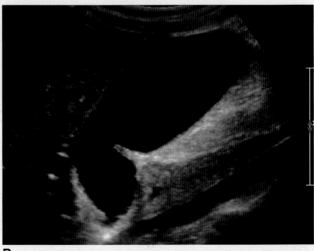

A

B

FIGURE 8-13 Transverse (**A**) and longitudinal (**B**) images of a junctional fold.

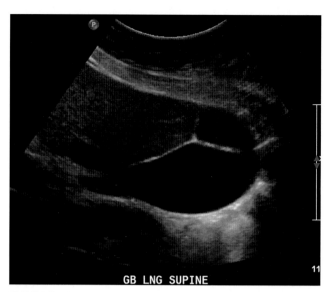

FIGURE 8-14 Longitudinal sonogram of a phrygian cap, located at the fundus of the gallbladder.

pain, and sometimes an enlarged gallbladder. Sonography may show enlarged intrahepatic ducts with a normal CBD, mimicking Caroli disease, or the ducts may appear to enter a cystic mass in the porta hepatis, mimicking a choledochal cyst. Although sonography may be difficult to interpret in this situation, it is still a good initial step, indicating that jaundice is caused by an anatomic biliary abnormality.[11]

Biliary Atresia

Biliary atresia is the most common type of obstructive biliary disease in infants and young children.[15] Destruction of the extrahepatic biliary system occurs because of inflammation and sclerosing cholangiopathy.[16] Progressive obliteration of the extrahepatic ducts and, in many instances, the gallbladder takes place. This obliteration extends into the proximal intrahepatic duct system, which usually remains patent in the first few weeks of life. The severity varies with the duration of involvement. Fibrosis and obliteration of the biliary tree progress distal to proximal.[17]

More than 50% of neonates have transient jaundice characterized by mild elevation of serum bilirubin, which resolves

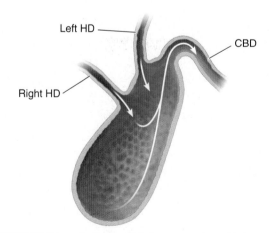

Left HD

Right HD

CBD

FIGURE 8-15 Schematic diagram of bile flow pattern (arrows) in interposition of the gallbladder. The sonographic appearance reveals dilated intrahepatic ducts adjacent to a normal or enlarged gallbladder with no dilatation of the common bile duct (CBD). Differential diagnosis includes choledochal cyst, gallbladder hydrops, and Caroli disease.[27] HD, hepatic duct.

spontaneously. Persistent or sudden-onset jaundice after the 1st and 2nd week of life may indicate a more serious abnormality, most commonly, biliary atresia or neonatal hepatitis. Less common causes include choledochal cysts, inspissated bile syndrome, enzyme deficiencies, metabolic abnormalities, hemolysis, hyperalimentation, and other congenital biliary anomalies.[11,17]

Biliary atresia is twice as common in males, whereas neonatal hepatitis is four times more common in females. It is important to distinguish biliary atresia from neonatal hepatitis because atresia may be treated surgically with a liver transplant or the Kasai procedure. The outcome is better with early surgical intervention. If surgical correction is not possible, death usually occurs within months; however, a few children survive several years.[4,17] Complications of untreated biliary atresia are cirrhosis, cholangitis, portal hypertension, malabsorption, and failure of biliary drainage.[16,17]

In normal neonates, the CHD is generally visible sonographically and measures no more than 1 mm. Intrahepatic duct dilatation combined with inability to visualize the CHD is suggestive of biliary atresia.[17] If only the cystic duct is obstructed, a hydropic gallbladder will develop.[4] Detection of both intrahepatic and extrahepatic dilatations excludes atresia and indicates obstruction (choledochal cyst, inspissated bile, and biliary calculi).[17]

Choledochal Cysts

There are five types of choledochal cysts, the most common being Type I, a fusiform dilatation of the CBD. Along with Type IV, Type I, has an abnormally long channel between the bile duct and pancreatic duct. The less common Type II is seen as true diverticula extending off the CBD. Type III is a duodenal choledochocele and Type IV is characterized by multiple cystic dilatations of the intrahepatic and extrahepatic ducts. Type V, Caroli disease (communicating cavernous ectasia), is a nonobstructive, saccular dilatation of communicating intrahepatic ducts.[2] Different causes of choledochal cysts have been cited, including congenital weakness of the duct wall, which results in the formation of a cystic structure, and angulation of the CBD, causing partial obstruction leading to dilatation and cyst formation.[4]

Clinically, the signs and symptoms include intermittent jaundice associated with colicky pain, failure to thrive, and sometimes a palpable subhepatic mass displacing the stomach and the duodenum.[4,18] Choledochal cysts are three to four times more common in females than in males, and often present early in life. Surgical management is recommended because of the increased incidence of malignant transformation that may occur later in life.[2]

Sonographically, choledochal cysts appear as a localized cystic mass separate from the gallbladder in the region of the porta hepatis or intrahepatically depending on the type (Fig. 8-16). To avoid mistaking a fluid-filled bowel loop for a choledochal cyst, the examiner should verify peristalsis.

ACQUIRED DISEASES

Biliary Sludge

Sludge represents precipitates formed in the bile. It consists of a collection of calcium bilirubinate, mucus, and lesser amounts of cholesterol crystals within viscous bile that contains high concentrations of mucus and other proteins.[19]

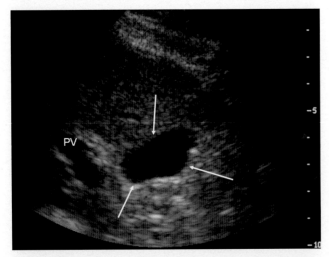

FIGURE 8-16 Longitudinal image in postcholecystectomy patient. A choledochal cyst is seen at the porta hepatis *(arrows)*. *PV*, portal vein.

The pathogenesis, clinical significance, and ultimate prognosis of sludge remain uncertain. Sludge alone can produce biliary symptoms such as the classic pain of gallstones, and it can also be associated with other complications. Therefore, sludge associated with biliary pain can be a significant finding. The presence of sludge implies the formation of a precipitate and should not be regarded as normal. Sludge is sometimes a precursor to gallstone disease.[2,19]

Sludge may be caused by conditions such as prolonged fasting, total parenteral nutrition (TPN), bile stasis, pregnancy, rapid weight loss and recent surgery and in critically ill patients.[2,19]

Sonographically, sludge produces a homogeneous, low-amplitude, nonshadowing echo pattern that tends to layer dependently (Figs. 8-17A–D and 8-18A, B). True sludge often forms a fluid–fluid level that remains constant in longitudinal and transverse images. Sludge slowly moves with changes in patient position. Sludge can disappear and

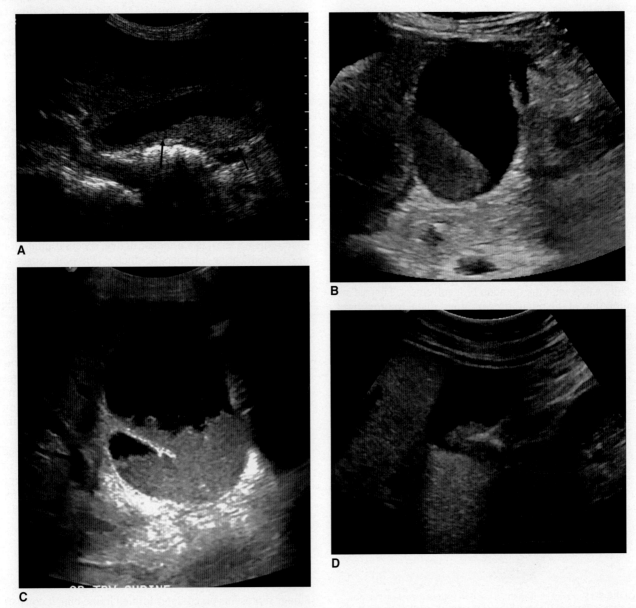

FIGURE 8-17 Varying sonographic appearances of sludge. **A:** Layering sludge *(arrows)* that is isoechoic to the liver. **B:** Sludge with adjacent pericholecystic fluid. **C:** More complex appearing sludge in a gallbladder with a junctional fold. **D:** Sludge tracking into the gallbladder neck.

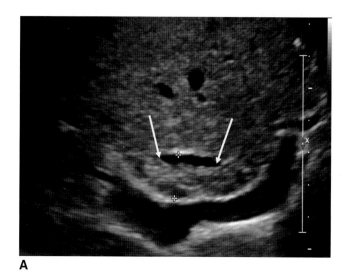

A

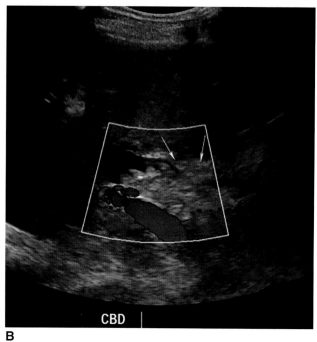

B

FIGURE 8-18 Sludge has a similar appearance within the bile ducts. **A:** Homogeneous, layering sludge *(arrows)* within the bile duct. Calipers denote bile duct. **B:** Sludge *(arrows)* filling the proximal portion of the bile duct.

reappear over time. Scattered brighter echoes within sludge may represent larger cholesterol crystals. If sludge completely fills the gallbladder (total bile sludging or hepatization of bile), it may be difficult to distinguish the echo-filled gallbladder from adjacent liver parenchyma (Fig. 8-19). Sludge may also lead to gallstones.[2,19]

Tumefactive sludge from long-standing biliary obstruction frequently does not layer but often resembles a polypoid mass that can mimic a gallbladder neoplasm (Fig. 8-20A, B). Color Doppler sonography can be useful in determining tumefactive sludge from a neoplasm.[20] Occasionally, mobile, round, echogenic, nonshadowing masses known as sludge balls are seen within the gallbladder.[19] Also, sludge may be found in conjunction with gallstones (Fig. 8-21).

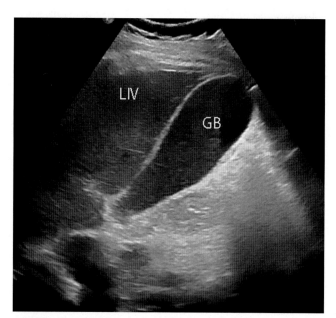

FIGURE 8-19 Hepatization of bile. Sludge in the gallbladder has the same echo texture as liver. *GB,* gallbladder; *LIV,* liver.

Using excessively high-gain settings fills the gallbladder with artifactual echoes, giving a false appearance of sludge. This artifactual pattern has a snowflake appearance, whereas true sludge has a defined, low-level pattern. Increased echogenicity of surrounding organs is another clue of too much gain. It is also important to distinguish sludge from the "false debris" echo pattern of slice thickness artifacts.

Cholelithiasis (Gallstones)

Gallstones can be large or small, single or multiple, symptomatic or silent. Gallstones are common worldwide with 2% to 10% of the population affected, with North America being near the 10% mark. The prevalence of gallstones is higher in females than in males.[2] Gallstones are occasionally seen in fetuses and children (Fig. 8-22A, B).[15,21]

The majority of stones contain a mixture of cholesterol, bilirubin, and calcium. Approximately 75% of the gallstones in the United States are primarily cholesterol, with black or brown pigment stones accounting for 25% to 30% (Fig. 8-23). Many factors are associated with gallstone formation. Supersaturation of bile with cholesterol, abnormal gallbladder emptying, and altered absorption contributes to cholesterol stone formation.[22,23]

The most common risk factors for cholelithiasis are female gender, obesity, age, pregnancy, and diabetes.[2] Other associated risks include ethnicity, genetics, diet, TPN, cirrhosis, rapid weight loss, ileal disorders (Crohn), and various medications.[21]

The majority of patients with gallstones are asymptomatic, with most found during routine abdominal scanning. Patients with symptoms, however, generally present with right upper quadrant (RUQ) pain that is steady, occurs after meals, or radiates to the upper back, shoulder, or epigastric area. The patient may also have nausea or vomiting.[24] Pertinent laboratory values may include an elevated alkaline phosphatase and mildly elevated AST and ALT levels, when the cystic duct or CBD is obstructed.[8]

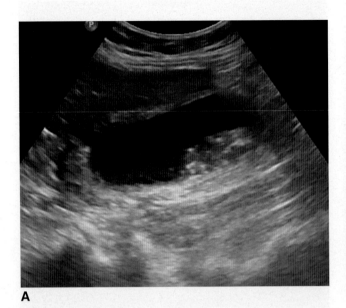

A

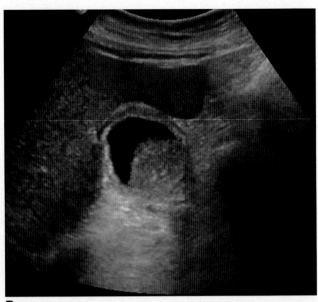

B

FIGURE 8-20 Sonogram shows tumefactive sludge within the gallbladder. **A:** The sludge balls moved from the gallbladder neck to the body as the patient changed position. **B:** A larger collection of tumefactive sludge.

Prognosis and treatment of cholelithiasis can vary depending on the frequency and severity of the attacks as well as the size of the stones. Small calculi tend to be more troublesome because they may exit the gallbladder and cause ductal obstruction.[24] Cholelithiasis may take a benign course, and a low-fat diet may be sufficient treatment in some cases. Persistent symptoms may require surgical intervention, either laparoscopic or open cholecystectomy, to provide definitive treatment of gallstones.[21] Percutaneous cholecystostomy may assume a limited role in elderly

patients and patients at high risk. Surgical cholecystostomy to remove stones has been performed, but cholecystectomy is often necessary subsequently because of the high recurrence rate.[25] Sonography is the modality of choice for monitoring stones in these patients.[2]

The classic sonographic appearance of a gallstone is a mobile, gravity-dependent, echogenic foci within the gallbladder lumen that casts a posterior acoustic shadow (Fig. 8-24A–F).[5] If the proper technique and transducer are used, virtually all calculi over 5 mm can be accurately diagnosed. If less than 2 to 3 mm, stones can be more difficult to visualize. However, small stones are typically multiple and described as "gravel," thereby making detection easier (Fig. 8-25A, B).[19] Small gallstones that are located within the cystic duct or in the neck of the gallbladder can be more difficult to visualize.[5] The majority of gallstones produce "clean" shadows with distinct margins because they are highly reflective. The visualization of a clean shadow is dependent on gain settings, transducer position and frequency, harmonics, focusing, and compound imaging.[2] Cholesterol stones or polyps can demonstrate reverberations and comet tail artifacts because of the rigidity and physical characteristics of cholesterol. Other causes of echogenic foci with reverberation and comet tail artifacts within the RUQ include air in the biliary tree, surgical clips in the gallbladder bed, gas in an intrahepatic abscess, drainage catheters, emphysematous cholecystitis, lead pellets, focal hepatic calcifications, and scars.

As the patient changes position, gallstones should roll to the most dependent portion of the gallbladder (Fig. 8-26A, B). Stones that do not demonstrate mobility may be polyps, stones impacted in the gallbladder neck, or stones adherent to the gallbladder wall (Fig. 8-27A, B).

There are many possible technical, anatomic, and diagnostic pitfalls of cholelithiasis (Table 8-1). Again, meticulous scanning in multiple planes using a variety of techniques, patient positions, and transducer frequencies is crucial for accurate diagnosis and proper patient management.

FIGURE 8-21 Transverse image of the gallbladder with sludge and gallstones.

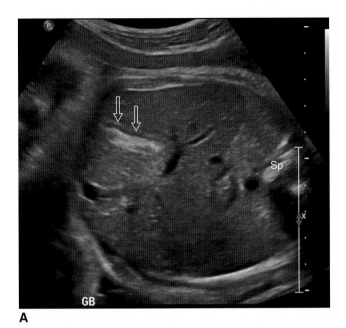

A

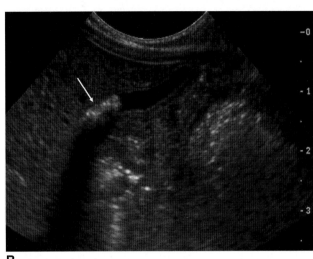

B

FIGURE 8-22 Fetal and neonatal gallstones. **A:** Fetal gallstones in the third trimester. Gallstones within the fetal gallbladder *(arrow)* do not always create a shadow. **B:** Stones with shadowing *(arrow)* within the neck of the gallbladder in this neonate. *Sp,* spine.

With careful technique, the wall–echo–shadow (WES) triad or double-arc shadow sign may be seen (Fig. 8-28A, B). The first arc or curved echogenic line represents the thickened gallbladder wall. The second arc is from the surface of the stone followed by posterior acoustic shadowing.[1,2] With chronic disease, the gallbladder may be so contracted that it is difficult to visualize sonographically. Air-filled bowel loops in the RUQ may create shadowing, which can be mistaken for a contracted gallbladder with stones. The differential diagnosis for chronic cholecystitis is adenomyomatosis and gallbladder carcinoma.[26]

Acute Cholecystitis

In up to 95% of cases, acute cholecystitis or inflammation of the gallbladder results from impacted stones within the neck of the gallbladder or the cystic duct.[5,19,20,27] It is the most common inflammatory condition of the gallbladder.[27] Inflammation may result in necrosis, ulceration, swelling, and edema.[5] Various degrees of bacterial infection occur with acute cholecystitis, leading to potential complications.[8]

Clinically, the signs and symptoms of cholecystitis are indistinguishable and somewhat nonspecific. Patients present with RUQ pain, positive Murphy sign, nausea, vomiting, distention, fever, a palpable RUQ mass, and/or jaundice.[8,20,28] These symptoms can be confused with acute pancreatitis, perforated peptic ulcer, liver abscess, or acute alcoholic hepatitis.[8] Laboratory results can also be nonspecific, possibly showing serum liver transaminase, leukocytosis, hyperbilirubinemia, or elevated alkaline phosphatase.[29] Approximately 20% of patients with cholelithiasis will develop acute cholecystitis; however, only 20% to 35% of patients with RUQ pain will have acute cholecystitis.[5,20]

On sonogram, a positive sonographic Murphy sign, wall thickening, and gallstones are signs of acute cholecystitis. Pericholecystic fluid and, at times, a hydropic gallbladder can also be seen.[5,20] Together, the findings of cholelithiasis and a positive sonographic Murphy sign are highly suggestive of acute cholelithiasis. Gallbladder wall thickening and pericholecystic fluid are considered secondary signs.[27] Color or power Doppler imaging may also be helpful in diagnosing acute cholecystitis by detecting hyperemia and an enlarged cystic artery (Fig. 8-29A–F).[2]

FIGURE 8-23 Pathogenesis of cholesterol gallstones is a multifactorial process. (Reprinted with permission from Rubin E, Rubin R. The liver and biliary system. In: Rubin E, Gorstein F, Rubin R, et al, eds. *Rubin's Pathology: Clinicopathologic Foundations of Medicine*. 4th ed. Lippincott Williams & Wilkins; 2005:804.)

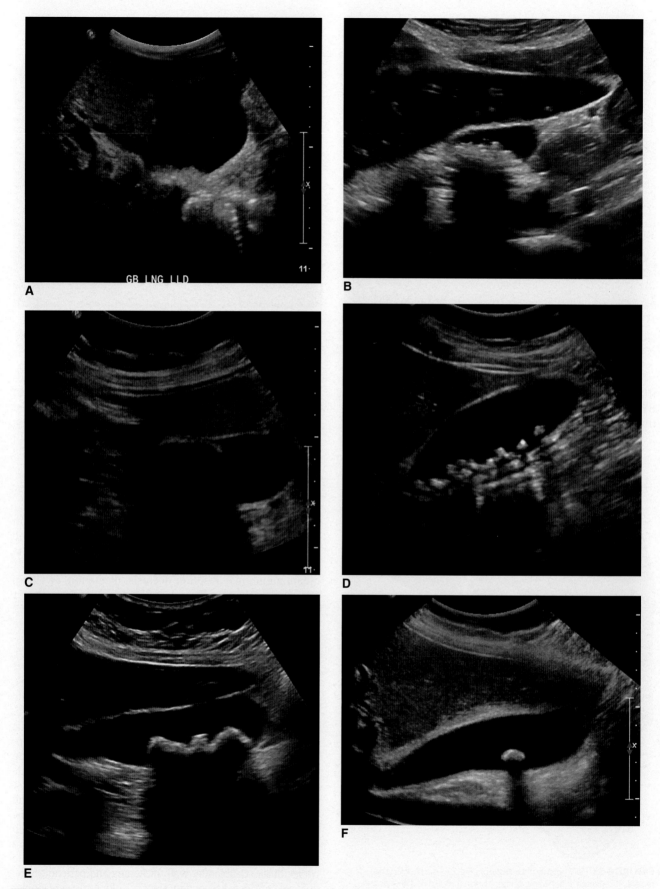

GB LNG LLD

A

B

C

D

E

F

FIGURE 8-24 Varying appearances of gallstones. **A:** Classic sonographic appearance of a gallstone within the fundus. **B:** Mixture of shadowing stones along with sludge. **C:** Single, large stone. **D:** Multiple, shadowing, dependent stones within the gallbladder. **E:** Layering, irregularly shaped stones. **F:** Single, small, shadowing stone.

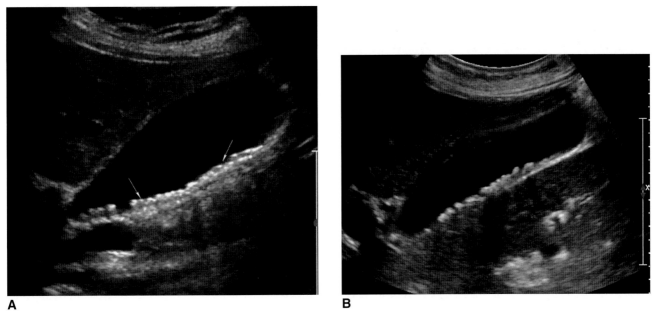

FIGURE 8-25 Gravel. **A:** The thin layer of numerous small stones *(arrows)* in this longitudinal image of the gallbladder could be mistaken for bowel gas with shadowing just behind the gallbladder, but the small stones were observed to move within the gallbladder lumen. **B:** Longitudinal image showing gravel in another patient.

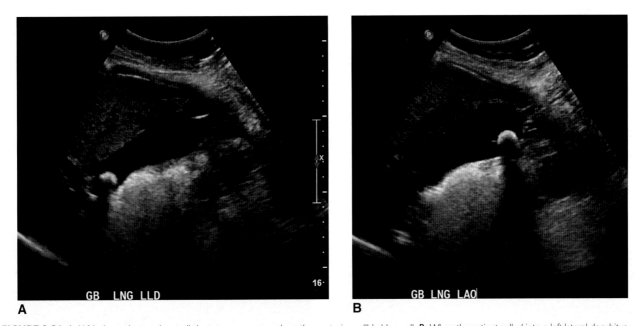

FIGURE 8-26 A: With the patient supine, a distinct stone was seen along the posterior gallbladder wall. **B:** When the patient rolled into a left lateral decubitus position, the stone rolled to the fundus.

One thought is to manage the patient medically because 60% of acute cases resolve spontaneously, and surgery should be saved until the acute attack has subsided. The preferred approach is to perform a cholecystectomy within the first several days of the onset of symptoms because early surgical intervention results in fewer complications and lower costs.[20,30] In patients with severe acute cholecystitis who are poor surgical candidates, are very ill, or are elderly, sonographically guided aspiration and percutaneous drainage of the gallbladder or antibiotic therapy is an alternative.[29] The pathophysiologic events of acute cholecystitis represent a dynamic process. Time is needed for these changes to occur. As a result, the clinical onset may precede the appearance of sonographic signs by as much as 12 to 24 hours.[31]

The major complications of acute cholecystitis include emphysematous cholecystitis, gangrenous cholecystitis, empyema, and perforation of the gallbladder.[19] The differential diagnosis of acute cholecystitis is broad and consists of pneumonia, pancreatitis, choledocholithiasis, hepatitis, liver abscess or neoplasm, peptic ulcer disease, and heart disease.[20]

Acute Acalculous Cholecystitis

In approximately 5% to 14% of acute cholecystitis cases, gallstones are not present. This is referred to as acute

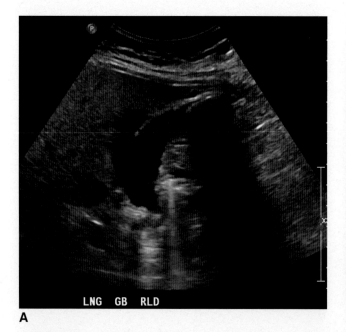
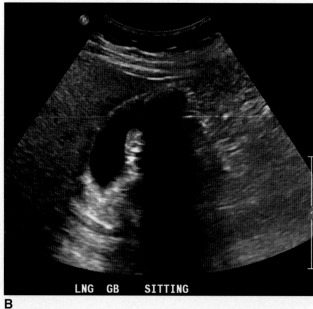

FIGURE 8-27 A: Longitudinal image of a stone stuck in the fundus of the gallbladder. Despite moving the patient in additional positions **(A)** patient in right lateral decubitus. **B:** Patient sitting, the stone was not mobile. The patient was also placed in supine and left lateral decubitus.

TABLE 8-1	**Pitfalls in Identifying Cholelithiasis**
False Positive	

- Bowel gas or ligamentum teres
- Junctional folds or valves of Heister
- Edge shadowing or other artifacts
- Scarring or surgical clips

False Negative

- Using inappropriate technique, transducer frequency, focal zone, or gain settings
- Stones within the phrygian cap or Hartman pouch
- Mistaking a thin layer of stones for bowel gas
- Small stones

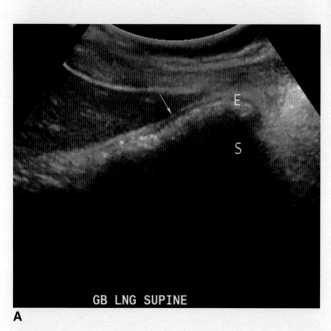
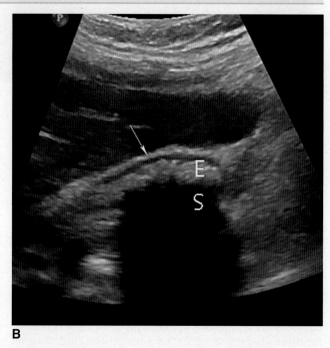

FIGURE 8-28 A: Longitudinal image of a wall–echo–shadow (WES) triad. **B:** With chronic disease, the wall can be difficult to visualize but was identified after careful evaluation. *Arrow*, gallbladder wall; *E*, echo from stone; *S*, shadow.

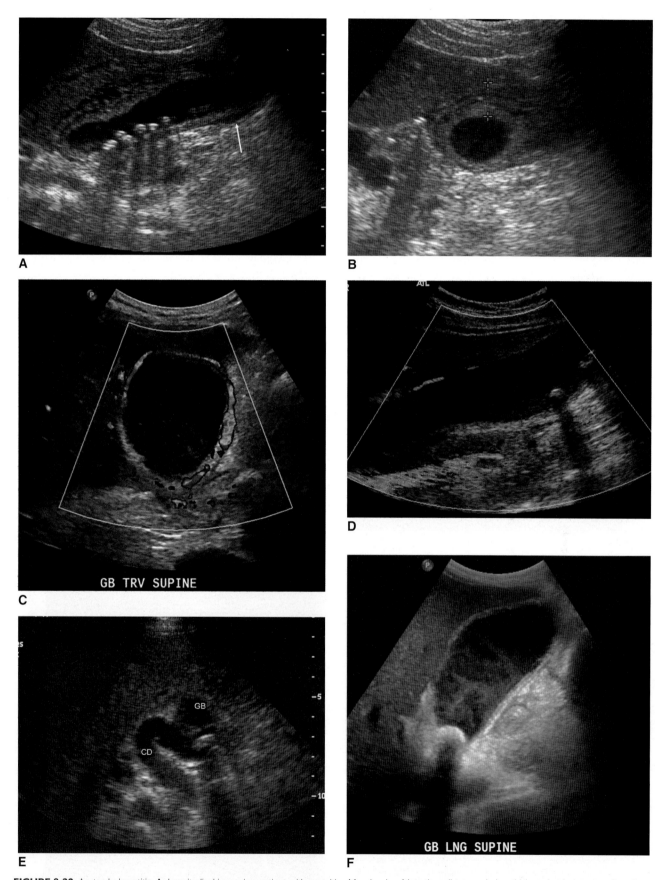

FIGURE 8-29 Acute cholecystitis. **A:** Longitudinal image in a patient with a positive Murphy sign. Note the gallstones, sludge, thickened, edematous wall, and pericholecystic fluid *(arrow)*. **B:** Transverse image of another patient with acute cholecystitis and thickened wall *(calipers)*. **C:** Hydropic gallbladder and increased color Doppler flow in a patient with positive Murphy sign, sludge, and acute cholecystitis. **D:** Longitudinal image of acute cholecystitis, stone, sludge, and increased Doppler flow. **E:** Acute cholecystitis causing dilatation of the cystic duct *(CD)*. **F:** Acute cholecystitis with a stone stuck in the gallbladder neck. *GB*, gallbladder.

acalculous cholecystitis (AAC).[5] A combination of stagnant bile and direct vascular changes may be responsible for AAC. High concentrations of stagnant bile can be directly toxic and cause overdistension of the gallbladder, leading to vascular compromise. Viscous stagnant bile can also act as a functional obstruction of gallbladder outflow, providing an excellent pathway for secondary bacterial invasion. Direct vascular changes, such as clotting, occur with severe burns and trauma. This leads to selective thrombosis of vessels supplying the gallbladder, followed by ischemia, necrosis, secondary bacterial involvement, infection, and possibly perforation through the gallbladder wall.[28,32,33]

The majority of acalculous cholecystitis cases occur in patients in the intensive care unit. There are multiple other causes of AAC, including trauma, surgery, severe burns, sepsis, long-term TPN, prolonged fasting, diabetes, and HIV.[2,5,19,20,29]

Clinically, the signs and symptoms of acalculous cholecystitis are indistinguishable and somewhat nonspecific. Patients often present with RUQ pain and a positive Murphy sign. Other symptoms include nausea, vomiting, distention, fever, and a palpable RUQ mass.[8,28] Symptoms of AAC can occur 24 hours to 50 days after the initial event but usually occur within 2 weeks.[32] Because of the difficultly in diagnosis, acalculous cholecystitis has a high morbidity and mortality rate.[20]

Sonographically, the gallbladder is often distended with a thickened wall and internal debris or sludge.[5] Wall thickening with hypoechoic areas within the wall and pericholecystic fluid can also be seen.[19,29] Diagnosis, however, is often difficult because of the absence of gallstones. Also, the patient's mental status (i.e., patient is sedated) hinders the evaluation of a positive Murphy sign (Fig. 8-30A–D).[5]

There are two schools of thought regarding the treatment of acute cholecystitis. Mortality rates from AAC far exceed

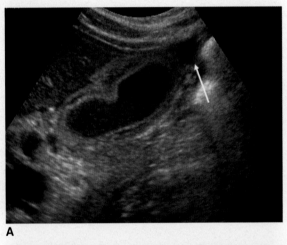

A

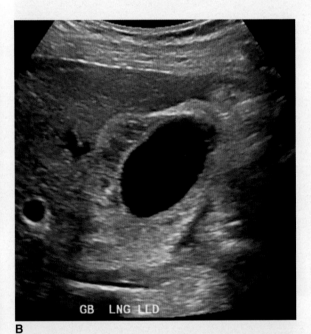

GB   LNG LLD

B

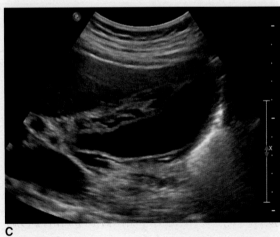

C

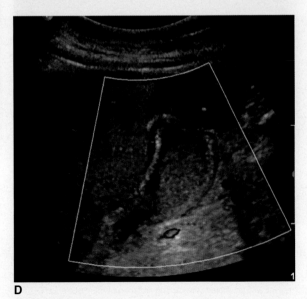

D

FIGURE 8-30 Acute acalculous cholecystitis. **A:** Thickened gallbladder wall, sludge, and pericholecystic fluid *(arrow)* are seen in this longitudinal image. The patient had right upper quadrant pain, nausea, and vomiting. **B:** Transverse image showing a thickened gallbladder wall in this patient with acute acalculous cholecystitis. **C:** Longitudinal image in a patient with a positive Murphy sign and fever. The gallbladder wall is thickened and edematous. **D:** Longitudinal image in an ICU patient. Thickened wall and a large amount of sludge is visualized.

those from acute calculous cholecystitis. This could be due to several factors, such as the lack of clinical and laboratory specificity in the diagnosis of AAC.[28,34] Gangrene of the gallbladder can also occur in patients with AAC. Again, early diagnosis and treatment is the best way to avoid or minimize complications.[5]

Complicated Cholecystitis

Patients with acute cholecystitis are at risk for developing empyema, gallbladder perforation, gangrenous cholecystitis, or emphysematous cholecystitis.[5,19]

Empyema

Empyema or suppurative cholecystitis, pus in the gallbladder, typically occurs in diabetic patients. The pus-filled gallbladder resembles sludge on a sonogram. Patients present with symptoms comparable to cholecystitis, including fever, chills, and RUQ pain. Signs of sepsis can be present. A magnetic resonance image (MRI) or a percutaneous needle aspiration of the gallbladder is helpful to distinguish pus from sludge.[19,29] Patients with empyema are treated with cholecystectomy and IV antimicrobial therapy.[29]

Gallbladder Perforation

Two to 11% of patients with acute cholecystitis will have a gallbladder perforation.[35] Typically, perforations occur in the fundus because of chronic inflammation and low amount of blood flow to this area.[2,5] With an acute perforation, the bile leak will cause peritonitis; however, acute perforations are uncommon. Subacute perforations, which are more common, result in an abscess formation. The abscesses can occur in or around the gallbladder or liver or within the peritoneal cavity.[5] Gallbladder perforation is a life-threatening condition with high mortality rates (12% to 42%) that have not improved despite medical advances. Age, delay in treatment, and sepsis are the main factors contributing to a high mortality rate.[35]

Clinically, patients present with RUQ pain, nausea, vomiting, and fever. Laboratory work may reveal an increased WBC and abnormal liver function tests.[36] On sonogram, a complex fluid collection (abscess), irregular gallbladder wall, gallstones, inflammatory changes within the gallbladder fossa, and a focal defect of the gallbladder wall can also be seen.[5,19,37,38] Defects are typically focal and small; however, they can be large and involve a considerable portion of the wall (Fig. 8-31A, B). Computed tomography (CT) may be helpful in determining wall defects.[38] In order to avoid sepsis, an early cholecystectomy should be performed.[37] Despite imaging advancements, early identification by ultrasound or CT is difficult, with only fair sensitivity.[35]

Gangrenous Cholecystitis

Gangrenous cholecystitis is caused by absent blood supply or infection. The gallbladder wall becomes ischemic and eventually necrotic.[5,20] Approximately 2% to 38% of acute cholecystitis cases will develop into gangrenous cholecystitis.[20] Clinically, patients are acutely ill, and a positive sonographic Murphy sign is present in one-third of patients; however, a positive sign may not be present because of nerve damage and, therefore, the patient presents with diffuse versus localized pain.[5,29] Laboratory work may reveal an increased WBC.[29]

Sonography is often nonspecific in the diagnosis of gangrenous cholecystitis. A thickened, irregular gallbladder wall with both hyperechoic and hypoechoic striations is also suggestive of gangrenous cholecystitis.[5] Intraluminal membranes from sloughing off the walls and fibrous strands may be visualized on sonography. Gas within the gallbladder wall, or lumen, an absent gallbladder wall, or an abscess may also be seen.[20] Gallbladder perforation occurs early or late in the course of acute cholecystitis (Fig. 8-32A–D).[39]

Because of the increased mortality and morbidity rates, early cholecystectomy and IV antimicrobial therapy are advised if gangrenous cholecystitis is suspected.[19,20,29]

Emphysematous Cholecystitis

Emphysematous cholecystitis, a rare form of acute cholecystitis, is a condition in which gas-forming bacteria invade

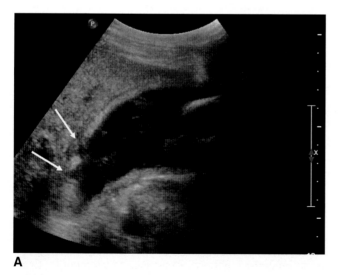
A

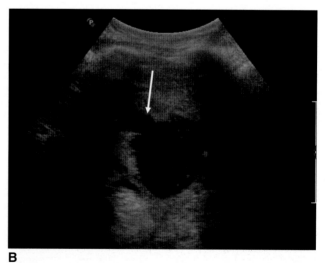
B

FIGURE 8-31 Longitudinal (**A**) and transverse (**B**) images in a patient with gallbladder perforation. The defect seen on the anterior wall (*arrows*) is better demonstrated in the transverse section. Debris is also located within the gallbladder lumen.

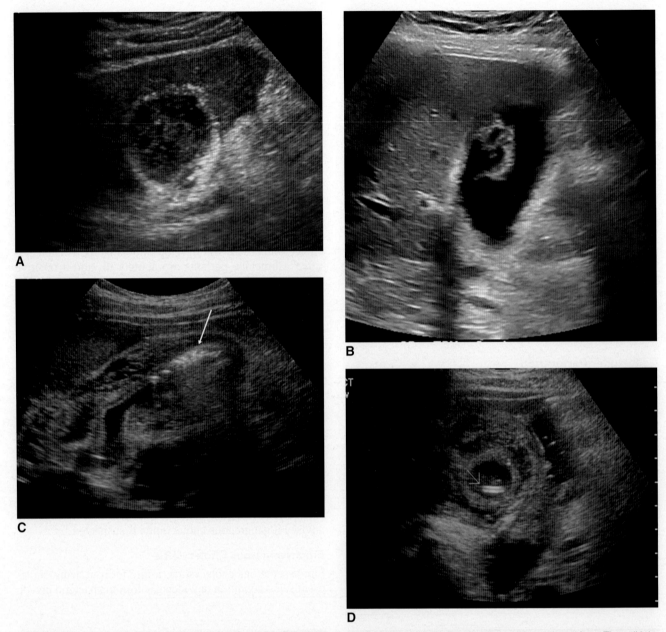

FIGURE 8-32 Gangrenous cholecystitis. Transverse (**A**) and longitudinal (**B**) images in an acutely ill patient with right upper quadrant pain and fever. The wall is irregularly thickened. **C:** Longitudinal image in the latter stages of gangrenous cholecystitis. Air *(arrow)* is seen within the fundus of the contracted gallbladder. The wall is also thickened and edematous. **D:** A stent *(arrow)* was placed within the gallbladder in this patient with gangrenous cholecystitis. The patient was acutely ill and unable to have a cholecystectomy. Note the thick gallbladder wall and ascites.

the gallbladder wall, lumen, pericholecystic spaces, and on occasion the bile ducts. This condition is more common in men, and as many as 40% of cases are associated with diabetes. Many cases do not contain gallstones; however, they are more common in acute cases. Patients present with sudden progressive RUQ pain, fever, nausea, and vomiting. Patients with emphysematous cholecystitis are likely to develop a gangrenous gallbladder or abscess formation. Gallbladder perforation can also occur.[2,5,29,40] Emphysematous cholecystitis is fatal in about 15% of cases.[2]

Sonographically, gas bubbles are prominent, non–gravity-dependent, and change with patient position. Air appears as echogenic foci within the gallbladder's wall or lumen, causing the gallbladder wall to appear echogenic. Ring-down or comet tail artifacts are also seen.[2,20] This may make it difficult to visualize the gallbladder with emphysematous cholecystitis sonographically. Common features that help differentiate gangrenous cholecystitis from a porcelain gallbladder are that a porcelain gallbladder occurs in the wall, is smooth, and has a homogeneous shadow. With emphysematous cholecystitis, the near-field echoes tend to be dimpled and are not smooth as seen in the porcelain gallbladder (Fig. 8-33A–D). A CT or noncontrast radiography can be performed to distinguish air from calcification.[29,40]

In critical patients, percutaneous cholecystostomy and IV antimicrobial therapy can be used as a temporary treatment. Emphysematous cholecystitis is considered a surgical emergency and should be treated with cholecystectomy.[20,29]

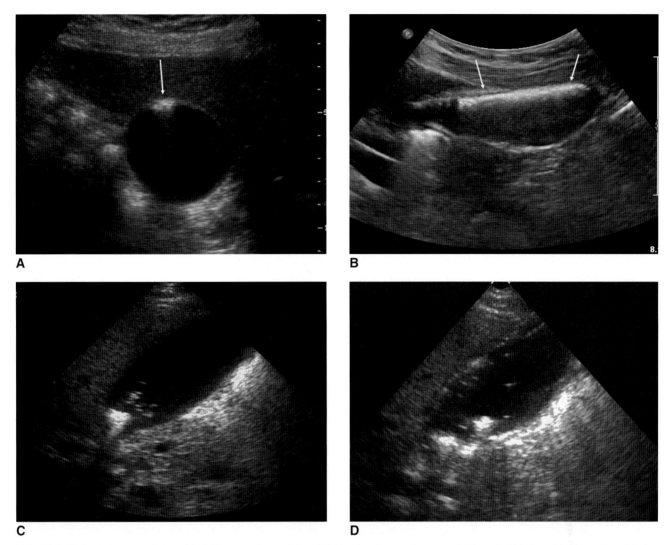

FIGURE 8-33 Emphysematous cholecystitis. **A:** Transverse image of the gallbladder showing a small amount of air *(arrow)* within the gallbladder wall in a diabetic patient. **B:** Longitudinal image in a different patient with a larger amount of air *(arrows)* in the wall. With emphysematous cholecystitis, air can be seen within both the wall and gallbladder lumen. **C:** With the patient supine, air within the gallbladder is seen at the neck. **D:** When the patient rolls into a left decubitus position, the air moves out of the neck and swirls within the gallbladder lumen.

Chronic Cholecystitis and Associated Conditions

Chronic cholecystitis, a common form of symptomatic gallbladder disease, is virtually always associated with stones.[29] By definition, there is chronic inflammation of the gallbladder wall, and it is often incidentally found on sonography.[5,26] Repeated acute attacks produce a series of inflammatory changes that result in thickening and fibrosis of the gallbladder wall as well as contraction of the gallbladder.[5,29]

Chronic cholecystitis affects women more frequently than men, and it occurs most often in the elderly.[26] The patient tends to have intolerance to fatty or fried foods, possibly associated with intermittent nausea and vomiting. There is often moderate RUQ and epigastric pain, which may radiate to the scapula. These attacks may be frequent or years apart. The patient, however, can also be asymptomatic.[2,3,8] Alkaline phosphates, AST, and ALT levels may be elevated. If jaundice is present, the direct bilirubin value is also

elevated. It is possible for an attack of acute cholecystitis to be superimposed on underlying chronic disease, in which case, some clinical and sonographic features of both entities could be present.[3,8]

Without cholecystectomy, complications sometimes arise from untreated chronic cholecystitis. Bouveret syndrome, or gallstone ileus, is a complication that occurs when a biliary-enteric fistula forms between the gallbladder and the duodenum. Large stones can erode through the gallbladder wall and into the duodenal bulb, where they become impacted in the duodenal lumen. There, the stone may cause gastric outlet obstruction (gastric dilatation) or distal bowel obstruction in the ileum, colon, or rectum, or it may be passed spontaneously. This condition should be considered, especially in women older than 60 years with symptoms of upper intestinal obstruction as well as gallbladder disease.[41,42] Another possible complication of untreated cholecystitis is Mirizzi syndrome in which a gallstone becomes impacted in the gallbladder neck or cystic duct, exerting pressure on the adjacent common duct.[29]

The sonographic features of chronic cholecystitis are a small, contracted gallbladder with stones and an evenly thickened, fibrous echogenic wall. A stone is often lodged within the neck (Fig. 8-34A–D).[26]

A porcelain gallbladder occurs when all or part of the gallbladder wall is calcified (Fig. 8-35A, B). It is a relatively rare manifestation of chronic cholecystitis, and it is more common in men.[5,19] It is associated with a high incidence of gallbladder carcinoma.[2,19] Sonographically, a single echogenic line representing the calcified wall is seen. All or part of the wall may be calcified. If the wall is strongly calcified, a posterior shadow is also seen, which can obscure the gallbladder. Differential diagnosis consists of gallstones or emphysematous cholecystitis.[2,5] CT or noncontrast radiography may assist in the diagnosis of porcelain gallbladder.[19]

Gallbladder Wall Thickening

The gallbladder wall is thickened, when it measures greater than 3 mm.[2,24] Approximately 50% of patients with acute cholecystitis will have gallbladder wall thickening. The nonfasting patient will also have a thickened gallbladder wall.[19] There are several other causes of gallbladder wall thickening including adenomyomatosis, gallbladder carcinoma, hepatic congestions, congestive heart failure, hypoalbuminemia, hypertension, and infections including hepatitis, pancreatitis, and HIV (Pathology Box 8-1).[5,19,20] Wall thickening alone is still a nonspecific finding, and further research is needed to determine whether analysis of specific morphologic features will help differentiate acute cholecystitis (Fig. 8-36A–E).[27]

Cholestasis and Pregnancy

Intrahepatic cholestasis occurs during the second and third trimesters of pregnancy and resolves shortly after delivery. The patient presents with pruritus. Laboratory values show elevated alkaline phosphatase, serum transaminase, and bile acids. Even though it is a benign condition for the mother, the fetus is at risk for prematurity, dysrhythmia, distress, or intrauterine death. By sonography, gallstones may be detected; however, there is no ductal dilatation.[16,43,44]

Gallbladder Neoplasms

Benign

Gallbladder polyps are masses that extend from the gallbladder musoca. They are present in 0.3% to 12% of healthy

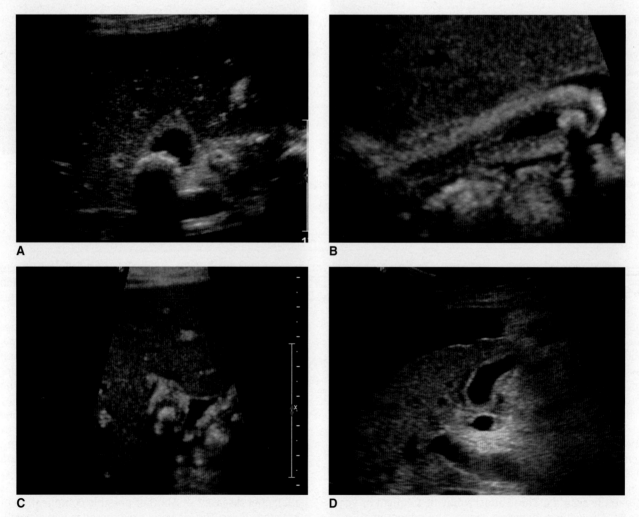

FIGURE 8-34 Chronic cholecystitis. **A:** Longitudinal image in a patient with continued right upper quadrant pain. A stone is seen within the neck of a contracted gallbladder. The stone did not shift even though the patient moved into multiple positions. **B:** Longitudinal and (**C**) transverse images demonstrate thickened gallbladder wall, stone, and ascites. **D:** In a patient with chronic cholecystitis, cirrhosis, and ascites, a contracted gallbladder is seen on the sonogram.

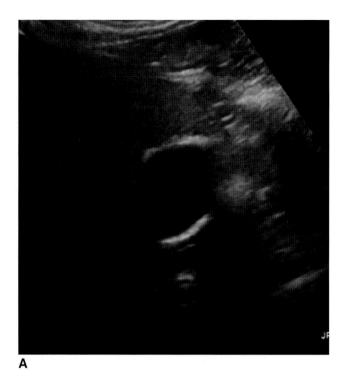

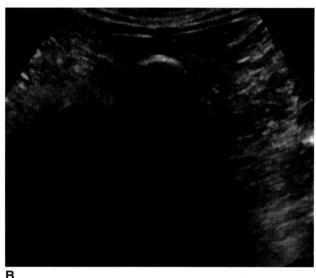

A   **B**

FIGURE 8-35 Porcelain gallbladder. **A:** Transverse image showing a calcified anterior and posterior wall. **B:** In the same patient, at times, the anterior calcified wall is strongly calcified and the posterior wall cannot be seen.

PATHOLOGY BOX 8-1
Causes of Gallbladder Wall Thickening

Intrinsic Causes

Acute cholecystitis

Chronic cholecystitis

Gangrenous cholecystitis

Emphysematous cholecystitis

Adenomyomatosis

Polyp

Gallbladder carcinoma: primary or metastatic

Gallbladder torsion

Extrinsic Causes

Right-sided heart failure

Alcoholic liver disease

Hepatitis

AIDS

Sepsis

Hypoalbuminemia

Renal failure

Ascites (benign)

Multiple myeloma

Portal node lymphatic obstruction

Systemic venous hypertension

Gallbladder wall varices

Physiologic Causes

Contracted gallbladder after eating

---

individuals. Because of the use of abdominal ultrasound for various unrelated indications, gallbladder polyps are found in 0.3% to 12% of healthy individuals. Polyps are often asymptomatic and are incidentally found on imaging studies.[45] Unlike cholelithiasis, polyps do not have any association with gender, age, or obesity.[46]

The majority of gallbladder polyps are composed of cholesterol and are considered benign; however, early stage gallbladder cancers can present as polyps. Although rare, polyps can be classified as adenomas.[45,46] Adenomas are pedunculated, well-circumscribed lesions within the gallbladder that typically measure less than 2 cm.[45,47] When large, adenomas may become more heterogeneous. Polyps greater than 1 cm are suggestive of malignancy.[47] Malignant potential in a polyp can be as high as 27%.[45]

The majority of polyps are caused by chronic inflammation, hyperplasia of the gallbladder wall, or lipid deposits.[48] Polyps are fixed, nonmobile lesions that do not display a posterior shadow. They can be single or multiple (Fig. 8-37A–D).[47] Care should be taken to not misdiagnose a polyp as sludge, gallstones, or a malignant lesion.[36,45] Treatment involves removal of polyps greater than 1 cm if the patient is over 50 years old. Any polyp that is growing, even when less than 1 cm, should be removed because of the increased risk of malignancy.[5,48,49] Moreover, the gallbladder should be removed in the setting of polyps and primary sclerosing cholangitis (PSC).[49,50]

Malignancies

The vast majority of gallbladder malignancies are adenocarcinomas and predominately affect women with an average age of 72.[50,51] The remaining small percentage is composed

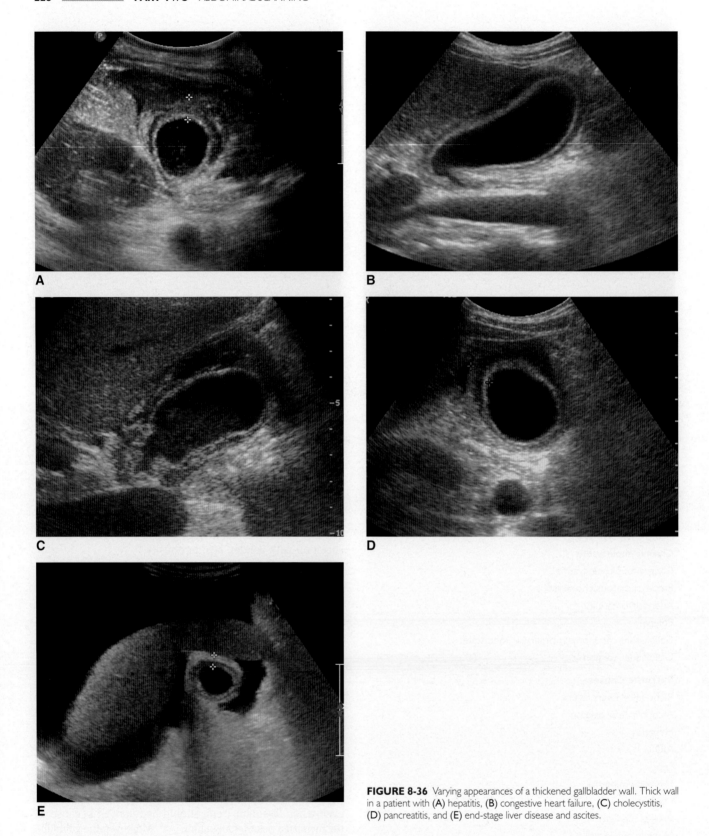

FIGURE 8-36 Varying appearances of a thickened gallbladder wall. Thick wall in a patient with (**A**) hepatitis, (**B**) congestive heart failure, (**C**) cholecystitis, (**D**) pancreatitis, and (**E**) end-stage liver disease and ascites.

of wall tumors, metastases, and lymphoma. Even though gallbladder cancer is uncommon, it is the fifth most common malignancy of the digestive system. The primary risk factors are chronic cholecystitis and cholelithiasis; however, rapidly growing polyps and a porcelain abgladder are also well-documented risks for developing gallbladder cancer.[5,24,52,53]

Other risk factors include PSC, ductal anomalies, and choledochal cysts.[5] Gallstones are present in as many as 95% of cases, and a porcelain gallbladder is seen in approximately 25% of gallbladder cancers.[51,54]

Gallbladder carcinoma can metastasize to the liver, lymph nodes, CHD, and other surrounding organs.[53] Intraductal

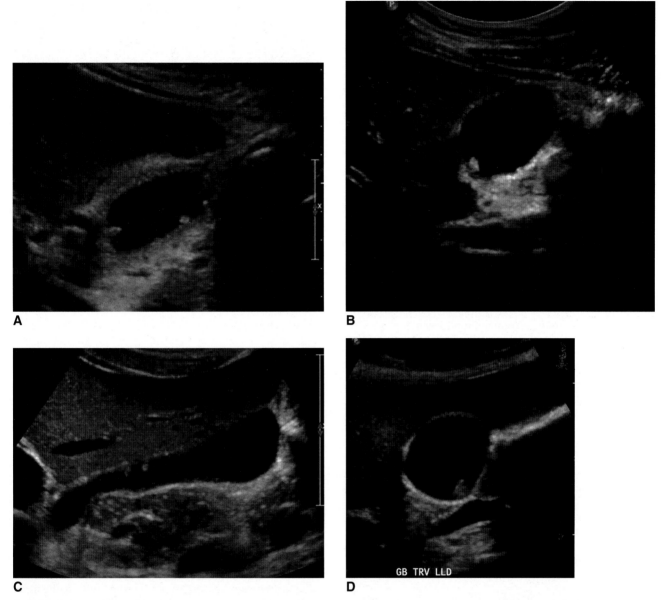

A

B

C

D

FIGURE 8-37 Polyps can be small, large, single, or multiple **(A–D)**. Careful evaluation is needed to ensure that polyps are not mistaken for gallbladder folds or sludge balls.

spread occurs in at least 4% of cases and can clinically mimic pancreatic or bile duct tumors. Gallbladder cancer is often difficult to detect in its early stages, because patients may be asymptomatic or present with the signs and symptoms of cholelithiasis or cholecystitis. In addition, there are no laboratory alternatives to assist in early diagnosis. In the late stages of gallbladder carcinoma, patients will have jaundice, malaise, or weight loss.[51,53] The majority of gallbladder carcinomas are found incidentally during routine cholecystectomy. Despite imaging advancements, only 50% of gallbladder carcinomas are diagnosed preoperatively.[55] Cholecystectomy should be performed if metastasis has not yet occurred. The 5-year survival rate for primary gallbladder carcinoma is less than 5%.[49]

If gallbladder carcinoma is diagnosed by sonography, it is typically in the advanced stage. At this point, a heterogeneous, irregular-shaped mass replaces the gallbladder. Tumefactive sludge or sludge balls can mimic a malignant gallbladder mass.[5,9,53] Direct invasion into the liver, irregular wall thickening, or a poorly defined polypoid mass may also be seen (Fig. 8-38A, B). In addition, a gallbladder mass greater than 1 cm, wall thickening greater than 1 cm, or disruption of the gallbladder wall should increase suspicion of malignancy.[5,53] Gallstones encased in tumor are also a sign of gallbladder carcinoma.[53] Color Doppler imaging may be useful to establish the internal vascularity that is often present in malignancies.[56] Contrast-enhanced sonography may also be beneficial to differentiate benign from malignant masses.[9] Differential diagnosis for gallbladder cancer includes hepatocarcinoma, cholangiocarcinoma, and metastases. On the other hand, the benign differential diagnosis includes cholecystitis, polyps, and inflammatory and noninflammatory diseases. When a gallbladder malignancy is suspected, it is imperative to search the entire abdomen for other signs of malignancy such as liver metastases, vascular invasion, biliary dilatation, porta hepatis nodes, retroperitoneal adenopathy, or ascites.[53]

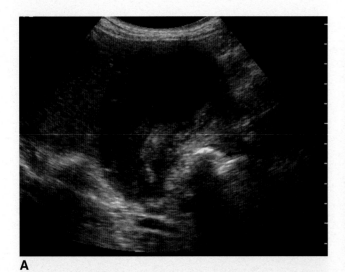

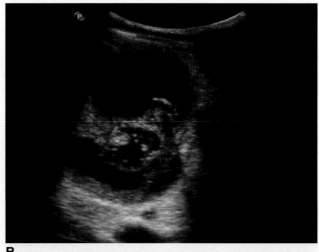

FIGURE 8-38 Gallbladder carcinoma. **A:** Echoes completely fill the gallbladder lumen. A stone *(arrow)* was seen at the posterior portion of the gallbladder. Note the irregularly thickened, heterogeneous gallbladder wall. **B:** A heterogeneous mass extending from the gallbladder wall represents gallbladder carcinoma.

Melanoma is the most common tumor to metastasize to the gallbladder. Even with therapy, melanoma metastasis to the gallbladder carries a poor prognosis; however, long-term survival is occasionally seen.[57,58] Melanoma metastasis to the gallbladder is not associated with cholelithiasis, which differs from gallbladder cancer. Sonographic findings, however, are similar to asymmetric wall thickening and solitary or multiple masses within the gallbladder. Treatment of metastatic melanoma to the gallbladder is cholecystectomy.[59]

Other blood-borne metastases to the gallbladder can occur from the lungs, kidneys, and esophagus. Metastases from the stomach, pancreas, and bile ducts can reach the gallbladder by direct invasion. Malignancy of the liver, ovary, and colon can also metastasize to the gallbladder. Primary gallbladder cancer is strongly associated with stones and inflammatory gallbladder disease; however, metastatic disease is completely independent of cholelithiasis and cholecystitis.[27,55]

Hyperplastic Cholecystoses

Hyperplastic cholecystoses are a group of benign, noninflammatory conditions that are both degenerative and proliferative. They include adenomyomatosis, cholesterolosis, neuromatosis, fibromatosis, and lipomatosis.[3]

Adenomyomatosis is a common condition characterized by excessive proliferation of the surface epithelium, with gland-like formations and outpouchings of the mucosa into or through a thickened muscle layer. These pouches, or diverticula, are called Rokitansky–Aschoff sinuses.[60,61] There are three forms of adenomyomatosis: (1) diffuse, involving the entire gallbladder; (2) segmental, in which the proximal, middle, or distal one-third is involved circumferentially; and (3) localized, the most common type, confined almost exclusively to the fundus.[19] It is more common in women, and patients generally present with RUQ pain. The sonographic appearance includes focal or diffuse wall thickening; small, round, anechoic spaces in the gallbladder wall represent Rokitansky–Aschoff sinuses and echogenic foci spaced at varying intervals in the gallbladder wall. These echogenic foci display acoustic shadowing or comet tail reverberation artifacts with a twinkle artifact on color Doppler.[19,60,61]

Gallstones are also common (Fig. 8-39A–D).[60] Diagnosis is often made by sonography; however, adenomyomatosis can be misdiagnosed as gallbladder carcinoma, emphysematous cholecystitis, or chronic cholecystitis.[60,61]

Cholesterosis is characterized by lipid-laden macrophages that deposit within the gallbladder wall. Cholesterol polyps make up approximately 20% of these deposits; however, they represent 50% of all gallbladder polyps.[5] It occurs more frequently in women than in men.[4] The lesions may be diffuse, with no impairment of gallbladder function, or localized single or multiple polypoid lesions, which may be pedunculated and interfere with function.[3] A diffuse form of cholesterolosis is known as a "strawberry gallbladder" (Fig. 8-40). At gross examination, the mucosa is bright red with areas of yellow fat. There is no malignant association with this process.[46]

Neuromatosis and fibromatosis are rare proliferations of nerve and fibrous tissue, respectively. Lipomatosis is an excessive buildup of fat layers in the gallbladder wall. These three processes may or may not interfere with gallbladder function and are often not visualized sonographically.[3]

The hyperplastic cholecystoses are often asymptomatic, but when symptoms do occur, they often mimic those of cholelithiasis. Stones may or may not be present. Laboratory values are usually normal unless function is impaired. The risk of malignancy is low. Cholecystectomy should be considered in symptomatic patients.[3]

These lesions may not be detected sonographically, but when visible, the appearance can vary. Fixed polypoid lesions or a small misshapen gallbladder may be seen.[3]

Miscellaneous Gallbladder Pathology

An enlarged, distended, palpable, and nontender gallbladder in a jaundiced patient is referred to as a Courvoisier gallbladder. It occurs when there is obstruction of the CBD, typically owing to a malignant neoplasm at the pancreatic head.[62] With any distal mass, dilation begins with the gallbladder, followed by the common duct, and finally the intrahepatic tree. Upon removal of the obstructing mass, the gallbladder decompresses actively (because of its contractile muscle), whereas the ducts passively return to normal in reverse order.[63]

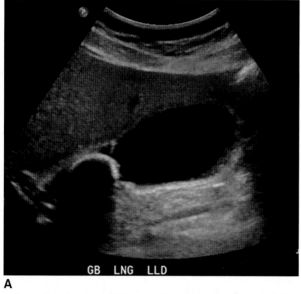

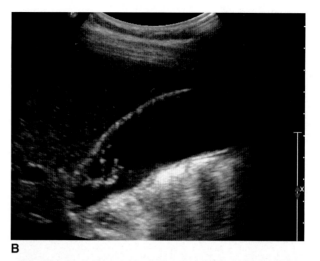

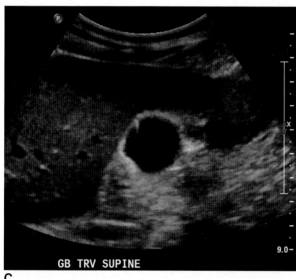

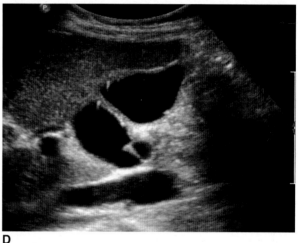

FIGURE 8-39 Adenomyomatosis. **A:** Thickened wall with echogenic foci and comet tail artifact near the neck of the gallbladder. **B:** Adenomyomatosis throughout the majority of the anterior gallbladder wall. Sludge was also seen. **C, D:** Comet tail artifacts are seen at the body of the gallbladder representing adenomyomatosis.

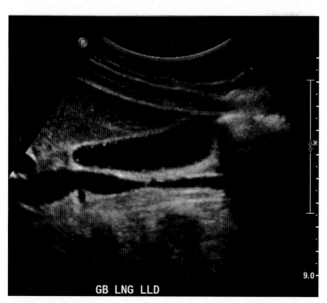

FIGURE 8-40 Strawberry gallbladder. Longitudinal image of the gallbladder demonstrating multiple small, nonshadowing foci consistent with cholesterolosis.

A hydropic gallbladder is abnormally distended and filled with thick bile, mucus, or pus. The most common cause of hydropic gallbladder is a stone obstructing the gallbladder neck or cystic duct. There are numerous other causes including hyperalimentation, a variety of infections, and any obstruction of the CBD or cystic duct. The obstruction leads to gradual reabsorption of the bile despite continued accumulation of secretions from the gallbladder wall. The patient may be asymptomatic or present with RUQ pain, nausea, and vomiting; a palpable mass; and the symptoms of the underlying pathology. Sonographically, the gallbladder is rounded, distended, measures greater than 4 cm in AP diameter, and may have stones (Fig. 8-41A, B).[64]

Hydatid cysts of the gallbladder are rare. Parasitosis, caused by *Echinococcus granulosus*, enters the gallbladder through the cystic duct via the liver. The gallbladder can also become affected if there is an intrabiliary rupture of a cyst or a direct rupture of a cyst into the gallbladder. A primary hydatid cyst of the gallbladder is rare. On sonography, the appearance is described as a "cyst within a cyst."[65]

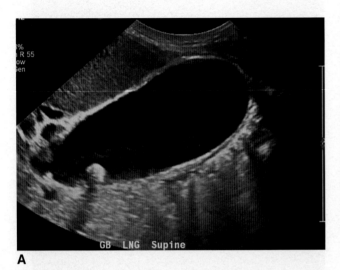

A

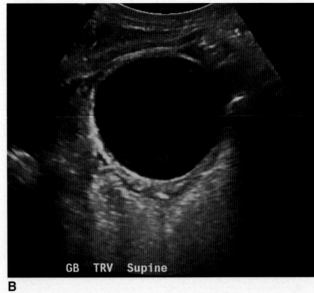

B

FIGURE 8-41 Hydropic gallbladder. Longitudinal (**A**) and transverse (**B**) images in a patient with right upper quadrant pain, nausea, vomiting, and a palpable mass. The gallbladder measured greater than 4 cm in the anteroposterior diameter. Sludge, stone, and a thickened gallbladder wall were also noted.

Torsion, or volvulus, of the gallbladder is rare, but its incidence may be increasing possibly owing to the increase in life expectancy. It can occur at all ages but is more common in elderly patients. It is three times more frequent in women than in men. The cause is uncertain but is thought to be lengthening of the gallbladder mesentery in old age that allows the gallbladder to be free floating on a pedicle. Vigorous bowel peristalsis, a mobile gallbladder fundus, gallstones, atherosclerosis of the cystic artery, and kyphosis have all been implicated as predisposing or contributing factors. Pathologically, the walls of the twisted gallbladder become thickened, edematous, and hemorrhagic. Gangrene or a palpable mass may be present. The sonographic features include gross wall thickening and a distended tender gallbladder.[20,66,67] Color Doppler imaging may be helpful to visualize the cystic artery. Gallstones are seldom present. The appearance and laboratory values are often nonspecific. Sonography is the modality of choice; however, CT, magnetic resonance cholangiopancreatography (MRCP), and hepato-iminodiacetic acid (HIDA) scans can be helpful. The diagnosis of torsion is seldom made preoperatively. The treatment is immediate cholecystectomy.[67]

The Postcholecystectomy Patient

In postcholecystectomy patients, the gallbladder fossa is commonly filled with bowel loops, although closer examination may reveal echogenic foci with reverberations and/or shadows representing surgical clips. Occasionally, postoperative evaluation of the gallbladder fossa may demonstrate fluid collections. These range from asymptomatic, simple anechoic collections to complex abscesses with the associated clinical presentation (Pathology Box 8-2).

Controversy exists over whether the size of the common duct should increase after the gallbladder is removed. Some indicate that the duct may increase in caliber because it becomes a floppy, passive tube from previous episodes of inflammation, or as the result of surgical exploration of the duct at

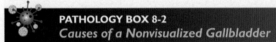

PATHOLOGY BOX 8-2
Causes of a Nonvisualized Gallbladder

Patient is nonfasting
Postcholecystectomy
Contracted gallbladder with stones (chronic cholecystitis)
Congenitally absent gallbladder
Porcelain gallbladder
Hepatization of gallbladder
Mirizzi syndrome or gallstone ileus
Gallbladder neoplasms completely filling lumen
Ectopic gallbladder
Emphysematous gallbladder
Overlying bowel
Residual barium in nearby bowel

the time of cholecystectomy. Another theory is the duct may act as a reservoir for bile in the absence of the gallbladder.[68] Although some studies state that a normal postcholecystectomy common duct can measure up to 11 mm, others consider it dilated if it exceeds 6 mm in maximum intraluminal AP diameter. Yet another study suggests that the extrahepatic bile duct may measure 1 mm larger than expected after a cholecystectomy.[69] Rescanning 30 to 45 minutes after a fatty meal may help determine whether obstruction truly exists. Fatty meals stimulate biliary flow and relax the sphincter of Oddi. If a normal or slightly dilated duct enlarges after a fatty meal or if an abnormally large duct fails to shrink, CBD obstruction is strongly indicated. After a fatty meal, healthy, nondilated, patent ducts should decrease slightly in caliber if they change at all. A slight decrease in diameter virtually excludes obstruction.[68,70] Fatty meals are especially useful to confirm that an asymptomatic patient with equivocal or mildly prominent ducts has normal function.[70]

Postcholecystectomy syndrome is not a true syndrome; however, it refers to the recurrence of preoperative symptoms, particularly biliary colic. Incomplete relief may be caused by an error in the original diagnosis of gallbladder disease. Retained common duct stones, biliary strictures, and chronic pancreatitis are the most frequent causes. Others include an excessive cystic duct stump, sphincter of Oddi spasms, biliary tract carcinomas, an amputation neuroma, and adhesions constricting the CBD.[62]

Bile Duct Obstruction

Bile duct obstruction, either intrahepatic or extrahepatic, causes a direct interference with the flow of bile (Fig. 8-42A–E). The obstruction can be from an intrinsic or extrinsic cause such as stones, benign or malignant tumors, and strictures.[5] Causes of biliary obstruction depend on the location. Intrahepatic biliary obstruction can be caused by PSC or any space-occupying mass within the liver. Obstruction at the porta hepatis can be caused by cholangiocarcinoma, PSC, gallbladder cancer, or metastatic tumors. Biliary obstruction at the pancreas includes causes such as pancreatic cancer, pancreatitis, choledocholithiasis, or cholangiocarcinoma.[6] A previous episode of obstruction or inflammation with loss of elasticity or an ampullary dysfunction may also cause the duct to dilate.[68]

Clinically, the patient will present with RUQ pain, jaundice, and fever. In the obstructed patient, bilirubin or alkaline phosphatase can be elevated.[5] A duct can also appear normal despite abnormal laboratory values. This is more likely to occur in patients with fibrosed or infiltrated livers because the hardened, noncompliant liver prohibits the ducts from dilating. Conversely, a duct can be abnormal even though laboratory values are normal.[70] Duct size can also change sporadically because it is part of a dynamic system that responds as obstructions occur and resolve.[69]

By sonography, the bile ducts should be measured inner wall to inner wall (Fig. 8-6).[5] The use of color Doppler imaging is essential to distinguish bile ducts from small hepatic vessels.[2,53] The CHD is considered dilated if the internal diameter measures greater than 6 mm or CBD measures greater than 8 mm.[69] Again, there is currently debate over whether the bile duct increases with age or after a cholecystectomy. Intrahepatic ducts measuring greater than 2 mm in diameter or more than 40% of the adjacent portal vein are considered dilated.[2,5] Additional sonographic criteria for intrahepatic dilatation include (1) the parallel channel sign (double-barrel sign), representing the dilated duct running anterior to its accompanying portal vein or hepatic artery; (2) irregular, jagged walls and branching patterns of the ducts (compared with smooth walls and smooth bifurcations of the portal venous system); and (3) stellate confluence of dilated ducts converging toward the porta hepatis (Fig. 8-43A–D).[1,56,71]

Sonography is also an important tool in locating the level and cause of obstruction (Fig. 8-44A, B). The findings depend on the type and location of the obstruction (dilatation may be intrahepatic, extrahepatic, or both).[1] With any type of blockage, the duct becomes dilated proximal to the obstruction.[6] For example, if the obstruction is at the porta hepatis, the intrahepatic ducts will become dilated, but the duct between the porta hepatis and pancreas will be normal.[2] With real-time scanning, it is easier to trace the extent of ductal dilatation. It is also important to note whether obstruction is focal or diffuse. The entire course and caliber of the duct must be examined for dilatation (Table 8-2). It is also important to note the duct at the obstruction. If the duct tapers at the obstruction, it is typically a benign process. If, however, the duct ends abruptly, there is an increased association with malignancy. It is also important to evaluate the ductal wall. Diffuse wall thickening is associated with cholangitis, whereas focal thickening is seen with stones, pancreatitis, and pancreatic carcinoma.[6]

Other conditions that can mimic dilated intrahepatic biliary radicles are Caroli disease (communicating cavernous ectasia of the intrahepatic ducts), enlarged hepatic arteries, cavernous transformation of the portal vein, and intrahepatic arteriovenous malformations.[56,71]

Choledocholithiasis

Stones within the bile duct are the most common pathology of the biliary tract.[5,6] Common duct stones are usually formed in the gallbladder, and then pass into the CBD, where they may cause an obstruction (Fig. 8-45). After cholecystectomy, stones may be retained within the duct or they may form spontaneously. Choledocholithiasis may lead to cholangitis.[72]

Patients with choledocholithiasis may be asymptomatic unless obstruction occurs. Small stones may remain in the duct without obstructing or may pass silently out into the

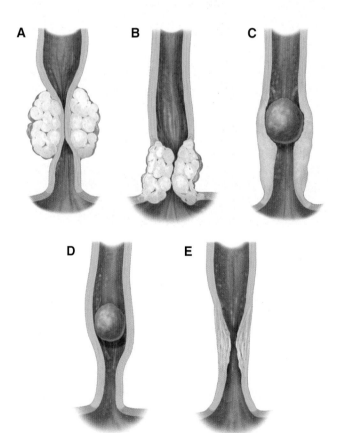

FIGURE 8-42 Types of extrahepatic biliary obstruction. **A–C**: Complete common bile duct obstructions and (**D, E**) incomplete obstructions. **A**: Extrinsic cancer fixing and compressing duct, (**B**) intrinsic cancer, (**C**) impacted stone with edema of duct, (**D**) ball-in-valve stone causing intermittent obstruction, and (**E**) stricture of duct.

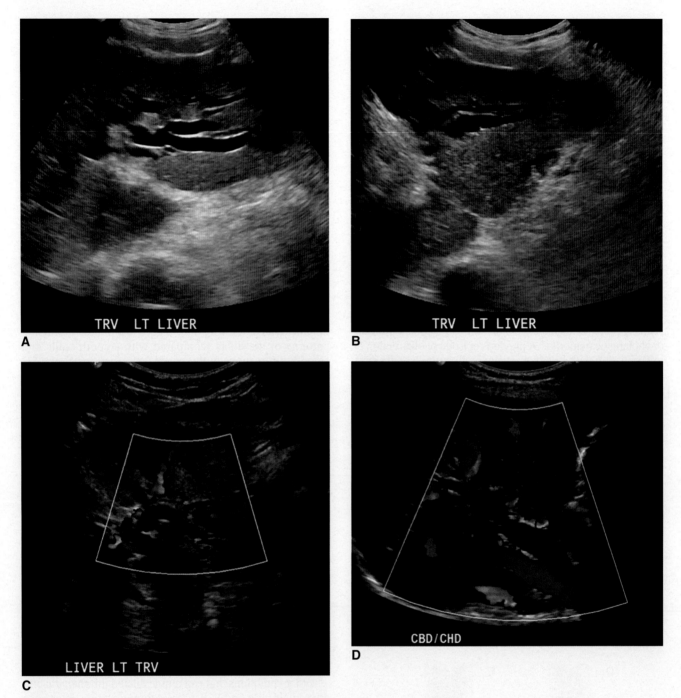

FIGURE 8-43 Dilated intrahepatic ducts. **A, B:** Parallel channel sign of dilated intrahepatic ducts. One channel represents the dilated duct and the other its accompanying portal vein. **C, D:** Stellate confluence of irregular branching channels represents dilated intrahepatic ducts.

bowel. The clinical symptoms of ductal stones may include RUQ pain, intermittent or persistent obstructive jaundice, and cholangitis. With obstruction, bilirubin, alkaline phosphatase, and transaminase values increase.[70] The patient may have temporary relief of symptoms if the stone passes into the duodenum or returns into the gallbladder.[24]

Common duct stones are found in 8% to 20% of patients undergoing cholecystectomy and 2% to 4% of patients following cholecystectomy.[6] Sonographically, stones can be visualized in dilated or nondilated ducts, although stones are typically easier to identify in the dilated duct. Bile duct

stones can create a shadow, be single or multiple, large or small, mobile, or stationary (Fig. 8-46A–D).[5,6] Small stones may be difficult to detect because of their location and bowel gas.[24] The duct can also be packed with stones, producing a broad acoustic shadow, making it difficult to differentiate the duct from surrounding bowel. If visualization of the duct is not optimal, transducer compression, suspension of breathing, or full inspiration can be used to displace the gas and improve visualization.[2] Other helpful techniques include harmonics, transducer pressure, and altering patient position.[5] If stones are visualized, an endoscopic retrograde

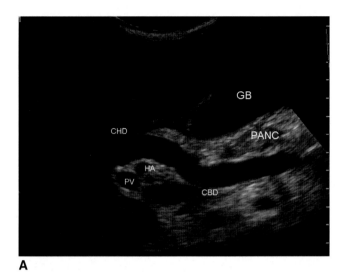

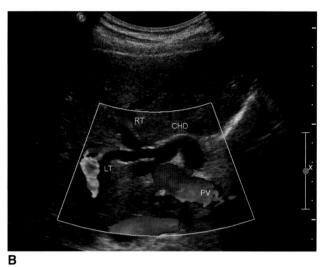

A **B**

FIGURE 8-44 Dilated common hepatic duct *(CHD)* and common bile duct *(CBD)*. **A:** Dilated CBD to the level of the pancreas. With an obstruction at the pancreas, the entire ductal system would be dilated. **B:** Dilated CHD at the porta hepatis. With an obstruction at the CHD, the right *(RT)* and left *(LT)* intrahepatic ducts would be dilated, but the CBD would remain normal. *GB,* gallbladder; *HA,* hepatic artery; *PANC,* pancreas; *PV,* portal vein.

TABLE 8-2 Defining the Level and Cause of Intrahepatic Biliary Dilatation
Causes of Intrahepatic Dilatation with a Normal CBD
• Proximal bile duct tumors (benign and malignant)
• Klatskin tumor
• Cholangitis (PSC)
• Tumors at the porta hepatis (adenopathy and metastases)
• Mirizzi syndrome
• Liver neoplasms compressing intrahepatic ducts
• Benign strictures
Causes of Intrahepatic Dilatation with a Dilated CBD
Choledocholithiasis
Carcinoma of pancreatic head
Pseudocyst obstructing CBD
Acute pancreatitis
Chronic pancreatitis
Choledochal cyst
Lymphadenopathy
Benign strictures
Ampullary tumors

CBD, common bile duct; PSC, primary sclerosing cholangitis.

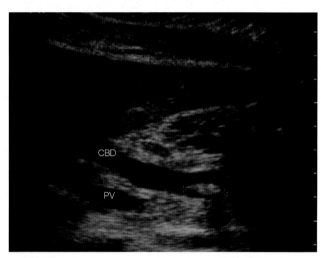

FIGURE 8-45 Choledocholithiasis. Bile surrounding the stone *(calipers)* makes visualization easier. *CBD,* common bile duct; *PV,* portal vein.

cholangiopancreatography (ERCP) is used for removal and treatment.[20] If the obstruction or stones are not identified sonographically, an MRCP or ERCP could be helpful (Figs. 8-47 and 8-48).[5]

Cholangiocarcinoma

Cholangiocarcinoma is a primary malignancy of the bile duct. The majority of these tumors are adenocarcinomas that grow slowly and may extend along the length of the CHD and CBD.[62] Cholangiocarcinomas may occur throughout the biliary tree; however, they are more common at the porta hepatis (Klatskin tumors).[5,6] Ampullary carcinomas may also include the distal portion of the CBD.[8,73]

Cholangiocarcinoma occurs equally in men and women, usually between 50 and 70 years of age.[8] Risk factors for developing cholangiocarcinoma include sclerosing cholangitis, choledochal cysts, and parasitic infections.[5] If detected early, the curative treatment for cholangiocarcinoma is surgery. However, the majority of patients present at the late stages. At this point, palliative treatment to prolong life is the goal.[74]

Signs and symptoms include marked icterus and a palpable gallbladder if the obstruction is distal to the cystic duct. Abdominal pain, anorexia, fatigue, weight loss, hepatomegaly, and ascites may be present.[68] A laboratory workup often reveals elevated serum bilirubin and alkaline phosphatase levels.[8,62]

By sonogram, ductal wall irregularity may be seen.[5,6] Tumors are typically small and are seldom seen by sonography; however, sonography is helpful in identifying the level of the ductal obstruction.[6] Cholangiocarcinomas vary in echogenicity from hypoechoic to hyperechoic. The portal vein should be evaluated for tumor involvement.[5] Other signs of malignancy such as liver metastases, ascites, and adenopathy should also be sought (Fig. 8-49A–D).

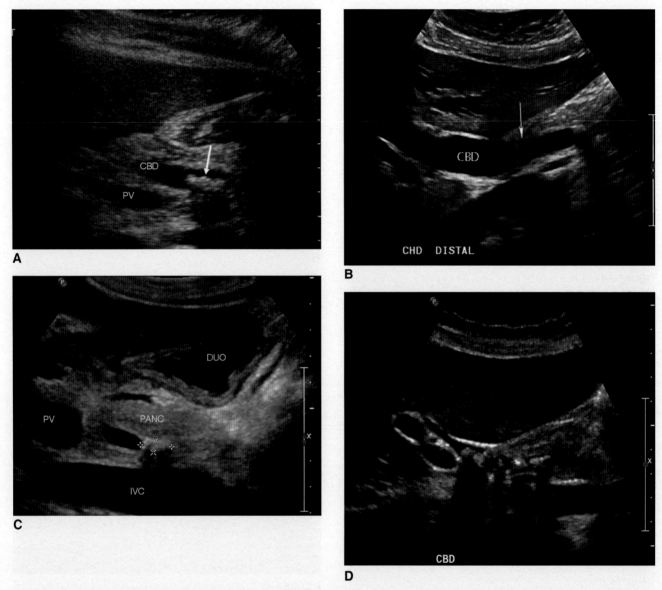

FIGURE 8-46 Choledocholithiasis. **A:** Large stone *(arrow)* in distal portion of dilated common bile duct *(CBD)*. **B:** Stone *(arrow)* in the distal *CBD*. **C:** Stone *(calipers)* at the distal CBD at the level of the pancreas. All of the stones have a distal shadow and cause dilatation proximal to the blockage. **D:** Multiple shadowing stones and within the *CBD* at the head of the pancreas. *DUO*, duodenum; *IVC*, inferior vena cava; *PANC*, pancreas; *PV*, portal vein.

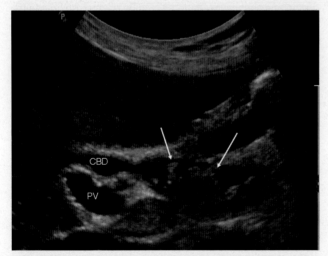

FIGURE 8-47 More heterogeneous mass *(arrows)* within the duct was proven to be sludge by endoscopic retrograde cholangiopancreatography evaluation. *CBD*, common bile duct; *PV*, portal vein.

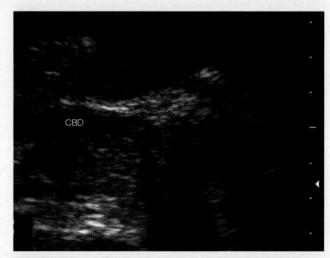

FIGURE 8-48 A mass within the duct can also cause obstruction. This heterogeneous mass *(calipers)* within the common bile duct *(CBD)* was an adenocarcinoma.

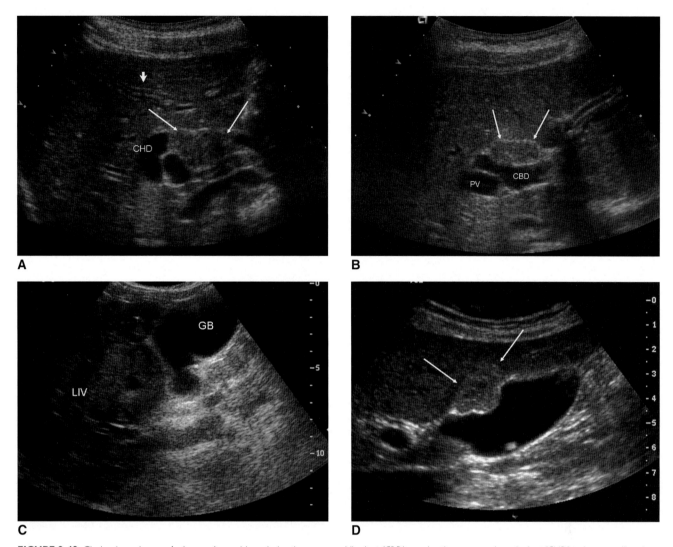

FIGURE 8-49 Cholangiocarcinoma. **A:** A mass *(arrows)* is replacing the common bile duct *(CBD)*, causing the common hepatic duct *(CHD)* to become dilated. The intrahepatic ducts are dilated as well *(arrowhead)*. **B:** In a different patient, the cholangiocarcinoma *(arrows)* is compressing the duct at the porta hepatis. **C:** Metastasis to the liver from cholangiocarcinoma. The liver is heterogeneous, which represents multiple masses. The gallbladder is prominent as well. **D:** In this case, a mass *(arrows)* is compressing the gallbladder. A sludge ball is present as well. *GB,* gallbladder; *LIV,* liver; *PV,* portal vein.

The list of differential diagnoses for cholangiocarcinoma is extensive. Other possible malignant intraductal tumors include hepatocellular carcinoma invading the bile duct, cystadenocarcinoma, metastases of melanoma to the bile ducts, lymphoma or other metastases in the porta hepatis simulating Klatskin tumors, and rhabdomyosarcomas.[73,75,76] Benign intraluminal tumors are very rare but include cystadenomas, papillomas, adenomas, granular cell myoblastomas, fibromas, neurinomas, leiomyomas, hamartomas, and lipomas.[73,76,77] Other causes of nonshadowing solid intraductal masses include material from a ruptured hydatid cyst, biliary sludge, blood clots, and nonshadowing calculi.[73,76] Extrinsic masses may also compress the duct externally and cause obstruction. Such masses include pseudocysts, adenopathy, lymphoma, or metastases in the porta hepatis region as well as pancreatic masses or inflammation.

Cholangitis

Cholangitis is a rare, chronic, inflammatory, and fibrosing disorder of the intrahepatic and extrahepatic biliary system. Primary sclerosing cholangitis (PSC) is idiopathic, chronic, and sometimes familial, whereas secondary sclerosing cholangitis (SSC) is due to a prior biliary infection.[5,50,78]

Patients with cholangitis may be asymptomatic or present with epigastric or RUQ pain, fatigue, pruritus, and jaundice. In the chronic stages, patient can progress to cirrhosis and liver failure. Patients are also at risk for cholangiocarcinoma.[5] There is also an increased risk for other carcinomas including hepatobiliary, hepatocellular, gallbladder, and pancreatic.[50] Laboratory tests may reveal an increased alkaline phosphatase value, elevated AST and ALT levels, increased WBC, and an increased direct bilirubin value (if jaundice is present).

The sonographic findings with cholangitis may include thickened and edematous duct walls that narrow the lumen, thus dilating the ducts proximally; however, diagnosis is difficult sonographically (Fig. 8-50A–C). The primary role of sonography in patients with cholangitis is to screen for cholangiocarcinoma. Cholangiography is typically the modality of choice to diagnose cholangitis, whereas a biliary drain is placed to treat acute cholangitis (Fig. 8-51).[6,79] For PSC, liver transplant is currently the only known cure.[78]

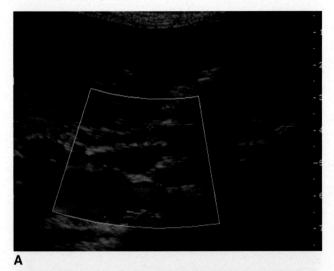

A

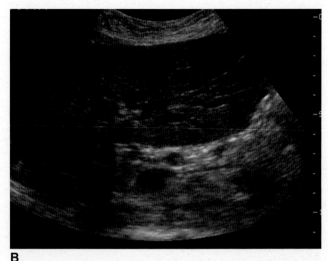

B

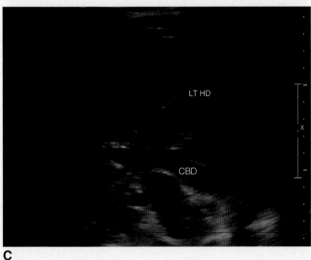

C

FIGURE 8-50 Primary sclerosing cholangitis. **A:** The common bile duct (*CBD*) walls (*calipers*) are thickened in this patient with primary sclerosing cholangitis. **B:** The thickened walls caused dilatation (stellate pattern) of the intrahepatic ducts. **C:** Dilated common bile and left hepatic duct (*LT HD*) are seen in this patient with cholangitis. Note the echogenic, irregular walls of the bile ducts.

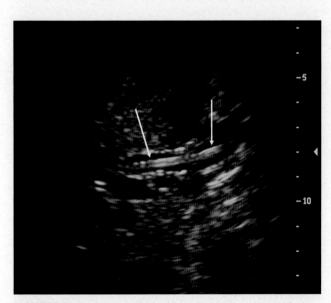

FIGURE 8-51 Echogenic parallel lines (*arrows*) within the common bile duct represent a biliary stent.

Other Biliary Tree Pathology

Pneumobilia, air in the biliary tree, results from an extended communication of the bile duct to the gastrointestinal (GI) tract. This may occur following surgery, liver transplant, stent placement, fistula, ERCP, infection, emphysematous cholecystitis, or biliary necrosis. Sonographically, the air produces mobile bright echoes with dirty shadowing that follow the branching of the portal venous tree[5] (Fig. 8-52A–D). It is important to determine whether the air is in the duct or the portal vein. Portal vein air is present with necrotic bowel.

Benign strictures of the extrahepatic bile ducts most often result from surgical trauma. The remaining cases are caused by blunt abdominal trauma or erosion of the duct wall by a gallstone, which is known as Mirizzi syndrome. Mirizzi syndrome occurs when a stone obstructs the cystic duct, causing inflammation and obstruction of the common duct.[5] Depending on the degree of obstruction, the patient may be asymptomatic, icteric, or present with symptoms similar to cholangitis. Sonographically, strictures can mimic the appearance of cholangitis with dilated ducts if significant occlusion is present.[8]

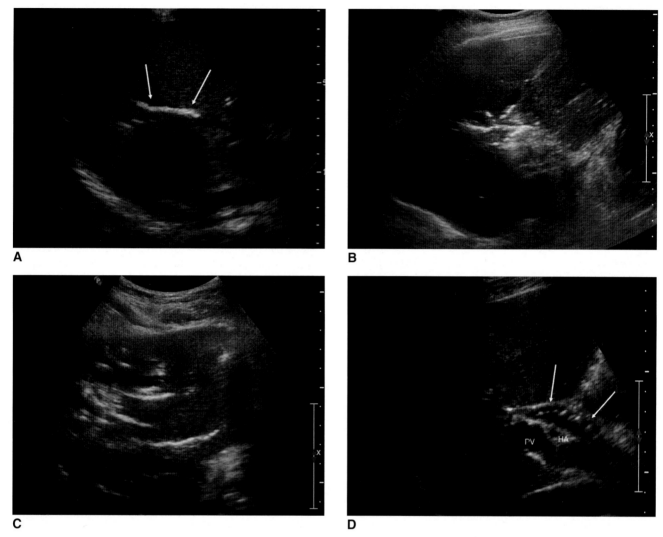

FIGURE 8-52 Pneumobilia. **A:** The echogenic air (arrows) and posterior dirty shadowing are seen in the right hepatic lobe. **B, C:** Diffuse, extensive air within the intrahepatic ducts follows the branching pattern of the ducts and portal venous tree. The air moved under real-time observation. **D:** Air (arrows) was seen within the common bile duct after a liver transplant. HA, hepatic artery; PV, portal vein.

Bilomas, collections of bile, can occur with laceration or rupture of the biliary tract and appear as upper abdominal fluid collections. Following liver transplant, bilomas are cystic areas that can be seen along the falciform ligament or ligamentum venosum. They can be associated with hepatic artery thrombosis (Fig. 8-53).[80]

In some areas of the world, larvae (liver flukes) may infest the liver, gallbladder, and biliary tree and may cause obstruction. Sonographically, the appearance will depend on the stage. It can range from nonspecific findings, such as hepatomegaly to linear structures (worms) within the bile ducts or gallbladder. Movement may also be seen.[2]

AIDS Cholecystopathy

AIDS cholecystopathy was originally described in 1986. With the use of highly active antiretroviral medication, it has become rare in the Western world. It can, however, still be seen in patients with advanced immunosuppression

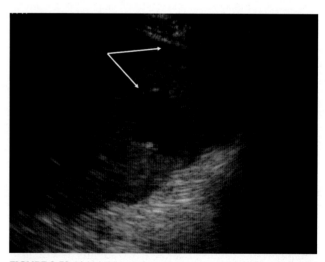

FIGURE 8-53 Multiple bilomas (arrows) were seen in this postliver transplant patient. Hepatic artery thrombosis was also seen.

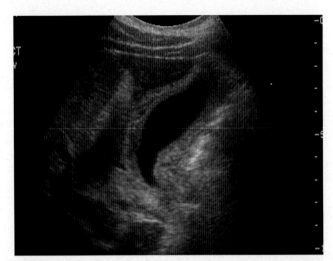

FIGURE 8-54 Longitudinal image in a patient with elevated liver function tests demonstrates a markedly thickened gallbladder wall, which is a common finding in AIDS cholecystopathies.

or in patients living in developing countries.[81] Cytomegalovirus or cryptosporidiosis have been responsible for biliary tract abnormalities and may lead to acalculous cholecystitis.[27]

Patients can present with RUQ pain, fever, diarrhea, weight loss, and hepatomegaly. ALP is also five to seven times the normal limit.[81]

Ultrasound is the key modality to screen for gallbladder and biliary pathology in HIV patients. Gallbladder wall thickening and pancreatic, extrahepatic, and intrahepatic ductal dilation or strictures can be seen (Fig. 8-54).[2,27,81] HIV cholangitis is listed as a secondary form of sclerosing cholangitis.[81]

CORRELATION OF OTHER RELATED DIAGNOSTIC IMAGING PROCEDURES

Plain, noncontrast abdominal radiographs can reveal calcified gallstones (but only 15% contain sufficient calcium to be visualized), air in the biliary tree, porcelain gallbladder, gas-containing calculi (characteristic stellate appearance of gas collections), and mass effects distorting the abdominal organs.[8,34]

Oral cholecystography (OCG) is a rarely utilized radiography examination that requires the patient to ingest iodinated contrast medium. The examination was used to document gallbladder function, wall thickening, or strictures.[61]

Barium-contrast radiographic examinations such as a GI series may confirm the presence of biliary-enteric fistulas (i.e., gallstone ileus) because the barium refluxes into the biliary tree.[42]

Percutaneous transhepatic cholangiography and drainage (PTCD) is an invasive procedure performed under x-ray guidance. It is used for the diagnosis and treatment of malignant and benign biliary disease. It can, however, deliver significant radiation exposure to the patient and interventional team. Percutaneous transhepatic cholangiography (PTC) can used before PTCD to directly visualize the bile ducts. The use of PTCD and PTC is now decreasing because of advancements in endoscopic retrograde biliary drainage and MR cholangiography.[82]

Scintigraphy examinations, such as the HIDA scan, are utilized to evaluate for ductal patency, chronic cholecystitis, and acute cholecystitis. It is a functional test to determine if the cystic duct is patent, thus ruling out acute cholecystitis. It will also demonstrate the major bile ducts and excretion of the tracer into the duodenum. Consequently, obstructive choledocholithiasis can also be diagnosed. Scintigraphy is used to evaluate acute gallbladder pathology; however, sonography has replaced scintigraphy in the majority of clinics.[20] For investigation of the gallbladder and biliary tree, nuclear medicine is approximately 85% accurate, but it can generate false-positive results. It does, however, only provide an isolated view in the workup of acute RUQ pain.[8,20,83,84] Also, it is a long exam, often taking up to 4 hours.[20]

ERCP is a test to evaluate biliary dilatation.[48] ERCP requires the insertion of an endoscope through the esophagus and stomach into the duodenum. At this point, radiopaque contrast material can be injected retrograde through the ampulla of Vater to opacify the pancreatic and biliary ducts for radiographic visualization. ERCP may be therapeutic as well as diagnostic because common duct stones can be effectively removed endoscopically via sphincterotomy or stent placement can be performed. Although it is an effective imaging procedure for biliary disorders, ERCP has definite risks, contraindications, and complications.[8,85,86] Owing to potential risks, ERCP should be limited to those who are at high risk for recurrent choledocholithiasis or in the setting of diagnosed biliary disease.[85]

MRCP is gaining an increased role in detecting choledocholithiasis and other acute biliary diseases.[20,24,48] Gallstones and choledocholithiasis are best visualized on T2-weighted images, whereas gallbladder inflammation is seen on T1-weighted images.[19] Wall thickening, pericholecystic fluid, and inflammatory changes can also be seen.[29]

CT can provide information on the biliary system, if additional imaging is needed following a sonography examination.[20] Dilated bile ducts, intrahepatic and extrahepatic masses, choledocholithiasis, large gallstones, thickened gallbladder wall, pericholecystic fluid, and porcelain gallbladder may be detected by CT.[19,48] CT is also helpful in diagnosing gallbladder perforation and abscess.[10] CT can provide a global overview; however, it is inferior to sonography for diagnosing gallstones and other biliary pathology.[19,20,30]

Positron emission tomography (PET) has a role in diagnosing malignant conditions of the gallbladder and biliary tree, such as cholangiocarcinoma. PET is typically used alongside MRI, CT, and ultrasound. PET may be useful to identify metastatic or recurrent disease.[87]

Intraductal ultrasound (IDUS) is also used to evaluate ductal pathology sonographically. IDUS uses a high-frequency probe that is inserted into the duct during an ERCP.[48] It can be used to evaluate malignant biliary structures and cholangiocarcinoma.[73]

Endoscopic ultrasound (EUS) is commonly used to evaluate ductal pathology sonographically. A small transducer is attached to an endoscope and is introduced into the duodenum. At this level, the bile duct can be visualized.[79] Small stones are more likely to be detected on EUS than conventional abdominal sonography.[24] EUS is safe and produces superior images of the bile duct. Because benign versus malignant biliary pathology is difficult to determine, a fine-needle aspiration can also be performed during EUS. Even though conventional sonography or CT evaluates the majority of gallbladder masses, EUS is a new resource that will continue to be used.[48]

SUMMARY

- The normal, distended pear- or teardrop-shaped gallbladder is located in the main lobar fissure between the right and left hepatic lobes.
- Laboratory tests helpful in evaluating pathophysiology of the biliary tract include WBC, AST, ALT, LDH, alkaline phosphatase, and bilirubin.
- Sonography is the primary modality of choice to evaluate for RUQ pain or a positive sonographic Murphy sign indicating pain.
- Sonographic imaging of the gallbladder and biliary tree is accurate, quick, painless, noninvasive, inexpensive, and carries no risk of ionizing radiation.
- Sonography, along with clinical and laboratory values, is needed to perform an accurate diagnosis of RUQ pain.
- As imaging technology continues to develop, sonography will continue to play an important role in the diagnostic evaluation and management of gallbladder and biliary disease.

REFERENCES

1. Odwin CS, Fleischer AC. Abdominal sonography. In: Odwin CS, Fleischer AC, eds. *Lange Review for the Ultrasonography Examination*. 4th ed. McGraw Hill Company; 2012:205–322.
2. Khalili K, Wilson SR. The biliary tree and gallbladder. In: Rumack CM, Levine D, eds. *Diagnostic Ultrasound*. Vol 1. 5th ed. Elsevier Mosby; 2018:165–209.
3. Anderhub B. *A Clinical Guide*. Mosby; 1995.
4. Netter FH. *The CIBA Collection of Medical Illustrations*. Vol 3 (Digestive System), Part III (Liver, Biliary Tract, and Pancreas). 2nd ed. CIBA Pharmaceutical Company; 1964.
5. Rubens DJ. Ultrasound imaging of the biliary tract. *Ultrasound Clin*. 2007;2:391–413.
6. Baron RL, Tublin ME, Peterson MS. Imaging the spectrum of biliary tract disease. *Radiol Clin North Am*. 2002;40:1325–1354.
7. Dodds WJ, Groh WJ, Darweesh RM, Lawson TL, Kishk SM, Kern MK. Sonographic measurement of gallbladder volume. *AJR Am J Roentgenol*. 1985;145:1009–1011.
8. Apstein MD, Hauser SC, Ostrow JD, et al. Liver biliary tree and pancreas. In: Stein JH, ed. *Internal Medicine*. 4th ed. Mosby; 1994.
9. Inoue T, Kitano M, Kudo M, et al. Diagnosis of gallbladder diseases by contrast-enhanced phase-inversion harmonic ultrasonography. *Ultrasound Med Biol*. 2007;33:353–361.
10. Hata K, Aoki S, Hata T, Murao F, Kitao M. Ultrasonographic identification of the human fetal gallbladder in utero. *Gynecol Obstet Invest*. 1987;23:79–83.
11. Stringer DA, Dobranowski J, Ein SH, Roberts EA, Daneman A, Filler RM. Interposition of the gallbladder—or the absent common hepatic duct and cystic duct. *Pediatr Radiol*. 1987;17:151–153.
12. Doyle TC. Flattened fundus sign of the septate gallbladder. *Gastrointest Radiol*. 1984;9:345–347.
13. Lev-Toaff AS, Friedman AC, Rindsberg SN, Caroline DF, Maurer AH, Radecki PD. Multiseptate gallbladder: incidental diagnosis on sonography. *AJR Am J Roentgenol*. 1987;148:1119–1120.
14. Kidney M, Goiney R, Cooperberg PL. Adenomyomatosis of the gallbladder: a pictorial exhibit. *J Ultrasound Med*. 1986;5:331–333.
15. Riddlesberger MM Jr. Diagnostic imaging of the hepatobiliary system in infants and children. *J Pediatr Gastroenterol Nutr*. 1984;3:653–664.
16. Rutherford AE, Pratt DS. Cholestasis and cholestatic syndromes. *Curr Opin Gastroenterol*. 2006;22:209–214.
17. Green D, Carrol BA. Ultrasonography in the jaundiced infant: a new approach. *J Ultrasound Med*. 1986;5:323–329.
18. Taylor LA, Ross AJ. Abdominal masses. In: Walker WA, Durie PR, Hamilton JR, Walker-Smith J, eds. *Pediatric Gastrointestinal Disease Pathophysiology, Diagnosis, Management*. Vol 1. BC Decker Inc.; 1991.
19. Gore RM, Yaghmai V, Newmark GM, Berlin JW, Miller FH. Imaging benign and malignant disease of the gallbladder. *Radiol Clin North Am*. 2002;40:1307–1323.
20. Hanbidge AE, Buckler PM, O'Malley ME, Wilson SR. From the RSNA refresher courses: imaging evaluation for acute pain in the right upper quadrant. *Radiographics*. 2004;24:1117–1135.
21. Stinton LM, Shaffer EA. Epidemiology of gallbladder disease: cholelithiasis and cancer. *Gut Liver*. 2012;6:172–187.
22. Bouchier IA. Gallstone: formation and epidemiology. In: Blumgart LH, ed. *Surgery of the Liver and Biliary Tract*. Vol 1. 2nd ed. Churchill Livingston; 1994:555–556.
23. Jones RS, Jones BT. Cholecystitis and cholelithiasis. In: Rakel RE, ed. *Conn's Current Therapy: 1994*. WB Saunders Company; 1994.
24. Portincasa P, Moschetta A, Petruzzelli M, Palasciano G, Di Ciaula A, Pezzolla A. Gallstone disease: symptoms and diagnosis of gallbladder stones. *Best Pract Res Clin Gastroenterol*. 2006;20:1017–1029.
25. Laffey KJ, Martin EC. Percutaneous removal of large gallstones. *Gastrointest Radiol*. 1986;11:165–168.
26. Sato M, Ishida H, Konno K, et al. Segmental chronic cholecystitis: sonographic findings and clinical manifestations. *Abdom Imaging*. 2002;27:43–46.
27. Runner GJ, Corwin MT, Siewert B, Eisenberg RL. Gallbladder wall thickening. *AJR Am J Roentgenol*. 2014;202:W1–W12.
28. Lin KY. Acute acalculous cholecystitis: a limited review of the literature. *Mt Sinai J Med*. 1986;53:305–309.
29. Smith EA, Dillman JR, Elsayes KM, Menias CO, Bude RO. Cross-sectional imaging of acute and chronic gallbladder inflammatory disease. *AJR Am J Roentgenol*. 2009;192.188–196.
30. Trowbridge RL, Rutkowski NK, Shojania KG. Does this patient have acute cholecystitis? *JAMA*. 2003;289(1):80–86.
31. van Weelde BJ, Oudkerk M, Koch CW. Ultrasonography of acute cholecystitis: clinical and histological correlation. *Diagn Imaging Clin Med*. 1986;55:190–195.
32. Beckman I, Dash N, Sefczek RJ, et al. Ultrasonographic findings in acute acalculous cholecystitis. *Gastrointest Radiol*. 1985;10:387–389.
33. Munster AM, Goodwin MN, Pruitt BA Jr. Acalculous cholecystitis in burned patients. *Am J Surg*. 1971;122:591–593.
34. Becker CD, Vock P. Appearance of gas-containing gallstones on sonography and computed tomography. *Gastrointest Radiol*. 1984;9:323–328.
35. Ausania F, Guzman Suarez S, Alvarez Garcia H, Senra del Rio P, Casal Nuñez E. Gallbladder perforation: morbidity, mortality and preoperative risk prediction. *Surg Endosc*. 2015;29:955–960.
36. French DG, Allen PD, Ellsmere JC. The diagnostic accuracy of transabdominal ultrasonography needs to be considered when managing gallbladder polyps. *Surg Endosc*. 2013;27:4021–4025.
37. Konno K, Ishida H, Sato M, et al. Gallbladder perforation: color Doppler findings. *Abdom Imaging*. 2002;27:47–50.
38. Sood BP, Kalra N, Gupta S, et al. Role of sonography in the diagnosis of gallbladder perforation. *J Clin Ultrasound*. 2002;30(5):270–274.
39. Date RS, Thrumurthy SG, Whiteside S, et al. Gallbladder perforation: case series and systematic review. *Int J Surg*. 2012;10(2):63–68.
40. Bernstein D, Soeffing J, Daoud YJ, Fradin J, Kravet SJ. The obscured gallbladder. *Am J Med*. 2007;120:675–677.
41. Fitzgerald EJ, Toi A. Pitfalls in the ultrasonographic diagnosis of gallbladder diseases. *Postgrad Med J*. 1987;63:525–532.
42. Maglinte DD, Lappas JC, Ng AC. Sonography of Bouveret's syndrome. *J Ultrasound Med*. 1987;6:675–677.
43. Bacq Y. Intrahepatic cholestasis of pregnancy. *Clin Liver Dis*. 1999;3(1):1–13.
44. Rioseco AJ, Ivankovic MB, Manzur A, et al. Intrahepatic cholestasis of pregnancy: a retrospective case-control study of perinatal outcome. *Am J Obstet Gynecol*. 1994;170(3):890–895.
45. Sarkut P, Kilicturgay S, Ozer A, Ozturk E, Yilmazlar T. Gallbladder polyps: factors affecting surgical decision. *World J Gastroenterol*. 2013;19(28):4526–4530.
46. Mellnick VM, Menias CO, Sandrasegaran K, et al. Polypoid lesions of the gallbladder: disease spectrum with pathologic correlation. *Radiographics*. 2015;35:387–399.

47. Park JY, Hong SP, Kim YJ, et al. Long-term follow up of gallbladder polyps. *J Gastroenterol Hepatol*. 2009;24:219–222.

48. Mishra G, Conway J. Endoscopic ultrasound in the evaluation of radiologic abnormalities of the liver and biliary tree. *Curr Gastroenterol Rep*. 2009;11:150–154.

49. Aldouri AQ, Malik HZ, Waytt J, et al. The risk of gallbladder cancer from polyps in a large multiethnic series. *Eur J Surg Oncol*. 2009;35:48–51.

50. Leung UC, Wong PY, Roberts RH, Koea JB. Gall bladder polyps in sclerosing cholangitis: does the 1-cm rule apply? *ANZ J Surg*. 2007;77:355–357.

51. Miller G, Jarnagin WR. Gallbladder carcinoma. *Eur J Surg Oncol*. 2008;34:306–312.

52. Hsing AW, Gao YT, Han TQ, et al. Gallstones and the risk of biliary tract cancer: a population-based study in China. *Br J Cancer*. 2007;97:1577–1582.

53. Rodríguez-Fernández A, Gómez-Río M, Medina-Benítez A, et al. Application of modern imaging methods in diagnosis of gallbladder cancer. *J Surg Oncol*. 2006;93:650–664.

54. Weiner SN, Koenigsberg M, Morehouse H, Hoffman J. Sonography and computed tomography in the diagnosis of carcinoma of the gallbladder. *AJR Am J Roentgenol*. 1984;142:735–739.

55. Graff AE, Lewis SL, Bear JR, Van Echo DC, Dainer HM. Gallbladder carcinoma, the difficulty of early detection: a case report. *Cureus*. 2016;8(2):e493.

56. Jeffrey RB, Ralls PW. Gallbladder and bile ducts. In: Jeffrey RB, Ralls PW, eds. *Sonography of the Abdomen*. Raven Press; 1995.

57. Katz SC, Bowne WB, Wolchok JD, Busam KJ, Jaques DP, Coit DG. Surgical management of melanoma of the gallbladder: a report of 13 cases and review of the literature. *Am J Surg*. 2007;193:493–497.

58. Samplaski MK, Rosato EL, Witkiewicz AK, Mastrangelo MJ, Berger AC. Malignant melanoma of the gallbladder: a report of two cases and review of the literature. *J Gastrointest Surg*. 2008;12:1123–1126.

59. Martel JP, McLean CA, Rankin RN. Melanoma of the gallbladder. *Radiographics*. 2009;29:291–296.

60. Yoon JH, Cha SS, Han SS, Lee SJ, Kang MS. Gallbladder adenomyomatosis: imaging findings. *Abdom Imaging*. 2006;31:555–563.

61. Stunell H, Buckley O, Geoghegan T, O'Brien J, Ward E, Torreggiani W. Imaging of adenomyomatosis of the gallbladder. *J Med Imaging Radiat Oncol*. 2008;52:109–117.

62. Way LW. Biliary tract. In: Way LW, ed. *Current Surgical Diagnosis and Treatment*. 10th ed. Appleton & Lange; 1994:537–566.

63. Van Gansbeke D, de Toeuf J, Cremer M, Engelholm L, Struyven J. Suprahepatic gallbladder: a rare congenital anomaly. *Gastrointest Radiol*. 1984;9:341–343.

64. Krebs CA, Giyanani VL, Eisenberg RL. Biliary system. In: Krebs CA, Giyanani VL, Eisenberg RL, eds. *Atlas of Disease Process*. Appleton & Lange; 1993:51–83.

65. Yeola-Pate M, Banode PJ, Bhole AM, Golhar KB, Shahapurkar VV, Joharapurkar SR. Different locations of hydatid cysts. *Infect Dis Clin Pract*. 2008;16:379–384.

66. Quinn SF, Fazzio F, Jones E. Torsion of the gallbladder: findings on CT and sonography and role of percutaneous cholecystectomy. *AJR Am J Roentgenol*. 1987;148:881–882.

67. Lemonick DM, Garvin R, Semins H. Torsion of the gallbladder: a rare cause of acute cholecystitis. *J Emerg Med*. 2006;30(4):397–401.

68. Willson SA, Gosink BB, vanSonnenberg E. Unchanged size of dilated common bile duct after a fatty meal: results and significance. *Radiology*. 1986;160:29–31.

69. Matcuk GR Jr, Grant EG, Ralls PW. Ultrasound measurements of the bile ducts and gallbladder: normal ranges and effects of age, sex, cholecystectomy, and pathologic states. *Ultrasound Q*. 2014;30:41–48.

70. Simeone JF, Butch RJ, Mueller PR, et al. The bile ducts after a fatty meal: further sonographic observations. *Radiology*. 1985;154:763–768.

71. Wing VW, Laing FC, Jeffrey RB, Guyon J. Sonographic differentiation of enlarged hepatic arteries from dilated intrahepatic bile ducts. *AJR Am J Roentgenol*. 1985;145:57–61.

72. Kondo S, Isayama H, Akahane M, et al. Detection of common bile duct stones: comparison between endoscopic ultrasonography, magnetic resonance cholangiography, and helical-computed-tomographic cholangiography. *Eur J Radiol*. 2005;54:271–275.

73. Robledo R, Prieto ML, Perez M, Camúñez F, Echenagusia A. Carcinoma of the hepaticopancreatic ampullar region: role of US. *Radiology*. 1988;166:409–412.

74. Singh P, Patel T. Advances in the diagnosis, evaluation and management of cholangiocarcinoma. *Curr Opin Gastroenterol*. 2006;22:294–299.

75. Geoffray A, Couanet D, Montagne JP, Leclère J, Flamant F. Ultrasonography and computed tomography for diagnosis and follow-up of biliary duct rhabdomyosarcomas in children. *Pediatr Radiol*. 1987;17:127–131.

76. Subramanyam BR, Raghavendra BN, Balthazar EJ, Horii SC, LeFleur RS, Rosen RJ. Ultrasonic features of cholangiocarcinoma. *J Ultrasound Med*. 1984;3:405–408.

77. Marchal GJ, VanHolsbeeck M, Tshibwabwa-Ntumba E, et al. Dilatation of the cystic veins in portal hypertension: sonographic demonstration. *Radiology*. 1985;154:187–189.

78. MacFaul GR, Chapman RW. Sclerosing cholangitis. *Curr Opin Gastroenterol*. 2006;22:288–293.

79. Van Erpecum KJ. Complications of bile-duct stones: acute cholangitis and pancreatitis. *Best Pract Res Clin Gastroenterol*. 2006;20(6):1139–1152.

80. Muradali D, Chawla T. Organ transplant. In: Rumack CM, Wilson SR, Charboneau JW, Levine D, eds. *Diagnostic Ultrasound*. Vol 1. 4th ed. Elsevier Mosby; 2011:639–706.

81. Tonolini M, Bianco R. HIV-related/AIDS cholangiopathy: pictorial review with emphasis on MRCP findings and differential diagnosis. *Clin Imaging*. 2013;37:219–226.

82. Morita S, Kitanosono T, Lee D, et al. Comparison of technical success and complications of percutaneous transhepatic cholangiography and biliary drainage between patients with and without transplanted liver. *AJR Am J Roentgenol*. 2012;199:1149–1152.

83. Coletti PM, Ralls PW, Lapin SA, Siegel ME, Halls JM. Hepatobiliary imaging in choledocholithiasis. A comparison with ultrasound. *Clin Nucl Med*. 1986;11:482–486.

84. Dykes EH, Wilson N, Gray HW, McArdle CS. The role of 99mTc HIDA cholescintigraphy in the diagnosis of acute gallbladder disease: comparison with oral cholecystography and ultrasonography. *Scott Med J*. 1986;31:170–173.

85. Suarez AL, LaBarre NT, Cotton PB, Payne KM, Coté GA, Elmunzer BJ. An assessment of existing risk stratification guidelines for the evaluation of patients with suspected choledocholithiasis. *Surg Endosc*. 2016;30(10):4613–4618.

86. Chau EM, Leong LL, Chan FL. Recurrent pyogenic cholangitis: ultrasound evaluation compared with endoscopic retrograde cholangiopancreatography. *Clin Radiol*. 1987;38:79–85.

87. Srinivasa S, McEntee B, Koea JB. The role of PET scans in the management of cholangiocarcinoma and gallbladder cancer: a systematic review for surgeons. *Int J Diagn Imaging*. 2015;2:1–9.

CHAPTER 9

The Pancreas

KELLIE A. SCHMIDT

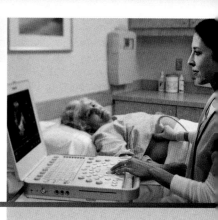

OBJECTIVES

- Describe pancreatic surface anatomy, vascular supply, and the common relational landmarks.
- Discuss the most common pancreatic congenital anomalies to include pancreas divisum, annular pancreas, and ectopic pancreas.
- Identify the endocrine and exocrine functions of the pancreas.
- Correlate laboratory values and clinical indications associated with pancreatic abnormalities, disease, and pathology.
- Explain the sonographic evaluation of the pancreas to include patient preparation and protocol and demonstrate completing the examination procedure.
- Differentiate normal from the varying sonographic appearances associated with pancreatic disease or pathology.
- Describe the pathology, etiology, clinical signs and symptoms, and sonographic appearance for congenital diseases, inflammatory diseases, neoplastic diseases, and nonneoplastic cystic lesions.

KEY TERMS

acute pancreatitis

chronic pancreatitis

pancreatic carcinoma

phlegmon

pseudocyst

GLOSSARY

acini cells cells that perform exocrine functions secreting digestive enzymes

alpha cells cells that perform endocrine functions secreting glucagon

amylase enzyme that digests carbohydrates

beta cells cells that perform endocrine functions secreting insulin

delta cells cells that perform endocrine function secreting somatostatin

endocrine secreting into blood or tissue

exocrine secreting into a duct

glucagon hormone secreted by the alpha cells that functions to increase activity of phosphorylase

insulin hormone secreted by beta cells that functions to increase the uptake of glucose and amino acids by most body cells

islets of Langerhans endocrine portion of the pancreas made up of alpha cells and beta cells, which is the source of insulin and glucagon; also called pancreatic islet

lipase fat-digesting enzyme

phlegmon diffuse inflammatory reaction to infection spreading along fascial pathways, producing edema and swelling

pseudocyst an abnormal or dilated cavity resembling a true cyst but not lined with epithelium

somatostatin hormone secreted by delta cells that functions to regulate insulin and glucagon production

Sonographic imaging of the pancreas is often fraught with technical limitations, specifically overlying bowel gas. Although sonography may identify some pancreatic lesions, its primary use is often to identify abnormalities of other organs associated with pancreatic disease.

ANATOMY

The pancreas is a nonencapsulated structure that lies obliquely in the anterior portion of the retroperitoneum. It consists of three main portions: the head, body, and tail. The head is located to the right and inferior to the body and tail. It has the largest anteroposterior (AP) dimension of the gland and is bordered by the C-loop of the duodenum[1] (Fig. 9-1).

Extending posterior and medial from the head is a curved projection of pancreatic tissue, the uncinate process. The uncinate process lies anterior to the inferior vena cava and posterior to the superior mesenteric vein (SMV). The body and tail of the pancreas are bounded anteriorly and superiorly by portions of the stomach, duodenum, and left lobe of the liver.

The body of the pancreas lies anterior to the aorta, superior mesenteric artery (SMA), and left renal vein. Between these vessels and the body of the pancreas, the splenic vein may be identified as it courses from the spleen, toward its confluence with the SMV.

The neck of the pancreas lies just anterior to this confluence, where the SMV and splenic vein merge to form the portal vein. In many patients, the left lobe of the liver lies between the body and the anterior abdominal wall. Branches of the celiac axis—namely the hepatic, left gastric, and splenic arteries—course along the superior border of the body.

The tail of the pancreas extends from the body into the left anterior pararenal space. Bordered posteriorly by the splenic vein, it frequently extends to the splenic hilum.

The tail is bordered anteriorly by the stomach and laterally by the left kidney. Because of its proximity to the stomach, the pancreatic tail is often obscured by gas on sonography.

The parenchyma of the pancreas consists of small groups of acini, which secrete digestive enzymes, clustered in multiple lobules, each surrounding a tributary duct. The smaller ducts merge into increasingly larger ducts, subsequently emptying into the main pancreatic duct, the duct of Wirsung. Enzymes secreted by the pancreas are carried by the main pancreatic duct into the alimentary tract via the ampulla of Vater. Near the ampulla, the main pancreatic duct merges with the distal common bile duct to form a single perforating channel into the duodenum (Fig. 9-2). A smaller accessory duct, the duct of Santorini, branches from the main pancreatic duct and perforates into the duodenum separately from the ampulla.[2]

Wedged within the acinar lobules are groups of endocrine cells known as the islets of Langerhans. These clusters contain various types of cells that release hormones directly into the bloodstream and lymph system. This allows them to be distributed throughout the body, where they stimulate other organs or functional tissues.

Blood supply to the pancreas is provided by branches of the splenic artery and the pancreaticoduodenal arteries. The superior pancreaticoduodenal artery arises from the gastroduodenal artery and perfuses the head of the pancreas. The gastroduodenal artery arises from the common hepatic artery and perforates the pancreatic parenchyma along the superior aspect of the head.[3] The body and tail sections of the pancreas are perfused by the inferior pancreaticoduodenal artery, which arises from the SMA. Branches of this and the splenic artery enter the pancreas at numerous points along the body and tail.[4]

Congenital Anomalies

Congenital anomalies of the pancreas are rare, but do exist. Pancreas divisum is the most common congenital anomaly, occurring in approximately 4% to 14% of the population.[5] It results from a failure of fusion of the dorsal and ventral pancreatic buds during embryologic development (Fig. 9-3). This variant results in anomalous drainage of the pancreatic ducts, but it is usually not associated with any significant sequelae.[5]

An annular pancreas is another congenital anomaly in which the head of the pancreas surrounds the second portion of the duodenum (Fig. 9-4). It occurs more frequently in males and has been associated with complete or partial atresia of the duodenum. Annular pancreas is associated with other congenital abnormalities in up to 70% of affected infants.[6] This includes duodenal stenosis or atresia, Down syndrome, tracheoesophageal fistula, gastrointestinal anomalies, and congenital heart disease.[6,7]

Ectopic pancreatic tissue may also occur. The reported incidence ranges from 0.5% to 13.7%.[8] In this setting, pancreatic tissue grows in other organs. This usually occurs in the walls of the stomach, duodenum, large or small intestine and rarely in the gallbladder, spleen, or liver. Ectopic pancreatic structures may be comprised of acinar and ductal elements. Because they are functional deposits of pancreatic tissue, they are susceptible to developing acute pancreatitis or tumor.

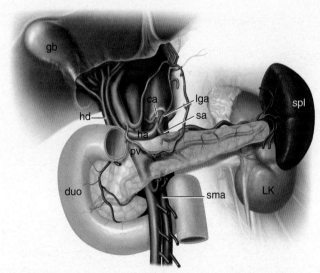

FIGURE 9-1 Diagram showing the normal relationship of the pancreas to the prevertebral vessels and surrounding upper abdominal organs. *ca*, celiac axis; *duo*, duodenum; *gb*, gallbladder; *ha*, proper hepatic artery; *hd*, common hepatic duct; *lga*, left gastric artery; *LK*, left kidney; *pv*, main portal vein; *sa*, splenic artery; *sma*, superior mesenteric artery; *spl*, spleen.

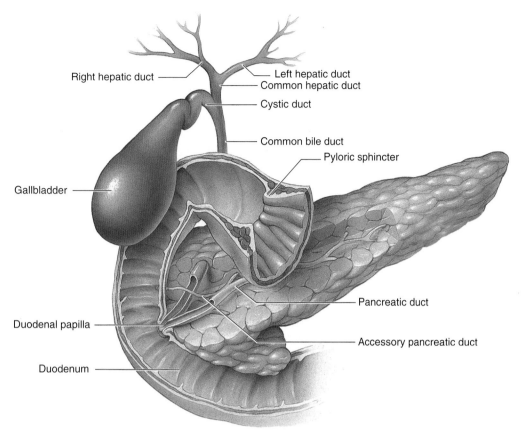

FIGURE 9-2 Diagram showing the relationship of the common bile duct and main pancreatic duct as they merge and enter the ampulla of Vater. (Asset provided by Anatomical Chart Co.)

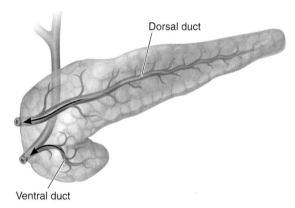

FIGURE 9-3 Diagram showing pancreas divisum. The smaller ventral duct *(arrow)* drains the head and uncinate process of the pancreas, whereas the larger dorsal duct drains the rest of the pancreatic gland. (Reprinted with permission from Blackbourne LH. *Advanced Surgical Recall.* 2nd ed. Lippincott Williams & Wilkins; 2004.)

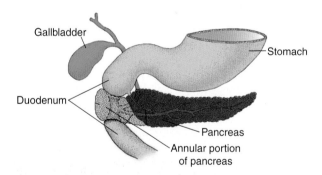

FIGURE 9-4 Diagram of an annular pancreas. The head of the pancreas wraps around the duodenum and blocks or impairs the flow of foodstuffs to the rest of the intestine.

PHYSIOLOGY

The pancreas is responsible for both endocrine and exocrine functions.

Endocrine Function

The endocrine function of the pancreas consists of hormone production, which occurs in the islets of Langerhans.

Specialized cells, referred to as alpha, beta, and delta cells, are contained within the islets of Langerhans. Each is responsible for the production of specific hormones. The majority of these cells are beta cells, which produce insulin. Insulin aids in the metabolism of carbohydrates. By facilitating the transport of glucose across cell membranes, insulin increases the energy available for normal physiologic functions. It also influences the metabolism of proteins and fats. Insulin is released by the pancreas via a negative feedback mechanism. When the blood glucose level rises above a certain level, believed to be 100 mg/dL, the beta cells immediately secrete insulin.[9] When the blood glucose level falls, insulin secretion decreases. Other factors influencing insulin secretion include autonomic nervous system responses, the release of other endocrine hormones, and certain drugs.[10] Abnormalities of insulin secretion result in impairment of metabolic functions throughout the body. Diabetes results from an imbalance between insulin secretion and the metabolic needs of the body.

Glucagon, secreted by alpha cells within the islets of Langerhans, is another important hormone. It functions primarily in the liver and aids in conversion of glycogen into glucose, or usable energy. As with insulin, blood glucose levels initiate the release of glucagon.

Delta cells comprise the smallest component and are responsible for producing somatostatin, a hormone involved with regulating the production of insulin and glucagons.

Exocrine Function

The exocrine function of the pancreas is to secrete enzymes, commonly referred to as pancreatic juice, that aid in food breakdown and digestion. These secretions accumulate in small intercellular spaces and the acini cells and are eventually transported to the duodenum via the excretory ducts. Chemical analysis of pancreatic juice shows that in addition to digestive enzymes, it consists of water and inorganic salts such as potassium, sodium, and calcium.

The enzymes secreted by the pancreas are amylase, lipase, trypsinogen, and chymotrypsinogen—all of which are essential to the digestion and absorption of essential nutrients. Amylase breaks down complex carbohydrates into usable sugars; lipase is an enzyme that breaks down fats; and trypsinogen and chymotrypsinogen are preproteolytic enzymes that reduce proteins to their component amino acids. Additionally, some of these substances play an important role in the pathogenesis of pancreatic disease, especially in pancreatitis. The preproteolytic enzymes in the normal pancreas are inert. It is postulated that an inhibiting factor is secreted by the same cells that secrete exocrine enzymes. This inhibiting factor prevents trypsinogen and chymotrypsin from autodigesting the protein in the cell walls of the pancreas. With injury or disease, the inhibiting factor is unable to prevent the activation of proteolytic enzymes, which spill out into the surrounding parenchyma. Once the process begins, it can advance rapidly, each bursting cell releasing yet more digestive juice, reducing normal tissue to amorphous fluid.[11] Another component of pancreatic juice is the alkaline substance bicarbonate, which neutralizes the acidic gastric enzymes and triggers the action of the otherwise inert pancreatic enzymes in the duodenum. The pancreas is capable of secreting about 1,500 mL of pancreatic fluid per day.[12]

LABORATORY VALUES

Amylase

Amylase is an enzyme essential in the digestion of carbohydrates. The level of amylase within the blood is a useful laboratory test when diagnosing pancreatic disease. In a diseased pancreas, disintegrating acinar cells release their digestive enzymes into the organ's parenchyma, and ultimately into the capillaries that supply the diseased area.

Amylase levels can be accessed with either serum or urine analysis. Normal values vary from laboratory to laboratory.

Serum amylase is considered elevated when the value is three or more times the normal reference range.[13] Levels usually begin to increase within 5 to 8 hours following the first onset of clinical symptoms.[14] They usually reach a maximum level within the first 1 to 2 days of disease onset, and often persist until the underlying cause is treated.[15] Amylase elevation is also associated with pancreatic duct obstruction, pancreatic malignancy, and biliary disease. Other non–pancreas related processes may also cause an increased amylase level, such as perforated ulcers, bowel obstruction, and some cancers, but it is not commonly used to monitor these entities. With chronic pancreatitis, it is not uncommon for amylase levels to be normal or only slightly elevated.

An increased amylase level in the urine may lag behind the onset of an increased serum amylase. Additionally, in the setting of pancreatitis, urine amylase may remain elevated for up to 7 days after serum values have returned to normal. Elevation of the serum amylase without concurrent elevation of the urinary amylase value may represent a pathologic process not related to pancreatic disease such as decreased renal function.[16] Drugs such as aspirin, diuretics, alcohol, and oral contraceptives may also cause an increased amylase level.

A decreased amylase value has been associated with permanent damage to the pancreas, as well as hepatitis and cirrhosis of the liver.[17,18] The diagnosis of acute pancreatitis is often based on clinical symptoms rather than laboratory values.[19]

Lipase

Lipase is a fat-splitting enzyme excreted by the pancreas. It is released into the bloodstream in increased quantities in the setting of inflammatory, and occasionally neoplastic, pancreatic disease. With acute pancreatitis, lipase levels may be 5 to 10 times the normal reference range. Lipase levels increase rapidly within 3 to 6 hours of onset, peak at 24 hours, and remain elevated for 1 to 2 weeks.[19] Lipase elevation also occurs in patients with obstruction of the pancreatic duct, pancreatic carcinoma, acute cholecystitis, cirrhosis, and severe renal disease.[20] Drugs associated with an increased lipase value include codeine, indomethacin, and morphine.

Fat Excretion

Fecal fat excretion values reflect the amount of undigested fat molecules passing through the alimentary tract. Increased fecal fat (steatorrhea) is symptomatic of pancreatitis. Other abnormalities may also result in an increased discharge of fat into fecal matter, including celiac disease, inflammatory bowel disease, or short bowel syndrome. However, fat excretion is increased significantly in pancreatic disease.[21] Weight loss and oily stool are often associated with pancreatic steatorrhea.

Bilirubin and Liver Function Tests

An elevation of bilirubin and other liver function values may also occur with pancreatic disease.[22] This is due to the close anatomic relationships between the liver and biliary system with the pancreas. Pathologic processes in one structure may cause disease in the other. Neoplasia or inflammatory enlargement of the head of the pancreas frequently causes stenosis or complete obstruction of the distal common bile duct. In such cases, total serum bilirubin values are increased. Conversely, biliary duct disease, such as calculi and subsequent inflammation, may spread to the pancreas. Altered biliary and hepatic function values may suggest an underlying pancreatic process.

SONOGRAPHIC EVALUATION

Indications

The pancreas is usually sonographically evaluated as part of a complete abdominal sonography examination. Common indications include epigastric pain, abdominal pain, abdominal distension, or jaundice. Patients with abnormal laboratory values or a prior history of acute or chronic pancreatitis may also be referred for sonography. Sonography is not considered the best imaging test to evaluate for pancreatic disease or neoplasm, but it may be very useful in identifying secondary signs of a pancreatic process such as dilated biliary ducts, fluid collections, and gallstones.

Preparation

Preparation for pancreatic sonography attempts to minimize the amount of gas in the stomach and duodenum by having the patient refrain from eating or drinking anything for 8 to 12 hours prior to the examination. Pancreatic sonography is contraindicated for patients who have undergone gastroscopic examination within 6 hours because large amounts of air are introduced into the stomach during this procedure. The head of the pancreas is intimately related to the duodenum. Gas present here as well as the overlying transverse colon may easily obscure visualization.

It is also recommended that the pancreas be the first organ evaluated when performing a complete sonographic evaluation of the abdomen. This is because patients are often asked to perform deep inspiration during the course of the examination. This often improves visualization of abdominal organs by displacing them caudally. However, it also increases the amount of air within the bowel, which in turn obscures visualization of the pancreas.

Transverse Imaging

In the transverse plane, the pancreas is identified as a crescent-shaped structure draping over the prevertebral vessels (Figs. 9-5 and 9-6). It has been described variously as horseshoe-, dumbbell-, or comma-shaped.[23] Normally, its echogenicity is equal to or greater than that of the liver, depending on the patient's age and body habitus.[24] Fat deposition in the interlobular areas accounts for the varying degrees of echogenicity and in some settings may cause contour alterations.[25] Children normally have less pancreatic fat than adults, so a hypoechoic pancreas in a pediatric patient is a normal finding.[26] In the adult population, a hypoechoic pancreas represents an abnormal finding.[1]

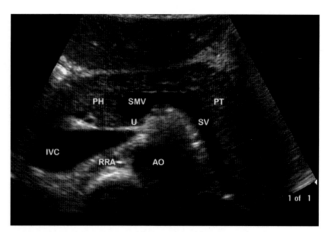

FIGURE 9-5 Transverse image of the normal pancreas draping over the prevertebral vessels. *AO*, aorta; *IVC*, inferior vena cava; *PH*, pancreatic head; *PT*, pancreatic tail; *RRA*, right renal artery; *SMV*, superior mesenteric vein; *SV*, splenic vein; *U*, uncinate process. (Image courtesy of Philips Medical Systems, Bothell, WA.)

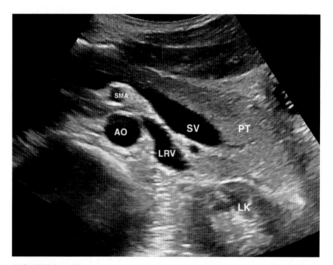

FIGURE 9-6 Transverse image of the normal pancreas with a fully visualized pancreatic tail. *AO*, aorta; *LK*, left kidney; *LRV*, left renal vein; *PT*, pancreatic tail; *SMA*, superior mesenteric artery; *SV*, splenic vein.

The main pancreatic duct, the duct of Wirsung, is frequently visualized sonographically in normal patients.[27,28] It appears as an echogenic lucency bordered by two parallel linear echoes traversing the body of the pancreas[29] (Fig. 9-7). In the normal population, the pancreatic duct diameter is usually 3 mm or less.[4] The normal pancreatic duct mean diameter has been found to measure 3 mm in the head, 2.1 mm in the body, and 1.6 mm in the tail.[4] The contour of the duct walls should be smooth without any areas of focal dilatation.[30] Color Doppler is useful in distinguishing the pancreatic duct from surrounding vascular structures.

The accessory pancreatic duct, the duct of Santorini, is not commonly seen. The duct of Santorini drains the head of the pancreas.

The dimensions of the pancreas are best assessed using a true transverse plane of section. It is important to align the transducer so that the incident beam intersects the pancreas perpendicular to its transverse axis. This is usually a slight obliquity, with the head of the pancreas slightly lower than the tail.

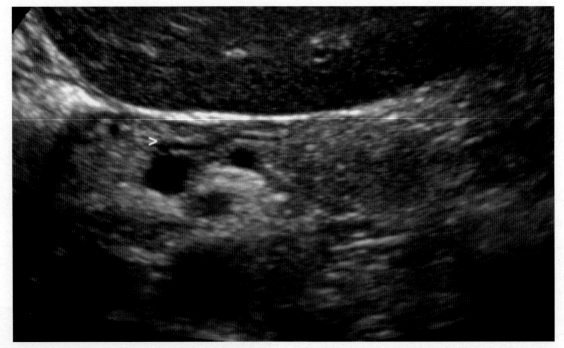

FIGURE 9-7 Transverse image of the pancreas showing a normal main pancreatic duct *(arrowhead)*. The duct of Wirsung.

Pancreatic size can vary considerably from individual to individual.[4] The head of the pancreas is the widest portion of the gland, with the normal AP dimension measuring between 2 and 3.5 cm[3] (Fig. 9-8). The body of the pancreas is narrower and normally measures between 2 and 3 cm[23] (Fig. 9-9). The tail may be difficult to image from a projection that provides a true AP measurement; but in the normal gland, it measures 1 to 2 cm[31] (Fig. 9-10). A child's pancreas is smaller than an adult's, but relative to other upper abdominal organs such as the liver and kidneys, it may appear larger. Size, texture, and contour are all important considerations in identifying pancreatic disease.

In the transverse plane, the common bile duct should be seen in cross section entering the head of the pancreas.

Longitudinal Imaging

On a longitudinal section, the pancreas is identified as an ovoid or circular structure lying anterior to the prevertebral vessels (Fig. 9-11). From a slightly oblique longitudinal section, the common bile duct may be seen entering the pancreatic head (Fig. 9-12). Anterior to the bile duct, the gastroduodenal artery is visualized. The neck of the pancreas appears as a narrow structure just anterior to the confluence of the

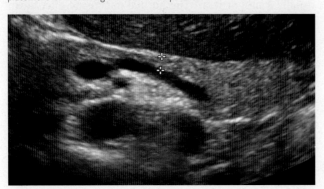

FIGURE 9-8 Transverse image of the pancreas showing normal caliper placement for measuring the head of the pancreas.

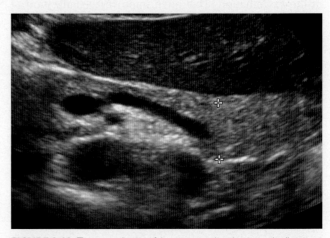

FIGURE 9-9 Transverse image of the pancreas showing normal caliper placement for measuring the body of the pancreas.

FIGURE 9-10 Transverse image of the pancreas showing normal caliper placement for measuring the tail of the pancreas.

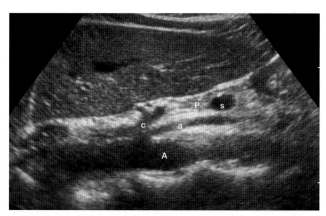

FIGURE 9-11 Longitudinal image of the normal pancreas *(P)* lying anterior to the prevertebral vessels. *A*, aorta; *a*, superior mesenteric artery; *c*, celiac axis; *s*, splenic vein.

SMV and the splenic vein. The body can be seen anterior to the SMA and posterior to the left lobe of the liver. In a true longitudinal section through the left anterior pararenal space, the tail appears thicker than the other portions because it is being transected as it dips posteriorly.

Examination Technique

The sonographic examination usually begins with the patient supine. Using the left lobe of the liver as a window, the transducer is aligned in a transverse position, just below the xiphoid process. A slight caudal angulation is applied, and the transducer position is adjusted so that the prevertebral vessels are identified. Instructing the patient to take a deep breath usually enhances the liver's usefulness as an acoustic window. During deep inspiration, the liver and diaphragm move inferiorly and over the pancreas. Because the head of the pancreas usually sits below the body and tail, rotating the probe counterclockwise a few degrees may permit visualization of the entire organ in a single image; however, additional acoustic windows may be necessary to image the various portions of the pancreas. In most patients with adequate preparation, the head and body of the pancreas are visualized 70% to 77% of the time.[10]

The pancreatic tail is often difficult to see. Bordered anteriorly by the stomach and splenic flexure of the colon, it is frequently obscured by air that has accumulated in the lumen of one or both of these organs. The tail of the pancreas is visualized in only 37% of patients on routine sonographic examination.[10] There are alternative approaches to imaging the tail using various acoustic windows. By rotating the patient into the right lateral decubitus or prone position, the examiner can attempt to image through the left lateral or posterior intercostal spaces. In using the lateral approach, it should be remembered that the plane of section is now coronal with the near field representing lateral and the far field representing medial.[32] With the patient prone, the tail of the pancreas may be seen anterior to the left kidney. Although this approach produces limited results, it may be useful when other approaches have failed.[33]

Another technique involves having the patient drink approximately 200 to 300 mL of water.[34] The patient is then examined either upright or in the left lateral decubitus position, depending on which position provides the best acoustic window. Most examiners prefer to begin with the upright position, because air in the stomach rises above the water to lodge in the fundus.

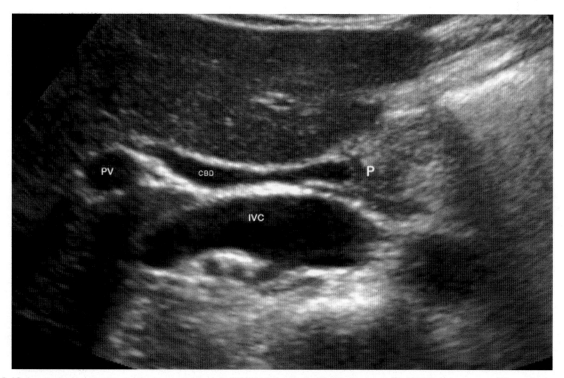

FIGURE 9-12 Longitudinal image showing the common bile duct *(CBD)* entering the head of the pancreas *(P)*. *IVC*, inferior vena cava; *PV*, portal vein.

PATHOLOGY

Congenital Diseases

Cystic Fibrosis

Cystic fibrosis is the most common lethal genetic defect in the Caucasian population.[35] It is characterized by a dysfunction of epithelial chloride transport that affects multiple organs, including the lungs, liver, intestine, reproductive tract, and the pancreas. Cystic fibrosis is the major cause of pancreatic exocrine failure in children. This results in decreased enzyme production, which, in turn, leads to improper digestion of food and liquids. Approximately 85% to 90% of children with cystic fibrosis suffer from pancreatic insufficiency.[35,36] Recurrent acute and chronic pancreatitis can occur in this population and may even precede the diagnosis of cystic fibrosis by several years. Steatorrhea is also seen in affected patients.[35] On sonography, the affected pancreas will appear hyperechoic and small. Hypoechoic areas representing pancreatic fibrosis may be seen. Small cysts and calcifications may also be present. Gallstones and liver disease are also common.

Inflammatory Diseases

Acute Pancreatitis

In acute pancreatitis, all or part of the pancreas is inflamed. Biliary tract disease and excessive alcohol intake are the two most common causes. Gallstones are seen in approximately 40% to 70% of patients with acute pancreatitis.[1] Pancreatitis can be attributed to other various conditions (Table 9-1).

Acute pancreatitis is characterized by an edematous, enlarged gland; subsequently, there is a breakdown of the pancreatic architecture (Fig. 9-13). It is believed that blockage of the pancreatic ductules leads to a release of digestive enzymes, which lyse cell walls.[10] Duct obstruction can be caused by biliary reflux, duodenal reflux, or hypersecretion of pancreatic enzymes. As the cell walls are destroyed by proteolytic digestive enzymes, more enzymes are released into the interstitial spaces, precipitating further destruction. Lipolytic enzymes, which break down fat, also effect changes in the internal morphology of the pancreas. Necrosis of blood vessel walls may cause hemorrhage into or around the pancreas. In 30% of cases, pancreatic enlargement and decreased parenchymal echogenicity owing to interstitial edema may be seen along with ill-defined hypoechoic/

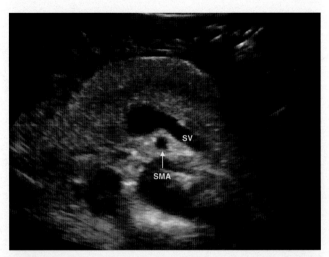

FIGURE 9-13 Transverse image of the pancreas in a patient with acute pancreatitis. The pancreas is edematous and enlarged. *SMA*, superior mesenteric artery; *SV*, splenic vein.

hyperechoic areas representing edema or hemorrhage.[37] Although alcohol and biliary tract pathology, especially gallstones, are the most common predisposing factors, abdominal trauma, drugs, viral infections, and many other causes exist.[38]

Acute pancreatitis is frequently a self-limiting disease often lasting less than one week; however, a number of complications can occur. Pancreatic abscess may result from a localized suppurative process that results in pus collecting in or around the gland. Fluid collections in the pancreatic parenchyma break through the thin-walled connective tissue layer surrounding the organ and spill into surrounding areas. Most frequently, this fluid accumulates in the anterior pararenal space, although it may extend posteriorly to a potential space behind the renal fascia.[39–41] Pancreatic abscess is frequently associated with a left-sided pleural effusion and splenomegaly resulting from splenic vein thrombosis.[42] In phlegmonous pancreatitis, the inflammatory reaction spreads to the soft tissues surrounding the pancreas. A phlegmon is an inflammatory process that spreads along fascial pathways, producing edema and swelling. Other complications of acute pancreatitis include dehydration resulting from fluid loss, subsequent renal failure, pulmonary edema, and the development of chronic pancreatitis. Death may occur in a small percentage of patients from accompanying sepsis.[43] Complications of acute pancreatitis are varied. The course and prognosis of the disease depend on the severity of the complications and the underlying cause.

Clinically, the patient presents with sudden onset of severe abdominal pain, usually localized in the epigastrium or upper quadrants, often radiating to the back. The pain reaches a maximum within minutes or a few hours after onset of the disease and persists until the inflammation subsides. Characteristic of the pain associated with pancreatitis is the relief obtained by sitting up or bending at the waist. Nausea and vomiting are frequently present, and a mild fever may develop within the first few days. Serum amylase concentration increases to its maximum value within 24 hours after onset and gradually returns to normal over 3 to 10 days. An elevated white blood cell count (leukocytosis), proteinuria, and elevated bilirubin value may be present. Serum lipase

TABLE 9-1	Causes of Pancreatitis
Abdominal surgery	
Alcoholism	
Certain medications	
Cystic fibrosis	
Gallstones	
High calcium levels in the blood	
High triglyceride levels in the blood	
Infection	
Injury to the abdomen	
Metabolic disorders	
Obesity	
Pancreatic cancer	

concentration also increases and remains elevated longer than that of serum amylase.

Sonographically, an inflamed pancreas appears enlarged and hypoechoic, although in some cases, it may appear normal.[4] Additionally, the enlargement may be focal or diffuse. The pancreatic duct may appear enlarged secondary to obstruction.[44]

The echotexture of the pancreas may be hypoechoic owing to edema, and the borders of the gland may appear irregular. Care must be taken in young patients whose pancreas may normally appear less echogenic to differentiate it from a diseased organ. In children, acute pancreatitis presents similar to an adult, with decreased echogenicity and increased AP diameter.[26] In children, diffuse or focal enlargement of the pancreas is generally a more reliable indicator of disease than altered echogenicity.[26] On ultrasound, a more indicative feature of acute pancreatitis in children is dilation of the pancreatic duct.[26]

Occasionally, when biliary calculi are the precipitating factor in acute pancreatitis, small stones may make their way through the ductal system and into the pancreatic duct. These may be seen sonographically as highly echogenic foci within a dilated duct (Fig. 9-14).

Pancreatic pseudocysts, encapsulated collections of the by-products of tissue destruction, are common findings with severe disease. The incidence of pseudocysts in acute pancreatitis ranges from 5% to 16%.[45] The occurrence of pseudocysts in chronic pancreatitis ranges from 20% to 40%.[45] Pseudocysts arise in about half of patients with severe disease and form more than 75% of cystic lesions of the pancreas.[46] Sonography may be used to follow pseudocyst maturation and, when necessary, to guide drainage. Although pseudocysts can occur anywhere in the abdominal cavity, they are most frequently found in or around the pancreas itself, especially in the area of the tail (Fig. 9-15). Hemorrhage

of a pseudocyst may occur as a result of tissue necrosis (Fig. 9-16) and, if blood loss is significant, emergency surgical intervention may be indicated. Secondary infection of a pseudocyst may necessitate drainage.[45] Pseudocysts may contain pancreatic juice, blood, pus, and/or inflammatory by-products.[39]

Because pseudocysts are a frequent complication of acute pancreatitis, any cystic-looking structures in the region of the pancreas should be carefully evaluated. They can have a varied sonographic appearance. Variations include smooth-bordered and entirely cystic to poorly marginated, seemingly solid masses with no posterior acoustic enhancement.[47] Septa or debris may be seen within and free fluid may be found in the retroperitoneal compartments.[40] The walls may be thin and smooth, or thick and irregular. Sonography is an excellent modality for detecting and following pseudocysts. Its reported accuracy is 96%, owing to displacement of gas-containing bowel by the mass.[31]

Endoscopic sonography may be useful in the early diagnosis of acute pancreatitis. The procedure, which can be performed at the bedside noninvasively, often allows a more diagnostic evaluation of the pancreas because gas obscuration is not a factor. An enlarged pancreas with normal echogenicity is commonly visualized in patients with edematous pancreatitis. Focal hypoechoic areas representing intrapancreatic fluid collections may be seen if necrotizing pancreatitis is present. Computed tomography (CT) and magnetic resonance imaging are also utilized to make a final diagnosis and delineate the extent of disease.

Chronic Pancreatitis

Chronic pancreatitis results from repeated bouts of acute pancreatitis. Progressive interlobular fibrosis, destruction, and atrophy of functioning tissue results. In the early stages, gross anatomic changes may be absent. As the disease

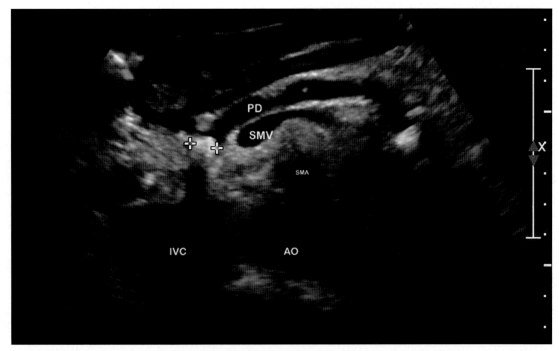

FIGURE 9-14 Transverse image of the pancreas in a patient with acute pancreatitis resulting from a pancreatic duct stone *(calipers)*. The pancreatic duct *(PD)* is dilated secondary to obstruction. *AO*, aorta; *IVC*, inferior vena cava; *SMA*, superior mesenteric artery; *SMV*, superior mesenteric vein.

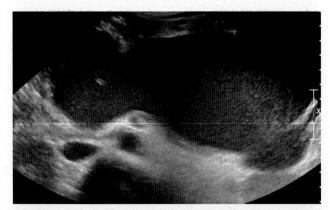

FIGURE 9-15 Transverse image of a large pancreatic pseudocyst.

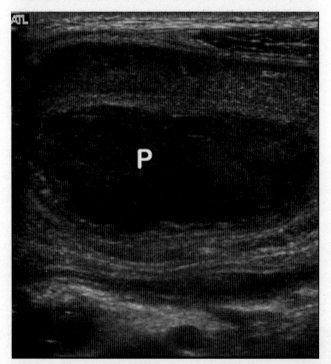

FIGURE 9-16 Pancreatic pseudocyst (P) containing internal debris consistent with hemorrhage. (Image courtesy of Philips Medical Systems, Bothell, WA.)

progresses, the gland becomes small and atrophic. Calculi may be found within the pancreatic duct system, and cystic formations are common. Intraparenchymal fluid collections are frequently seen.[10]

The prognosis for chronic pancreatitis is best when the causative agent can be removed, as in chronic cholecystitis, or alcohol-induced disease. Chronic pancreatitis may also occur in patients with hypercalcemia or hyperlipidemia. Chronic pancreatitis has been linked to an increased risk of developing pancreatic cancer. The risk of developing pancreatic cancer with a history of chronic pancreatitis is 1.8% after 10 years and 4.0% after 20 years.[48]

In chronic pancreatitis, clinical symptoms include persistent epigastric pain radiating to the left lumbar region, nausea, vomiting, flatulence, and weight loss. Paralytic ileus, a malfunction of the nerves and muscles in the intestine, is a common complication. Jaundice may also be present. During exacerbation of acute inflammatory disease, which frequently occurs in chronic relapsing pancreatitis, serum amylase and bilirubin levels may be elevated.

The sonographic findings in chronic pancreatitis are varied. Because gross anatomic changes may not occur in the course of this disease, sonography may not detect abnormalities. In cases where anatomic changes have occurred, however, sonographic evaluation most frequently reveals heterogeneous increased echogenicity secondary to fibrotic and fatty changes (Fig. 9-17). The pancreas may be enlarged with irregular borders, and the pancreatic duct may be dilated (Fig. 9-18). A sonographic hallmark of chronic pancreatitis is the presence of calcifications within the parenchyma, which appear sonographically as bright reflections that may or may not cast a posterior acoustic shadow[49] (Figs. 9-19 and 9-20). Reported complications associated with chronic relapsing pancreatitis include changes in parenchymal texture, glandular atrophy, glandular enlargement, focal masses, dilation and beading of the pancreatic duct (often with intraductal calcifications), venous thrombosis, and pseudocysts.[4]

Neoplastic Disease

Malignant tumors of the pancreas rank as the fourth leading cause of cancer-related deaths in the United States.[50] Early diagnosis is associated with a slightly better prognosis, but because many pancreatic malignancies do not produce symptoms until late in the disease, early detection is uncommon. Tumors most commonly occur in men older than 30 years of age and are approximately 50% to 90% more common in black males.[51] Risk factors include a family history of pancreatic cancer, smoking, high-fat diet, chronic pancreatitis, diabetes, and cirrhosis of the liver.

Because of its dual role as an exocrine and endocrine gland, the pancreas is unique in cellular structure and physiologic function. Tumors may be classified according to the cell of origin.[52,53] Neoplasms of exocrine origin comprise the largest group of pancreatic tumors and include the single most common malignant lesion: adenocarcinoma.[54] Adenocarcinomas account for 85% of all pancreatic malignancies.[54] The frequency of these lesions is 60% to 70% in the head, 15% in the body, and 15% in the tail.[51] Adenocarcinoma is one of the most lethal of all malignancies, with an overall 5-year survival rate of 9%.[54] Anatomically, these lesions vary in size and gross appearance. Some are well-circumscribed, solid, ovoid masses, whereas others infiltrate surrounding pancreatic parenchyma so diffusely that the pancreas appears as a matted mass of tumor. Some small carcinomas that arise in the ampulla of Vater may be very difficult to detect sonographically. Tumors in the pancreatic head usually spread into the duodenum and compress the common bile duct and ampulla of Vater. Mechanical obstruction of the biliary tract causes dilatation of the ducts and frequently the gallbladder. A markedly distended and clinically palpable gallbladder, commonly referred to as a Courvoisier gallbladder, is easily visualized sonographically and is a reliable indicator of a lesion in the pancreatic head.[55]

Other exocrine lesions of the pancreas are rare. These various types of exocrine neoplasms account for more than 75% of all pancreatic cancers (Pathology Box 9-1).

Tumors of endocrine origin are referred to as neuroendocrine tumors or islet cell tumors. These are far less common

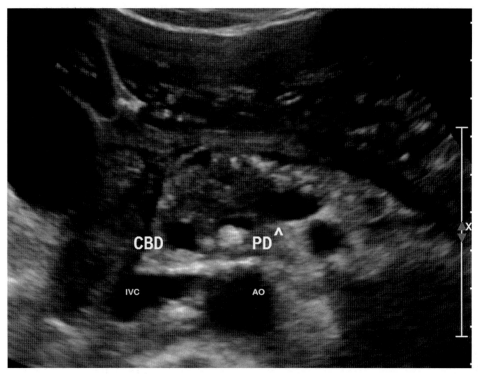

FIGURE 9-17 Transverse image of the pancreas in a patient with chronic pancreatitis. The parenchyma of the pancreas is heterogeneous secondary to fibrotic and fatty changes. The common bile duct *(CBD)* and pancreatic duct *(PD^)* are dilated. *AO*, aorta; *IVC*, inferior vena cava.

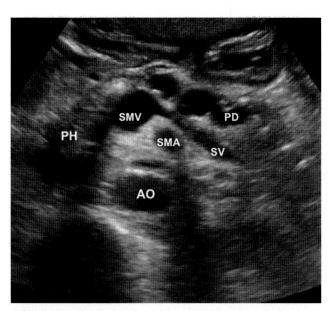

FIGURE 9-18 Transverse image of the pancreas in a patient with chronic pancreatitis. Calcifications are seen in the pancreas. The pancreatic duct *(PD)* is dilated. *AO*, aorta; *PH*, pancreatic head; *SMA*, superior mesenteric artery; *SMV*, superior mesenteric vein; *SV*, splenic vein.

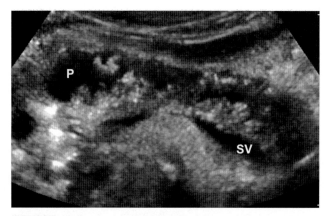

FIGURE 9-19 Transverse image of the pancreas in a patient with chronic pancreatitis. Calcifications are seen throughout the parenchyma of the pancreas. In addition, there is an accompanying pseudocyst *(P)*. *SV*, splenic vein.

than exocrine neoplasms and account for about 1% to 5% of all pancreatic cancers. Insulinomas and gastrinomas are the most common types of endocrine tumors (80%).[4] Neuroendocrine neoplasms may produce hormones that can make an individual symptomatic. Insulinomas produce large amounts of insulin, and gastrinomas produce gastrin. Most endocrine tumors are solid and are often very small, making them difficult to detect with sonography. These tumors can be singular or multiple and are more common in the body or tail of the pancreas.

Solid Neoplastic Lesions

Sonographically, solid pancreatic tumors are generally hypoechoic, but they can vary in echogenicity and echotexture.[1] The borders may be well defined (Fig. 9-21), but more often, they appear as poorly marginated, complex masses most commonly involving the pancreatic head[56–58] (Fig. 9-22). Color Doppler imaging will often show increased vascularity to areas of tumor (Fig. 9-23). Because pancreatic carcinoma is rarely detected early in the disease process, by the time the patient is referred for diagnostic imaging procedures, the neoplasm has usually spread. Enlarged lymph nodes in the porta hepatis and in the para-aortic region indicate nodal metastasis. Inflammation of

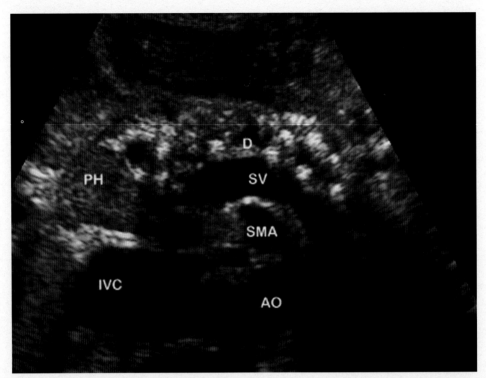

FIGURE 9-20 Transverse image of the pancreas in a patient with chronic pancreatitis. Calcifications are seen throughout the body and tail of the pancreas. *AO*, aorta; *D*, pancreatic duct; *IVC*, inferior vena cava; *PH*, pancreatic head; *SMA*, superior mesenteric artery; *SV*, splenic vein. (Image courtesy of Philips Medical Systems, Bothell, WA.)

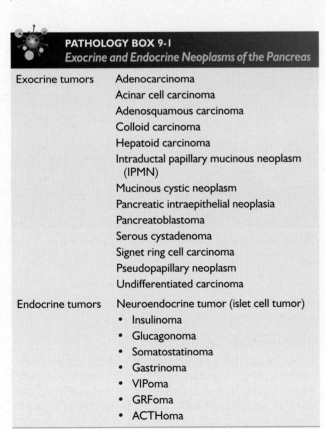

PATHOLOGY BOX 9-1
Exocrine and Endocrine Neoplasms of the Pancreas

Exocrine tumors	Adenocarcinoma
	Acinar cell carcinoma
	Adenosquamous carcinoma
	Colloid carcinoma
	Hepatoid carcinoma
	Intraductal papillary mucinous neoplasm (IPMN)
	Mucinous cystic neoplasm
	Pancreatic intraepithelial neoplasia
	Pancreatoblastoma
	Serous cystadenoma
	Signet ring cell carcinoma
	Pseudopapillary neoplasm
	Undifferentiated carcinoma
Endocrine tumors	Neuroendocrine tumor (islet cell tumor)
	• Insulinoma
	• Glucagonoma
	• Somatostatinoma
	• Gastrinoma
	• VIPoma
	• GRFoma
	• ACTHoma

or sitting upright may alleviate the pain. Jaundice occurs if the lesion produces biliary obstruction, and weight loss is common. Symptoms usually occur late in the disease. Laboratory results are generally nonspecific for pancreatic disease. Serum amylase and lipase values are occasionally elevated, steatorrhea does not occur in the absence of jaundice, and occult blood may be detected in stool when the tumor involves the ampulla of Vater.[59]

Additionally, tumors in the head of the pancreas may cause obstructive jaundice, in which case, the common bile and intrahepatic ducts may appear dilated (Fig. 9-24). If the neoplasm is very small, the only sonographic indicator of an intrapancreatic abnormality may be the blunt termination of a dilated common bile duct in the head of the pancreas (Fig. 9-25).

Endoscopic ultrasound is considered the best imaging method for detecting small-diameter pancreatic masses, with a sensitivity of 92% to 100%, specificity of 89% to 100%, and accuracy of 86% to 99%.[60] Endoscopic ultrasound has been shown to have better accuracy in diagnosing pancreatic tumors than conventional CT and should be performed when there is suspicion of pancreatic cancer without a definite mass seen on CT scan. Endoscopic ultrasound-guided fine needle aspiration has become a beneficial modality of diagnosing solid pancreatic lesions. This version of imaging is also the most sensitive means for detecting venous and gastric invasion.[61,62] In addition to better imaging, newer antitumor therapies are being developed and researched, such as antitumor agents, brachytherapy, and ablations.[63]

Cystic Neoplastic Lesions

The majority of pancreatic tumors are solid, and cystic tumors account for approximately 2% to 10% of all pancreatic neoplasms.[64] Malignant cystic tumors account for 1% of pancreatic malignancy.[4] When a fluid-filled structure is seen in or around

the pancreas is a common sequela in carcinomatosis, and the remainder of the organ may appear enlarged and hypoechoic.[59] The patient with pancreatic carcinoma commonly presents with vague, diffuse pain located in the epigastrium that radiates to the back. As with acute pancreatitis, leaning forward

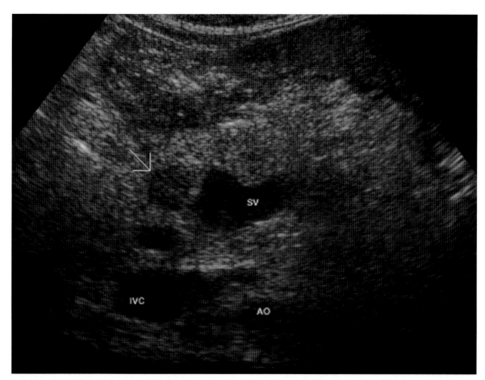

FIGURE 9-21 Transverse image of the pancreas with a well-circumscribed neoplasm *(arrow)* within the head of the pancreas. *AO*, aorta; *IVC*, inferior vena cava; *SV*, splenic vein.

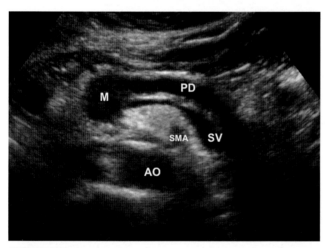

FIGURE 9-22 Transverse image of the pancreas showing a complex mass *(M)* within the pancreas consistent with neoplasm. The pancreatic duct *(PD)* is dilated. *AO*, aorta; *SMA*, superior mesenteric artery; *SV*, splenic vein.

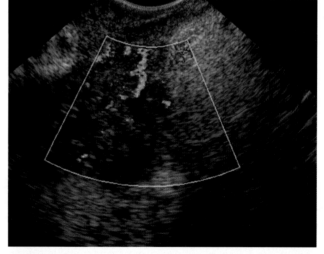

FIGURE 9-23 Color and spectral Doppler image showing blood flow within a pancreatic neoplasm.

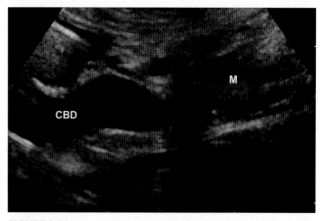

FIGURE 9-24 Large malignant mass *(M)* within the head of the pancreas causing obstruction of the common bile duct *(CBD)*.

the pancreas, the most likely diagnosis is a pseudocyst. Differentiation from a tumor can be made by analyzing laboratory results, which will most likely demonstrate inflammatory disease. In the absence of clinical suspicion of acute or chronic pancreatitis, cystic neoplastic disease must be considered.[65] Cystic neoplastic lesions consist of serous cystadenomas, mucinous cystic neoplasms, intraductal papillary mucinous neoplasms (IPMN), and solid pseudopapillary neoplasms.

Serous cystadenoma, previously known as microcystic adenoma, is typically a benign tumor and occurs more commonly in women.[66] These lesions represent about one-third of all pancreatic cystic neoplasms.[66] They occur more frequently in the head of the pancreas. On ultrasound, these lesions appear well circumscribed and loculated and may contain calcifications. Morphologically, these tumors have thin, well-defined, fibrous capsules containing multiple cysts

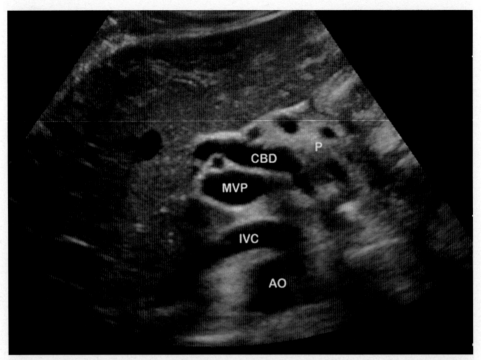

FIGURE 9-25 Longitudinal image showing a dilated common bile duct (*CBD*) ending bluntly in the pancreatic head (*P*) of a patient with pancreatic cancer. The pancreatic parenchyma was heterogeneous although no discrete mass was identified. *AO*, aorta; *IVC*, inferior vena cava; *MVP*, main portal vein.

of varying size.[66] In lesions where cysts are only a couple of millimeters in size (microcysts), the tumor appears solid owing to the innumerable interfaces.[66]

Mucinous cystic adenomas are a benign tumor, but can progress into a cancerous lesion. Resection for these tumors is recommended and usually yields an excellent prognosis for survival in which patients often do not need any follow-up.[67] Mucinous cystadenomas are located in the body and tail region of the pancreas.[67] Virtually all of these lesions occur in women.[67] Sonographically, they appear as solitary, unilocular, well-circumscribed round or lobular cysts (about 80%) that can range in dimensions (1 to 36 cm).[68]

IPMN arises from the pancreatic ducts, usually in the head of the pancreas, and produces mucin. These tumors have the potential to become malignant, with malignant transformation occurring in 25% to 70% of cases, of which 15% to 43% are invasive.[69] This tumor occurs more commonly in elderly males.[68] Ductal dilation is a distinguishable feature of IPMN on ultrasound. Findings include lobulated dilation of the branching ducts, diffuse dilation of the branch ducts, diffuse dilation of the main pancreatic duct, and intraductal papillary tumors.[4] IPMNs may be solitary or multiple and can be highly variable in appearance (grape-like multicystic, unilocular, or finger-like).[68]

Solid pseudopapillary neoplasms are rare with low malignant potential and a great prognosis.[70] These tumors occur more commonly in young women and often arise in the pancreatic head and tail.[68] They are well-circumscribed masses that demonstrate variable degrees of internal hemorrhage, cystic degeneration, and there may be associated calcifications.[70] Larger lesions often possess a combination of solid, cystic, and pseudopapillary tissue patterns.[68]

Primary cystic neoplasms have a variable sonographic appearance. Again, 85% to 90% of cystic masses in the pancreatic bed are related to inflammatory disease.[71] Other noninflammatory cystic lesions of the pancreas include polycystic disease and cystic fibrosis.

Nonneoplastic Cystic Lesions

Polycystic Disease

Polycystic disease is an autosomal dominant disease characterized by the presence of multiple small cysts in the kidney; liver; and, less commonly (10%), the pancreas.[72] Patients present with a family history of polycystic disease or are being worked up for hypertension, renal insufficiency, or pyelonephritis. The slowly multiplying and enlarging cystic masses eventually destroy the normal pancreatic tissue. The vast majority of patients with polycystic disease, however, succumb to renal failure well before the pancreas is physiologically affected. The finding of well-defined cystic lesions in the pancreas should alert the sonographer to the possibility of polycystic disease. In such cases, the liver and kidneys should be evaluated for the presence of multiple cysts. In the absence of renal or hepatic cysts, the diagnosis of polycystic disease cannot be made; instead, one of the abovementioned inflammatory or neoplastic lesions should be considered.

Von Hippel–Lindau Disease

Von Hippel–Lindau disease is an autosomal dominant disorder that involves the central nervous system. Pancreatic lesions may develop in 35% to 77% of patients with von Hippel–Lindau and most of them present as benign cysts.[73] Pancreatic neuroendocrine tumors have been reported to occur in 17% of patients with this disease[73] (Fig. 9-26). Pancreatic carcinoma has also been reported.[73] Peripheral calcifications may also occur in the pancreas.

Additional Pathologic Assessment

Other means of sonographic evaluation may prove useful in characterizing pancreatic tumors. The first of these imaging techniques is elastography. Elastography is the assessment of the stiffness of the pancreas. The two types

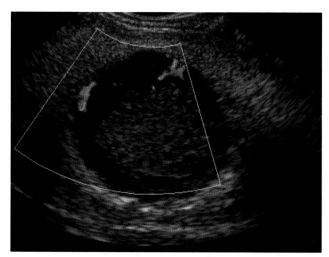

FIGURE 9-26 Pancreatic neuroendocrine tumor in a patient with von Hippel–Lindau disease. Blood flow is appreciated within the mass with color Doppler image. (Image courtesy of Philips Medical Systems, Bothell, WA.)

of elastography are strain elastography and shear wave elastography. Strain elastography is a qualitative technique where a comparison is performed and relative stiffness differences of the pancreatic tissue are displayed by colors.[74] Shear wave measures the speed of the propagation waves traveling within a tissue, giving a quantitative number.[74] Elastography is a useful technique to characterize small solid pancreatic lesions and also to evaluate the extent of pancreatic disease. Limitations of elastography include differences in acquisition techniques and suboptimal visualization of the entire pancreatic gland.

A second tool for assessment of the pancreas is contrast-enhanced ultrasound. Contrast-enhanced ultrasound involves intravenous injection of air-filled microbubbles into systemic circulation.[75] Real-time imaging is used to observe the contrast-enhanced phases (arterial, portal/venous, and late phases).[76] This provides accuracy in perfusion studies, allowing the visualization of the pancreatic lesion microvasculature.[76] Pancreatic tumors and pancreatic diseases have different vascularization patterns in contrast-enhanced ultrasound.

SUMMARY

- The pancreas is a nonencapsulated structure, with an oblique lie in the anterior portion of the retroperitoneum, and with three main portions (the head, body, and tail).
- Congenital anomalies of the pancreas are rare, with pancreas divisum being the most common.
- The pancreas is responsible for both endocrine (secreting into blood or tissue) and exocrine functions (secreting into a duct).
- Serum amylase is one of the most useful laboratory values for the diagnosis of pancreatic disease.
- Other values to monitor include lipase, fat excretion, bilirubin, and liver function tests.
- Patient preparation is an attempt to minimize the amount of gas in the stomach and duodenum by having the patient refrain from eating or drinking 8 to 12 hours prior to the examination.

- The pancreas examination includes evaluating the pancreas by taking images and obtaining measurements in both the transverse and longitudinal sections.
- Cystic fibrosis is the most common lethal genetic defect resulting in multiple pancreatic pathologies.
- Inflammatory pancreatic diseases include both acute and chronic pancreatitis.
- Pancreatic pseudocysts are frequent complications of acute pancreatitis.
- Neoplastic pancreatic diseases include both solid and cystic neoplastic lesions.
- Polycystic disease and von Hippel–Lindau diseases are autosomal dominant.
- Although sonography may not be considered as the primary imaging modality in evaluation of the pancreas, it is useful in detecting some lesions, particularly in an unsuspecting population.
- Sonography can aid in diagnosis-associated causes of pancreatic disease including biliary and hepatic abnormalities.

REFERENCES

1. Stevens KJ, Lisanti C. Pancreas imaging. In: *StatPearls* (Internet). StatPearls Publishing; 2020.
2. Soufi M, Yip-Schneider MT, Carr R, et al. *Intraductal* papillary mucinous neoplasia originating from the accessory (Santorini) duct: a rare entity. *Am Surg.* 2020:1–3. doi:10.1177/0003134820956337
3. Hagen-Ansert SL. The pancreas. In: Hagen-Ansert SL, ed. *Textbook of Diagnostic Sonography*. Vol 1. 8th ed. Elsevier; 2018:305–335.
4. Winter P, Sun MRM. The pancreas. In: Rumack CM, Levine D. *Diagnostic Ultrasound*. Vol 1. 5th ed. Elsevier; 2017:210–255.
5. Bogveradze N, Hasse F, Mayer P, et al. Is MRCP necessary to diagnose pancreas divisum? *BMC Med Imaging.* 2019;19:33.
6. Aleem A, Shah H. Annular pancreas. In: *StatPearls* (Internet). StatPearls Publishing; 2020.
7. Skandalakis JE. The pancreas. In: Skandalakis J, Gray S, eds. *Embryology for Surgeons*. Williams and Wilkins; 1994:336–404.
8. Zhang P, Wang M, Bai L, Zhuang W. A unique case of ectopic pancreas presenting jejunal malignance. *J Surg Case Rep.* 2019;7:rjz217.
9. Dietrich CF, Braden B. Sonographic assessments of gastrointestinal and biliary functions. *Best Prac Res Clin Gastroenterol.* 2009;23(3):353–367.
10. Nealon WH, Bhutani M, Riall TS, Raju G, Ozkan O, Neilan R. A unifying concept: pancreatic ductal anatomy both predicts and determines the major complications resulting from pancreatitis. *J Am Coll Surg.* 2009;208(5):790–799.
11. Uchida K, Yazumi S, Nishio A, et al. Long-term outcome of autoimmune pancreatitis. *J Gastroenterol.* 2009;44(7):726–732.
12. McGuckin E, Cade JE, Hanison J. The pancreas. *Physiology.* 2020;21(11):604–610.
13. Brown TT, Prahlow JA. Postmortem serum amylase and lipase analysis in the diagnosis of acute pancreatitis. *Acad Forensic Pathol.* 2018;8(2):311–323.
14. Batra HS, Kumar A, Saha TK, Misra P, Ambade V. Comparative study of serum amylase and lipase in acute pancreatitis patients. *Indian J Clin Biochem.* 2015;30(2):230–233.
15. Kim YS, Chang JH, Kim TH, Kim CW, Kim JK, Han SW. Prolonged hyperamylasemia in patients with acute pancreatitis is associated with recurrence of acute pancreatitis. *Medicine (Baltimore).* 2020;99(3):e18861.
16. Lam R, Muniraj T. Hyperamylasemia. In: *StatPearls* (Internet). StatPearls Publishing; 2020.
17. Clark LR, Jaffe MH, Choyke PL, Grant EG, Zeman RK. Pancreatic imaging. *Radiol Clin North Am.* 1985;23(3):489–499.
18. Smotkin J, Tenner S. Laboratory diagnostic tests in acute pancreatitis. *J Clin Gastroenterol.* 2002;34(4):459–462.
19. Ismail OZ, Bhayana V. Lipase or amylase for the diagnosis of acute pancreatitis? *Clin Biochem.* 2017;50(18):1275–1280.

20. Smith RC, Southwell-Keely J, Chesher D. Should serum pancreatic lipase replace serum amylase as a marker of acute pancreatitis? *ANZ J Surg.* 2005;75(6):399–404.

21. Azer SA, Sankararaman S. Steatorrhea. In: *StatPearls* (Internet). StatPearls Publishing; 2020.

22. Keller J, Aghdassi AA, Lerch MM, Mayerle JV, Layer P. Tests of pancreatic exocrine function—clinical significance in pancreatic and non-pancreatic disorders. *Best Pract Res Clin Gastroenterol.* 2009;23:425–439.

23. Mittlestaedt CA. *Abdominal Ultrasound.* Churchill Livingstone; 1987.

24. Majumder S, Philip N, Takahashi N, Levy MJ, Singh VP, Chari ST. Fatty pancreas: should we be concerned? *Pancreas.* 2017;46(10):1251–1258.

25. Marks WM, Filly RA, Callen PW. Ultrasonic evaluation of normal pancreatic echogenicity and its relationship to fat deposition. *Radiology.* 1980;137:475–479.

26. Restrepo R, Hagerott HE, Kulkarni S, Yasrebi M, Lee EY. Acute pancreatitis in pediatric patients: demographics, etiology, and diagnostic imaging. *AJR Am J Roentgenol.* 2016;206(3):632–644.

27. Didier D, Deschamps JP, Rohmer P, Lassegue A, Ottignon Y, Weill F. Evaluation of the pancreatic duct: a reappraisal based on a retrospective correlative study by sonographic and pancreatography in 117 normal and pathologic subjects. *Ultrasound Med Biol.* 1983;9:509–518.

28. Weinstein DP, Weinstein BJ. Ultrasonic demonstration of the pancreatic duct: an analysis of 41 cases. *Radiology.* 1979;130:729–732.

29. Ohto M, Saotome N, Saisho HH, et al. Real-time sonography of the pancreatic duct: application to percutaneous pancreatic ductography. *AJR Am J Roentgenol.* 1980;134:647–650.

30. Bryan PJ. Appearance of the normal pancreatic duct: a study using real-time ultrasound. *J Clin Ultrasound.* 1982;10:63–68.

31. Pochammer KF, Szekessy T, Frentzel-Beyme B, et al. Cranio-caudad dimension of the pancreatic head. *Radiology.* 1985;155:861–868.

32. Lawson TL, Berland LL, Foley WD. Coronal upper abdominal anatomy: technique and gastrointestinal applications. *Gastrointest Radiol.* 1981;6:115–121.

33. Goldstein HM, Katragadda CS. Prone view ultrasonography for neoplasms of the pancreatic tail. *AJR Am J Roentgenol.* 1978;131:231–236.

34. Okaniwa S. How does ultrasound manage pancreatic diseases? Ultrasound findings and scanning maneuvers. *Gut Liver.* 2020;14(1):37–46.

35. Gillespie CD, O'Reilly MK, Allen GN, McDermott S, Chan VO, Ridge CA. Imaging the abdominal manifestations of cystic fibrosis. *Int J Hepatol.* 2017;2017:5128760.

36. Singh VK, Schwarzenberg SJ. Pancreatic insufficiency in cystic fibrosis. *J Cyst Fibros.* 2017;16(2):70–78.

37. Türkvatan A, Erden A, Türköğlu MA, Seçil M, Yener Ö. Imaging of acute pancreatitis and its complications. Part 1: acute pancreatitis. *Diagn Interv Imaging.* 2015;96(2):151–160.

38. Chatila AT, Bilal M, Guturu P. Evaluation and management of acute pancreatitis. *World J Clin Cases.* 2019;7(9):1006–1020.

39. Donovan PJ, Sanders RC, Siegelman SS. Collections of fluid after pancreatitis: evaluation by computed tomography and ultrasonography. *Radiol Clin North Am.* 1982;20:653–665.

40. Raptopoulos V, Kleinman PK, Marks S. Renal fascial pathway: posterior extension of pancreatic effusions within the anterior pararenal space. *Radiology.* 1986;158:367–374.

41. Zerem E. Treatment of severe acute pancreatitis and its complications. *World J Gastroenterol.* 2014;20(38):13879–13892.

42. Zaleman M, Van Gansbeke D, Matos C, Engelholm L, Struyven J. Sonographic demonstration of portal venous system thrombosis secondary to inflammatory disease of the pancreas. *Gastrointest Radiol.* 1987;12:114–121.

43. Leppäniemi A, Tolonen M, Tarasconi A, et al. 2019 WSES guidelines for the management of severe acute pancreatitis. *World J Emerg Surg.* 2019;14:27.

44. Burrowes DP, Choi HH, Rodgers SK, Fetzer DT, Kamaya A. Utility of ultrasound in acute pancreatitis. *Abdom Radiol (NY).* 2020;45(5):1253–1264.

45. Misra D, Sood T. Pancreatic pseudocyst. In: *StatPearls* (Internet). StatPearls Publishing; 2020.

46. Shruti M, Bertran-Rodriguez CE, Ishani S. Pancreatic pseudocysts in patients with acute and chronic pancreatitis, trends, and clinical outcomes of hospitalization: insights from a national inpatient database. *Am J Gastroenterol.* 2019;114:41–42.

47. Laing FC, Gooding GA, Brown T, Leopold GR. Atypical pseudocysts of the pancreas: an ultrasonographic evaluation. *J Clin Ultrasound.* 1979;7:27–32.

48. Lalwani N, Mannelli L, Ganeshan DM, et al. Uncommon pancreatic tumors and pseudotumors. *Abdom Imaging.* 2015;40(1):167–180.

49. Javadi S, Menias CO, Korivi BR, et al. Pancreatic calcifications and calcified pancreatic masses: pattern recognition approach on CT. *AJR Am J Roentgenol.* 2017;209:77–87.

50. Siegel RL, Miller KD, Fuchs HE, et al. Cancer statistics, 2021. *CA Cancer J Clin.* 2021;71(1):7–33.

51. McGuigan A, Kelly P, Turkington RC, et al. Pancreatic cancer: a review of clinical diagnosis, epidemiology, treatment and outcomes. *World J Gastroenterol.* 2018;24(43):4846–4861.

52. Cubilla AL, Fitzgerald PJ. Classification of pancreatic cancer (non-endocrine). *Mayo Clin Proc.* 1979;54:449–458.

53. Larsson L. Endocrine pancreatic tumors. *Human Pathol.* 1978;9:401–416.

54. Rawla P, Sunkara T, Gaduputi V. Epidemiology of pancreatic cancer: global trends, etiology and risk factors. *World J Oncol.* 2019;10(1):10–27.

55. Agrawal S, Vohra S. Simultaneous Courvoisier's and double ducts signs. *World J Gastrointest Endosc.* 2017;9(8):425–427.

56. Koenigsberg P. Focal lesions of the pancreas. *Semin Roentgenol.* 1985;20:3–21.

57. Shawker TH, Garra BS, Hill MC, et al. Spectrum of sonographic findings in pancreatic carcinoma. *J Ultrasound Med.* 1986;5:169–175.

58. Shawker TH, Linzer M, Hubbard VS. Chronic pancreatitis: the diagnostic significance of pancreatic size and echo amplitude. *Radiology.* 1985;154:568–574.

59. Niccoloni DG, Graham JH, Banks PA. Tumor-induced acute pancreatitis. *Gastroenterology.* 1976;71:142–145.

60. Yousaf MN, Chaudhary FS, Ehsan A, et al. Endoscopic ultrasound (EUS) and the management of pancreatic cancer. *BMJ Open Gastroenterol.* 2020;7(1):e000408.

61. Helmstaedter L, Riemann JF. Pancreatic cancer-EUS and early diagnosis. *Langenbecks Arch Surg.* 2008;393:923–927.

62. Figueiredo FA, Giovannini M, Monges G, et al. Pancreatic endocrine tumors: a large single–center experience. *Pancreas.* 2009;38(8):936–940.

63. Moutinho-Riberio P, Liberal R, Macedo G. Endoscopic ultrasound in pancreatic cancer treatment: facts and hopes. *Clin Res Hepatol Gastroenterol.* 2019;43(5):513–521.

64. Xiao S, Ye Z. Pancreatic cystic tumors: an update. *J Pancreatol.* 2018;1(1):2–18.

65. Freeny PC, Weinstein CJ, Taft DA, Allen FH. Cystic neoplasms of the pancreas: new angiographic and sonographic findings. *Am J Roentgenol.* 1978;131:795–802.

66. Dababneh Y, Mousa OY. Pancreatic serous cystadenoma. In: *StatPearls* (Internet). StatPearls Publishing; 2020.

67. Bojanupu S, Kasi A. Pancreatic mucinous cystadenoma. In: *StatPearls* (Internet). StatPearls Publishing; 2020.

68. Bollen TL, Wessels FJ. Radiological workup of cystic neoplasms of the pancreas. *Visc Med.* 2018;34:182–190.

69. Buscail E, Cauvin T, Fernandez B, et al. Intraductal papillary mucinous neoplasms of the pancreas and European guidelines: importance of the surgery type in the decision-making process. *BMC Surg.* 2019;19:115.

70. Dinarvand P, Lai J. Solid pseudopapillary neoplasm of the pancreas: a rare entity with unique features. *Arch Pathol Lab Med.* 2017;141(7):990–995.

71. Wolfman NT, Ramquist NA, Karstaedt N, Hopkins MB. Cystic neoplasms of the pancreas: CT and sonography. *Am J Roentgenol.* 1982;138:37–40.

72. Sonavane AD, Amarapurkar DN, Amarapurkar AD. Polycystic pancreas. *ACG Case Rep J.* 2016;3(3):199–201.

73. Zhi X, Bo Q, Zhao B, Sun D, Li T. Von hippel-lindau disease involving pancreas and biliary system. *Medicine (Baltimore).* 2017;96(1):e5808.

74. Dietrich CF, Hocke M. Elastography of the pancreas, current view. *Clin Endosc.* 2019;52(6):533–540.

75. Ran L, Zhao W, Zhao Y, Bu H. Value of contrast-enhanced ultrasound in differential diagnosis of solid lesions of pancreas (SLP). *Medicine (Baltimore).* 2017;96(28):e7463.

76. D'Onofrio M, Gallotti A, Principe F, Mucelli RP. Contrast-enhanced ultrasound of the pancreas. *World J Radiol.* 2010;2(3):97–102.

CHAPTER 10

The Spleen

TANYA D. NOLAN

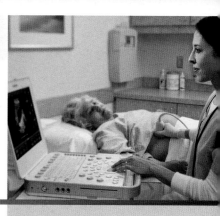

OBJECTIVES

- Describe the normal anatomy and function of the spleen.
- Describe the normal vasculature of the spleen.
- List the common causes of splenomegaly.
- Demonstrate the scanning techniques used to image the spleen.
- Identify the sonographic appearance and etiology of benign focal lesions of the spleen including splenic cyst, abscess, infarct, hematoma, and hemangioma.
- Discuss the sonographic findings of lymphoma, leukemia, and metastases of the spleen.
- Identify technically satisfactory and unsatisfactory sonographic examinations of the spleen.

GLOSSARY

erythrocyte red blood cell; contains hemoglobin and is responsible for transporting oxygen

erythropoiesis process of red blood cell production; occurs in the fetal spleen from the fifth to sixth month of fetal life after which the bone marrow assumes the function

hematocrit laboratory value of the percentage of blood volume made up of red blood cells; can be low in cases of anemia, blood loss, and leukemia

infarct tissue death caused by an interruption of blood supply

leukocyte white blood cell; main function is to protect against and fight infection in the body

leukocytosis elevated white blood cell count usually owing to infection

leukopenia decreased white blood cell count; can be a result of many factors including viral infection and leukemia

A thorough sonographic examination of the left upper quadrant (LUQ) includes the spleen. Because of its asymmetric shape and its location behind the ribs, the spleen can be difficult to orient, align, and elongate appropriately. Radionuclide imaging and computed tomography (CT) are often used to image the spleen; however, sonography is effective in characterizing splenic masses, evaluating splenic size and echotexture, identifying and characterizing palpated LUQ masses, monitoring the course of splenic trauma, and locating intraperitoneal blood collections.

EMBRYOLOGY AND NORMAL ANATOMY

During the fifth week of embryology, the spleen develops from the mesenchymal cells located between the layers of the dorsal mesentery. The spleen is not considered an endodermal derivative of the primitive gut although it does share an arterial supply with the foregut organs. The spleen moves from its original median position toward the LUQ as the stomach rotates and the mesogastrium develops.[1]

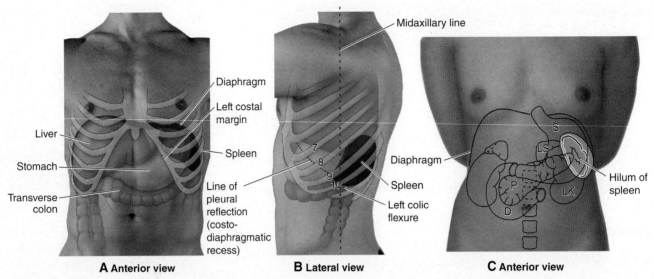

FIGURE 10-1 The spleen in relationship to surrounding organs and structures. *D*, duodenum; *LK*, left kidney; *LS*, lesser sac; *P*, pancreas; *S*, stomach.

Eventually, splenic mesenchymal cells differentiate to form splenic pulp, connecting tissues, and the splenic capsule.

The spleen is an intraperitoneal, ovoid organ entirely covered by peritoneum except at a small bare area at the hilum through which the splenic artery, splenic vein, and efferent lymphatic vessels pass. The spleen is a delicate and vulnerable organ, and its long axis parallels the ninth to eleventh ribs[2] (Fig. 10-1). The spleen is bordered anteriorly by the stomach; medially by the left kidney, splenic flexure

of the colon, and pancreatic tail; and posteriorly by the diaphragm, pleura, left lung, and ribs[1,3] (Fig. 10-2). When imaging the spleen, the neighboring organs and structures may create indentations and impressions on its visceral surface that may simulate masses.[3] Therefore, knowledge of the normal variants of the spleen is essential in preventing a misdiagnosis.

Although the spleen has some mobility, the organ does not normally extend inferiorly beyond the left costal margin. As

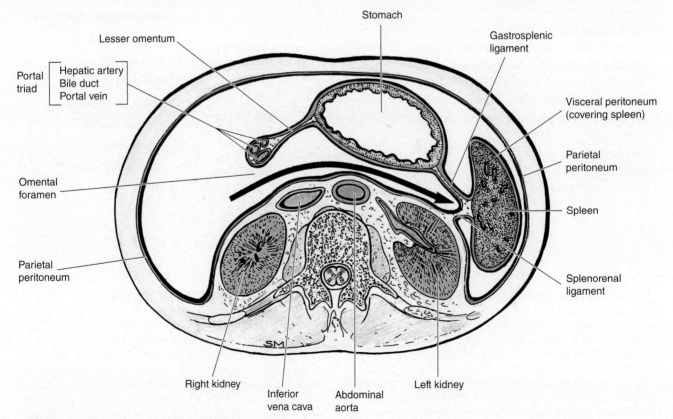

FIGURE 10-2 Cross section of the abdomen at the level of the hilus of the spleen.

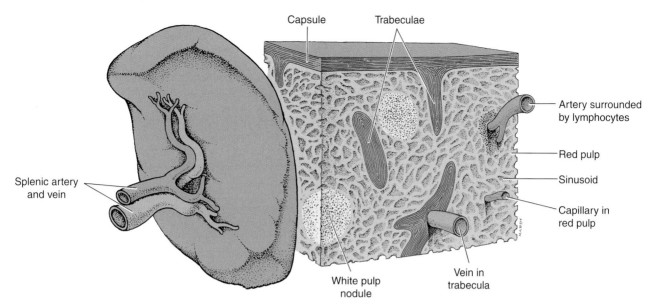

FIGURE 10-3 Schematic of the cellular structure of the spleen.

a result, clinically palpating the spleen through the anterior lateral wall is difficult without significant enlargement of the organ.[2] Moderate evidence suggests that palpation may be beneficial in supporting the diagnosis of splenomegaly, but this clinical examination cannot accurately rule out alternative conditions and must be correlated with diagnostic imaging.[4]

At the hilus, the splenic arteries and veins are covered by the mesentery of the lienorenal ligament, which also houses the tail of the pancreas. The lienorenal and gastrosplenic ligaments attach the spleen to the left kidney and greater curvature of the stomach, respectively.[2,3] The phrenicocolic ligament is not directly attached to the spleen; however, it supports the inferior end of the organ. The lienorenal, gastrosplenic, and phrenicocolic ligaments work together to stabilize the spleen and hold it loosely in position. Laxity of peritoneal attachments allows for hypermobility or wandering of the spleen.[5]

The average spleen measures 12 cm in length, less than 8 cm in anteroposterior dimension, and less than 4 cm in transverse dimension.[6,7] In children, spleen length increases with age and is correlated with body parameters (height, weight, and body surface area). The formula used to determine spleen size in children is $5.7 + 0.31 \times$ age (years). Infants who are 3 months or younger should have a spleen less than 6 cm in length. The adult splenic size is commonly compared to that of a person's fist and weighs less than 150 g.[8,9] Splenic size and weight vary based on age, gender, and nutritional status. The normal spleen is smaller in women, decreases in volume and size with advancing age, and increases in size during digestion.[2,9] It has been reported that 3D sonographic visualization and measurement of the spleen volume have a moderate-to-high agreement when compared with CT volumetry.[10]

Overall, the spleen has the greatest amount of lymphoid tissue within the human body.[1] A fibrous capsule composed of dense fibroelastic connective tissue surrounds the spleen and is thickened at the splenic hilum. Strands of connective tissue project from the splenic capsule and divide the spleen into several compartments. These communicating compartments are filled with splenic lymphoid tissue termed *splenic pulp*, which function to filter the peripheral blood[2,8] (Fig. 10-3). The presence of white and red splenic pulp within the spleen make its texture soft and sponge-like. The white pulp is clustered around splenic arterioles and activates immune response when antigens and their antibodies are present within the blood.[1,7] The red pulp consists of a network of blood-filled venous sinuses and reticular splenic cords, termed the *Cords of Billroth*. The red pulp is dedicated to seizing foreign particles and old, damaged, or mutated erythrocytes.[1] Venous sinuses also act to store more than 300 mL of blood depending upon the systematic blood pressure. When the blood pressure drops, venous sinuses are constricted and may eject as much as 200 mL of blood into the venous circulation in an effort to restore blood volume.[7,8]

The highly vascular spleen receives its arterial blood from the splenic artery, a branch of the celiac axis (Fig. 10-4). This artery courses along the superior pancreatic border

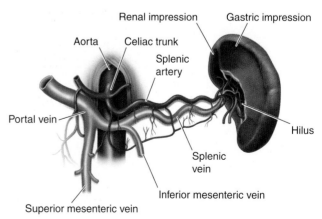

FIGURE 10-4 Circulation of the spleen, including the splenic vein and splenic artery.

and divides into the superior and inferior terminal branches before entering the splenic hilum. Within the hilum, the splenic artery divides into six or more segmental branches before separating into several minor arterioles within the spleen.[2,3,6] These arterioles may be visible as small echogenic lines passing through the splenic parenchyma.[11] The intrasplenic arterial branches do not anastomose or communicate to create collateral flow. Without collateral flow, the spleen is at increased risk for infarction. Small branches of the segmental arteries provide blood to the white pulp before flowing into the venous sinusoids. This blood is then transported by pulp veins through splenic trabeculae to the splenic vein.[6] Eventually, the splenic vein is joined by the inferior mesenteric vein and travels posterior to the tail and body of the pancreas. The splenic vein then unites with the superior mesenteric vein posterior to the neck of the pancreas to form the hepatic portal vein.[2,3,6]

VARIANTS OF NORMAL

There are numerous congenital variations of the spleen.[1] Several studies divide broad-spectrum splenic anomalies associated with heterotaxia syndrome into asplenia and polysplenia. Heterotaxy is related to a disruption in the normal embryologic development of left–right symmetry. This condition results in abnormal organ positions, situs, and/or arrangement.

Asplenia is the congenital absence of the spleen, also known as Ivemark syndrome.[1,6] Splenic aplasia may be diagnosed in cases of congenital absence, surgical removal, or atrophy resulting from arterial or venous occlusions.[12] Asplenia is associated with right-sided morphology of the heart and lungs. Often, the patient's lungs are trilobed, and both main bronchi are located above the main pulmonary arteries.[13] Other congenital malformations associated with asplenia include cardiovascular anomalies, situs ambiguous complexes, and visceral heterotaxia.[6,14] The major causes for mortality and morbidity among patients with congenital asplenia are related to cardiac malformations.[14]

Splenic hypoplasia is characterized by a small pathologic spleen with reduced function resulting from abnormal development or parenchymal involution.[14] Often, acquired hyposplenia is caused by sickle cell anemia. Some suggest that functional hyposplenism may be underdiagnosed as an immunodeficiency condition in children. Hyposplenic patients are at increased risk to develop solid tumors and vascular, autoimmune, and thrombolytic diseases. The major cause of mortality and morbidity among patients with hyposplenia is pneumococcal sepsis.[1]

Polysplenia is characterized by the presence of multiple smaller spleens, of similar size.[1,13] In cases of polysplenia, there is a left-sided dominance in lung and cardiac morphology.[6] Often, patients with polysplenia demonstrate bilobed lungs with the main bronchi found below the pulmonary arteries. Other associated anomalies include visceral heterotaxia, malrotations of the intestine, short pancreas, inferior vena cava (IVC) anomalies, cardiac defects, and biliary atresia.[13]

An accessory spleen is a common anatomic variant seen in approximately 10% to 30% of the population. Accessory (supernumerary) spleens occur when a portion of splenic tissue separates itself from the main body of the spleen and is found in an ectopic position.[1,15] Most accessory spleens are small and measure approximately 2.0 cm.[16] Approximately 75% of accessory spleens are found near the splenic hilum or gastrosplenic ligament (Fig. 10-5). The other 20% are located within the tail of the pancreas where they may be mistaken for hypervascular pancreatic tumors. Only 5% occur along the splenic artery and in the gastrosplenic, splenocolic, or gastrocolic ligament.[1,15] Differentiating accessory spleens from pancreatic masses or from hilar lymph nodes may be difficult unless it is possible to trace their blood supply to the splenic artery. Sonographically, accessory spleens present as round, mildly echogenic, and homogeneous with posterior enhancement.[17] Following splenectomy, an accessory spleen may assume the function and size of the removed organ. In cases of hematologic disorders, residual splenic tissue and accessory spleens present after laparoscopic splenectomy may lead to a relapse.[1,18] Rarely, accessory spleens undergo

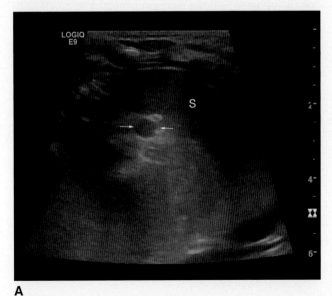

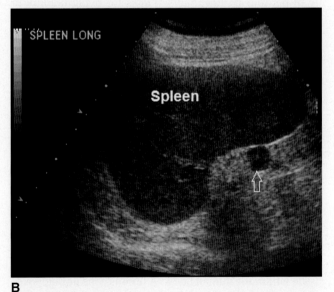

A

B

FIGURE 10-5 Accessory spleen. **A:** Small accessory spleen (arrows) is seen in the splenic hilum (S). **B:** On a different patient, an accessory spleen (arrow) is visualized in the splenic hilum. (**A:** Courtesy of GE Healthcare, Wauwatosa, WI; **B:** Courtesy of Natalee Braun, Ogden, UT.)

torsion or infarction clinically associated with acute LUQ pain. In most cases, accessory spleens are of no clinical consequence.[6,17]

The wandering or ectopic spleen is a rare occurrence and is a spleen that migrates from its normal LUQ position to another location within the abdomen or pelvis. Wandering spleen is associated with a loss or a weakening of supporting ligaments.[6,19] Developmental ligamental laxity occurs when there is an incomplete fusion of the dorsal mesentery with the posterior peritoneum or secondary to hormonal changes and maternal influences during pregnancy. With age, laxity may be related to splenomegaly, trauma, extreme weight loss, weak abdominal muscles, and gastric distension. Because the wandering spleen lacks its normal peritoneal attachments, this variant is associated with a high incidence of splenic torsion and infarction.[1,20]

Clinically, patients with a wandering spleen may present as asymptomatic or have varying degrees of abdominal pain. Sonographers should extensively examine the left side of the patient from the thorax to the pelvis in cases where the normal spleen is not imaged in its anatomic position. Contrast-enhanced CT is the imaging modality of choice in the diagnosis of wandering spleen. However, variable echo patterns in sonography combined with duplex Doppler and color flow imaging are sensitive in demonstrating a lack or absence of blood flow secondary to splenic artery torsion.[19–21] The preferred treatment for wandering spleen is splenopexy wherein a surgeon repositions the spleen in the LUQ to prevent torsion of the splenic vessels and preserve splenic function.[21]

PHYSIOLOGY

The spleen is an organ of mystery and perplexity for physiologists. Although the spleen is rarely the primary site of disease, it is often involved in inflammatory, hematopoietic, and metabolic disorders associated with immune and hematologic diseases. Functions of the spleen overlap those of other body organs, making it possible for a person to live without a spleen. However, studies completed on individuals with splenic absence have given some indication to the importance of its function. For example, patients who underwent splenectomy often suffered from leukocytosis, decreased circulating iron, decreased immune response, and an increased presence of circulating morphologically defective blood cells.[8,9,22] Physiologically, the four major functions of the spleen include reserving, filtering, producing, and defending blood products.[7,8] Within the spleen, the red pulp is dedicated to filtration, the white pulp is dedicated to adaptive immunity, and the perifollicular zone—located between red and white pulp—acts to connect both functions.[23]

Functions of the Spleen

Reservoir and Filter

The spleen acts as a reservoir for blood because a small volume of the blood entering the terminal capillaries of the spleen continues to circulate and enter highly distensible venous sinuses. This blood reservoir is crowded with red blood cells (RBCs) and platelets that may be used to provide a transfusion-type response when the body is stressed by hemorrhage.[8] The majority of circulating blood, however, will pass through the hyperpermeable capillary walls into the red pulp for the purpose of filtration.[7,8]

Destruction of Red Blood Cells and Microorganisms

Approximately 5% of cardiac output is filtered every minute by the spleen.[23] Within the red pulp, resident macrophages ingest and destroy unwanted debris; microorganisms; and old, damaged, or dead blood cells, particularly erythrocytes. Phagocytosed erythrocytes are catabolized, and the freed iron is stored in the macrophage cytoplasm or released back into the blood plasma.[8,23,24] Ferritin, the iron protein complex, may be routed to the bone marrow and used to synthesize new hemoglobin whereas the broken down erythrocytes aid in the formation of bile pigments.

Defective cells, such as spherocytes, sickle cells, and thalassemic cells, are removed from circulation as they travel through the sinus walls. These cells lack the biconcave shape of normal RBCs, and the removal process is termed *splenic culling*. RBCs that contain an unwanted granule, or even a parasite, are not culled. Rather, these nuclear fragments or membrane inclusions are milked from the erythrocytes, and the cleansed RBCs are returned to normal circulation. This process is referred to as *splenic pitting*.[23,25]

Erythropoiesis

The spleen is responsible for erythropoiesis from approximately the fifth to the sixth months of fetal life. With age, the bone marrow assumes this primary function, but the spleen retains its capacity to produce RBCs throughout an adult's life. The spleen's hematopoietic functions can be regained if chronic anemia develops or bone marrow parenchyma is lost.[8,24]

Defense Against Disease

Lymphoid organs function as sites of proliferation, differentiation, or function of lymphocytes and mononuclear phagocytes.[8] The white pulp, within the spleen, produces lymphocytes and plasma cells needed to form antibodies. There are many different types of lymphocytes including the T cells, B cells, and plasma cells.[8,25] As a secondary defense, the spleen is able to phagocytose bacteria bypassed by the lymph nodes.

Laboratory Values

Normally, there are approximately 5,000 to 10,000 white blood cells (WBCs) per microliter of blood. Leukocytosis occurs when the leukocyte count is higher than normal.[8,24] When a physiologic stressor is present, leukocytosis is a normal response and may indicate the presence of inflammation, infection, hemorrhage, carcinoma, and/or acute leukemia. In contrast, an abnormally low level of WBCs is referred to as *leukopenia*. A decrease in leukocyte counts below 1,000 per mm³ increases a patient's risk for disease. Patients with counts below 500 per mm³ are in jeopardy for serious life-threatening infections. Leukopenia may result from radiation therapy, chemotherapeutic agents, systemic lupus erythematosus, vitamin B$_{12}$ deficiency, cortisol treatment, and anaphylactic shock. Leukopenia has also been associated with hypersplenism, viral infections, leukemia, aplastic anemia, and diabetes mellitus.[8,24]

A laboratory hematocrit indicates the percentage of blood volume occupied by RBCs. The volume of RBCs circulating within the body is greatly influenced by the spleen's sequestering and destructive function. Abnormal findings in the level of hematocrit result from altered erythropoiesis, anemias, hemorrhage, Hodgkin disease, and/or leukemia.[8,24]

Abnormal laboratory tests, history of infectious disease, LUQ pain, and a palpable enlarged spleen are all clinical manifestations and indications for a sonographic examination of the spleen.[1,7]

NORMAL SONOGRAPHIC APPEARANCE AND TECHNIQUE

The normal echogenicity of the spleen is comparable with that of the liver and equal to or slightly hyperechoic to the kidney when the tissues are evaluated at the same distance from the transducer.[6] Splenic parenchyma is homogeneous with low to mid-level echoes, which are usually disrupted only by the arteries and veins in the area of the hilus (Fig. 10-6). Within the splenic hilum, the splenic artery, and its bifurcations, along with convergence of the splenic veins are visualized. Differentiation between these vessels is difficult without the evaluation of their Doppler signals[6,9] (Fig. 10-7).

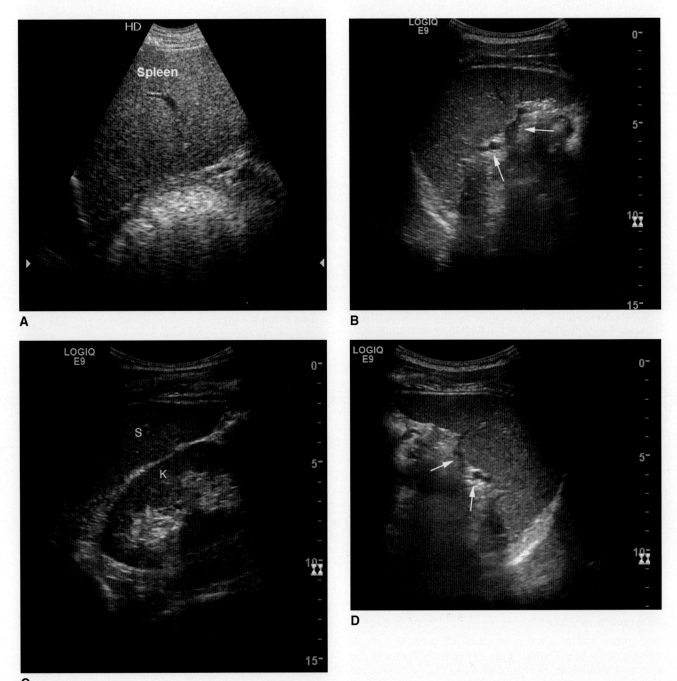

FIGURE 10-6 Normal spleen. **A** and **B:** Longitudinal scan of a normal spleen. The splenic vessels are visible at the hilus *(arrows)*. **C:** Longitudinal section lateral to the hilus of the spleen *(S)* outlines the splenic contour and shows its relationship to the left kidney *(K)*. **D:** Transverse scan of a normal spleen. The vessels are visible at the hilus *(arrows)*. (**A:** Courtesy of Philips Medical System, Bothell, WA; **B–D:** Courtesy of GE Healthcare, Wauwatosa, WI.)

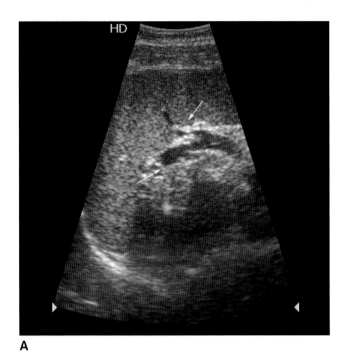

A

B

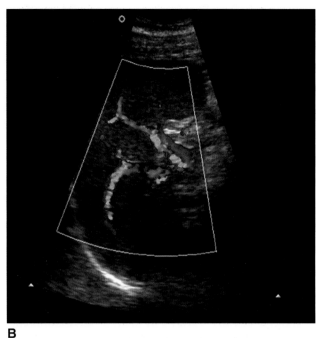

C

FIGURE 10-7 Color and spectral Doppler images. **A:** Longitudinal image of the normal spleen. Splenic vessels are visible at the splenic hilus *(arrows)*. **B:** Color Doppler image demonstrating splenic vessels at the splenic hilum. **C:** Pulsed Doppler waveform indicates the presence of the splenic arterial flow above the baseline and venous flow below the baseline. (Images courtesy of Philips Medical System, Bothell, WA.)

Examination of the spleen requires a creative manipulation of the transducer and the patient. The spleen may be imaged with the patient in supine or right lateral decubitus positions. Commonly, the transducer will be placed between left intercostal spaces in a coronal plane. However, subcostal imaging may also be effective among some patient populations.[9,26] When patients are placed in the right lateral decubitus position, the patients are brought closer to the scanning sonographer and their left arm may be raised over their head to assist in separating the ribs for better transducer access.[1,26] Rolling the patient toward the sonographer supports an ideal ergonomic position. When scanning, sonographers should maintain good posture and abduct the shoulder no more than 30 degrees from the body.[27] Patients may also assist the sonographer in obtaining appropriate images by varying their respiration to optimize the image window. A large inspiration depresses the diaphragm and moves the spleen inferiorly away from bony thorax. On the other hand, when the patient expires, the image excludes the left lung base and may be helpful in eliminating acoustic shadowing.[9,26]

According to the American Institute of Ultrasound in Medicine (AIUM) practice parameters, images of the long axis and transverse planes of the spleen should be acquired. Orthogonal views are used to evaluate borders, record longitudinal measurement, and demonstrate left kidney and pleural spaces.[28] A 3.5- to 5-MHz mid-frequency transducer with a small footprint is generally used to image the spleen. If necessary, a linear array transducer may be used to increase image detail, but there is a slight disadvantage in scanning the intercostal space with a larger transducer footprint. A smaller transducer head makes intercostal scanning more feasible.[1,6,9]

Longitudinal imaging sections of the spleen should include the hilus with its blood vessels and several representational parenchymal images. Additionally, the left hemidiaphragm and the interface with the left kidney should be well demonstrated. The longest axis of the spleen and anteroposterior dimensions may be measured in this orientation. After evaluating and obtaining images of the spleen in longitudinal sections, the transducer should be rotated 90 degrees for transverse imaging. If a volumetric index is required, the organ should be measured in transverse orientation at its widest point.[29] Gain settings, focal zone placement, and depth should demonstrate a homogenous and uniform spleen. Harmonic and compound imaging may be used to improve the quality of the image and detect subtle lesions. Common scanning pitfalls include mistaking the fluid-filled stomach, adrenal mass, or pancreatic mass as a splenic mass or the left lobe of the liver as a hematoma. When a mass is present in the LUQ or when the spleen is enlarged, visualization of the organ is often accomplished from an anterior approach. A spleen surrounded by free intraperitoneal fluid or associated with a pleural effusion is best visualized from an anterolateral approach.[9]

Owing to the normal variations in splenic shape and size, length is the dimension primarily monitored for splenic enlargement. In 95% of adults, the normal spleen length is less than 12 to 13 cm, the breadth less than 8 cm, and the thickness less than 4 cm. A long axis greater than 12 cm is generally taken to indicate enlargement.[1,6,9,29] Splenic enlargement may alter the echogenicity of the organ. For example, decreased echogenicity may be indicative of lymphoma, whereas increased echogenicity may suggest the presence of myelofibrosis or infection.[29]

Spectral and Color Doppler

Spectral and color Doppler are valuable tools in evaluating the splenic and perisplenic vasculature. Abnormalities in the direction and flow of splenic vessels are indicative of pathology. Common pathologies include portal hypertension, with or without collateral vessels; splenic vein thrombosis; and aneurysms of the splenic artery. Absence of flow in areas of the splenic parenchyma is associated with avascular lesions, such as cysts or necrosis. Additionally, color Doppler imaging may illuminate hypoechoic vascular lesions easily overlooked with gray scale imaging.[29]

Contrast-Enhanced Ultrasound

Contrast-enhanced ultrasound (CEUS) has proven to be a cost-effective, safe, and accurate means to identify and characterize splenic trauma, injury, and solid focal splenic lesions. CEUS utilizes an intravenous contrast agent composed of microbubbles that in real-time demonstrate vascular architecture and contrast enhancement in comparison with adjacent tissues. Contrast enhancement is determined over the time-contrast washes in and washes out of the region of interest, and it is characterized by the changes documented over different vascular phases.[30] In cases of splenic trauma, active splenic bleeds were characterized by fountain-like jets of contrast enhancement or irregular areas adjacent to the spleen that persisted in the late parenchymal phase. Pseudoaneurysm was suspected when a round or oval area of contrast enhancement with distinct margins presented during the arterial phase and isoechogenicity demonstrated in the delayed phase.[31] A differentiation in contrast enhancement within focal splenic lesions was compared and effective in determining whether a splenic lesion was benign or malignant in 98% of cases.[32]

Shear Wave Elastography

Shear wave elastography measures the elasticity of tissues by producing a radiofrequency force impulse that propagates transversely oriented shear waves. These waves travel through surrounding tissue and relay information about their biomechanical quality.[33] Shear wave elastography has been used to measure the stiffness in spleen parenchyma. Spleen stiffness has been reported more commonly among patients with splenomegaly and may be beneficial in predicting its etiology.[34] However, spleen stiffness added no value in conjunction with liver stiffness to the prediction of esophageal varices related to portal hypertension.[35]

DISEASES OF THE SPLEEN

Changes in size, echogenicity, blood flow, and morphology of the spleen are used as evidence of pathologic changes affecting the spleen.[1,6,9,26,29]

Splenomegaly

One of the most common splenic abnormalities observed in sonography is enlargement of the spleen.[6] Generally, if the lower splenic edge is palpated below the left costal margin at the end of inspiration, the spleen is enlarged approximately three times its normal size.[2] Splenomegaly may cause symptoms of LUQ fullness or pain associated with the stretching of the splenic capsule and suspensory ligaments, lower extremity edema, and increased pressure on the adjacent organs—particularly the stomach and intestines. Additionally, the patient may present with ascites, portal hypertension, jaundice, lymphadenopathy, fever, or hemorrhage.[1,2,6]

When imaging, a good rule of thumb is that the spleen should not extend below the left margin of the left kidney. An enlarged spleen fills the abdominal cavity, extends into the pelvis, and has increased vascularity at the splenic hilum. The spleen may measure up to 20 cm in length with minimal-to-moderate enlargement. A severely enlarged spleen is reported to be 21 to 29 cm in length, and a grossly enlarged spleen is greater than 30 cm in length[29] (Fig. 10-8). Although the spleen parenchyma is very homogeneous, it may change in its echogenicity when enlarged. It is not possible to differentiate between the pathologic causes of splenic enlargement.[9]

A wide range of pathologic processes may produce splenomegaly. Diseases related to the classification of splenomegaly are broadly categorized as inflammatory, infectious, congestive, infiltrative, hematologic, metabolic, and traumatic[1,8,29] (Table 10-1). Causes include, but are not limited to, heart failure, cirrhosis, portal hypertension, red blood cell abnormalities, portal splenic thrombosis, cystic fibrosis, malignancy, and HIV/AIDS.[36]

Hypertension

A common cause of splenomegaly is portal congestion secondary to liver cirrhosis. In cirrhosis, nodular parenchymal regeneration and fibrosis result in a reduction of blood flow and portal obstruction. Increased pressure within the portal venous system reverses normal flow through the

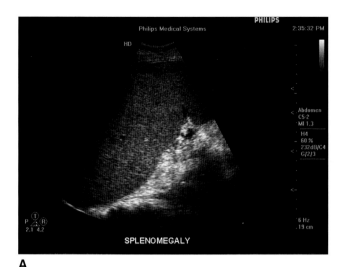

A

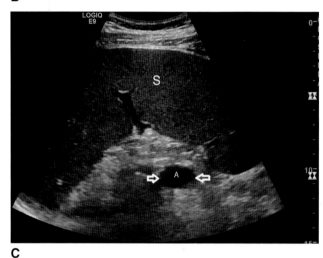

B

C

FIGURE 10-8 Splenomegaly. **A:** The enlarged spleen fills the abdominal cavity and extends into the pelvis. **B:** Splenomegaly and associated left kidney. **C:** Enlarged spleen *(S)* is seen with an accessory spleen *(arrows)* near the splenic hilum.

TABLE 10-1	**Disease Category or Pathologic Process Causing Splenomegaly**
Disease Category	**Pathologic Process**
Congestive	Portal hypertension
Hematologic	Thalassemia, hereditary spherocytosis, autoimmune hemolytic anemia, sickle cell disease (in early stage)
Infiltrative	Leukemia, Hodgkin lymphoma, non-Hodgkin lymphoma
Metabolic	Gaucher disease, Niemann–Pick disease
Chronic inflammatory conditions	Sarcoid, tuberculosis, malaria
Hematopoietic malignancies	Acute lymphocytic leukemia, chronic myelogenous leukemia, CLL, agnogenic myeloid metaplasia
Trauma	Parenchymal hematoma, subcapsular hematoma

CLL, chronic lymphocytic leukemia.

portal and splenic veins toward the liver.[37] The reversal of blood flow and damping of normal respiratory variation in venous Doppler signals are common indications for portal hypertension. As pressure increases, the portal vein becomes enlarged and tortuous, and collateral vessels open between the portal veins and the systemic veins where the pressure is considerably lower. Collateral varices appear within the splenic hilus, retroperitoneum, and gastrohepatic ligament (Fig. 10-9). The most common varice is the splenorenal collateral that transports blood from the splenic vein to the left renal vein before terminating at the IVC. A recanalized umbilical vein in the ligamentum teres within the liver is also indicative of portal hypertension.[9,38] Sonographically, small, echogenic parallel lines, termed "reflective channels," within the splenic parenchyma have been used as a diagnostic criterion for differentiating splenomegaly caused by acute systemic infections, hemolytic anemias, infiltrative processes, and portal hypertension. Color Doppler images of these channels prove whether they are vascular in nature and whether blood flow is present. The echogenic walls are caused by dilated sinusoidal veins with collagen in their walls. These channels should be differentiated from splenic calcifications owing to tuberculosis, histoplasmosis, and calcified infarcts of sickle cell disease.[1,39]

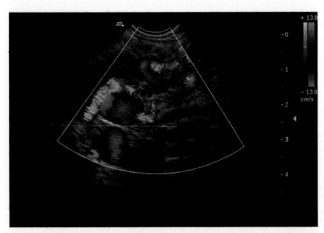

FIGURE 10-9 Splenic varices. Dilated tortuous splenic varices secondary to portal hypertension. (Image courtesy of Philips Medical System, Bothell, WA.)

Blood Disorders

Red blood cell abnormalities, including hereditary spherocytosis and hemoglobin defects, also cause vascular congestion that results in reticuloendothelial hyperplasia and splenomegaly. Polycythemia vera is a rare blood disease in which the bone marrow creates a surplus of red cells, white cells, and platelets. This excess of blood products increases the viscosity of blood and reduces profusion leading to an enlarged spleen.[40]

Hemolytic anemia refers to disorders where RBCs are destroyed faster than they are created. Intrinsic hemolytic anemias are often inherited, such as sickle cell anemia and thalassemia. Sickle cell disease is characterized by RBCs with altered plasticity and shape. These changes, like other hematologic disorders, increase the blood's viscosity and the risk for vessel occlusions and splenic infarcts. The presentation of sickle cell disease varies based on the chronicity of the disease. A life-threatening complication of sickle cell disease is acute splenic sequestration, which is marked by quickly advancing anemia and compromised circulation. During this crisis, large amounts of blood are rapidly pooled within the liver and spleen, the spleen suddenly enlarges, and a sharp decrease in the patient's hematocrit is promptly observed.[9,36] Because the spleen can hold as much as one-fifth of the body's blood supply at one time, mortality rates may increase up to 50% owing to cardiovascular collapse.[8]

Malignancies

Malignancies affecting splenic size include leukemia, lymphoma, hemangiosarcoma, and metastatic spread from other primary cancers. Malignancies cause splenic enlargement because malignant cells diffusely infiltrate the splenic parenchyma, causing the spleen to appear nodular or miliary. Additionally, affected bone marrow may fail to maintain its hematopoietic capabilities, causing the spleen to swell as it resumes its blood production capabilities. Last, both lymphoma and leukemia increase granulomatous inflammation resulting in the expansion of white pulp.[6,8,40]

Acquired Immunodeficiency Syndrome

Infections affecting splenic size may be systemic or focal. Systemic infections include mononucleosis, tuberculosis, histoplasmosis, schistosomiasis, sarcoidosis, and candidiasis.

Focal infections include parasitic infections and abscess.[40] HIV is frequently accompanied by opportunistic infections and lymphoma, which affect the spleen as well as other abdominal viscera and the retroperitoneum. Most commonly, HIV-seropositive patients present with an enlarged spleen, with or without associated adenopathy within the splenic hilus.[41] Tuberculosis, lymphoma, and Kaposi sarcoma appear as hypodense nodular implants within the splenic parenchyma. *Candida, Pneumocystis jirovecii,* or *Mycobacterium avium* may demonstrate numerous punctuate nonshadowing calcifications typical of granulomatous disease within the spleen, liver, kidneys, and adrenal glands.[9]

Metabolic Diseases

Metabolic diseases affecting splenic size include Gaucher disease, Niemann–Pick disease, amyloidosis, histiocytosis, and hemochromatosis, and diabetes mellitus. In patients with metabolic disorders, the spleen may be distended owing to the presence of macrophages, vascular compromise, and excessive metabolic elements unique to each disease process. For example, patients with Gaucher or Niemann–Pick diseases cannot metabolize fats. Lipids begin to build up within the organs, including the spleen, and diffuse nodules are demonstrated on sonographic images representing focal areas of fibrosis and infarction.[1,8] Amyloidosis patients create and store abnormal proteins. Histiocytosis patients have an excessive quantity of immune cells, and hemochromatosis patients have too much iron. In cases of diabetes mellitus, patients reveal vascular infarcts secondary to diabetes-induced small vessel atherosclerosis.[40]

Splenic Lesions

A variety of lesions are found within the spleen. These include true or primary cysts, secondary or pseudocysts, infarctions, granulomas, abscesses, primary benign and malignant neoplasms, and metastases (Table 10-2).

Cysts

Cysts in the spleen may be congenital or acquired. Cysts arising from the epithelial or endothelial lining are considered primary or true cysts. Primary cysts account for about 10% of all benign nonparasitic splenic cysts and predominantly occur in children. Usually, primary cysts are asymptomatic unless they are large in size and compress adjacent organs.[42] True cysts are often solitary and unilocular, but in 20% of cases, true cysts can be multiple and multilocular.[40]

Secondary or acquired cysts may develop in association with inflammation, trauma, or parasitic infestations. Secondary cysts are often complex and may include internal echoes and wall calcifications. Posttraumatic or splenic pseudocysts account for approximately 80% of all splenic cysts and are often in sequelae to hematomas. In their development, a capsule of fibrous tissue envelopes a subcapsular or intraparenchymal hematomas wherein the contents may liquefy and resolve. Traumatic pseudocysts only require treatment if they become large and symptomatic. However, hemorrhagic collections are important to monitor because a delayed splenic rupture may occur as a result of the trauma in approximately 50% of patients. A splenic rupture is a life-threatening event in which the splenic capsule bursts and blood spills out into the abdominal cavity. Additionally, it

TABLE 10-2 Sonographic Characteristics of Disease Category or Process That Produces Focal or Diffuse Lesions

Sonographic Appearance	Disease Category or Process
FOCAL LESIONS	
Splenic cysts	
Anechoic, well-defined walls, enhanced sound transmission	Congenital
Sharply demarcated wall, multilocular internal structure representing daughter cyst, mural calcifications	Acquired echinococcal (hydatid)
Large cysts, dense, clearly defined walls	Epidermoid or epithelial
May not have well-defined wall, mural calcifications	Posttraumatic or postinflammatory pseudocysts
Single or multiple simple cysts	Polycystic kidney disease lymphangioma, extension of pancreatic pseudocyst
Abscesses	
Usually multiple, range from anechoic with well-defined borders to echo-filled and septate, gas creates dirty shadowing, air–fluid or fluid–fluid level might be visible	Bacterial endocarditis, diverticulitis, osteomyelitis, pelvic or other infection
Infarcts	
Well-demarcated, wedge-shaped, or round, hypoechoic in acute phase; more echogenic in later stage; measures 1–2 cm and usually located in periphery with apex pointing medially	Bacterial endocarditis, tumor embolization, hemoglobinopathy, myeloproliferative disorders, leukemia, lymphoma, vasculitis (SLE, polyarteritis nodosa)
Hematoma	
Isoechoic to echogenic mass within parenchyma, which may become hypoechoic as hematoma resolves, may demonstrate fluid–fluid level, may produce splenomegaly	Trauma, coagulation disorder
Fractured spleen may appear only as enlarging spleen with normal echogenicity; blood might be found in pelvis, flanks, Morrison pouch, lesser and greater sacs; subcapsular hematoma may appear as normal spleen, or hypoechoic, or echogenic mass adjacent to clearly defined capsule; pericapsular hematoma may efface smooth contour of splenic capsule.	Ruptured spleen secondary to trauma or enlargement
Echogenic lesions	
Sometimes with hypoechoic areas and accompanying splenomegaly	Primary benign and malignant neoplasms and metastases, abscesses, hematomas
DIFFUSE CHANGES	
Calcifications	
Echogenic foci with varying degrees of acoustic shadowing	Sequelae of granulomatous disease such as histoplasmosis or tuberculosis, from previous hematoma or infarction, cysts
Hypoechoic nodules	
Irregular, multiple hypoechoic parenchymal masses; occasionally hyperechoic lesions	Hodgkin and non-Hodgkin lymphoma, benign (i.e., hemangioma, hematoma, isolated lymphangioma) and malignant neoplasms (metastases)

SLE, systemic lupus erythematosus.

is important to distinguish between pseudocysts and other benign or malignant cysts because treatment options vary based on their etiology.[6,26]

Parasitic cysts are common among the benign cysts that present worldwide. These cysts are overwhelmingly echinococcal (hydatid) in origin, attributable to *Echinococcus multilocularis* or *Echinococcus granulosus*.[43] Patients may present with LUQ pain, fever, and an elevated WBC. Sonographically, hydatid cysts have varied appearance from simple and centrally anechoic to complex, depending on the stage of the disease. Some complexities imaged result from

hydatid sand, enfolded membranes, and eggshell calcifications. Most cysts demonstrate well-defined posterior walls and acoustic enhancement[9] (Fig. 10-10).

Lymphangiomas are rare, noncancerous, slow-growing, protein-filled complex cystic masses resulting from lymphatic malformations or obstructions. These cystic masses are most often found in children, and they can involve the spleen focally or diffusely.[6,7] Many patients suffer from lymphangiomatosis of the skin, lung, bone, and viscera. It is important to differentiate between lymphangiomas and hemangiomas, which have similar appearance. Sonographically,

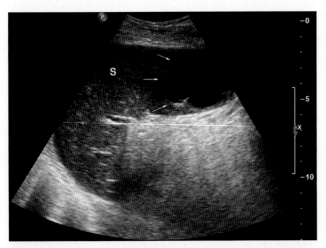

FIGURE 10-10 Splenic cyst. Longitudinal scan of the spleen *(S)* demonstrating a simple, anechoic, intraparenchymal cyst *(arrows)*. (Image courtesy of Philips Medical System, Bothell, WA.)

lymphangiomas often appear as multiseptated cystic masses with possible echogenic calcifications.[9,44]

Abscesses

Abscesses often result from the hematologic spread of infection.[6] Common causes of splenic abscess are endocarditis, septicemia, and trauma.[9] Diagnosis of splenic abscess may be hampered by clinical symptoms that are often absent or very subtle. A delayed diagnosis increases the mortality rate in patients with abscess because of an increased risk for splenic rupture. Nonspecific symptoms related to splenic abscess include LUQ pain, high-grade fever, vomiting, and referred pain to the chest or shoulder.[6,45]

Typically, abscesses have a complex appearance with mixed echogenic properties that are difficult to distinguish from metastatic lesions or hematomas. Often, the border of an abscess is ill-defined, thickened, and irregular. When gas is present in the lesion, characteristic high-level echoes, ring-down artifact, and dirty shadowing are often observed.[9] Additionally, an air–fluid level demonstrating when the transducer is held in a posterior or posterolateral position is helpful in diagnosis.

Immunocompromised patients are most susceptible to fungal and microbacterial microabscesses, which present as target lesions or small hypoechoic nodules. With advanced pharmacology, splenectomy is rarely a treatment for abscess. Rather, sonography-guided fine needle aspiration of the abscess may be used in concert with strong broad-spectrum intravenous antibiotics as treatment.[1,9,46]

Infarcts

Infarcts in the spleen are secondary to a wide range of pathologic causes, including blood disorders, atheromatous disease, diabetes, congenital abnormalities, and neoplasm.[6] The two most prevalent risk factors for splenic infarcts are hematologic and cardioembolic disease. A splenic infarct results from an occlusion of a segment of the splenic artery. Parenchymal necrosis occurs because intrasplenic arterial branches fail to anastomose and provide compensatory blood flow.[47]

Splenic infarction may present without symptoms or with acute LUQ pain that worsens with deep inspiration. Laboratory values may indicate anemia, leukocytosis, and elevated lactate dehydrogenase. Sonographically, splenic infarcts appear as well-demarcated, hypoechoic, wedge-shaped, or rounded areas along the splenic periphery with diminished Doppler flow (Fig. 10-11). The echogenicity of the infarct is

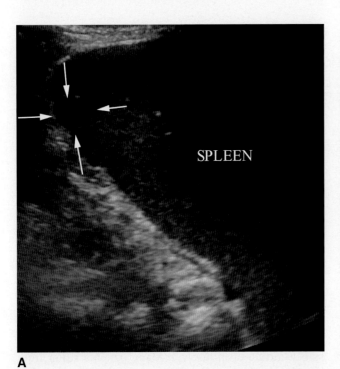

A

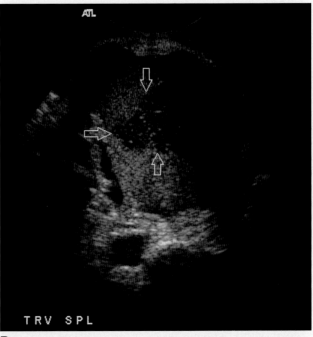

B

FIGURE 10-11 Splenic infarct. **A:** A longitudinal plane displays a small wedge-shaped area located at the periphery representing a small infarct *(arrows)*. **B:** In a different pediatric patient with a history of left upper quadrant pain, this transverse plane shows a large, wedge-shaped splenic infarct *(open arrows)*. After the examination, it was discovered she had leukemia. (Images courtesy of Robert DeJong, Baltimore, MD.)

related to the age of the infarct. During the inflammatory phase, the infarct is hypoechoic, corresponding to edema, inflammation, and necrosis. Later, fibrosis and shrinkage supervene, and the parenchyma is hyperechoic.[6,47] A key sonographic indication for infarct is the "bright band sign." This sign calls attention to the avascular defect and is seen as two or more linear specular reflectors oriented parallel or nearly parallel to each other. These parallel reflectors will be demonstrated perpendicular to the sound beam, within the splenic parenchyma, on multiple sonographic images.[47,48]

Infarcts are a rare cause of splenic rupture; however, the area should be monitored for advancing subcapsular hemorrhage, free peritoneal blood, and/or expanding areas of liquefaction. Few, if any, features distinguish infarct from other sources of focal splenic disease, including small abscesses, metastatic disease, and lymphoma.[6,9]

Trauma, Hematoma, and Rupture

The spleen is the most frequently damaged organ in cases of blunt abdominal trauma. Patients may present clinically with hypovolemic shock and LUQ pain. Blunt abdominal trauma is associated with high mortality rates owing to rapid liver, spleen, and major blood vessel exsanguination. Injuries to the bowel or pancreas often lead to abdominal sepsis. The spectrum of injuries to the spleen includes shattered spleen, fragmentation, disruption of hilar vessels, parenchymal lacerations, capsular tears, and contusions.[9] A definitive exclusion of splenic hematomas following abdominal trauma is vital because these blood collections can rupture through the splenic capsule shortly following the traumatic incidence. In 50% of cases, splenic rupture occurs within 1 week of injury, resulting in hemoperitoneum or hemoretroperitoneum.[40]

Because sonography is portable, highly sensitive to free peritoneal fluid, and may be performed quickly, the modality is well suited for point-of-care imaging in a trauma setting. However, CT is the definitive modality because it can globally depict the body's organs and its cavities. CT is also sensitive in showing vascular injury and the extension of parenchymal lesions.[9] When sonography is utilized, the spleen may appear normal if there is a small, fresh hematoma. Alternately, the spleen can present as a heterogeneous mass if there are extensive parenchymal injuries. The appearance of a hematoma using ultrasound is variable based on the age of the bleed. Blood may initially appear isoechoic, making the identification of acute trauma difficult. Over time, blood collections evolve in appearance from echogenic to anechoic, possibly with pseudocyst formation[6,36] (Fig. 10-12).

Prior to rupture, a subcapsular hematoma often demonstrates a double outline because accumulated blood is caught between the capsule and the splenic parenchyma.[9] When the spleen is demonstrated as enlarging and heterogeneous, these dynamic and complex sonographic changes are indicative of splenic rupture (Fig. 10-13). In case of rupture, the sonographer should examine the pelvis, Morrison pouch, and the flanks of the patient for intraperitoneal hemorrhage. Hemoperitoneum is often indicated as a complex fluid found within the lesser and greater sac on both sides of the gastrosplenic ligament. Early identification and regular follow-up of patients with splenic injury are important because of possible delayed rupture. Currently, patients with splenic trauma are treated conservatively to reduce the risk of infection arising from splenectomy.[1,9,26]

Rarely, the spleen may spontaneously rupture. Abnormalities that have been associated with a spontaneous rupture include Hodgkin disease, infectious mononucleosis, pneumonia, chickenpox, polycythemia rubra vera, and agnogenic myeloid metaplasia. As a consequence of splenic rupture, splenosis can occur in which the splenic tissue is transplanted within the peritoneal cavity. Deposits may be found along the small intestine, omentum, parietal peritoneum, colon, mesentery, and diaphragm. These implants cannot be differentiated from accessory spleens. Most of these masses do not produce symptoms and are in areas not readily accessible by sonography.[6]

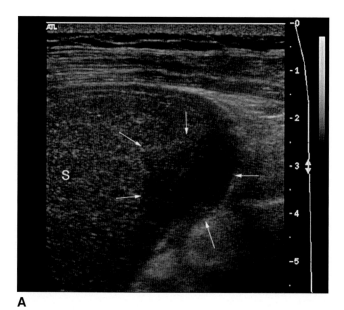
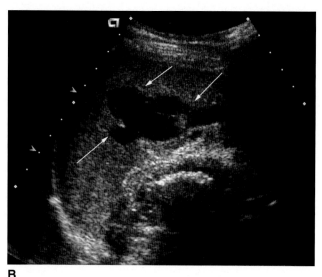

A   **B**

FIGURE 10-12 Hematoma. **A:** Longitudinal scan of the spleen (S) demonstrating a resolving splenic hematoma (arrows). **B:** Longitudinal image of the spleen in a patient 6 months post–blunt abdominal trauma demonstrating a resolving hematoma (arrows). (**A:** Courtesy of Philips Medical System, Bothell, WA.)

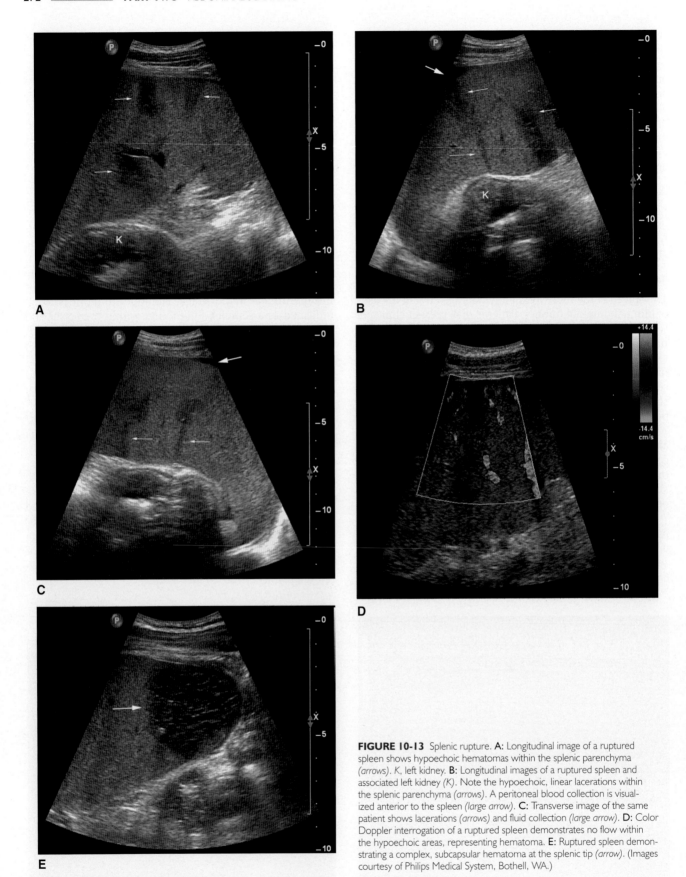

FIGURE 10-13 Splenic rupture. **A:** Longitudinal image of a ruptured spleen shows hypoechoic hematomas within the splenic parenchyma *(arrows)*. *K*, left kidney. **B:** Longitudinal images of a ruptured spleen and associated left kidney *(K)*. Note the hypoechoic, linear lacerations within the splenic parenchyma *(arrows)*. A peritoneal blood collection is visualized anterior to the spleen *(large arrow)*. **C:** Transverse image of the same patient shows lacerations *(arrows)* and fluid collection *(large arrow)*. **D:** Color Doppler interrogation of a ruptured spleen demonstrates no flow within the hypoechoic areas, representing hematoma. **E:** Ruptured spleen demonstrating a complex, subcapsular hematoma at the splenic tip *(arrow)*. (Images courtesy of Philips Medical System, Bothell, WA.)

Splenic Calcification

Splenic calcifications are generally an incidental finding and may occur in association with a wide variety of hematologic, infective, malignant, and vascular conditions.[49] Calcifications in the spleen appear echogenic and may demonstrate varying degrees of acoustic shadowing. Multiple hyperechoic calcifications appear as a "starry sky."[26] Often, calcifications are the sequelae of granulomatous disease—most commonly histoplasmosis, tuberculosis, or extrapulmonary *P. jirovecii*. Calcifications may also result from a previous infarction or hematoma. Splenic artery calcification is common and should not be confused with calcification in a lesion. If a neoplasm is not present, splenic calcifications are considered benign[6,9] (Fig. 10-14).

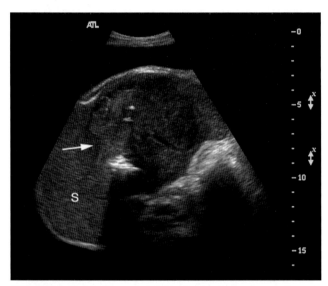

FIGURE 10-14 Splenic mass. Longitudinal image of a complex splenic mass with calcifications *(arrow)*. (Image courtesy of Philips Medical System, Bothell, WA.)

Malignant Neoplasms

Lymphoma

The most common malignant disease to affect the spleen is lymphoma, including Hodgkin and non-Hodgkin lymphoma.[6] Lymphoma is a primary malignancy of the lymphatic system; however, both Hodgkin and non-Hodgkin lymphoma are primary splenic lymphomas. Clinically, patients may present with nodal enlargement, fever, fatigue, weight loss, coughing, pressure, and congestion. Often, laboratory results demonstrate an elevated white blood count and anemia.[1,50] Sonographically, lymphomas may present as isolated hypoechoic masses with poorly defined margins or, in cases of diffuse involvement, the entire parenchyma of the spleen may demonstrate several tumor-like nodules resulting in a heterogeneous appearance[1,6,9,26] (Fig. 10-15). In the past, diffusely infiltrated spleens have escaped detection, but the rate of identification has increased markedly with echo-enhancing contrast media and harmonic imaging.[29] Current treatments for lymphomas include radiation therapy, chemotherapy, and bone marrow transplantation.[40]

Leukemia

Leukemia is a primary malignancy of the bone marrow, lymph nodes, and spleen. Among adults in the western hemisphere, chronic lymphocytic leukemia (CLL) is the most prevalent hematologic malignancy.[51] Patients with leukemia are primarily males who present with anemia, elevated WBC, excessive bruising, fatigue, recurrent infections, and pallor.[40] Splenic involvement may occur during the active stages of the disease or during remission. The red pulp is primarily involved and diffusely infiltrated with low-level nodular neoplastic cells; therefore, discrete or focal nodules are uncommon. Splenomegaly may be the only sonographic finding.[51,52]

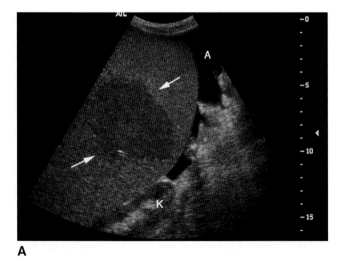

A

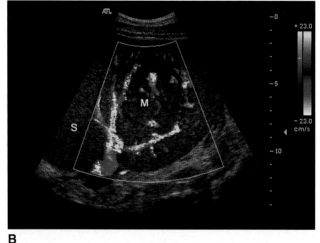

B

FIGURE 10-15 A: Hypoechoic intraparenchymal splenic mass *(arrows)* with associated ascites (A). Left kidney (K) is compressed owing to splenomegaly. **B:** Color Doppler of the splenic mass (M) demonstrating blood flow within the hypoechoic lesion. (Images courtesy of Philips Medical System, Bothell, WA.)

Angiosarcoma

Angiosarcomas are a rare aggressive primary malignant vascular neoplasm.[9,53] This type of malignancy occurs most among patients 50 to 60 years of age. Patients may exhibit an LUQ mass, pain, malaise, fever, anemia, and weight loss.[40] The prognosis for a patient diagnosed with angiosarcoma is very poor with a mortality rate of 70% within 6 months of the diagnosis.[1,9,53] Sonographically, angiosarcomas present with a heterogeneous splenic texture, single or multiple complex masses, and splenomegaly (Fig. 10-16). Solid components of these tumors may also demonstrate an increase in Doppler blood flow.[9]

Metastatic Lesions

Metastasis is defined as the transfer of primary cancerous lesions to another organ.[40] Despite its rich blood supply, metastasis to the spleen is relatively uncommon. Metastatic involvement of the spleen by carcinoma is usually seen in advanced cases of the disease when the carcinoma has already metastasized or directly invaded other visceral organs. Metastatic spread to the spleen is most common with melanoma, breast, colorectal, and ovarian carcinomas.[54] Overall, melanoma is the most frequent metastatic lesion of the spleen. Sonographically, metastatic lesions may vary in appearance, demonstrating hypoechoic, hyperechoic, anechoic, or heterogeneous qualities. However, most metastatic lesions found within the spleen demonstrate a "bull's-eye" appearance with a hypoechoic halo[6,9] (Fig. 10-17). There is no consistent correlation between the sonographic appearance of the lesions and the histologic type of primary tumor. Fine needle biopsy is a safe and efficient method of diagnosing splenic nodules and is necessary for a definitive diagnosis.[55]

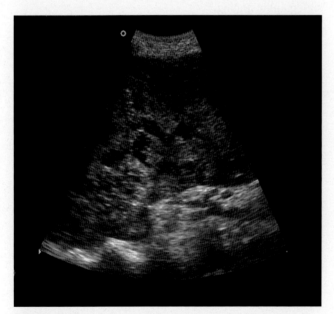

FIGURE 10-16 Angiosarcoma. Diffusely abnormal spleen demonstrating mixed echogenicity consistent with angiosarcoma. (Image courtesy of Philips Medical System, Bothell, WA.)

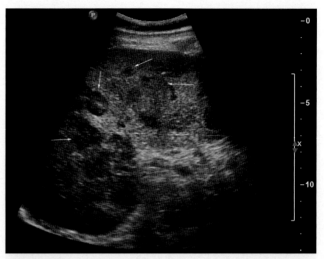

FIGURE 10-17 Metastases. Longitudinal image of the spleen demonstrating multiple solid, hypoechoic masses characteristic of metastases. Many of the masses demonstrate a "bull's-eye" appearance with a hyperechoic center and a hypoechoic rim *(arrows)*. (Image courtesy of Philips Medical System, Bothell, WA.)

Benign Neoplasms

Hemangioma

Hemangiomas are the most common benign vascular neoplasm of the spleen most often affecting men 20 to 50 years of age.[1,6,9] Hemangiomas are generally isolated phenomena, but they may occur in association with Klippel–Trenaunay–Weber syndrome or hemangiomatosis.[6,9] Sonographically, splenic hemangiomas appear similar to liver hemangiomas. These neoplasms measure less than 4 cm and have variable echogenicity with calcifications. Owing to the complex appearance, differential diagnoses may include hydatid cyst, abscess, and metastases. Duplex Doppler and color Doppler techniques may be useful in demonstrating blood flow within the hypoechoic areas of parenchyma, helping distinguish between hemangiomas and infarctions, which are usually avascular (Fig. 10-18). Symptoms are often secondary to rupture or compression of adjoining structures.[6,9] Complications of hemangiomas include spontaneous splenic rupture, anemia, thrombocytopenia, portal hypertension, and malignant degeneration.[36]

Hamartoma

Hamartomas, also referred to as splenomas, are a rare vascular proliferation tumor composed of varying mixtures of tumor tissue and normal splenic tissue.[1,6,56] Hamartomas are often associated with syndromes such as Wiskott–Aldrich syndrome and may grow larger in women than in men.[6,56] Clinically, a patient may present with pancytopenia, anemia, and thrombocytopenia.[6] However, most hamartomas are asymptomatic.[1] Sonographically, hamartomas are homogeneous, solid, and well defined with variable echogenicity.[1,6,9,56] These tumors may also demonstrate hypervascularity when evaluated with Doppler imaging.[6,9]

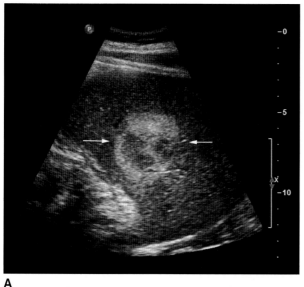

A

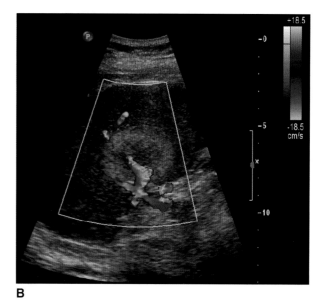

B

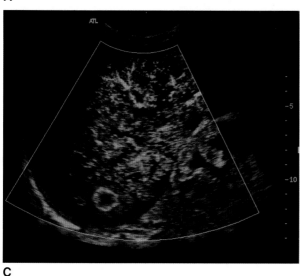

C

FIGURE 10-18 Splenic hemangioma. **A:** Transverse image of the spleen demonstrates a focal, echogenic lesion consistent with a splenic hemangioma (*arrows*). **B:** Color Doppler investigation of the splenic hemangioma. **C:** Splenic hemangioma imaged using contrast enhancement and power Doppler imaging. (Images courtesy of Philips Medical System, Bothell, WA.)

SUMMARY

- The spleen is an intraperitoneal organ located in the LUQ of the abdomen.
- In the adult, the spleen measures approximately 12 to 13 cm in length and is surrounded by a fibrous capsule.
- The spleen functions as a reservoir for blood, removes old and abnormal RBCs from circulation, and plays a role in the body's immunity.
- Small accessory spleens are a normal variant typically found in the splenic hilum or along the gastrosplenic ligament.
- Splenic ptosis, or wandering spleen, occurs because the supporting ligaments of the spleen are lax and allow the spleen to migrate along the left side from the thorax to the pelvis, making it susceptible to torsion and infarction.
- Splenomegaly is the most common sonographically observed splenic abnormality and is diagnosed when the spleen measures greater than 13 cm in length.
- Splenomegaly results from several causes, including portal hypertension, infection, metabolic and hematologic disorders, trauma, and infiltrative processes such as leukemia and lymphoma.
- Splenic cysts are either congenital or acquired. Acquired cysts can be parasitic, postinflammatory, or traumatic.
- Splenic abscesses are complex lesions with mixed echogenicity and are often a result of infection spreading through the bloodstream.
- Acute splenic infarcts are well-defined, hypoechoic, wedge-shaped, or round areas seen along the periphery of the spleen.
- The spleen is frequently injured in cases of blunt abdominal trauma. Fractures of the splenic capsule, parenchymal lacerations, and splenic hematomas are common.
- In a trauma setting, an enlarging, heterogeneous spleen suggests a ruptured spleen.
- In Hodgkin and non-Hodgkin lymphoma, involvement of the spleen may appear normal, may have focal hypoechoic or hyperechoic masses, or may be diffusely enlarged.

REFERENCES

1. Varga I, Babala J, Kachlik D. Anatomic variations of the spleen: current state of terminology, classification, and embryological background. *Surg Radiol Anat.* 2018;40(1):21–29. doi:10.1007/s00276-017-1893-0
2. Moore K, Dalley A, Agur A. *Clinically Oriented Anatomy.* 7th ed. Lippincott, Williams, & Wilkins; 2014.
3. Kelley L, Peterson C. *Sectional Anatomy for Imaging Professionals.* 3rd ed. Elsevier Mosby; 2013.
4. Stewart KR, Derck AM, Long KL, et al. Diagnostic accuracy of clinical tests for the detection of splenomegaly. *Phys Ther Rev.* 2013;18(3):173–184.
5. Jones B, Callahan J, Cole A, et al. The case of the wandering spleen. *J Diagn Med Sonogr.* 2012;29(3):130–132. doi:10.1177/8756479312472392
6. Gross S. Left upper quadrant pain. In: Henningsen C, Kuntz K, Youngs DJ, eds. *Clinical Guide to Sonography. Exercises for Critical Thinking.* Elsevier Mosby; 2014:88–100.
7. Davis K, Curry R. The spleen. In: Curry R, Tempkin BB, eds. *Sonography: Introduction to Normal Structure and Function.* Elsevier Mosby; 2016:295–307.
8. McCance K, Huethe S. *Pathophysiology: The Biologic Basis for Disease in Adults and Children.* 7th ed. Elsevier Mosby; 2014.
9. Vos P, Mathieson J, Cooperberg P. The spleen. In: Rumack CM, Wilson SR, Charboneau JW, eds. *Diagnostic Ultrasound.* 4th ed. Elsevier Mosby; 2011.
10. Hidaka H, Nakazawa T, Wang G, et al. Reliability and validity of splenic volume measurement by 3-D ultrasound. *Hepatol Res.* 2010;40:979–988.
11. Tempkin BB. Spleen scanning protocol. In: Tempkin BB, ed. *Sonography Scanning: Principles and Protocols.* Elsevier Mosby; 2015:203–220.
12. Sucandy I, Polavarapu H, Pezzi C. Hypoplasia of the spleen: review of pathogenesis, diagnosis, and potential clinical implications. *N Am J Med Sci.* 2015;7(8):368–370.
13. Low J, Williams D, Chaganti J. Polysplenia syndrome with agenesis of the dorsal pancreas and preduodenal portal vein presenting with obstructive jaundice—a case report and literature review. *Br J Radiol.* 2011;84:219–222.
14. Bhalla K, Singh J, Yadav J, et al. Asplenia syndrome in a neonate: a case report. *J Clin Diagn Res.* 2016;10(6):5–6.
15. Landmann A, Johnson J, Webb K, et al. Accessory spleen presenting as acute abdomen: a case report and operative management. *J Pediatr Surg Case Rep.* 2016;12:9–10.
16. Sadro CM, Lehnert B. Torsion of an accessory spleen: case report and review of the literature. *Radiol Case Rep.* 2013;8(1):1–4.
17. George M, Evans T, Lambrianides A. Accessory spleen in pancreatic tail. *J Surg Case Rep.* 2012;11:1–2. doi:10.1093/jscr/rjs004
18. Kirshtein B, Lantsberg S, Hatskelzon L, et al. Laparoscopic accessory splenectomy using intraoperative gamma prove guidance. *J Laparoendosc Adv Surg Tech A.* 2007;17(2):205–208.
19. Lombardi R, Menchini L, Corneli T, et al. Wandering spleen in children: a report of 3 cases and a brief literature review underlining the importance of diagnostic imaging. *Pediatr Radiol.* 2014;44:279–288. doi:10.1007/s00247-013-2851-6
20. Perin A, Cola R, Favretti F. Accessory wandering spleen: report of a case of laparoscopic approach in an asymptomatic patient. *Int J Surg Case Rep.* 2014;5:887–889.
21. Fonseca A, Ribeiro M, Contrucci O. Torsion of a wandering spleen treated with partial splenectomy and splenopexy. *J Emerg Med.* 2013;44(1):33–36. doi:10.1016/j.jemermed.2011.06.146
22. Kristinsson S, Gridley G, Hoover R, et al. Long-term risks after splenectomy among 8,149 cancer-free U.S. veterans: a cohort study with up to 27 years follow-up. *Haematologica.* 2013;113(28):7804–7809. doi:10.1073/pnas.1606751113
23. Brousse V, Buffet P, Rees D. The spleen and sickle cell disease: the sick(led) spleen. *Br J Haematol.* 2014;166:165–176. doi:10.1111/bjh.12950
24. Tortora G, Derrickson B. *Principles of Anatomy and Physiology.* 13th ed. Biological Sciences Textbooks; 2012.
25. Bronte V, Pittet M. The spleen in local and systemic regulation of immunity. *Immunity.* 2013;39(5):806–818.
26. Hofer M. *Ultrasound Teaching Manual: The Basics of Performing and Interpreting Ultrasound Scans.* 3rd ed. Thieme Publishers; 2013.
27. Alshuwaer TA, Gillman F. Prevention of shoulder injuries in sonographers: a systematic review. *JDMS.* 2019;35(5):1–21. doi:10.1177/8756479319850140
28. American Institute of Ultrasound in Medicine. (2017). AIUM practice parameter for the performance of an ultrasound examination of the abdomen and/or retroperitoneum. Accessed January 3, 2022. https://www.aium.org/resources/guidelines/abdominal.pdf
29. Stephensen SR. Palpable left upper quadrant mass. In: Sanders R, ed. *Clinical Sonography: A Practical Guide.* 5th ed. Lippincott, Williams, & Wilkins; 2016:466–479.
30. Dietrich CF, Averkiou M, Nielsen MB, et al. How to perform contrast-enhanced ultrasound. *Ultrasound Int Open.* 2018;4(1):E2–E15.
31. Tagliati C, Argalia G, Marco Giuseppetti G. Contrast-enhanced ultrasound performance in predicting blunt splenic injuries requiring only observation and monitoring. *Med Ultrson.* 2019;21(1):16–21.
32. Lerchbaumer MH, Tobias K, Ernst-Michael J, et al. Vascular pattern and diagnostic accuracy of contrast-enhanced ultrasound (CEUS) in spleen alterations. *Clin Hemorheol Microcirc.* 2020;75(2):177–188.
33. Davis L, Baumer T, Van Holsbeeck M. Clinical utilization of shear wave elastography in the musculoskeletal system. *Ultrasonography.* 2019;38(1):2–12.
34. Yalcin K, Demir BC. Spleen stiffness measurement by shear wave elastography using acoustic radiation force impulse in predicting the etiology of splenomegaly. *Abdom Radiol.* 2020;46(2):609–615.
35. Sindhu N, Koteshwar P, Shetty S. Point shear wave elastography of the spleen in predicting the presence of esophageal varices in cirrhosis: liver stiffness vs. spleen stiffness. *JDMS.* 2020;36(2):95–101.
36. Burns J, Willis A, Wybo J, Ladis-Michalek JM. *Abdominal Sonography Including Superficial Structures.* SDMS; 2009.
37. Boyer T, Habib S. Big spleens and hypersplenism: fix it or forget it? *Liver Int.* 2015;35(5):1492–1498.
38. Toreno F, Kuntz K. Diffuse liver disease. In: Henningsen C, Kuntz K, Youngs DJ, eds. *Clinical Guide to Sonography.* 2nd ed. Elsevier Mosby; 2014:27–40.
39. Owen C, Meyers P. Sonographic evaluation of the portal and hepatic systems. *J Diagn Med Sonogr.* 2006;22:317–328.
40. Naymagon L, Pendurti G, Billett H. Acute splenic sequestration crisis in adult sickle cell disease: a report of 16 cases. *Hemaglobin.* 2015;39(6):375–379.
41. Nong H, Wu F, Su N, et al. Ultrasound guided biopsy: a powerful tool in diagnosing AIDS complications. *Radiol Infect Dis.* 2015;2(3):123–127.
42. Ingle S, Chitra H, Patrike S. Epithelial cysts of the spleen: a mini-review. *World J Gastroenterol.* 2014;20(38):13899–13903.
43. Tarahomi M, Otaghvar HA, Ghayifekr N, et al. Primary hydatid cyst of umbilicus, mimicking an umbilical hernia. *Surgery.* 2016;1–3.
44. Ioannidis I, Kahn A. Splenic lymphangioma. *Arch Pathol Lab Med.* 2015;139(2):278–282.
45. Faruque A, Qazi S, Arhad M, et al. Isolated splenic abscess in children, role of splenic preservation. *Pediatr Surg Int.* 2013;29(8):787–790.
46. McKinney E. Splenic abscess detection and monitoring using sonography. *J Diagn Med Sonogr.* 2012;28(4):168–172.
47. Ricci Z, Oh S, Stein M, et al. Solid organ abdominal ischemia, part 1: clinical features, etiology, imaging findings, and management. *Clin Imaging.* 2016;40(4):720–731.
48. Llewellyn M, Jeffrey B, DiMaio M, et al. The sonographic "bright band sign" of splenic infarction. *J Ultrasound Med.* 2014;33(6):929–938.
49. Cummins K, Westall G, Grigoriadis G. Numerous Howell-Jolly bodies in a patient with idiopathic splenic calcification. *Br J Haematol.* 2015;169(6):767.
50. Van Vliet J. Primary diffuse large B cell lymphoma of the spleen. *J Diagn Med Sonogr.* 2010;26(3):147–149.
51. Bassuner KJ, Kirkpatrick DL, Northrup M, Connors JP. Multiple targetoid lesions in the spleen: sonographic findings of chronic lymphocytic leukemia and their relation to effective staging. *JDMS.* 2015;31(4):243–246.
52. Siegel M. *Pediatric Sonography.* 4th ed. Wolters Kluwer; 2011.
53. Xu L, Zhang Y, Hong Z, et al. Well-differentiated angiosarcoma of spleen: a teaching case mimicking hemangioma and cytogenic analysis with array comparative genomic hybridization. *World J Surg Oncol.* 2015;13:300.
54. Sardenberg R, Pinto C, Bueno C, et al. Non-small cell lung cancer stage IV long-term survival with isolated spleen metastasis. *Ann Thorac Surg.* 2013;95(4):1432–1434.
55. Olson M, Atwell T, Harmsen W, et al. Safety and accuracy of percutaneous image-guided biopsy of the spleen. *Am J Roentgenol.* 2016;206(3):655–659.
56. Thipphavong S, Duigenan S, Schindera S., et al. Nonneoplastic, benign, and malignant splenic disease: cross-sectional imaging findings and rare disease entities. *Am J Roentgenol.* 2014;203(2):315–322.

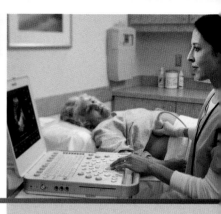

CHAPTER 11

The Gastrointestinal Tract

BARBARA HALL-TERRACCIANO

OBJECTIVES

- Understand the anatomy of the gastrointestinal tract, including the five sonographic layers of the bowel wall.
- Define the process for sonographic evaluation of the gastrointestinal tract, including examination preparation and technique.
- Know the transabdominal and endoluminal approaches include the endovaginal and the endorectal ultrasound approach as well as the choice of the transducer for the examination.
- Describe the esophagus, stomach, small bowel, appendix, and colon.
- Discuss disorders of the esophagus, stomach, small bowel, appendix, and colon that can be sonographically visualized.

GLOSSARY

appendicolith fecolith or calcification found in the appendiceal lumen

atonic without muscular tone

Crohn disease inflammatory bowel disease causing chronic inflammation of the gastrointestinal tract

duodenal web complete or incomplete obstruction at the duodenum because of membranous web or intraluminal diverticulum

dysphagia difficulty swallowing

elastography technique for identifying changes in elasticity of soft tissue resulting from diseases processes

endoluminal within the lumen of a tubular organ such as the gastrointestinal tract

endoscope (sonoendoscope) flexible lighted tube with high-frequency sound waves that produce images of the digestive tract walls and lining in addition to adjacent structures such as lymph nodes, major blood vessels, pancreas, liver, and chest

endosonography sonography done using an ultrasound transducer attached to an endoscope

esophagogastroduodenoscopy (EGD) endoscopic procedure to depict the esophagus, stomach, and first portion of the duodenum

glucagon agent used to achieve bowel aperistalsis

graded compression technique where transducer is slowly and firmly compressed against the abdominal wall to displace inferior structures, generally bowel loops

gut digestive tract

H. pylori (Helicobacter pylori) bacteria that live in the digestive tract causing sores/ulcers, which may evolve into cancer

KEY TERMS

adenocarcinoma

appendiceal abscess

appendicitis

carcinoid tumor

Crohn disease

diverticulosis

duodenal ulcer

gastric carcinoma

gastric dilatation

gastric ulcer disease

gastritis

gastrointestinal stromal tumor

hematoma

intussusception

leiomyoma

leiomyosarcoma

lymphoma

mucocele

peptic ulcer

small bowel edema

small bowel obstruction

squamous cell carcinoma

ulcerative colitis

volvulus

(continued)

hematochezia discharge of fresh (bright red) blood through the anus

ileus failure of the intestine to propel its contents because of diminished motility

ligament of Treitz suspensory ligament at the level of the duodenal junction

McBurney point point over the right side of the abdomen that is one-third of the distance from the anterior superior iliac spine to the umbilicus

Ménétrier disease rare condition of the stomach where overgrowth of mucous cells in the membrane lining results in large gastric folds leading to decreased or absent acid production

midaxillary line vertical line from the midaxilla toward the iliac crest

optical endoscopy rigid or flexible tube with a fiberoptic light source designed to investigate the inside of bowel, organs, and lung structures

peristalsis rhythmic dilatation and contraction that propels the contents of the gastrointestinal tract

peritonitis inflammation of the covering of the peritoneum that covers and supports abdominal organs

polyp growth on a stalk protruding from mucous membranes

ulcer an erosion in the mucosal layer of the wall of the gastrointestinal tract; frequently located in the stomach or duodenum

volvulus abnormal twisting of the intestines that can lead to obstruction, gangrene, perforation, and peritonitis

Zollinger–Ellison syndrome rare condition of secreting tumors (gastrinomas) forming in the pancreas or duodenum causing abnormally increased stomach acid

The gastrointestinal (GI) tract, also known as the alimentary canal, includes the lips, mouth, pharynx, esophagus, stomach, small intestine, appendix, and colon through to the anus. Sonographic examination of the GI tract began in the 1980s using endoscopic ultrasonography (EUS) and the transabdominal approach. Forty years later, those methods, as well as the endorectal and endovaginal approaches, are still utilized. All methods have continued to gain diagnostic importance because of technical equipment advancements and increased sonographer GI exposure, which has led to indispensable experience and diagnostic accuracy. At its inception, GI ultrasound was not often performed by sonographers because of the difficulty in evaluating the GI structures by an inexperienced operator; however, continued sonographer exposure to GI studies has contributed to expanded use of this modality. Technical advances in ultrasound systems have included options such as harmonic imaging, beam steering, and speckle reduction in addition to high-resolution transducers, which also increase the visualization of GI structure and added diagnostic accuracy. GI sonography is extremely useful and appreciated in countries where access to expensive testing—such as endoscopy, computerized tomography (CT), magnetic resonance imaging (MRI), and positron emission tomography (PET)—is limited and in areas where contrast studies are commonly performed.

SONOGRAPHIC GASTROINTESTINAL EXAMINATION TECHNIQUE

Real-time transducers provide the sonographic equivalent of fluoroscopy. Peristaltic activity visible on real-time

examinations is impossible to capture on still images but can be acquired with cine clips. Movement of the GI tract is invaluable to the sonographer who is evaluating its function and ruling out an anomaly. Peristalsis of the bowel is expected, and when viewed by an experienced sonographer, it can help with a diagnosis.

Although the GI tract is not usually the primary focus of an abdominal sonogram, clinicians value GI information when abnormalities are discovered that may be the cause of abdominal symptoms. Incidental information, such as excessive or no peristaltic activity, increased intraluminal fluid contents, suspected bowel dilatation, and inflammation, is critical to making an accurate diagnosis. A targeted GI ultrasound can provide information about the GI tract, in many cases, similar to a CT and MRI.

Three classes of sonographic exam performed on the GI tract are transabdominal, transvaginal/transrectal, and endoluminal sonography/endoscopic ultrasonography (EUS). Transabdominal sonography is the traditional method, often used as a screening procedure to evaluate abdominal or pelvic pain and cause of fever, rebound tenderness, and palpable abdominal mass by evaluating the bowel wall thickness (BWT) and the pattern of echogenicity, vascularity, and mobility. Other reasons for GI ultrasound include follow-up of a previous GI sonography exam; abnormal laboratory data; or the results from radiography, CT, MRI, and/or PET.

Endoluminal sonography is not widely used by general sonographers. It is performed by endosonographers and gastroenterologists using specialized endoscopes. The endoscope or linear endoscope is specially designed with a sonographic transducer at its tip, which produces sonographic images from within the lumen and directly adjacent to the GI wall. An optical endoscope evaluates the lumen with a light. Endoluminal sonographic examinations are directed specifically at the bowel or surrounding structures. The coupling of sonography and endoscopy has allowed physicians to better visualize and stage cancers within or adjacent to the GI tract and to evaluate the depth of lesions within the intestinal wall. Transesophageal, transduodenal, and transgastric sonographic evaluations can detect abnormalities in the pancreatobiliary system, paraluminal and intramural lesions including lymphadenopathies, ascites, and lesions in the left liver lobe; and reasons for rectal bleeding, diarrhea, hematochezia, bowel obstruction, and change of bowel habit. Linear endoscopes have brought a new landscape to EUS because of their ability to track a needle in real time across the image plane into a target lesion. This is known as endoluminal ultrasound with fine needle aspiration (EUS-FNA). The electronic instruments also permit the use of Doppler technology to assess vascular flow.[1] Endosonography has been performed primarily on the upper GI tract: the esophagus, stomach, and duodenum. The method of examination is similar to conventional upper GI endoscopy. Following the usual premedication, the sonoendoscope is introduced into the esophagus with the patient in the left lateral decubitus position. When the lesion is identified visually, it can be examined with the attached sonographic transducer. EUS-FNA has now become part of the diagnostic and staging algorithm for the evaluation of benign and malignant diseases of the GI tract and its bordering organs.[1] Its uses within the GI tract include esophageal, gastric, duodenal, colon, and rectum. Lymph nodes related to lung cancer can be biopsied via the esophagus. Structures inferior to the esophagus and adjacent to the intestines such as pancreas, adrenal gland, gallbladder, bile duct, liver, kidney, and lung can be biopsied. Muscles of the inferior rectum and anal canal can be examined for fecal incontinence.

Endovaginal sonography (EVS), used to evaluate the prostate gland, is also suitable for evaluating the rectal wall and perirectal area and can be used to stage rectal tumors. Endovaginal transducers can locate and document the appendix in females and are especially helpful in the case of large body habitus.[2] The same transducer visualizes portions of the inferior small intestine and colonic haustra.

Patient Preparation

Patient preparation for transabdominal sonography depends on the physician's order. If the examination requisition for a GI ultrasound examination includes abdominal organs such as liver, gallbladder, pancreas, bile ducts, kidneys, and aorta, the patient should be advised to fast for 8 hours before the examination to ensure distention of the gallbladder and to minimize stomach gas. Morning studies are recommended to decrease intraluminal air, peristaltic motion, and patient hunger. The organs should be documented first, followed by the GI tract. Prior to examination of the stomach and duodenum, the patient can drink 10 to 40 oz of water through a straw to improve visualization. Having the patient drink fluid also helps in evaluating the mucosa and peristalsis of the jejunum and ileum. Oral fluid is contraindicated if the patient has GI obstruction or ileus or is scheduled for upper GI barium studies. Note that examinations can be performed in emergencies without preparation.

For transabdominal examination of the colon, no special preparation is necessary, except for the rare occasion during pelvic sonography when a water enema is required to establish the position of the rectosigmoid colon. Laxatives should be avoided prior to a GI ultrasound study. Osmotic laxatives cause water retention in the colon. Stimulant laxatives increase digestive movements. Both may contribute to abnormal sonographic results.

Before endorectal sonography, a cleansing enema may be helpful so that fecal material is not confused with mucosal lesions. EVS does not usually require bowel cleansing, although if the area of interest is obscured by intraluminal air or solid contents, a cleansing enema is recommended.

Limitations

Sonographic examination of the GI tract can be difficult because gas in the tract can obscure details of the bowel wall and lumen as well as structures deep into the bowel such as the pancreas and the periaortic area of the retroperitoneum or masses. Fluid or feces in the bowel lumen can be perceived as disease. Large patient body habitus may influence transducer selection. A high-frequency transducer should be utilized to obtain high-resolution images when possible. Obese patients often require a lower-frequency transducer for deeper penetration, which offers a lower-resolution image. Other limitations include the inability to continuously view the entire small bowel and, as with any sonographic examination, operator dependence.

Transducer Selection

Ultrasound examination of the GI tract usually benefits from the use of at least two different transducers. A low-frequency convex transducer in the range of 1 to 6 MHz is used to obtain initial GI views and for large habitus patients. A high-frequency linear probe ranging from 5 to 17 MHz will examine the bowel wall and evaluate superficial findings discovered with the low-frequency transducer. First, the abdomen is scanned by means of the convex low-frequency transducer, in order to visualize deeper structures and detect grossly abnormal pathologies, such as significant thickening of the intestinal wall, bowel dilatation, and the presence of fistulae or abscesses. This is followed by a linear higher-frequency transducer, for detailed evaluation of the intestinal wall, which requires extra time and patience by the ultrasound operator.[3] Endovaginal and endorectal sonography are utilized to view layers of the rectum and stage rectal tumors, GI stroma tumors, inflammatory bowel disease, intestinal endometriosis, diverticulitis, appendicitis, bowel mass, and Crohn disease (CD) among others.

Patient Position

Examination of the intestinal tract begins with the patient comfortably relaxed in a supine position so as not to tense the abdominal wall.[4] Flexing the left knee, especially when the knee is supported by a medical extremity wedge, alleviates back discomfort. The transducer is held maintaining contact with the patient's skin to gauge pressure, while the left hand is free to optimize image characteristics on the ultrasound system. A systemic approach in examining the whole intestine is encouraged.[4]

ANATOMY OF THE BOWEL WALL

The GI tract is an approximately 30-foot muscular tube of varying diameter, originating at the lips and terminating at the anus (Fig. 11-1). The layers of the bowel wall are similar throughout the GI tract, with the esophagus having four layers and the rest of the GI tract having five layers.

Described anatomically, the innermost layer is the echogenic epithelium (mucosal surface). Within the esophagus, the innermost layer is composed of stratified squamous cells. In the stomach and bowel, this layer is composed of simple and columnar cells. Some of these cells are modified for digestive activities. The plasma membrane of the cells is adapted to perform certain functions: microvilli enhance the absorptive area, goblet cells secrete mucus, and cells with cilia oscillate to aid in digestion. Deep into the epithelium is a hypoechoic mucosal layer that consists of the *lamina propria*, which in the esophagus is a loose areolar tissue and elsewhere is a glandular tissue, and the *muscularis mucosa*, which is immediately below the lamina propria and is very thin and smooth. Just above and below the muscularis mucosa are scattered patches of lymphoid tissue. Below the muscularis mucosa is a looser areolar tissue, called the *submucosa*. It is the thickest layer and is echogenic. Deeper yet lies the hypoechoic *muscularis propria*, also known as the *muscularis externa*. This structure consists of an inner circumferential layer and an outer longitudinal layer of smooth muscle. The final layer of the wall is the echogenic *serosa*, a thin epithelial layer on the periphery of the bowel.

When using ultrasound frequencies in the range of 5 to 17 MHz, the wall of the intestine can be seen well and exhibits five different layers that correspond well to the histologic layers (Fig. 11-2A). The layered wall structure changes with disease.[4] The five layers from interior to exterior are as follows:

- an inner hyperechoic layer—commonly this represents the border between the digestive fluid and the mucosa;
- a hypoechoic layer—usually thin, this represents the mucosa, lamina propria, and lamina muscularis;
- a hyperechoic layer—the submucosa;
- a hypoechoic layer—the muscular layer; its thickness depends upon the segment of the digestive tract; and
- an outer hyperechoic layer—the serous layer, the border to the peridigestive fat.[5]

Thus, the sonographic structure of the bowel is usually described with five layers: three echogenic layers separated by two hypoechoic ones (Fig. 11-2B–D).[5] Using high-frequency transducers, the muscularis mucosa and the two layers of the muscularis propria can be resolved as well. Visualizing the layers of the bowel wall is useful in detecting certain pathologic conditions that follow. A transabdominal approach demonstrates bowel wall layers with less definition than endoluminal sonography.

Gut Interrogation

GI ultrasound should examine the BWT, wall changes, vascular anomalies, motility, and symmetry of thickness. BWT is the measurement most consistently reported in diagnostic and activity trials.[4] The measurement should include the outer hyperechoic layer to the inner hyperechoic layer and be performed with mild compression. Transducer compression of the bowel wall will reduce thickness and can make it challenging to distinguish wall layers. Some wall thickening is nonspecific, which may make it difficult or impossible to diagnose disease processes, although the finding must be evaluated. Focal, irregular, and asymmetrical thickening of the bowel wall suggests malignancy.[6]

ESOPHAGUS AND ESOPHAGOGASTRIC JUNCTION

Normal Anatomy of the Esophagus

The esophagus is a fibromuscular hollow tube positioned between the pharynx and stomach cardia within the thorax.

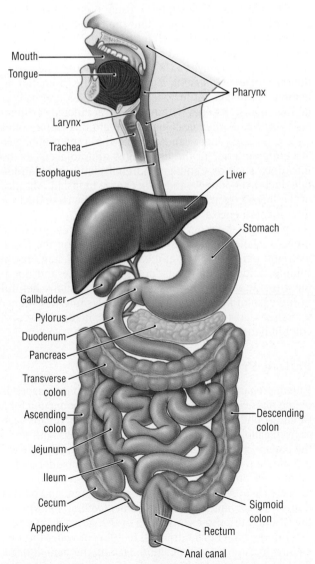

FIGURE 11-1 Gastrointestinal tract. An anatomic anterior view of the gastrointestinal tract from the lips/mouth to the anus. (Reprinted with permission from Agur AMR, Dalley AF II. *Grant's Atlas of Anatomy*. 14th ed. Wolters Kluwer; 2017.)

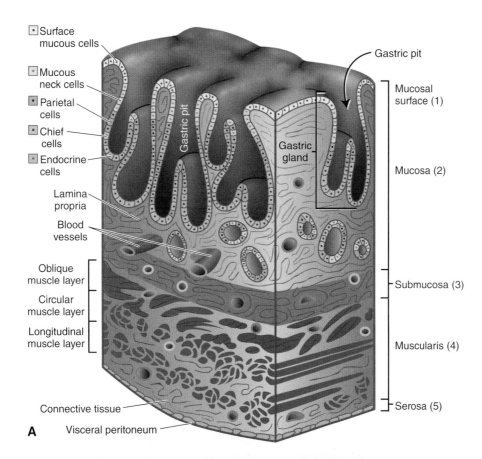

Surface mucous cells

Mucous neck cells

Parietal cells

Chief cells

Endocrine cells

Lamina propria

Blood vessels

Oblique muscle layer

Circular muscle layer

Longitudinal muscle layer

Connective tissue

Visceral peritoneum

Gastric pit

Gastric gland

Mucosal surface (1)

Mucosa (2)

Submucosa (3)

Muscularis (4)

Serosa (5)

A

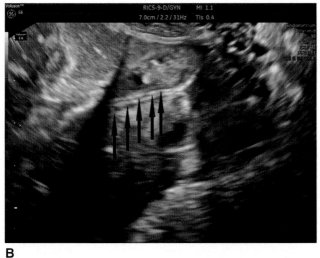

B

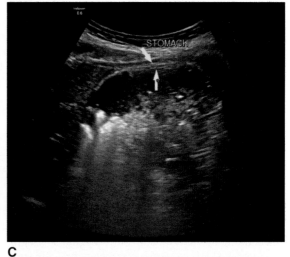

C

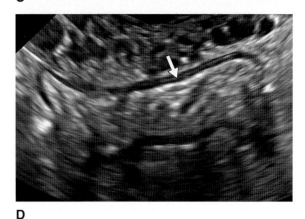

D

FIGURE 11-2 Bowel wall. **A:** Drawing of the gastric wall layers. The corresponding sonographic layers are numbered: mucosal surface (1); mucosa (lamina propria and muscularis mucosa) (2); submucosa (3); muscularis propria, which anatomically has a longitudinal muscle layer and a circular muscle layer (4); and serosa (5). **B:** Endocavity image of the five bowel layers (arrows). (Image courtesy of Barbara Hall-Terracciano.) **C:** Sonographic image of the fluid-filled stomach demonstrates the five sonographically visible bowel wall layers (arrows): three echogenic and two hypoechoic layers. (Images courtesy of Doña Ana Community College Diagnostic Medical Sonography program, Las Cruces, NM.) **D:** Five bowel wall layers depicting normal wall anatomy. The arrow should be positioned 2 mm to the anterior surface. The outer and innermost echogenic layers are not depicted compared to endoscopic sonography. (Image courtesy of Barbara Hall-Terracciano)

It is approximately 10 inches long. The superior width of the tube is 1.4 cm, with the distal width reaching 2 cm. Unlike the GI tract distal to the esophagus, it is composed of four layers: inner mucosa, submucosa, muscularis propria, and outer adventitia. It does not have a serosal layer. The mucosa is stratified squamous epithelium covering the entire lumen. The submucosa is a thick layer that connects the mucosa to the muscular layer. The muscular portion is made of longitudinal and circular muscle fibers. The outermost layer is adventitia composed of fibrous tissue that connects with the pharynx superiorly and with the stomach distally.

Sonographic Technique

A sonoendoscope is often utilized to assess the esophagus because this imaging method is able to view the entire lumen. Transabdominal sonography can depict most of the tubular structure in a supine patient using the thyroid as an acoustic window for the superior portion and the heart as an acoustic window with the transducer adjacent to the left sternum for the midportion. The inferior portion, esophagogastric junction, and stomach can be visualized transabdominally when using the left liver lobe as an acoustic window (Fig. 11-3A, B). The esophagogastric junction is within the superior abdomen (epigastric region) posterior to the left liver lobe and anterior to the aorta. An abdominal transducer should be placed inferior to the xiphoid and angled superiorly to locate the junction. Giving an erect patient water to drink may ensure transabdominal views of the entire esophagus. Layers of the esophageal wall and surrounding mediastinal structures will be seen best intraluminally. EUS provides an accurate evaluation of the depth of tumor invasion and the extent of lymph node involvement. PET is used to detect early esophageal cancer. MRI is adept at locating early esophageal lesions as well as detecting and staging wall invasion. CT detects lesions and can also search for spread of invasive disease. Barium swallow studies show esophageal lining anomalies, but are unable to determine the depth of wall invasion.

Sonographic Esophageal Wall Dimensions

Normal adult esophageal and esophagogastric junction single wall thickness is reported as 2 to 5 mm. Esophageal wall thickness may differ depending on contraction and dilatation. Acute conditions such as esophageal spasm, esophagitis, hematoma, and perforation can cause abnormal wall thickness measurement variations of the esophagus. Irregular measurements may be caused by a transient or acute condition. Focal causes for wall thickness include tumor, hernia, varices, and mucocele and are more likely to be long-lasting.

Disorders of the Esophagus

Carcinoma

Esophageal cancer is rare with an incidence of about 1% in the United States.[7,8] The most common esophageal cancers are squamous cell carcinoma or, less commonly, adenocarcinoma per the Cleveland Clinic, Memorial Sloan Kettering Cancer Center, and the Mayo Clinic, among others. Squamous cell carcinoma is common in the upper and mid-esophagus, whereas adenocarcinoma mostly affects the distal portion. Both types affect men more than

women, usually in those over 25 years of age (mostly over 65 years of age).[7,8] The lesions begin as raised longitudinal plaque-like or polypoid areas, which quickly enlarge circumferentially; subsequently, strictures form and dysphagia develops. Because the esophagus lacks a serosa, extension into the surrounding mediastinum is unimpeded. Currently, about 20% of patients survive 5 years after diagnosis based on an average of localized, regional, and distant stages.[7] Survival rates over 5 years are attributed to early detection.

Other Tumors of the Esophagus

Rare malignant tumors of the esophagus:
- carcinosarcoma, mucoepidermoid carcinoma, adenoid cystic carcinoma
- lymphoma
- glomangiomas

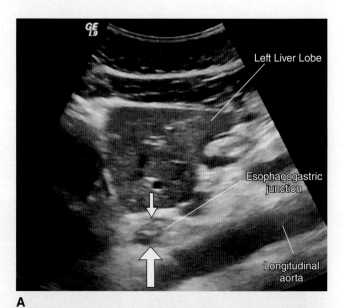

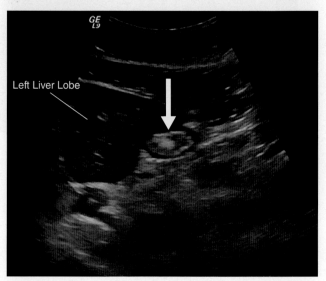

FIGURE 11-3 Esophagogastric junction. **A:** The esophagogastric junction is positioned posterior to the left liver lobe in this sagittal view (*arrows*). **B:** A target view of the stomach is seen adjacent to the left liver lobe (*arrow*). (Images courtesy of Doña Ana Community College Diagnostic Medical Sonography program, Las Cruces, NM.)

Benign tumors of the esophagus:
- polyp, granular cell tumor
- adenoma
- papilloma (malignant potential)
- leiomyoma

Sonographic tumor findings:
- wall deviations and disruptions
- wall thickening
- lesions with a polypoid, smooth-walled, vascular, or lobulated nature
- mass with isoechoic, cystic, partially cystic, or heterogeneous appearance

Disorders of the Esophagogastric Junction

The esophagogastric junction can be evaluated with endosonography or, if the left lobe of the liver is large enough, with transabdominal sonography. The esophagogastric junction can be seen posterior to the left lobe and anterior to the abdominal aorta.[5] A variety of abnormalities, including hiatal hernia, esophageal varices, anomalous motility, and tumors similar to those of the esophagus, can be demonstrated.

STOMACH

Normal Anatomy of the Stomach

The stomach is the expanded part of the alimentary tract and normally lies in the left upper quadrant of the abdomen. The fundus is medial to the spleen and anterior to the left kidney. The body and antrum of the stomach lie posterior or inferior to the left lobe of the liver, anterior to the pancreas, and medial to the gallbladder and porta hepatis.[5] The antrum and body of the stomach often appear as a target-like structure inferior to the left lobe on longitudinal sonograms. Both hypo- and hyperechoic contents as well as air shadows can be seen (Fig. 11-4A–D). If the left hepatic lobe is large enough, the gastroesophageal junction can also be visualized as a target-like structure just below the diaphragm and just to the left of the spine. Gas, mucus, or

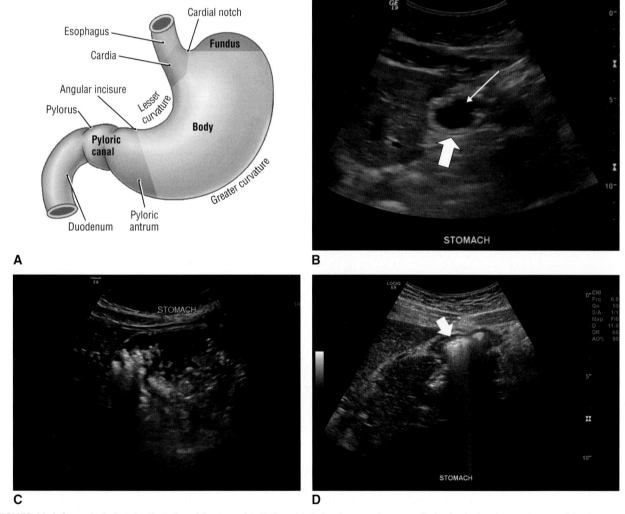

FIGURE 11-4 Stomach. **A:** Anterior illustration of the stomach with these labeled regions: esophagus, cardia, fundus, body antrum, pylorus, and duodenum. (Reprinted with permission from Agur AMR, Dalley AF II. *Grant's Atlas of Anatomy*. 14th ed. Wolters Kluwer; 2017.) **B:** Transverse view of the stomach demonstrating target-like view. *Short arrow* shows hyperechoic mucosa. *Long arrow* shows hypoechoic contents. (Image courtesy of Doña Ana Community College Diagnostic Medical Sonography program, Las Cruces, NM.) **C:** Stomach with swirling fluid (hypoechoic) and solid (echogenic) contents. (Image courtesy of Barbara Hall-Terracciano.) **D:** Stomach displaying air with shadowing. Note the *arrow* is positioned at the anterior stomach wall in the correct location for acquiring an accurate measurement. (Image courtesy of Doña Ana Community College Diagnostic Medical Sonography program, Las Cruces, NM.)

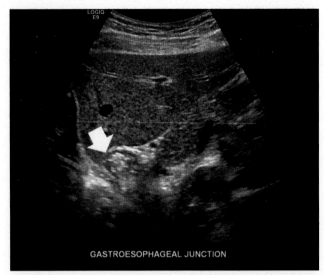

FIGURE 11-5 Gastroesophageal junction. *Arrow* points to circular junction of the esophagus and stomach. (Image courtesy of Doña Ana Community College Diagnostic Medical Sonography program, Las Cruces, NM.)

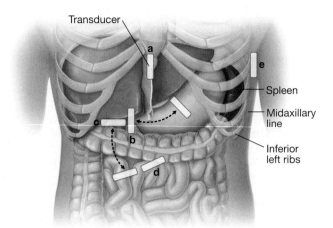

FIGURE 11-6 The illustration displays the recommended transducer position to acquire the best sonographic visualization of the stomach.

fluid may fill the center of the stomach (Fig. 11-5). Often, when fluid is present in the stomach, the rugal folds and posterior wall structure can be seen.

Sonographic Technique

Within the GI tract, the stomach has the most potential for a sonographic diagnosis. The layers of the GI tract wall are thicker here than anywhere else and nearly always can be visualized transabdominally in the normal patient. A few special techniques are occasionally helpful. If uncertainty exists whether a cystic structure in the left upper quadrant represents the stomach, giving the patient a few sips of water through a straw produces a sparkling or swirling pattern in the stomach as the water flows. A recommendation to view the stomach also includes giving the patient 500 to 800 mL (approximately 20 to 30 oz) of plain water to allow filling of the cavity followed by sonographic exploration 10 to 15 minutes after the water ingestion.[5] This allows air bubbles to diffuse from the water, which removes artifact that may be suspicious of disease. Usually, the stomach contains some air when the patient is supine. Follow the suggested transducer positions in Figure 11-6 to examine the stomach.

Placing a patient in the right lateral decubitus position moves fluid into the antrum and pyloric region of the stomach, as well as the duodenum, which provides better visualization. Some studies suggest that the antrum and body are viewed best with a semi-erect patient. Turning the patient into the left lateral decubitus position often improves visualization of the fundus.

If a solid-looking mass is suspected to be in the stomach, or when detailed evaluation of the gastric mucosa is required, the patient should be examined first with minimal stomach contents and again after water ingestion in the upright, left lateral decubitus, supine, and right lateral decubitus positions, thus demonstrating most of the gastric mucosa. Some investigators recommend giving 1 mg of glucagon intravenously before the patient drinks the water to ensure retention of the fluid in the stomach—this should produce 30 to 60 minutes of gastric distention.

Examination of the stomach can be done with a 3.5 or 5 MHz transducer. The gastric wall should be examined with a 5 or 7.5 MHz transducer. The examination should begin at the distal esophagogastric junction at the level of the cardia portion of the stomach, moving into the fundus, body, antrum (most consistently identified portion), pylorus, and then duodenum. Use the left lobe of the liver to identify the esophagogastric junction, then move toward the spleen intercostally to identify the cardia and fundus. A second option is to scan sagittally near the midaxillary line superior to inferior. Note that the cardia and fundus are deep and that air is usually positioned in this region, as well as the body of the stomach, causing limitations. The stomach body is visualized inferior to the left anterior ribs. The anterior wall is usually seen, although the posterior wall may be obscured by air. Examine the antrum with the patient in a supine position. It is viewed well sagittally adjacent to the left liver lobe and the pancreas. Again, with the patient in a supine position, the pylorus is located by finding the gallbladder, then adjusting the transducer in an oblique fashion longitudinally. The pylorus is located medial and posterior to the gallbladder.

Upper GI radiographic studies and EUS are commonly performed to search for anomalies of the stomach walls and its function. Gastric ultrasound via the abdominal method displays differing appearances depending on fasting and ingestion of fluid versus solids. The antrum can appear flat to oval in shape with a fasting patient. Upon fluid ingestion, a glittery appearance will be seen as the fluid and air whirl in the stomach lumen. Once the fluid separates from the air, a hypoechoic interface will be seen with air (brighter), and the interface will change when the patient moves to different positions. Ring-down artifacts will be visualized when air moves within the stomach. Food in the stomach lumen appears similar to a whiteout snowstorm. CT, MRI, and PET are not routinely used imaging modalities for gastric assessment.

Sonographic Stomach Wall Dimensions

If the stomach is not distended, its wall should measure approximately 3 to 6 mm thick. When the stomach is distended to a diameter of 8 cm or more, the wall should measure 2 to 4 mm. Bowel abnormalities and thickening are caused by infiltrative and inflammatory processes, infection, edema, ischemia, or neoplastic invasion. In general, the criterion for abnormal thickening of the gastric wall is a thickness of greater than 5 mm.[6] The wall is also considered abnormal if a normal-appearing portion is visualized adjacent to a significantly thicker section.

Disorders of the Stomach

Gastric Dilatation

Many disorders can cause the stomach to dilate (see Fig. 11-5). Gastric outlet obstruction (a dilatation) is a clinical syndrome that can manifest with a variety of symptoms, including abdominal pain, postprandial vomiting, early satiety, and weight loss. It is caused by either a benign or malignant mechanical obstruction or a motility disorder interfering with gastric emptying. Anatomically, the mechanical obstruction can be at the distal stomach, pyloric channel, or duodenum, and it can be intrinsic or extrinsic to the stomach.[9] Acute dilatation can occur after surgery, because of adhesions blocking the small bowel, tumor, ulcer, pyloric muscle hypertrophy, or after placement of a body cast. It is not clear whether this dilatation is caused by reflex paralysis of gastric motility or obstruction of the duodenum by the superior mesenteric artery impinging on it. Tumor or ulcers may obstruct the gastric outlet. Pyloric muscle hypertrophy is rare in adults, but when it does occur, it is usually associated with gastritis or ulcer. Other factors contributing to dilatation of the stomach are diabetes mellitus, scleroderma, or surgical vagotomy, which may bring about gastric dilatation as a complication of neuropathy. Observation of gastric peristalsis can be made using an abdominal imaging approach to differentiate atonic from obstructive dilatation, but the distinction may be impossible in many cases because of rigidity of the stomach wall, often seen in tumor infiltration and gastric ulcer disease and the uncoordinated peristaltic waves seen in neuropathic conditions. Volvulus is another rare cause of gastric dilatation.

Gastritis

Gastritis is inflammation of the gastric mucosa caused by several conditions, including infection, drugs, stress, and autoimmune phenomena.[10] It can be classified based on the site of involvement and as acute or chronic. Chronic gastritis is caused by several factors and may present as enlarged rugal folds with generalized thickening of the mucosal layer of the wall (Fig. 11-7A, B). This thickening may accompany either increased acid production, as in Zollinger–Ellison syndrome, or decreased acid production, as in Ménétrier disease. Chronic gastritis may also demonstrate hyperplastic and inflammatory polyps. Another variation is atrophic gastritis, in which the mucosa is thinned. This may be difficult to see sonographically, but it is considered a precursor of gastric carcinoma.

Ulcer Disease

Peptic ulcer disease (PUD) is characterized by discontinuation of the inner lining of the GI tract because of gastric acid secretion or pepsin. It extends into the muscularis propria layer of the gastric epithelium. It usually occurs in the stomach and proximal duodenum. It may involve the lower esophagus, distal duodenum, or jejunum.[11] The ulcers mostly appear along the antral portion of the lesser curvature. Sonographically, there may be major wall thickening, usually caused by marked edema of the submucosa, with milder thickening of the gastric mucosa (Fig. 11-8A, B). Typically, the mucosa is undercut at the edge of a benign ulcer. A malignant ulcer, by contrast, should show more "heaping up" of the margin of the ulcer. The bowel layers adjacent to the ulcer may be obliterated in either benign or malignant ulcers. Ulcers can be detected sonographically, particularly if they are large, but often, they are only suggested by focal or generalized edema of the wall. EUS can detect defects, such as ulceration, in the gastric wall required to diagnose superficial ulcerations of the mucosal lining, as well as behind the base of the defect. It is helpful in differentiating benign from malignant gastric ulcers. CT of the abdomen with contrast is of limited value in the diagnosis of PUD itself but is helpful in the diagnosis of its complications like perforation and gastric outlet obstruction.[11]

Complications of PUD, gastric or duodenal, include anterior or posterior perforation. Usually, anterior perforation results in free intraperitoneal air and, often, subsequent peritonitis, which may appear sonographically as ascites, loculated ascites, or dense debris in the peritoneal space. Some reports describe the appearance of free air in the peritoneal region as an increase in echogenicity of a peritoneal stripe with multiple reflective artifacts and a comet tail appearance. Care must be taken to differentiate this from bowel gas. Thickening of the bowel serosa may be observed because of peritoneal irritation and reactive edema. Generalized peritoneal infection or localized abscess may also result. The chief complication of posterior duodenal perforation is

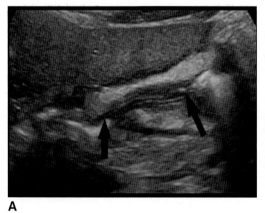
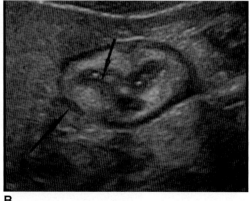

A   **B**

FIGURE 11-7 Gastritis. **A:** Longitudinal view of the distal stomach wall showing thickening (arrows). **B:** Transverse image of the same inflamed stomach wall demonstrating a thickened hypoechoic mucosal and submucosal layer (arrows). (Images courtesy of Dr. Taco Geertsma, UltrasoundCases.info.)

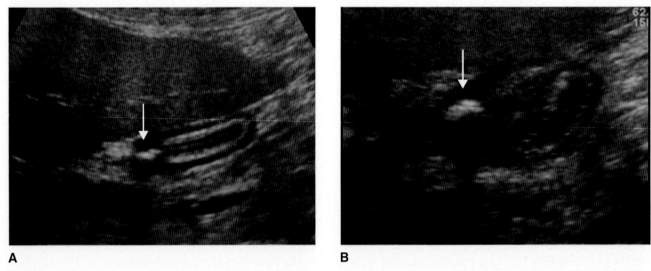

FIGURE 11-8 Gastric ulcer. **A, B:** Longitudinal images demonstrate the gastric antrum in a patient with an air-filled benign gastric ulcer (*arrow*). (Images courtesy of Dr. Taco Geertsma, UltrasoundCases.info.)

bleeding. Bleeding from an ulcer can be slow and go unnoticed or can cause life-threatening hemorrhage. Ulcers that bleed slowly might not produce symptoms until the person becomes anemic. Bleeding that occurs more rapidly might show up as melena, a jet black, very sticky stool, or even a large amount of dark red or maroon blood in the stool. People with bleeding ulcers may also vomit. This vomit may look like red blood or "coffee grounds."[12] Other symptoms might include "passing out" or feeling light-headed. Posterior perforation of the stomach may result in pancreatitis.

Gastroduodenal Crohn Disease

CD is an idiopathic inflammation that starts in the submucosa and spreads to all layers of the bowel wall. This disease is chronic and usually occurs in young adults. Although this disease may affect any part of the GI tract, the terminal ileum is the most common site.[13] It is rare in the stomach

and duodenum; approximately 2% to 8% of patients have stomach or duodenal involvement. Because the entire wall is involved at diagnosis, the sonographic appearance is that of a nonspecific hypoechoic target lesion if the lumen is viewed transversely (Fig. 11-9A–E). Chronic inflammation is seen as hypervascular echoes in the wall. Followup ultrasound examinations may be used often for patients diagnosed with CD. Continued interrogation of the GI walls for abscess and thickness are necessary during and following treatment of the condition. Advanced carcinoma, lymphoma, hematoma, abscess, colitis, and tuberculosis can appear similar to CD (Fig. 11-10A–D).

Other Inflammatory Conditions

Infection of the stomach can display marked thickening of the stomach wall and swelling of the gastric rugae, a condition called *phlegmonous gastritis*. Most cases are caused by

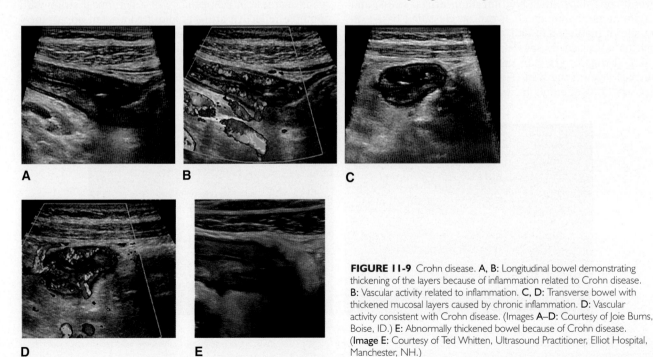

FIGURE 11-9 Crohn disease. **A, B:** Longitudinal bowel demonstrating thickening of the layers because of inflammation related to Crohn disease. **B:** Vascular activity related to inflammation. **C, D:** Transverse bowel with thickened mucosal layers caused by chronic inflammation. **D:** Vascular activity consistent with Crohn disease. (Images **A–D:** Courtesy of Joie Burns, Boise, ID.) **E:** Abnormally thickened bowel because of Crohn disease. (**Image E:** Courtesy of Ted Whitten, Ultrasound Practitioner, Elliot Hospital, Manchester, NH.)

FIGURE 11-10 Bowel with disease appearing similar to Crohn disease. **A:** Stomach cancer. **B:** Bowel lymphoma. **C:** Bowel abscess. **D:** Colitis. (Images courtesy of Dr. Taco Geertsma, UltrasoundCases.info.)

bacteria such as α-hemolytic streptococci; *Staphylococcus*, *Escherichia coli*, *Clostridium welchii*, *H. pylori*, and *Proteus* species have also been found. Peritonitis occurs in 70% of cases. When gas-forming organisms such as *E. coli* or *C. welchii* are the cause, small gas bubbles may form in the gastric wall—this is a type of emphysematous gastritis. Swallowing a corrosive substance is a more common cause of emphysematous gastritis.

Gastric Cancer

Gastric or stomach cancer is an inclusive term for common cancers affecting the stomach. The incidence of gastric cancer has declined in the United States and represents approximately 1.5% of all new U.S. cancer cases detected annually.[14] The 5-year survival rate for localized gastric cancer (no cancer spread outside the stomach) is 69% and the 5-year survival rate for regional gastric cancer (cancer spread to nearby structures/lymph nodes) is 31% in the United States.[15] Stomach cancer is much more common in other parts of the world, particularly in less developed countries. It is the fifth most common neoplasm and the third most deadly worldwide.

Adenocarcinoma

Adenocarcinoma is the most common type of cancer of the stomach. It accounts for 90 to 95% of gastric cancers.[16] This cancer type originates in the glandular tissue known as epithelial tissue. The stomach is lined with a mucous membrane composed of columnar epithelial cells and glands. Gastric carcinoma invades the submucosa and muscularis propria (Fig. 11-11A, B). These cells are prone to inflammation, known as gastritis, which can lead to peptic ulcers and, ultimately, gastric cancer. Expect sonographic appearance to demonstrate hypoechoic localized or diffuse thickening of the walls because of the invasion by the cancer or polypoid lesions.

Gastric adenocarcinomas are primarily classified as cardia and noncardia based on their anatomic site; they arise in the region adjoining the esophageal–gastric junction and, thus, share epidemiologic characteristics with esophageal adenocarcinoma. Noncardia cancer, also known as distal stomach cancer, is more common and arises in the lower portion of the stomach.[16] Most gastric cancers spread primarily toward the serosa of the gastric wall. Some gastric tumors arise in the margin of a long-standing benign peptic ulcer.

Gastric Cancer Staging

Staging procedures for cancers of the stomach can include radiologic imaging, laparoscopy, laboratory testing, EUS, CT, PET, MRI, and abdominal ultrasound. These procedures help diagnose and determine the extent of the disease.

Tumor, node, and metastasis (TNM) staging is the common way to determine the invasiveness of gastric cancer. There are varying, although very similar, grading methods. The following is one example of gastric cancer staging options:
- Tumor (T)
  - TX: unable to assess
  - T0 or Stage 0: high grade, severely abnormal cells in the inner stomach lining, a defined lesion is not seen

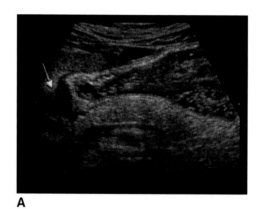

A

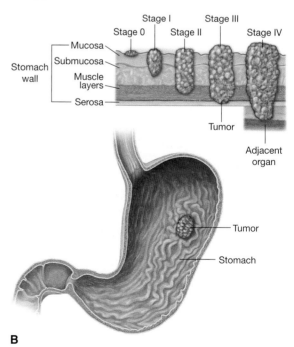

B

FIGURE 11-11 A: Adenocarcinoma of the lesser curvature of the stomach with irregular thickened wall *(arrow)*. (Image courtesy of Dr. Taco Geertsma, UltrasoundCases.info.) **B:** As illustrated, there are five stages of invasion with the progression of gastric carcinoma.

- T1 or Stage 1: tumor involvement of the lamina propria, muscularis, or submucosa (inner layers)
- T2 or Stage 2: tumor involvement of the muscularis propria (muscle layer)
- T3 or Stage 3: tumor advancement through layers of the muscle into the connective tissue (outer layer)
- T4 or Stage 4: tumor has progressed through the stomach layers into surrounding structures
  - Nodes (N)
    - NX: lymph nodes cannot be assessed
    - N0: no cancer spread to the adjacent lymph nodes
    - N1: cancer spread to one to two adjacent lymph nodes
    - N2: cancer spread to three to six adjacent lymph nodes
    - N3: cancer spread to seven or more lymph nodes
  - Metastasis (M)
    - MX: metastasis cannot be assessed
    - M0: no cancer spread
    - M1: cancer spread to other body regions

Lymphoma

Lymphoma is a cancer that usually begins in the lymph and node structures. Primary gastric lymphoma (PGL) is the most common extranodal non-Hodgkin lymphoma and represents a wide spectrum of disease, ranging from indolent low-grade marginal zone lymphoma or mucosa-associated lymphoid tissue lymphoma to aggressive, diffuse, large B-cell lymphoma.[17] The incidence rate of this type of lymphoma is low, accounting for less than 5% of gastric malignancies.[18] The cells of origin are lymphocytes located just above and below the muscularis mucosa, usually at the antrum and body of the stomach. Endosonography characteristically reveals this involvement as well as a tendency for the tumor to spread laterally following the muscularis mucosa rather than vertically through the layers of the wall as in gastric carcinoma (Fig. 11-12A, B). Endoscopic appearances of PGL are ulcerated lesions, polypoidal lesions, thickened gastric folds, and erosions.[18] By transabdominal sonography, the thickened, hypoechoic gastric wall and the marked rugal thickening may be revealed. Sonographically, gastric

carcinoma is sometimes more echogenic than lymphoma, and in infiltrative lesions, all layers are more equally involved than in lymphoma.

Gastric Lymphoma Staging

Lymphoma diagnostic procedures may include radiologic imaging, CT, PET, MRI, as well as abdominal ultrasound. The involvement of primary GI lymphoma often requires CT, MRI, PET, laboratory testing, bone marrow aspiration, and biopsy or EUS for staging. The procedures guide clinicians toward a diagnosis and aid in the determination of the extent of disease. There is staging agreement among many authorities regarding the grading of primary lymphoma.

Stage 1: confined to GI tract
Stage 2: extending in the abdomen from the primary GI site
Stage 2E: penetration of serosa to involve adjacent organs or tissues
Stage 4: disseminated extranodal involvement or concomitant supradiaphragmatic nodal involvement (17)

Gastrointestinal Stromal Tumor

Gastrointestinal stromal tumors (GISTs) belong to a category of GI mesenchymal tumors that can have benign qualities or malignant potential. They start from the interstitial cells of Cajal and aid in digestive motility. Even though this is a rare stomach tumor, it is the most common site for GISTs. Approximately 60% are gastric in location and the second most prevalent site is the small bowel, occurring at a rate of about 30%. The anorectum, colon, and esophagus can be affected by GIST formation, but these locations are much less common. This smooth muscle tumor arises from the muscularis propria and is, therefore, primarily exophytic, usually with an appearance similar to the sonographically familiar uterine fibroid. GISTs mostly appear as a homogeneous hypoechoic mass, but they can be difficult to differentiate sonographically or histologically from their benign counterpart, the leiomyoma, because they can also display a heterogeneous appearance (Fig. 11-13A–C).[19] A tumor smaller than 2 cm is usually not cancerous, although it should be resected because of its potential to become malignant.

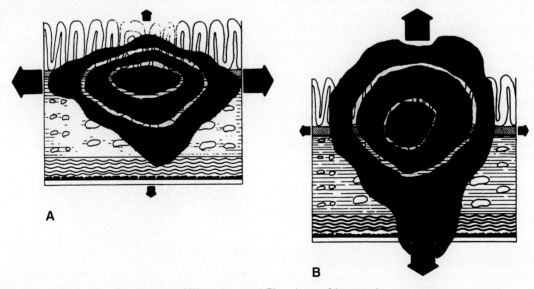

A

B

FIGURE 11-12 Gastric tumor invasion. Growth pattern of **(A)** lymphoma and **(B)** carcinoma of the stomach.

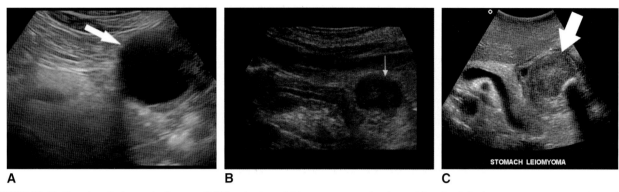

FIGURE 11-13 Gastrointestinal stromal cell tumors (*GISTs*) and a stomach leiomyoma comparison image. Note the similar heterogeneous texture and smooth contour. **A:** Malignant gastrointestinal stromal tumor of the fundal stomach (*arrow*). **B:** GIST of the dorsal antral wall of the stomach and anterior pancreas (*arrow*). (Images courtesy of Dr. Taco Geertsma, UltrasoundCases.info.) **C:** Leiomyoma of the stomach antrum (*arrow*). (Image courtesy of Susan R. Stephenson, Salt Lake City, UT.)

Researchers state that all GISTs will become malignant if left to evolve. Hemorrhage and cystic degeneration can occur with this type of tumor.

GISTs are discovered with radiologic testing, similar to tests that diagnose gastric cancer and gastric lymphoma. A defined diagnosis for these tumors requires biopsy and pathology testing.

Other Malignant Gastric Lesions

- carcinoid
- hemangioendothelioma
- hemangiopericytoma
- Kaposi sarcoma
- liposarcoma, myxosarcoma
- fibrosarcoma
- secondary tumors

Sonographic findings:
- wall invasion, ulcerating lesion
- wall thickening
- polypoid lesion
- hypoechoic lesion
- vascular lesion
- smooth-walled intraluminal filling defect

Benign Gastric Tumors

Benign gastric tumors are rare and most are asymptomatic. Hyperplastic polyps and gastric adenomas are polypoid masses arising from the gastric mucosa; adenomas seem to have some malignant potential. Other types of tumors arise from the submucosal or muscle layer and spare the mucosa unless surface ulceration develops. Lipomas are generally echogenic. Smooth muscle tumors may show a typical swirled texture if they are large enough.

SMALL BOWEL

Normal Anatomy

The small bowel is a tubular structure approximately 20 feet in length and approximately 1 inch in diameter. It is divided into three sections: the proximal, mid-level jejunum, and distal ileum. These sections of bowel begin at the pyloric sphincter and terminate at the ileocecal valve and have the same five bowel wall layers described earlier. The inner mucosal layer is the absorptive surface. Dr. Kerckring

(1640–1693) was acknowledged for discovering and describing the inner mucosal small bowel layer known as mucosal folds, valvulae conniventes, Kerckring folds/valves, or plicae circulares. Villi and microvilli that protrude from these folds increase the surface area, allowing for increased absorption and secretion. If the small bowel is distended with fluid, the valvulae conniventes of the mucosa and other layers of the bowel wall are usually visible transabdominally.[4]

The duodenal bulb, the first portion of the duodenum, normally lies to the right of the gastric antrum, anterosuperior to the pancreatic head, and medial to the gallbladder. It is the shortest portion, beginning at the pylorus and ending at the medial side of the neck of the gallbladder. The second portion of the duodenum, the descending duodenum, bends inferiorly to the right of the pancreatic head and continues parallel with and to the right of the spine. Next, it bends to the left, extending inferior to the pancreas and passing between the superior mesenteric artery anteriorly and the aorta posteriorly, forming the third portion referenced as the transverse duodenum. The fourth section, the ascending duodenum, extends superiorly and to the left, posterior to the stomach. The jejunum begins at the duodenal–jejunal flexure, which is frequently referenced as the ligament of Treitz (Fig. 11-14).

The jejunum, the mid-section, the ileum, and the distal portion of the small bowel lie in the central portion of the abdomen, inferior to the liver and stomach and superior to the urinary bladder. There is no marked delineation between the two sections of bowel. These two sections are suspended by mesentery, which allows mobility of the tubular bowel. The jejunum makes up 40% of this portion of bowel. It has a thicker wall and wider lumen than the ileum. The ileum is the longest section and is positioned in the right inferior abdomen.

Sonographic Technique

Small bowel loops should be examined with the patient supine and in a relaxed position. A methodical approach is necessary in order to thoroughly examine the entire bowel starting at the right inferior abdomen near the ileocecal valve. Situate the transducer in a transverse position and travel superiorly along the ascending colon until the superior bowel is reached, then move directly and slightly left, scanning inferiorly to the distal bowel. Continue this "up-and-down"

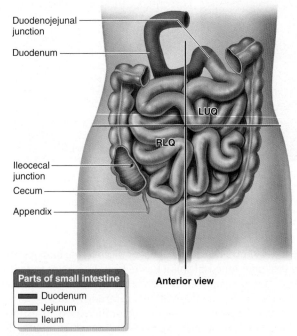

FIGURE 11-14 The illustration presents an anterior view of the small bowel. The jejunum begins at the duodenal–jejunal flexure and the ileum ends at the cecum. There is no clear external line of demarcation between the jejunum and the ileum and the term *jejuno-ileum* is often used. *LUQ*, left upper quadrant; *RLQ*, right lower quadrant. (Reprinted with permission from Moore KL, Dalley AF II, Agur AMR. *Clinically Oriented Anatomy.* 7th ed. Wolters Kluwer; 2014.)

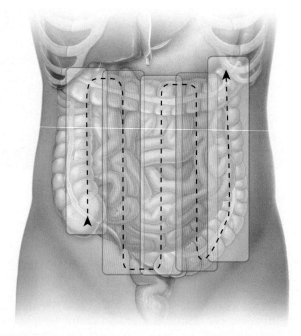

FIGURE 11-15 Illustration of recommended scanning technique for the jejunum and ileum. Place the transducer transversely in the right lower quadrant/pelvis and move superiorly to the region of the hepatic flexure of the colon. Slide the transducer left slightly and scan distally to the point of the inferior small bowel. Continue the "up-and-down" method, moving slightly left each pass until the entire bowel is viewed.

pattern until the entire small bowel is examined, using caution to overlap the movements (Fig. 11-15).

The duodenum requires additional imaging in a C-shaped pattern with the transducer kept in the transverse position to the bowel length. Start at the pylorus and continue through the terminal ascending duodenum. See Figure 11-14.

The small bowel is best visualized by examining both before and after ingestion of water (Fig. 11-16A, B). Drinking fluid may enhance visualization of the mucosa of the duodenum, jejunum, and ileum and demonstrate peristalsis. The best time to view the small bowel depends on the transit time of the fluid within the bowel. The valvulae conniventes, the folds in the inside bowel wall from which the

microscopic villi protrude, can sometimes be demonstrated (Fig. 11-17A–D). If ileus or obstruction is present, however, ingesting fluid by mouth is not recommended.

MRI and CT enterography display detailed images of the small bowel. The two modalities also stage cancerous processes. PET is utilized to diagnose, stage, and evaluate the patient's response to cancer treatments.

Sonographic Small Bowel Wall Dimensions

The normal luminal thickness for small bowel is 1 to 2 mm, although a thickness of 3 to 5 mm is considered normal in collapsed bowel if the wall is symmetrical (Fig. 11-18A, B). As with the entire GI tract, evaluate for wall thickness, wall

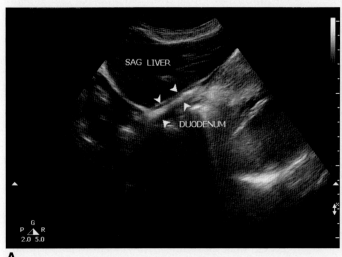

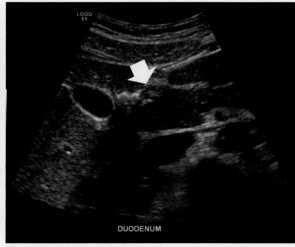

FIGURE 11-16 Duodenum. **A:** *Arrows* point to the duodenum currently empty of contents. **B:** Normal duodenum demonstrating filling. The hyperechoic "bright" central canal of the duodenum demonstrates water peristalsing through the superior part *(arrow)*. (Images courtesy of Barbara Hall-Terracciano.)

FIGURE 11-17 Small bowel demonstrating wall conniventes. **A:** Longitudinal image of normal, nondistended small bowel *(arrows).* (Image courtesy of Barbara Hall-Terracciano.) **B:** Longitudinal image of edematous small bowel. Note the presence of fluid-filled "pockets" at the conniventes *(arrow).* (Image courtesy of Dr Taco Geertsma, UltrasoundCases.info.) **C, D:** Transverse images of normal, nondistended small bowel demonstrating valvulae conniventes *(arrows).* (Images courtesy of Barbara Hall-Terracciano.)

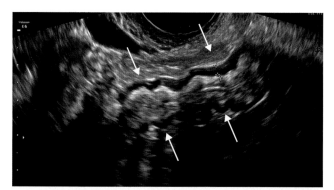

A

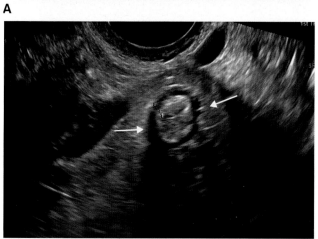

B

FIGURE 11-18 Small bowel. **A:** The longitudinal small bowel displays both the anterior and posterior wall in an ideal position for wall thickness measurement, see *arrows* and *calipers.* **B:** A transverse view of small bowel *(arrows)* displays *calipers* measuring the normal wall thickness. (Images courtesy of Barbara Hall-Terracciano.)

symmetry, adjacent structures such as lymph nodes or masses, motility, changes to the wall, lumen, and vascular patterns.

Disorders of the Small Bowel

Duodenum

Duodenal Ulcer

PUD refers to the clinical presentation and disease state that occurs when there is a disruption in the mucosal surface at the level of the stomach or first part of the small intestine, the duodenum. Duodenal ulcers are part of a broader disease state categorized as PUD. Ulceration occurs from damage to the mucosal surface that extends beyond the superficial layer.[20] Duodenal ulcers occur more frequently than other ulcers, causing intermittent pain in the epigastric region, usually 2 to 3 hours after ingesting a meal. According to multiple studies that have evaluated the prevalence of duodenal ulcers, they are estimated to occur in about 5% to 15% of the Western population.[20]

Duodenal ulcers occur in the first portion of the duodenum 95% of the time and most of those are within 3 cm of the pylorus. They are usually less than or equal to 1 cm in diameter and display air (Fig. 11-19).[20] Complications include bleeding, perforation causing abdominal air, and narrowing and obstruction of the duodenum or outlet of the stomach. Perforation explains findings of free intraperitoneal gas (pneumoperitoneum) positioned inferior to the anterior abdominal wall, near the duodenum, and in perihepatic spaces. Free fluid can be seen near the perforation site.

Ultrasound can detect marked wall thickening and hyperechoic regions representing air within the bulb. It can also localize gas collections, leading to an accurate diagnosis. Imaging with cine loop detects and records discharge of fluid and air bubbles at the perforation. Historically, double-contrast barium studies of the stomach and duodenum were performed to determine anomalies such as wall lesions. Although CT may or may not detect small or early perforations, because of its inconspicuous nature, it will

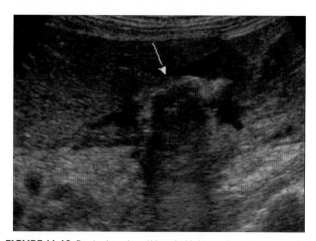

FIGURE 11-19 Peptic ulceration. Although this image demonstrates peptic ulcer disease of the antrum, it depicts the typical air-filled ulcerated crater appearance that is found within the affected bowel wall, including the duodenum. *Arrow* is directed at air-filled ulcer crater of the wall. (Image courtesy of Dr. Taco Geertsma, UltrasoundCases.info.)

easily detect superior abdominal free air and peritonitis, suggesting perforated ulceration. Upright chest radiography can help detect free intraperitoneal air below the diaphragm, suggestive of bowel perforation. Some patients will require esophagogastroduodenoscopy, which will allow a detailed examination of the bowel epithelium.

Other Duodenal Conditions

- duodenitis
- adenocarcinoma and carcinoma
- GIST (similar to stomach GIST)
- diverticulum
- stricture
- duodenal web

Sonographic findings:

- wall deviations
- wall erosions[21]
- thickening of folds[21]
- nodules or nodular folds[21]
- bulb deformity[21]
- solid lesions with a polypoid, smooth-walled, vascular, or lobulated nature
- mass with isoechoic, cystic, partially cystic, or heterogeneous appearance
- dilated stomach or proximal duodenum

- dilated proximal duodenum
- hyperechoic linear echoes within the duodenum.

Jejunum and Ileum

This region of bowel should be examined first without food or fluid intake, followed by water ingestion if tolerated and allowed. High resolution transabdominal transducers visualize loops in the small bowel with and without fluid and gassy distentions. This region of bowel should be smaller than 3 cm in diameter and be pliable on palpation. If fluid is present in the loops, the valvulae conniventes should be visible. The intestinal loops are easily visualized when ascites is present. Peristaltic motion should be seen in the normal bowel.[5]

Ileus

The *ileus* is also called acute intestinal pseudo-obstruction and is characterized by failure of the intestine to propel its contents because of diminished motility. The causes leading to pathology of the ileus are numerous and include peritonitis, spinal fracture, renal colic, acute pancreatitis, bowel ischemia, myocardial infarction, surgery, medications, hypokalemia, and infection. The pathologic appearance on a sonogram is a distended small bowel with either air or fluid (Fig. 11-20A–D). Peristalsis within the bowel is

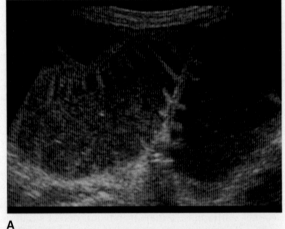

A

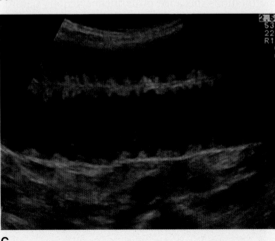

C

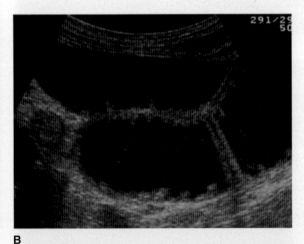

B

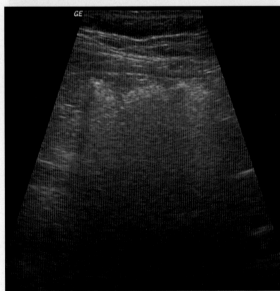

D

FIGURE 11-20 Ileus. **A–C:** Longitudinal images demonstrate dilated fluid-filled bowel loops in a patient with ileus. **D:** Radiograph of the abdomen demonstrates dilated bowel loops consistent with ileus. (Images courtesy of Dr. Taco Geertsma, UltrasoundCases.info.)

inhibited. The normal bowel is usually less distended than when it is obstructed.

Obstruction

Jejunal and ileal obstruction has multiple causes. Adhesions, inflammation, neoplastic lesions, volvulus, intussusception, and luminal obstruction (such as fecal impaction) are common (Fig. 11-21A–D). Typically, the bowel loops are perfectly round in cross section, and peristalsis can vary from none to markedly increased. The valvulae conniventes are often visible, as seen in Figure 11-17A–D.

In volvulus, the twisted, dilated loop appears C-shaped when viewed longitudinally and often contains only fluid, no air. Intussusception is the telescoping of a proximal segment of the GI tract into an adjacent distal segment. This rare form of bowel obstruction occurs infrequently in adults (Fig. 11-22A, B).[22] The majority of cases in children are idiopathic, and pathologic lead points are identified in only 25% of cases involving children. Intussusception is unusual in adults, and the diagnosis is commonly overlooked. In the majority of cases in adults, a pathologic cause is identified.[23] The bowel appears as concentric circles when seen in a transverse plane, which results in an identifiable bowel

lesion in about three-fourths of adults with this condition. The longitudinal view demonstrates mesentery seen as an echo-rich layer between two multilayered structures known as the sandwich sign.[4]

Hematoma

Hematoma of the bowel may result from trauma, ischemia, medication, or a hematologic abnormality such as hemophilia, Henoch–Schönlein purpura, anaphylactoid purpura, or thrombocytopenic purpura (Fig. 11-23). Traumatic hematoma occurs most commonly in the duodenum because it is fixed in position and less able to move out of harm's way. In adults, a common cause of bowel hematoma is anticoagulant therapy. The most frequent cause of bowel ischemia is arterial obstruction. Sonographically, bowel hematoma is seen as nonspecific wall thickening of variable echogenicity. The thickening may be eccentric, and the mesentery may be involved. Often, there is thickening of the mucosal folds and dilated bowel loops.[4]

Edema

Swelling of the valvulae conniventes can be caused by hypoproteinemia, which may be because of cirrhosis, kidney

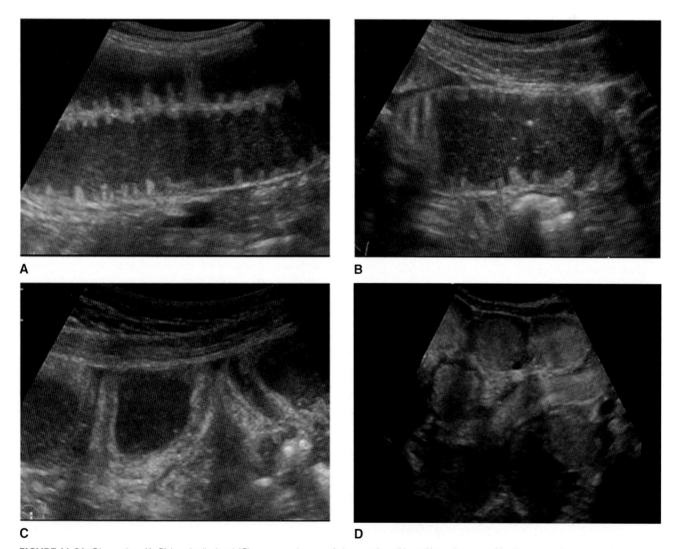

A

B

C

D

FIGURE 11-21 Obstruction. **(A, B)** Longitudinal and **(C)** transverse images of obstructed small bowel loops because of fecal impaction. Note that the loops are fluid filled and perfectly round in the transverse image. The valvulae conniventes are well seen in **(A)** and **(B)**. **D:** Multiple loops of small bowel demonstrate heterogeneous content retention caused by an obstructing colon tumor. (Images courtesy of Dr. Taco Geertsma, UltrasoundCases.info.)

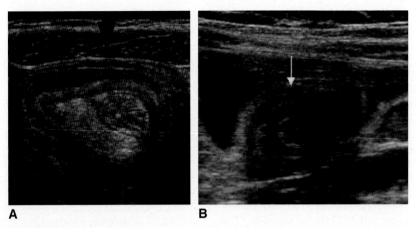

A   B

FIGURE 11-22 Intussusception. **A, B:** Transverse small bowel images demonstrate multiple concentric layers *(arrows)* telescoping into the next segment, consistent with intussusception. (Images courtesy of Dr. Taco Geertsma, UltrasoundCases.info.)

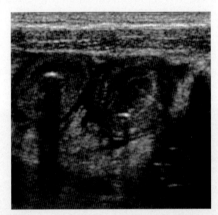

FIGURE 11-23 Bowel wall thickening with hypervascularity and free abdominal fluid in a patient with Henoch–Schönlein purpura is related to wall hematoma. (Image courtesy of Dr. Taco Geertsma, UltrasoundCases.info.)

disease, or protein loss from the GI tract, as may occur in Ménétrier disease, Whipple disease, intestinal lymphangiomatosis, inflammatory bowel disease, and GI tumors. The blockage of mesenteric lymph channels, angioneurotic edema, and abetalipoproteinemia can also cause thickening of small bowel mucosal folds (Fig. 11-24). Edema is visualized by wall thickening and hyperemia.

Small Bowel Crohn Disease

CD of the small bowel, also known as regional enteritis or Crohn enteritis, is a form of inflammatory bowel disease, presenting with chronic diarrhea (possibly bloody) and

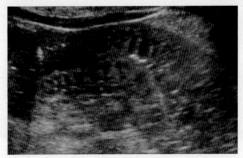

FIGURE 11-24 Small bowel edema. Angioedema in a patient demonstrating small bowel wall thickening and ascites. (Image courtesy of Dr. Taco Geertsma, UltrasoundCases.info.)

abdominal pain. It is a common reason for performing sonography of the small bowel and is a common nonspecific cause of small bowel inflammation. The inflammation starts in the submucosa and becomes transmural, often with granulomatous features. The frequency with which bowel sections are affected varies with the small bowel, particularly ileum, affected in 70% to 80% of cases, the small and large bowel affected in 50% of cases, and only the large bowel affected in 15% to 20% of cases.[24]

BWT is an important indicator of the disease; CD usually has significant bowel wall thickening, from 5 to 15 mm.[25] The "target" sign, corresponding to remarkable BWT, is visible as a strong echogenic center surrounded by a hypoechoic border.[26] Other abnormal bowel findings specific to ultrasound are altered echogenicity, hypervascularity, loss of the normal visible stratification, dilatation, and stenosis (see Fig. 11-9A–E). Complications include stenosis, abscess, perforation, interloop abscess, effusion, infiltration, ulceration, dilatation, and fistulation (Fig. 11-25A–D).

Small Bowel Cancer

The most common primary neoplastic lesions of the small bowel, in order of occurrence, are smooth muscle tumors (sarcoma), adenocarcinomas, carcinoid tumors, lymphoma, and GISTs. The bowel may also be involved as a part of multisystem lymphoma. When primary and multisystem lymphomatous involvements of the GI tract are combined, lymphoma is the most common neoplasia of the small bowel.

Sarcoma

A leiomyosarcoma is the common sarcoma, or smooth muscle tissue cancer, of the small bowel. It occurs in the ileum most often. The lesion is hypoechoic and can display a homogeneous or heterogeneous appearance, often with edge shadowing.

Adenocarcinoma

Primary adenocarcinoma of the small bowel may be present as either a constricting circumferential lesion or as a polypoid heterogeneous lesion. The lesions may range from 1 to 10 cm in diameter.

Carcinoid

The primary tumor in small bowel carcinoid is typically only up to 3.5 cm in size and slow growing (Fig. 11-26A–D).

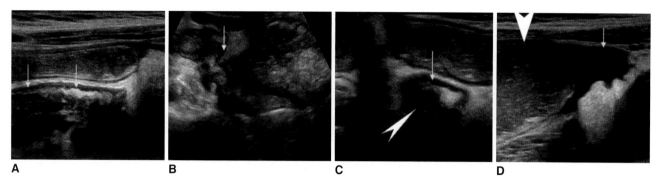

FIGURE 11-25 Crohn disease. **A:** A sagittal view of the small bowel demonstrates thickened bowel wall and effusion *(arrows)*. **B:** *Arrow* is directed at stenosis caused by wall thickening or extrinsic pressure. **C:** Transverse view of the bowel demonstrates a "target" sign *(arrowhead)* with wall thickening *(small arrow)*. **D:** The small bowel is dilated *(arrowhead)* and demonstrates stenosis *(arrow)*. (Images courtesy of Dr. Taco Geertsma, UltrasoundCases.info.)

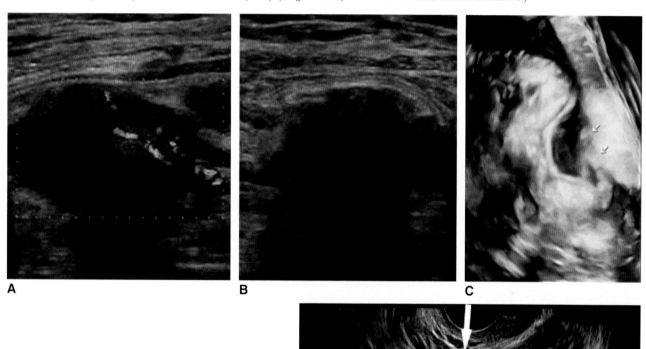

FIGURE 11-26 Small bowel carcinoid. **A:** Carcinoid with a hypoechoic vascularized mass in continuation with the small bowel and liver and lymph node metastases. **B:** Carcinoid with a hypoechoic mass in continuation with the bowel wall demonstrating irregular borders and posterior shadowing. **C:** Small bowel, ileum, with invasive cancerous lesion *(arrows)*. **D:** Cancerous lesion of image C in 3D format *(arrow)*. (Images **A** and **B:** Courtesy of Dr. Taco Geertsma, UltrasoundCases.info. Images **C** and **D:** Courtesy of Barbara Hall-Terracciano.)

Metastases, commonly to the mesentery, liver, and lymph nodes, often exceed the size of the primary neoplasm. The sonographic appearance is a circumscribed, hypoechoic, vascularized mass.

Gastrointestinal Stromal Tumors

GISTs are the most common tumor of the GI tract found typically in the stomach and mid-distal small bowel. As mentioned earlier, they are homogeneous, hypoechoic, and exophytic to the structure they are related to (see Fig. 11-13A, B).

Lymphoma

Lymphoma of the small bowel is usually part of a systemic involvement, most frequently by non-Hodgkin lymphoma (including Burkitt, undifferentiated, and histiocytic lymphoma). Fifty percent of patients with Hodgkin disease, however, also show involvement of the GI tract eventually. Sonographically, the bowel wall is irregular, thickened, and hypoechoic (see Fig. 11-10B). Mass involvement may appear as a target lesion. The mesenteric nodes may also be affected without involvement of the bowel wall (Fig. 11-27A, B).

Benign Small Bowel Tumors

Leiomyoma

Leiomyoma is the most common benign tumor of the small bowel—it looks like leiomyomas elsewhere, including in the uterus. The tumor arises from the muscularis propria and

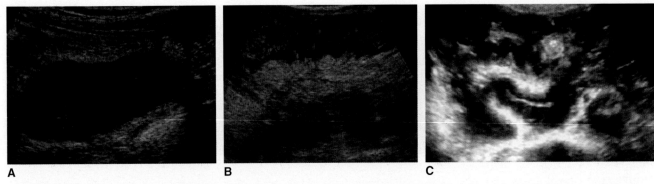

A   **B**   **C**

FIGURE 11-27 Small bowel lymphoma. **A:** Non-Hodgkin disease in the ileocecal bowel region with a hypoechoic, vascularized, well-defined mass. **B:** B-cell lymphoma with an irregular hypoechoic thickening of the bowel wall and hypervascularization. **C:** B-cell lymphoma with tumorous thickening of the bowel wall. (Images courtesy of Dr. Taco Geertsma, UltrasoundCases.info.)

is usually eccentrically located in the wall. Leiomyosarcomas can appear identical to larger leiomyomas, but larger tumors and tumors with central necrosis are more likely to be malignant (Fig. 11-28).

Other Benign Small Bowel Tumors

Adenomas, lipomas, hemangiomas, and neurofibromas are other benign tumors that can arise in the small bowel. Metastatic malignancies, especially from melanoma and carcinomas of the lung, kidney, and breast, occur as either single or multiple intramural or intraluminal masses. These metastases may appear similar to smooth muscle tumors or lymphoma. Carcinoid tumors are discussed in the next section.

Other Jejunal and Ileal Conditions

- jejunal and ileal atresia
- ischemia
- lymphoma
- adenocarcinoma
- carcinoid tumor
- angioedema
- lipoma
- enteritis
- diverticulosis
- ischemia
- intussusception
- leiomyosarcoma

Sonographic findings are:
- hypervascularized tumor or bowel wall
- hyperechoic, ovoid, smooth delineated lesions
- wall thickening

- enlarged adjacent lymph nodes
- intra- or extraluminal lesion
- perforation
- ascites
- inward pouching lesions with thick hyperechoic walls, hyperechoic centers, posterior shadowing
- bowel dilatation
- narrowing of bowel circumference

VERMIFORM APPENDIX

Normal Anatomy of the Appendix

The vermiform appendix is a compressible tubular structure attached to the cecum with a closed blind-ending distal tip that does not display peristalsis (Fig. 11-29A, B). It should measure no greater than 6 mm in diameter, and the hypoechoic portion of the wall should measure no more than 2 mm thick (Fig. 11-18A, B). Although the normal appendix may be difficult to visualize, if ascites, gangrene, perforation, abscess, hyperemia, or inflammation is present, it can be easily seen.

Sonographic Technique

The sonographic examination of the right lower quadrant (RLQ) begins with identifying the superior right colon, which is then followed downward to the cecum. By placing steady pressure on the transducer (graded compression), one can displace gas-filled bowel loops to search for the appendix, near the cecum and terminal ileum. A normal appendix can be identified in some persons, whereas the diseased appendix can be visualized consistently using one or more of the following methods:
- Locate the McBurney point (Fig. 11-30).
- Place the probe in the right upper quadrant over the ascending colon with the probe indicator toward the patient's right. Sliding inferiorly down to the RLQ will reveal the cecum/terminal ileum and ultimately the appendix.[27]
- Place the transducer directly over the point of maximal tenderness, as indicated by the patient.[27]
- Graded compression is applied to image the right colon; firm pressure is applied to bring the abdominal wall in contact with the psoas muscle every 1 cm.[27] Obscuring bowel loops will be displaced, allowing for viewing of the cecum, terminal ileum, and appendix.

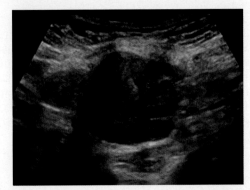

FIGURE 11-28 Leiomyosarcoma of the small bowel. This tumor appears similar in contour and texture to a leiomyoma of the uterus. (Image courtesy of Dr. Taco Geertsma, UltrasoundCases.info.)

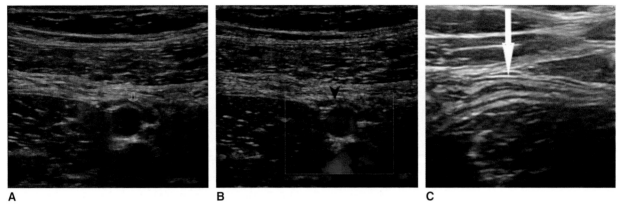

FIGURE 11-29 Normal appendix. **A:** Longitudinal normal appendix *(arrowhead)*. **B:** Same longitudinal normal appendix *(arrowhead)* with color Doppler interrogation. **C:** Normal tubular appendix *(arrow)*. (Images **A** and **B:** Courtesy of Doña Ana Community College Diagnostic Medical Sonography program, Las Cruces, NM. Image **C:** Courtesy of Dr. Taco Geertsma, UltrasoundCases.info.)

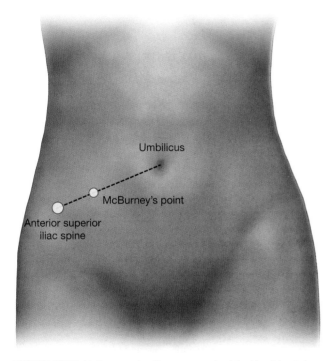

FIGURE 11-30 McBurney point. The area over the right side of the abdomen that is one-third of the distance from the anterior superior iliac spine to the umbilicus is the McBurney point. This area is where the appendix is attached to the cecum.

- Endovaginal approach may be combined with the transabdominal approach to increase the success rate of diagnosis in female patients.[2]
- Changing patient positioning starting from supine imaging, moving to left posterior oblique followed with imaging, then returning to supine and again imaging may increase the detection rate of the appendix.[28]

The abdominal sonographic examination is performed with a 5 to 12 MHz transducer searching the region of pain first without compression followed by the graded compression technique. This method may help the sonographer to locate the area of maximum tenderness.

In EVS, the transducer is placed in closer proximity to the appendix, increasing the visibility and clarity of the structure and therefore increasing the diagnostic yield of the study. An additional benefit of this study is the ability to review other organs in the female pelvis and possibly diagnose causes for the patient's symptoms.[2]

Color flow and power Doppler imaging can add valuable information in the diagnosis of appendicitis. The increase in blood flow in the appendix may be patchy or may involve the entire appendix. Flow imaging is particularly helpful in equivocal cases in which the appendix is visualized but is normal or nearly normal; in this situation, a lack of flow on power Doppler suggests the appendix is normal, whereas increased flow suggests mild appendicitis. In appendicitis cases that are clearly abnormal on grayscale sonography, little or no power Doppler flow suggests wall ischemia and impending rupture. Retrocecal appendicitis may be easier to identify using flow imaging.

Although it was initially believed that any appendix visualized sonographically was abnormal, it is now clear that the normal appendix can be identified. It is also becoming clear that some cases of appendicitis can resolve without surgery, perhaps to recur later.

Sonographic Appendix Wall Dimensions

The visualization of a noncompressible appendix greater than 6 mm in diameter with mucus in the appendiceal lumen and with associated focal pain over the appendix is sufficient to establish the diagnosis of unruptured appendicitis (Fig. 11-31A, B). The appendiceal lumen is often distended and filled with mucus but in some cases of appendicitis, the lumen is nondistended and appendiceal wall thickening is the primary finding. But in some cases of appendicitis, the lumen is nondistended and appendiceal wall thickening is the primary finding. Always examine the entire structure, proximal to the distal tip, as it may be inflamed without change occurring to the proximal portion. Loss of defined inner luminal layers indicates inflammatory, gangrenous, or ulcerative transformation. Retrocecal appendices are particularly difficult to visualize sonographically; therefore, additional techniques such as patient position change or endovaginal approach are indicated if possible. A calcified appendicolith is a strong indicator of appendicitis, even if a dilated appendiceal lumen is not seen (Fig. 11-31C, D). Hyperemia is often noted because of inflammation of the appendiceal wall. Note that appendiceal enlargement may be due to other disease circumstances, such as peptic ulcer with perforation or CD.

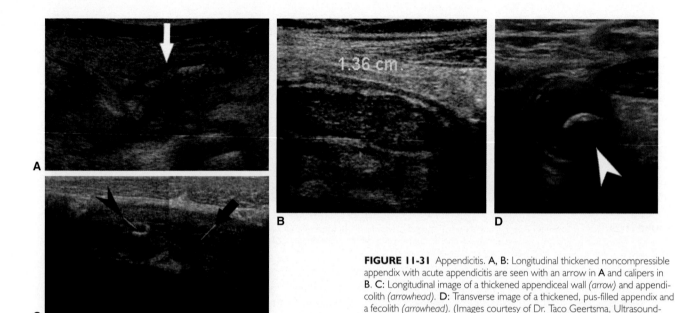

FIGURE 11-31 Appendicitis. **A, B:** Longitudinal thickened noncompressible appendix with acute appendicitis are seen with an arrow in **A** and calipers in **B**. **C:** Longitudinal image of a thickened appendiceal wall *(arrow)* and appendicolith *(arrowhead)*. **D:** Transverse image of a thickened, pus-filled appendix and a fecolith *(arrowhead)*. (Images courtesy of Dr. Taco Geertsma, Ultrasound-Cases.info.)

Disorders of the Appendix

Appendicitis

Appendicitis is an inflammation of the vermiform appendix usually caused by obstruction of the orifice. It is a common surgical emergency of the abdomen and occurs most often between the ages of 5 and 45 with a mean age of 28. Males have a slightly higher predisposition of developing acute appendicitis compared to females, with a lifetime incidence of 8.6% for men and 6.7% for women.[29] Appendicitis has generally been considered a clinical diagnosis, characterized initially by general periumbilical pain associated with leukocytosis, fever, and sometimes nausea. A common symptom is localized pain in the RLQ with point tenderness over the appendix and signs of peritoneal irritation such as rebound tenderness. Rebound tenderness and pain located over the McBurney point is considered a positive McBurney sign and is a clinical indicator of appendicitis (see Fig. 11-30).

There is variation in the clinical presentation of appendicitis; many cases do not exhibit the classical RLQ symptom. Other indications include abdominal swelling, appetite loss, constipation, and RLQ pain with walking or coughing. CT diagnostic accuracy of appendicitis is considered superior to that of sonography, but sonography is highly effective in the evaluation of acute appendicitis. Ultrasound is less expensive and avoids ionizing radiation. Color and power Doppler techniques add increased diagnostic reliability during an ultrasound examination. MRI is used to search for and evaluate the appendix, especially in the pregnant female and indeterminate appendiceal ultrasound examinations.

The chief complication of appendicitis is abscess formation or generalized peritonitis. Appendiceal rupture is not required for these complications to arise, as pathogens may travel through the intact wall. When the appendix has ruptured, it is much more difficult to visualize because the lumen is no longer distended and the anatomy is distorted by surrounding inflammation and adjacent abscess. Appendiceal abscesses may be echogenic because organisms in the colon

may form gas within them. Gas in a tubo-ovarian abscess can mimic this finding, but is less common. Characteristically, appendiceal abscesses are at the cecal tip or in the pericolic gutter, but sometimes, they occur between small bowel loops medially, where they are much more difficult to find sonographically. The small bowel loops may be thickened because of inflammation from the adjacent abscess.

Power Doppler imaging can help differentiate between bowel wall thickening because of abscess and bacterial ileocolitis; in the case of abscess, the increased blood flow will be greatest on the serosal surface of the bowel adjacent to the abscess, whereas the blood flow will be greatest in the mucosa in the case of ileocolitis. Fluid collections near the appendix can be examined in a similar way; if increased blood flow is detected in omentum and peritoneum around the fluid, abscess must be suspected.

Sonographic findings supportive of the diagnosis of appendicitis include the following:
- aperistaltic, noncompressible, dilated appendix (>6 mm outer diameter)
- appears round when compression is applied
- hyperechoic appendicolith with posterior acoustic shadowing
- distinct appendiceal wall layers
  - implies non-necrotic (catarrhal or phlegmon) stage
  - loss of wall stratification with necrotic (gangrenous) stages
- echogenic prominent pericecal and periappendiceal fat
- periappendiceal hyperechoic structure: amorphous hyperechoic structure (usually >10 mm) seen surrounding a noncompressible appendix with a diameter above 6 mm
- periappendiceal fluid collection
- target appearance (axial section)
- periappendiceal reactive nodal prominence/enlargement
- wall thickening (3 mm or above)
  - mural hyperemia with color flow Doppler increases the specificity
  - vascular flow may be lost with necrotic stages

- alteration of the mural spectral Doppler envelope
  - may support diagnosis in equivocal cases
  - a peak systolic velocity greater than 10 cm/s suggested as a cutoff
  - a resistive index (RI) measured above 0.65 may be more specific[28]

Appendicolith (Fecolith)

An appendicolith is a calcified deposit within the lumen of the appendix and may be caused by calcified fecal matter known as a fecolith. Fecoliths are stony pieces of feces obstructing the appendiceal lumen. Both the appendicolith and fecolith are usually smaller than 1 cm and can cause inflammation, abscess, and hyperemia. This obstructing structure displays posterior shadowing (see Fig. 11-31D).

Mucocele

Mucocele, distension of the appendix by mucus, is an uncommon lesion, found in 0.25% of appendectomies (Fig. 11-32A, B). It is slightly more common in men than in women. RLQ pain resembling appendicitis is the most common symptom, although some patients may be asymptomatic. Mucoceles are classified into three groups: focal or diffuse hyperplasia, mucinous cystadenoma, and mucinous cystadenocarcinoma. Only the last is considered to have malignant potential. Mucocele rupture can cause massive accumulation of gelatinous ascites, called *pseudomyxoma peritonei*. If the mucocele is the mucinous cystadenocarcinoma variety, ascites is malignant and the patient has a poorer prognosis. An association has been noted between mucoceles and the presence of one or more colon tumor(s).

Sonographically, the mucocele appears as a purely cystic or complex mass up to 7 cm in diameter, demonstrating through transmission posteriorly and located in the RLQ. This lesion may be difficult to differentiate from ovarian cysts, mesenteric cysts, omental cysts, duplication cysts, renal cysts, or even abdominal abscess.

Neuroendocrine Tumors

Neuroendocrine tumors (NETs), previously known as carcinoid tumors, of the appendix are unusual, but are the most common primary tumor of the appendiceal tip from subepithelial neuroendocrine cells.[30] They are mostly asymptomatic and are typically located only because of findings involving appendicitis. NETs arise from the subepithelial neuroendocrine cells lying on the *lamina propria mucosae* and the submucosal layer of the appendix wall. This tumor is usually benign if smaller than 1 cm, but it can have histologic features of malignancy, especially if measurements exceed 1 cm. Local invasiveness is a good indicator of the degree of malignancy. Most appendiceal NETs are benign.

Sonographically, these tumors appear as sharply marginated hypoechoic small masses without acoustic enhancement. Appendiceal carcinoids are NETs that classically arise at the appendiceal tip. They have a more benign course than other GI carcinoids, rarely metastasizing, with a 5-year survival rate of greater than 90%.[29]

Other Disorders of the Appendix

Sonographic detection of adenocarcinoma of the appendix has been reported (Fig. 11-33). The clinical presentation may be similar to that of acute appendicitis. CD of the appendix can occur as an isolated condition or more commonly with CD of the colon or ileum. The sonographic appearance of these conditions is nonspecific.

Bacterial Ileocolitis and Mesenteric Adenitis

When an abnormal appendix is not visualized sonographically, a search for other sonographic abnormalities in the RLQ will sometimes show other GI findings. Enlarged lymph nodes adjacent to the cecum may be observed. RLQ lymphadenopathy without associated appendicitis is termed *mesenteric adenitis* and is the most common diagnosis at surgery if the appendix is normal. Abnormal lymph nodes are rounder in outline than normal nodes, and they must be greater than 4 mm in anteroposterior diameter to be considered abnormal (Fig. 11-34A, B).

In some cases, the ileum, cecum, or both may show mild wall thickening as well as lymphadenopathy. *Yersinia*, *Campylobacter*, or *Salmonella* bacteria may be cultured from the stool in some of these patients. Bacterial ileocolitis is usually a self-limited disease that does not require surgery.

COLON AND RECTUM

Normal Anatomy of the Colon and Rectum

The colon usually lies in the periphery of the abdomen, laterally on the right and left, and superiorly along the liver

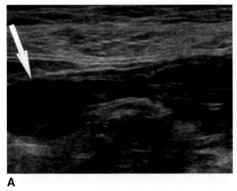
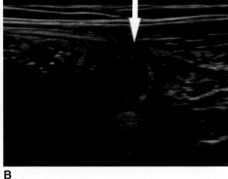

A   **B**

FIGURE 11-32 Appendix mucocele. **A:** Longitudinal thickened appendix *(arrow)* without signs of an acute appendicitis that proved to be a mucus-filled appendix with chronic inflammation. **B:** Transverse image of the appendix demonstrating a thickened mucus-filled structure consistent with mucocele *(arrow)*. (Images courtesy of Dr. Taco Geertsma, UltrasoundCases.info.)

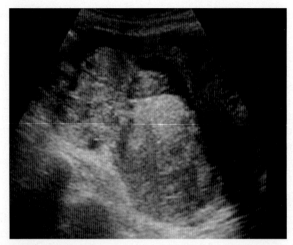

FIGURE 11-33 Appendix adenocarcinoma. Appendiceal mucinous carcinoma demonstrating a large complex mass. (Image courtesy of Dr. Taco Geertsma, UltrasoundCases.info.)

margin in the upper abdomen (see Fig. 11-1). Because the colon hosts gas-producing bacteria, it is more often distended with gas than the rest of the bowel. Its customary position, its larger diameter, and its characteristic haustral folds best seen at the ascending and transverse colon, which are up to 3 to 5 cm apart, can frequently help identify the colon (Fig. 11-35A–D).

Sonographic Technique

No special techniques are available for evaluating the colon. A normal person usually has more air in the colon than in the small bowel, and the colon's larger diameter and prominent haustral indentations are often identifiable. A fluid-filled colon is unusual, generally indicating diarrhea or obstruction. The examiner may sometimes have difficulty differentiating a solid mass in the colon from a small bowel lesion. It is helpful to know where the colon is usually located and to note the greater amount of air in the colon. Figure 11-36 demonstrates the recommended scanning pattern and transducer position when examining the colon.

Endoluminal examinations of the rectum and anus should be performed in both the axial and longitudinal directions if possible because this allows better evaluation of the layers of the bowel wall involved, the extent of invasion of any tumor that may be present, and evidence of local lymphadenopathy.

Sonographic Colon, Rectum, and Anus Wall Dimensions

The colon wall should measure 4 to 9 mm thick when not distended, and 2 to 4 mm when the colon is distended to a diameter of 5 cm or more. The rectum and anal wall thickness is similar to the wall dimensions of the colon.

Disorders of the Colon

Obstruction

The colon is usually partially filled with gas and, when colonic obstruction occurs, the obstructed loop is likely to be gas filled. This makes colon obstruction easy to diagnose radiographically and difficult to diagnose sonographically, although dilated loops of bowel may be identified. Although a specific diagnosis is not always possible, the location of the dilated loop may give some clues. Cecal volvulus is manifested by dilatation of the right colon only. Sigmoid volvulus shows maximum dilatation in the central abdomen. Diverticulitis with obstruction usually causes dilatation of the left, and perhaps the entire, colon, and an obstructing rectal carcinoma appears similar.

Colon Crohn Disease (Form of Inflammatory Bowel Disease)

CD of the colon, also known as regional or granulomatous colitis, produces signs identical to CD of the small bowel (Fig. 11-37A, B). It tends to be a transmural inflammation, potentially developing fistulae and pericolonic abscesses. Multiple separate areas of the colon may be involved; the right colon is a frequent site, and associated ileal involvement is common. Initially, the disease is limited to the mucosa; as the disease progresses, the entire bowel wall is involved with linear longitudinal and circumferential ulcers extending deep into the bowel wall, predisposing to fistulae. Inflammation also extends into the mesentery and over time leads to chronic fibrotic change and stricture formation.[24] Typically, the bowel layers in the colon wall are

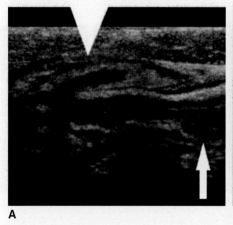

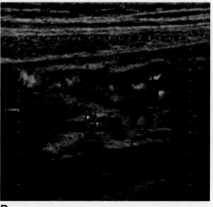

A   B

FIGURE 11-34 Ileocolitis. Mesenteric lymph nodes. **A:** Thickened ileocecal valve *(arrowhead)* related to ileocolitis with reactive mesenteric lymph nodes *(arrow).* **B:** Hypervascularity of the ileocecal wall. (Images courtesy of Dr. Taco Geertsma, UltrasoundCases.info.)

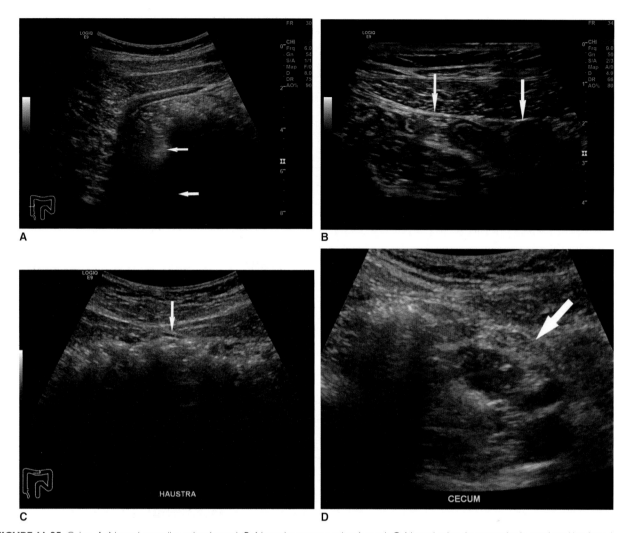

FIGURE 11-35 Colon. **A:** Normal ascending colon *(arrows)*. **B:** Normal transverse colon *(arrows)*. **C:** Normal colon demonstrating haustral marking *(arrow)*. **D:** Normal cecum *(arrow)*. (Images courtesy of Doña Ana Community College Diagnostic Medical Sonography program, Las Cruces, NM.)

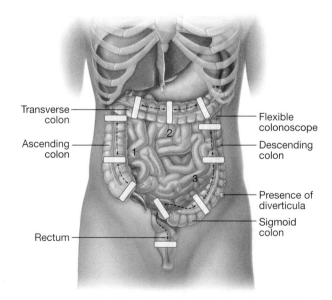

FIGURE 11-36 The illustration of the colon displays the anatomy and the recommended transducer position to acquire the best sonographic visualization of the colon.

not visible. Inflammatory activity, reflected by excess blood flow in the bowel wall, is shown on color Doppler imaging (see images in Fig. 11-25). Common complications include abscess formation, fistula, lumen stenosis, wall thickening, intramural edema, ulceration, decreased peristalsis, obstruction, and adhesions.

Ulcerative Colitis (Form of Inflammatory Bowel Disease)

Ulcerative colitis is a chronic inflammatory disease that causes ulceration of the colonic mucosa, usually starting in the rectum and then spreading to the sigmoid colon and superiorly. The cause is not known, but a hypersensitivity or autoimmune mechanism is suspected. Unlike Crohn colitis, ulcerative colitis does not skip some areas, leaving them unaffected, but spreads in a continuous pattern (Table 11-1). Patients with ulcerative colitis are at high risk of developing a particularly virulent form of colon carcinoma. The bowel wall appears thickened and is usually hypoechoic, although sometimes, the layers of the bowel wall are visible sonographically (Fig. 11-38A–C).

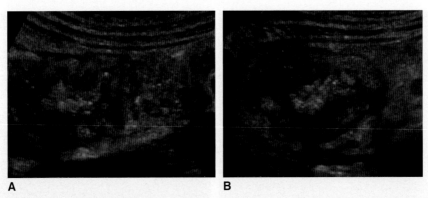

A   **B**

FIGURE 11-37 Crohn diseased colon. **A:** Thickening of the ascending colon wall in a longitudinal view. **B:** Thickening of the transverse ascending colon wall. (Images courtesy of Dr. Taco Geertsma, UltrasoundCases.info.)

TABLE 11-1 **Differences of Crohn Disease and Ulcerative Colitis**	
Crohn Disease	**Ulcerative Colitis**
• Inflammation of the entire GI tract • Affects all bowel wall layers • Affects portions (patches) of the GI tract, most commonly distal small bowel	• Inflammation of the rectum, possibly extending superiorly • Mucosal involvement • May extend throughout the bowel

GI, gastrointestinal.

Diverticular Disease

Diverticulosis is an acquired condition in which small hernias of the mucosa (diverticula) form through the muscular layer of the colon. The rectosigmoid colon is most often affected. This condition, which is associated with a low bulk diet, affects more than 50% of people older than 50 years in Western countries. Diverticulosis is usually asymptomatic and can be visualized with ultrasound if air fills the outpouched diverticula, especially if use of linear array probe is tolerated by patient habitus. The affected diverticula are characterized as bright bowel outpouchings (also referred to as bowel bright "ears") showing some degree of acoustic shadowing because of the presence of gas or inspissated feces.[31] If one or more diverticula become filled with inspissated fecal material and then become inflamed, diverticulitis results (Fig. 11-39A–C). Often, there is also inflammatory

thickening of the bowel wall and edema. Other abnormal discoveries include areas of echogenic and noncompressible fat at the diverticular region and organized collections suggesting abscess.[31] Pericolic abscesses may form because of diverticular rupture or transmural spread of infection. Sonographically, these abscesses appear as masses adjacent to the colon. They may be hypoechoic or may contain gas.

Colorectal Cancer

Colorectal cancer was the third most common cancer with 1.8 million new cases in 2018.[32] It is the second leading cause of cancer death in men and women in the United States.[33] Lung and breast cancers were the most common cancers worldwide, each contributing 12.3% of the total number of new cases diagnosed in 2018.[32] The majority of colon cancer develops in the rectum, followed by the sigmoid region and the rest of colon at the same rate. Transabdominal sonography demonstrates a large colon cancer as a nonspecific hypoechoic heterogeneous target lesion (Fig. 11-40A–E). Smaller polypoid lesions are much more difficult to identify because of gas or fecal material in the colon.

With high-frequency endorectal probes, the rectum can be imaged in transverse and longitudinal planes and can demonstrate the layers of the rectal wall. Endorectal ultrasound can be used to determine whether a tumor extends beyond the rectal wall in staging (Fig. 11-41A, B). Staging of colorectal carcinoma can be defined by characteristics including the depth of tumor penetration through the rectal

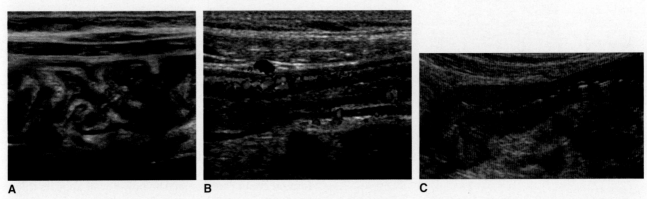

A   **B**   **C**

FIGURE 11-38 Ulcerative colitis. **A:** Longitudinal colon with a thick hypervascular wall. This patient was diagnosed with pancolitis, a severe form of colitis that involves the entire colon *(arrows)*. **B:** Hypervascularized thickened colon wall diagnosed with ulcerative colitis in a teenage female. **C:** Thick-walled colon because of ulcerative disease. Notice the haustra may be prominent or absent. (Images courtesy of Dr. Taco Geertsma, UltrasoundCases.info.)

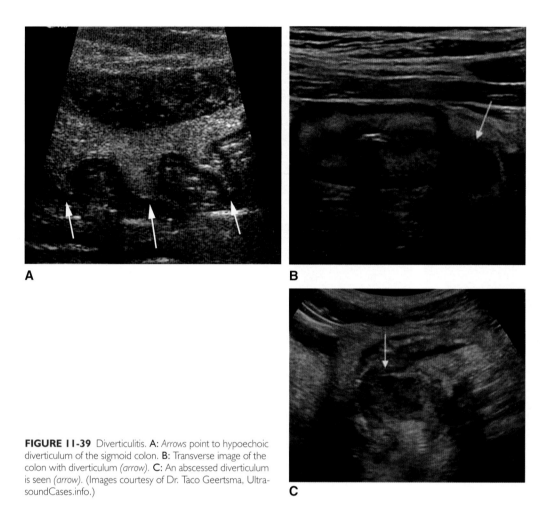

FIGURE 11-39 Diverticulitis. **A:** *Arrows* point to hypoechoic diverticulum of the sigmoid colon. **B:** Transverse image of the colon with diverticulum *(arrow)*. **C:** An abscessed diverticulum is seen *(arrow)*. (Images courtesy of Dr. Taco Geertsma, UltrasoundCases.info.)

wall, lymph node involvement, and presence of distant metastatic disease.

Colorectal Cancer Staging (American Joint Committee on Cancer: Simplified)

- Tumor (T)
- TX: unable to assess
- T0: no evidence of primary tumor
- Stage 0: early stage with mucosal involvement only
- Stage 1: tumor involvement of the submucosa and possibly muscularis propria
- Stage 2: tumor advancement through outer layers of the colon and possibly attachment into adjacent tissue or organs. No lymph node involvement or spread to distant sites.
- Stage 3: tumor is same as stage 2. Lymph nodes are involved. There is no distant site association.
- Stage 4: cancer may or may not have penetrated the bowel wall. It may or may not have spread to lymph nodes. There is spread to a distant organ, distant lymph nodes, or the peritoneum.

Preoperative staging is used to determine bowel wall involvement as well as to decide between excision techniques and postsurgical treatments. Staging modalities include endorectal ultrasound if appropriate, CT enterography, PET, and MRI enterography. Endorectal ultrasound is cost-effective but is limited to the inferior colon, whereas the previously mentioned modalities do not have the same limitations.

Lymphoma

Lymphoma is a rare tumor of the colon. It appears similar to lymphoma of the small bowel; a hypoechoic lesion—annular, eccentric, or diffusely involving the bowel wall—may be observed.

Other Disorders

Inflammatory Disorders

Other inflammatory colon conditions that may result in colon wall thickening include ischemia, amebiasis, shigellosis, tuberculosis, pseudomembranous colitis, radiation colitis, endometriosis, and pancreatitis. In ischemic colitis, little or no flow is detectable with power Doppler imaging (Fig. 11-42).

Irritable Bowel Syndrome

Irritable bowel syndrome (IBS) is a chronic painful condition causing recurrent diarrhea with a mucus discharge and alternating constipation. Affected individuals suffer from nausea, noncardiac chest pain, sporadic heartburn, and abdominal bloating. A lack of characteristic imaging features and no diagnostic biomarkers make IBS difficult to recognize. It is

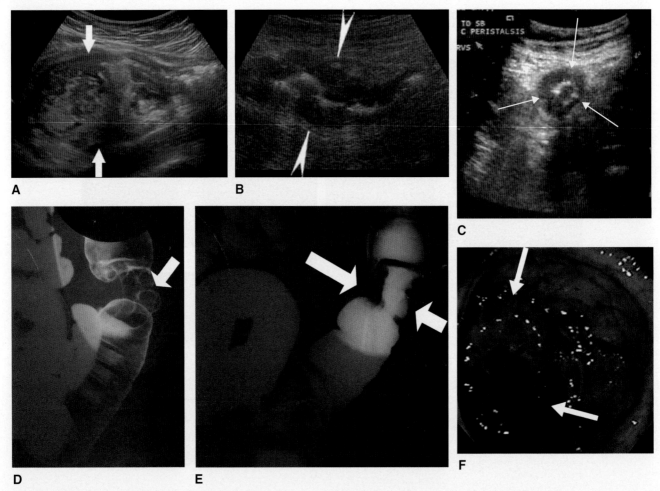

FIGURE 11-40 Colon carcinoma. **A:** Ascending colon with a cancerous mass *(arrows).* **B:** Descending colon cancer. Note thickened hypoechoic irregular contoured walls *(arrowheads).* **C:** Transverse mass seen at the *arrows,* diagnosed as moderate- to well-differentiated invasive adenocarcinoma of the sigmoid colon in a 36-year-old female. **D, E:** Air contrast barium enema displaying the same sigmoid colon lesion *(arrows)* seen in image **C. F:** Surgical image of the cancerous lesion. (Incidentally, the sigmoid colon cancer diagnosis in this patient led to family member testing. One member was diagnosed with rectal cancer, another with colon cancer, and a third with precancerous polyps. The patient and three family members were treated using multiple methods to include chemotherapy and surgery.) (Images **A** and **B:** Courtesy of Dr. Taco Geertsma, UltrasoundCases.info. Images **C–F:** Courtesy of Cheryl Vance, San Antonio, TX.)

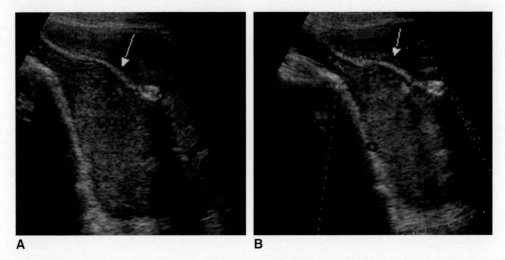

FIGURE 11-41 Rectal mass. A large carcinoma of the rectum *(arrow)* is demonstrated **(A)** without and **(B)** with blood flow. (Images courtesy of Dr. Taco Geertsma, UltrasoundCases.info.)

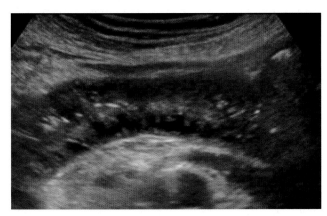

FIGURE 11-42 Ischemic bowel. Affected bowel wall shows thickening and increased echogenicity. (Image courtesy of Dr. Taco Geertsma, Ultrasound-Cases.info.)

ileus; in an adult, it is known as distal intestinal obstructive syndrome. Decreased peristalsis results in the normally thick meconium in an infant or a combination of meconium and fecal matter in an adult, lacking the ability to maneuver through the bowel. Ultrasound imaging demonstrates thickened wall, dilatation, wall hypervascularization, intussusception, thick intraluminal contents, and lymph node enlargement.

Benign Tumors

The same lesions seen in the small bowel can also involve the colon: leiomyomas, polyps, lipomas, fibromas, and hemangiomas. Polyps begin as benign mucosal outgrowths (Fig. 11-44). They can progress to carcinoma.

SONOGRAPHIC EVALUATION

Although sonography is not likely to replace GI barium studies, CT enterography, MRI enterography, endoscopy, or colonoscopy of the GI tract—nor is it likely to replace CT, MRI, or endoscopy in staging of GI malignancies—its role in the evaluation of abdominal disorders continues to advance. The sonographic signs of GI lesions are summarized in Table 11-2. Sonography has the unique ability to visualize the layers of the bowel wall, by transabdominal, endorectal, endovaginal, or endoscopic ultrasound, which is often useful in the diagnosis or staging of GI lesions.

often diagnosed based on symptoms only. Figure 11-43A–C demonstrates a portion of colon affected by IBS.

Cystic Fibrosis

Cystic fibrosis affects the bowel, mostly the terminal ileum or proximal large intestine by obstructing, which can result in rupture and sepsis. In an infant, this is called meconium

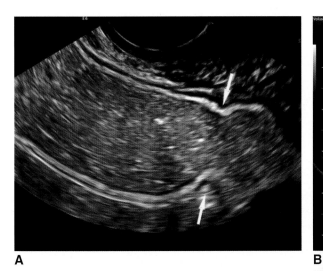

A

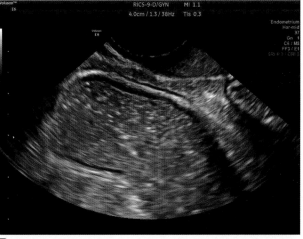

B

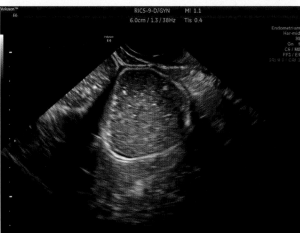

C

FIGURE 11-43 Irritable bowel. **A:** Longitudinal widened colon with narrowing (arrows), indicative of irritable bowel. **B:** Longitudinal widened colon with heterogeneous contents, similar to (**A**). **C:** Transverse widened colon displaying effects of irritable bowel. (Images courtesy of Barbara Hall-Terracciano.)

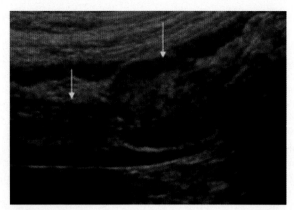

FIGURE 11-44 Benign colon polyp. Colon polyp on a stalk *(arrows)*. (Image courtesy of Dr. Taco Geertsma, UltrasoundCases.info.)

Additionally, the use of sonographic endoscopy to direct biopsy and needle aspiration of GI lesions is developing as a valuable diagnostic tool.

SPECIAL DIAGNOSTIC TECHNIQUES

Contrast agents have been and are currently being studied for use and for sonographic visualization of the GI tract more prominently in European countries compared with the United States. Contrast-enhanced endoluminal sonography is used to differentiate malignant from benign masses, assess depth of cancer invasion of the GI tract walls, examine fistulas, and determine vascular flow to differentiate fibrous from inflammatory strictures and study inflammatory bowel disease, among others. Contrast agents were used initially as Doppler signal enhancers, including in contrast-enhanced EUS examinations.

Both color Doppler and power Doppler imaging can be used, especially for regions with very low flow volumes, where the unenhanced signal is very weak or the signal-to-noise ratio is very poor. Highly vascularized bowel wall and lesions can be determined with Doppler imaging based on the signal intensity. This contributes to determining inflamed and uninflamed regions of bowel, as well as assisting with the determination of benign versus malignant lesions.

TABLE 11-2 Sonographic Appearance of Gastrointestinal Lesion

Appearance	Lesion
Target or pseudokidney sign (circumferential hypoechoic thickening of the bowel wall)	Lymphoma, intussusception, nonspecific inflammation, chronic ulcerative colitis, regional enteritis, hematoma, metastatic tumor
Focal hypoechoic lesions in the submucosa of the stomach	Neuroma, fibroma, gastric cysts, varices, ectopic pancreas
Focal hyperechoic lesions in the submucosa of the stomach	Ectopic pancreas, lipoma
Focal defect in the gastric mucosa with the mucosal layer preserved to the edge of the ulcer	Benign gastric ulcer
Defect in the gastric mucosa with indistinct mucosal layer at the ulcer edge	Benign or malignant ulcer
Focal hypoechoic lesions of the muscularis propria (exophytic)	Leiomyoma, leiomyosarcoma, metastatic tumor
Large cystic lesions	Obstruction, ileus, volvulus, mucocele
Thickening of the valvulae in the small bowel	Cirrhosis, renal disease, Ménétrier disease, Whipple disease, lymphangiomatosis, abetalipoproteinemia, inflammatory diseases
Mild thickening of the colon wall (<1 cm)	Chronic ulcerative colitis, regional enteritis, diverticulitis, pseudomembranous colitis, amebiasis, shigellosis, radiation colitis
Multiple concentric rings of bowel wall on transverse view, folded layers on longitudinal view	Intussusception

Elastography is used to indicate and define bowel wall lesions. The ability to discern bowel-related fibrosis from inflammation using elastography also aids in the diagnosis of inflammatory bowel disease.

SUMMARY

- The GI tract is, essentially, a 30-foot muscular tube, originating at the mouth and terminating at the anus.
- Sonography of the GI tract can either be performed transabdominally or endoluminally.
- Real-time sonography permits the visualization of peristaltic activity, which is helpful in identifying the GI tract and evaluating its function.
- When examining the abdomen, the patient should have nothing by mouth for about 8 hours whenever possible; however, if the stomach and duodenum are to be further examined, the patient can drink 10 to 40 oz of water through a straw to improve visualization.
- Having the patient drink fluid also helps in examining the stomach and jejunum and ileum mucosa and peristalsis.

- Before endorectal sonography, a cleansing enema may be helpful so that the fecal material is not confused with mucosal lesions.
- The layers of the esophagus are as follows: mucosa layering the lumen, submucosa, muscularis propria, and the outermost adventitia.
- The layers of the bowel wall are similar from the stomach to the anus: (1) a hyperechoic inner layer—the border between the digestive fluid and the mucosa; (2) a hypoechoic layer—usually thin, represents the mucosa, lamina propria, lamina muscularis; (3) a hyperechoic layer—the submucosa; (4) a hypoechoic layer—the muscular layer, and its thickness depends on the segment of the digestive tract; and (5) an outer hyperechoic layer—the serous layer, the border to the peridigestive fat.

- The sonographic structure of the bowel is usually described by five layers: three echogenic layers separated by two hypoechoic ones.
- Sonographic endoscopy has demonstrated excellent sensitivity and specificity in the staging of esophageal cancer, particularly in the advanced stages.
- The stomach normally lies in the left upper quadrant of the abdomen with the fundus medial to the spleen and anterior to the left kidney and the body and antrum posterior or inferior to the left lobe of the liver, anterior to the pancreas, and medial to the gallbladder and porta hepatis.
- The antrum and body of the stomach often appear as a target-like structure inferior to the left lobe on longitudinal sonograms.
- If the stomach is not distended, the bowel wall should measure 2 to 6 mm thick; however, when the stomach is distended to a diameter of 8 cm or more, the wall should measure 2 to 4 mm.
- Chronic gastritis may present as enlarged rugal folds with generalized thickening of the mucosal layer of the wall.
- Peptic ulcers most often occur in the antral portion of the lesser curvature and may appear sonographically as a focal or generalized edema of the wall.
- Gastric carcinoma arises from the mucosa of the stomach, invading the submucosa and muscularis propria.
- Ileus is characterized by failure of the intestine to propel its contents owing to diminished motility and may be caused by peritonitis, spinal fracture, renal colic, acute pancreatitis, bowel ischemia, myocardial infarction, surgery, medications, hypokalemia, cystic fibrosis, and infection.
- Sonographically, ileus presents as distended bowel with either air or fluid, although usually less distended than with obstruction, with normal to increased peristalsis.
- Small bowel obstruction also has many causes, such as adhesions, inflammatory masses, neoplastic lesions, volvulus, intussusception, and luminal obstruction (such as fecal impaction).
- Sonographically, with small bowel obstruction, the bowel loops are typically perfectly round in cross section, and peristalsis can vary from none to markedly increased.
- In volvulus, the twisted, dilated loop appears C-shaped when viewed longitudinally and often contains only fluid, no air.
- Intussusception is a telescoping of the bowel into itself, and in adults it is most commonly associated with an identifiable bowel lesion. Sonographically, intussusception appears as a nonspecific target lesion or as a mass with multiple concentric rings when viewed transversely.
- CD is the most common nonspecific inflammation of the small bowel with inflammation starting in the submucosa and becoming transmural; the ileum is most often affected, but the colon, jejunum, and stomach may also be affected.
- Sonographically, the most obvious finding in CD is a hypoechoic thickening of the bowel wall and mesentery.
- The normal appendix is a long tubular structure that is seen extending from the cecum and should measure no more than 6 mm in diameter, and the hypoechoic part of the wall should be no more than 2 mm thick.
- Appendicitis is usually associated with obstruction of the appendiceal lumen; although it may occur in any age group, young adults are most often affected.
- Appendicitis presents clinically as periumbilical pain that moves to the RLQ with rebound tenderness, leukocytosis, fever, and sometimes nausea.
- Sonographically, appendicitis appears as a noncompressible appendix greater than 6 mm with mucus and possible appendicolith in the appendiceal lumen.
- Complications of appendicitis include perforation and abscess.
- Mucocele rupture can cause massive accumulation of gelatinous ascites, called pseudomyxoma peritonei.
- The colon usually lies in the periphery of the abdomen, laterally on the right and left, and superiorly along the liver margin.
- The colon wall should measure 4 to 9 mm thick when not distended and 2 to 4 mm when the colon is distended to a diameter of 5 cm or more.
- Ulcerative colitis is an inflammatory disease confined to the colonic mucosa and submucosa that starts in the rectal region and, as the disease progresses, extends up the left colon and may eventually involve the entire colon. Unlike Crohn colitis, ulcerative colitis does not skip some areas—leaving them unaffected—but spreads in a continuous pattern.
- Colon carcinoma is the third leading cause of death from cancer—after carcinoma of the lung and breast—and appears sonographically as a hypoechoic target lesion.
- The accuracy of bowel ultrasound is limited by operator expertise.

REFERENCES

1. Cazacu IM, Luzuriaga Chavez AA, Saftoiu A, et al. A quarter century of EUS-FNA: progress, milestones, and future directions. *Endosc Ultrasound*. 2018;7:141–160.
2. Hobbs J. Diagnostic imaging of appendicitis with supplementation by transabdominal and transvaginal sonography. *J Diagn Med Sonogr*. 2015;31(6):345–351.
3. Andrzejewska M, Grzymislawski M. The role of intestinal ultrasound in diagnostics of bowel diseases. *Prz Gastroenterol*. 2018;13(1):1–5. doi:10.5114/pg.2018.74554
4. Atkinson N, Bryant R, Dong Y, et al. How to perform gastrointestinal ultrasound: anatomy and normal findings. *World J Gastroenterol*. 2017;23(38):6931–6941. doi:10.3748/wjg.v23.i38.6931
5. Sporea I, Popescu A. Ultrasound examination of the normal gastrointestinal tract. *Med Ultrason*. 2010;12(4):349–352.
6. Fernandes T, Oliveira M, Castro R, Araújo B, Viamonte B, Cunha R. Bowel wall thickening at CT: simplifying the diagnosis. *Insights Imaging*. 2014;5(2):195–208. doi:10.1007/s13244-013-0308-y
7. American Cancer Society. Cancer Facts & Figures. Accessed March 2020. https://www.cancer.org
8. American Cancer Society. Esophagus cancer—early detection, diagnosis, and staging—tests for esophageal cancer. Accessed March 20, 2020. www.cancer.org/cancer/esophagus-cancer/detection-diagnosis-staging/how-diagnosed.html
9. Kumar A, Annamaraju P. Gastric outlet obstruction. In: *StatPearls* [Internet]. StatPearls Publishing; 2022.

10. Vakil N. *Overview of Gastritis*. Merck Manual Professional Version. 2020. Merck & Co., Inc. Kenilworth, NJ. Accessed April 25, 2022. https://www.merckmanuals.com/professional/gastrointestinal-disorders/gastritis-and-peptic-ulcer-disease

11. Malik T, Gnanapandithan K, Singh K. Peptic ulcer disease. In: *StatPearls* [Internet]. StatPearls Publishing; 2020. https://www.ncbi.nlm.nih.gov/books/NBK534792/

12. Caufield S, Schafer T. *Peptic Ulcer Disease*. American College of Gastroenterology; 2012.

13. Sander RC, Hall-Terracciano B, Lunsford B. Right lower quadrant pain. In: Sander RC, Hall-Terracciano B, eds. *Clinical Sonography: A Practical Guide*. Wolters Kluwer; 2016.

14. National Cancer Institute, Surveillance, Epidemiology, and End Results Program. 2020. https://seer.cancer.gov/

15. American Cancer Society. Stomach cancer. Early detection, diagnosis, and staging. Stomach cancer survival rates. https://cancer.org/cancer/stomach-cancer.html

16. Rawla P, Barsouk A. Epidemiology of gastric cancer: global trends, risk factors and prevention. *Prz Gastroenterol*. 2019;14(1):26–38. doi:10.5114/pg.2018.80001

17. Juarez-Salcedo L, Sokol L, Chavez JC, Dalia S. Primary gastric lymphoma, epidemiology, clinical diagnosis, and treatment. *Cancer Control*. 2018;25(1):1073274818778256. doi:10.1177/1073274818778256

18. Malipatel R, Patil M, Rout PP, et al. Primary gastric lymphoma: clinicopathological profile. *Euroasian J Hepatogastroenterol*. 2018;8(1):6–10. doi:10.5005/jp-journals-10018-1250

19. Chan K. What's the mass? The gist of point-of-care ultrasound in gastrointestinal stromal tumors. *Clin Pract Cases Emerg Med*. 2018;2(1):82–85. doi:10.5811/cpcem.2017.12.36375

20. Ocasio Quinones G, Woolf A. Duodenal ulcer. In: *StatPearls* [Internet]. StatPearls Publishing; 2020. https://www.ncbi.nlm.nih.gov/books/NBK557390/

21. Weerakkody Y. Duodenitis. Accessed October 8, 2021. https://radiopaedia.org/articles/41233

22. Potts J, Samaraee A, El-Hakeem A. Small bowel intussusception in adults. *Ann R Coll Surg Engl*. 2014;96(1):11–14.

23. Vo N, Sato T. Intussusception in children. In: *UpToDate*. Wolters Kluwer; 2020.

24. Gaillard F, Glick Y. Crohn disease. Accessed October 8, 2021. https://radiopaedia.org/articles/6791

25. Maffe G, Brunetti L, Formagnana P, Corazza GR. Ultrasonographic findings in Crohn's disease. *J Ultrasound*. 2015;18(1):37–49.

26. Casciani E, De Vincentiis C, Polettini E, et al. Imaging of the small bowel: Crohn's disease in paediatric patients. *World J Radiol*. 2014;6(6):313–328.

27. Chao A, Gharahbaghian L. *Tips and Tricks: Ultrasound in the Diagnosis of Acute Appendicitis. Emergency Ultrasound*. American College of Emergency Physicians; 2020.

28. Jacob D, Jones J. Acute appendicitis. Accessed October 8, 2021. https://radiopaedia.org/articles/922

29. Jones MW, Lopez RA, Deppen JG. *Appendicitis*. In: *StatPearls* [Internet]. StatPearls Publishing; 2021. Updated August 6, 2021. https://www.ncbi.nlm.nih.gov/books/NBK493193/

30. Knipe H, Bell D. Appendiceal carcinoid. Accessed October 8, 2021. https://radiopaedia.org/articles/41519

31. Jones J, Weerakkody Y. Colonic diverticulitis. Accessed October 8, 2021. https://radiopaedia.org/articles/6201

32. Worldwide Cancer Data. Global cancer statistic for the most common cancers in the world. Accessed October 8, 2021. https://www.wcrf.org/dietandcancer/worldwide-cancer-data/

33. Colorectal Cancer Alliance. Know the facts. 2020. Accessed October 8, 2021. https://www.ccalliance.org/

CHAPTER 12

The Kidneys

M. ROBERT DEJONG AND JEANINE RYBYINSKI

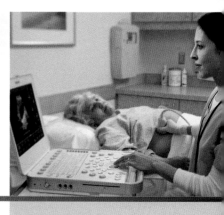

OBJECTIVES

- Discuss the normal anatomy of the kidneys including vasculature.
- Describe the microscopic internal renal anatomy to include the glomerulus and nephrons.
- Discuss the physiology of the upper urinary system.
- List the common laboratory function tests for the kidneys and what an abnormal value may indicate.
- Recognize sonographic anatomy of the upper urinary tract.
- Discuss the routine scanning protocol of the kidneys.
- Describe the sonographic appearance of the various cystic lesions of the kidneys.
- Describe the sonographic appearance of common benign and malignant solid masses of the kidneys.
- List some of the causes for hydronephrosis and the sonographic appearance of each grade.
- List common causes, and describe the sonographic appearance of kidney stones.
- Discuss the sonographic appearance of medical renal disease, and list common causes for medical renal disease and renal failure.
- Describe the sonographer's role in native renal biopsies.

GLOSSARY

acoustic enhancement a localized area of increased echo brightness behind a structure of low attenuation; also called posterior enhancement or enhanced through transmission

acoustic shadow caused by a dense structure, usually containing calcium, of high attenuation that absorbs the sound beam causing a black area that does not contain any echoes underneath the structure

acute kidney injury (AKI) a rapid or abrupt decrease in renal function based on lab values and urine output; previously called acute renal failure (ARF)

blood urea nitrogen (BUN) a blood test that measures the amount of urea nitrogen in the blood. It helps determine kidney function

chronic kidney disease (CKD) a long-term process that damages the kidneys, causing renal failure; previously called chronic renal failure (CRF)

contralateral the other side of the body

KEY TERMS

acoustic shadow

acute tubular injury (ATI)

adenoma

autosomal dominant polycystic kidney disease

angiomyolipoma

blood urea nitrogen (BUN)

column of Bertin

cortex

creatinine

dromedary hump

duplicated or bifid collecting system

ectopic kidney

emphysematous pyelonephritis

enhancement

estimated glomerular filtration rate (eGFR)

extrarenal pelvis

glomerulus

horseshoe kidney

hydronephrosis

junctional parenchymal defect

kidney stones or calculi

lymphoma

medical renal disease

nephrocalcinosis

(continued)

nephron

oncocytoma

parenchyma

pyelonephritis

pyonephrosis

renal agenesis

renal cell carcinoma

renal cyst

renal failure

renal pelvis

sinus

subcapsular hematoma

transitional cell carcinoma

creatinine a blood test that measures the level of creatinine in the blood. It helps determine kidney function along with BUN

cyst a round structure of smooth, thin-walled tissue that contains fluid

estimated glomerular filtration rate (eGFR) an estimate of how well the kidneys are working and can determine if kidney disease is present and what stage. It measures the kidneys' ability to filter toxins or waste from blood

Gerota fascia a fibrous connective tissue that encapsulates the kidneys and adrenal glands; also known as the renal fascia

glomerulus a ball-shaped structure that make up the nephron and involved in the filtration of the blood. Plural form is glomeruli

hematuria when there is blood in the urine and can be referred to as either gross hematuria, when the blood is visible in the urine, or microscopic hematuria, when blood can only be seen under a microscope

hypernephroma another term for renal cell carcinoma

hypertension, or high blood pressure, is when the force of the blood pushing against the walls of the blood vessels is at a higher pressure than normal

ipsilateral on the same side of the body

nephrectomy surgical removal of a kidney

nephron the functional unit in the kidney that consists of a glomerulus and a tubule, through which the glomerular filtrate passes to become urine by removing waste and excess substances and fluid

nephropathy refers to kidney disease

nephrotoxic anything or any substance that can damage the kidneys

oliguria when there is a low output of less than 400 mL of urine in 24 hours, oligio—little, uria—urine, little urine

proteinuria when there is protein in the urine

renal pelvis an area in the center of the kidney where urine collects to be funneled into the ureter

septation a tissue partition inside a cyst

According to the National Institute of Diabetes and Digestive and Kidney Disease, 1 in 3 people with diabetes and 1 in 5 people with high blood pressure have kidney disease. Nearly 786,000 people in the United States are living with end-stage renal disease (ESRD), with 71% on dialysis and 29% with a kidney transplant. Despite the prevalence of the disease, as many as 9 in 10 people are unaware that they have chronic kidney disease (CKD).[1]

Sonography is generally the first imaging test to evaluate the kidneys when renal disease is suspected because neither radiation nor nephrotoxic contrast is needed. Both computed tomography (CT) and magnetic resonance imaging (MRI) contrast agents can damage the kidneys and possibly cause the patient to acquire acute kidney injury (AKI). A renal sonogram provides the nephrologist or physician information about renal length, cortical thickness, the echogenicity of the renal cortex, and if pathology is present. If further information is needed, the patient will be sent for a CT scan or a MRI scan.

Renal sonograms may be challenging to perform. Sonographers must have a good understanding of anatomy, physiology, and pathophysiology of the organs scanned. With this knowledge, the sonographer has the information needed to adjust the protocols, if necessary. In addition, the sonographer should be able to evaluate lab reports, physical examination findings, and any operative or imaging reports. This information assists the sonographer in anticipating potential findings, especially as typically the minimal amount of clinical information is on the order. All sonographic images are evaluated regarding the demonstration of appropriate anatomy, technical settings, measurements, and vascularity. Image optimization ensures the best patient care and potential for diagnosis.

This chapter discusses the upper third of the urinary system, which comprises the kidneys and the proximal ureters. Chapter 13 discusses the lower third of the urinary system, including the distal ureters, urinary bladder, and the urethra, and Chapter 20 reviews the pediatric urinary system. Chapter 6 discusses renal Doppler examinations, Chapter 24 renal transplants, and Chapter 26 sonography-guided interventional procedures, including renal biopsies.

ANATOMY

Often having an understanding of how the organs are developed can assist the sonographer in understanding variations in anatomy, congenital anomalies, and other organ systems that may be affected.

Embryology [1–3]

The urinary system begins its development along with the reproductive system as they develop from the same origin, often described as the urogenital ridge. This is why anomalies in one system may have associated anomalies in the other system. The urogenital ridge will form during the fourth week of gestation and divide into the nephrogenic cord, to form the urinary tract, and the gonadal ridge, to form the reproductive tract. The correct development of the urinary tract is through a complex interaction between embryonic tissues, the mesonephric duct, the ureteric duct, and the metanephric blastema. A disruption of this intricate process through either a genetic or environmental cause can result in congenital anomalies of the urinary system, including renal agenesis, multicystic dysplastic kidney (MCDK), or infantile polycystic kidney disease (PKD). What follows is very basic information on the embryology of the kidneys, and the reader is encouraged to read more detailed information about the formation of the urinary system.

The kidneys will develop in three morphologic stages called the pronephros, the mesonephros, and the metanephros. The pronephros is the earliest nephric stage and is a transitory, nonfunctional structure that disappears by the fourth week of gestation. Pronephros is derived from Greek and means before kidney. Its purpose is not well understood, but it is thought that it might provide a structure for the mesonephros. The mesonephros forms just caudal to the pronephros and develops into the mesonephric tubules and the mesonephric duct, also known as the Wolffian duct. This structure provides partial function, whereas the kidney continues to develop and completely regresses by the 12th week of gestation. The Wolffian duct will regress in females and become Gartner duct that can form a cyst called a Gartner duct cyst, which is usually located along the anterolateral wall of the proximal third of the vagina. They can sometimes be identified on an endovaginal examination. In males, the Wolffian duct develops into parts of the male reproductive system, including the epididymis, vas deferens, seminal vesicles, and the ejaculatory duct. In females, the mesonephric duct develops into the paramesonephric duct, or Müllerian duct, which develops into the female reproductive system, including the uterus and the cervix. In males, the Müllerian duct will regress and become the appendix testes. The ureteric bud comes off the mesonephric duct and develops into the different parts of the collecting system, such as the calyces, collecting ducts, renal pelvis, and ureter. The ureteropelvic junction (UPJ) is the last to canalize and is the most common site of obstruction in congenital hydronephrosis. During the fifth week of gestation, the metanephros phase begins, and the metanephric mesoderm will form the excretory parts of the kidneys that form the nephrons, glomerulus, Bowman capsule, and the convoluted tubules (Pathology Box 12-1). Note that the collecting system and the parenchyma develop from two

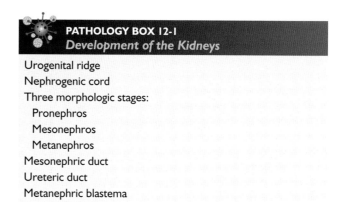

PATHOLOGY BOX 12-1
Development of the Kidneys

Urogenital ridge
Nephrogenic cord
Three morphologic stages:
 Pronephros
 Mesonephros
 Metanephros
Mesonephric duct
Ureteric duct
Metanephric blastema

different sources. The kidneys become functional at about 12 weeks of gestational age. Nephrogenesis, development of the kidney, will continue through 32 to 36 weeks of gestational age.

The kidneys initially develop in the pelvic region where they lie close together in the sacral region. As the fetus grows and the abdomen enlarges, the kidneys are drawn apart and ascend to their final position in the abdomen around T12–L3. During this ascent, the kidneys will rotate 90 degrees, causing the hilum, which initially faces ventrally, to face medially. This ascent process occurs between 6 and 9 weeks of gestational age. While in the pelvis, the kidneys will receive their blood supply from the common iliac arteries. As the kidneys ascend, they are vascularized by a succession of transient, higher arteries off the abdominal aorta that corresponds to the level of the kidneys, until the kidneys reach their final position and the main renal arteries are formed. These lower vessels should regress as they become unnecessary, but if they persist, they become accessory renal arteries.

Location and Size[3–8]

The normal urinary system consists of two kidneys, two ureters, the urinary bladder, and the urethra. The kidneys are in the retroperitoneum on either side of the vertebrae. The ureters take the urine from the kidney to the urinary bladder, where it is stored temporarily until it is excreted from the body through the urethra. The left kidney is located at about the level of T12–L3, whereas the right kidney is slightly lower in the abdomen owing to the larger size of the liver (Fig. 12-1A). The left kidney will be slightly higher, superior, in the abdomen and more toward the back, posterior, then the right kidney. The kidneys lie on the posterior abdominal wall on the quadratus lumborum muscle on either side of the spine in the perineal space of the retroperitoneum (Fig. 12-1B, C). The long axis of the kidney is in an oblique plane parallel to the lateral border of the psoas muscle. It is not in a sagittal plane. The upper pole of the kidney is more medial and lies more posterior than the lower pole. This is why the lower pole of the kidney tilted up toward the skin surface (Fig. 12-2).

Renal length gives an approximation of renal function; therefore, it is important for the sonographer to measure the kidneys carefully. Kidney size has been correlated with the patient's height, age, and body mass index (BMI). The size

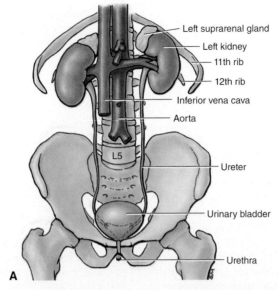

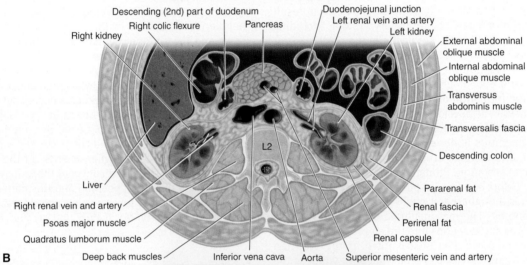

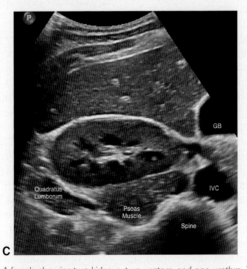

FIGURE 12-1 Anatomy of the urinary system. **A:** A female showing two kidneys, two ureters, and one urethra. The main difference between a male and female urinary system is the urethra in a male is longer. *Note:* The suprarenal gland is another name for the adrenal gland. **B:** An anatomic transverse image of the kidneys in their retroperitoneal location surrounded by the renal capsule and both perirenal and pararenal fat. Note the surrounding structures and their relationship to the kidneys. **C:** Transverse image of the right kidney showing the kidney and its relationship to the psoas and quadratus lumborum muscles. *GB*, gallbladder; *IVC*, inferior vena cava.

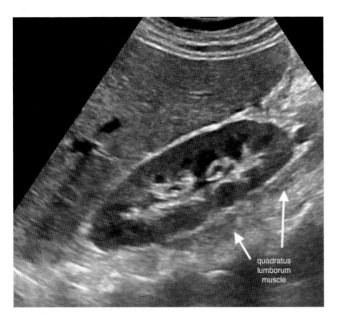

FIGURE 12-2 Longitudinal image of the right kidney showing the tilt of the kidney with the upper pole deeper in the image and the lower pole closer to the surface. This image also demonstrates a Riedel lobe of the liver.

the renal hilum in a transverse plane that is perpendicular to the long axis of the kidney. The two measurements should be at a right angle to one another (Fig. 12-3B). The kidneys are slightly larger in men, and the left kidney is usually slightly longer than the right. The difference between the two normal kidneys should be within 15 mm if the right kidney is smaller and 10 mm if the left kidney is smaller. The rule of thumb that is commonly used in sonography is that the kidneys should be within 2 cm of each other in length. If one kidney is more than 2 cm or shorter by at least 2 cm in length, when compared with the other kidney, the sonographer needs to try and determine the cause. The potential reasons for this discrepancy in size are discussed later in this chapter. When a kidney is removed, the remaining kidney will start to grow again and increase in size, called hypertrophy, to compensate for assuming the function of the other kidney, measuring greater than 12 to 13 cm in length. As people age, their kidneys tend to shrink. Therefore, a 9.5-cm kidney in an 80-year-old woman may be normal, whereas in a 26-year-old, it would be small.

The cortical thickness is measured from the base of the pyramid to the capsule and is normally between 6 and 10 mm. If the pyramids are difficult to see, the parenchymal thickness can be measured, instead of measuring from the edge of the sinus echo to the capsule and should be between 15 and 20 mm (Fig. 12-4). Cortical thickness appears to be closely related to estimated glomerular filtration rate (eGFR), and studies have shown that in patients with a low eGFR, their cortical thickness is reduced in size. Some nephrologists use the cortical thickness over the renal length measurement to determine the severity of renal failure as well as to follow the patient for progression of the disease.

of the kidneys is roughly the size of the patient's fist. In adults, the normal kidney is approximately 10 to 14 cm long in males and 9 to 13 cm long in females. A general number used is renal length is between 9 and 12 cm. The kidneys measure about 5 to 7 cm in width, 3 to 5 cm in thickness, and weigh approximately 120 to 170 g (Fig. 12-3A). The width and thickness measurements are measured at the level of

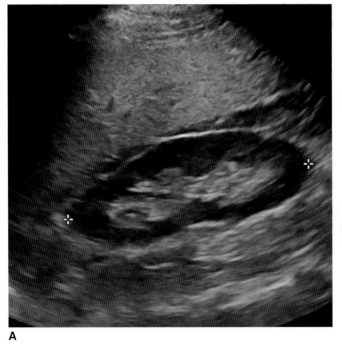

A

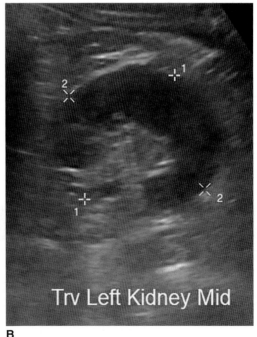

B

FIGURE 12-3 Standard renal measurements. **A:** Longitudinal image of the right kidney demonstrating how to correctly measure the length of the kidney. **B:** Transverse image of the left kidney at mid pole demonstrating the transverse measurement (calipers 1) and the thickness measurement (calipers 2). (Images courtesy of T. Whitten.)

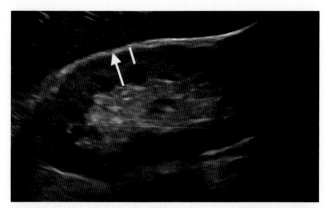

FIGURE 12-4 Image demonstrating how to measure cortical thickness (*solid line*) and parenchymal thickness (*arrow*).

Another sonographic method to evaluate the kidney for renal failure is by obtaining a renal volume. Renal volume can be used to help assess renal function, especially in patients with CKD, because renal volume will decrease with a decrease in renal function. Renal volume is a more sensitive indicator of declining renal function as opposed to a single linear measurement. It is calculated by measuring the three axes of the kidney and using the formula for an ellipsoid:

$$\text{Volume} = \text{length} \times \text{width} \times \text{thickness} \times \pi/6$$

An easier version to use for calculation is volume = length × width × thickness × 0.523 (where $\pi/6 = 3.14/6 = 0.523$). Some ultrasound (US) units can calculate the renal volume from the three measurements when the volume tool is activated. Because the kidney is not a true ellipse, renal volumes are underestimated using this method. A normal renal volume is between 110 and 190 mL in men and between 90 and 150 mL in women (Pathology Box 12-2). Renal volumes calculated using a 3D transducer and 3D software have been shown to be more accurate when compared with renal volumes obtained using MRI.

Obtaining accurate renal length measurements is very important for patient care as medical decisions are made based on these measurements. It is important when measuring the length of the kidney to ensure that the full length of the kidney is being accurately measured, as it is easy to oblique the transducer and foreshorten the length, creating a false measurement. Look at the cortex as it should be about the same thickness as it surrounds the sinus echoes. Check the individual measurements of each kidney and compare the measurements between the kidneys to make sure that they make sense. The difference in size between the two kidneys should be less than 2 cm, and the measurements should be repeated if the difference is greater than 2 cm and a reason for the discrepancy cannot be determined. Sometimes, the lower pole may be hard to define due to a rib shadow or overlying bowel gas. A kidney that measures less than 9 cm is usually abnormal, so if a measurement is less than 9 cm, it is important to reevaluate the image, especially if the other kidney is a normal size. If the sinus echoes touch or are near the border of a pole, then the measurement will be inaccurate as this image has been captured in an oblique plane. If seeing the lower pole border is difficult due to a rib shadow, try using a sector transducer as it can get between the ribs and show both the borders of the kidney. It is acceptable for the rib shadow to go through the middle of the kidney when obtaining a length measurement. If the issue is bowel gas, try placing the transducer closer to the scanning table and angling anteriorly toward the kidney. If that does not work, turn the patient into an oblique or decubitus position. A last resort is to turn the patient into a prone position. Sometimes, pathology can interfere or mask the poles of the kidney, and the sonographer will need to make their best judgment on how to measure the length of the kidney. This will involve using the border of the mass to represent the pole of the kidney (Fig. 12-5A–H). There will be a slight variation in measurements between sonographers, called intervariability, and between repeated measurements from the same sonographer, called intravariability. If you realize that the sonographer on the prior study measured incorrectly, do not try to make your measurements match theirs, as this is very poor patient care. The radiologist, supervisor, or manager should directly discuss scanning errors with the employee that measured incorrectly. It is important for sonographers to remain professional and resist discussing errors or mistakes of colleagues among staff because this leads to a hostile working environment.

Renal Anatomy[3–9]

The kidney is bean shaped with a convex lateral border, a concave medial border, an upper pole, and a lower pole. The kidney is divided into the renal parenchyma, which consists of the renal cortex and the medulla, and the renal sinus (Fig. 12-6A, B). The renal cortex lies under the capsule and contains Bowman capsule, the glomerulus, and the proximal and distal convoluted tubules of the nephron. It is in the renal cortex where filtration occurs. The medulla is the inner portion of the renal parenchyma and contains the loop of Henle, which is where reabsorption takes place. The renal medulla consists of 7 to 14 renal pyramids, which are separated from each other by an inward extension of the renal cortex called a renal column or column of Bertin, through which the blood vessels pass. On average, there are eight renal pyramids in each kidney. The renal pyramids along with the surrounding cortical tissue create one lobe of the kidney. The arcuate arteries, which are located at the base of the pyramids, separate the medulla from the cortex and are termed the corticomedullary junction. The apex of the pyramid, called the renal papilla, fits into the cup-like

PATHOLOGY BOX 12-2
Normal Renal Measurements

Length	Men: 10–14 cm
	Women: 9–13 cm
	General number: 9–12 cm
Width	5–7 cm
Thickness	3–5 cm
Cortical thickness	6–10 mm
Parenchymal thickness	15–20 mm
Volume	Men: 110–190 mL
	Women: 90–150 mL

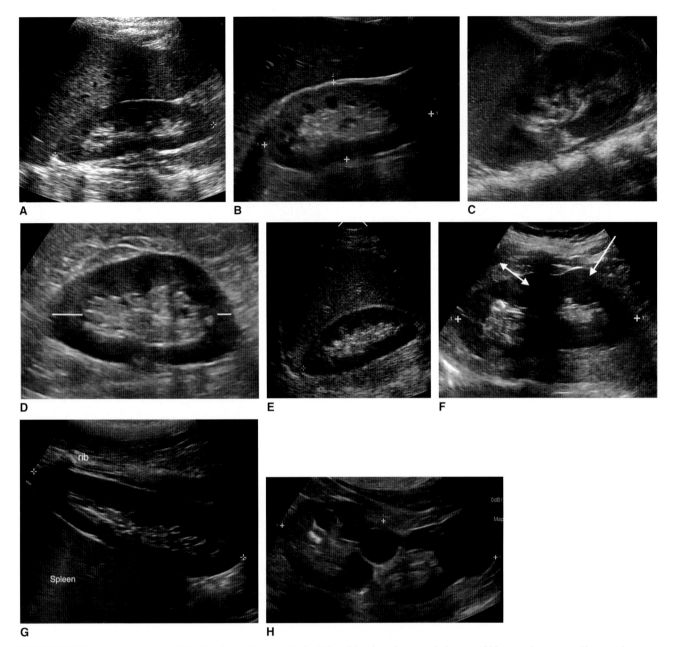

FIGURE 12-5 Renal measurements. **A:** Good technique in measuring the kidney. Note how the cortex is the same thickness at the upper and lower poles. There is a slight rib shadow through the middle of the kidney, which is acceptable for measuring purposes. **B:** In this image, the lower pole is obscured by the rib. The sonographer may sometimes "guess" where the lower pole should be, as in this case. Try following the curve of the kidney on both the anterior and posterior surfaces and determine where they would meet to form the lower pole. Note that the echogenicity of the kidney is brighter than the liver, which is compatible with medical renal disease, and the prominent pyramids. **C:** Note that the sinus echoes are touching the lower pole, indicating that this is an oblique image and not a true longitudinal and should not be used for a length measurement. This is the left kidney that has a dromedary hump. **D:** On this image, the cortical thickness of the lower pole is thinner than the upper pole, indicating that the image has been frozen in an oblique plane and should not be used to measure the length of the kidney. **E:** This image was obtained using a sector array transducer, which easily fits between the ribs because of its small footprint and allows good visualization of both the upper and lower poles. **F:** Here the rib shadow does not interfere with measuring the length of the kidney; however, the area under the rib must be evaluated. The *double-headed arrow* points to the rib shadow, and the single arrow to a solid renal mass. **G:** In this image, the patient is prone. A rib shadow is seen in the upper pole; however, it is not obscuring the border. **H:** There are multiple cysts in the kidney with a large cyst replacing the lower pole. Because the lower pole is not seen, the border of the cyst served as the lower pole. It would not be proper to guess where the lower pole border is inside the cyst as it would be hard to duplicate its location on follow-up examinations.

cavity of a minor calyx to collect the urine. There are between 7 and 14 minor calyces, which converge to form the two to three major calyces. Urine flows from a minor calyx into a major calyx and then into the funnel-shaped renal pelvis, which narrows to form the ureter at the UPJ. The renal sinus is a cavity located within the medial aspect of the kidney and contains blood vessels, the renal pelvis, and fat. Renal parenchyma surrounds the centrally located, hyperechoic renal sinus, which abuts the columns of Bertin without a connective tissue interface (Fig. 12-7). On the medial border of the kidney is an indentation called the renal hilum, which is where the renal arteries, nerves, lymphatics, and

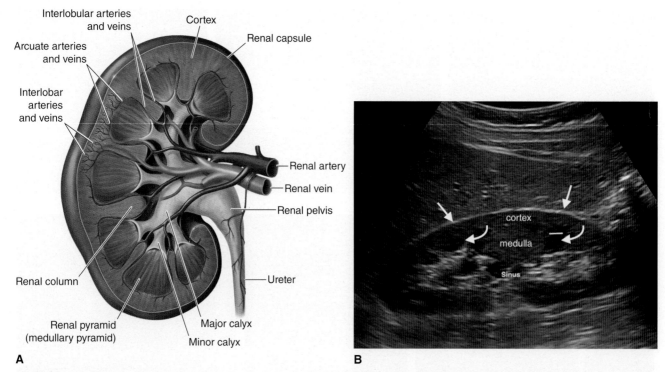

FIGURE 12-6 Renal anatomy. **A:** Interior view of the kidney demonstrating the different parts of renal anatomy, including renal vasculature. **B:** Image of a normal kidney identifying various parts of renal anatomy. The *solid line* indicates the area of the corticomedullary junction at the top of the pyramid. *Curved arrows* indicate renal pyramids, and *straight arrows* indicate Gerota fascia.

fat enter the kidney and the renal veins and ureter leave the kidney. The renal veins are anterior to the renal arteries, and the ureter is posterior to the renal vessels (Fig. 12-8A, B). The kidneys are surrounded by an inner fibrous capsule, a middle layer of perinephric fat, an outer layer of fibrous connective tissue that also surrounds the adrenal gland, and, finally, an outer layer of pararenal fat. The innermost layer is the fibrous renal capsule, which covers the surface of the kidney and goes between the kidney and the adrenal gland to provide support to the renal tissue and protection from infection. There is not any adipose tissue found between the renal parenchyma and the renal capsule. The renal capsule is covered by a layer of perirenal fat, called the adipose capsule or renal fat pad, which helps support

the kidney and is a protective layer acting as a shock absorber (Fig. 12-9A–C). The next layer anchors the kidneys to the surrounding structures and is the perirenal fascia, which is a collagen-filled, fibrous connective tissue that envelops the kidney, the adrenal gland, and the perirenal fat to form the perirenal space. The perirenal fascia divides into two layers that pass in front of and behind the kidney. The anterior and posterior fascial leaflets fuse, closing off the perirenal space from the rest of the retroperitoneum. The anterior perirenal fascia is called Gerota fascia, which separates the perinephric fat from the paranephric fat (Pathology Box 12-3). It is named after Dr. Dimitrie Gerota, an anatomist and the first Romanian radiologist and later urologist after losing his hand to radiodermatitis. The posterior renal fascia is a fibrous sheath covering the posterior side of the kidney and the perinephric space and is called Zuckerkandl fascia, named after the Hungarian Zuckerkandl brothers who worked together at The University of Vienna. Emil was an anatomist and surgeon, and Otto was a urologist. Emil described the posterior fascia in 1883 in a paper but did not recognize the anterior fascia. In 1895, Dr. Gerota described the anterior fascia and named the posterior fascia after Emil Zuckerkandl. The posterior pararenal space of the retroperitoneum is posterior to the Zuckerkandl fascia. Over time, the Zuckerkandl name has been forgotten and most people refer to both fasciae as Gerota fascia. Finally, there is another layer of fat, called the pararenal fat. The fatty layers are important in protecting and holding the kidneys in their normal position. When the amount of fatty tissue around the kidney rapidly decreases owing to rapid weight loss, it may cause a ureter to become kinked, causing hydronephrosis.

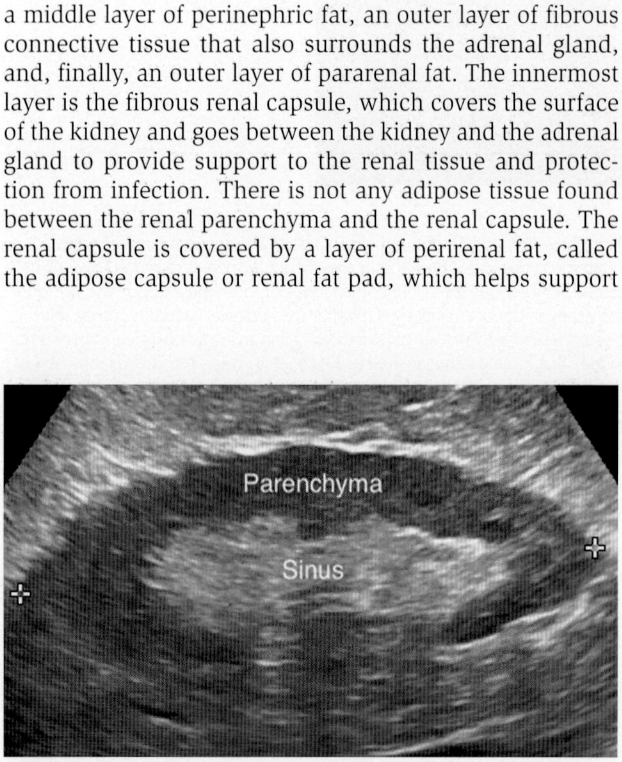

FIGURE 12-7 Image of a normal kidney identifying the parenchyma and the echogenic sinus.

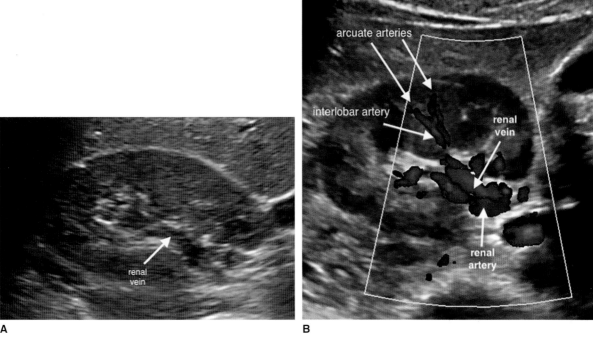

A **B**

FIGURE 12-8 Renal vasculature. **A:** Transverse image at the level of the renal hilum. The *arrow* is pointing to the renal vein, which can often be seen on the gray-scale image owing to its larger size. A color Doppler image of the area should be obtained to verify that it is the renal vein. **B:** Color Doppler image showing the renal vein in *blue* and the renal artery and its segmental branches in *red*. An interlobar artery is seen going between the pyramids and ending at the arcuate arteries, which demarcates the corticomedullary junction. The interlobar vein is seen next to the artery. Flow past the arcuate arteries is not seen because of the color velocity scale being too high.

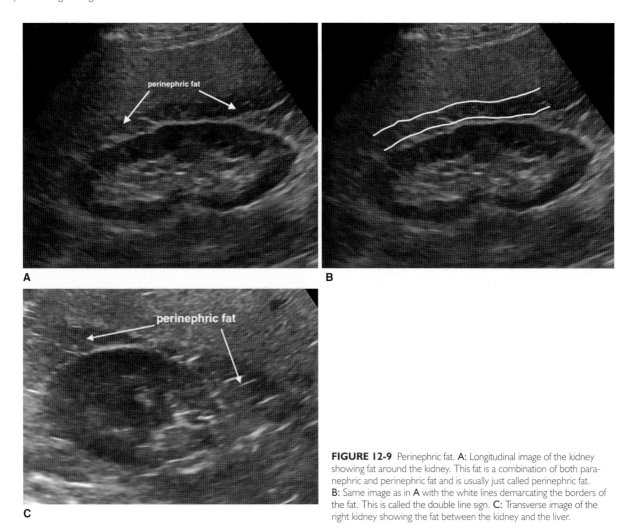

A **B**

C

FIGURE 12-9 Perinephric fat. **A:** Longitudinal image of the kidney showing fat around the kidney. This fat is a combination of both para-nephric and perinephric fat and is usually just called perinephric fat. **B:** Same image as in **A** with the white lines demarcating the borders of the fat. This is called the double line sign. **C:** Transverse image of the right kidney showing the fat between the kidney and the liver.

Vascular Anatomy[3–9]

The kidneys receive their blood supply from the renal arteries, which arise from the lateral borders of the aorta, at around the level of L1–2, just distal to the superior mesenteric artery (SMA). Approximately 20% to 30% of the cardiac output enters the renal arteries. They are the first lateral branches off the aorta, and their long axis is best seen in a transverse plane. The renal arteries are approximately 4 to 6 cm in length and 5 to 6 mm in diameter and are located posterior to the renal veins (Fig. 12-10). Because the aorta lies to the left of the midline, the right renal artery (RRA) is longer than the left and travels posterior to the inferior vena cava (IVC) on its way to the kidney (Fig. 12-11A, B). The left renal artery (LRA) is more superior in location and courses posterior to the left renal vein (LRV) (Fig. 12-12). The main renal artery supplies branches to the adrenal gland, ureter, perinephric tissue, and the renal capsule as it

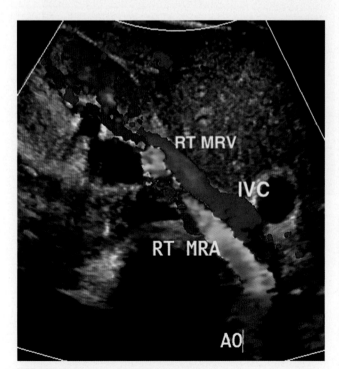

FIGURE 12-10 Transverse image showing the renal arteries coming off the aorta. *IV*, inferior vena cava; *LRA*, left renal artery; *LRV*, left renal vein; *RRA*, right renal artery, *SMA*, superior mesenteric artery.

approaches the renal hilum. The renal artery branches are an example of anatomic end arteries, which means that there is no communication between the arteries so that if one arterial branch becomes thrombosed or damaged, the renal parenchyma supplied by that vessel will become necrotic. The renal artery supplies blood to the five segments of the kidney: superior or apical, anterior superior, anterior inferior, inferior, and posterior. As the renal artery approaches the renal hilum, it divides into anterior and posterior segmental arteries, with the anterior branch receiving approximately 75% and the posterior branch approximately 25% of the blood flow. The first division of the renal artery is the posterior branch that passes behind the renal pelvis to become the posterior segmental artery. This branch supplies blood to a large portion of the posterior kidney. The main renal artery continues as the anterior branch, and at the renal hilum, it divides into the four anterior branches: the apical, upper, middle, and lower segmental branches. The apical segmental artery will supply blood to the anterior and posterior surfaces of the upper pole. The lower anterior segmental artery will supply blood to the anterior and posterior surfaces of the lower pole. The upper and middle segmental arteries supply blood to the remainder of the anterior surface. The segmental arteries then course through the renal sinus and branch into the lobar arteries. As the lobar arteries reach the minor calyces, they further divide into the interlobar arteries, which run between the pyramids, supplying them with blood. At the base of the pyramids, the interlobar arteries bend to form the incomplete arches of the arcuate arteries, indicating the true corticomedullary junction. The arcuate arteries travel across the top of the renal pyramids and give rise to the cortical radiate arteries, which were formerly known as interlobular arteries. The cortical radiate arteries come off the side of the arcuate artery at right angles and are arranged radially over the basal surface of the pyramids, perpendicular to the renal surface (Fig. 12-13). The cortical radiate arteries pass through the cortex as they divide to form the afferent arterioles. The afferent arterioles send the blood into a high-pressure capillary bed called the glomerulus where filtration takes place. The blood exits the glomerulus through the efferent arterioles. The efferent arterioles form a second capillary network around the tubule, which is called the peritubular capillaries, which empty their blood into a small network of venules that converge to become the cortical radiate veins. The blood next travels to the arcuate veins and then the interlobar veins, which form the main renal vein. Note that there are no segmental veins. The renal veins emerge from the renal hilum to enter the side wall of the IVC at about the level of L2 (Pathology Box 12-4). The right renal vein is typically about 3 to 4 cm in length as it is right next to the IVC, whereas the LRV is about 6 to 7 cm in length. The renal veins have a diameter of 10 to 12 mm. The LRV courses between the SMA and the aorta to reach the IVC (Fig. 12-14A–C). The LRV receives venous blood from the left adrenal vein, left gonadal (ovarian, testicular) vein, and the inferior phrenic vein. The right renal vein does not receive venous blood from other veins. The

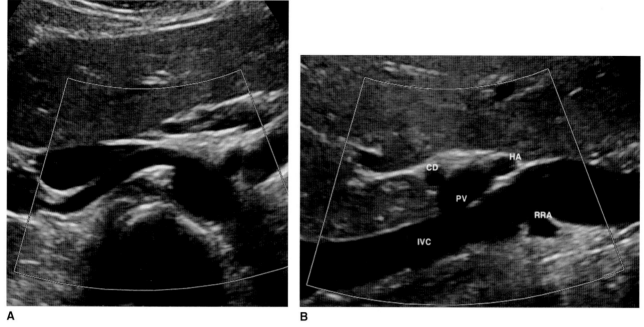

A　　　　　　　　　　　　　**B**

FIGURE 12-11 Surrounding vasculature. **A:** Grayscale image using a feature called Clarify™ that "cleans up" the noise inside vessels. This image shows the origin of the right renal artery off the aorta (*Ao*) as it passes posterior to the IVC. **B:** Longitudinal image of the IVC using Clarify™ showing a small circle posterior to the IVC, which is the right renal artery (*RRA*). Anterior to the IVC is the "Mickey Mouse" sign of the portal triad. *CD*, common duct; *HA*, hepatic artery; *IVC*, inferior vena cava; *PV*, portal vein.

nutcracker syndrome is when the LRV, the nut, is compressed between the SMA and the aorta, the nutcracker. Some patients may be asymptomatic, whereas others have hematuria, flank, or abdominal pain. Two common variants of the LRV are a retroaortic LRV, where the vein courses posterior to the aorta, and a circumaortic LRV, where both a retroaortic LRV and a normal renal vein pass anterior to the aorta (Fig. 12-15).

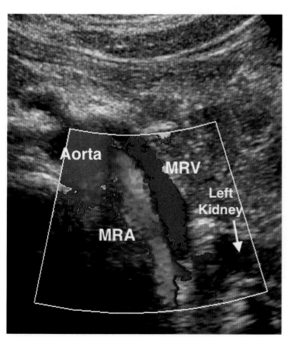

FIGURE 12-12 Color Doppler image of the left main renal artery (*MRA*, in *red*) and main renal vein (*MRV*, in *blue*) from a supine approach. Note that the left kidney is visible and the short length of the artery. The vein is superior to the artery. The color velocity scale was inverted from BART (*blue* away, *red* toward) so that the artery, which is going away from the transducer, is encoded with *red*.

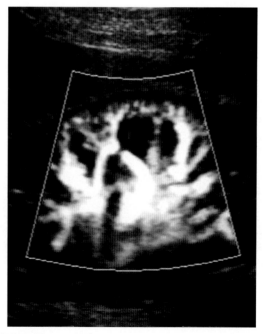

FIGURE 12-13 A power Doppler image showing normal perfusion of the kidney. Note the exceptional detail of the individual arteries even at the level of the cortical radiate arteries. When flow is seen all the way to the capsule, this is called cortical blush. Just like the spleen, there is no communication between branches.

PATHOLOGY BOX 12-4
Renal Vascular Anatomy

Abdominal aorta—brings blood from the heart to the abdomen

Main renal artery—branch of the aorta that comes off its side wall

Segmental arteries—usually five branches of the renal artery that brings blood to the different parts of the kidney. They course through the renal sinus and branch into the lobar arteries

Lobar arteries—When they reach the minor calyces, they divide into the interlobar arteries.

Interlobar arteries—They run between the pyramids and at the base of the pyramid they bend to form the incomplete arches of the arcuate arteries, which indicates the corticomedullary junction.

Arcuate arteries—They travel across the top of the renal pyramids and give rise to the cortical radiate arteries.

Cortical radiate arteries—These arteries come off the side of the arcuate artery at right angles and pass through the cortex to divide and form the afferent arterioles.

Afferent arterioles—These arterioles send the blood into a high-pressure capillary bed called the glomerulus.

Glomerulus—It is where filtration takes place.

Efferent arterioles—The efferent arterioles receive oxygenated blood from the glomerulus.

Peritubular capillaries—Capillary network that interacts with the tubule.

Venules—The venules receive blood from the peritubular capillaries and start the journey to the main renal vein.

From here the veins run alongside their same named arteries.

Cortical radiate veins—These veins receive the blood from the venules.

Arcuate veins—Receive the blood from the cortical radiate veins.

Interlobar veins—Receive the blood from the arcuate veins and form the main renal vein.

Main renal vein—Takes the unoxygenated blood away from the kidney and back to the heart.

IVC—The renal veins empty into the IVC, which takes the blood back to the heart.

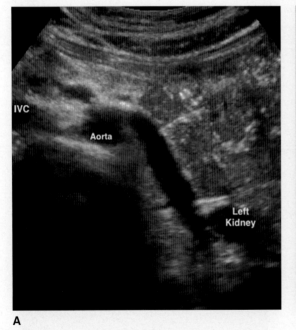

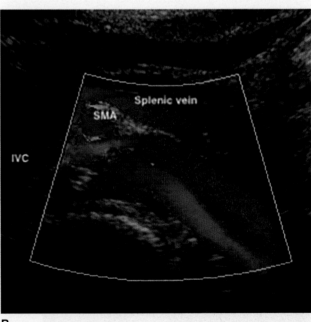

A   **B**

FIGURE 12-14 Renal veins. **A:** Transverse image from a supine position demonstrating the main left renal vein (*LRV*) from the kidney to the level of the aorta. As the renal veins are larger in diameter than the artery, it is easily seen on the grayscale image. **B:** *Blue* is toward the transducer, and *red* is away from the transducer. The LRV starts as *blue* because flow is toward the transducer. At mid aorta, the vein turns downward toward the inferior vena cava (*IVC*) and is now red because flow is now away from the transducer.

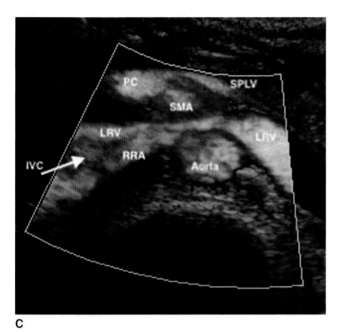

C

FIGURE 12-14 (*continued*) **C**: Power Doppler image of the LRV and surrounding vasculature. The increased resolution of power Doppler allows each vessel to be seen with no bleeding over as can be seen with color Doppler. With color Doppler, the right renal artery (*RRA*) and LRV are side by side going in the same direction, sometimes making it difficult to separate them, but each vessel is seen individually with power Doppler. *PC*, portal confluence; *SMA*, superior mesenteric artery; *SPLV*, splenic vein.

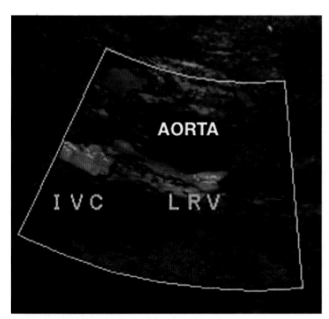

FIGURE 12-15 Color Doppler image of a retroaortic left renal vein (*LRV*). *IVC*, inferior vena cava.

PHYSIOLOGY AND MICROSCOPIC ANATOMY[3,6–12]

The kidneys play an important role in keeping our body functioning properly by removing and excreting waste products and regulating the amounts of electrolytes in the body. They are responsible for regulating blood pressure by removing excess water from the body as the kidneys need

the correct pressure to work properly. The kidneys ensure that the makeup and volume of the fluids in the body are correct by controlling the chemical balance of the blood and regulating the body's level of sodium, potassium, and calcium. The kidneys control the pH levels of the blood by maintaining an acid–base balance. The kidney is an endocrine organ and secretes several hormones, to maintain normal functioning of the body. If the kidney is not functioning properly, it will affect the entire body, causing organs, especially the liver and heart, to not function properly. The following are some of the hormones the kidneys produce and their function.

1. Erythropoietin is produced when oxygen levels in the blood are low, which signals the bone marrow to produce mature red blood cells (RBCs) to maintain healthy oxygen levels in our body.
2. Vitamin D is essential for several body functions. Vitamin D in an inactive form needs to be changed by the kidneys before it can act within the body. Active vitamin D stimulates the uptake of calcium from food, which is important for the maintenance of healthy bones.
3. Renin regulates angiotensin and aldosterone levels, called the renin–angiotensin system, and together they control blood pressure. If the kidneys are not functioning properly, they can release too much renin, causing vasoconstriction, retaining extra fluid, and increasing the blood pressure, which can lead to hypertension.

The formation of urine involves the following three processes: glomerular filtration, tubular reabsorption, and tubular secretion. Approximately 1,100 to 1,200 mL of blood passes through the kidneys every minute, with more than 90% of the blood going to the nephrons and only a small amount supplying the kidney's nutritional needs. One-third of the nephrons must function correctly, or the person will need to be on dialysis.

The nephron is the functional unit of the kidney, and each kidney has about 1 million nephrons. The functions of the nephron are to control blood concentration and volume by removing water and solutes as needed, help regulate blood pH, and remove toxic wastes. A nephron is composed of the renal corpuscle and renal tubules (Fig. 12-16A). The renal corpuscle is made up of Bowman capsule, a cup-like structure, and a tuft of capillaries called the glomerulus that sits inside it. The renal tubule is a long, convoluted structure that emerges from the glomerulus and is divided into three parts. The glomerulus and convoluted tubules of the nephron are in the cortex of the kidney, whereas the collecting ducts are in the pyramids of the medulla. The first part of the renal tubule is called the proximal convoluted tubule because it is near the glomerulus. The second part is called the loop of Henle, as it forms a loop with a descending and ascending limb that goes through the renal medulla. The third part of the renal tubule is called the distal convoluted tubule and is only found in the renal cortex and empties its filtrate into collecting ducts that line the medullary pyramids. Nephrons are classified into two types. Most of the nephrons are the cortical nephrons, which start high in the cortex and have a short loop of Henle that does not penetrate deeply into the medulla. Whereas the juxtamedullary nephrons start low in the cortex near the medulla and have a long loop of Henle that penetrates deeply into the renal medulla (Fig. 12-16B).

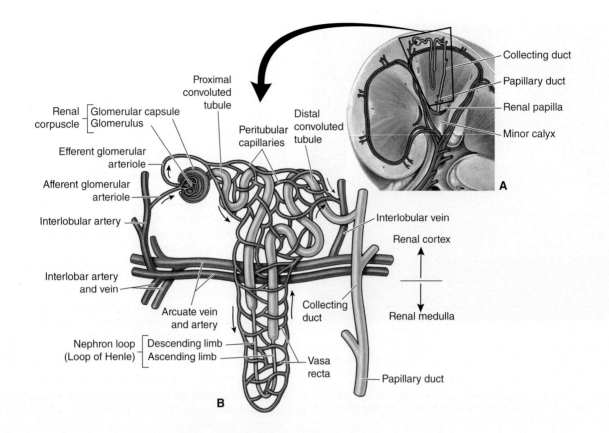

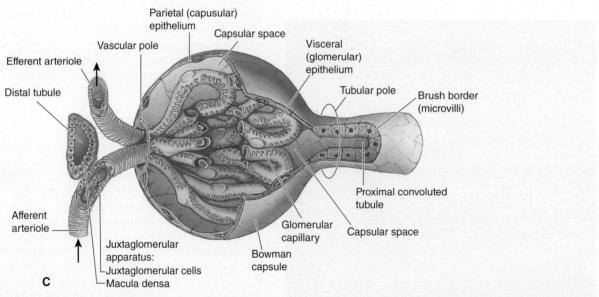

FIGURE 12-16 Nephron. **A:** Illustration of a nephron showing its relationship with the cortex and medulla. **B:** A detailed image of a nephron showing the various vessels and tubes and how they interact with one another. The *black arrows* show the flow of blood from the arterial to the venous side. The yellow tube is the path that urine follows. Recall that the interlobular vessels are now called the cortical radiate vessels. **C:** A diagram showing how blood enters the capillaries of the glomerulus through the afferent arteriole and exits via the efferent arteriole. (A hint to remember is that they are alphabetical.) The beginning of urine, called the filtrate at this point, exits the glomerulus via the proximal convoluted tubule.

What follows is basic information on how urine is made, and the reader is encouraged to read a more detailed explanation. Urine is formed by the filtration of blood in the nephron, where substances needed by the body are returned to the blood, whereas waste products and excessive water pass into the collecting ducts as urine. Blood enters the glomerulus via the afferent artery, which comes off the cortical radiate artery. Unlike most capillary beds, the glomerular capillaries will drain into the efferent arterioles rather than venules. The glomerular capillary hydrostatic pressure is affected by the afferent and efferent arteriolar resistance, which is the pressure exerted by fluid on the capillary walls of the glomerulus to provide the force for filtration. As blood pressure increases, it causes the hydrostatic pressure to

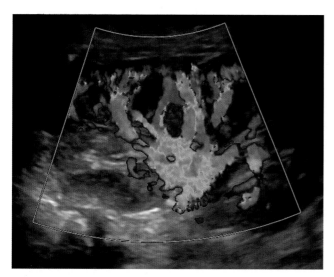

FIGURE 12-17 A color Doppler image showing intrarenal arteries (*red*) and intrarenal veins (*blue*). This patient has a fatty liver, so the echogenicity of the renal parenchyma is reduced.

increase as well. This causes an increase in the GFR, which increases the amount of water and solutes in the filtrate. The glomerulus is an intertwined group of capillaries and is responsible for filtering the blood. Glomerulus comes from the Latin "glomus," meaning ball of yarn as the capillaries look like a ball of yarn. The walls of the glomerulus act like a sieve, as they have tiny little holes called fenestrae that allow the smaller molecules of wastes and water to pass into Bowman capsule, whereas the larger molecules of proteins and blood cells will stay in the blood. The small molecules are forced through the fenestrae by the hydrostatic pressure within the glomerulus. The waste products and excessive water pass into Bowman capsule, which funnels these products, called the filtrate, into the proximal tubule. Blood then exits the glomerulus and flows into the efferent arterioles and passes into a set of peritubular capillaries, which follow the collecting tubule (Fig. 12-16C). The interaction between the peritubular capillaries and the tubules returns needed substances to the blood and removes wastes. As the fluid moves through the tubule, the peritubular capillaries reabsorb most of the water, along with nutrients that the body needs. The remaining fluid and wastes in the tubule become urine which drains from the collecting tubule into a minor calyx, which, in turn, empties into a major calyx, then into the renal pelvis, and finally into the ureter to drain the urine into the bladder. Back in the nephron, the blood enters a renal venule and begins the journey to the main renal vein following in reverse the path that the arterial blood used (Fig. 12-17).

SONOGRAPHIC ANATOMY AND NORMAL SONOGRAPHIC APPEARANCE[4-8,13]

The position of the kidney can vary slightly from patient to patient. The right kidney is posterior to the liver, whereas the left kidney is posterior to the spleen. The upper poles of the kidneys are partially protected by the 11th and 12th ribs. Once the location of the kidneys has been determined,

the contour and internal architecture are evaluated. The contour of a normal kidney should appear smooth. The internal renal has specific sonographic characteristics as described in the following sections.

Renal Capsule

The renal capsule appears sonographically as a bright reflector surrounding the kidney. It is a specular reflector and is only seen when imaged perpendicular to the sound beam (Fig. 12-18).

Renal Cortex

The renal parenchyma is best appreciated on a longitudinal view of the kidney and will demonstrate the cortex and the medullary pyramids. The renal cortex extends from the renal capsule to the bases of the pyramids and into the spaces between them, the columns of Bertin. The normal adult renal cortex is homogeneous with the echogenicity of the cortex less than, hypoechoic, or equal to, isoechoic, to that of the adjacent liver. Studies have shown that the cortex may appear isoechoic to the liver in adults with normal renal function. As the spleen is more echogenic than the liver, a normal left kidney will always be less echogenic than the spleen (Fig. 12-19A). In order to correctly compare the right kidney against the liver, it must be a normal echogenicity. Fatty livers will be markedly increased in echogenicity, and there will be a big difference in echogenicity between the two organs (Fig. 12-19B). Livers with hepatitis can cause the kidney to appear echogenic because of the decreased echogenicity of the liver (Fig. 12-19C, D). When the renal cortex is more echogenic than the liver, this is abnormal and is discussed later in this chapter.

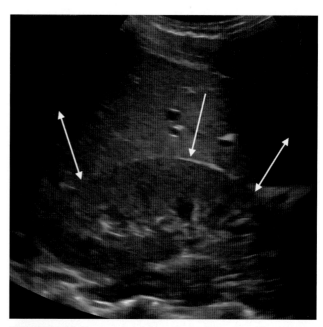

FIGURE 12-18 The *arrow* is pointing to Gerota fascia where it is echogenic as it is perpendicular to the sound beam. The *double-headed arrows* are pointing to where the echogenic line disappears. The upper pole seems to blend in with the liver parenchyma.

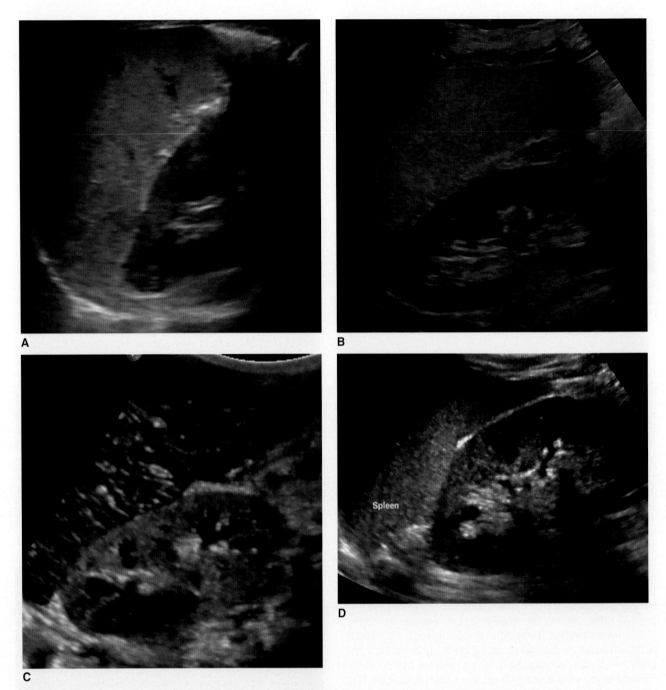

FIGURE 12-19 Kidney echogenicity. **A:** An image demonstrating that the left kidney is less echogenic than the spleen. It is acceptable to show just the upper pole of the left kidney for the comparison shot when it is difficult to show the entire left kidney. **B:** Note how the echoes in the kidney are reduced in echogenicity due to the increased attenuation of the fatty liver. **C:** This patient has hepatitis as seen by the increased echogenicity of the portal triads. To see the parenchyma of the kidney, the overall gain is increased, causing the kidney to appear more echogenic than the liver. **D:** Same patient as in C showing the normal relationship between the spleen and the left kidney, verifying that the echogenicity of the right kidney is normal.

Renal Medulla

Posterior to the cortex is the inner portion of the renal parenchyma, which is called the medulla and contains the renal pyramids. The renal pyramids are uniform in distribution and in size and shape. The broader base of each pyramid faces the cortical area, and its apex or papilla points toward the renal pelvis. Sonographically, the medullary pyramids are cone or triangle shaped and are hypoechoic relative to the renal cortex and can be seen in about 50% of normal adults. The pyramids are more visible when the kidney cortex is echogenic (Fig. 12-20).

Renal Sinus

The renal sinus is the central portion of the kidney and contains the major and minor calyces, the renal pelvis, renal vessels, fat, nerves, and lymphatics. The fat in the sinus

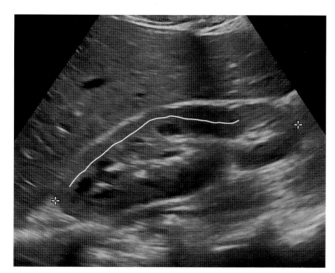

FIGURE 12-20 Longitudinal of the right kidney demonstrating several pyramids and the medulla tissue between them. The white line represents the border between the cortex and the medulla. This kidney is slightly more echogenic than the liver.

PATHOLOGY BOX 12-6
The Ureter

1. 25–35 cm in length
2. 3–4 mm in diameter
3. Common places where stones can get stuck:
   a. UPJ
   b. Where it crosses over the iliac vessels
   c. UVJ

is an extension of the perirenal fat. The renal sinus will appear as an oval highly echogenic structure in the center of the kidney. This bright echogenicity is not because the renal sinus is a dense structure but is caused by the multiple interfaces from fat, the calyces, renal pelvis, vessels, and lymphatics. The normal renal sinus should be more echogenic than both the normal renal cortex and the normal liver. The renal cortex is the least echogenic structure in the upper abdomen, whereas the renal sinus is the most echogenic structure (Pathology Box 12-5).

Renal Pelvis

The normal renal pelvis is not seen with US unless it is dilated. If the patient is well hydrated, the renal pelvis may sometimes be seen as a lighter gray echo pattern inside the echogenic renal sinus.

Ureter

From the renal pelvis, urine flows into the ureters, which are approximately 25- to 30-cm long and 3 to 4 mm in diameter. The smooth muscle wall of the calyces, pelvis, and ureters contracts rhythmically and propels urine by peristalsis to the bladder where it is stored. The ureter is not seen sonographically unless it is dilated. When dilated, the proximal ureter can be seen, leaving the kidney. There are three areas

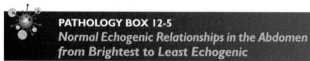

PATHOLOGY BOX 12-5
Normal Echogenic Relationships in the Abdomen from Brightest to Least Echogenic

1. Renal sinus
2. Pancreas
3. Spleen
4. Liver
5. Renal cortex

along the course of the ureter where it narrows, allowing a stone to become stuck: at the UPJ, as the ureter enters the pelvis and crosses over the common iliac artery bifurcation, and at the ureterovesical junction (UVJ), which is the most common place (Pathology Box 12-6).

RENAL FUNCTION TESTS[7,14,15]

One of the most common requests for a renal sonogram is elevated blood urea nitrogen (BUN) and creatinine, especially on patients in a hospital. However, there are other laboratory values that the sonographer should understand. Because the sonogram is of the kidneys, there will be both blood and urine lab tests to evaluate. Fortunately, it is not necessary to know the range of normal values because the report will give the range of normal values used by that lab along with high or low values highlighted on the report (Pathology Box 12-7).

Blood Tests

1. BUN measures the amount of urea nitrogen in the blood. It is usually ordered along with creatinine to help evaluate renal function. Urea nitrogen is a normal waste product in the blood that comes from the breakdown of protein from food during digestion.

   The formation of urea begins in the liver. Proteins that are used by the cells of the body produce ammonia. Ammonia is highly toxic and cannot be allowed to accumulate. In the liver cells, carbon dioxide reacts chemically with the ammonia and produces urea. Urea is next released into the bloodstream as a small water-soluble molecule. It is filtered out by the kidneys and excreted in the urine. BUN increases in renal failure, renal parenchymal disease, obstructive uropathy, congestive heart failure (CHF), dehydration, hemorrhage, and eating a high-protein diet. Values can decrease in liver failure, overhydration, pregnancy, and not consuming enough protein. BUN can also increase with age.

2. Creatinine is a waste product produced by the muscles from the breakdown of the compound creatine and is removed from the blood by the kidneys, primarily by glomerular filtration, and eliminated from the body in the urine. It is more sensitive than BUN to evaluate renal function. The amount of creatinine produced depends on body size and muscle mass, and therefore, creatinine levels can be slightly higher in men. Increased creatinine can be caused by glomerulonephritis, acute

PATHOLOGY BOX 12-7
Renal Blood and Urine Tests

Renal blood tests

1. BUN measures the amount of urea nitrogen in the blood. Used to help determine renal function
   a. Increases in
      i. Renal failure
      ii. Parenchymal disease
      iii. Urinary obstruction
      iv. Decreased blood flow
      v. Dehydration
   b. Decreases in
      i. Liver failure
      ii. Overhydration
      iii. Pregnancy
      iv. With age
2. Creatinine is a waste product from the breakdown of the compound creatine produced by the muscles. It is removed from the blood primarily by glomerular filtration and eliminated in the urine. It is more sensitive than BUN to evaluate renal function.
   a. Increases in
      i. Glomerulonephritis
      ii. ATI
      iii. Diabetics
      iv. Urinary obstruction
      v. Decreased blood flow
      vi. Certain medications such as Bactrim, Zantac, Tagamet, Keflex, and chronic or excessive use of NSAIDs
   b. Decreased values are not a concern for renal function

3. eGFR
   a. Accurate indicator of kidney function as it measures how well the glomeruli are filtering the blood.
   b. Decreases when there is decreased blood flow to the glomerulus, urinary obstruction, and primary renal disease.
   c. Increases values are not a concern.

Urine tests

1. Proteinuria occurs when protein or albumin is passing through the glomerulus or tubules and is ending up in the urine.
   a. Causes include
      i. Diabetes
      ii. Hypertension
      iii. Glomerulonephritis
      iv. Nephrotic syndrome
      v. Overuse of NSAIDs
      vi. Renal vein thrombosis
2. Hematuria is when there are RBCs in the urine. The bleeding can happen anywhere in the urinary system.
   a. Causes include
      i. UTI
      ii. Pyelonephritis
      iii. Kidney stones
      iv. Prostate enlargement
      v. Post–kidney biopsy complication
      vi. TCC
      vii. Renal vein thrombosis
      viii. Cystitis

---

tubular injury (ATI), complication of diabetes, blocked urinary tract, and certain medications such as Bactrim, Zantac, Tagamet, Tricor, cephalosporin antibiotics such as Keflex, and chronic or excessive nonsteroidal anti-inflammatory drug (NSAID) use. It is uncommon to have low levels of creatinine and is usually not a cause for concern. Increased BUN and creatinine levels in the blood indicate decreased renal function.

3. BUN/creatinine ratio. When the BUN levels are compared with the creatinine levels, it gives a better understanding of kidney function and is known as the BUN/creatinine ratio. The BUN/creatinine ratio is useful to help differentiate between acute and chronic renal disease. An increase in BUN/creatinine ratio can be caused by renal disease, such as AKI, dehydration, gastrointestinal (GI) bleeding, hyperthyroidism, CHF, and certain antibiotics and corticosteroids. This ratio can also increase with age and decreasing muscle mass. A low BUN/creatinine ratio can be caused by advanced liver disease, renal failure, hypothyroidism, and diets poor in protein.

4. eGFR is a calculation of the GFR and provides a more accurate indicator of kidney function. It is the volume of fluid filtered from the glomerular capillaries into Bowman capsule per unit time. It is calculated from a formula based on the creatinine serum test and other factors including age and gender. GFR is a measure of functional renal mass and is influenced by glomerular capillary hydrostatic pressure and renal blood flow. It indicates how well the glomerular filtration process is working and can be used to help determine the stage of kidney disease so that the best treatment can be determined. The eGFR can decrease with primary renal disease, decreased renal perfusion, or obstructive renal disease. Patients with renal artery stenosis can be at risk of having a decreased eGFR due to the reduction of blood to the glomerulus. An eGFR score below 60 mL/min/1.73 m^2 (milliliters of cleansed blood per minute per body surface) suggests kidney disease, and an eGFR below 15 mL/min/1.73 m^2 indicates ESRD and the patient needs to be started on dialysis. eGFR can decrease with age. This is one lab value where the higher the number, the better the outcome.

5. An increase in RBCs can be seen in patients with renal cell carcinoma (RCC). A low RBC count, which can cause anemia, can be seen in chronic renal disease.

6. An increase in white blood cells (WBCs) can be seen in patients with an infection or inflammatory process such as pyelonephritis and has been seen in patients with kidney stones. A low WBC count has been associated with CKD in the elderly.

Urine Tests

1. Proteinuria is when there is a high amount of protein in the urine and is an indication of an underlying disease that needs to be determined. Normally, the plasma proteins are too large to go through the filtration process in the glomerulus. The smaller proteins, usually albumin, that pass through the glomerulus are reabsorbed by the tubules. Proteinuria occurs when either the glomeruli or tubules in the kidney are damaged. When there is kidney damage, the protein that goes through the filter is not reabsorbed back into the blood but passes into the urine. The most common cause of proteinuria is seen in patients with diabetes or hypertension. Other causes include patients with glomerulonephritis, nephrotic syndrome, or certain medications, especially NSAIDs, and patients with renal vein thrombosis. Some patients may have temporary proteinuria, particularly in younger people after exercise or during an illness, patients who are dehydrated, and patients who are under emotional stress. Proteinuria due to exercise usually resolves in 24 hours. Persistent high levels of protein in the urine may indicate kidney disease. Low levels of protein in the urine are normal.

2. Albuminuria is when there is too much albumin protein in the urine. Because albumin is a type of protein and the main protein found in proteinuria, the two terms are used interchangeably, although they are not the same thing. Other proteins can be found in proteinuria, whereas albumin is the only protein in albuminuria. Because albumin molecules are small, they are among the first protein to pass through the filtration process and end up in the urine. When the kidneys are functioning properly, there should be no albumin seen in the urine. Albuminuria is the earliest indicator of glomerular disease and is seen with cardiovascular disease. The most common cause is diabetes and can be an early indicator of diabetic nephropathy. Other causes include hypertension, cirrhosis, heart failure, and lupus.

3. Microalbumin/creatinine ratio is usually used to screen people who are at higher risk for kidney disease. The test measures the albumin and creatinine in a urine sample collected randomly, as opposed to a timed collection, and an albumin-to-creatinine ratio is calculated. An albumin-to-creatinine ratio is calculated by dividing albumin concentration in milligrams by creatinine concentration in grams. Creatinine is released into the urine at a constant rate, and its level in the urine is an indication of urine concentration. This property of creatinine allows its value to be used to correct for urine concentration when measuring albumin in a random urine sample. This provides a more accurate indication of the how much albumin is in the urine. If the albumin-to-creatinine ratio shows albumin in the urine, the patient may be tested again to confirm the results. If the results continue to show albumin in urine, it is suggestive of early-stage kidney disease. If the test results show high levels of albumin, it is suggestive of renal failure.

4. Hematuria is when there are blood cells in the urine. *Hematuria* may be defined as microscopic hematuria, when the blood cells are only seen with a microscope, and gross hematuria, when the blood in the urine can be seen with the eye. Blood can come from the kidneys or other parts of the urinary tract. Hematuria is a symptom and not a disease, and the treatment is dictated by the cause. Causes of hematuria include a urinary tract infection (UTI), pyelonephritis, kidney stones, prostate enlargement, post–kidney biopsy complication, kidney trauma, bladder or kidney transitional cell carcinoma (TCC), renal vein thrombosis, and cystitis. Medications such as aspirin, Coumadin, or Plavix can cause hematuria. Intense exercise or sustained aerobic exercise can be the source of hematuria, and often, the urine clears up in a few days. Runners are most often affected. Sometimes, the cause of hematuria cannot be identified.

SONOGRAPHIC SCANNING TECHNIQUE[4,7,8]

Sonographers will need to select the correct transducers, patient positions, technical controls, and protocol. It is important for the sonographer both to attend the patient and to scan properly to reduce their scanning-related risks for musculoskeletal (MSK) injuries.

Patient Preparation

No patient preparation is needed for a renal sonogram. If the bladder needs to be imaged, then it must contain urine and the patient should drink 16 to 24 ounces of fluid about 30 minutes before the examination. If an abdominal study is also ordered, then the patient will need to be NPO (nothing by mouth) for 6 to 8 hours.

Transducer

The most common transducer to use is a curved linear-array transducer of the appropriate frequency for the size of the patient. Common frequencies used are in the 1 to 6 MHz range. To scan between the ribs, a sector transducer may be utilized. Scanning is usually performed with harmonics turned on, but this can cause penetration issues, especially on patients with fatty livers. If the echoes in the far field are absent or washed out, owing to the overall gain being increased, turn harmonics off and evaluate the image. It may be a more diagnostic image without using harmonics. Sometimes, the sonographer may need to take two images, one with and one without harmonics, to have images with the best resolution and an image with proper penetration (Fig. 12-21A, B). Compound imaging is another control that can be used to help reduce artifacts in the image. Sometimes, it may interfere with the acoustic shadow or enhancement artifacts. Always try scanning with these controls on and off to see which gives the better image.

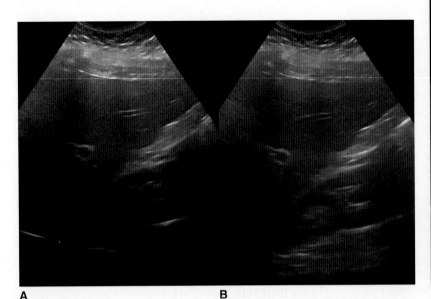
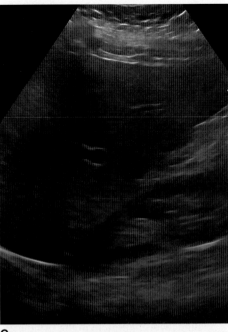

A   **B**   **C**

FIGURE 12-21 Technical settings. **A:** This patient has a fatty liver with the image obtained using harmonics and no other adjustments made. The vascular structures in the liver are full of echoes, and there are no echoes in the far field of the liver and in the renal parenchyma. **B:** The same patient with the overall gain increased to see the far-field echoes and the time gain compensation adjusted to help balance the image. Echoes in the kidney parenchyma are seen, but the vascular structures still have echoes inside them. The overall image looks grayed out. **C:** This is the same patient with harmonics turned off. The parenchymal echoes in the liver and kidney are now seen, and cystic structures remain echo free. Overall, this is a much better image than image **B.** Harmonics does not always improve the image but can degrade it.

Patient Position

The native kidneys are scanned in a supine position to start, using the liver and spleen as acoustic windows. Usually, the transducer is placed subcostal on the side of the patient aiming toward the midline, making the imaging plane is a variation of a coronal plane. Images may also be obtained from an intercostal approach. Usually, both approaches are needed. If the kidneys are not adequately seen from a supine position, then a posterior oblique position can be tried. If one or the other kidney is still not very well seen, then scanning the kidney from a right or left lateral decubitus view may allow better visualization of the kidney. If the kidneys are still not optimally seen, scanning them with the patient in a prone position can often visualize them as there will be no issue with the ribs or bowel gas. When scanning in a prone position, a pillow or a rolled sheet can be placed under the abdomen at the level of the kidneys to help increase the space between the iliac crest and the ribs. This is a good position to scan newborns. Because turning a patient into a prone position can be difficult, one work around is while the patient is in a decubitus position, place the transducer on the back of the patient as if they were in a prone position (Fig. 12-22). It may take scanning the patient in a variety of positions to properly evaluate the entire kidney.

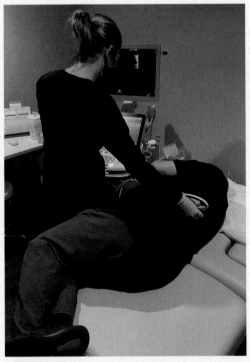

FIGURE 12-22 The patient is in a right lateral decubitus, or left side up, position with the transducer perpendicular to the skin at the level of the left kidney.

Transducer Positions

The long axis of the kidney is in an oblique plane, so the transducer will also need to be in an oblique plane. When the patient is supine, the kidneys are closer to the stretcher as they are retroperitoneal organs and located in the back of the patient. Having the transducer in the middle of the side of the patient is typically not a good spot to see the kidney. The transducer should be near the stretcher and angled toward the abdominal wall, until the kidney is seen. (Sometimes, the sonographer's hand is resting on the stretcher to see the kidney.) If the upper pole is not well seen owing to the angle of reflection issues, moving the transducer up toward the head and scanning between the ribs will give a better angle and the upper pole can be better appreciated (Fig. 12-23A, B). In transverse images, the upper pole can be obtained between the ribs, the mid from either an intercostal approach, especially the left kidney, or a subcostal approach and the lower poles from a subcostal approach (Fig. 12-24A–C).

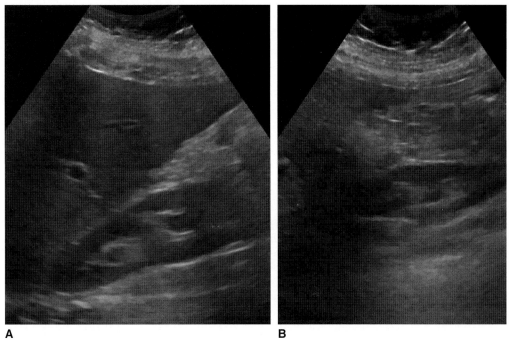

A **B**

FIGURE 12-23 Approaches to visualize the long kidney. **A:** Using an intercostal approach, the upper pole and middle of the kidney are well demonstrated. The lower pole has some bowel interference and is not visualized well. **B:** This image is obtained from a subcostal approach, and the upper half of the kidney is not seen due to bowel gas. The lower pole is best seen from this approach. The sonographer should image the kidney with both intercostal and subcostal approaches.

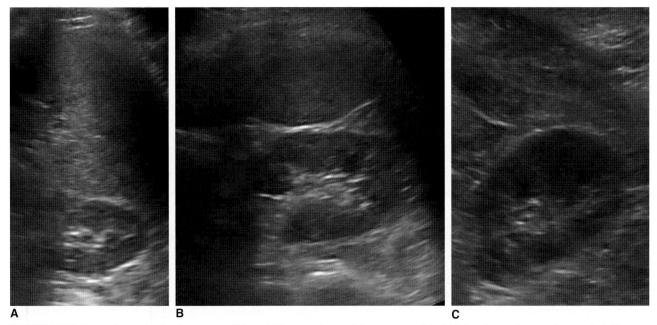

A **B** **C**

FIGURE 12-24 Approaches to visualize the transverse kidney. **A:** Transverse image of the upper pole of the left kidney from an intercostal approach. **B:** Transverse image of the mid pole of the left kidney from an intercostal approach. **C:** Transverse image of the lower pole of the left kidney from a subcostal approach.

Breathing Technique

When the patient is scanned from a subcostal approach, a deep inspiration will bring the kidneys down from under the ribs. When scanning from an intercostal approach, the goal is to get the kidney in a good position between the ribs. This can take trying a variety of breathing styles, including having the patient in quiet breathing, which is letting the patient breath normally or in a full or partial expiration. On some patients, a combination of breathing styles and approaches may be needed. For example, to see the upper pole of the kidney, an intercostal approach is used with the patient is in full expiration, whereas the lower pole is best seen from a subcostal approach with the patient in a deep inspiration.

Bladder Images

This section discusses when to include the bladder as part of the examination. The anatomy and pathology of the bladder is discussed in Chapter 13.

In some departments, a renal sonogram always includes longitudinal and transverse images of the bladder, whereas in other departments, it is only scanned when clinically indicated. To evaluate the bladder, there needs to be some urine inside of it.

When there is bilateral hydronephrosis, the bladder should be scanned to see if it is too full and causing the hydronephrosis. If the patient has a full bladder, ask them to take their time and empty their bladder fully. (Some patients will quickly empty their bladder but not fully because they do not want to hold up the room.) After the bladder is emptied, the kidneys should then be rescanned to evaluate if the hydronephrosis stayed the same or went away. If there is still some degree of hydronephrosis present, recheck the bladder to evaluate how full it is.

When there is hematuria clinically, images of the bladder should be obtained to evaluate if the bladder is the source of the bleeding. Kidney stones, blood clots, tumors, or thickened bladder walls caused by cystitis can all be the causes of the hematuria.

If there is a concern for kidney stones, color Doppler should be used to evaluate the bladder for ureteral jets. The speed of the urine leaving the ureter is fast enough to produce a Doppler shift, and the jet can be appreciated with color Doppler as a sudden burst of color in the bladder toward the transducer (Fig. 12-25). Normally, ureteral jets should occur twice or more per minute and should be symmetric with color Doppler in a healthy individual. The jets are directed upward and toward the contralateral side crossing the midline. A nonobstructive stone is suspected with a weak jet or when color constantly "dribbles" out of the ureteral orifice. If a color jet is not visualized, then obstruction should be suspected, especially if multiple jets have been seen on the contralateral side.

Doppler

This section discusses when to add color and spectral Doppler to the examination. Renal arterial and venous Doppler examinations are discussed in Chapter 6.

Color and spectral Doppler may need to be added to a routine renal US for various reasons, such as patients with

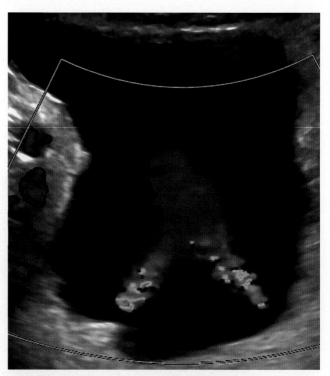

FIGURE 12-25 A good example of bilateral bladder jets indicating that there is no obstruction present. In some patients, it may be necessary to take an image of each jet.

pyelonephritis, medical renal disease, and evaluation of a renal mass. The renal preset should be used over a general or abdominal one. A renal preset optimizes the US machine, especially the Doppler settings, for the kidneys, whereas the general or abdominal presets are optimized for the liver (Fig. 12-26A, B). The sonographer should adjust the color velocity scale and color gain to appropriate settings to allow for good visualization of flow inside the kidney and in the main renal vessels.

The following paragraphs of this section discuss scenarios when color and spectral Doppler would be appropriate to include with a routine renal examination. It should be noted that adding color and spectral Doppler to an examination does not automatically allow the sonographer to upcharge to a more expensive renal Doppler study that was not originally ordered. The billing or coding department should be consulted as up-charging inappropriately puts the department at risk for being fined for fraudulent coding.

Some departments might require a color Doppler image with or without a spectral Doppler waveform of the main renal artery and vein at the hilum of the kidney to assess inflow and outflow in all studies. Some clinicians just want to know that there is flow to the kidney and flow leaving the kidney. In some patients, the renal vein may be prominent or dilated, which could mimic hydronephrosis. Color Doppler should be used to investigate this area of dilatation to show if it is a vein (Fig. 12-27A–E).

The resistive index (RI) is an arterial measurement that is obtained from the interlobar artery and relates to renal vascular resistance and is influenced by the amount of diastolic flow. This measurement reflects the condition of the vascular bed where blood flow is traveling.

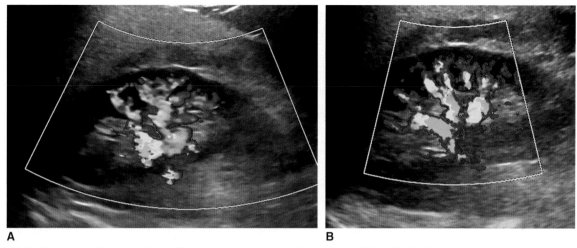

FIGURE 12-26 Renal presets. **A:** Flow inside the kidney using a general setting. The flow is very "blobby" looking because color is bleeding outside the border of the vessel. **B:** Same kidney using the renal preset. Note the difference in the appearance of the renal vessels. When using the renal preset, the vessels are more defined and flow is seen out to the capsule.

The RI is determined by the following equation:

$$RI = \text{peak systole} - \text{end diastole/peak systole}$$

The RI is calculated by the US unit and is determined by the sonographer placing the calipers at peak systole and end diastole. An RI does not require the use of angle correction. The normal kidney should have an RI between 0.6 and 0.7. A RI greater than 0.7 is suggestive of increased vascular pressure, resistance, or compliance inside the kidney. It is important to properly measure the signal as it is easy to mistake noise or mirror artifact for diastolic flow (Fig. 12-28A–E). Observing the color Doppler pattern will help determine when end diastole occurs. If the color is flashing, that is, the arterial

flow completely disappears in diastole, then there is no flow in end diastole and the RI is 1. If the arterial flow just about disappears and end-diastolic flow is minimal, then the RI will be greater than 0.8. If the arterial flow is seen very well during diastole, then the RI will be normal, less than 0.7. End-diastolic flow is correctly measured right before the next systolic upstroke as this represents the end of the diastolic cycle. End-diastolic flow should not be measured where diastolic flow stops if it is before the systolic upstroke. Some common examples when an RI should be measured in a kidney include patients with medical renal disease, those with AKI, those with CKD, and patients with hypertension caused and not caused by renal artery stenosis.

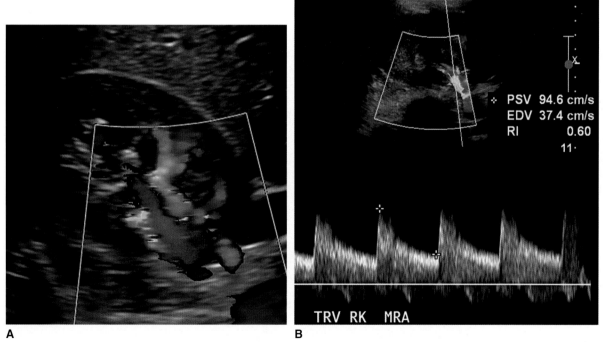

FIGURE 12-27 Color and spectral Doppler. **A:** Color Doppler image of the right kidney at the hilum showing a normal main renal artery (*MRA*) and main renal vein. **B:** Spectral Doppler of the MRA with a low resistive signal and a velocity of 94.6 cm/sec and a resistive index (*RI*) of 0.60.

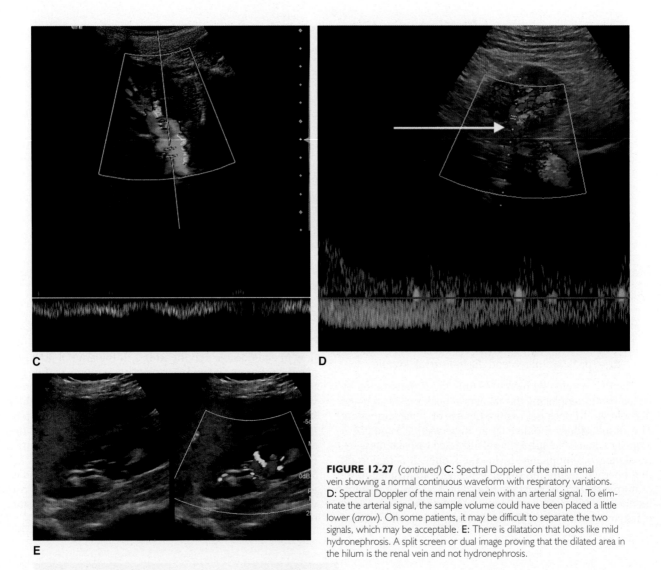

FIGURE 12-27 *(continued)* **C:** Spectral Doppler of the main renal vein showing a normal continuous waveform with respiratory variations. **D:** Spectral Doppler of the main renal vein with an arterial signal. To eliminate the arterial signal, the sample volume could have been placed a little lower *(arrow)*. On some patients, it may be difficult to separate the two signals, which may be acceptable. **E:** There is dilatation that looks like mild hydronephrosis. A split screen or dual image proving that the dilated area in the hilum is the renal vein and not hydronephrosis.

A color or power Doppler image of the entire kidney should be obtained to show perfusion in patients with AKI or CKD to evaluate for flow inside the kidney (Fig. 12-29). Patients who have pyelonephritis need a perfusion image to look for areas of flow voids that might be caused by early abscess formation. A common reason is to show perfusion in a "pseudotumor" on a patient with a dromedary hump or fetal lobulations to show that these areas have normal perfusion (Fig. 12-30A–C). A renal mass will not demonstrate perfusion but flow on the border of the mass and sometimes specs of color inside the mass.

An uncommon reason is when one kidney is unexpectedly found to be very small, less than 6 cm, to document for renal artery occlusion by showing a lack of flow in the kidney (Fig. 12-31).

Color Doppler can be helpful in identifying small stones as it produces what is called the twinkling artifact that is caused by the calcium in the stone. Any bright echoes in the kidney should be investigated with color Doppler.

The twinkling artifact does not occur with every stone nor does seeing the artifact always mean that it is caused by a stone (Fig. 12-32A–C).

RENAL PROTOCOL[8]

The following suggested protocol is based on the current protocol, at the time of publication, found on the American Institute of Ultrasound in Medicine (AIUM) or the American College of Radiology (ACR) website. Besides the AIUM and ACR, the Society for Pediatric Radiology (SPR) and the Society of Radiologists in Ultrasound (SRU) have worked together to create this protocol. The renal protocol is found in the document entitled *Practice Parameter for the Performance of an Ultrasound Examination of the Abdomen and/or Retroperitoneum.*

Vascular protocols can be found on the ACR website and the Intersocietal Accreditation Commission Vascular Testing (IAC VT) website. These protocols are free, and

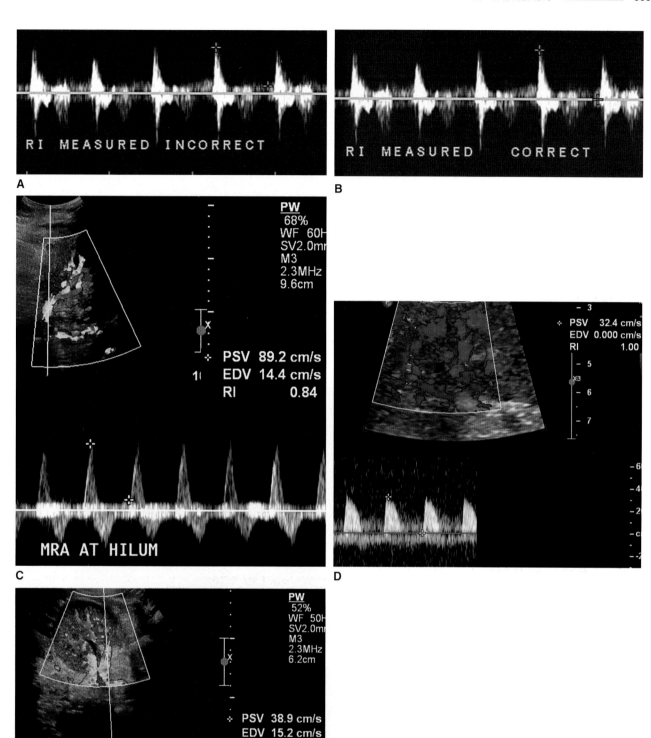

FIGURE 12-28 Diastolic flow. **A:** The end-diastolic flow on this spectral Doppler signal is measuring flow from an adjacent vessel. Note how the systolic flow is a bright white signal and the diastolic flow is gray. Closely evaluating the false diastolic flow, the signal can be seen going through the systolic signal. **B:** Same signal with the diastolic flow being properly measured at the baseline as there is no diastolic flow at the end of diastole. **C:** An example of noise being measured for diastolic flow. Here the signal can be seen going in front of the systolic signal. This is a biphasic arterial signal, and these signals and triphasic signals do not have flow at the end of diastole. **D:** A properly measured end diastole despite the signal being seen through diastole. This is a monophasic arterial signal, and they do not have end-diastolic flow. The signal appears to be a mirror image artifact of the venous flow. **E:** An example of a properly measured normal signal. *MRV,* main renal vein.

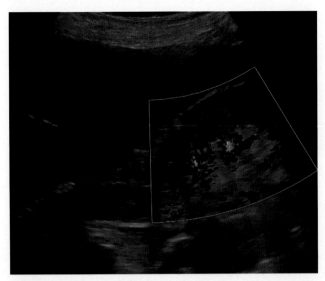

FIGURE 12-29 A color Doppler image of a patient with an echogenic kidney due to an acute kidney injury from computed tomography contrast agent demonstrating the poor flow in the kidney.

you do not have to be a member of the organization to download them. They can be found on each organization's website and should be reviewed annually for any changes. This is important as current protocols are what accreditation reviewers will use to judge your examinations. The following required images are a small representation of what a sonographer sees while scanning. The images should be sufficient and technically accurate to provide the interpreting physician the information needed to make a correct diagnosis. All pathology must be documented in at least two planes. Some departments may require a video clip through each kidney.

Before starting the examination, the sonographer should take the time to look at the patient's medical history, any imaging reports, and the appropriate lab values. Remember for the kidney to check both blood and urine lab values, which should only take a few minutes. Make sure that the room is prepared and that all needed transducers and supplies are handy. Before scanning, introduce yourself, and explain the sonogram including what they should expect during the examination,

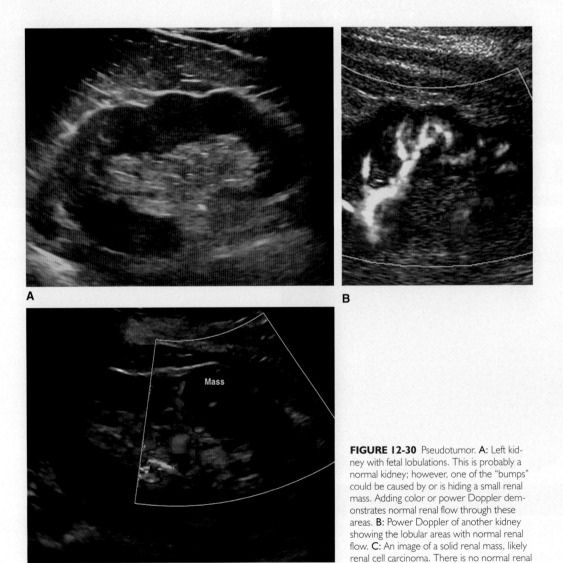

FIGURE 12-30 Pseudotumor. **A:** Left kidney with fetal lobulations. This is probably a normal kidney; however, one of the "bumps" could be caused by or is hiding a small renal mass. Adding color or power Doppler demonstrates normal renal flow through these areas. **B:** Power Doppler of another kidney showing the lobular areas with normal renal flow. **C:** An image of a solid renal mass, likely renal cell carcinoma. There is no normal renal perfusion seen inside the mass.

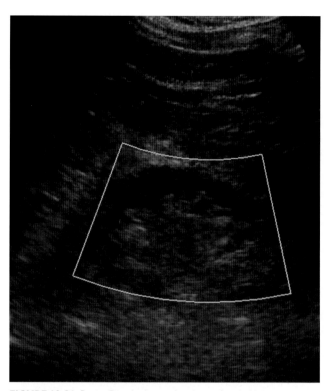

FIGURE 12-31 Power Doppler image showing no flow inside an unexpected small kidney compatible with renal artery occlusion. Patients usually do not feel anything when this occurs, and if the other kidney is functioning normally, lab values and urine output are not affected.

breathing requirements, the different positions that may be needed, and how long the examination will take. Ask the patient if they have any questions and their understanding of why they are having the test. Now, you are ready to start scanning!

Longitudinal Images

A long-axis image of the middle of the kidney measuring the longest length of the kidney and the renal cortical thickness. One to two longitudinal images of the kidney documenting from midline to its lateral border. One to two longitudinal images of the kidney documenting from midline to its medial border. An image demonstrating the liver and right kidney together and the spleen and left kidney together for parenchymal comparison (Fig. 12-33A–E).

Transverse Images

A transverse image at the mid pole of the kidney, with the transducer angled to be perpendicular to the kidney. Note that the current AIUM/ACR/SRU/SPR protocol does not require a transverse or an anteroposterior (AP) (or height) measurement, but some departments still may require these measurements. The department can add to a protocol, but they cannot delete any required images. Next one to two transverse images of the kidney documenting from the upper pole to the mid kidney and one to two transverse images of

the kidney documenting from the mid kidney to the lower pole (Fig. 12-34A–E).

Additional Images

Some departments might require a color Doppler and spectral Doppler waveform of the main renal artery and vein at the hilum (Fig. 12-35A–C). Some protocols may require images of the bladder and images of bladder jets on all patients. Images to determine postvoid residual volume are not routinely documented unless these images are requesting by the physician (Fig. 12-36) (Pathology Box 12-8).

ANATOMIC VARIATIONS[4,7,8,13,16,17]

At times, the kidney or renal sinus will not demonstrate their normal US appearance. However, these kidneys may have normal lab values and normal urine output and will be in their proper anatomic position. In these cases, the kidneys are called normal variants (Pathology Box 12-9).

Dromedary Hump

The dromedary hump is a common variation of kidney shape and is caused by the splenic impression onto the superolateral mid pole of the left kidney. It is called a dromedary hump because it resembles the hump of a dromedary camel. Sonographically, it appears as a focal bulge in the mid-pole region, giving the kidney a more triangular shape. This area will have the same echo texture as the surrounding kidney tissue (Fig. 12-37). A dromedary hump is considered a renal pseudotumor as it may mimic the appearance of a renal mass. To differentiate between the two, interrogating the area with color or power Doppler will demonstrate normal parenchymal flow patterns, whereas a renal mass will show peripheral flow around the mass with possibly scattered flow inside (Fig. 12-38A–C).

Persistent Fetal Lobulations

Embryologically, the kidneys originate as distinct lobules that will fuse together as they develop. When these lobules do not fuse and there is incomplete fusion of the developing renal lobules, this is termed *persistent fetal lobulations*. This gives the kidney a bumpy contour or outline, as opposed to a smooth, flat, and continuous one. Persistent fetal lobulations have been described as indentations or a scalloped appearance of the renal outline between the renal pyramids (Fig. 12-39). Like the dromedary hump, fetal lobulations are considered pseudotumors and can be worrisome for a renal mass. Color or power Doppler should be used to document normal parenchymal flow underneath these "bumps" (Fig. 12-40A, B).

Columns of Bertin

Columns of Bertin are a normal variant where there are double layers of renal cortex between the renal pyramids, thus widening the space between them. They are named after Exupere Joseph Bertin, a French anatomist, who first

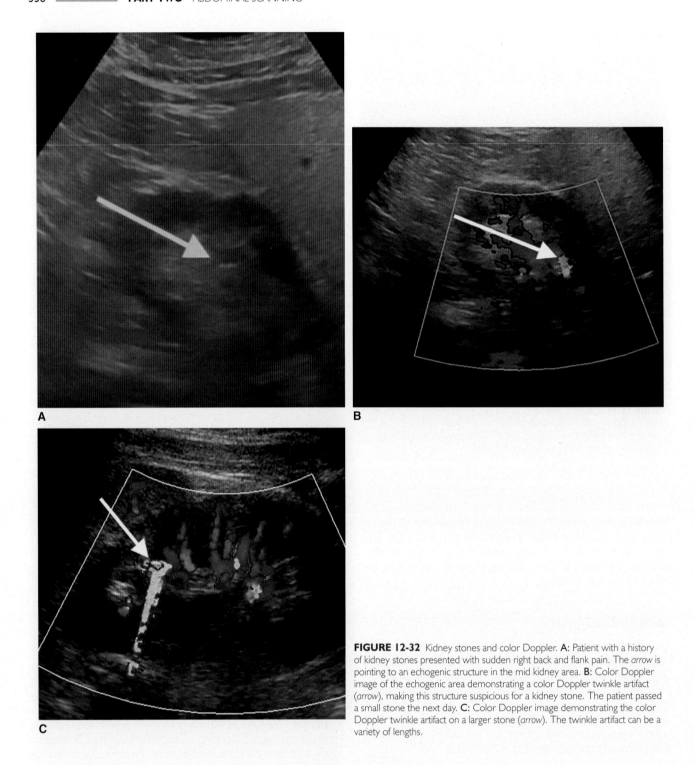

FIGURE 12-32 Kidney stones and color Doppler. **A:** Patient with a history of kidney stones presented with sudden right back and flank pain. The *arrow* is pointing to an echogenic structure in the mid kidney area. **B:** Color Doppler image of the echogenic area demonstrating a color Doppler twinkle artifact (*arrow*), making this structure suspicious for a kidney stone. The patient passed a small stone the next day. **C:** Color Doppler image demonstrating the color Doppler twinkle artifact on a larger stone (*arrow*). The twinkle artifact can be a variety of lengths.

described them in 1744. Columns of Bertin are not hypertrophic tissue but occur because of an incomplete fusion of the fetal lobes, causing two adjacent septa to become a large column with double the thickness. Columns of Bertin are present in approximately 50% of the population, with 20% being bilateral.

Sonographic criteria include indentation of the renal sinus, continuous with the adjacent renal cortex, and have the same echogenicity as that of the cortex. They can present with varying depths within the medullary substance of the kidneys and are usually located at the junction of the upper and middle thirds of the kidney. They have been described

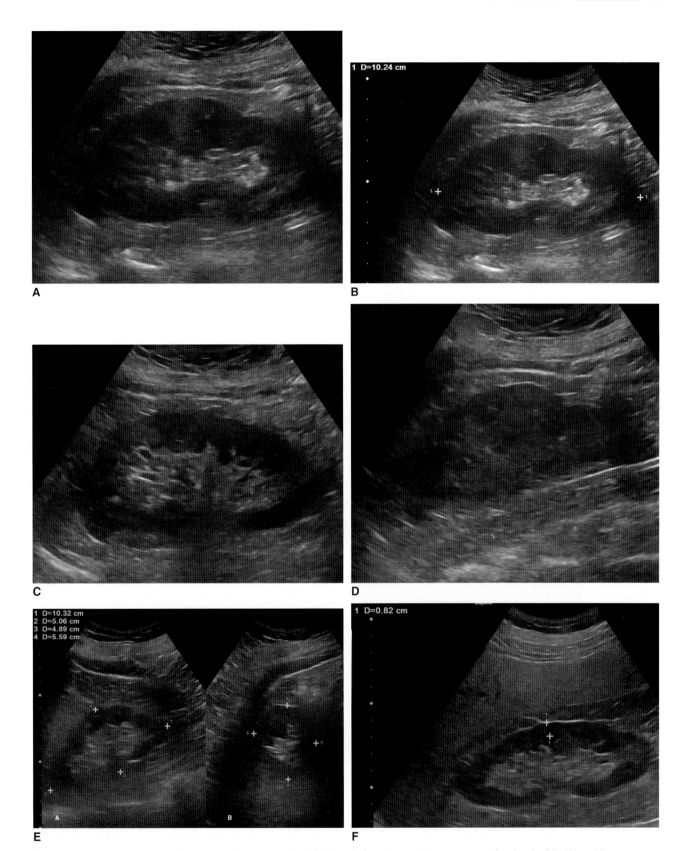

FIGURE 12-33 Longitudinal images. **A:** Long axis of the length of the left kidney. **B:** Same image with measurement of the length of the kidney. Measurements are best if both poles can be seen. **C:** The transducer is now angled medially to see the medial aspect of the kidney. In this image, the sinus echoes are well seen and may extend to the posterior border of the kidney. **D:** The transducer is now angled laterally to see the lateral aspect of the kidney. In this image, mostly parenchyma is seen. **E:** Both longitudinal and transverse kidney measurements (*calipers*) demonstrated within a dual screen. **F:** Longitudinal kidney demonstrating the measurement (*calipers*) of its cortical thickness.

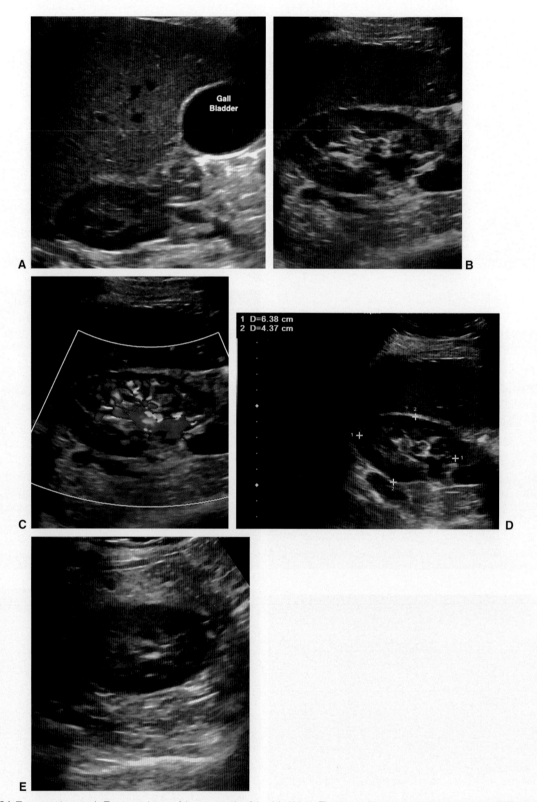

FIGURE 12-34 Transverse images. **A.** Transverse image of the upper pole of the right kidney. The sinus echoes are just coming in to view. **B.** Transverse image of the mid pole of the right kidney. There is some dilatation present which could be hydronephrosis or vessels. **C.** Color Doppler of the mid pole of the right kidney proving that the dilated area is the renal vein. The sonographer should always investigate dilation with color or power Doppler. **D.** Transverse and AP measurements at the mid pole. Since the kidney is often tilted, the transducer must be angled to be perpendicular to the kidney for accurate measurements. **E.** Transverse image of the lower pole of the right kidney.

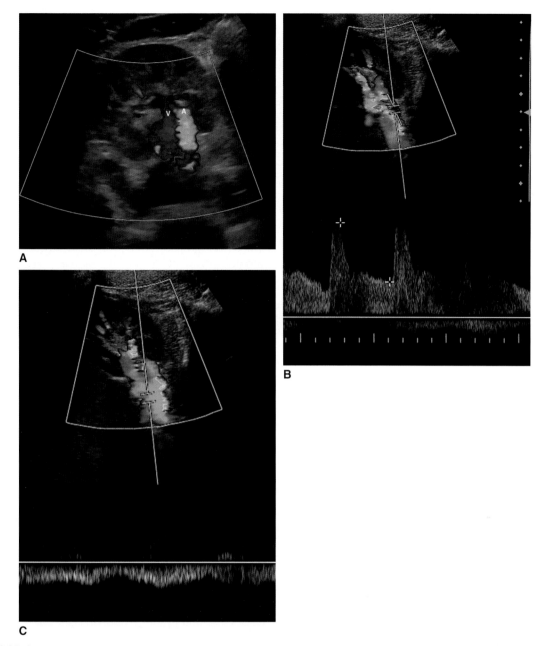

FIGURE 12-35 Color and spectral Doppler of the hilum. **A:** Color Doppler of the main renal artery (A) and main renal vein (V) at the hilum. **B:** Spectral Doppler of a normal main renal artery showing forward flow in diastole compatible with a low resistance signal. **C:** Spectral Doppler of a normal main renal vein showing normal phasic flow.

as a renal pseudotumor; however, the echogenicity of the column is isoechoic and continuous with the renal cortex (Fig. 12-41). Columns of Bertin may indent deep into the renal sinus and mimic a duplicated collecting system; however, a transverse scan through the column will demonstrate the echogenic sinus at the bottom (Fig. 12-42).

Junctional Parenchymal Defect

A junctional parenchymal defect is a fusion defect usually seen in the upper pole of the right kidney, although there

are reports in the literature of it being seen in the lower pole and in the left kidney. The defect is due to a partial fusion at the junction of two embryonic parenchymatous masses called ranunculi, which is where the term *junctional parenchymal defect* originates. On US, it is seen as a triangular or linear echogenic structure, which extends from the capsule to the renal sinus, near the junction of the upper and middle poles. The extension of perirenal fat into the defect causes it to be echogenic. A junctional parenchymal defect has no clinical significance and is discovered incidentally during an abdominal US or CT (Fig. 12-43).

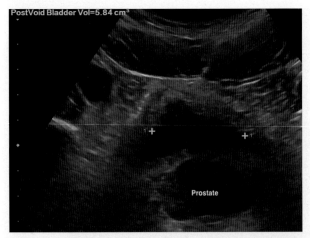

FIGURE 12-36 Most ultrasound units will automatically calculate the bladder volume when all three measurements of the bladder (length, anteroposterior, and width) are completed. Prevoid and postvoid volumes will be differentiated.

Extrarenal Pelvis

An extrarenal pelvis is an anatomic variant where part of the renal pelvis is located outside the renal hilum. It appears dilated as opposed to the intrarenal pelvis, which is surrounded by sinus fat that helps to keep it compressed. It is found in approximately 10% of the population. Patients will be asymptomatic, and it is usually an incidental finding on US or CT. An extrarenal pelvis is best appreciated in a mid-pole transverse image as a midline longitudinal image will show no evidence of hydronephrosis. When the transducer is aimed at the medial aspect of the kidney, the fluid will be seen extending outside the renal border (Fig. 12-44A–D). Sonography will demonstrate a cystic area lying partially or entirely outside the renal pelvis on a transverse mid-pole image. Transverse images of the upper and lower poles will be normal. Care should be taken not to mistake an extrarenal pelvis for hydronephrosis by noting lack of dilated calyces

---

PATHOLOGY BOX 12-8
Renal Protocol

Before the examination:

1. Check patient's medical history
2. Check appropriate imaging reports
3. Check appropriate blood and urine lab values
4. Prepare room
   a. Clean sheet and pillowcase or whatever is used to cover the table and pillow to protect the patient
   b. Transducers
   c. Supplies such as step stool, gel, something to use to protect the patient's clothing as needed, blanket or sheet to cover patient, and something to clean the gel off the patient.
5. Before scanning
   a. Introduce yourself
   b. Explain the sonogram including what they should expect during the examination
   c. Breathing requirements
   d. Different patient positions that may be needed
   e. How long the examination will take
   f. If they have any questions
   g. Why they are having the test.

6. Longitudinal images
   a. Long-axis image measuring the longest length of the kidney and the renal cortical thickness
   b. 1–2 longitudinal images from midline to lateral border
   c. 1–2 longitudinal images from midline to medial border
   d. An image demonstrating liver/right kidney and spleen/left kidney
7. Transverse images
   a. Mid pole of the kidney with transducer angled to be perpendicular to the kidney
      i. Transverse and AP measurements optional
   b. 1–2 transverse images from upper pole to mid kidney
   c. 1–2 transverse images from mid kidney to lower pole
8. Optional images
   a. Color Doppler of main renal artery and vein at hilum
   b. Spectral Doppler waveform of main renal artery and vein at hilum
   c. Images of bladder

PATHOLOGY BOX 12-9
Normal Variants

1. Dromedary hump
   a. Prominent focal bulge on lateral border of the left kidney, which gives the kidney a more triangular shape
2. Fetal lobulations
   a. When the embryologically lobules do not fuse together after birth causing the outline of the kidney to have a scalloped or bumpy appearance. Can occur in either kidney.
3. Hypertrophied column of Bertin
   a. Incomplete fusion of fetal lobes that causes a large column with increased thickness and varying depths within the medullary substance. Sonographically, double layers of renal cortex are seen between the renal pyramids with the same echogenicity as that of the cortex.

4. Junctional parenchymal defect
   a. Fusion defect due to a partial fusion at the junction of two embryonic ranunculi. Sonographically seen as an echogenic line, due to extension of the perirenal fat, near the junction of the upper and middle poles.
5. Extrarenal pelvis
   a. Anatomic variant where part of the renal pelvis is outside the renal hilum and is best appreciated in a transverse image. There will be no hydronephrosis on a midline image.
6. Renal sinus lipomatosis
   a. A benign condition of an accumulation of excessive fat within the renal sinus and appears as an enlarged echogenic central sinus that is usually less echogenic than the normal renal sinus.

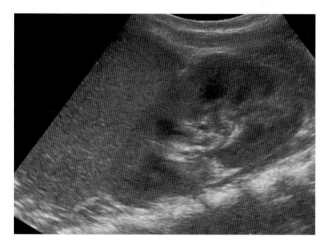

FIGURE 12-37 An image of the spleen showing how it "molds" or imprints itself on the left kidney causing the distortion of the renal shape.

or a hydroureter. As there will be a normal midline image of the kidney that does not show any hydronephrosis, it should be easy not to confuse an extrarenal pelvis for hydronephrosis.

Renal Sinus Lipomatosis

Renal sinus lipomatosis refers to a condition when there is an accumulation of excessive fat within the renal sinus. It is usually found in patients in their sixth or seventh decade, who are obese, or have had exposure to steroids. Renal sinus lipomatosis has no clinical significance, and patients are asymptomatic with normal urine output and renal function tests. It is usually bilateral and found incidentally. Sonographically, it is seen as an enlarged echogenic central sinus that is usually less echogenic than a normal renal sinus, and what appears to be cortical

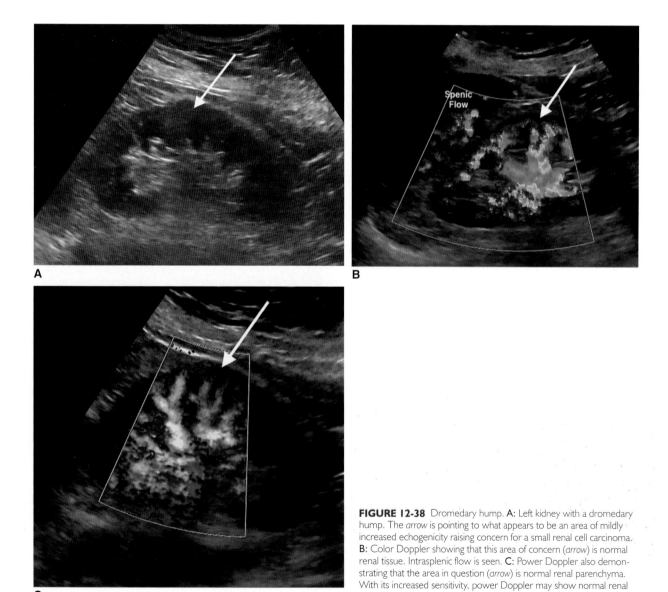

FIGURE 12-38 Dromedary hump. **A:** Left kidney with a dromedary hump. The *arrow* is pointing to what appears to be an area of mildly increased echogenicity raising concern for a small renal cell carcinoma. **B:** Color Doppler showing that this area of concern (*arrow*) is normal renal tissue. Intrasplenic flow is seen. **C:** Power Doppler also demonstrating that the area in question (*arrow*) is normal renal parenchyma. With its increased sensitivity, power Doppler may show normal renal perfusion best when imaging technically difficult patients.

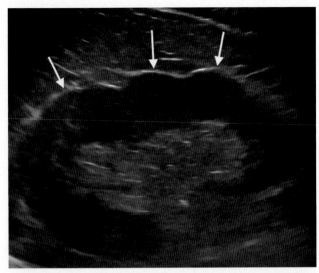

FIGURE 12-39 Image showing the scalloped edges or bumpy look (*arrows*) on a kidney with fetal lobulations.

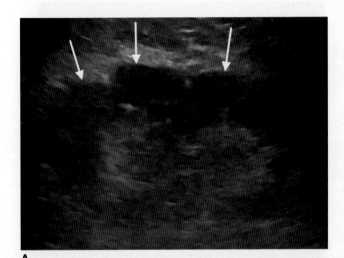

A

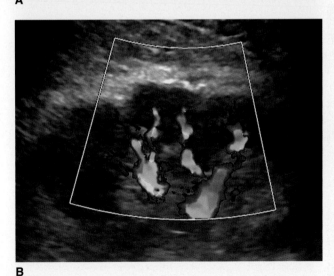

B

FIGURE 12-40 Fetal lobulations. **A:** Kidney demonstrating fetal lobulations (*arrows*). **B:** A color Doppler image showing flow in the tissue under the lobulation.

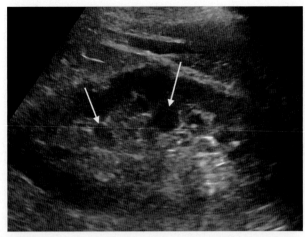

FIGURE 12-41 Columns of Bertin (*arrows*) in a patient who also has a dromedary hump.

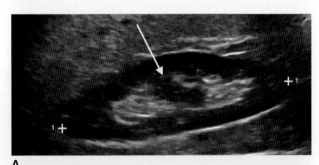

A

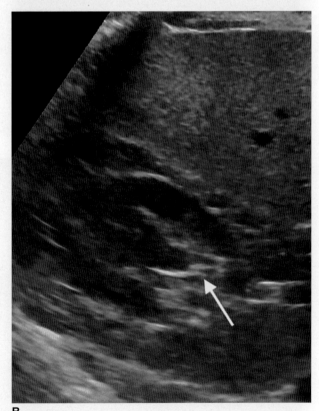

B

FIGURE 12-42 Columns of Bertin. **A:** The *arrow* is pointing to a column of Bertin that appears to split the sinus echoes in half. **B:** A transverse image in the plane of the *arrow* in Figure 12-42 showing sinus echoes at the bottom of the column (*arrow*).

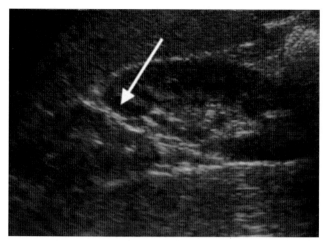

FIGURE 12-43 A junctional parenchymal defect highlighted by an echogenic line (*arrow*).

thinning, due to the widening of the sinus echoes. These patients may also have a fatty pancreas, which appears as a bright, echogenic pancreas, that has no clinical significance (Fig. 12-45A, B).

CONGENITAL ANOMALIES[3,6,7,15,16]

The World Health Organization (WHO) defines *congenital anomalies* as structural or functional anomalies that occur during intrauterine life. WHO describes causes and risk factors as follows: although approximately 50% of all congenital anomalies cannot be linked to a specific cause, there are some known genetic, environmental, and other causes or risk factors. Congenital renal anomalies can be a kidney in the wrong place in the body, missing, on the same side of the body, or joined together. Some of the following anomalies may also be repeated in the pediatric section (Pathology Box 12-10).

Renal Agenesis

Renal agenesis is the failure of a kidney and ureter to develop and has a 3:1 male predominance. Bilateral renal agenesis is also known as Potter syndrome and is usually detected in utero. Because the fetus has no kidneys, it does not produce urine that causes oligohydramnios, and a fetal US is ordered. It is not considered compatible with life with pulmonary hypoplasia as the leading cause of death. People born with unilateral renal agenesis will have compensatory

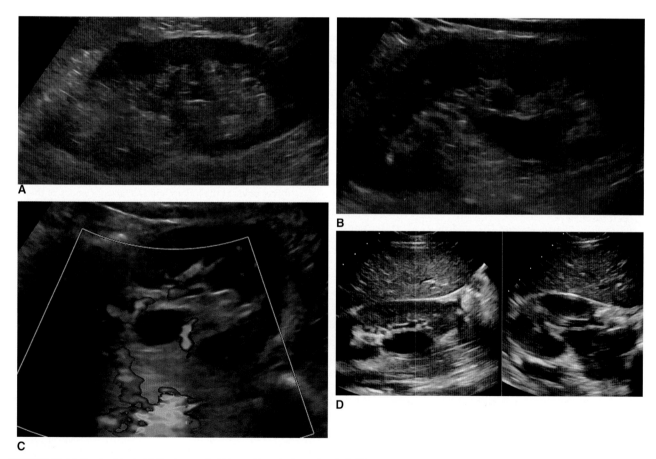

FIGURE 12-44 Renal pelvis. **A:** Midline image of a kidney with no hydronephrosis. **B:** The transducer is angled medially and is showing some fluid that should not be mistaken for hydronephrosis. **C:** Transverse image at the mid pole demonstrating fluid compatible with an extrarenal pelvis. Color Doppler was used to verify that the cystic area was not a prominent renal vein. **D:** This feature, called X-Plane™, allows sonographers to use the longitudinal image to construct the transverse image. This image is demonstrated through the medial aspect of the kidney. The white line shows where the transverse image is being obtained, nicely demonstrating the extrarenal pelvis in both planes simultaneously.

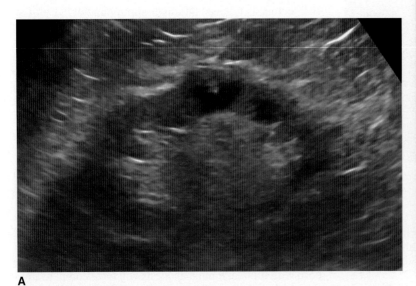

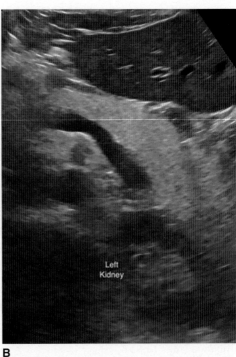

Left
Kidney

A   **B**

FIGURE 12-45 Lipomatosis. **A:** Image of a patient with sinus lipomatosis demonstrating a decrease in the echogenicity and widening of the sinus echoes. **B:** The pancreas of the patient in **A** showing the bright echo texture of the pancreas that also has fatty infiltration.

PATHOLOGY BOX 12-10
Congenital Anomalies

1. Renal agenesis
   a. Failure of a kidney or kidneys to develop. Bilateral renal agenesis is usually incompatible with life and is usually suspected on a prenatal US from the lack of amniotic fluid. A patient with unilateral renal agenesis will have normal urine output and normal renal lab values, and the remaining kidney will hypertrophy, measuring larger than normal. Unilateral renal agenesis is often discovered incidentally if it was not diagnosed on the prenatal sonogram or at birth.

2. Ectopic kidney
   a. An ectopic kidney is when a kidney does not ascend to its normal position in the upper abdomen. Failure to visualize a kidney in the renal fossa should prompt a search in the pelvic area, especially when the contralateral kidney is normal in size. Pelvic kidneys are usually asymptomatic and are found incidentally by US or CT.
   b. Scanning tip: When only one kidney is found and it is normal in size, somewhere is a second kidney. However, if the kidney is enlarged, there is only one kidney in the body.

3. Crossed ectopic kidney
   a. In crossed renal ectopia, both kidneys are found on the same side of the body.

4. Horseshoe kidney
   a. Two distinct functioning kidneys connected at their lower poles by an isthmus of functioning renal parenchyma that crosses anterior to the aorta. The IMA stops their ascent, causing them to be just superior to the umbilicus. The renal pelvis of the kidneys will be rotated anteriorly.

5. Duplicated collecting system
   a. It is caused by an incomplete fusion of the upper and lower poles of the kidney and will have variations of the ureter and pyelocalyceal system. It affects the left kidney more often than the right, is bilateral in 15%–20% of patients, and is more common in women. With complete duplication, the ureter draining the lower pole inserts laterally into the bladder trigone, has a short intravesical segment, and is more prone to reflux. The upper pole ureter inserts medially and inferiorly to the lower pole ureter and can have a ureterocele, causing obstruction of the upper pole. On sonography, a duplicated collecting system appears as two distinct echogenic renal sinuses that are separated by normal parenchymal tissue. The kidney is larger than normal, usually measuring greater than 13 to 14 cm in length.

hypertrophy of the contralateral kidney, which is caused by hypertrophic growth of the proximal tubule, causing an increase in the renal cortex and, therefore, an overall increase in size of the kidney, not just its length. Having

only one kidney does not affect urine output or renal lab values. US will demonstrate the hypertrophied kidney and an empty renal fossa on the contralateral side. Unilateral renal agenesis can be verified by identifying only one ureteral

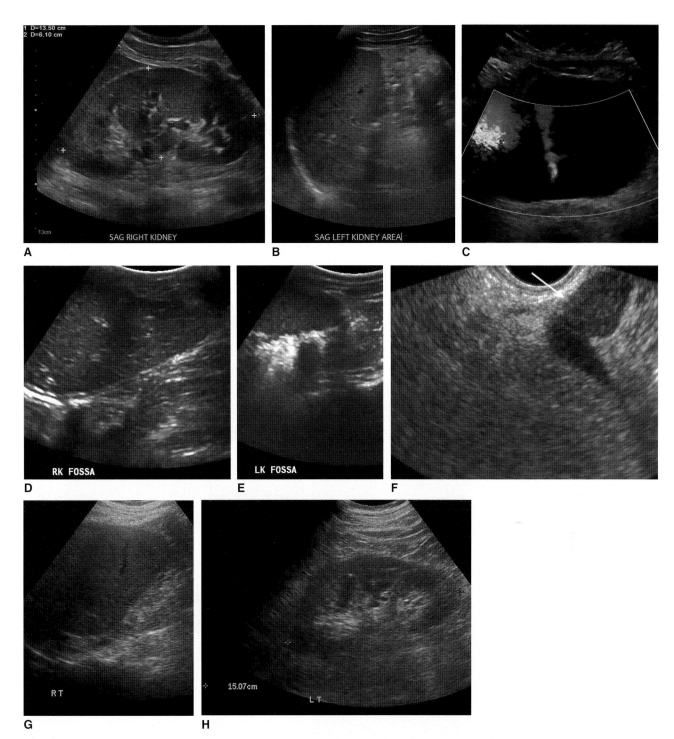

FIGURE 12-46 Renal agenesis. **A:** Longitudinal image of the right kidney that is larger than usual. **B:** An image of the left upper quadrant (*LUQ*) on the same patient showing the absence of the left kidney. **C:** A good way to verify the absence of a kidney is to look for bladder jets. This is the same patient demonstrating a right ureteral jet. A left urine jet was never visualized. **D:** Image of the right upper quadrant (*RUQ*) verifying the absence of the right kidney in a newborn who was suspected to have bilateral renal agenesis by the fetal ultrasound. **E:** Image of the LUQ verifying the absence of the left kidney. The baby did not survive. **F:** The *arrow* is pointing to a single left seminal vesicle found incidentally on an endorectal ultrasound. **G:** The ipsilateral renal fossa showing the absence of the right kidney. **H:** The hypertrophied contralateral kidney on the same patient.

jet in the bladder. In cases of bilateral renal agenesis, both renal fossae will be empty.

Patients with unilateral renal agenesis have an incidence of associated genital malformations, such as ipsilateral seminal vesicle agenesis in men and uterus didelphys and blind or atretic hemivagina in women (Fig. 12-46A–F).

When an anomaly of the reproductive tract is discovered, it would be beneficial for the sonographer to obtain one longitudinal image of each kidney to document the presence of one or both kidneys. Interestingly, because US was not widely available before the early to mid-1980s, people over the age of 40 to 50 with only one kidney were probably born with an MCDK that regressed and was absorbed by the body because MCDK is more common than renal agenesis. MCDK is discussed in greater depth within the pediatric section.

Ectopic Kidney

An ectopic kidney is when a kidney does not completely ascend to its normal position in the upper abdomen. During fetal development, the kidneys begin to develop in the pelvic area near the bladder. As they continue to develop, they migrate to their normal position in the retroperitoneum. However, one of the kidneys may stop anywhere along the path of ascension or it can remain in the pelvis. Failure to visualize a kidney in the renal fossa, when the contralateral kidney is normal size,

should prompt a search for the other kidney starting in the pelvic area (Fig. 12-47A–C). Pelvic kidneys are usually asymptomatic and are found incidentally by US or other imaging modalities. Pelvic kidneys may be felt as a pelvic mass, and a physician might request a pelvic sonogram, especially on a female patient. The most common associated abnormality is vesicoureteral reflux. Other urinary problems include a kidney infection or urinary stones. Like a horseshoe kidney, a pelvic kidney can be prone to injury from contact sports.

Scanning Tip: When only one kidney is found in the upper abdomen, there is a clue to tell you whether there is just one kidney in the body or if there is another kidney located in an ectopic position. A single functioning kidney will become larger in all dimensions, termed *hypertrophy*, to compensate for its increased workload. Imaging an enlarged

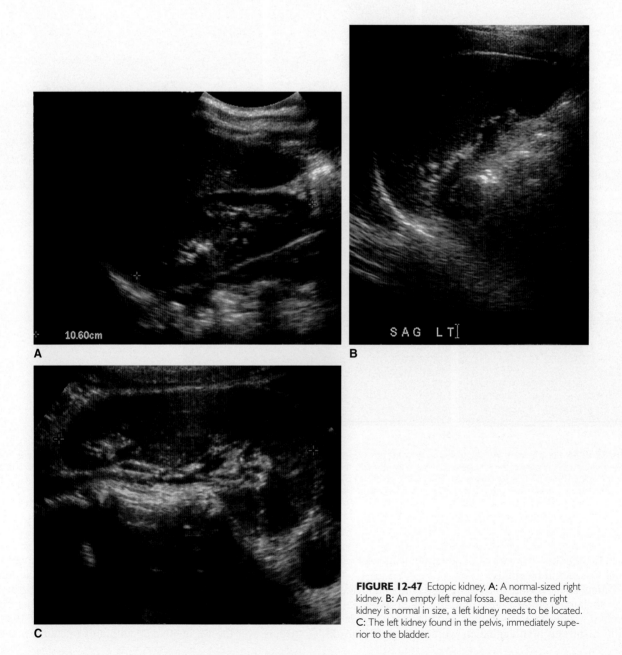

FIGURE 12-47 Ectopic kidney, **A:** A normal-sized right kidney. **B:** An empty left renal fossa. Because the right kidney is normal in size, a left kidney needs to be located. **C:** The left kidney found in the pelvis, immediately superior to the bladder.

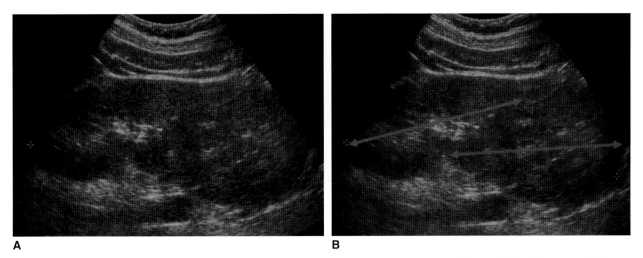

A **B**

FIGURE 12-48 Crossed ectopia. **A:** A long-axis image from the left side of the abdomen showing what could be a duplicated kidney. There was no kidney on the right side, and a more careful evaluation determined that this was crossed ectopia. **B:** The double-headed *arrows* define the borders of the two kidneys.

kidney decreases the likelihood that another kidney exists. On the other hand, if it is found that kidney is of normal in size, it is likely that another kidney is located somewhere within the body, and every effort should be made to find its location.

Crossed Ectopic Kidney

In crossed renal ectopia, both kidneys are found on the same side of the body. There is an estimated incidence of around 1 out of 1,000 births, with a 2:1 male-to-female ratio. In 85% to 90% of cases, the upper pole of the ectopic kidney will be fused to the lower pole of the other kidney, although fusion may occur anywhere. It is three times more common for both kidneys to be on the right side, a left-to-right ectopia. Each kidney keeps their own vessels and ureters, and the ureter of the ectopic kidney will cross the midline to enter the bladder at its proper location. Crossed renal ectopia is usually asymptomatic and found incidentally on imaging. It can be sonographically difficult to differentiate the two kidneys (Fig. 12-48).

Horseshoe Kidney

A horseshoe kidney is the most common type of renal fusion anomaly affecting approximately 0.25% of the population, with a male preponderance of 2:1. It consists of two distinct functioning kidneys on either side of the midline, with 95% of the kidneys connected at their lower poles by an isthmus of functioning renal parenchyma. This fusion causes the kidneys to form a U shape, like a horseshoe, hence the name.

The inferior mesenteric artery (IMA) stops the kidneys in their ascent, causing them to stop just superior to the umbilicus. This isthmus crosses the midline of the body anterior to the aorta. The arterial blood supply can come off the aorta or the iliac artery. Patients with a horseshoe kidney are often asymptomatic and found incidentally, although these patients are prone to hydronephrosis, infections, stones, and vesicoureteral reflux. Patients may be referred to US for the evaluation of a pulsatile abdominal mass to rule out an abdominal aortic aneurysm (AAA), as

the aorta transmits its pulsations through the renal tissue to the surface of the body, allowing them to be felt. This pulsation is the classic clinical sign of an AAA. Because these kidneys are "out in the open" and not protected by the ribs or fat layers, they are more prone to injury, and it is recommended that people with a horseshoe kidney refrain from playing rough contact sports. Sonographically, these kidneys will rarely look like a kidney as the renal pelvis is malrotated and faces anteriorly. There is also a band of tissue connecting the two kidneys. The upper pole can be defined, but the lower pole does not have an identifiable end point, and measurements are approximated as to where the sonographer believes best represents the "lower pole" as it is not defined (Fig. 12-49A–C). This can cause discrepancies in measurements between studies as each sonographer chooses what they believe is the best end point to measure or tries to determine where to measure based on prior images.

Duplicated Collecting System

A duplicated collecting system, also known as a duplex collecting system, is the most common congenital anomaly of the urinary system and is defined as one kidney with two separate, noncommunicating renal pelvises as opposed to just one. It is caused by an incomplete fusion of the upper and lower poles of the kidney with variations in the ureter and pyelocalyceal system. A duplicated collecting system is bilateral in 15% to 20% of patients, is found in the left kidney more often than the right, and is more common in women. A complete duplication occurs when the two separate collecting systems each have their own ureter and ureteral opening into the bladder. The ureter draining the lower pole inserts laterally into the bladder trigone, has a short intravesical segment, and is more prone to reflux. The upper pole ureter inserts medially and inferiorly to the lower pole ureter and can have a ureterocele, causing obstruction of the upper pole. An incomplete duplication is when there are two separate collecting systems with separate ureters that join, called a bifid ureter, before entering the bladder through a single ureteral opening. It is difficult for US to differentiate

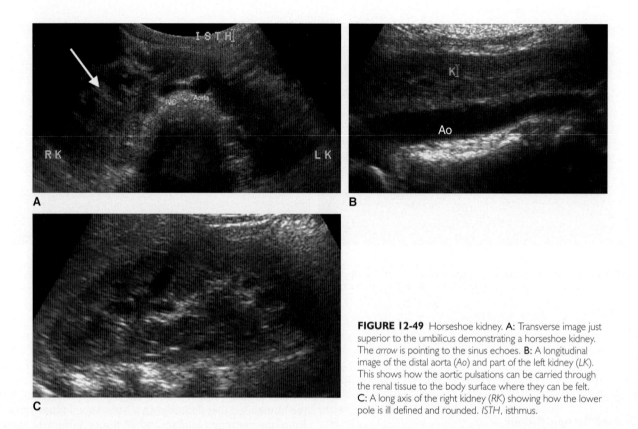

FIGURE 12-49 Horseshoe kidney. **A:** Transverse image just superior to the umbilicus demonstrating a horseshoe kidney. The *arrow* is pointing to the sinus echoes. **B:** A longitudinal image of the distal aorta (*Ao*) and part of the left kidney (*LK*). This shows how the aortic pulsations can be carried through the renal tissue to the body surface where they can be felt. **C:** A long axis of the right kidney (*RK*) showing how the lower pole is ill defined and rounded. *ISTH*, isthmus.

between a complete and incomplete duplication, especially if no ureterocele is present. A duplicated collecting system is usually an incidental finding as the patient is usually asymptomatic and there are no issues with renal function and urine output. Symptomatic patients can present with infection, reflux, or obstruction, and any complications are usually related to the abnormal implantation of the ureters. Patients with incomplete duplicated collecting systems have less symptoms. With sonography, a duplicated collecting system appears as two distinct echogenic renal sinuses that are separated by normal parenchymal tissue. The kidney is larger than normal, measuring greater than 13 to 14 cm in length. Transverse scans will confirm this anomaly by observing the disappearance and reappearance of the renal sinus echoes while scanning from the upper to the lower pole. If there is hydronephrosis in the upper pole, the bladder should be evaluated for a ureterocele. A ureterocele is an abnormal dilatation of the distal ureter and can herniate into the bladder. On US, a ureterocele will appear as a round, cyst-like structure projecting into the bladder, usually near the vesicoureteral junction (Fig. 12-50A–I).

CYSTIC RENAL MASSES[4,7,8,13,18–23]

Renal masses are characterized as either solid, cystic, or complex cystic. This section discusses cystic and complex cystic masses, and the following section discusses solid masses.

US often finds unknown pathology in a patient, including kidney cysts. Usually, these unexpected cysts are found on the right kidney as sonograms of the right upper quadrant (RUQ) are much more common than full abdominal or left

upper quadrant (LUQ) sonograms. When a cyst is found on the right kidney, some departments will require images of the left kidney to evaluate it for cysts. Sometimes, a patient may be referred from CT or MRI for more information about the characteristics of a cystic lesion. Cysts can occur in the renal cortex or in the renal sinus and can include simple cysts, complicated cysts, and atypical cysts. All cysts need to be evaluated with color Doppler to ensure that the "cyst" is not vascular pathology, such as a renal artery aneurysm or pseudoaneurysm (PSA). This section discusses only renal cystic disease found in adults.

Cortical Cysts

A renal cyst is a benign mass of uncertain etiology that contains serous fluid and has an epithelial lining. These cysts can be acquired or congenital, focal or multifocal, and unilateral or bilateral. Simple cysts are cortical in location, and larger cysts can distort the renal contour. Renal cysts are thought to be present in about 5% of the general population, in about 25% of people older than 40 and in about 50% of people over the age of 50. The number, location, and size of renal cysts can increase with age. Most patients with renal cysts are asymptomatic; however, some patients may experience flank pain or hematuria that is caused by distention of the cyst wall or bleeding into the cyst. Renal cysts are unusual in children, with a frequency of less than 1%.

A simple cyst is characterized by sonography when it meets all of the following criteria:
- Circular or oval in shape
- Smooth, thin walls

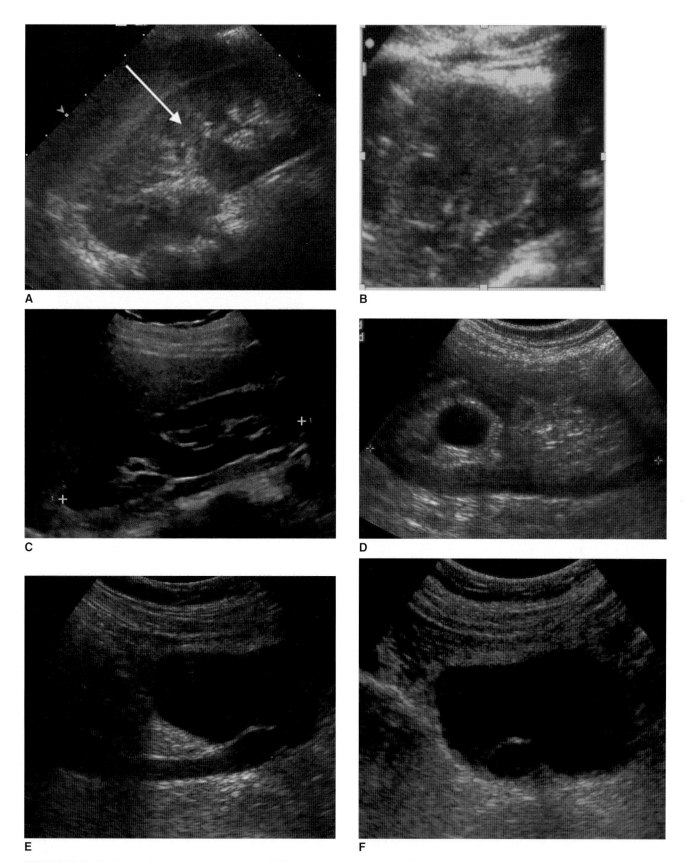

FIGURE 12-50 Duplicated collecting system. **A:** A duplicated kidney with the *arrow* pointing to the break between the two poles. **B:** A transverse image in plane with the *arrow* showing all parenchyma and no sinus echoes. **C:** A duplicated kidney with hydronephrosis in both poles. **D:** A left duplicated kidney with hydronephrosis in the upper pole. **E:** Longitudinal image of the bladder showing the dilated ureter and ureterocele from the upper pole moiety. **F:** Transverse image of the bladder showing the ureterocele.

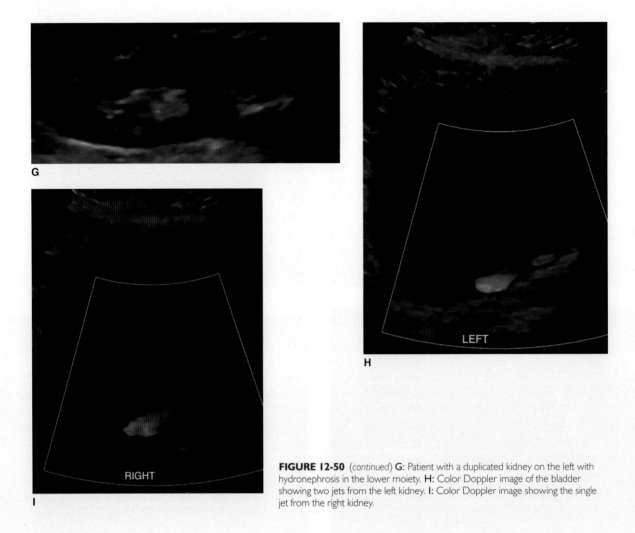

FIGURE 12-50 *(continued)* **G:** Patient with a duplicated kidney on the left with hydronephrosis in the lower moiety. **H:** Color Doppler image of the bladder showing two jets from the left kidney. **I:** Color Doppler image showing the single jet from the right kidney.

- Lack of internal echoes (anechoic)
- Well-defined back wall
- Posterior acoustic enhancement, which is increased brightness of the echoes under the cyst due to the sound beam passing through a low attenuative structure such as fluid (Pathology Box 12-11)

Cysts are typically discovered incidentally while scanning the patient for other reasons. The sonographer should note the location of the cyst and measure its size in all three dimensions. When there are multiple cysts, some departments may have the sonographer measure all the cysts, whereas others just the largest. To measure the cyst, using the dual-image function can be helpful so that all three measurements are on the same image. This is especially helpful when there are multiple cysts and allows the sonographer to ensure that they are measuring the same cyst as they go from longitudinal to transverse planes. Some cysts can be missed on longitudinal images but are seen on a transverse image, when located along the lateral margin. The sonographer will need to go back and find the cyst in the longitudinal plane and measure its length and AP dimensions. An image of the cyst with color Doppler should be obtained to prove that the cystic lesion is not vascular. Larger cysts can compress the renal tissue and obscure the normal kidney (Fig. 12-51A–I).

Some simple renal cysts may show internal echoes from reverberations, slice thickness artifacts, noise, and other artifacts. It is important for the sonographer to recognize that these echoes are artifacts and to try and eliminate them. Here are some technical hints to try and clean up the cyst:

1. Activate harmonic and compound imaging as both technologies help to reduce artifacts.
2. If the cyst is deep in the body, turning off harmonics may help clean up the cyst. The harmonic sound beam is affected by attenuation, and deeper structures may require increased overall gain, causing system noise to be seen inside the cyst.
3. Try different frequencies by adjusting the frequency electronically or by cycling between PEN (penetration),

PATHOLOGY BOX 12-11
Criteria for a Simple Cyst

a. Circular or oval in shape
b. Smooth, thin walls
c. Lack of internal echoes
d. Well-defined back wall
e. Acoustic enhancement

GEN (general), and RES (resolution) depending on what the manufacturer uses. Remember to cycle through normal and harmonic frequencies.

4. Change transducer types. Most examinations will probably be performed with a curved linear array. Changing to a sector transducer allows scanning between the ribs. The way a sector transducer interacts with tissue can be different than the way a curved linear array does, and this may reduce or eliminate any artifacts.

5. Turn the patient into different positions such as an oblique or a decubitus (Pathology Box 12-12).

Real internal echoes within a cyst can be caused by hemorrhage or infection, and these cysts are now termed *complex cysts* and are discussed later in this chapter.

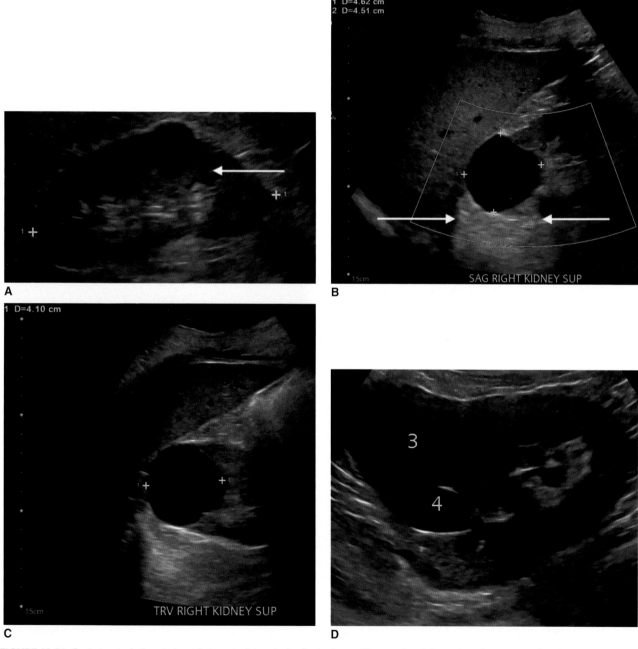

FIGURE 12-51 Cortical cysts. **A:** A cortical cyst that meets all the criteria of a simple cyst. The *arrow* is pointing to the enhancement artifact. **B:** Longitudinal image of a cyst in the upper pole. The length (calipers 1) and anteroposterior dimensions (calipers 2) are measured. The annotation identifies the scanning plane and location of the cyst. The area between the *arrows* demonstrates enhancement. Color Doppler was used to verify it was cystic. (Some sonographers will use sag as opposed to long for long axis or longitudinal. The kidney is not in a sagittal (*SAG*) plane but an oblique plane. The better annotation is long.) Some sonographers use the term superior (*SUP*) pole, and others upper pole. Either is correct, and the term used is a personal preference of the sonographer, although some departments may determine which term to use. **C:** Transverse (*TRV*) image of the same cyst with the width of the cyst being measured. **D:** A kidney with multiple cysts. Here the sonographer is numbering the cysts for reference. This can be helpful on follow-up studies to ensure the same cyst is being measured.

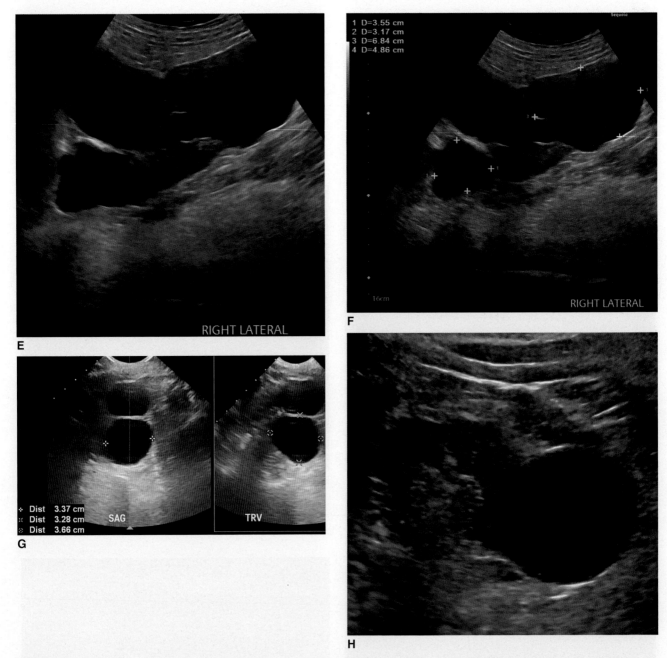

FIGURE 12-51 *(continued)* **E:** Longitudinal image of the kidney along its lateral aspect showing multiple cysts. **F:** Same kidney measuring the cysts. Calipers 1 and 2 are measuring the smaller cyst in the upper pole, and calipers 3 and 4 the larger cyst in the lower pole. It is important to confirm that this plane represents the largest length of the cysts. **G:** An X-Plane™ image using this feature to measure a cyst in all three planes on one image. This is how a dual or side-by-side image appears. **H:** While scanning TRV, an unexpected cyst is found that was not seen on the longitudinal images. The cyst is very lateral, with most of the cyst not in the kidney making it easy to miss.

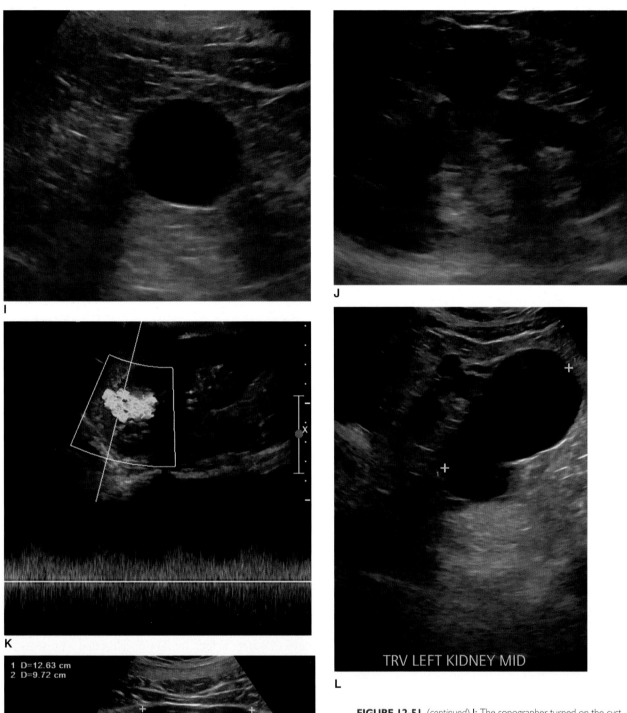

I

J

K

L

TRV LEFT KIDNEY MID

M

1 D=12.63 cm
2 D=9.72 cm

FIGURE 12-51 (*continued*) **I:** The sonographer turned on the cyst to obtain a longitudinal image of the cyst by angling the transducer very laterally from mid kidney. No renal tissue is seen, and enhancement is demonstrated. **J:** An exophytic cyst of the mid pole of the left kidney. The majority of the cyst is outside the kidney. **K:** Color Doppler showed that this was not a cyst, but an arteriovenous fistula (*AVF*) caused by a renal biopsy. The Doppler waveform is compatible with an AVF as it is very turbulent, and the signal is pulsatile with good diastolic flow. There is aliasing seen due to the high-flow state. **L:** A kidney cyst easily mistaken for the gallbladder. **M:** A 12-cm cyst in the lower pole. Very little kidney tissue is seen. The *arrows* are outlining the kidney. The *dotted arrow* is pointing to a reverberation artifact. The *curved arrow* is pointing to slice thickness artifact. Both of these artifacts are commonly seen in cystic structures, and the sonographer needs to be able to identify them and, when possible, eliminate them. Some tips to eliminate these artifacts are found in Pathology Box 12-12.

PATHOLOGY BOX 12-12
Tips on "Cleaning" up a Cyst

a. Activate both harmonic and compound imaging as they reduce artifacts in an image.

b. If the cyst is deep in the body, try turning off harmonics.

c. Try different frequencies by adjusting the frequency electronically or by cycling between PEN (penetration), GEN (general), and RES (resolution).

d. Try different transducer types.

e. Turn the patient into different positions.

f. Lower the overall gain as long as it does not remove needed echoes.

g. If the machine still has time gain compensation (TGC) pods, adjust the ones at the level of the artifact to see if that can help, being careful not to remove needed echoes.

Parapelvic and Peripelvic Cysts

Cysts that involve the renal pelvis are either a parapelvic cyst or a peripelvic cyst, depending on where they originate, and can be referred to as a renal sinus cyst. They are both benign cysts, and most patients are asymptomatic. They occasionally may cause pain, hematuria, or the parapelvic cyst hydronephrosis. The parapelvic cyst originates in the adjacent renal parenchyma and extends into the renal sinus. They are usually single and look like a simple renal cortical cyst, just deeper in the kidney and pushing into the renal sinus echoes. The peripelvic cyst originates within the renal sinus itself and is not a true cyst as it does not contain serous fluid, but most contain lymphatic fluid. A peripelvic cyst is spherical in appearance, are usually bilateral, can cause obstruction, and usually remain unchanged in size on follow-up examinations. It is important not to confuse a peripelvic cyst with hydronephrosis as there will be a lack of communication to a calyx and a normal proximal ureter (Fig. 12-52A–E).

Complex Renal Cysts[4,7,8,13,18–22]

A renal cyst must show all the signs of a simple cyst; otherwise, it is termed a *complicated or complex cyst*. These cysts will exhibit one or more of the following characteristics: septations, thick walls, calcifications, internal echoes, or mural nodularity. Most of the time, these internal echoes are caused by protein content, hemorrhage, or infection. When an imaging study demonstrates a complex cyst, it becomes important to determine whether it is malignant. A complex renal cyst needs a contrast-enhanced CT to help determine whether it is a benign complex cyst or a malignant cyst. Recently, contrast-enhanced ultrasound (CEUS) has shown to be reliable in differentiating a complex versus a malignant cyst. CEUS can be an alternative for CT as it avoids the use of nephrotoxic contrast agents and ionizing radiation.[23–25]

Proteinaceous Cysts

A proteinaceous cyst contains a thick protein fluid inside. They are not malignant and do not require surgery. If clinically indicated, they could be followed (Fig. 12-53).

Hemorrhagic Cysts[24]

A hemorrhagic cyst occurs in about 6% of simple cysts. Hemorrhage can occur in a preexisting simple cyst, or it can form from the liquefaction of a traumatic hematoma within the kidney parenchyma. A hemorrhagic cyst could be the result of the cyst increasing in size, trauma, or the patient has a predisposition to bleeding. As a hemorrhagic cyst resolves, they develop features such as calcification, thickening of the wall, and septations, giving it the appearance of a complex cyst. Depending on the age of the bleed, hemorrhagic cysts can vary in their sonographic appearance from anechoic to complex masses, with or without acoustic enhancement. These complex hemorrhagic cysts will require further imaging to rule out a malignancy as they have a similar appearance to a malignant cyst. If there is no evidence of malignancy by MRI, CT, or CEUS, then a hemorrhagic cyst can be followed with a US examination.

Infected Cysts

A simple renal cyst can become infected by hematogenous dissemination of bacteria, or a renal abscess may resolve into a cyst. An infected simple cyst accounts for 2.5% of all complications and is not usually incidental because there is a clinical history of symptoms suggesting an infection that includes fever, chills, elevated WBC count, and a UTI. On US, infected renal cysts are characterized by thickened walls and have a fluid–fluid level. Some cysts may contain gas.

Septations[24–27]

Septations in cysts can be caused by hemorrhage, infection, or malignancy. A benign septated cyst will have thin, smooth septations that have a thickness of less than 1 mm. Sonographic characteristics of benign septa in a cyst include that they are very thin, are few in number, and will attach to the cyst wall without any thickened elements. Thin septations are better detected by US than CT. When a cystic mass contains one or more thick septations that are thicker than 1 to 2 mm and has solid elements or nodules at the wall attachment, this cyst must be considered malignant. The septations and nodules should be investigated with color or power Doppler to look for flow because that represents the neovascularity seen in malignant cysts. To help distinguish complex cysts from malignant cysts, a CT, MRI, or CEUS can be ordered to further investigate the cyst (Fig. 12-54A–I).

The Bosniak classification system was developed in 1986 by Morton A. Bosniak, a radiologist from New York, to help categorize cystic renal masses. This system was based on imaging characteristics using contrast-enhanced CT and placed cysts into five categories with the primary goal to help differentiate nonsurgical from surgical lesions. The Bosniak system is a scale of increasing probability of a malignant cystic RCC based upon imaging features of the renal cyst. It is not intended to be used alone to determine management of complex cystic lesions, but to be used along with clinical findings and current clinical practice and guidelines.

A Bosniak 1 or 2 cyst is a benign cyst that does not need follow-up.

A Bosniak 2F cyst needs to be followed.

A Bosniak 3 or 4 cyst needs to be removed.

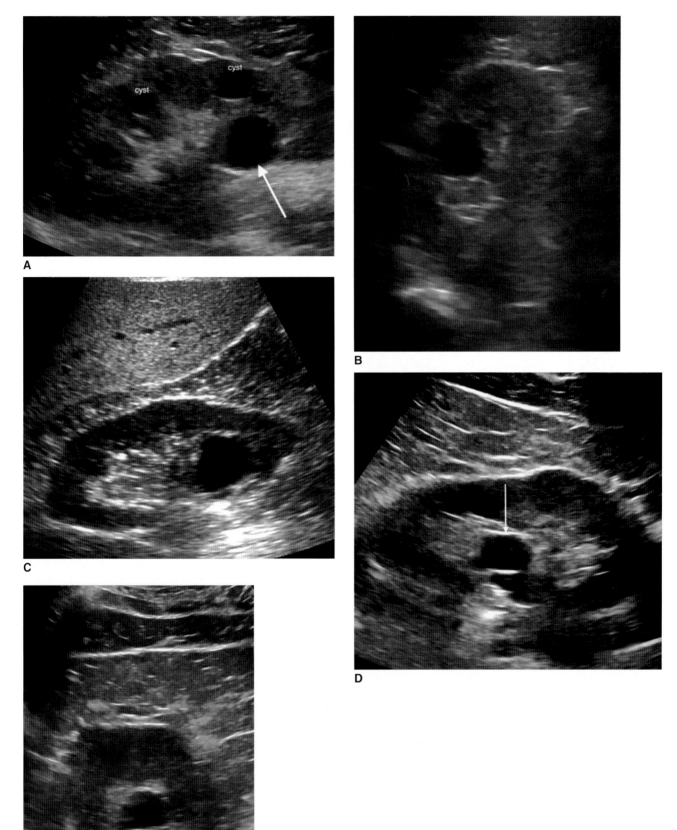

FIGURE 12-52 Parapelvic and peripelvic cysts. **A:** An image of a kidney with multiple cysts. There are two cortical cysts. The *arrow* is pointing to a parapelvic cyst that plunges deeply into the sinus echoes. **B:** A transverse image of a parapelvic cyst that extends about halfway into the sinus echoes. **C:** A peripelvic cyst in the lower pole that exhibits acoustic enhancement. **D:** A peripelvic cyst (*arrow*) in the mid pole of the kidney. The cyst is encompassed by the echogenic sinus echoes and is well defined and circular in shape, so it is not hydronephrosis. **E:** A transverse image of the peripelvic cyst proving that it is a peripelvic cyst.

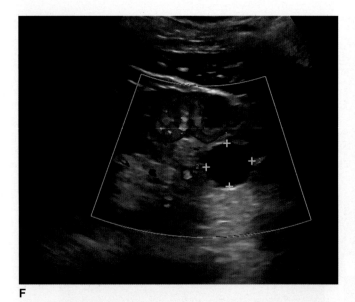

F

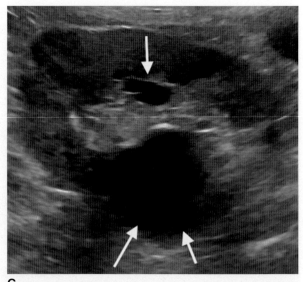

G

FIGURE 12-52 *(continued)* **F:** A color Doppler image of a peripelvic cyst showing that this is a cyst. **G:** The two *arrows* are pointing to a parapelvic cyst and the single arrow to a peripelvic cyst.

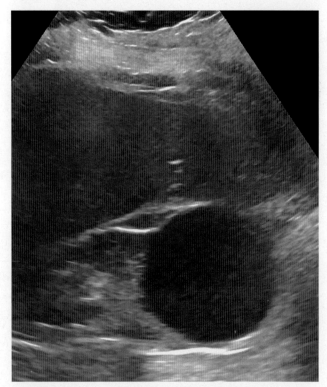

FIGURE 12-53 A cyst in the lower pole of the right kidney. To see the low-level echoes better inside the cyst, the overall gain is turned up, causing brightening of all echoes. This is likely a proteinaceous cyst as it remained unchanged at a 6-month follow-up.

The system was not intended to be used by US or MRI. The use of US to characterize renal cysts using the Bosniak classification remains controversial as US does not always demonstrate the neovascularization of the septations and nodules needed to place it in the proper category.

Original Criteria of Bosniak renal cyst classification system

- Bosniak 1: criteria of a simple cyst. No workup is needed. The risk of malignancy is 0%.

- Bosniak 2: mildly complex cyst with thin septa and calcifications. The risk of malignancy is 0%.
- Bosniak 2F: moderately complex cyst that requires follow-up to demonstrate stability. Also applied to a totally intrarenal cyst that is greater than 3 cm. Follow-up recommended in 6 to 12 months. The risk of malignancy is about 5%.
- Bosniak 3: indeterminate complex cyst with thick, irregular septations and cyst wall, thick nodular calcifications, and wall nodularity. Treatment includes partial nephrectomy or ablation. The risk of malignancy is about 55%.
- Bosniak 4: very complex cyst with gross irregular thick cyst wall and septa. Treatment includes partial or total nephrectomy. The risk of malignancy is about 100%.

Owing to its poor predictive value, the original system referred some benign cysts to surgery, whereas some malignant cysts were not. Therefore, a new Bosniak classification, called version 2019, was proposed to increase the accuracy of malignancy in a cystic renal mass and now includes MRI criteria. The 2019 update is very CT and MRI specific, and the criteria that can be used with US remains the same as the original criteria. Because CEUS increases the sensitivity in the detection of blood flow, in 2020, the European Federation of Societies for Ultrasound in Medicine and Biology (EFSUMB) proposed a CEUS-adapted Bosniak cyst classification system using the same five categories. One difference between the US chart and the CT and MRI charts is that the US chart discusses grayscale characteristics and when CEUS needs to be used, whereas CT and MRI charts are solely contrast based. Hopefully, because US contrast is not nephrotoxic and there is no radiation, the medical community will start to use CEUS more and use CT and MRI on technically challenging patients or to clarify CEUS findings.

Calcifications

The presence of calcifications in a cyst is a nonspecific finding. Calcifications in renal cysts may be fine and linear, or amorphous and thick. Thin calcifications in the cyst wall or

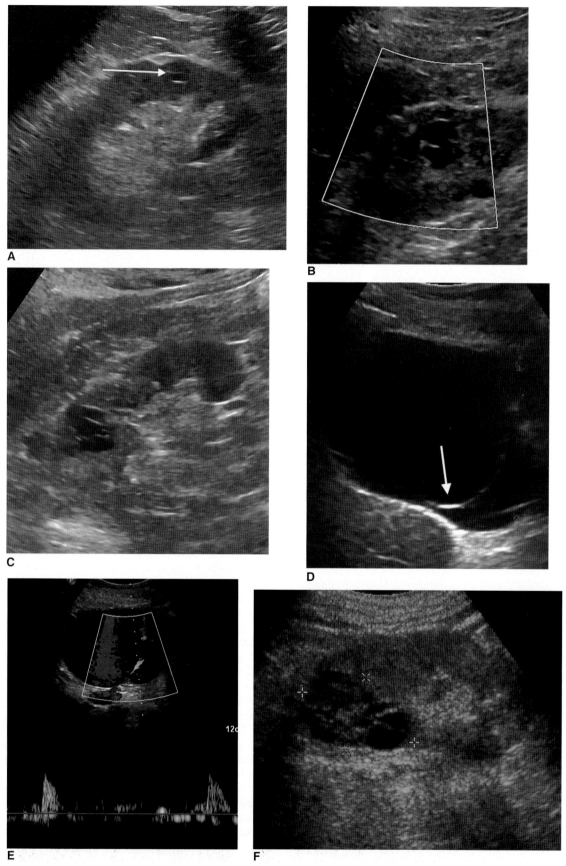

FIGURE 12-54 Septations. **A:** A cyst with a thin, single septation (*arrow*). **B:** Transverse image with color Doppler showing no flow within the septations. **C:** A cyst with multiple thin septations. **D:** A large cyst with two thin septations. The *arrow* is pointing to a calcification within the septation. **E:** Color Doppler demonstrates an arterial waveform within the septation. The cyst had benign characteristics, except for its size. Finding arterial flow in the septation changed the diagnosis to a cystic renal cell carcinoma. **F:** A very complicated cyst with multiple thick septations and mural nodules.

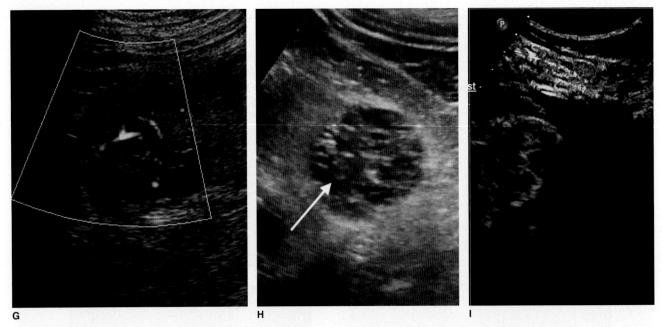

G   H   I

FIGURE 12-54 (*continued*) **G:** Power Doppler showed flow within septations and the nodule that were compatible with a cystic renal cell carcinoma. **H:** A complicated cyst with multiple septations and calcifications. **I:** A contrast-enhanced ultrasound showed flow in the septations and nodules compatible with a cystic renal cell carcinoma.

in a septation are usually a benign feature. Thick, irregular, amorphous calcifications are more concerning for malignancy, and further imaging is needed. Calcifications may not be dense enough to be identified on a CT examination.

A milk-of-calcium cyst is a viscous colloidal suspension of calcium salts that gravitates to the most dependent portion of a calyceal diverticulum that has lost communication with the collecting system, or within a simple renal cyst. The etiology of milk of calcium is unclear; however, it may be related to obstruction or infection. They are more common in the upper pole of the kidneys. Patients are typically asymptomatic. They are an incidental finding that does not require treatment unless the patient becomes symptomatic.

Sonographically, a milk-of-calcium cyst shows dependent echogenic material. A milk-of-calcium cyst may demonstrate a comet-tail artifact, or posterior shadowing may be seen (Fig. 12-55A–C).

Autosomal Dominant Polycystic Kidney Disease[4,7,13,28–30]

PKD is a genetic condition that causes the growth of numerous cysts in the kidneys. The kidneys lose their ability to filter waste from the blood, leading to renal failure. There are two inherited forms of PKD: autosomal dominant PKD, also called adult PKD (ADPKD), which is the most common type. In autosomal dominant PKD, if one of the parents carries the disease gene, the child has a 50/50 chance of inheriting the disease. The other type is autosomal recessive PKD, or infantile PKD, where both parents must have and pass along the gene mutation for the child to be affected. This type will be discussed in the pediatric chapter.

ADPKD is an inherited autosomal dominant trait and is the most common kidney disorder passed down through family members. Once diagnosed with ADPKD, US will be used to screen family members who would be at risk. ADPKD

affects 1 in every 1,000 to 2,000 people and is found in all races, occurring equally in both men and women. ADPKD always affects both kidneys. The kidneys are normal at birth, and over time, they start to develop multiple cysts. By the age of 30, approximately 68% of patients will have visible cysts on their kidneys by US, and eventually, all patients will demonstrate multiple cysts on their kidneys.

ADPKD is characterized by enlarged kidneys that contain multiple cysts that vary in size and are found in both the renal cortex and the medulla. The cysts can grow large enough to obliterate the renal sinus. In some patients, the normal renal parenchyma is replaced with multiple cysts and the kidneys lose their characteristic renal shape. Because these cysts only involve a portion of the nephron, renal function is maintained for the first fourth to fifth decades of the patient's life. Over time, the enlarging cysts increase the size of the kidney by up to four times its normal size. The damages caused by these enlarging cysts and the increase in the kidney size become irreversible and lead to progressive renal failure. Patients are usually asymptomatic until they start to develop either hypertension or renal failure. ADPKD is the fourth leading cause of kidney failure and causes about 5% of all renal failure and is responsible for 10% to 15% of patients on dialysis. By the age of 60 years, approximately 50% of patients with ADPKD will have ESRD.

Several conditions associated with ADPKD include cysts in other organs, with the liver being the most common organ affected. Other organs include the spleen, pancreas, thyroid, ovaries, seminal vesicles, and prostate. The most serious complication of ADPKD is a cerebral berry aneurysm, which can cause a subarachnoid hemorrhage. When compared with the general population, the risk of a patient with ADPKD developing a brain aneurysm is approximately fivefold greater. Some other complications include aortic dissection, abnormalities of the heart valves, and colon diverticulosis.

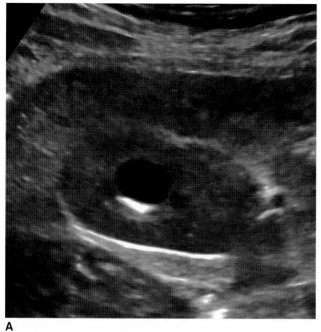

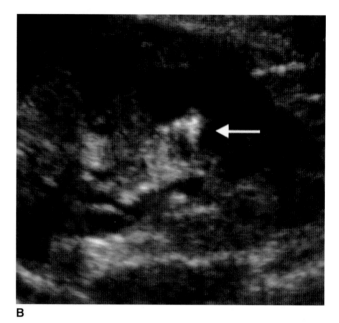

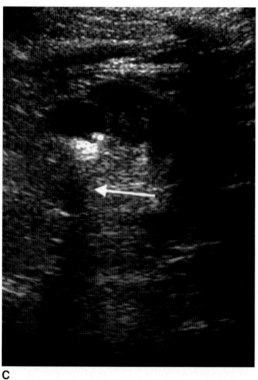

FIGURE 12-55 Milk-of-calcium cyst. **A:** Transverse image of a milk-of-calcium cyst demonstrating the echogenic material at the dependent portion of the cyst. **B:** The *arrow* is pointing to a comet-tail artifact, a type of reverberation artifact, caused by the echogenic material inside the cyst. **C:** The *arrow* is pointing to an acoustic shadow caused by the echogenic material inside the cyst. It is important not to mistake a milk-of-calcium cyst for a kidney stone because shadowing is seen.

Clinical symptoms of ADPKD include flank or abdominal pain, which is the most common complaint; hypertension; palpable mass; hematuria; and renal insufficiency. Patients with ADPKD also have a high incidence of kidney stones. Complications from ADPKD include infection, hemorrhage, rupture of a cyst, and renal obstruction.

Sonographically, both kidneys are enlarged, with numerous cysts in the kidney. The kidneys usually do not have their normal renal contour or shape as it is distorted by the multiple cysts. Sonographic signs of complications include a thickened cyst wall, internal echoes with a fluid–debris or a

fluid–fluid level inside the affected cyst(s), hydronephrosis, and free fluid in the abdomen. Once ADPKD is identified, the liver, pancreas, and spleen should be scanned for any evidence of involvement (Fig. 12-56A–F).

Acquired Cysts[4,7,13,30]

Acquired cystic kidney disease (ACKD) is a condition that occurs in the native kidneys of patients with ESRD, especially those patients who are on either renal or peritoneal dialysis. About 60% of patients who are on dialysis for

2 to 4 years and 90% of patients who are on dialysis for 8 years or more will develop ACKD. ACKD is characterized by three or more cysts, ranging from 0.5 to 3 cm, in both kidneys involving both the renal cortex and the medulla. Some cysts can develop before dialysis, suggesting that the cysts are not only due to dialysis. The causes of the cysts in ACKD are not fully understood and are hypothesized to be a result of the build-up of waste products in the kidneys. ACKD affects men more than women, and patients are usually asymptomatic. Hemorrhage into cysts is common and, when it occurs, can cause flank pain. Unlike ADPKD, ACKD is not a genetic disorder and there is no association of cysts in other organs. ACKD can be distinguished from ADPKD as the kidneys are small in size. One concerning

complication of ACKD is that the patient can develop an RCC, which occurs in 4% to 10% of patients. The longer a person is on dialysis, the higher their risk of developing an RCC. RCC is found predominantly in men, with a male-to-female ratio of 7:1, compared with 2:1 in the general population. With sonography, the native kidneys are small and echogenic and contain several small cysts. There will be internal echoes within the cyst if there is a hemorrhage (Fig. 12-57A–C).

von Hippel–Lindau Disease[4,7]

von Hippel–Lindau (vHL) disease is an inherited autosomal dominant disease in which patients develop multiple benign

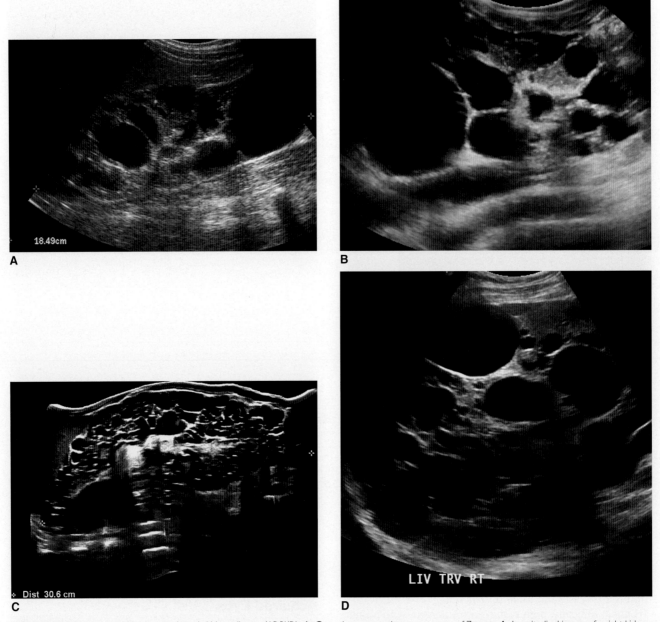

FIGURE 12-56 Autosomal dominant polycystic kidney disease (*ADPKD*). **A–C** are the same patient over a span of 7 years. **A:** Longitudinal image of a right kidney in the early stages of ADPKD measuring 18.5 cm in length. There are numerous cysts seen of various sizes with cortex seen and the kidney shape preserved. **B:** A follow-up examination 3 years later because of flank pain. The kidney is now larger with bigger cysts. The length was estimated at 24 cm. **C:** A follow-up examination 4 years later because of the onset of renal failure. To appreciate the length of the kidney, the extended field-of-view feature was used so that the length of the kidney could be obtained, which now measures at least 30 cm. In 7 years, the kidney almost doubled in size. **D:** An image of a liver affected by ADPKD.

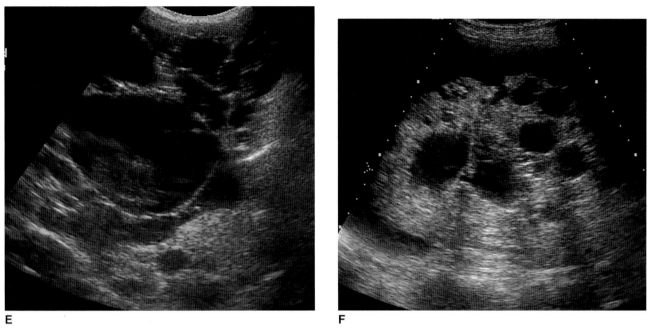

E   F

FIGURE 12-56 *(continued)* **E:** An image of a spleen that is affected by ADPKD. **F:** A rare image of a pancreas that is affected by ADPKD.

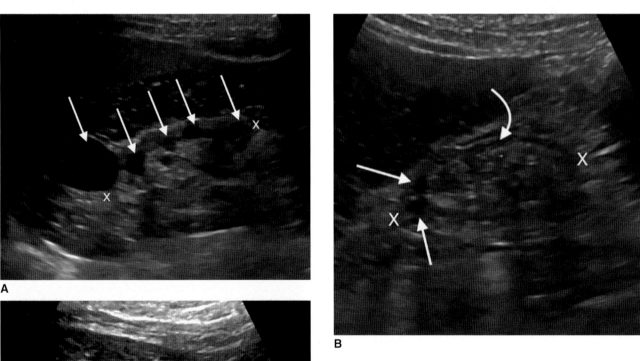

A

B

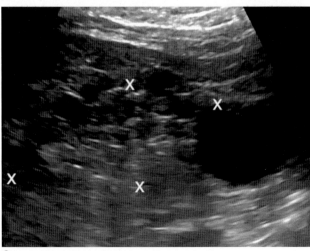

C

FIGURE 12-57 Acquired cystic kidney disease. **A:** The kidney of a patient who has been on dialysis for 4 years. The kidney is between the Xs, and the *arrows* are pointing to the cysts. **B:** The kidney of a patient who has been on dialysis for 6 years. The kidney is between the Xs, and the *curved arrow* is identifying the very thin cortex. The *arrows* are pointing to the cysts. **C:** The kidney of a patient who has been on dialysis for 2 years. There are cysts of various sizes with very little cortex seen. The kidney is between the Xs. You can see by these examples how it can be difficult to find the kidney with their reduced cortex, prominent sinus, and the various cysts. (Images courtesy of J. Guse.)

and malignant tumors that affect various organs. vHL disease is named after a German ophthalmologist, Eugen von Hippel (1867 to 1939), who described a rare disorder of the eye, angiomatosis of the retina, and Arvid Vilhelm Lindau (1892 to 1958), a Swedish pathologist who described the association between angiomatosis of the retina and hemangioblastomas of the central nervous system and called it angiomatosis of the central nervous system. In 1964, the disease was renamed von Hippel–Lindau disease. Symptoms of vHL disease will vary among patients as it depends on the location of the tumors. Most patients are diagnosed with their first tumor in early adulthood. Patients with vHL will have a sonogram to evaluate their kidneys for cysts and RCC. US can also look for tumors in other organs, such as the adrenal gland and pancreas. Cortical renal cysts are a common finding in patients with vHL. RCC occurs in about 70% of individuals with vHL disease and are diagnosed at an earlier age than the general population. RCCs on these patients are usually multifocal and bilateral and are one of the leading causes of death.

SOLID RENAL MASS[4,7,13,31]

Renal masses cause a distortion of the normal renal tissue, and detecting them depends on its echogenicity, size, and location. Solid renal masses can be either benign or malignant. A benign tumor is a localized growth of cells that does not spread to other parts of the body. A malignant tumor is a cancer, and its cells can grow and spread to other parts of the body. The word *cancer* is derived from the Latin word for *crab*. Hippocrates first described cancer as having a central body with the tendency to reach out and spread like "the arms of a crab." Cancer is a term used for abnormal cells that divide without control and have no known purpose in the physiologic function of the body. Cancers can invade other organs, which is called metastatic disease, and reoccur after surgically removal.

What is the difference between the terms mass, tumor, nodule, neoplasm, lesion, and cancer? These terms appear to describe the same thing, so are they interchangeable? The term *mass* describes any overgrowth of tissue and can be either benign or malignant. *Tumor* is Latin for swelling and is a general term that can be applied to something that is either benign or malignant. The terms *tumor and cancer* are sometimes used interchangeably, which is misleading as a tumor is not always malignant. A nodule is a growth or lump that can be malignant or benign. The word *neoplasm* is used to describe any new abnormal growth and is classified as benign or malignant. The word neoplasm comes from the Greek *neo*, meaning new, and *plasia*, meaning tissue or cells, so neoplasm literally means new tissue. The term *lesion* describes an area of abnormal tissue that is either benign or malignant. All of these terms, mass, tumor, nodule, lesion, and neoplasm, can be used to describe either benign or malignant growths, thus the confusion. Cancer is the only term that can be used to describe a malignancy.

Most renal masses are incidental findings that are found by US or CT when the patient is having the test for an unrelated reason. With US, renal tumors are usually discovered on a US for the gallbladder or liver; therefore, most unsuspected tumors are discovered on the right kidney. The goal of imaging is to try and differentiate an RCC from a benign mass, although this is difficult with most masses. The sonographic appearance of most solid renal masses is similar, and it is difficult to determine whether the mass is benign or malignant, even with CT and MRI; therefore, all solid renal masses are considered malignant. Most benign tumors are thought to have the possibility of becoming malignant and may be treated as a malignancy.

Solid renal masses may be detected with US as they can distort the outline of the kidney. Some masses will grow away from the surface of the kidney and are called exophytic masses, whereas endophytic tumors will grow inward and are usually infiltrative. The ability of US to see a renal tumor will depend on its echogenicity and size. Larger tumors appear more isoechoic or hypoechoic to the normal renal cortex and are usually found as they distort the normal renal shape or inner architecture. Larger masses have a higher risk of being malignant and a higher risk of metastatic disease. With the increase in imaging resolution, small renal masses (SRMs) are being detected more frequently. *Small renal masses* are defined as a renal neoplasm 4 cm or less in its greatest dimension and include angiomyolipomas (AMLs), adenomas, oncocytomas, and RCCs. An SRM will have a slow growth rate of 1 to 3 mm per year. About 25% of all SRMs are benign. Most SRM are echogenic, making it difficult to determine whether the mass is benign or malignant. Only a fat-containing AML, using CT criteria, can be confidentially diagnosed. Some patients may be a candidate for a percutaneous renal mass biopsy, usually by US, to help with management decisions. Small tumors less than 4 cm usually do not grow rapidly or metastasize and can be monitored with active surveillance, which is defined as monitoring of a renal tumor size by serial imaging, usually contrast CT. Patients who are the poor surgical candidates may undergo focal ablation either by cryoablation, freezing the cells to destroy them, or by radiofrequency (RF) ablation, destroying the cells with heat. Active surveillance is a treatment option in patients with multiple comorbidities or who are not the good candidates for surgery. Another option is called watchful waiting where the patient does not receive routine imaging and treatment is not indicated until symptoms appear; however, curative treatment is not the goal. Signs of an SRM being malignant include a growth rate greater than 5 mm per year, the diameter becomes greater than 4 cm, or there is evidence of metastatic disease. US is helpful with SRM as it can distinguish cysts from hypovascular solid tumors seen on CT and can better visualize septations in complex cystic lesions.

Benign Masses[4,7,13,32]

About 20% of renal tumors are benign. The three most common benign masses are adenoma, oncocytoma, and AML. Benign epithelial tumors include adenoma and oncocytoma, and mesenchymal tumors include, but are not limited to, AML. There is a lot of variation in the literature as to what is the most common solid benign renal mass; however, as a sonographer, it does not matter which one is more common as all masses should be worked up the same way. Adenomas and oncocytomas can look the same on US, and both have a similar sonographic appearance to an RCC. Because a renal adenoma can be histologically indistinguishable from an RCC, and a renal oncocytoma has similar cellular features as a granular RCC, both are thought to have the potential for malignant transformation and are, therefore, treated with surgery or ablation depending on the state of the patient's health.

Adenoma[32–34]

Adenomas are usually less than 2 cm in size and are rarely larger than 3 cm. Larger tumors can cause a localized bulge of the renal capsule and can distort the collecting system as well as interfere with the normal function of the kidneys. Adenomas can be single or multiple masses and are found immediately below the renal capsule within the renal cortex. They are usually asymptomatic; however, larger tumors can cause painless hematuria. Adenomas can be classified as precancerous, and many doctors choose to surgically remove them to prevent the possibility of them becoming malignant in the future. Adenomas are more common in older patients and patients with ESRD, who have a higher incidence of their adenoma becoming malignant. The sonographic appearance of an adenoma is a solid mass that can be hyperechoic to hypoechoic to the normal renal cortex and hypovascular with color Doppler (Fig. 12-58A–C).

Oncocytoma[32,33–35]

An oncocytoma is a relatively benign renal tumor that occurs in the cortex. They are bilateral in 13% of patients and are

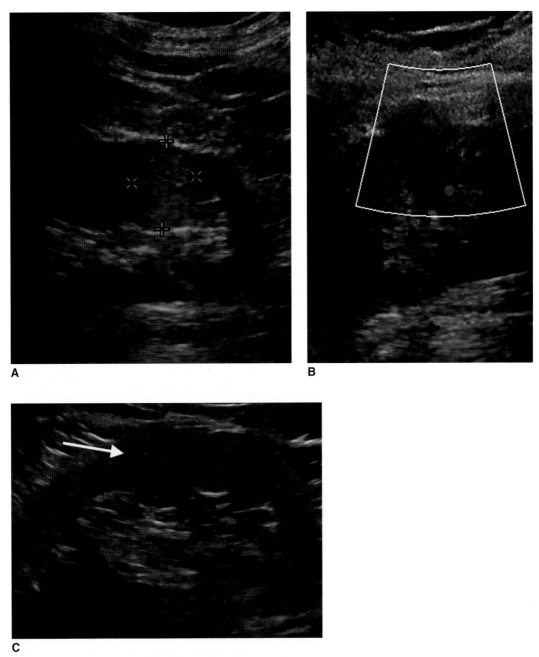

A

B

C

FIGURE 12-58 Adenomas. **A:** An echogenic adenoma right under the capsule in the lower pole. **B:** A larger adenoma that has distorted the renal capsule. This adenoma is hypoisoechoic to the parenchyma. The bulge brought the mass to the attention of the sonographer. Color Doppler shows no flow inside the mass. **C:** The *arrow* is pointing to a subtle hypoechoic adenoma that is indenting both the capsule and the sinus echoes. The capsule distortion is not as noticeable as the previous example.

found in 32% of patients with an RCC. They occur more often in men and are usually found in patients in their sixties or older. Oncocytomas can vary in size and have been reported to be as large as 20 cm. Oncocytomas are not unique to the kidneys and can occur in other organs, with the salivary glands being a common site. Patients are typically asymptomatic, but symptoms of pain and hematuria have been reported. Oncocytomas share the same origin as chromophobe RCCs and, therefore, have overlapping histologic and imaging features. There have been reported cases of hybrid lesions consisting of both oncocytic and chromophobe RCC elements with rare cases of liver metastases. Even with a biopsy of the mass, it can be difficult to differentiate an oncocytoma from an RCC because an RCC can also have oncocytic elements. A definitive diagnosis of oncocytoma can only be made with surgery. The main clinical difficulty is distinguishing it from an RCC, as imaging and histology can be very similar.

By imaging, an oncocytoma is a well-circumscribed mass with a central stellate scar, which can be difficult to visualize on imaging. The *central stellate scar* refers to a central zone of fibrous connective tissue with bands radiating toward the periphery, causing it to resemble a star. Unfortunately, the central stellate scar is not a unique feature and is only seen in about one-third of oncocytomas, and some RCCs have what appears to be a central scar. Owing to this difficulty in making a definite diagnosis that the mass is an oncocytoma, they are usually resected.

Sonographically, oncocytomas can be hypoechoic to hyperechoic, homogeneous and have a well-defined wall. The stellate scar appearance is usually difficult to see with US; however, when the scar is seen, especially in larger lesions, it is hypoechoic. Sometimes, using one of the B-color maps can help bring it out. Color Doppler may demonstrate flow in the periphery and strip-like signals within the mass. Unfortunately, the US appearance of an oncocytoma can vary, making it difficult to separate it from an RCC (Fig. 12-59A–D).

Angiomyolipoma[32,35–37]

Also known as a renal hamartoma, AMLs are benign tumors located within the renal cortex. It is composed of blood vessels (angio), smooth muscle cells (myo), and fat cells (lipo), and the tumor can vary in the amount of each cell type. AMLs are strongly associated with tuberous sclerosis, which is a genetic disease, and these tumors are usually small, multiple, and bilateral. In patients without tuberous sclerosis, AML most often occurs in middle-aged women. The majority of AMLs are found in the right kidney. Most patients are asymptomatic, but symptoms can include a palpable mass, pain, and hematuria. The main clinical concern of a patient with an AML is spontaneously hemorrhage, which can be fatal. The patient may present with acute flank pain due to a spontaneous hemorrhage. If an AML is greater than 4 cm in size, it may be resected with a partial nephrectomy or undergo embolization to reduce the risk of hemorrhage. A definitive diagnosis of an AML can be made with CT if it contains macroscopic fat.

An AML is the brightest of all the renal masses because of the amount of fat in the tumor. AMLs are round or oval, well circumscribed, homogeneous; do not exhibit a hypoechoic rim; and are very hyperechoic when compared with the renal cortex. Its echogenicity will depend on the proportions of fat, smooth muscle, and vascular cells that make up the AML. If there is more muscle or vascular cells and less fat cells in the tumor, it may be more heterogeneous. A heterogeneous AML can also be seen if there is hemorrhage and necrosis. If an AML contains too little fat, called a fat-poor AML, it can be harder to differentiate from a small RCC on CT. A renal sonogram may be ordered to try and help differentiate an SRM from an AML that was found on a CT scan. Patients may be followed up with US to watch for any changes in the AML, which may indicate that it is an RCC, and monitor growth to determine the need for an intervention (Fig. 12-60A–D).

Malignant Masses[38–40]

Cancers within the kidney are termed *kidney or renal pelvis* cancers. According to the American Cancer Society, the 2022 estimates for kidney and renal pelvic cancer in the United States were about 79,000 new cases, accounting for about 4% of all new cancer cases, of which 50,290 are men and 28,710 are women. About 13,920 people will die from this disease, accounting for about 2.3% of all cancer deaths, of which 8,960 are men and 4,960 are women.

As stated previously, most renal masses are detected incidentally during a US or CT scan, and all solid renal masses are treated as if they are malignant. There are no blood or urine tests that raise a suspicion for RCC nor are there any tumor markers. The various types of adult kidney and renal pelvis cancers include RCC, which is the most common type accounting for about 85% of kidney cancers; urothelial or TCC, accounting for 5% to 10%; sarcoma, which is rare; and lymphoma. Malignant tumors can spread from the original tumor and form new tumors in other parts of the body, called metastatic disease, either by direct extension to nearby organs or to distant sites via the vascular and lymphatic system.

There are many different types of RCC, and the type is determined by the cells that are seen under a microscope. Knowing which type of cell makes up the tumor helps to plan treatment. The most common cell type is clear cell. Clear cell RCC is usually referred to as *conventional* RCC as it is the most common type, accounting for 80% of all RCC cases. It is called clear cell as the cells in the tumor look like clear bubbles under the microscope. Papillary RCC makes up about 15% of all RCCs. Renal medullary carcinoma is a rare form of non–clear cell carcinoma that affects young adults, almost exclusively with sickle cell disease or trait, who has the gene, but not the disease. It is a very aggressive cancer, and most patients usually present with metastases at the time of diagnosis. About 5% of people with RCC will have the chromophobe subtype. This rare cancer looks similar to clear cell RCC but tends to be larger and has other different microscopic features. Chromophobe RCC tends to be a less aggressive type of RCC, even though these tumors grow quite large before they metastasize.

Renal Cell Carcinoma[4,7,8,13,35,38–42]

An RCC is also called a hypernephroma, renal adenocarcinoma, or renal or kidney cancer. The modified 2016 WHO classification defines over 14 types of RCCs. The following factors may raise a person's risk for RCC: smoking,

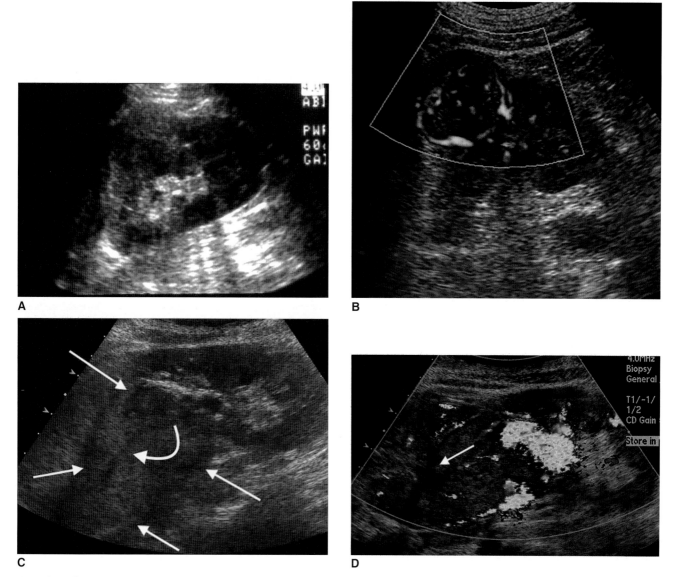

FIGURE 12-59 Oncocytomas. **A:** Longitudinal image of an adenoma on the mid pole of the kidney. Sonographically, this image looks like a renal cell carcinoma. **B:** Power Doppler demonstrates flow in the periphery, and the *arrow* is pointing to the strip-like signals within the mass. This is typically not the vasculature of a renal cell carcinoma seen with color or power Doppler. **C:** A large oncocytoma is seen arising from the posterior surface of the upper pole. The bottom of the mass is off the image. The *arrows* are outlining the mass as the wall is not demonstrated well because of specular reflectors. The curved area is pointing to the central stellate scar. **D:** Color Doppler image showing flow in the periphery and the strip-like flow within the mass. The bottom of the mass is now seen. The *arrow* is pointing to the central stellate scar.

which is the most important risk factor doubling the risk; being overweight; high blood pressure, especially in men, although it is not known whether the increased risk is due to the hypertension itself or the medicines used to treat it; and taking certain pain medicines for a long time, such as acetaminophen, aspirin, and other NSAIDs. Patients with RCC are more likely to present with symptoms caused by their metastatic disease than by the primary tumor. The classic triad of flank pain, hematuria, and flank mass is uncommon and only presents in about 10% of patients. The frequency of the individual components of the classic triad is asymptomatic hematuria, 60%; flank pain, 40%; and palpable mass in the flank or abdomen, 25%. A person with an RCC may have one or more of the following symptoms: a lump or swelling in the kidney area or abdomen; lower

back pain or pain in the side, called flank pain, that does not go away; feeling tired; and unexpected weight loss.

RCC has no predilection for the left or right kidney or a preference in pole location. RCC originates in the proximal renal tubular epithelium and accounts for 5% of adult cases of cancer in men and 3% in women. According to the American Cancer Society, the 2021 estimates for kidney and renal pelvis cancer in the United States were about 76,080 new cases, accounting for about 4% of all new cancer cases, of which 48,780 are men and 27,300 are women. About 13,780 people will die from this disease, accounting for about 2.3% of all cancer deaths, of which 8,790 are men and 4,990 are women. These numbers include all the various types of kidney and renal pelvis cancers. Kidney and renal pelvis cancers are the sixth

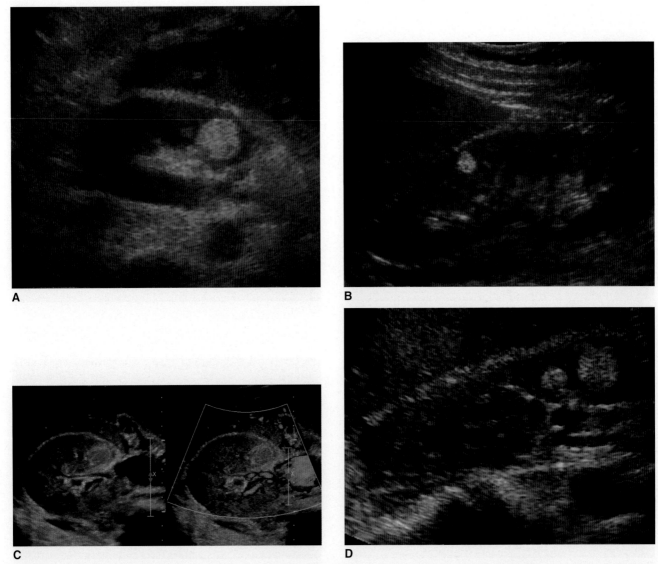

FIGURE 12-60 Angiomyolipomas. **A:** Transverse image of a very bright, echogenic mass in the kidney compatible with an angiomyolipoma. **B:** Longitudinal image showing a small echogenic angiomyolipoma. **C:** Transverse image of the kidney of an angiomyolipoma that has less fat in it. making it not as echogenic as the previous examples. This angiomyolipoma is also heterogeneous. Power Doppler shows that there is no flow in the mass. **D:** Longitudinal image along the lateral aspect of the kidney showing two angiomyolipomas.

most common cancer in men and the ninth most common cancer in women, with breast cancer being the most common cancer in women, except for skin cancers, and prostate cancer being the most common cancer in men, except for skin cancers. Most people are diagnosed with a kidney and renal pelvis cancer between the ages of 65 to 74 years. RCC is rare in people under the age of 45. As you can tell from the abovementioned statistics, kidney and renal pelvis cancer is more common in men than in women. People who have been on long-term dialysis may develop a cystic type of RCC, and up to 60% of people with vHL syndrome can develop clear cell RCC and have a higher incidence of multiple and bilateral masses. People with ACKD will have more bilateral, multifocal, and papillary RCC than the general population, and patients who are younger than 40 years are at a much higher risk to have bilateral tumors. RCC can metastasize via the bloodstream or by lymphatic dissemination. RCC typically metastasizes

to the following organs in order from the most affected to the least affected: the lung, which accounts for 45% of all metastases; bone; lymph nodes; the liver; adrenal glands; and the brain, which accounts for 8% of all metastases. RCC can metastasize to the other kidney in 10% to 15% of patients and is considered a metastatic tumor and not a primary. Once an RCC is discovered, the patient will need a CT or MRI to look for metastatic disease to help stage the tumor. US cannot be used for staging as it cannot evaluate the lungs for metastatic disease.

The 5-year survival rate for kidney and renal pelvis cancer will depend on the cell type and if it is confined to the kidney or has spread. Tumors confined to the kidney have a 5-year survival rate of 93%; if it has spread locally, 70%; or if there are distal metastases, a 5-year survival rate of 13%. A 5-year survival rate means that people who have cancer are, on average, about 80% as likely as people who do not have cancer to live for at least 5 years after being diagnosed.

The main goal in treating an RCC is to remove the cancer and to protect renal function. Treatment will depend on the stage and grade of the tumor, the patient's age, and overall health. Surgical resection remains the only known curative treatment for a localized RCC and is the most common treatment. Surgical options include a partial or radical nephrectomy, and the surgery can be an open surgery, meaning an incision is made, or by laparoscopic or robotic methods. A partial nephrectomy is performed usually when the tumor is contained in the kidney, and only the tumor is excised, leaving the rest of the normal kidney untouched. A radical nephrectomy is more commonly performed and includes removing the entire kidney, Gerota fascia, the perirenal fat, and, sometimes, the ipsilateral adrenal gland. There is also the possibility of ipsilateral lymph node dissection. The perirenal fat is removed as it may be involved with the cancer. If the adrenal gland is abnormal on a CT scan, it will be removed, although some surgeons may still opt to remove it even if it is normal on CT. The remaining kidney on a patient who had a radical nephrectomy will eventually hypertrophy, that is enlarge, to compensate for the extra work it now performs. Unfortunately, approximately 20% to 30% of patients after a nephrectomy will go on to develop metastatic disease.

Not every patient will have surgery and may enter into what is called active surveillance if their mass is less than 4 cm and if the surgeon is not 100% convinced that the mass is malignant. With active surveillance, the patient will be seen at specified intervals for tests and will usually have a chest X-ray looking for metastatic lung disease and a CT or US scan of the kidney. The goal is to monitor any progression or changes of the mass. Other treatment options include chemotherapy, cold or hot ablation, radiation therapy, and immunotherapy, or the patient may decide to enter a clinical trial, which are research programs to evaluate new medical treatments, new chemotherapy, and new immunotherapy drugs. Current clinical trials and their locations can be found at www.cancer.gov. Ablation is usually performed on patients who are not the good candidates for surgery. US may be used to guide ablation procedures and sometimes as part of the postprocedural imaging to evaluate for reoccurrence. Targeted therapy and immunotherapy may be used on patients with metastatic disease. Immunotherapy works with the patient's own immune system to attack the cancer. Targeted therapy uses drugs to attack the cancer cells without damaging healthy cells. Some drugs will prevent blood flow to the tumor, which basically starves the tumor, causing it to shrink.

A solid RCC on US can be hyperechoic, isoechoic, or hypoechoic to the surrounding normal renal parenchyma, and homogeneous or heterogeneous, with larger tumors being heterogeneous due to internal hemorrhage and necrosis. The majority of RCCs will be isoechoic, whereas RCCs of less than 4 cm, an SRM, are often hyperechoic, making them difficult to differentiate from an AML. The most common appearance is isoechoic, and the sonographer needs to be on the lookout for distortion or bulge on the normal renal contour or a bulge into the central renal sinus. Most masses will be large enough to easily see. A suspicious area will need to be evaluated with color Doppler looking for an area of abnormal flow patterns in the cortex, as this may indicate where the tumor is located. Abnormal flow patterns can be seen with other pathology such as pyelonephritis, so it is not specific to RCC; however, the patient's history will help determine the reason for the abnormal flow. The presence of calcifications in the mass is considered suspicious for RCC. Macroscopic calcifications may be seen in some RCCs and can have a variety of appearances, including punctate, curvilinear, central, or peripheral. A hypoechoic rim, which represents a vascular pseudocapsule, may be seen with grayscale. It is thought that the pseudocapsule that surrounds the mass is composed of a large number of fibrous tissue and capillaries that are between the normal renal tissue and the RCC. Vascularity of the RCC may be seen in up to 92% of cases, demonstrating the basket sign and/or vessels within the tumor that represent neovascularity, which are new blood vessels. Spectral Doppler waveforms will show high systolic and high end-diastolic flow with a low RI (Fig. 12-61A–K).

A strength of US is in determining if the mass is solid or cystic. A small percentage of all RCCs will have a cystic appearance, and the septations need to be investigated with color and power Doppler to determine whether they have flow within them. A multilocular cystic RCC will show thick internal septations, which measure greater than 2 mm, are nodular, and may contain calcifications. A unilocular cystic RCC will have internal echoes with thick, irregular walls that may have calcifications (see Fig. 12-54E–I).

When a solid renal mass is found, the ipsilateral, the same side, renal vein must be evaluated from the kidney to the IVC, as well as the IVC itself. Extension of an RCC into the renal vein occurs in up to 24% of patients, and tumor thrombus may extend into the IVC in up to 10% of cases. Invasion of the IVC is more common with the right kidney because of the shorter length of the vein. Color Doppler is used to evaluate the renal vein by either documenting a normal patent vein or seeing low-level echoes inside the vein, which represents a tumor thrombus. A tumor thrombus is not a blood clot but is the RCC growing inside the vein, making this at least a stage T3 cancer. This tumor thrombus needs to be evaluated with color Doppler to look for color signals inside the thrombus and, if seen a waveform, needs to be obtained to document the arterial flow in the vein, which represent feeding vessels (Fig. 12-62A, B).

Transitional Cell Carcinomas[4,7,13,43,44]

TCCs are malignant tumors that arise from the lining of the renal pelvis, calyces, ureter, and bladder and account for 8% to 10% of all renal cancers. They are also called urothelial carcinomas. In all, 90% to 92% of renal pelvis cancers are TCCs, and the remaining 10% are squamous cell carcinomas (SCCs). TCC of the renal pelvis is histologically the same as a TCC of the bladder. Upper urinary tract urothelial tumors may be multifocal and, in 2% to 10% of cases, bilateral. The major cause of urothelial cancer is cigarette smoking. Other risk factors include taking aristolochic acids, which is found in certain herbal products; people with chronic kidney stones or infections; and occupational exposure to toxins used in rubber, paint, and dye factories. These primary renal tumors become clinically apparent within a relatively short time because their growth causes fragmentation, producing noticeable but painless hematuria in 60% of cases. They are small and usually not palpable but may block urinary outflow, causing hydronephrosis. These tumors are invasive

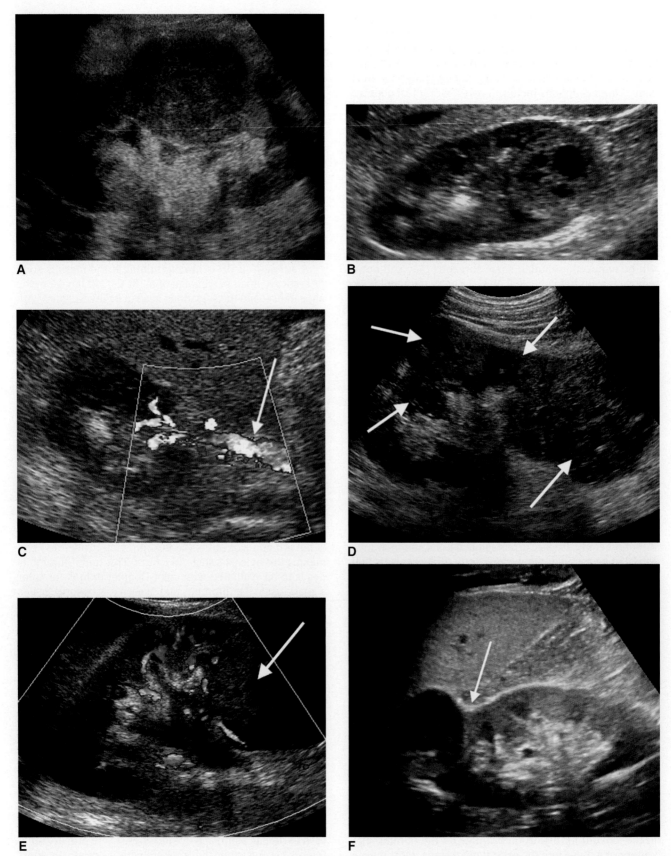

FIGURE 12-61 Renal cell carcinoma (*RCC*). **A:** Hyperechoic, large RCC arising from the anterior mid pole. **B:** RCC in the lower pole with cystic areas. **C:** Same patient showing that the main renal vein (*arrow*) is patent. This is a mandatory image whenever a solid renal mass is found. **D:** The *arrows* are pointing to multiple renal masses, which were RCC. This patient had von Hippel–Lindau syndrome. **E:** Color Doppler of an RCC demonstrating flow around the periphery called the basket sign. The *arrow* is pointing to the mass. **F:** An RCC in the upper pole of the kidney. The *arrow* is pointing to the kidney capsule as it encompasses the mass. Note how the mass touches the sinus echoes.

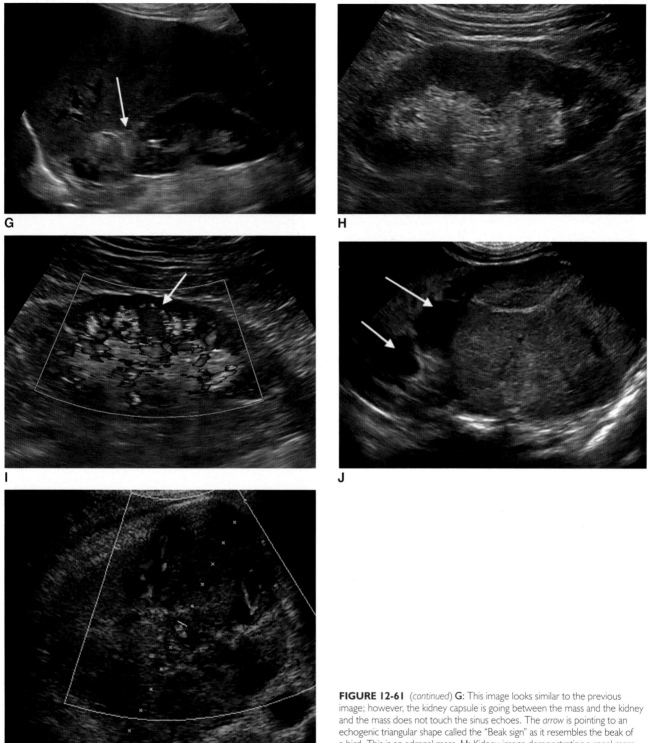

FIGURE 12-61 (*continued*) **G:** This image looks similar to the previous image; however, the kidney capsule is going between the mass and the kidney and the mass does not touch the sinus echoes. The *arrow* is pointing to an echogenic triangular shape called the "Beak sign" as it resembles the beak of a bird. This is an adrenal mass. **H:** Kidney image demonstrating a renal mass. **I:** The *arrow* is pointing to this small isoechoic mass, which did not distort the renal capsule. Color Doppler outlines the mass. **J:** A very large RCC that takes up half the kidney. The *arrows* are pointing to hydronephrosis cause by the mass. **K:** A biopsy of a renal mass that was diagnosed as papillary renal cell carcinoma. There are no characteristics of a papillary RCC to distinguish it from a clear cell RCC by ultrasound.

without the bulky mass, infiltrating the wall of the pelvis and calyces.

TCC, just like RCC, is much more common in men and is typically diagnosed between the ages of 60 and 70 years. Renal pelvis tumors rarely occur before the age of 40.

Patients who have a TCC of the renal pelvis have a 30% to 50% chance of developing a bladder TCC, whereas patients with a bladder TCC have a 2% to 3% chance of developing a TCC in the renal pelvis. TCCs of the renal pelvis are bilateral in 2% to 4% of patients. There is no preference

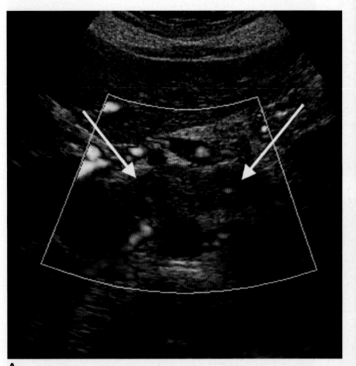

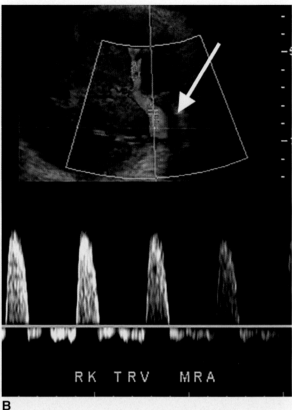

A

B

FIGURE 12-62 Extension of renal cell carcinoma (*RCC*). **A:** Power Doppler was used to evaluate thrombus-like material within in the renal vein. The *arrows* are pointing to areas of flow inside this left renal vein that has been invaded by renal cell carcinoma. This finding advances the grade of the cancer. Spectral Doppler signals, not shown, were arterial. **B:** The renal vein was not visualized on this patient with RCC. The *arrow* is pointing to the vein that was full of tumor thrombosis. A diagnostic sign of renal vein thrombosis is a biphasic arterial signal. *MRA*, main renal artery.

between the right and left kidney, nor is there any location preference. The majority of patients present with gross painless hematuria, which is the most common presenting symptom, and a smaller percent with microscopic hematuria. Up to one-third of patients present with flank pain, caused by the gradual obstruction of the collecting system, or acute renal colic, especially if passing blood clots. These symptoms are characteristic of a renal stone and are typically the reasons that the US is ordered. A small percentage of patients will be asymptomatic, making these tumors rarely an incidental finding. The majority of renal pelvis TCCs are low-stage papillary neoplasms and have a good prognosis. The infiltrating type will often invade into the renal parenchyma. The most common sites for metastases are the liver, bone, and lungs. The 5-year survival rate after surgery will depend on the stage of the disease, with those having distant metastasizes 0%. Patients with tumors that have penetrated through the urothelial wall or have distant metastases usually cannot be cured with currently available forms of treatment. Fortunately, the majority of TCC are low grade, and the prognosis for the patient is good, with a 5-year survival of over 90%, following surgical removal.

There are different treatments depending on the grade of the tumor and the health of the patient. The traditional treatment of an upper tract TCC is a total nephroureterectomy, which involves removing the kidney and the entire length of the ureter including its insertion into the bladder. A nephroureterectomy gives the best chance of completely getting rid of the TCC. Other types of treatment include chemotherapy, for patients with metastatic disease, and radiation therapy, which is rarely used to treat TCC, except for palliative care in controlling pain on patients with advanced disease. Unlike an RCC, a patient who is discovered to have a renal pelvis TCC needs their bladder evaluated. If a TCC is suspected by US, the patient will be sent for a CT or MRI scan for further evaluation.

A TCC of the renal pelvis typically appears as a solid, homogeneous mass in the renal pelvis, causing a separation of the echogenic renal sinus echoes. There may be some focal hydronephrosis caused by the mass and some vascularity seen inside the mass with color Doppler. TCC may invade the adjacent renal parenchyma as an infiltrating mass not affecting the normal renal contour unlike an RCC (Fig. 12-63A–E). With this sonographic appearance, it may be difficult to distinguish a TCC from an RCC. Unlike an RCC, a TCC rarely invades the renal vein. These findings may also be associated with blood clots and fungus balls. Here knowing the patient's history is helpful because if the patient has a history of trauma or a renal biopsy, these findings would be more compatible with a blood clot, or if the patient has fungemia, then a fungal ball should be suspected.

Squamous Cell Carcinoma[4,7,45]

SCC of the renal pelvis is a rare neoplasm and is the second most common malignant urothelial tumor after TCC.

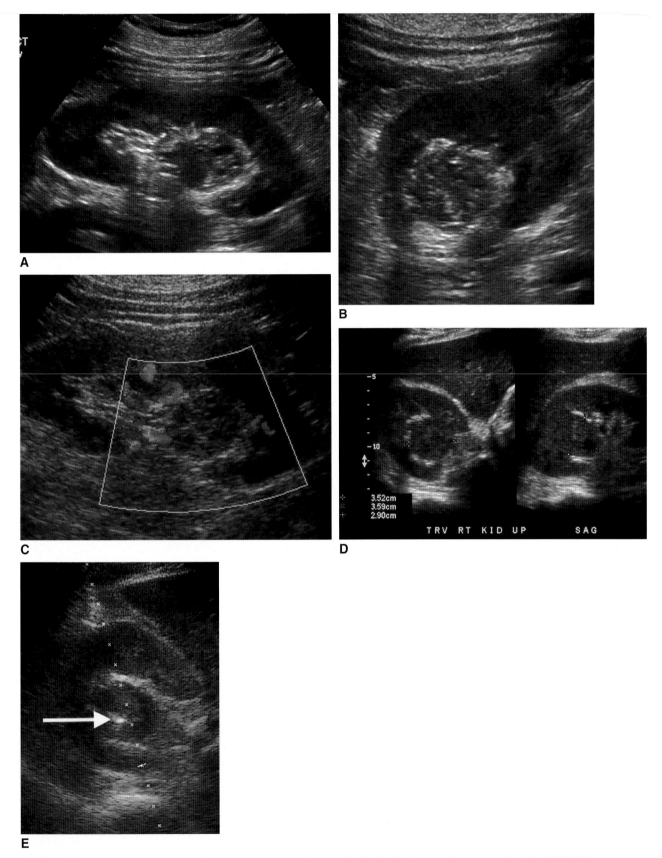

FIGURE 12-63 Transitional cell carcinoma (*TCC*). **A:** Longitudinal image of a mass visualized inside the sinus echoes compatible with a TCC. **B:** Transverse image showing TCC surrounded by the bright white sinus echoes. **C:** Color Doppler of the TCC that does not demonstrate flow. **D:** Transverse and longitudinal images of a mass in the upper pole (*UP*) of the kidney. The sinus echoes do not completely surround the mass as it is spreading into the cortex. **E:** A biopsy of the TCC mass. The *arrow* is pointing to the needle tip. The *dotted line* is the projectory of the needle when using a biopsy guide. Surgery for the TCC confirmed that the cancer had started to spread into the parenchyma. *KID*, kidney; *SAG*, sagittal; *TRV*, transverse.

It represents less than 1% of malignant renal tumors. The most common cause is chronic irritation from kidney stones, usually from a staghorn. Other risk factors include chronic pyelonephritis, exposure to endogenous and exogenous chemicals, and vitamin A deficiency. Patients may present with flank or abdominal pain, microscopic or gross hematuria, weight loss, or a palpable abdominal mass. Renal SCC is higher in individuals who have a horseshoe kidney. Patients typically present at an advanced stage and have a poor prognosis, with a 5-year survival rate reported at less than 10%. It is very rarely diagnosed preoperatively because of its rarity and inconclusive lab results and radiology findings. Treatment is surgical resection, which is rarely curative, and chemotherapy or radiation is usually ineffective.

Renal SCC is seen sonographically as a diffusely enlarged kidney where the normal architecture is not seen; however, it has maintained its kidney or reniform shape. In most patients, a stone is seen, usually a staghorn, with hydronephrosis caused by the stone. On some patients, a large mass in the renal pelvis may be the sonographic finding. Enlarged local lymph nodes may be seen. US findings are nonspecific, and findings are similar to chronic inflammatory conditions, such as xanthogranulomatous pyelonephritis (XGP) or other neoplasms of the kidney. The patient will need a CT and/or an MRI examination to further investigate the mass and the abdomen, but both modalities may have inconclusive results, and the diagnosis will be made at surgery.

Metastatic Renal Tumors[4,7,13,41,46,47]

When a cancer spreads to another part of the body and grows, it is called a metastasis. Nearly all types of cancer have this ability. When this happens, it is called metastatic cancer. The cells of the metastatic mass are the same cells as the primary cancer and are not the cells of the invaded organ. For example, if a person has a primary lung cancer and malignant masses are found in the kidney, these masses will be referred to as metastatic lung cancer and not kidney cancer.

The kidneys are a common site for metastatic disease. The most common sites where metastases occur are, in order, lymph nodes, lungs, liver, brain, bones, adrenals, peritoneum, pleura, and the kidneys. Metastases to the kidneys are seen in 7% to 12% of patients with a malignancy and indicate that the cancer is in an advanced stage, which, unfortunately, is associated with a poor prognosis. Tumor cells are spread to the kidneys through the blood, hematogenous route, or via the lymphatic system. The majority of metastatic tumors will be found in the cortex, with the renal pelvis rarely involved. The two most common cancers that metastasize to the kidneys are melanomas and lung. Other sites include breast, stomach, GI, and pancreas. It is possible for a patient who has an RCC in one kidney to metastasize to the contralateral kidney. Renal metastases are rarely found before the primary mass has been identified. Metastases can appear several years after the primary tumor has been identified, even if it was surgically removed. If a renal mass is discovered in a patient with a known primary tumor, a biopsy of the mass is needed to determine whether the mass is a primary RCC or a metastatic mass to help plan treatment options. Any new renal mass found in a patient with advanced cancer is more likely a metastatic mass than

a primary one. When there is no known primary, the mass is treated like an RCC. Patients are usually asymptomatic, and their current renal functions are not affected. The most common presenting symptoms are flank pain, hematuria, and weight loss. Treatment is usually based on the primary cancer.

Sonographically, metastatic disease to the kidneys has a variety of appearances and can present as a solitary mass, multiple masses, or a diffusely infiltrating mass. They may be hyperechoic, isoechoic or hypoechoic, homogeneous or heterogeneous and can be unilateral or bilateral. A solitary metastasis will be indistinguishable from an RCC. Multiple metastases can appear as small, poorly marginated, hypoechoic masses. Melanoma metastatic lesions to the kidneys can appear as micrometastases and are usually small, multiple, asymptomatic, and bilateral. Infiltrating renal metastases have a subtle appearance with US and can cause the kidney to be enlarged, but not lose its shape. Sometimes, a B-color map will help bring out subtle pathologies (Fig. 12-64A, B).

A CT scan is more commonly ordered for any follow-up imaging examinations of the abdomen in patients with a known cancer. A CT scan can evaluate the entire abdomen, along with the kidneys, and can give a better picture of the full extent of any metastatic disease.

Lymphoma[4,7,13,47–49]

Primary renal lymphoma is a very rare disease and is defined as lymphoma involving the kidney without prior lymphatic disease beyond the kidney. It typically needs to be diagnosed with a biopsy. Therefore, this section discusses secondary renal lymphoma (SRL), which is more commonly seen.

The kidneys are the most common abdominal organ that is affected by non-Hodgkin lymphoma. It is seen when there is widespread nodal or extranodal lymphoma. The kidneys do not contain lymphoid tissue, and involvement is by either a hematogenous spread, the most common, or as direct extension via the retroperitoneal lymphatic channels. SRL has been reported in both pediatric and adult patients. Presenting symptoms can include flank pain, palpable abdominal mass, or hematuria. SRL can be either unilateral or bilateral, have solitary or multiple focal masses, or present as diffuse bilateral enlarged kidneys, nephromegaly, without any focal lesions.

Sonographically, lymphoma can be single or multiple masses that can be either anechoic or hypoechoic in appearance. Because there are few internal reflectors, lymphoma lesions can simulate renal cysts. It is, therefore, very important for the sonographer to document a lack of acoustic enhancement to show that the lesions are solid masses and not cysts. The overall gain should be increased to look for low-level echoes, being careful not to call artifacts real echoes. Lymphoma is commonly seen in both kidneys as multiple nodules. Lymphomas have very little internal vascularity with color or power Doppler. With infiltrating lymphoma, the kidney may be enlarged but keeps its reniform shape. There have been some reports that the tumor can invade the renal sinus and destroy the sonographic appearance of the echogenic, central complex. However, the sonographic appearances of renal lymphoma can be nonspecific, and further imaging with a contrast-enhanced CT is needed (Fig. 12-65A, B) (Pathology Box 12-13).

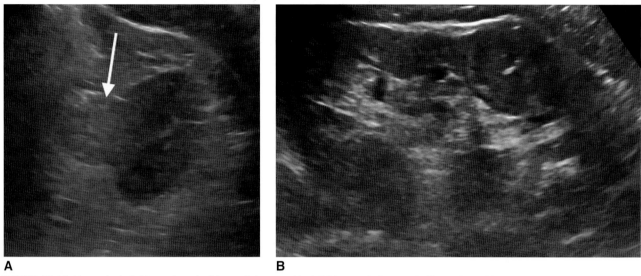

FIGURE 12-64 Metastasis. **A:** Solid mass (*arrow*) off the medial aspect of the left kidney at the lower pole. Biopsy showed this to be a lung metastatic lesion. This mass was challenging to demonstrate because of its location beyond the lower pole, and it could not be identified well within the sagittal plane. **B:** A renal cell carcinoma that metastasized to the contralateral kidney. Patient was 4 years past their nephrectomy.

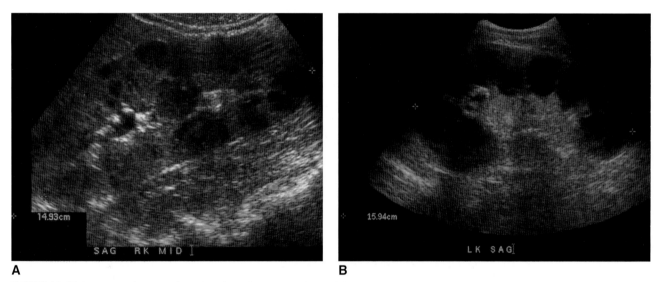

FIGURE 12-65 Lymphoma. **A:** Image of an enlarged right kidney containing multiple hypoechoic areas compatible with the patient's history of lymphoma. **B:** An enlarged kidney with diffuse infiltration of lymphoma. The lymphoma presents itself as hypoechoic and almost cystic masses resembling pyramids and involving most of the cortex.

Renal Mass Biopsies[50,51]

According to the American Urology Association (AUA), a renal mass biopsy should be performed when the mass is suspected to be hematologic, metastatic, inflammatory, or infectious, or whenever it may influence management. It is also recommended that multiple core biopsies be performed and are preferred over fine-needle aspiration (FNA) biopsies. When a patient is being treated with ablation, establishing a diagnosis of cancer before treatment is important. Most biopsies are being performed on SRM so that patients and physicians can use the results from the biopsy to make informed decisions about treatment and to decrease treatment on benign tumors. A positive biopsy result has a high accuracy rate, whereas a benign biopsy result does not ensure that the mass is benign. Some biopsies may be indeterminate and need to be repeated.

Renal masses can be easily biopsied under US guidance. It is best to use a needle guide when performing a biopsy on a renal mass, especially an SRM. The patient should be positioned so that the renal mass is accessible. For the left kidney, the needle should not pass through the spleen due to its friable nature. The patient's position could include oblique, decubitus or even prone, with the decubitus position usually the best approach. It is usually difficult to biopsy the renal mass with the patient in a supine position as it would be difficult for the person performing the biopsy to see the entrance to the needle guide. Both FNA and cores may be obtained, which will result in the need to change the needle guide from the smaller FNA, usually a 20 or 22 g, to the larger 18 or 16 g core needle. The sonographer can have a variety of duties, depending on the radiologist, including locating the mass, determining the best approach, using sterile techniques to place the sterile cover over the

PATHOLOGY BOX 12-13
Renal Masses

1. Cysts
   a. Cortical cysts
      i. Cysts in the cortex that have all the signs of a simple cyst. (Refer to Pathology Box 12-11)
   b. Parapelvic
      i. Originate in adjacent renal parenchyma and extends into renal sinus
   c. Peripelvic
      i. Originate within the renal sinus
      ii. Is not a true cyst as it does not contain contains lymphatic fluid
   d. Complicated cysts
      i. Cysts that contain septations or low-level echoes
   e. ADPKD
      i. Multiple cysts of various sizes in both kidneys
      ii. Usually, the kidney shape is not appreciated
      iii. Kidneys are very increased in size
      iv. Check liver, spleen, and pancreas for cysts
   f. ACKD
      i. Occurs in native kidneys of patients with ESRD
      ii. Characterized by three or more cysts, ranging from 0.5 to 3 cm, in both kidneys
      iii. Involves both renal cortex and medulla
2. Benign solid masses
   a. Adenoma
      i. Usually 2–3 cm in size
      ii. Hyperechoic to hypoechoic to the normal renal cortex and hypovascular
   b. AML
      i. Composed of blood vessels (angio), smooth muscle cells (myo), and fat cells (lipo)
      ii. The cell types can vary in the amount of each type
      iii. Round or oval, well circumscribed, homogeneous
      iv. Very echogenic
         1. The brightest of all the renal masses
   c. Oncocytoma
      i. Can vary in size and as large as 20 cm
      ii. Well circumscribed with a central stellate scar
      iii. Hypoechoic to hyperechoic, homogeneous, well-defined wall
      iv. Scar is hypoechoic if seen
      v. Color Doppler may demonstrate flow in the periphery and strip-like signals within the mass
3. Malignant masses
   a. RCC
      i. Hyperechoic, isoechoic, or hypoechoic to surrounding renal parenchyma
      ii. Homogeneous or heterogeneous, with larger tumors being heterogeneous due to internal hemorrhage and necrosis
      iii. Can distort renal capsule
      iv. Renal vein of that kidney needs to be checked for tumor thrombosis
   b. TCC
      i. Arise from the lining of the renal pelvis
      ii. More common in the bladder
      iii. Solid, homogeneous mass in the renal pelvis
   c. Metastatic tumors
      i. Primary includes melanomas of the lung, breast, stomach, GI, pancreas, and contralateral kidney
      ii. Usually in the cortex
      iii. Similar appearance to an RCC
   d. Lymphoma
      i. Affected by non-Hodgkin lymphoma
      ii. Solitary or multiple focal hypoechoic masses

transducer and cord, putting the needle guide onto the transducer and inserting the correct sized guide, making sure that the angle chosen on the unit matches the angle on the transducer when multiple angle approaches are available, potentially holding the transducer during the biopsy, and cleaning the transducer and performing high-level disinfection (HLD) according to the manufacturer's guidelines. The sonographer can also be a great source of encouragement to the patient (Fig. 12-66A–C).

Contrast-Enhanced Ultrasound and Elastography[24,42,52–54]

Currently, there is a lot of research to determine how CEUS and elastography can help with determining whether a renal mass is benign or malignant.

CEUS is a technique in which a contrast medium consisting of gas microbubbles is administered intravenously (IV) providing information on the micro-circulation, unlike Doppler that provides information on the macro-circulation.

The contrast medium currently used for CEUS, at the time of writing this section, has only been approved for use in the liver by the U.S. Food and Drug Administration (FDA). Performing a CEUS of the kidneys is considered using the agent off-label. Off-label means using something for a use other than what has been approved by the FDA. Both CT and MRI use their contrast agents routinely off-label. Depending on the hospital, it may be necessary to have the patient sign a consent form, indicating that they are aware of the off-label use. A major advantage of CEUS is that it can be safely used in patients with renal insufficiency unlike CT and MRI contrast, as both are known to be nephrotoxic, that is, they can damage the kidneys. Recently, CEUS has shown promising results in differentiating benign lesions, such as AMLs and oncocytomas. US contrast agents are used extensively around the world; therefore, much of the information of CEUS and its benefits come from Canada, Europe, and Asia. CEUS looks promising in helping to differentiate benign tumors from an RCC. The reader is encouraged to read articles on how CEUS is helpful in assessing kidneys and other organs (Fig. 12-67).

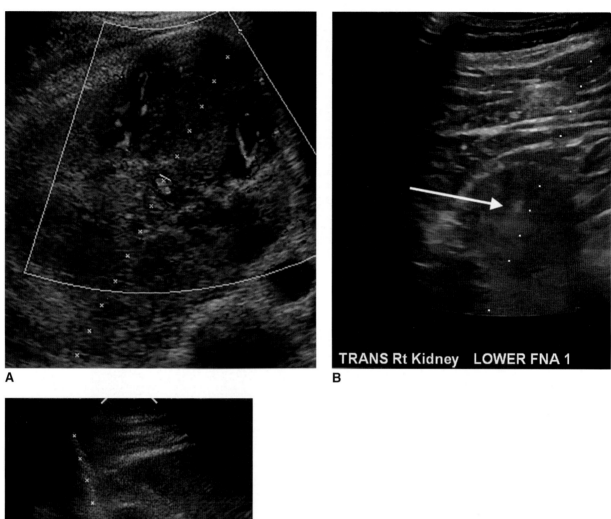

A

B

TRANS Rt Kidney   LOWER FNA 1

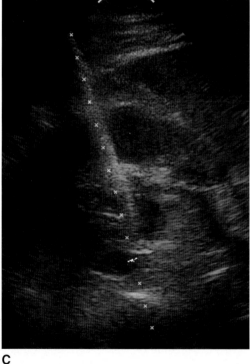

C

FIGURE 12-66 Renal mass biopsy. **A:** Biopsy of a mass that turned out to be a metastatic renal cell carcinoma (*RCC*). The *dotted line* is the needle path when using a biopsy guide. **B:** The first pass of a renal biopsy. The *arrow* is pointing to the 20 to 22 g spinal needle tip. This mass on a patient with colon cancer turned out to be a second primary of RCC. **C:** A core biopsy of the transitional cell carcinoma in Figure 12-63E. The *solid white line* behind the dotted needle indicates the path of the 16 to 18 g core needle. *FNA*, fine-needle aspiration; *Rt*, right; *TRANS*, transverse.

Elastography uses special software to measure the velocity of the shear waves generated by the tissue as the sound beam passes through. The stiffer the tissue, the faster the velocity will be in that tissue. This technique can differentiate between soft or hard tissue and is displayed as a color or grayscale map that overlays the B-mode image. Elastography may be able to differentiate between malignant and benign tissues as preliminary data have shown that the values for malignant masses were higher than the values for benign renal masses. It is hoped by using elastography on incidentally found renal masses that it will decrease the need for biopsies or CT when the findings are suggestive of a benign lesion. The reader is encouraged to learn about the various uses for elastography (Fig. 12-68).

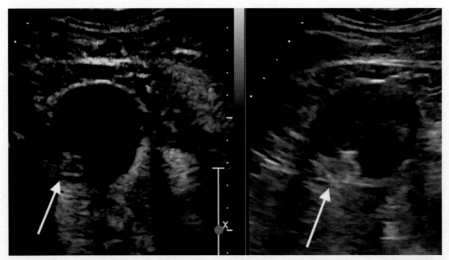

FIGURE 12-67 A complex cystic mass with a solid nodule on the posterior wall (*arrow*). Using contrast-enhanced ultrasound, flow is seen in the nodule suggestive of a cystic renal cell carcinoma. The pathology was affirmed.

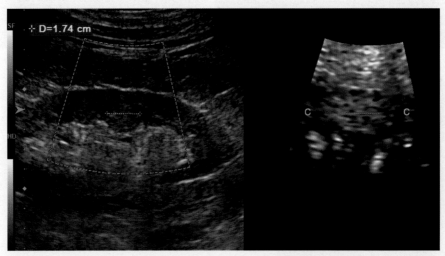

FIGURE 12-68 Elastography. An elastography study on a small renal cell carcinoma (*RCC*) identified by calipers within an elastography Q-box (*dotted box*). Note the difference in the stiffness of the mass (*calipers*) and the surrounding cortex (*C*) in the zoomed image on the right screen. The elastography scale is on the far left of the dual screen. In using this scale, the RCC has softer tissue when compared with the cortex. *HD*, hard; *SF*, soft.

HYDRONEPHROSIS[4,7,13,55–58]

Hydronephrosis means the condition of (osis) water (hydro) in the kidney (neph) and is dilatation of the renal calyces and pelvis, the pelvicalyceal system, with urine, or simply stated, dilatation of the collecting system. If the ureter is dilated, it is called hydroureter. When both are dilated, it is called hydronephroureterosis. Usually, when there is hydronephrosis, the ureter will be dilated. The patient may or may not have symptoms with hydronephrosis. The main symptom is pain, either in the back, flank, abdomen, or pelvis. Pain is frequently present with acute obstruction due to distention of the collecting system and the pressure on the renal capsule as the kidney swells up.

A common order for a renal sonogram is elevated BUN and creatine. The information that the ordering physician wants to know is if there is hydronephrosis. If there is no hydro, then the elevation is caused by parenchymal disease, such as nephrotic syndrome or glomerulonephritis.

To evaluate the kidneys for hydronephrosis, or hydro as it is commonly called, is probably the most common reason a renal sonogram is ordered. US can determine in most patients if hydro is present and the severity. Hydronephrosis causes internal pressure in the kidney and can lead to impaired renal function and, possible, renal failure. Even though urine flow is obstructed, the kidney will continue to make urine, causing the calyces to continue to distend, the renal pelvis to dilate, and the pressure inside the kidney to build up. Within the kidney, the degree of dilation will be limited by the renal parenchyma, whereas the ureters as they continue to dilate will become tortuous as they enlarge. The longer the patient has hydronephrosis, the more prone the kidneys are to develop an infection, a kidney stone, renal scarring, and AKI, or if they have had hydro for an extended time, CKD. A chronically dilated system can lead to cortical atrophy that progresses to the point at which only a thin rim of parenchyma is seen and there is permanent nephron loss.

Obstructive uropathy is when the flow of urine is blocked and cannot drain through the urinary tract, causing hydronephrosis. The cause of obstructive uropathy can occur anywhere along the urinary tract from the kidneys to the urethra. Some causes of intrinsic obstructive uropathy are kidney stones, blood clots, strictures, and tumors. Some causes of extrinsic obstructive uropathy are pregnancy, pelvic masses, fibroid uterus, retroperitoneal fibrosis, and an enlarged prostate. The common causes of obstructive uropathy in an adult are different than those of pediatric patients. For neonates and children, the cause is usually an anatomic abnormality, such as posterior urethral valves, ureteral stricture, and UVJ, or UPJ, pathology. In young adults, kidney stones are the most common cause; in adult men, it is an enlarged prostate termed *benign prostatic hypertrophy* (BPH), and in adult women pelvic masses. With obstructive uropathy, the cause of the obstruction will be "downstream" from the renal pelvis. If the ureter is dilated, the cause will be right past where the dilatation stops. When there is bilateral hydronephrosis, there is an outlet obstruction not allowing the urine to leave the body. As the obstruction is in a central location, it will cause both kidneys to "back-up." Bilateral hydro can be caused by BPH, posterior urethral valves, neurogenic bladder, prune belly syndrome, or a very full bladder. Therefore, it is important to always image the bladder and do a postvoid longitudinal image of each kidney to evaluate if the hydronephrosis has disappeared or if it has stayed the same. Other causes of hydro such as a pelvic mass or pregnancy may or may not cause bilateral hydro, typically they do not. Only when there is something blocking the passage of urine through the urethra and out of the body, there will be consistent bilateral hydro. The process of obstruction is that it always starts in the renal pelvis, progresses to the major calyces, then the minor calyces, and finally there is cortical thinning.

Dilation of the renal pelvis does not always mean that an obstruction is present, and nonobstructive causes of hydro include reflux, infection, and patients with diabetic nephropathy. Another cause is diseases that increase urine production, called urine volume overload, and the body cannot get rid of the urine fast enough. Some of these diseases include nephrogenic diabetes, vesicoureteral reflux, and primary polydipsia. Polydipsia is a condition where there is excess consumption of fluids, causing polyuria, which is production of abnormally large volumes of diluted urine, and ultimately hyponatremia, which is low sodium levels. The term *pelvicaliectasis*, renal pelvis and calyces, may be used when there is dilatation of the renal pelvis and the calyces and there is no obstruction. Some patients will have what is called fullness of the renal pelvis or mild pelviectasis, renal pelvis only. This can be a normal transient finding, especially if the patient's bladder is full. With these patients, there is minimal splaying of the renal pelvis. It is important to interrogate the renal pelvis with color Doppler to ensure that it is not renal vessels causing the "dilatation."

Hydronephrosis is usually treated by addressing the underlying cause. A kidney stone can pass by itself, or it might require some type of intervention, such as lithotripsy or surgery. When pregnancy is the issue, the kidney will return to normal after delivery. Fibroids may need surgery to relieve the pressure on the ureter or ureters. Some type of intervention will be needed on a prostate with BPH to relieve the pressure on the urethra. Whatever the cause, the treatment should be prompt to improve renal function and avoid any permanent damage to the kidney. In cases of severe hydronephrosis, urine may need to be drained from the bladder using a catheter or the patient may need a percutaneous nephrostomy, which is typically performed in interventional radiology (IR) by a radiologist. With the patient prone, the dilated renal pelvis is located and marked using US. Then a special catheter is inserted under US guidance into the renal pelvis and hooked up to a draining bag to relieve the hydronephrosis.

The sonographic appearance of hydronephrosis will vary by the degree of obstruction, with splaying or spreading of the central echo complex by urine. This will be seen by sonography as an anechoic oval area, which is the urine, surrounded by the echogenic sinus echoes. The individual calyces may be seen depending on the amount of dilatation. The sonographer should attempt to scan the ureters and the bladder, making sure that it is not overdistended. When the ureters are dilated, they are easier to visualize. As stated, postvoid images are needed to look for any changes in the hydronephrosis after voiding. Hydronephrosis can be classified as mild, moderate, or severe by sonography. In mild hydronephrosis, there is mild dilatation of the renal sinus. As the hydronephrosis increases, the individual calyces will be seen, and the proximal ureter is seen leaving the kidney. With moderate hydronephrosis, the renal sinus and calyces are dilated, the calyces lose their distinction, and the entire renal sinus is completely dilated, while the renal cortex is preserved. The proximal portion of the ureter is seen as it leaves the kidney. Cortical involvement will help differentiate moderate from severe hydronephrosis. In severe hydronephrosis, there is significant dilatation of the renal pelvis and calyces causing the cortex to be thin, called cortical thinning, due to the increased pressure within the renal sinus. There can also be renal atrophy over time (Fig. 12-69A–H) (Pathology Box 12-14). In cases of severe obstruction, a pelvicalyceal rupture can occur. With sonography, a perinephric fluid collection develops due to the extravasation of the urine. However, if the patient is very symptomatic, they will go straight to CT.

Spectral Doppler is used in the evaluation of hydronephrosis as it can help differentiate between obstructive and nonobstructive hydronephrosis. The sonographer should measure the RI of the interlobar arteries. Remember that a normal value is less than or equal to 0.7. In obstructive hydro, the RI is usually greater than 0.8, because of the increased pressure from intrarenal vasoconstriction. With nonobstructive hydro, the RI should be normal. A reminder is that the RI is an angle-independent measurement, which means you do not use angle correction. The US unit will automatically calculate the RI. It is important to really evaluate the diastolic aspect of the signal so as not to measure noise or mirror artifact as this will increase the RI value and can lead to a false diagnosis, such as having an abnormal value measure as a normal value. An RI difference between the kidneys of greater than 0.1 has been shown to be a sign of unilateral obstruction.

False-positive diagnoses of hydronephrosis include extrarenal pelvis, prominent vessels in the hilum, a full bladder, and parapelvic or peripelvic cysts. Except for a full bladder as the cause, none of the others will look like a completely

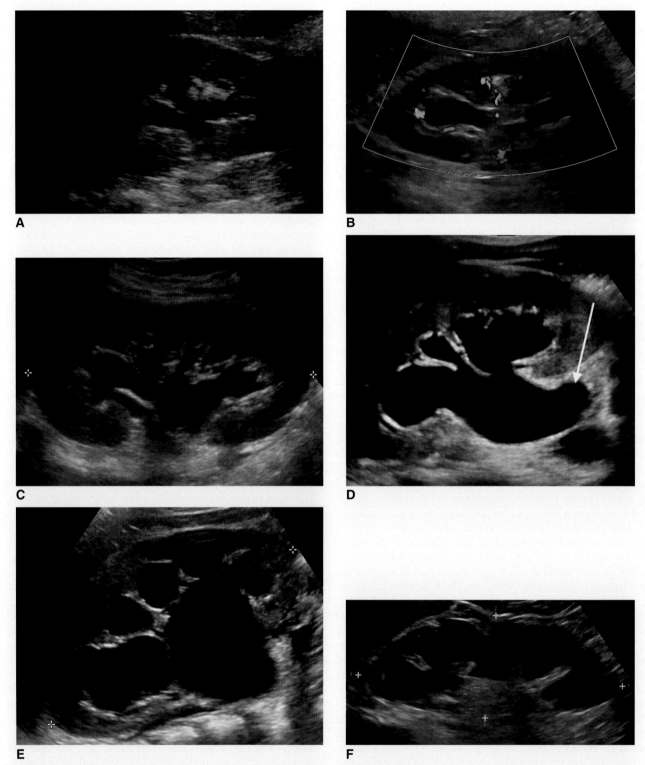

FIGURE 12-69 Hydronephrosis. **A:** Mild dilatation of the renal pelvis reported as mild pelviectasis. **B:** Color Doppler confirms mild hydronephrosis with only the renal pelvis dilated. **C:** The major calyces are dilated and reported as mild-moderate or moderate hydronephrosis. **D:** The dilatation now includes the minor calyces compatible with moderate hydronephrosis. The *arrow* is pointing to the proximal ureter. **E:** Severe obstruction and cortical thinning. This is called the "bear claw" sign. The proximal ureter is not seen because this was a ureteropelvic junction obstruction from the proximal ureter swelling and causing a stricture from a ureteroscopy. **F:** Very severe hydronephrosis with very little cortex seen. The kidney is normal in size.

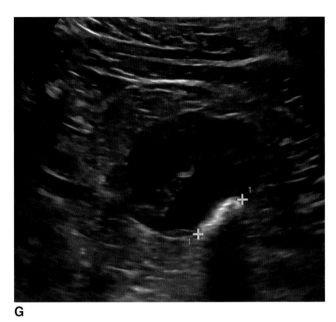

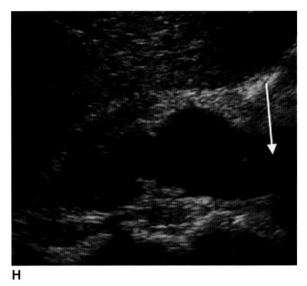

G

H

FIGURE 12-69 *(continued)* **G:** Transverse image of the kidney in F showing that the cause of the obstruction is a kidney stone. Likely recent as the kidney is normal in size. **H:** A small, atrophic kidney with severe hydronephrosis and cortical thinning from a long-standing obstruction. The *arrow* is pointing to the proximal ureter.

PATHOLOGY BOX 12-14
Degrees of Hydronephrosis

1. Mild/Grade I
   a. Mild dilatation of the renal pelvis (pelviectasis) with no dilatation of the calyces
   b. Moderate/Grade II
      i. Sometimes called mild-moderate. The major calyces are dilated (caliectasis)
   c. Moderate/Grade III
      i. Minor calyces are now dilated
   d. Severe/Grade IV
      i. Significant dilatation of the renal pelvis and the calyces with cortical thinning.

---

dilated renal pelvis, but they usually look like as if only a part of the renal pelvis is dilated. Because the renal pelvis is an open structure, it would be difficult to have only a portion dilated.

As stated at the beginning of the chapter, one of the most common requests for a renal sonogram is for elevated BUN and creatinine. The goal of US is to evaluate the kidneys for hydronephrosis, renal size, and echo texture. If hydronephrosis is present, the patient may require intervention. If hydronephrosis is not present, then the patient will be worked up for the cause of decreased renal function, which may include a US-guided biopsy of the kidney. This is discussed in more detail in "Medical Renal Disease" section.

KIDNEY STONES[4,7,13,57,59–68]

Kidney stones are one of the most common kidney diseases and affect more than 1 in 10 adults. They can also be referred to as *renal calculi*, which is the Latin word for pebble. Nephrolithiasis is derived from the Greek *nephros*, kidney, and *lithos* stone, so nephrolithiasis refers to stones in the kidney. Urolithiasis is derived from the Greek *ouron*, which means relating to urine and the urinary system, so urolithiasis refers to stones in the urinary system. Kidney stones are on the rise, and the number of people with kidney stones in the United States has increased from 3.2% in 1980 to 8.8% in the late 2000s. It is estimated that more than half a million people a year visit the emergency department for kidney stones with presenting symptoms that include hematuria, nausea and vomiting, and/or pain in the flank, groin, or abdomen. Nearly 19% of men and 9% of women will have a kidney stone in their lifetime. Kidney stones can develop at any time, although patients tend to present between the ages of 30 and 60 years, with the incidence of kidney stones increasing with age. White males between the age of 20 and 50 years have the highest occurrence. Patients who have had a stone have a recurrence rate of 50% or greater at 5 years and up to 80% at 10 years. Because of the high incidence of kidney stones, the southeastern part of the United States is referred to as the Stone Belt and runs parallel to what is called the Bible Belt. This is mainly due to the warm weather causing people to dehydrate, setting themselves up for a kidney stone. Interestingly, the state of North Carolina has the highest number of people with kidney stones.

Under certain conditions, substances that normally dissolve in urine, such as calcium, oxalate, and phosphate, precipitate out of the urine crystallize, stick together, and form a stone. This occurs when the urine is concentrated, usually from the person not drinking enough water and staying hydrated. Calcium stones are the most common type of kidney stone, and there are two types, calcium oxalate and calcium phosphate, which together account for 75% of stones, with calcium oxalate as the more common type. Many people who form a calcium-containing stone have a condition known as hypercalciuria, which is too much calcium in their urine. Even with normal amounts of calcium in the urine, calcium stones may form for other reasons. Calcium phosphate stones are less common than calcium oxalate stones and can form as a result of renal tubular acidosis, a disease in which the kidneys cannot properly remove acids from the blood, causing a serious condition called acidosis, which can lead to calcium deposits in the kidneys. Another type of stone that accounts for about 15% of stones is the struvite stone, which is composed of a mixture of magnesium, ammonium, phosphate, and calcium carbonate. These stones form as a result of infection, are often large, have branches, and grow fast, forming a staghorn calculus. Struvite stones are more common in women as they are more prone to UTIs. These stones will fill the calyx and need to be removed surgically or by extracorporeal shock wave lithotripsy (ESWL), referred to as *lithotripsy*, which is discussed later in this section. Uric acid is produced as the body metabolizes protein. When the pH of urine drops below 5.5, the urine can contain a lot of uric acid crystals, which can lead to the formation of stones. Uric acid stones account for 5% to 10% of stones and are more common in people who eat a large amount of protein, such as found in red meat. People with gout are also prone to uric acid stones. Kidney stones can vary in size, shape, and color. They can be as small as a grain of sand to several centimeters in size, be smooth, irregular, or jagged in shape. There is a wide variety of color among stones, including yellow, brown, tan, gold, and black. The color of kidney stones normally indicates the composition of the stone (Fig. 12-70). The size of a kidney stone will determine how quickly it will pass. Kidney stones can develop anywhere in the urinary system, but most develop in the kidney. Most stones are small and can travel down the ureter and pass out the urethra on their own.

A risk factor to develop stones is by not drinking enough water each day, especially if you live in a warm or

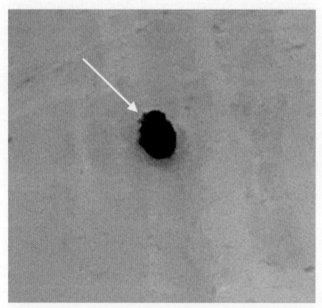

FIGURE 12-70 An enlarged image of a 0.3-mm kidney stone. Note the ragged border. The *arrow* is pointing to sharp edges.

hot climate, sweat a lot, and become dehydrated. A good example is cutting the lawn on a very hot and sunny day and not staying hydrated. Normal urine should be a very pale yellow, and dark yellow urine means that it is concentrated. Other risk factors that make one prone to developing kidney stones include eating a diet that is high in protein and salt, being overweight, surgeries on the digestive tract including gastric bypass, family history of kidney stones, reoccurring UTIs, being male, high uric acid levels, and diabetes. Another risk factor is having a diet that is high in oxalates, which is naturally found in many foods, including fruits and vegetables, nuts and seeds, grains, legumes, and tea, often a diet associated with vegetarians. Certain dietary supplements and medications can increase the risk of kidney stones, including vitamin C; dietary supplements; laxatives, especially when used excessively; calcium-based antacids; and certain medications used to treat migraines or depression. Usually, the cause of the kidney stone is idiopathic, which means of unknown cause.

Some stones stay in the kidney and do not cause any problems, and the patient is asymptomatic. Just like gallstones, kidney stones can be an incidental finding if it is not causing any symptoms, including hydronephrosis, and the patient may be unaware that they have a kidney stone. The initial clinical sign of a kidney stone is very extreme pain, on the side that has the stone. Most patients claim this is the worst pain that they have ever experienced, and according to some women, that includes childbirth. As the kidney stone travels down the ureter to the bladder, the patients will have renal colic, which is pain shooting from the kidney area down to the scrotum or labia. If it is small enough to make it to the bladder, it will be passed out of the body with the urine. Patients will be asked to strain their urine to capture the stone so that it can be analyzed. This will determine what is causing the kidney stones and to help form a plan to prevent their reoccurrence. When there is chronic obstruction, this can lead to progressive renal parenchymal damage and impaired renal function. One complication of a kidney stone is a spontaneous rupture of a renal calyx with extravasation of urine seen as a perinephric fluid collection.

The ureters are fibromuscular tubes that propel urine from the kidneys to the bladder by involuntary wave-like contractions. In an adult, the ureter is approximately 25 to 30 cm long and about 3 to 4 mm in diameter. The ureter is the smallest diameter structure of the urinary tract and is the area most prone to obstruction by a stone. There are three areas of narrowing in the ureter where a stone can get stuck and cause an obstruction. The first is where the ureter exits the kidney at the UPJ. The second place is where the ureter crosses over the iliac vessels, and the third place is where the ureter enters the bladder at the UVJ, which is the most common place they get stuck. When a stone is stuck in the ureter, it may be possible to follow the dilated ureter to the level of the stone. If the stone becomes stuck in the ureter, it will block the flow of urine, basically creating a dam, causing hydroureter and hydronephrosis (Fig. 12-71A–C). When a kidney stone is stuck in the ureter, it can cause severe pain in the back, flank pain, renal colic, vomiting, hematuria, fever, or chills. Hematuria may be gross hematuria, meaning it is visible to the eye and the urine is bloody, or microscopic hematuria, where the blood cells can only be

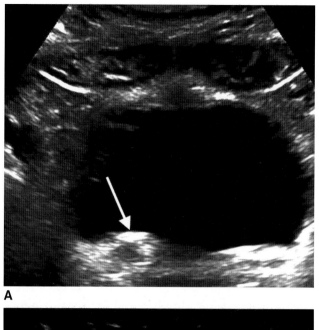

A

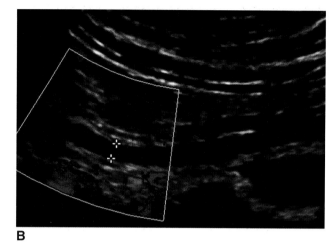

B

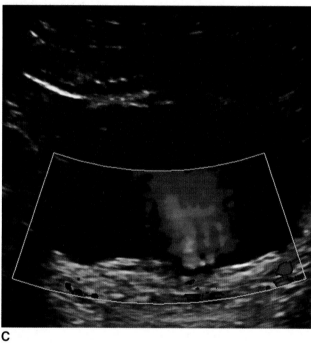

C

FIGURE 12-71 **A:** A stone (*arrow*) stuck at the ureterovesical junction (*UVJ*). **B:** The dilated ureter caused by the UVJ stone is seen mid abdomen. Care should be taken to not press too hard as that might collapse the ureter. **C:** Only a urine jet from the left kidney was seen compatible with complete obstruction of the right kidney.

seen under a microscope. The size of the stone is a major factor in whether it can pass on its own and how long it will take. Stones smaller than 4 mm can pass on their own about 80% of the time. Stones that are 4 to 6 mm around 50% will pass on their own, and the rest will require some type of intervention. Stones larger than 6 mm will probably need an intervention to be removed, as only around 1% to 2% will be able to pass on their own.

As long as the stone is not causing problems, especially hydro, the doctor will have the patient wait for it to pass on its own. They are usually given some type of pain medication as well as a drug to relax the muscles in the ureter to help pass the kidney stone more quickly such as tamsulosin, more commonly known by its brand name of Flomax™. Treatment for stones that cause obstruction depends on their size and their location. Treatments may include doing nothing and seeing if the stone will pass on its own, ESWL, percutaneous nephrolithotomy (PCNL), and ureteroscopic stone removal. ESWL is a noninvasive therapy that uses shockwaves targeted to the stone to break it up into smaller pieces, allowing the stone fragments to easily pass through the urinary system. Extracorporeal means from outside the body, shock wave that can be a sound beam, and lithotripsy from the Greek word *litho* meaning stone and *tripsy* meaning breaking. With ESWL, the shock wave causes a very rapid pressure increase, which is different from diagnostic US. The shock waves usually do not harm the normal tissue. When the shock wave strikes the stone, energy is lost and causes small cracks to form on the edge of the stone. As it exits, the stone more cracks occur. About

1,000 to 2,000 shock waves are needed to reduce the stone to small particles that will be able to pass through the ureter and urethra. The process generally takes about 1 hour, with some patients needing more than one session. To make the patient more comfortable, analgesics are given, and in some patients, a light or even general sedation may be needed. ESWL cannot be used on pregnant patients. After the procedure, some patients may experience hematuria, pain, and skin redness at the shock wave entry site. For stones in the ureter, a ureteroscope is placed through the urethra and bladder and guided up to the level of the stone to capture and remove the stone. If the stone is small, a basket device will be used to remove the stone. If the stone is large, or the diameter of the ureter is narrow, the stone will need to be broken into small pieces, usually done with a laser. Once the stone is broken into tiny fragments, they are removed. The ureteroscope will cause swelling of the ureter, and a ureteral stent is placed to allow the ureter to heal so that it does not form a stricture. It is usually removed in 5 to 10 days as an outpatient. Ureteroscopy is performed under general anesthesia. PCNL is a surgical procedure in which an opening is made in the flank to access the kidney. Under X-ray guidance, a thin telescopic instrument called a nephroscope is used to remove the stone from the kidney. The stone is either pulled out or broken into small pieces, by either a laser or a lithotripter, so it can be removed. PCNL is performed under general anesthesia and is usually used on large stones such as a staghorn calculus, which are usually unable to be removed by other methods.

The sonographic appearance of a renal stone is an echogenic structure with a posterior acoustic shadow. Stones smaller than 3 mm and uric acid stones do not cast an acoustic shadow. Some hints to help bring out an acoustic shadow include using harmonics, making sure that the focal zone, if the machine still uses them, is at the level of the stone; reducing the overall gain; and decreasing the dynamic range to make the image more contrast, which will accentuate the shadow. If the stone contains calcium, color Doppler may help verify that a nonshadowing echogenic structure in the kidney is a stone by producing a twinkling artifact. It was first described by Rahmouni et al. in 1996 for the detection of kidney stones.[69] Using color Doppler, it is seen as an area of rapidly alternating mixture of red and blue Doppler signals, resembling turbulent flow, behind the stone, like a comet-tail artifact. The cause of this artifact is not well understood but is thought to be a result of intrinsic noise from phase jitter within the Doppler processing components. Twinkling artifact is sensitive for the detection of small stones in the kidney that do not produce an acoustic shadow; however, not all stones will produce the twinkling artifact. Stones located at the UVJ, the most common place for a stone to become stuck, can be identified by seeing the twinkle artifact (Fig. 12-72A–K). The sonographer should not confuse renal artery calcifications for a kidney stone by observing the pulsations of the artery. CT has better sensitive than US in detecting stones as well as determining their location, and when stones are suspected, this is often the test of choice.

To determine whether a stone is completely or only partially obstructing the ureter, color Doppler can be used in the bladder to look for color jets from the boluses of urine entering the bladder. The color velocity scale, the pulse repetition frequency (PRF), should be set to look for a slow flow state. Color gain should be set just below the setting at which background noise is seen. To best visualize jets, the transducer is placed in a transverse position at the level of the trigone, which can be estimated by the landmarks of the seminal vesicles or mid-cervix. A Doppler shift is created by the urine that is ejected forcefully into the bladder through the vesicoureteral junction. The jet is described as a sudden burst of color in the bladder much like a geyser, lasting for a few seconds. Physiologic ureteral jets in well-hydrated patients will usually occur two or more per minute and will course anteromedially from the trigone. The duration of the jet varies, and there is usually a 30-second interval between jets. A complete obstruction shows the absence of the ureteral jet. However, jets are not always visualized, even on healthy patients, as the frequency of the jets may range from seconds to minutes. The hydration of the patient will also affect the presence and timing of the jets. Therefore, the absence of a ureteral jet does not always mean that there is an obstruction, but seeing a jet indicates that the ureter is patent. With a partial obstruction, there may be constant dribbling from the ureter. This continuous low-flow jet seen within the bladder is called the candle sign as the jet looks like a flame (Fig. 12-73A–C). Stones that are in the distal ureter can sometimes be seen using an endovaginal technique on women. The literature recommends waiting between 5 and 10 minutes without seeing a jet before deciding that there is a complete obstruction. This is a little unrealistic in today's scanning environment, and some departments stop waiting after seeing multiple jets on the contralateral side. There is some controversy about the value of color jets and not every lab will look for them.

NEPHROCALCINOSIS[4,7,13,70–73]

Nephrocalcinosis is a disease in which there is too much calcium, in the form of calcium phosphate and calcium oxalate, deposited in the kidneys, causing calcifications in the renal parenchyma. The underlying causes are hypercalcemia and hypercalciuria, which are caused by a variety of diseases including hyperparathyroidism, chronic glomerulonephritis, medullary sponge kidney (MSK), renal tubular acidosis, or any condition that leads to high levels of calcium in the blood or urine. It may also be caused by certain medications and supplements. Some patients will be asymptomatic or have symptoms related to the condition causing the nephrocalcinosis. The kidney prognosis will be determined by the underlying cause of the nephrocalcinosis. As there is some overlap in the causes of nephrocalcinosis and nephrolithiasis, the patient may have coexisting kidney stones. Nephrocalcinosis can eventually cause obstructive uropathy, which can result in kidney failure. Nephrocalcinosis is usually diagnosed incidentally and detected on an imaging study on a patient with normal kidney function. It can also be diagnosed when symptoms of renal failure, obstructive uropathy, or kidney stones develop. Treatment will include treating the underlying cause, if it is known, with the goal being to reduce symptoms and prevent more calcium from being deposited in the kidneys.

Renal medullary nephrocalcinosis is 20 times more common than cortical nephrocalcinosis and is usually a bilateral process. The most common cause of medullary

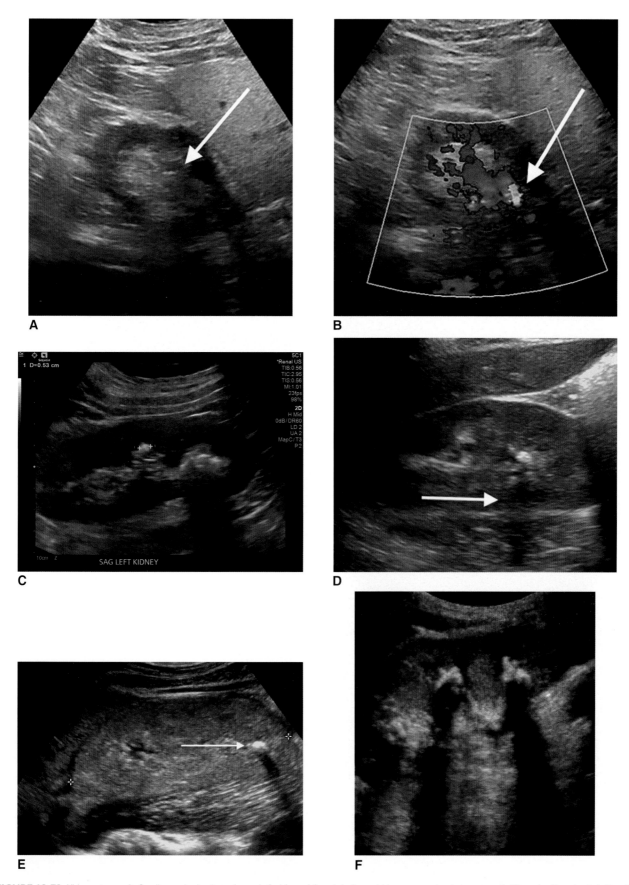

FIGURE 12-72 Kidney stones. **A:** Small, nonshadowing echogenic foci (*arrow*) found during a right upper quadrant sonogram. **B:** The color Doppler twinkle artifact that confirmed this was a small kidney stone. **C:** A uric acid stone that is not shadowing (calipers). The patient had a history of gout. A group of multiple stones did exhibit an acoustic shadow. **D:** An acoustic shadow (*arrow*) caused. **E:** A stone (*arrow*) casting an acoustic shadow in the lower pole of this echogenic kidney with medical renal disease. **F:** An image with harmonics of two stones casting a nice acoustic shadow exhibiting a clear shadow. The higher frequency of the harmonic beam is attenuated at a greater rate, allowing for a clean shadow.

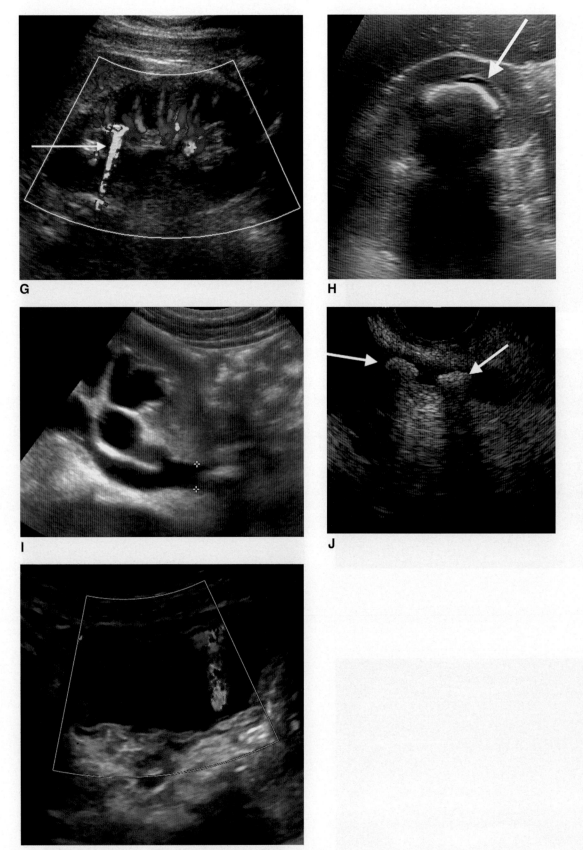

FIGURE 12-72 (*continued*) **G:** Color Doppler twinkle artifact (*arrow*) from a stone made of calcium in the kidney. **H:** A rim of hydronephrosis (*arrow*) caused by this large staghorn stone. **I:** A stone is seen beyond the calipers in the proximal portion of the ureter, causing hydronephrosis. **J:** Stones (*arrows*) in the distal ureter being imaged with a transvaginal approach and transducer. **K:** This patient had moderate hydronephrosis in the right kidney, and only the proximal ureter could be visualized. No stone was seen in the right UVJ. A urine jet is only seen from the left kidney as the right kidney was obstructed by a stone upstream not imaged by ultrasound. No visualization of the jet confirmed a complete obstruction.

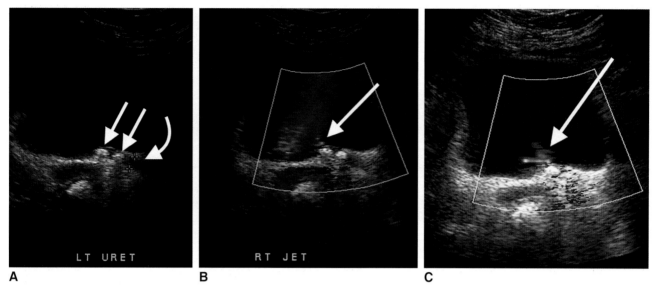

FIGURE 12-73 Kidney stones and bladder jets. **A:** The *arrows* are pointing to two stones at the ureterovesical junction. The *curved arrow* is pointing to the dilated ureter. **B:** A strong urine jet is seen from the right kidney. The small left jet (*arrow*) is nearly lost as it crosses the right jet. **C:** Small left jet (*arrow*) demonstrating a constant dribble out of the left ureter that is compatible with a nonobstructing stone. This is an example of the "candle sign."

nephrocalcinosis is hyperparathyroidism, followed by renal tubular acidosis. Other causes include MSK, chronic pyelonephritis, Cushing syndrome, and sickle cell disease. Medullary nephrocalcinosis will not affect the cortex. Normally by US, the renal pyramids are hypoechoic, but with medullary nephrocalcinosis, the renal pyramids are now echogenic and may or may not have shadowing, depending on the size of the calcifications (Fig. 12-74A–D).

Cortical nephrocalcinosis is usually bilateral and diffuse. The most common causes of cortical nephrocalcinosis are chronic glomerulonephritis and acute cortical necrosis. Other causes include hypercalcemic states associated with malignancy and taking excessive amounts of vitamin D_3, which results in hypercalcemia and hypercalciuria. Cortical nephrocalcinosis is located in the cortex, with the medullary pyramids being spared. On US, the cortex becomes echogenic, but typically does not cast an acoustic shadow (Fig. 12-75).

MEDULLARY SPONGE KIDNEY[4,7,74–78]

MSK is a condition where the medullary and papillary portions of the collecting ducts are dysplastic and dilated. Approximately 80% of patients will go on to develop medullary nephrocalcinosis. It is bilateral in 70% of patients and affects less than 0.5% to 1% of the general population and found in up to 12% of patients with renal calculi. The cortex of the kidney is normal and unaffected. It is a rare disorder that affects women slightly more than men. It was first recognized in 1939 by Lenarduzzi, a radiologist, and two of his colleagues at Padua University Hospital in Italy, Cacchi, a urologist, and Ricci, a pathologist, which is why it is also known as Lenarduzzi–Cacchi–Ricci disease. The exact cause of MSK is unknown and is believed to be a result of abnormal renal development in utero. There may also be a genetic component to the disease as recent evidence suggests an autosomal dominant gene expression.

MSK has a specific appearance that no other renal disease can mimic and characterized by cyst formation and dilatation of the medullary and papillary sections of the collecting ducts in one or more of the medullary pyramids. These dilations occur in the precalyceal collecting ducts, which are the terminal ducts of the nephrons. These precalyceal, or inner medullary collecting ducts (IMCDs), drain into progressively larger ducts called the ducts of Bellini, which drain the urine out of the renal papilla. In MSK, some of the IMCD are dilated and have outpouchings that are blind sacs, which look like cysts, that begins at the IMCD lumen and go nowhere. These dilated cysts give the kidney the appearance of a sponge. In these cysts, innumerable round tiny stones are found. Other IMCD are normal and are not dilated and do not have cystic outpouchings.

The diagnosis of MSK is suspected in patients presenting with a history of calcium-based kidney stones or a history of UTIs. People with MSK are usually asymptomatic unless they have UTIs or kidney stones. People with MSK typically pass twice as many stones per year as the average non-MSK person who forms stones. A symptom of MSK is the passing of small stones with urine. Although MSK is present from birth, symptoms do not occur until adolescence or in adults between the ages of 30 and 50 years. Women with MSK experience more stones, have more UTIs, and more complications than men. For patients with symptoms, treatment focuses on managing the symptoms and reducing the risk of complications as there is no cure for MSK.

Contrast CT urography is the test of choice to make a diagnosis of MSK. It is very difficult with sonography to distinguish between MSK and medullary nephrocalcinosis as they can coexist together. With MSK, there is a dilation of the renal collecting ducts, and US does not have the resolution to detect them. Sonography typically demonstrates echogenic medullary pyramids, which are seen whether or not medullary nephrocalcinosis is also present. In some patients, the kidneys may appear normal, especially if there are no

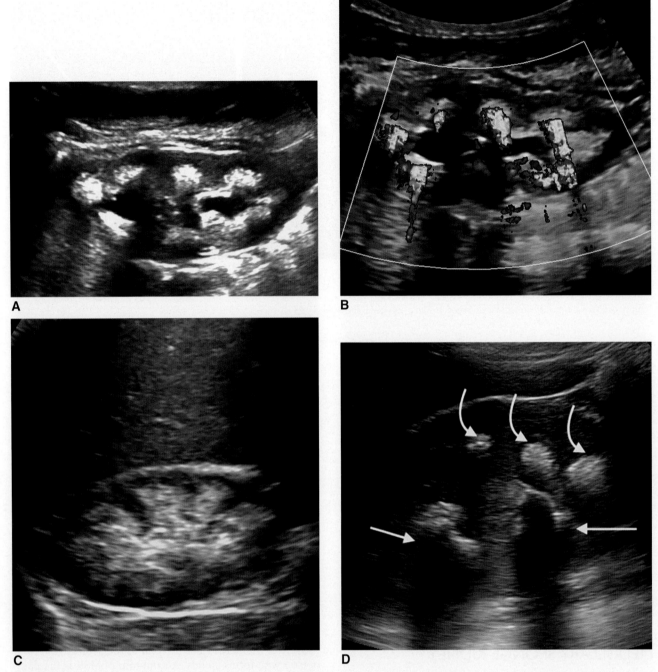

FIGURE 12-74 Nephrocalcinosis. **A:** The echogenic pyramids associated with medullary nephrocalcinosis. **B:** Twinkle artifact caused by the calcium in the echogenic pyramids. **C:** Another patient with medullary nephrocalcinosis where the pyramids are not as bright as the previous patient. **D:** The acoustic shadow (*straight arrows*) caused by staghorn stones. Note the irregular shape of these stones, especially on the right. The echogenic pyramids (*curved arrows*) are caused by nephrocalcinosis.

complications. The main role of US is to detect complications, such as kidney stones and hydronephrosis (Fig. 12-76A, B).

The future for diagnosing MSK and nephrocalcinosis continues to evolve using a high-definition ureteroscope, allowing urologists to see incredible detail inside the kidney. This has started redefining the definition of both nephrocalcinosis and MSK. Urologists feel that kidneys should only be labeled as having nephrocalcinosis once confirmed visually by ureteroscopy.

HEMATOMAS[79–86]

Hematomas of the kidneys can be from blunt trauma, more common, and those resulting from penetrating trauma by knife and gunshot wounds. Renal hematomas can occur with renal biopsies, interventional procedures, and surgery. Blunt injuries account for 90% to 95% of injuries and are mainly due to motor vehicle accidents. Other causes include falls, assaults, and contract sports.

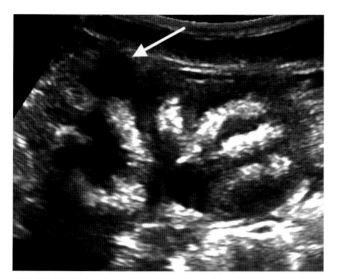

FIGURE 12-75 A patient with cortical calcinosis. Note how the areas of calcifications are rectangular in shape. The *arrow* is pointing to a kidney cyst.

The most important concern in the evaluation of a patient with blunt abdominal trauma is their hemodynamic stability. In the hemodynamically unstable patient, a rapid evaluation for hemoperitoneum can be accomplished by the emergency department doctors with a US FAST scan to look quickly for free fluid. FAST stands for Focused Assessment with Sonography for Trauma and is what is called a point-of-care (POC) US. It can be performed quickly on a trauma patient to identify intraperitoneal free fluid, which is assumed to be a hemoperitoneum, and can be an indication for an exploratory laparotomy. The FAST scan can be performed as the team works on the patient, including during resuscitation, and as various lines and catheters are being placed. The most injured organs in blunt abdominal trauma are, in order, the spleen, liver, retroperitoneum,

small bowel, kidneys, bladder, colorectum, diaphragm, and pancreas. Some references may have the liver as the most injured, with spleen the second. Renal injuries are estimated to occur in 1% to 5% of all abdominal traumas and are more commonly seen in males.

Microscopic or macroscopic hematuria is the most common sign of injury to the kidney. Most renal injuries are minor and include contusion, superficial laceration, and subcapsular and perinephric hematoma. Most forms of blunt trauma to the kidney may heal without treatment. Serious renal injuries from trauma are associated with multiorgan injuries. Significant injuries, such as a deep laceration or active hemorrhage, are more likely to need surgery. There have been reports of subcapsular renal hematomas caused by lithotripsy. The incidence of renal injuries increases with congenital anomalies, especially those kidneys not in their normal position such as a pelvic kidney and horseshoe kidneys, as well as patients with renal pathology such as cysts.

Trauma patients who are stable will go to CT as a CT scan is considered the gold standard to evaluate the severity of any abdominal and renal injury. CT is sensitive in identifying parenchymal lacerations and urinary extravasations, delineating segmental parenchymal infarcts, and determining the size and location of any surrounding retroperitoneal hematoma and/or associated intra-abdominal injuries. US can sometimes be the first imaging choice in evaluating a stable patient. Sonography is usually able to visualize the hemorrhage and hematoma, but it can be difficult to determine the cause. Depending on the findings, the patient may go on to have a CT scan. The US examination is performed using a convex-array transducer with a frequency appropriate for the size of the patient. The outcome of the US examination is influenced by the deep retroperitoneal position, the patient's body type, the sonographer's experience, and the patient's cooperation. A parenchymal renal injury can be difficult to separate from renal parenchyma as it is a slightly hyperechoic area

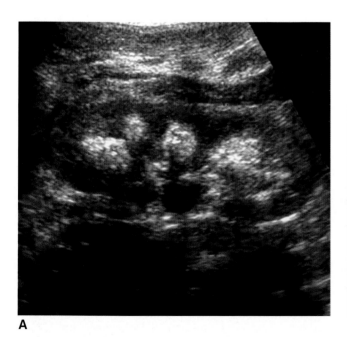

A

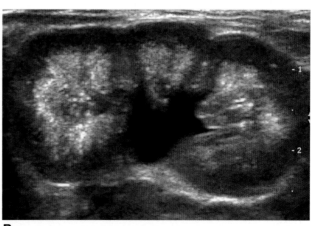

B

FIGURE 12-76 Medullary sponge kidney. **A:** A patient with medullary sponge kidney. Note the tiny bright echogenic dots inside the pyramids, which represent small calculi. The fluid is from an extrarenal pelvis. **B:** The same patient using a linear-array transducer and angled more medially to demonstrate the small calculi.

with no defined margins. US can show free fluid around the kidney, although it cannot differentiate between blood and urine and cannot always find the source of bleeding. Fresh subcapsular hematomas will be very echogenic as the body sends platelets and fibrin to stop the bleeding. It is important to evaluate the kidney with color and/or power Doppler to look for areas of viable tissue when there is a shattered kidney. One major use of US is with follow-up studies on patients with known trauma, thus reducing the radiation to the patient. Current research is evaluating CEUS and its use and role with trauma patients.

Renal hematomas develop from trauma, or they can occur spontaneously. A nontraumatic hematoma is called a spontaneous hematoma and is rare. They are usually caused by bleeding from renal tumors, with an AML being the most common cause. Other causes include vascular, inflammatory, cystic, and blood disorders. Patients taking anticoagulants, particularly warfarin, are at an increased risk for renal hemorrhage.

A renal hematoma can be subcapsular or perinephric. A subcapsular hematoma occurs right under the renal capsule, between the capsule and the renal parenchyma, and the cause of the hemorrhage is within the kidney. The renal capsule does not allow for expansion, and the accumulation of blood will compress the renal parenchyma. Flattening of the underlying renal parenchyma is more commonly found in subcapsular hematomas than in perinephric ones. In some cases, enlarging hematomas can compress the renal parenchyma, causing decreased perfusion of the kidney and hypertension, known as a Page kidney. The intrarenal arterial Doppler waveforms will have a decrease in diastolic flow with RI of less than 0.8. Once the hematoma has been drained or removed, a follow-up Doppler study should show normal diastolic flow in the intrarenal arteries with an RI of greater than 0.7. When a subcapsular hemorrhage breaks through the capsule, it forms a perinephric hematoma. A perinephric hematoma occurs between Gerota fascia and the renal capsule and usually does not deform the shape of the renal parenchyma. A hematoma within the perirenal space can become very large before pressure becomes sufficient to cause renal issues.

The most common clinical symptom of a renal hematoma is an acute onset of flank or abdominal pain. Other potential symptoms include hematuria, a palpable mass, decreasing blood pressure, signs of blood loss, and decrease in hemoglobin. The treatment of a subcapsular hematoma is aimed at maintaining renal function. Conservative management is the approach when the patient has two normal functioning kidneys and includes antibiotics, to prevent or treat an infection in the hematoma, control pain, and monitor vital signs. An abnormally low or dropping blood pressure is a sign of internal bleeding. When there is a possibility of loss of the kidney or the patient, aggressive management is needed and includes surgical evacuation or percutaneous drainage of the hematoma and, possibly, a total nephrectomy.

The sonographic appearance of a hematoma will have varying echo patterns depending on the age of the bleed. Acute hematomas are hyperechoic, but as the hematoma becomes organized, it will develop a complex and heterogeneous appearance. Eventually, it will liquify and become a seroma with an anechoic appearance like a cyst. Chronic hematomas may develop calcifications that can be located peripherally, centrally, or in a mixed pattern (Fig. 12-77A–D).

A percutaneous renal biopsy can create a subcapsular hematoma. Very few of these hematomas become clinically significant. A renal biopsy is used to help determine the cause of the patient's decline in renal function. The lower pole of the left kidney is biopsied with the patient prone as this provides the safest route. Usually, two cores are obtained, but more passes may be needed if a sample is poor. The potential for a hematoma to develop can occur after each pass, and the sonographer should evaluate the biopsy site looking for blood squirting out of the kidney with color Doppler. This is usually very easy to see as a red jet spurts out of the kidney. The resultant hematoma is going to be echogenic. The bleeding needs to be stopped for the safety of the patient. A quick and easy method is while watching with color Doppler, to apply pressure with the transducer used for the biopsy over the area of bleeding until the bleeding has visually stopped. The kidney will usually stop bleeding in about 5 minutes with constant pressure. To reduce a muscular skeletal injury, the sonographer should stand on a step stool with their arms straight, using both hands to hold the transducer and letting their body weight apply the pressure as opposed to their shoulders. After about 5 minutes, slowly ease up on pressure and see if the bleeding has stopped (Fig. 12-78A–E). If it has not, the sonographer might apply pressure for another 5 minutes with the request of the nephrologist. With primary responsibility to the patient, the nephrologist may also help to apply pressure. If the bleeding still has not stopped, the nephrologist will call IR to arrange for their help in stopping the bleeding. The patient will now go directly to IR, and the sonographer will continue to apply pressure to the site of bleeding. If the nephrologist feels that the patient is stable, they may instruct the sonographer to release the pressure at the time of transport. Once the patient has left the room, the sonographer will clean the transducer and room. The sonographer should perform the current recommendation of disinfection for equipment per the Occupational Safety and Health Administration (OSHA). A STAT portable renal US may be necessary to assess patients who initially left the department without signs of bleeding. These studies should be performed as quickly as possible. Clinically, a drop in a patient's blood pressure indicates that the patient is bleeding internally and could bleed to death if not corrected quickly. Occasionally, patients may be transferred to the operating room (OR) or IR before the sonographic examination can be completed. In this case, the patient's condition was deteriorating too quickly, and action had to be taken to ensure the patient's safety.

Acute Pyelonephritis[4,7,13,35,87–89]

Pyelonephritis, from the Greek *pyelo* (pelvis), *nephros* (kidney), and *itis* (inflammation), is when both the renal pelvis and parenchyma are inflamed. Acute pyelonephritis is a tubulointerstitial inflammation of the kidney and is the result of a bladder infection, most commonly caused by cystitis in women and prostatitis in men, which then ascends to the kidneys. About 60% of women and 12% of men will have at least one UTI during their lifetime. Acute pyelonephritis begins with colonization of the urethral

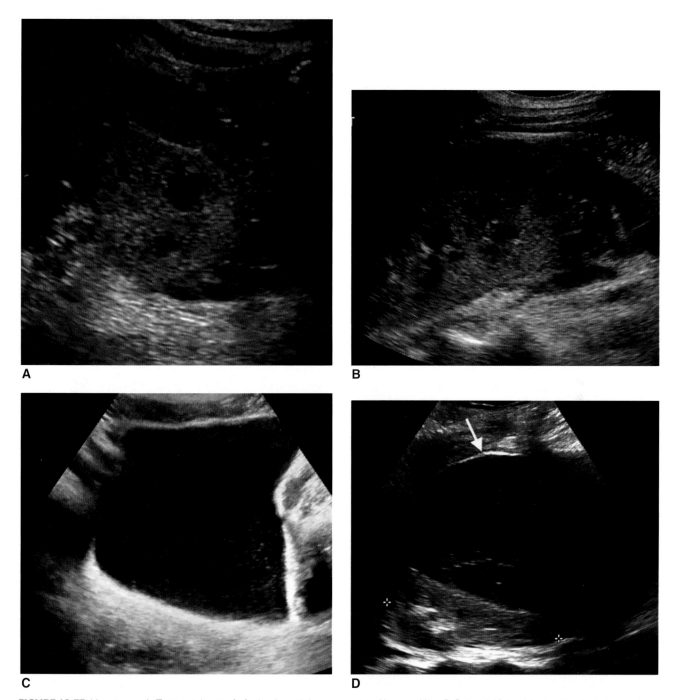

FIGURE 12-77 Hematomas. **A:** Transverse image of a fresh echogenic hematoma caused by an accident. **B:** Patient A 10 days later in which the hematoma is now a complicated cystic mass. **C:** Low-level echoes in the bladder compatible with hematuria. **D:** A large complex, subcapsular hematoma caused by lithotripsy of a staghorn calculus. The compressed page kidney is accompanied by hypertension and hematuria. The *arrow* is pointing to the renal capsule.

meatus or vaginal introitus by either uropathogens or fecal flora that travel by the urethra into the bladder. Normal urine contains water, salts, and waste products but is free of germs such as bacteria. Urine provides a good medium for bacteria to flourish in, especially *Escherichia coli*, commonly referred to as *E. coli*, causing a UTI. Emptying the bladder completely helps fight a bacterial infection. The bacteria then travel up the ureter to the collecting system and finally enter the renal tubules at the papillary tip, causing a purulent inflammation that extends up the tubule and into the renal interstitium with destruction of the parenchyma and the renal tubules. Acute pyelonephritis affects the cortex, sparing the glomeruli and vessels.

Pyelonephritis is most commonly caused by *E. coli*, a Gram-negative bacterium, which enters the urinary tract through the urethra. *E. coli* lives harmlessly in the GI tract but can cause serious infections when it gets into the urinary tract. The longer a urinary catheter is indwelling, the higher the risk of the patient developing bacteriuria, bacteria in the urine, which can lead to a UTI and pyelonephritis. Urinary tract obstruction caused by a kidney stone, usually a staghorn, can also lead to acute pyelonephritis. Acute

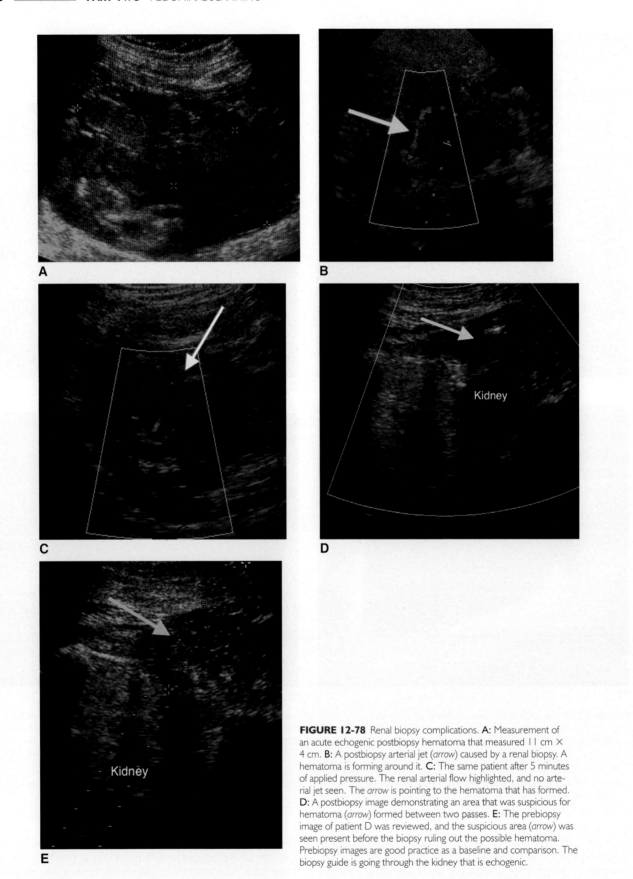

FIGURE 12-78 Renal biopsy complications. **A:** Measurement of an acute echogenic postbiopsy hematoma that measured 11 cm × 4 cm. **B:** A postbiopsy arterial jet (*arrow*) caused by a renal biopsy. A hematoma is forming around it. **C:** The same patient after 5 minutes of applied pressure. The renal arterial flow highlighted, and no arterial jet seen. The *arrow* is pointing to the hematoma that has formed. **D:** A postbiopsy image demonstrating an area that was suspicious for hematoma (*arrow*) formed between two passes. **E:** The prebiopsy image of patient D was reviewed, and the suspicious area (*arrow*) was seen present before the biopsy ruling out the possible hematoma. Prebiopsy images are good practice as a baseline and comparison. The biopsy guide is going through the kidney that is echogenic.

pyelonephritis is more commonly seen in women between the ages of 15 and 35 years and can occur in 1% to 2% of all pregnant women. Men are not as commonly affected until later in life when they have prostate enlargement,

BPH, causing urinary retention that increases the risk of developing a UTI. Statistics show that about 60% of women and about 12% of men will have at least one UTI during their lifetime. The Society of Uroradiology has proposed using acute pyelonephritis to describe acutely infected kidneys, eliminating the need for terms such as bacterial nephritis, lobar nephronia, renal cellulitis, lobar nephritis, renal phlegmon, and renal carbuncle.

Acute pyelonephritis can become an interstitial abscess and/or a perinephric abscess. A perinephric abscess is a serious condition with a mortality rate of 25% to 50%. A perinephric abscess is usually surgically drained, and the patient is placed on IV antibiotics. Acute pyelonephritis has other complications such as renal abscess, sepsis, papillary necrosis, acute renal failure (ARF), and emphysematous pyelonephritis (EPN), which is the most serious type of complication. A serious complication occurs when the infection gets into the blood becoming a urosepsis, which is a systemic inflammatory response that can lead to multiorgan dysfunction, failure, and even death. Urosepsis is a very serious condition with a mortality rate of 30% to 40%, which is why it is important to treat acute pyelonephritis quickly to prevent the progression to sepsis.

The classic triad presentation of acute pyelonephritis is fever, flank pain, and nausea or vomiting, but not all symptoms are always present. Patients may also have dysuria and urinary frequency and urgency. When a patient is febrile, the fever is often over 103°F or 39.4°C. Costovertebral angle tenderness will be over the affected kidney. People with acute pyelonephritis who have a high fever and elevated WBC count, leukocytosis, are admitted to the hospital for IV hydration and antibiotics.

Urine and blood tests are ordered to confirm the suspected diagnosis of acute pyelonephritis. A urinalysis will determine whether there is WBCs and/or RBCs present. Pyuria is a common finding, and the urine is sent to the lab for a urine culture to see what bacteria are growing to determine the type of antibiotic needed. It usually takes 1 to 3 days for the culture to grow. A complete blood cell count (CBC) is ordered to look for elevation in WBCs, elevated erythrocyte sedimentation rate, and elevated C-reactive protein levels. Elevation of both erythrocyte sedimentation and C-reactive protein occurs when there is inflammation somewhere in the body. A complete metabolic panel is used to evaluate creatinine and BUN levels to assess renal function.

Treatment for acute pyelonephritis is antibiotics both oral and IV, along with analgesics to control pain. NSAIDs work well to treat both pain and fever. Antibiotics may need to be adjusted based on the results of the urine culture. Overall, the majority of patients with pyelonephritis are managed as an outpatient, with most patients improving while on oral antibiotics.

Radiologic imaging is not required for diagnosis and treatment of uncomplicated patients. Imaging is only used when symptoms and laboratory abnormalities persist. Imaging is helpful in identifying renal and perirenal abscesses, stones, and hydronephrosis. The imagining study of choice for acute pyelonephritis is a contrast abdominal/pelvic CT as it provides anatomic and physiologic information and can characterize intrarenal and extrarenal pathology. US is the first choice when the examination needs to be done bedside or when radiation exposure is an issue, such as with pregnancy. Sonography can be used as an initial study to evaluate the urinary tract in patients with symptoms of pyelonephritis; however, interstitial nephritis is not well seen with grayscale images. Many patients with clinically

suspected pyelonephritis will have a negative sonographic examination. Findings of pyelonephritis that can be seen with US include changes in the echogenicity of the renal parenchyma due to edema, which will make the parenchyma more hypoechoic when compared with normal parenchyma. The kidney can be large and swollen with loss of corticomedullary differentiation. On some patients, the overall gain will need to be increased to see the parenchymal echoes. Hydronephrosis may be present, and sometimes, an abscess can be seen. The entire kidney should be evaluated with power or color Doppler, either the whole kidney at once or in segments, looking for regions of cortical perfusion defects, which may correspond to an area of infection or inflammation, despite the normal appearance on grayscale. These areas may represent early abscess formation. Because it is more sensitive, power Doppler is preferred as flow direction is not needed. With serial examinations of patients on antibiotics, the kidney should start to return to its normal sonographic appearance. On some patients, there may be residual areas of scarring (Fig. 12-79A–G).

The urinary bladder should always be imaged on patients with suspected pyelonephritis. Bladder wall thickness can be measured, residual volumes calculated, and the contents of the bladder can be evaluated looking for echoes floating around in the urine. In men, the prostate volume should be calculated looking for BPH, which may be causing some bladder outlet obstruction. The volume can be easily calculated by the US machine by activating volume measurement.

The role of CEUS on patients with suspected acute pyelonephritis looks promising and may equal contrast-enhanced CT. Other benefits of CEUS include that there is no radiation and that US contrast is not nephrotoxic unlike CT contrast.

Emphysematous Pyelonephritis[4,7,87,88,90]

EPN is an uncommon, severe complication of acute pyelonephritis caused by Gram-negative bacteria, most commonly *E. coli*. It is a necrotizing, causing necrosis, infection from acute multifocal bacterial nephritis, with extension of the infection through the renal capsule. EPN is characterized by the presence of gas in the renal parenchyma, collecting system, and perinephric space. The pathogenesis for gas formation is unclear. EPN occurs more frequently in diabetic patients, especially if it is uncontrolled, with women being more affected than men and occurs in the left kidney in about two-thirds of patients. Nondiabetic patients are either immunocompromised or have a urinary tract obstruction. EPN is life-threatening, primarily due to septic complications, with a mortality rate as high as 30% to 40% if not treated promptly. Patients who receive both medical and surgical management versus just medical management alone have a better prognosis. Patients with EPN are extremely ill and are usually in the intensive care unit (ICU). Treatment will depend on the severity of the disease. Although emergency nephrectomy has historically been the preferred treatment, a nephron-sparing approach is increasingly being favored with some patients only needing percutaneous drainage. IV antibiotics are used in mild cases. More advanced cases will drain any collections along with IV antibiotics, and more severe cases may need a nephrectomy. CT is the best diagnostic imaging modality as it can document enlarged

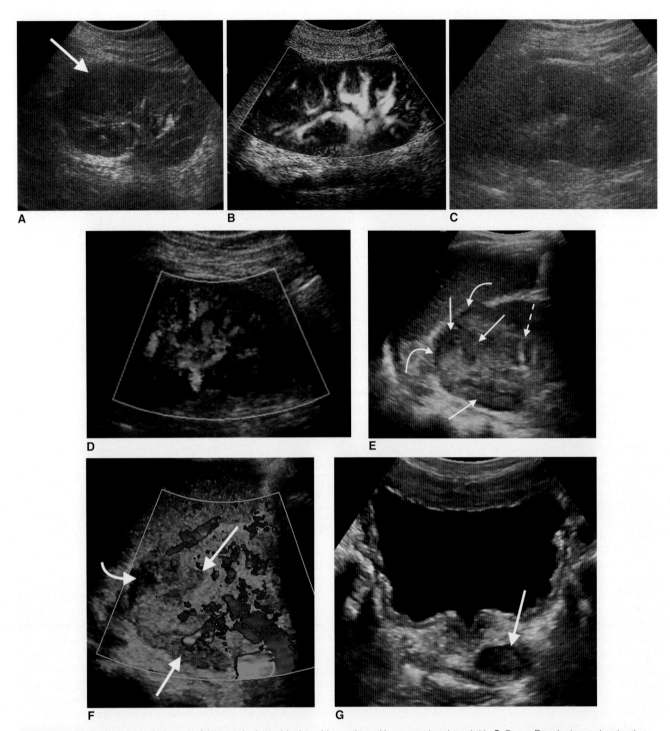

FIGURE 12-79 Pyelonephritis. **A:** An area of decreased echogenicity (*arrow*) in a patient with suspected pyelonephritis. **B:** Power Doppler image showing that the hypoechoic area has no flow compatible with pyelonephritis. **C:** A grayscale image on a patient who is suspected of having pyelonephritis. This is a technically difficult patient and there is no detail within the kidney. **D:** Color Doppler on this patient was surprisingly good and showed an area of flow void compatible with pyelonephritis. **E:** Small abscesses in the kidney (*straight arrows*) with accompanying gas within the collecting system (*dotted arrow*). Margins of an early perinephric abscess are also demonstrated (*curved arrows*). **F:** Color Doppler image of the same patient as **E** demonstrating intrarenal abscesses without flow (*straight arrows*). The abscess has broken through the capsule and is becoming a perinephric abscess (*curved arrow*). **G:** This is a pelvic image of the same patient as **E** and **F**. An abscess (*arrow*) in the prostate that is the source of the renal infection. Note the thickened bladder wall.

kidneys, destroyed renal parenchyma, intrarenal gas, fluid collections, focal necrotic areas, and any abscesses.

US demonstrates an enlarged kidney with echogenic foci, causing a ringdown artifact, representing gas inside the kidney, which can be located in the renal parenchyma, renal sinus, or both. When there is a lot of gas clumped together, "dirty shadowing" is seen, which is like an acoustic shadow, but instead of being echo free, it is filled with echoes, not allowing visualization of structures beneath it. In severe cases, when there is a significant amount of gas inside the kidney, the artifact may completely obscure the kidney, making visualization of the kidney very difficult or even impossible to see. It is the gas inside the kidney that limits the use of sonography (Fig. 12-80A–C).

Xanthogranulomatous Pyelonephritis[4,7,35,91–93]

XGP is, as the name suggests, a chronic granulomatous process that can result in a nonfunctioning kidney. The prefix xantho, is from the Greek meaning yellow, and refers to the replacement of corticomedullary tissue by yellow nodular areas of fatty tissue. XGP is a rare, serious, chronic inflammatory disorder that is associated with chronic nephrolithiasis and infection. These infections produce a chronic granulomatous inflammatory response and eventually destruction of the renal parenchyma, which can be replaced by lipid-laden foamy macrophages that gives a yellow color to the tissue. The most common organisms found with XGP are *E. coli* and *Proteus mirabilis*. XGP is typically unilateral and may be diffuse or focal, with the diffuse type more common involving the entire kidney. The inflammatory process can extend into the perinephric tissues and other organs.

Unilateral flank pain and fever are the most common presenting symptoms. Urinary symptoms, if present, can include dysuria, hematuria, and increased urinary frequency. XGP is seen in all age groups, including infants, but is most frequently seen in middle-aged to elderly patients. Women are twice as affected as men probably due to their increased incidence of UTIs and staghorn (struvite) kidney stones. There is also an increased incidence in patients with diabetes mellitus. Blood work often shows leukocytosis, anemia, and elevated C-reactive protein and erythrocyte sedimentation rate. Positive urine cultures may find *P. mirabilis* and *E. coli*. The clinical and imaging findings of XGP are a large staghorn calculus and hydronephrosis. Other findings can include UPJ obstruction, chronic interstitial nephritis, and calyceal stones. XGP can be confused with RCC, and a CT scan will confirm the diagnosis. Unfortunately, there are no conservative or medical therapies, and surgical nephrectomy is performed and is usually curative.

US findings include renal enlargement while keeping its kidney shape, lack of corticomedullary differentiation, and usually a staghorn calculus. The renal parenchyma can be replaced by cystic spaces, and there may be hypoechoic areas, which represent dilated calices or inflammatory masses. Perinephric fluid collections may be seen. Focal XGP will have one or more hypoechoic masses, often associated with a single calyx, and an obstructing stone. Focal XGP is seen in the renal cortex and does not communicate with the renal pelvis. It can be difficult to determine whether it is focal XGP, a malignancy, or an abscess by sonography. When sonographic findings suggest XGP, a CT is ordered as it can be more specific in determining the full extent

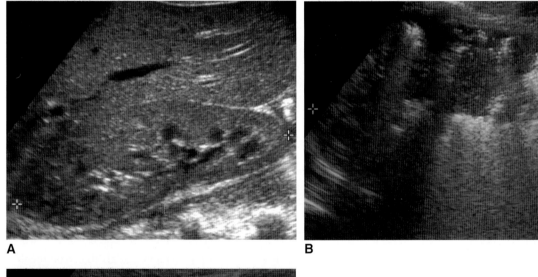

A   B

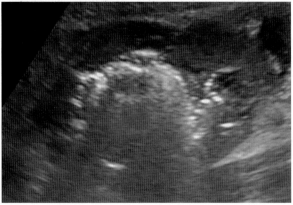

C

FIGURE 12-80 Emphysematous pyelonephritis. **A:** The normal right kidney of a patient in the medical intensive care unit. **B:** Grossly abnormal left kidney of the same patient containing air throughout the kidney indicative of emphysematous pyelonephritis. A large accumulation of air creates a "dirty" shadow in the mid-lower pole. **C:** Another patient with emphysematous pyelonephritis where the kidney shape and parenchyma are appreciated as the gas is located in the collecting system.

of XGP in the kidney and into the perirenal and pararenal spaces to help with surgical planning.

Chronic Pyelonephritis[4,35,94,95]

Chronic pyelonephritis is not reoccurring bouts of acute pyelonephritis. Chronic pyelonephritis is a complex renal disorder with chronic renal inflammation from tubulointerstitial inflammation caused by obstruction to the collecting system. These reoccurring and persistent renal infections cause deep segmental cortical scarring and clubbing of the pelvic calyces as the papillae retract into the scars. Many of the dilated tubules will contain colloid casts, which suggest the appearance of thyroid tissue, and are termed *thyroidization* of the kidney. Chronic pyelonephritis is most commonly caused by chronic vesicoureteral reflux, which leads to scarring of the kidneys, either unilateral or bilateral, from a superimposed infection, which is a secondary infection that is resistant to the treatment being used against the primary infection. These recurring episodes cause asymmetric scarring in the kidney, with areas of focal thinning caused by the fibrosis of the cortex and medulla. The renal changes may be unilateral or bilateral, but when bilateral, the kidneys are not equally damaged. When only one kidney is affected, the other kidney may undergo compensatory hypertrophy. Chronic pyelonephritis is a significant cause of renal failure and can lead to ESRD from the progressive renal scarring. Some patients can be asymptomatic if there is no acute infection; otherwise symptoms can include fever, malaise, and flank pain. Clinical signs include renal insufficiency and the development of hypertension. The diagnosis is made clinically and confirmed with imaging studies and lab tests. Once imaging has scanned the patient and the diagnosis of chronic pyelonephritis is made, repeat imaging is unlikely to find any new findings.

There is no specific treatment, as the damage to the kidneys is irreversible. Patients may also be followed up regularly with blood and urine tests and monitoring of their blood pressure. Even though there is no specific treatment for most patients, the patient's blood pressure will be controlled to help slow the progression. Surgery may be indicated to correct any obstruction or structural abnormalities, such as reflux, and a nephroureterectomy may be used to help address severe complications such as an abscess and organ dysfunction and to control UTIs and hypertension.

Diagnostic workup can include urine analysis for leukocyturia, proteinuria, and decreased urine concentration. Blood tests can show elevated creatinine and cystatin C, a protein that is produced by the cells in the body and regulated by the kidneys. A nuclear medicine static DMSA renal scintigraphy test is the most sensitive method for detecting scarring of the parenchyma. CT and US findings include renal scarring, atrophy and cortical thinning, caliceal clubbing, thickening and dilatation, and overall renal asymmetry. With US, a dilated blunt calix may be seen with an associated overlying cortical scar or atrophy (Fig. 12-81).

Renal and Perinephric Abscesses[35,96–99]

Renal and perinephric abscesses are complications of UTIs and acute pyelonephritis. When left untreated, acute pyelonephritis may develop into a renal abscess, which is a

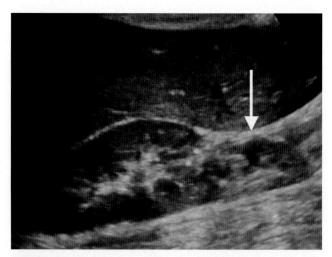

FIGURE 12-81 A thinned and abnormal lower pole (*arrow*) associated with chronic pyelonephritis. Note the loss of renal architecture inside the lower pole.

collection of pus within the kidney, especially patients who have diabetes, a urinary tract obstruction, or an infected kidney stone. A renal abscess is most commonly caused by Gram-negative bacteria such as *E. coli* and *Proteus*. It can also be caused by hematogenous seeding, usually by *Staphylococcus aureus*, with the bacteria spreading to the kidney tissue causing a renal abscess. A renal abscess will have symptoms that are similar to those seen in acute pyelonephritis and include fever, flank pain, abdominal pain, and dysuria. The diagnosis of a renal abscess should be considered in patients with an acute renal infection that fail to improve after 5 days of antibiotics.

A perinephric abscess is located between the kidney capsule and Gerota fascia and usually develops from acute pyelonephritis. Other causes include necrotic perirenal fat, the rupture of a renal abscess into the perirenal space from pyonephrosis. Perinephric abscesses are associated with patients who are diabetic and have kidney stones or patients with septic emboli. Men and women are equally affected, and patients with diabetes account for one-third of all perinephric abscess cases. Unlike a renal abscess, the symptoms of a perinephric abscess can have a slower onset and be unspecific. Patients may present with symptoms they have had for more than 1 week, such as a fever, flank pain, abdominal pain, night sweats, and chills.

A renal abscess occurs more frequently than a perinephric abscess. Leukocytosis is frequently observed in the setting of both renal and perinephric abscesses, and there may be elevation of erythrocyte sedimentation rate and C-reactive protein, which are the markers of infection. Blood culture may identify the type of bacteria. Urinalysis can show pyuria and proteinuria and can sometimes identify the bacteria, which can help determine the proper antibiotic.

Patients with a small renal abscess, less than 5 cm, are treated with antibiotics, and larger abscesses, greater than 5 cm, require image-guided percutaneous drainage and antibiotics. A sample of the pus is sent to the lab so that a Gram stain, a test used to detect the presence of bacteria, culture results, and antibiotic resistance testing, can determine the right antibiotic treatment. Some patients may need a nephrectomy if the kidney is severely infected.

Patients with a perinephric abscess will have a percutaneous drainage for both diagnostic and therapeutic purposes. As earlier, the pus will be sent to determine the proper antibiotic to use. If a percutaneous drainage is ineffective, a nephrectomy may be indicated, especially if the kidney severely infected.

CT is the diagnostic test of choice as it can determine the presence and the extent of a perinephric abscess. Usually, sonography is used to follow the progression of the abscess. Sonographically, a renal abscess presents as a round, hypoechoic complex mass with thick walls and acoustic enhancement. Other features can include internal mobile debris, septations, and gas that may cause "dirty shadowing." Doppler should show increased blood flow at the margins of the abscess as blood is sent to combat the infection. As there is no tissue inside the abscess, there will not be any internal flow. Sonographically, a perinephric abscess appears as a perirenal hypoechoic, complex collection and may have a fluid–debris level and contain gas. Sonography is usually the modality of choice, for both types of abscesses, to obtain a sample of the pus or for image-guided percutaneous draining (Fig. 12-82A–D).

Pyonephrosis[4,100-102]

Pyonephrosis comes from the Greek *pyon*, pus, and *nephros*, kidney, and is defined as infected hydronephrosis, which is when there is pus in an obstructed collecting system. Multiple infectious agents have been isolated in patients with pyonephrosis, including *E. coli*, *Enterococcus*, *Candida*, and *Staphylococcus*. Pyonephrosis may be caused by a variety of conditions that are caused by an ascending infection of

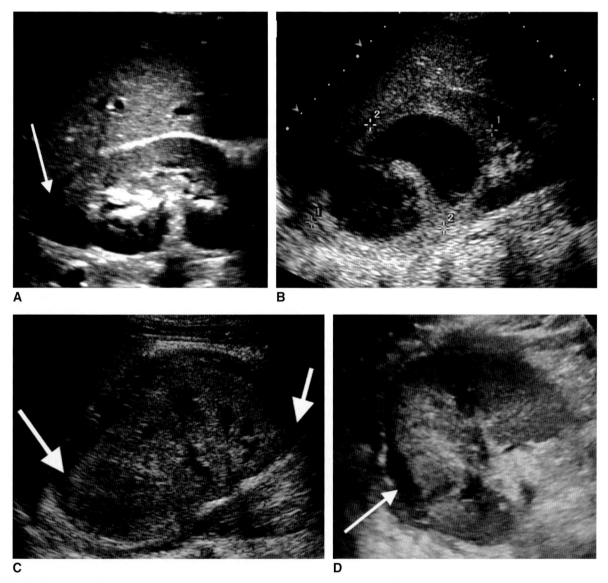

FIGURE 12-82 Abscesses. **A:** A complicated irregularly shaped fluid collection in the upper pole (*arrow*) that was determined to be an abscess. The gain was increased to show the low-level echoes inside the abscess. **B:** Two fluid collections are seen that contain low-level echoes. A sample was obtained and sent for culture to determine the best treatment. **C:** The borders (*arrows*) of a large perinephric abscess with septations. Note that there is a large hypoechoic area in the upper pole with a loss of definition in the sinus echoes. **D:** A transverse image of a different patient with a perinephric abscess (*arrow*). The lateral area of the kidney next to the abscess is more echogenic than usual.

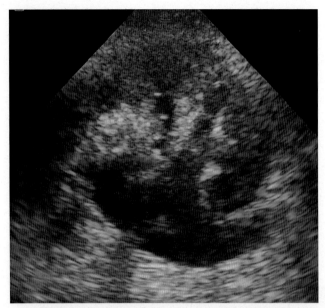

FIGURE 12-83 A patient appeared to have hydronephrosis. However, the internal echoes could not be cleared from the image, and the patient had cloudy urine. The bright white echoes within the calyces were compatible to gas, and the patient was diagnosed with pyonephrosis.

the urinary tract or from a bacterial pathogen in the blood. A kidney stone is the main cause in up to 70% of patients with pyonephrosis. Pyonephrosis can be the cause of a renal and perirenal abscess. It can also destroy the renal parenchyma and cause loss of renal function. If not recognized and treated promptly, pyonephrosis may progress to severe urosepsis swiftly, which is a true urologic emergency. Patients with pyonephrosis may present with a variety of clinical symptoms. from being asymptomatic to a history of fever, flank pain, a UTI, pyuria, and hydronephrosis. Lab values are nonspecific and show signs of infection. Pyonephrosis is suspected when the clinical symptoms of fever and flank pain are combined with the imaging evidence of a urinary tract obstruction, especially when debris in seen in the upper collecting system. A sample of the pus from a US-guided aspiration is sent for Gram stain and culture and can help to give a definitive diagnosis of pyonephrosis. Antibiotic therapy will be determined by the findings from either the blood, urine, or aspirated fluid cultures. Depending on the status of the patient and imaging findings, the patient may need an emergency percutaneous nephrostomy to drain the infected collecting system.

Sonographic findings suggestive of pyonephrosis are hydronephrosis with low-amplitude echoes and echogenic debris in the collecting system, which is the most consistent finding (Fig. 12-83). Other findings include fluid–fluid levels and gas with dirty shadowing within the collecting system. The presence of debris and layering of low-amplitude echoes in the hydronephrotic kidney are specific enough that their absence excludes pyonephrosis with a high degree of accuracy.

MEDICAL RENAL DISEASE[4,7,58]

Medical renal disease always affects both kidneys and is a catch all term used to describe the various disease processes that involve the parenchyma of the kidneys causing a decrease

in renal function. It can be caused by a variety of diseases, such as diabetic nephropathy, interstitial nephritis, ATI, acute glomerulonephritis, hypertensive nephropathy, and acquired HIV (human immunodeficiency virus) nephropathy. US is usually the first test a patient has with elevated BUN and creatinine levels to rule out hydronephrosis and to evaluate the echogenicity and length of the kidneys. It is important to obtain an accurate renal length as it is used to distinguish an acute from a chronic process. In a chronic process, the kidney will measure less than 9 cm. Echogenic kidneys can be a sign of renal disease, and this increase in echogenicity is believed to be caused by a deposition of collagen, fibrous tissue, inflammatory infiltrates, and proteinaceous casts. Currently, there are no sonographic criteria to determine what is causing the kidneys to be echogenic and they are given the diagnosis of medical renal disease. As this diagnosis lacks specificity, a biopsy, usually a US-guided one, is needed to determine the histologic cause of the patient's renal failure.

In order to compare the two organs, the liver and spleen must be normal for a valid comparison. The sonographer should obtain a color or power Doppler image to look for flow out to the capsule. The RI should be obtained on an intrarenal artery as it is affected by increased vascular resistance caused by parenchymal disease. In diseased kidneys, the RI will be elevated and greater than 0.7.

Acute Kidney Injury[4,7,58,103–106]

Acute kidney injury (AKI) is the preferred term replacing the older term acute renal failure (ARF). *Acute kidney injury* is defined as an abrupt or rapid decline in renal function over a few hours to a few days. This causes an accumulation of creatinine and urea in the blood, termed *azotemia*. Patients will present with a decrease in eGFR, and an increase in creatinine and BUN. The patient may or may not have a decrease in the amount of urine output. AKI causes both structural damage to the kidney and decreased function and is caused by inadequate renal perfusion due to severe trauma, illness, or surgery, or it can be caused by a rapidly progressive, intrinsic renal disease. AKI almost always occurs due to another medical condition such as sepsis, ischemia, or nephrotoxicity complicating recognition and treatment.

About 2% to 5% of patients will develop AKI while in the hospital. Up to 50% of patients in the ICU will develop AKI, with about 4% to 5% of these patients requiring dialysis. This is the reason that there are a lot of portable renal US ordered by the ICU doctors. AKI can be fatal, with a mortality rate 5.5 to 6.5 times higher than in similarly ill patients with normal renal function despite the use of dialysis. AKI is often reversible if it is found and treated quickly, with some patients recovering normal to near-normal renal function once treatment is finished. A renal biopsy may be needed to identify the intrarenal causes of AKI to help with treatment. People who have had AKI in the past are at an increased risk of developing CKD in the future.

The causes of AKI may be classified into three groups: prerenal, affecting 25% to 60% of patients; intrinsic renal, affecting 35% to 70% of patients; and postrenal causes, affecting 5% to 20% of patients. Prerenal and postrenal causes are due to extrarenal disease, which leads to decreased GFR.

If these pre- or postrenal conditions are not treated, they will cause renal cellular damage, and the patient is classified as intrinsic renal disease.

The clinical presentation and symptoms will usually come from the underlying disease. Some patients will have no symptoms, and AKI will be discovered incidentally through abnormal renal function values through either a basic metabolic panel (BMP) or a comprehensive metabolic panel (CMP).

Treatment of AKI is more supportive, that is, helping the kidneys to function, and includes treating the underlying clinical condition and removing any toxic products from the body. Occasionally, AKI can cause permanent loss of kidney function and is harder to reverse after damage to the kidneys has occurred. Patients with AKI are at a risk of developing a pleural effusion, with pulmonary complications as the single most significant risk factor for death.

Sonographically, AKI will show echogenic kidneys of normal size and normal cortical thickness (Fig. 12-84A–E).

Prerenal Causes[58,103]

Prerenal AKI represents the most common form and often leads to intrinsic AKI if it is not promptly corrected. Prerenal is caused by not enough blood flowing through the kidneys, called renal hypoperfusion, causing a decreased GFR as a normal GFR is dependent on adequate renal perfusion. Prerenal renal causes that can be seen with US are renal artery stenosis, which results in decreased perfusion, and renal vein thrombosis, which results in an increased pressure in the kidney. Other prerenal causes of AKI include sepsis, dehydration, heart failure, certain medications like angiotensin-converting enzyme (ACE) inhibitors or NSAIDs, and hepatorenal or cardiorenal syndrome.

Renal Causes[58,103–112]

Renal causes are caused by a process within the kidney. Diagnosing intrinsic renal causes of AKI can be challenging because of the wide variety of causes, which include glomerulonephritis, ATI, lupus, viruses, infections, certain antibiotics and medications, chemotherapeutic agents, and contrast agents used for imaging. Intrinsic renal causes are usually diagnosed with a renal biopsy.

Acute glomerulonephritis can cause both structural and functional changes and can be caused by infections, problems with the immune system, and sometimes the exact cause is unknown. Acute glomerulonephritis causes necrosis of the cellular elements in the glomeruli. The vascular elements, tubules, and interstitium become secondarily affected, resulting in enlarged, poorly functioning kidneys. Acute glomerulonephritis develops suddenly, typically after an infection. The patient may not have any symptoms, and it is diagnosed when blood tests are abnormal. Some patients may present with proteinuria, edema, hematuria, hypertension, oliguria, or nephrotic syndrome. Acute glomerulonephritis will progress to chronic glomerulonephritis in about 30% of adults and can eventually become renal failure. Glomerulonephritis is usually diagnosed with a kidney biopsy.

ATI is the new nomenclature now used in place of acute tubular necrosis (ATN) to define a sudden reduction in renal function. ATI is a medical condition causing the death of tubular epithelial cells that form the renal tubules of the kidneys, either by persistent hypoperfusion or by toxic injury, causing tubular dysfunction. It is the most common cause of AKI in hospitalized patients, responsible for 33% to 45% of all AKI cases. ATI is classified as either toxic or ischemic depending on the cause. Toxic ATI occurs when the tubular cells are exposed to a toxic substance and is called nephrotoxic ATI. Ischemic ATI occurs when the tubular cells do not get enough oxygen, causing cellular death due to their very high metabolism. Because the tubular cells can continually replace themselves, the overall prognosis for ATI is very good as long as the underlying cause is corrected. Recovery of renal function can occur within 7 to 21 days. Clinically, the patient may present with an acute decrease in their GFR and a sudden increase in serum creatinine and BUN. A urinalysis will show what is termed "muddy brown casts" from the epithelial cells and is diagnostic for AKI. ATI causes arterial vasoconstriction, which is reflected on Doppler findings by the reduced diastolic flow, which causes an elevated RI of greater than 8.0. Very severe cases may even demonstrate reverse diastolic flow, which can lead to a poor prognosis, with most of these patients not recovering their renal function.

Acute interstitial nephritis (AIN) is when the spaces between the kidney tubules, the interstitium, become inflamed, causing an acute deterioration in renal function. The most common symptom is a decrease in urine output, yet some patients may have an increase in urine output. Other symptoms include hematuria, hypertension, sudden weight gain from fluid, and fever. Over two-thirds of AIN cases are caused by an allergic reaction to drugs, called allergic interstitial nephritis, and infection-related AIN accounting for 5% to 10% of cases. Drugs that can cause AIN are usually from one of the following groups: antibiotics, proton-pump inhibitors for stomach acid control, and NSAIDS. AIN caused by long-term use of acetaminophen, aspirin, and NSAIDs is called analgesic nephropathy. Usually, renal failure will resolve when the drug is stopped. Usually, AIN is a short-term disorder. In rare cases, it can cause permanent damage, leading to CKD especially among elderly patients.

Nephrotic syndrome is not a specific disease but a group of symptoms that indicate that the kidneys are not working properly. These symptoms include proteinuria, hypoalbuminemia, low levels of the protein albumin in the blood, hyperlipidemia, high levels of cholesterol and other lipids in the blood, and edema. It is more common in men. The most common primary cause of nephrotic syndrome in adults is focal segmental glomerulosclerosis (FSGS), which can only be diagnosed with a kidney biopsy. Causes of FSGS include viruses, medications, obesity, hypertension, and vascular disease. Most people with FSGS will eventually develop kidney failure, despite treatment, and will be put on dialysis and possibly on the kidney transplant waiting list. After the kidney transplant, there is a chance that FSGS will return, causing the loss of the transplant. Most of the time, nephrotic syndrome happens because of secondary causes, with diabetes as the most common cause. Treatment for nephrotic syndrome includes treating the condition that is causing it and medication.

AIDS nephropathy is associated with both AKI and CKD. Abnormalities involve all components of the nephron with typical findings that include collapsing capillary loops, FSGS causing areas of scarring, microcystic tubular dilatation, and

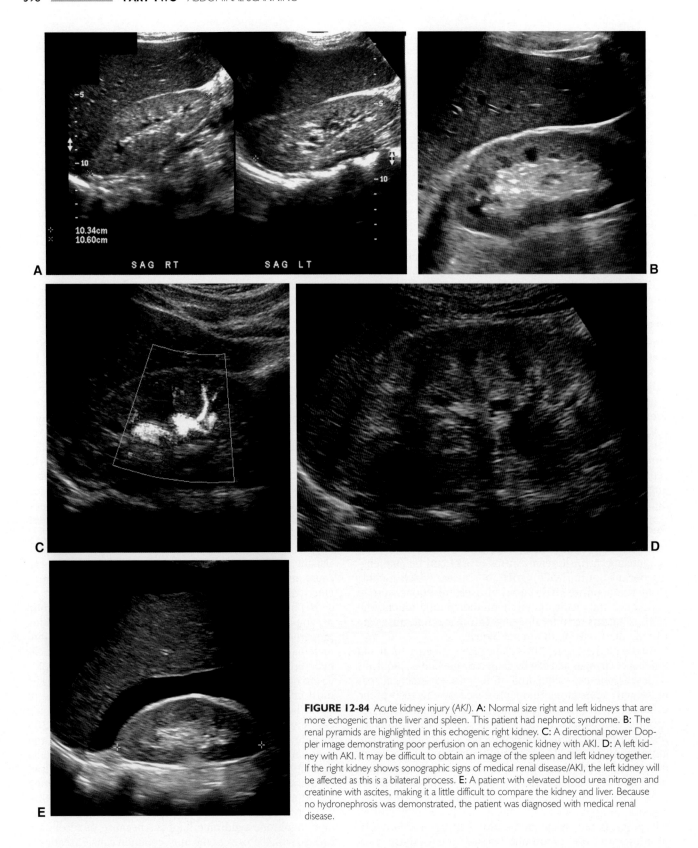

FIGURE 12-84 Acute kidney injury (*AKI*). **A:** Normal size right and left kidneys that are more echogenic than the liver and spleen. This patient had nephrotic syndrome. **B:** The renal pyramids are highlighted in this echogenic right kidney. **C:** A directional power Doppler image demonstrating poor perfusion on an echogenic kidney with AKI. **D:** A left kidney with AKI. It may be difficult to obtain an image of the spleen and left kidney together. If the right kidney shows sonographic signs of medical renal disease/AKI, the left kidney will be affected as this is a bilateral process. **E:** A patient with elevated blood urea nitrogen and creatinine with ascites, making it a little difficult to compare the kidney and liver. Because no hydronephrosis was demonstrated, the patient was diagnosed with medical renal disease.

prominent podocytes. AIDS nephropathy usually occurs in advanced HIV disease. The patient's prognosis is always poor, as it rapidly progresses to ESRD and death. A US of the kidneys will be ordered on these patients when they have elevated BUN and creatinine to look for hydronephrosis as the cause. US will demonstrate a greatly increased renal echogenicity, the brightest you will ever see, which is a fairly specific finding for AIDS patients, with a normal renal size. The increased echogenicity is thought to be caused by prominent interstitial expansion by the cellular infiltrate and the markedly dilated tubules, which contain voluminous casts (Fig. 12-85A–C). Do not confuse these kidneys

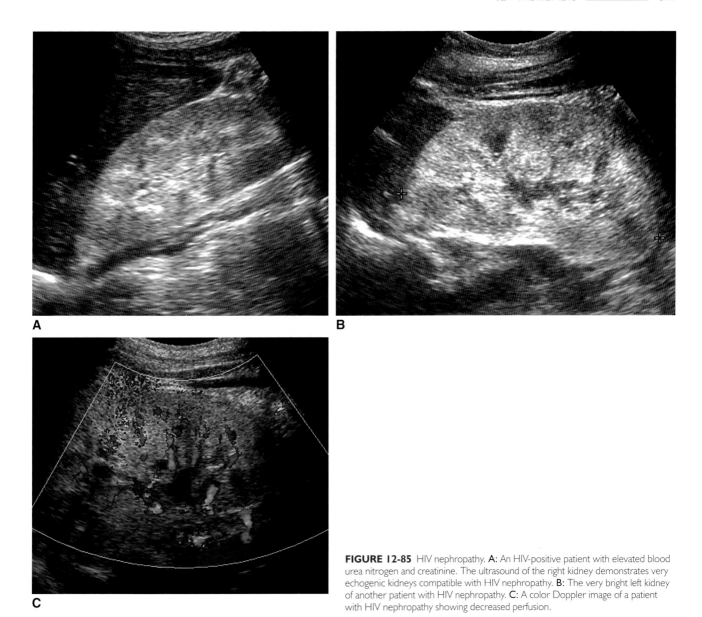

FIGURE 12-85 HIV nephropathy. **A:** An HIV-positive patient with elevated blood urea nitrogen and creatinine. The ultrasound of the right kidney demonstrates very echogenic kidneys compatible with HIV nephropathy. **B:** The very bright left kidney of another patient with HIV nephropathy. **C:** A color Doppler image of a patient with HIV nephropathy showing decreased perfusion.

with CKD, which also has bright kidneys, but not nearly as bright, as these patients will have small kidneys. AIDS nephropathy is the cause of the abnormal renal function tests, and in the author's experience, these patients very rarely had hydronephrosis.

Contrast induced AKI, also known as contrast induced nephropathy, is when a radiologic contrast agent injected into the vein is the cause of the patient getting AKI. It is one of the most common causes of AKI for patients who are in the hospital. Because they can affect kidney function, iodinated contrast agents and gadolinium, which have been linked to nephrogenic systemic fibrosis, should be used with caution on patients already diagnosed with AKI. The benefit of US contrast agents is that they are not nephrotoxic and do not affect the kidneys.

At the time of writing this chapter, the world is still in the midst of a pandemic caused by COVID-19, which has added a new cause of AKI. Studies have shown that between 25% and 40% of patients have proteinuria on hospital admission and that 30% to 50% of hospitalized patients will develop some form of AKI, with approximately 20% to 40% of patients admitted to the ICU. Proteinuria and hematuria are common findings in patients with COVID-19 AKI. Multiple causes and findings have been reported, including results from autopsies, such as systemic immune and inflammatory responses, decreased kidney perfusion, nephrotoxins from contrast agents and medications, renal microthrombi, local immunothrombosis causing hypoxia, and direct infection of the kidney tubules with SARS-CoV-2204-206 that induces cytoplasmic renal tubular inclusions. Autopsy studies have shown that ATI is the most common finding in kidneys of patients with COVID-19 AKI. US findings include increased or heterogeneous parenchymal echogenicity, possible loss of corticomedullary differentiation, preserved cortical thickness, decreased global perfusion, and elevated resistive indices, which are similar sonographic findings on any patient with AKI. Research continues on the effect of SARS-CoV-2204-206 on the kidneys.

Postrenal Causes[58,103–105,113–119]

Postrenal causes are not as common as renal causes and are caused by bilateral obstruction of the kidneys. Most causes of postrenal AKI can be diagnosed with US and include BPH, urologic or gynecologic tumors, bladder tumor, and a bladder that cannot empty, such as a neurogenic bladder. Prompt diagnosis followed by relief of the obstruction is important to improve renal function.

Chronic Kidney Disease

CKD has replaced the historic term chronic renal failure (CRF). According to the Centers for Disease Control and Prevention (CDC), there are approximately 37 million people who have CKD, but most people are yet to be diagnosed with it. CKD is the loss of renal function as a result of parenchymal disease that happens over a period of months to years. It is an irreversible disease that affects the function of the nephrons, causing a decreased GFR, decreased tubular function, and decreased reabsorption capabilities. CKD can lead to ESRD, which has a high morbidity and mortality rates. Because CKD is a progressive condition, sometimes treatment can help to slow down the decline in renal function. Fortunately, not all patients with CKD will end up with ESRD.

The two main causes of CKD are diabetes and hypertension, which together are responsible for up to two-thirds of patients with CKD. Other causes include glomerulonephritis, chronic pyelonephritis, renal vascular disease, BPH, polycystic renal disease, and repeated UTIs. CKD is more prevalent in the elderly population. Younger patients with CKD typically experience a progressive loss of renal function, whereas some patients over 65 years have a stable disease.

The guidelines define CKD as a decreased GFR of less than 60 mL/min/1.73 m² for at least 3 months. Whatever the underlying etiology, once the nephrons are damaged, there is a decrease in renal function. The nephrons begin a process of irreversible sclerosis that leads to a progressive decline in the GFR and, therefore, renal function. Patients with CKD may have symptoms that include leg swelling, loss of appetite, anemia, metal taste in the mouth, and confusion.

CKD is associated with an increased risk of cardiovascular disease and ESRD. When conservative management is no longer effective, the patient will need to be put on dialysis and potentially be placed on the renal transplant list, depending on the patient's age, related health issues, donor availability, and the patient's personal preference.

Sonographic findings are similar to AKI with echogenic kidneys, but the kidneys will be small measuring less than 9 cm and have cortical thinning. There may be poor visibility of the renal pyramids and the renal sinus. Some patients may have small cysts as described in "Acquired Cysts" section. Sonographic findings are not disease specific, and there is no correlation between the severity of disease and the kidney's echogenicity. Doppler findings will be elevated RIs of greater than 0.8 in the main and intrarenal arteries. With the possibility of reduced flow, the intrarenal vessels may be difficult to visualize. Power Doppler may be of help in these situations. Sonographically, a small, shrunken, echogenic kidney is diagnostic of ESRD. In addition to kidney length, assessment of the cortical thickness is helpful in distinguishing AKI from CKD. The cortex is normally about 1 cm thick, and the entire parenchyma measures about 1.5 cm. Thinning of the renal cortex commonly occurs in CKD and measures 6 mm or less (Fig. 12-86A–D). Some studies have shown that cortical thickness can be more sensitive than renal length in determining the progression of disease and should be used for follow-up care.

Because kidney length is especially important in distinguishing AKI from CKD, a clear understanding of "normal" kidney length is important. Studies of kidney length have revealed the following:

1. Normal kidney length is approximately 11 cm, with a normal range between 10 and 12 cm
2. The left kidney is longer than the right by about 0.3 cm

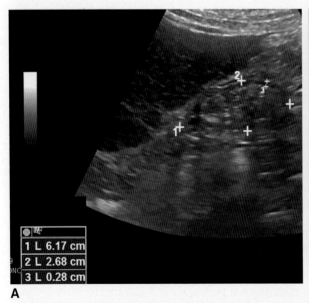

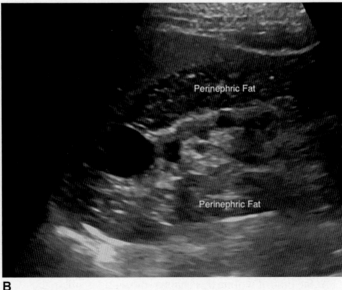

A   **B**

FIGURE 12-86 Chronic kidney disease (*CKD*). **A:** A patient with CKD with an echogenic kidney that measures 6.17 cm (*caliper 1*) in length, 2.68 cm in width (*caliper 2*) and with a cortical thickness of 0.28 cm (*caliper 3*). (Image courtesy of J. Guse.) **B:** An obese patient with a large layer of perinephric fat presented with chronic kidney disease related to diabetes. The kidney demonstrates multiple small cysts in the cortex and one larger cyst in the upper pole.

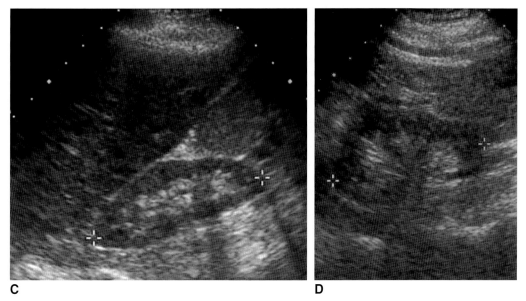

C
D

FIGURE 12-86 *(continued)* **C:** Small, echogenic right kidney in a patient with diabetic nephropathy. **D:** Small, echogenic left kidney in the same patient with diabetic nephropathy.

3. Women have smaller kidneys than men by about 0.5 cm
4. Kidney sizes less than 10 cm are unusual in people younger than age 60
5. Kidney length decreases with age beginning around age 60. This means that a 9.5-cm kidney probably represents CKD in a 30-year-old but may be normal for an 80-year-old. It is very important to carefully measure renal length and compare the lengths of the two kidneys. Any discrepancies between sides and one kidney that measures less than 9 cm should prompt the sonographer to reevaluate their measurements (Pathology Box 12-15).

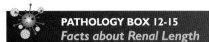

PATHOLOGY BOX 12-15
Facts about Renal Length

1. Normal kidney length approximately 11 cm
   a. Normal range between 10 and 12 cm
2. Left kidney is longer than right by about 0.3 cm
3. Women have smaller kidneys than men by about 0.5 cm
4. Kidney sizes less than 10 cm are unusual in people younger than 60 years
5. Kidney length decreases with age beginning around 60

SUMMARY

US plays an important role in evaluating the kidneys for a variety of pathology. It is cost-effective, accessible, can be performed portably, does not use radiation, has good patient acceptance, and can provide guidance for a variety of procedures. US can see kidneys that are normal, have congenital variants or anomalies, and a wide spectrum of pathology. US is typically the first imaging study for the kidneys. The sonographer needs to use all of their skills to give the patient the best study possible to save them from radiation and nephrotoxic contrast agents.

The future of renal US looks exciting with CEUS, elastography, new material and technology that creates the sound beam, and increased resolution and Doppler sensitivity. The reader is encouraged to read journal articles and attend local and national US meetings, including virtual meetings, to keep current on our evolving profession.

REFERENCES

1. National Institute of Diabetes and Digestive and Kidney Diseases. Kidney disease statistics for the United States. Accessed February 20, 2022. https://www.niddk.nih.gov/health-information/health-statistics/kidney-disease
2. Hill MA. Embryology: Renal system development. Accessed September 15, 2021. https://embryology.med.unsw.edu.au/embryology/index.php/Renal_System_Development
3. Carlson BM. *Human Embryology and Developmental Biology*. 6th ed. Elsevier:2018.
4. Drake R, Wayne Vogl A, Mitchell A. *Gray's Basic Anatomy*. 2nd ed. Elsevier:2017.
5. Tublin M, Levine D, Thurston W, Wilson SR. The kidney and urinary tract. In: Rumack C, Levine D, eds. *Diagnostic Ultrasound*. 5th ed. Elsevier; 2017.
6. Baba Y. Kidneys. Accessed February 7, 2021. https://radiopaedia.org/articles/kidneys?lang=us
7. Droual R. Urinary system. Accessed February 7, 2021. http://droualb.faculty.mjc.edu/Course%20Materials/Elementary%20Anatomy%20and%20Physiology%2050/Lecture%20outlines/urinary_system.htm
8. Weinberg K, Telegrafi S, Kozirovsky M. Urinary system. In: Hagen-Ansert S, ed. *Textbook of Diagnostic Ultrasonography*. 8th ed. Elsevier; 2017.
9. DeJong, MR. *Sonography Scanning: Principles and Protocols*. 5th ed. Elsevier; 2020.
10. Marieb EN, Hoehn K. *Human Anatomy and Physiology*. 11th ed. Pearson; 2019.
11. LibreTexts. Overview of urine formation. Accessed July 5, 2021. https://med.libretexts.org/Bookshelves/Anatomy_and_Physiology/

Book%3A_Anatomy_and_Physiology_(Boundless)/24%3A__Urinary_System/24.3%3A_Physiology_of_the_Kidneys/24.3A%3A_Overview_of_Urine_Formation

12. Lumen Learning. Renal blood flow and its regulation. Accessed July 5, 2021. https://courses.lumenlearning.com/cuny-kbcc-ap2/chapter/regulation-of-renal-blood-flow/

13. Bhatt S, Maclennan G, Dogra V. Renal pseudotumors. *AJR Am J Roentgenol.* 2007;188:1380–1387. Accessed July 7, 2021. https://www.ajronline.org/doi/full/10.2214/AJR.06.0920

14. Visible Body. Filtration, reabsorption, secretion: the three steps of urine formation. Accessed July 5, 2021. https://www.visiblebody.com/learn/urinary/urine-creation

15. National Kidney Foundation. Understanding your lab values. Accessed July 6, 2021. https://www.kidney.org/atoz/content/understanding-your-lab-values

16. LabTestsOnline. Accessed July 6, 2021. https://labtestsonline.org/tests-index

17. Keshavamurthy J. Developmental anomalies of the kidney and ureter. Accessed July 7, 2021. https://radiopaedia.org/articles/developmental-anomalies-of-the-kidney-and-ureter?lang=us

18. Hertzberg BS, Middleton WD. *Ultrasound: The Requisites.* 3rd ed. Elsevier; 2016.

19. Hartman DS, Choyke PL, Hartman MS. A practical approach to the cystic renal mass Accessed July 29, 2021. https://pubs.rsna.org/doi/full/10.1148/rg.24si045515

20. Botz B. Renal cyst. Accessed July 29, 2021. https://radiopaedia.org/articles/renal-cyst-1?lang=us

21. Hartman DS, Chesaru I. Cystic masses: ignore, follow, excise. Accessed July 29, 2021. https://radiologyassistant.nl/abdomen/kidney/cystic-masses

22. Garfield K, Leslie SW. Simple renal cyst. Accessed July 29, 2021. https://www.ncbi.nlm.nih.gov/books/NBK499900/

23. Sigmon DF, Sikhman R, Nielson JI. Renal cyst. Accessed July 29, 2021. https://www.ncbi.nlm.nih.gov/books/NBK470390/

24. Rometti M, Bryczkowsk C, Mirza MR. Hemorrhagic renal cyst. *JETem.* 2020;5(1):V1–V3. doi:10.21980/J8C92V. Accessed July 29, 2021.

25. Bennett J, Peterson C, Barr RG. Contrast-enhanced ultrasound of renal masses. *Appl Radiol.* 2020;49(6):10–16. Accessed July 29, 2021. https://www.appliedradiology.com/articles/contrast-enhanced-ultrasound-of-renal-masses

26. Qiu, X, Zhao Q, Ye Z, Meng L, Yan C, Jiang TA. How does contrast-enhanced ultrasonography influence Bosniak classification for complex cystic renal mass compared with conventional ultrasonography? *Medicine.* 2020;99(7):e19190. Accessed July 29, 2021. https://journals.lww.com/md-journal/FullText/2020/02140/How_does_contrast_enhanced_ultrasonography.81.aspx

27. Silverman SG, Pedrosa I, Ellis JH, et al. Bosniak classification of cystic renal masses, version 2019: an update proposal and needs assessment. *Radiology.* 2019;292:475–488. Accessed July 29, 2021. https://pubs.rsna.org/doi/pdf/10.1148/radiol.2019182646

28. Cantisani V, Bertolotto M, Clevert DA, et al. EFSUMB 2020 proposal for a contrast-enhanced ultrasound-adapted Bosniak cyst categorization—position statement. *Ultraschall Med.* 2021;42:154–166. © 2020. *Thieme.* Accessed July 29, 2021. https://www.thieme-connect.com/products/ejournals/pdf/10.1055/a-1300-1727.pdf

29. Bell DJ. Autosomal dominant polycystic kidney disease. Accessed July 29, 2021. https://radiopaedia.org/articles/autosomal-dominant-polycystic-kidney-disease-1?lang=us

30. Bennett WM, Rahbari-Oskoui FF, Chapman AB. Patient education: polycystic kidney disease (beyond the basics). Accessed July 29, 2021. https://www.uptodate.com/contents/polycystic-kidney-disease-beyond-the-basics

31. Ahmed S, Bughio S, Hassan M, Lal S, Ali M. Role of ultrasound in the diagnosis of chronic kidney disease and its correlation with serum creatinine level. *Cureus.* 2019;11(3):e4241. doi:10.7759/cureus.4241. Accessed September 21, 2021.

32. Algaba F. Renal adenomas: pathological differential diagnosis with malignant tumors. *Adv Urol.* 2008;2008:974848. Hindawi Publishing Corporation. doi:10.1155/2008/974848. https://www.hindawi.com/journals/au/2008/974848/

33. van Oostenbrugge TJ, Fütterer JJ, Mulders PFA. Diagnostic imaging for solid renal tumors: a pictorial review. *Kidney Cancer.* 2018;2(2):79–93. Accessed July 30, 2021. https://content.iospress.com/articles/kidney-cancer/kca180028

34. Radiology Key. Ultrasound of the renal tract. Accessed July 30, 2021. https://radiologykey.com/ultrasound-of-the-renal-tract/

35. Weerakkody Y, Knipe H. Chronic pyelonephritis. Accessed September 1, 2021. https://radiopaedia.org/articles/36717

36. AUA. Renal mass and localized renal cancer: AUA guideline. 2017. Accessed May 23, 2022 from https://www.auanet.org/documents/Guidelines/PDF/Renal-Mass-Guideline.pdf

37. Kinhirat S. Renal angiomyolipoma. Accessed July 30, 2021. https://radiopaedia.org/articles/renal-angiomyolipoma?lang=us

38. Vos N, Oyen R. Renal angiomyolipoma: the good, the bad, and the ugly. *J Belg Soc Radiol.* 2018;102(1):41. doi:10.5334/jbsr.1536. Accessed July 30, 2021.

39. American Cancer Society. About kidney cancer. Accessed July 31, 2021. https://www.cancer.org/cancer/kidney-cancer/about/what-is-kidney-cancer.html

40. National Cancer Institute. Cancer stat facts: kidney and renal pelvis cancer. Accessed July 31, 2021. https://seer.cancer.gov/statfacts/html/kidrp.html

41. Pandey J, Syed W. Renal cancer. In: *StatPearls [Internet].* StatPearls Publishing; 2021. Updated August 11, 2021. Accessed July 31, 2021. https://www.ncbi.nlm.nih.gov/books/NBK558975/

42. Niknejad MT. Renal cell carcinoma. Accessed July 31, 2021. https://radiopaedia.org/articles/renal-cell-carcinoma-1?lang=us

43. Sacco E, Pinto F, Totaro A, et al. Imaging of renal cell carcinoma: state of the art and recent advances. Accessed July 31, 2021. https://www.karger.com/Article/Pdf/322724

44. Niknejad MT. Transitional cell carcinoma (renal pelvis). Accessed August 1, 2021. https://radiopaedia.org/articles/transitional-cell-carcinoma-renal-pelvis

45. Browne RF, Meehan CP, Colville J, Power R, Torreggiani WC. Transitional cell carcinoma of the upper urinary tract: spectrum of imaging findings. *RadioGraphics.* 2005;25(6):1609–1627. Accessed August 1, 2021. https://pubs.rsna.org/doi/10.1148/rg.256045517#R16

46. Brits NF, Bulane S, Wadee R. Primary squamous cell carcinoma of the kidney: a case report and review of the literature. *Afr J Urol.* 2020;26:79. doi:10.1186/s12301-020-00088-9. Accessed August 1, 2021.

47. Zhou C, Urbauer DL, Fellman BM, et al. Metastases to the kidney: a comprehensive analysis of 151 patients from a tertiary referral centre. *BJU Int.* 2016;117(5):775–782. Accessed August 1, 2021. https://www.ncbi.nlm.nih.gov/pmc/articles/PMC4670601/

48. Cazacu SM, Săndulescu LD, Mitroi G, Neagoe DC, Streba C, Albulescu DM. Metastases to the kidney: a case report and review of the literature. *Curr Health Sci J.* 2020;46(1):80–89. Accessed August 1, 2021. https://www.ncbi.nlm.nih.gov/pmc/articles/PMC7323720/

49. Bokhari MR, Rana UI, Bokhari SRA. *Renal lymphoma.* In: *StatPearls [Internet].* StatPearls Publishing; 2021. Updated July 17, 2021. Accessed August 1, 2021. https://www.ncbi.nlm.nih.gov/books/NBK526034/

50. Sebastià C, Corominas D, Musquera M, Pano B, Ajami T, Nicolau C. Active surveillance of small renal masses. *Insights Imaging.* 2020;11:63. doi:10.1186/s13244-020-00853-y. Accessed November 22, 2021.

51. Sha M, Mumtaz F. Renal tumor biopsies: a shift towards improving outcomes in the management of small renal masses. In: Kommu SS, Gill IS, eds. *Evolving Trends in Kidney Cancer.* IntechOpen. 2020. doi:10.5772/intechopen.85781. Accessed November 22, 2021. https://www.intechopen.com/chapters/66738

52. Radiology Key. Renal mass biopsies. Accessed November 22, 2021. https://radiologykey.com/renal-mass-biopsy-2/

53. Keskin S, Güven S, Keskin Z, Özbiner H, Kerimoğlu Ü, Yeşildağ A. Strain elastography in the characterization of renal cell carcinoma and angiomyolipoma. *Can Urol Assoc J.* 2015;9(1–2):e67–e71. doi:10.5489/cuaj.2349. Accessed November 22, 2021. https://www.ncbi.nlm.nih.gov/pmc/articles/PMC4336040/

54. Gameraddin M. Ultrasound of the kidneys: application of doppler and elastography. In: Abdo Gamie SA, Mahmoud Foda E, eds. *Essentials of Abdominal Ultrasound. IntechOpen.* 2019. doi:10.5772/intechopen.85196. Accessed November 22, 2021. https://www.intechopen.com/chapters/66602

55. Ganeshan G, Iyer R, Devine C, et al. Imaging of primary and secondary renal lymphoma. *Am J Roentgenol.* 2013;201(5):W712–W719. Accessed August 1, 2021. https://www.ajronline.org/action/showCitFormats?doi=10.2214%2FAJR.13.10669

56. Lusaya DG, Lerma, EV. What is hydronephrosis and hydroureter? Accessed August 3, 2021. https://www.medscape.com/answers/436259-164717/what-is-hydronephrosis-and-hydroureter

57. Rishor-Olney CR, Hinson MR. Obstructive uropathy. In: *StatPearls [Internet]*. StatPearls Publishing; 2021. Updated July 7, 2021. Accessed August 3, 2021. https://www.ncbi.nlm.nih.gov/books/NBK558921/

58. Tamburrini S, Lugarà M, Iannuzzi M, et al. Pyonephrosis ultrasound and computed tomography features: a pictorial review. *Diagnostics*. 2021;11(2):331. doi:10.3390/diagnostics11020331. Accessed September 6, 2021.

59. Southgate SJ, Herbst MK. Ultrasound of the urinary tract. In: *StatPearls [Internet]*. StatPearls Publishing; 2021. Updated July 31, 2021. Accessed August 3, 2021. https://www.ncbi.nlm.nih.gov/books/NBK535381/

60. Khan SR, Pearle MS, Robertson WG, et al. Kidney stones. *Nat Rev Dis Primers*. 2016;2:16008. doi:10.1038/nrdp.2016.8. Accessed August 5, 2021. https://www.ncbi.nlm.nih.gov/pmc/articles/PMC5685519/

61. Schubbe M, Takacs E. Medical student curriculum: kidney stones. 2019. Accessed August 5, 2021. https://www.auanet.org/education/auauniversity/for-medical-students/medical-students-curriculum/medical-student-curriculum/kidney-stones

62. AMBOSS. Nephrolithiasis. Accessed August 5, 2021. https://www.amboss.com/us/knowledge/Nephrolithiasis/

63. Manzoor H, Saikali SW. Renal extracorporeal lithotripsy. In: *StatPearls [Internet]*. StatPearls Publishing; 2021. Updated July 31, 2021. Accessed August 5, 2021. https://www.ncbi.nlm.nih.gov/books/NBK560887/

64. McClain PD, Lange JN, Assimos DG. Optimizing shock wave lithotripsy: a comprehensive review. *Rev Urol*. 2013;15(2):49–60. Accessed August 5, 2021. https://www.ncbi.nlm.nih.gov/pmc/articles/PMC3784968/

65. Letafati M, Tarzamni MK, Hajalioghli P, Taheri SM, Vaseghi H, et al. Diagnostic accuracy of twinkling artifact sign seen in color Doppler ultrasonography in detecting microlithiasis of kidney. *Nephro-Urol Mon*. 2020;12(2):e102860. doi:10.5812/numonthly.102860. Accessed August 9, 2021. https://sites.kowsarpub.com/num/articles/102860.html

66. Dillman JR, Kappil M, Weadock WJ, et al. Sonographic twinkling artifact for renal calculus detection: correlation with CT. *Radiology*. 2011;259(3):911–916. Accessed August 9, 2021. https://pubs.rsna.org/doi/10.1148/radiol.11102128

67. Bacha R, Gilani SA, Manzoor I. Relation of color doppler twinkling artifact and scale or pulse repetition frequency. *J Med Ultrasound*. 2019;27:13–18. doi:10.4103/JMU.JMU_129_18. Accessed August 9, 2021. https://www.researchgate.net/publication/330852464_Relation_of_Color_Doppler_Twinkling_Artifact_and_Scale_or_Pulse_Repetition_Frequency

68. Hanafi MQ, Fakhrizadeh A, Jaafaezadeh E. An investigation into the clinical accuracy of twinkling artifacts in patients with urolithiasis smaller than 5 mm in comparison with computed tomography scanning. *J Family Med Prim Care*. 2019;8(2):401–406. doi:10.4103/jfmpc.jfmpc_300_18. Accessed August 9, 2021.

69. Rahmouni A, Bargoin R, Herment A, et al. Color doppler twinkling artifact in hyperechoic regions. *Radiology*. 1996; 199(1):269–271. doi: 10.1148/radiology.199.1.8633158

70. Sutijono D, Bomann JS, Moore CL, et al. Twinkle twinkle little stone: utilizing color Doppler in emergency ultrasound diagnosis of a ureterovesicular stone. *Crit Ultrasound J*. 2010;2:77–79. doi:10.1007/s13089-010-0039-y. Accessed August 9, 2021.

71. Shavit L, Jaeger P, Unwin RJ. What is nephrocalcinosis? *Kidney Int*. 2015;88(1):35–43. doi:10.1038/ki.2015.76. Accessed August 12, 2021. https://www.sciencedirect.com/science/article/pii/S2157161532151111

72. MedlinePlus. Nephrocalcinosis. Accessed August 12, 2021. https://emedicine.medscape.com/article/243911-overview

73. MedlinePlus. Nephrocalcinosis. Accessed August 12, 2021. https://medlineplus.gov/ency/article/000492.htm

74. National Center for Advancing Translational Sciences. Nephrocalcinosis. Accessed August 12, 2021. https://rarediseases.info.nih.gov/diseases/7177/nephrocalcinosis

75. Garfield K, Leslie SW. *Medullary sponge kidney*. In: *StatPearls [Internet]*. StatPearls Publishing; 2021. Updated Aug 12, 2021. Accessed August 14, 2021. https://www.ncbi.nlm.nih.gov/books/NBK470220/

76. Ghosh AK. Medullary sponge kidney. Accessed August 14, 2021. https://emedicine.medscape.com/article/242886-overview

77. National Order of Rare Disease. Medullary sponge kidney. Accessed August 14, 2021. https://rarediseases.org/rare-diseases/medullary-sponge-kidney/

78. Pisani I, Giacosa R, Giuliotti S, et al. Ultrasound to address medullary sponge kidney: a retrospective study. *BMC Nephrol*. 2020;21:430. doi:10.1186/s12882-020-02084-1. Accessed August 14, 2021.

79. Borofsky M. The diagnostic dilemma of medullary sponge kidney. Accessed August 14, 2021. https://kidneystones.uchicago.edu/the-diagnostic-dilemma-of-medullary-sponge-kidney/

80. Legome EL, Keim SM, Salomone JP, Udaeni J. Blunt abdominal trauma. Accessed August 17, 2021. https://emedicine.medscape.com/article/1980980-overview

81. Smith JK, Kenney PJ, Dheer AK, Lobera A. Imaging in kidney trauma. Accessed August 17, 2021. https://emedicine.medscape.com/article/379085-overview

82. CriticalCare Sonography. Trauma: right kidney laceration. Accessed August 17, 2021. https://www.criticalcare-sonography.com/2018/08/31/trauma-right-kidney-laceration/

83. Weerakkody, Y. Subcapsular perirenal hematoma. Accessed August 17, 2021. https://radiopaedia.org/articles/39804

84. Greco M, Butticè S, Benedetto F, et al. Spontaneous subcapsular renal hematoma: strange case in an anticoagulated patient with HWMH after aortic and iliac endovascular stenting procedure. *Case Rep Urol*. 2016;2016:2573476. doi:10.1155/2016/2573476. Accessed August 17, 2021.

85. Tuvell N, Sorrell K. Traumatic renal transplant subcapsular hematoma: diagnosis by duplex ultrasound. *J Vasc Ultrasound*. 2005;29(1):39–41. https://doi.org/10.1177/154431670502900106

86. Onur MR, Poyraz AK, Bozgeyik Z, Onur AR, Orhan I. Utility of semiquantitative strain elastography for differentiation between benign and malignant solid renal masses. *J Ultrasound Med* 2015;34:639–647. Accessed November 22, 2021. doi:10.7863/ultra.34.4.639

87. Barnard Health Care. Distinction between perirenal and subcapsular collections. *Dynamic Radiology*. Accessed August 19, 2021. https://www.barnardhealth.us/dynamic-radiology/distinction-between-perirenal-and-subcapsular-collections.html

88. Belyayeva M, Jeong JM. *Acute pyelonephritis*. In: *StatPearls [Internet]*. StatPearls Publishing; 2021. Updated July 10, 2021. Accessed August 24, 2021. https://www.ncbi.nlm.nih.gov/books/NBK519537/

89. Craig WD, Wagner BJ, Travis MD. Pyelonephritis: radiologic-pathologic review. *RadioGraphics*. 2008;28(1):255–276. Accessed August 24, 2021. https://pubs.rsna.org/doi/full/10.1148/rg.281075171

90. Fulop T. Acute pyelonephritis. Accessed August 24, 2021. https://emedicine.medscape.com/article/245559-overview

91. Shetty S. Emphysematous pyelonephritis (EPN). Accessed August 27, 2021. https://emedicine.medscape.com/article/2029011-overview

92. Gaillard, F., Morgan, M. Xanthogranulomatous pyelonephritis. Accessed August 30, 2021. https://radiopaedia.org/articles/9944

93. Jha SK, Aeddula NR. Pyelonephritis Xanthogranulomatous. In: *StatPearls [Internet]*. StatPearls Publishing; 2021. Updated July 6, 2021. Accessed August 30, 2021. https://www.ncbi.nlm.nih.gov/books/NBK557399/

94. Deem SG. Xanthogranulomatous pyelonephritis. Accessed August 30, 2021. https://emedicine.medscape.com/article/2050430-overview#a1

95. Lohr JW. Chronic pyelonephritis. Accessed September 1, 2021. https://emedicine.medscape.com/article/245464-overview

96. Manski D. Accessed September 1, 2021. http://urology-textbook.com/kidneys.html

97. Bass WR. Renal corticomedullary abscess. Accessed September 3, 2021. https://emedicine.medscape.com/article/440073-overview

98. Donaldson R. Renal abscess. Accessed September 3, 2021. https://wikem.org/wiki/Renal_abscess

99. Kim ED. Perinephric abscess. Accessed September 3, 2021. https://emedicine.medscape.com/article/439831-overview

100. Meyrier A. Renal and perinephric abscess. Accessed September 3, 2021. https://somepomed.org/articulos/contents/mobipreview.htm?30/5/30814?source=see_link#

101. Petersen AC. Pyonephrosis. Accessed September 6, 2021. https://emedicine.medscape.com/article/440548-overview

102. Cozman C, Smith S, Keoghane S. Pyonephrosis: is the kidney always doomed? *Urology News*. 2020;24(3). Accessed September 6, 2021. https://www.urologynews.uk/features/features/post/pyonephrosis-is-the-kidney-always-doomed

103. Faubel S, Patel NU, Lockhart ME, Cadnapaphornchai MA. Renal relevant radiology: use of ultrasonography in patients with AKI. *Clin J Am Soc Nephrol.* 2014;9(2):382–394. doi:10.2215/CJN.04840513. Accessed September 10, 2021. https://cjasn.asnjournals.org/content/9/2/382

104. Makris K, Spanou L. Acute kidney injury: definition, pathophysiology and clinical phenotypes. *Clin Biochem Rev.* 2016;37(2):85–98. Accessed September 10, 2021. https://www.ncbi.nlm.nih.gov/pmc/articles/PMC5198510/

105. Malkina A. Acute Kidney Injury (AKI). Accessed September 13, 2021. https://www.merckmanuals.com/professional/genitourinary-disorders/acute-kidney-injury/acute-kidney-injury-aki

106. Workeneh BT. Acute kidney injury. Accessed September 13, 2021. https://emedicine.medscape.com/article/243492-overview#a1

107. Mutnuri S. Acute tubular necrosis. Accessed September 13, 2021. https://emedicine.medscape.com/article/238064-overview#a1

108. Hanif MO, Bali A, Ramphul K. Acute renal tubular necrosis. In: *StatPearls [Internet].* StatPearls Publishing; 2021. Updated July 10, 2021. Accessed September 13, 2021. https://www.ncbi.nlm.nih.gov/books/NBK507815/

109. Wen Y, Yang C, Menez SP, et al. A systematic review of clinical characteristics and histologic descriptions of acute tubular injury. *Kidney Int Rep.* 2020;5(11):1993–2001. Accessed September 13, 2021. https://www.sciencedirect.com/science/article/pii/S2468024920315059

110. Salifu MO. HIV-associated nephropathy and other HIV-related renal disorders. Accessed September 13, 2021. https://emedicine.medscape.com/article/246031-overview#a1

111. Sivashankar M, Balagobi B, Perera ND, Ruvinda PGN. A case report of post-surgical page kidney due to extensive renal hematoma following percutaneous nephrolithotomy. *Int J Surg Case Rep.* 2021;86:106382. Accessed November 22, 2021. doi:10.1016/j.ijscr.2021.106382.

112. Sperati JC. Coronavirus: kidney damage caused by COVID-19. Accessed November 22, 2021. https://www.hopkinsmedicine.org/health/conditions-and-diseases/coronavirus/coronavirus-kidney-damage-caused-by-covid19

113. Legrand M, Bell S, Forni L, et al. Pathophysiology of COVID-19-associated acute kidney injury. *Nat Rev Nephrol.* 2021;17(11):751–764. doi:10.1038/s41581-021-00452-0. Accessed September 13, 2021.

114. Tancredi T, DeWaters A, McGillen KL. Renal ultrasound findings secondary to COVID-19 related collapsing focal segmental glomerulosclerosis—a case report. *Clin Imaging.* 2021;71:34–38. doi:10.1016/j.clinimag.2020.11.011. Accessed September 13, 2021. https://www.ncbi.nlm.nih.gov/pmc/articles/PMC7644181/

115. Workeneh, BT. What causes postrenal acute kidney injury (AKI)? Accessed September 13, 2021. https://www.medscape.com/answers/243492-167428/what-causes-postrenal-acute-kidney-injury-aki

116. National Kidney Foundation. Chronic Kidney Disease (CKD) Symptoms and causes. Accessed September 21, 2021. https://www.kidney.org/atoz/content/about-chronic-kidney-disease

117. Arora P. Chronic Kidney Disease (CKD). Accessed September 21, 2021. https://emedicine.medscape.com/article/238798-overview

118. Di Muzio, B, MacManus D. Chronic kidney disease. Accessed September 21, 2021. https://radiopaedia.org/articles/37533

119. Kanmaniraja D, Kurian J, Holder J, et al. Review of COVID-19, part 1: abdominal manifestations in adults and multisystem inflammatory syndrome in children. *Clin Imaging.* 2021;80:88–110. doi:10.1016/j.clinimag.2021.06.025. Accessed November 22, 2021. https://www.ncbi.nlm.nih.gov/pmc/articles/PMC8223038/

CHAPTER 13

The Lower Urinary Tract

CATHIE SCHOLL

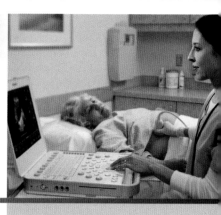

OBJECTIVES

- Describe the embryologic development, normal anatomy, and function of the lower urinary tract.
- Discuss the various sonographic techniques that can be used for evaluation of the lower urinary tract.
- Identify the normal sonographic appearance of the lower urinary tract and common anatomic variants.
- List clinical indications associated with lower urinary tract disease.
- Describe the sonographic appearance of congenital lower urinary tract abnormalities such as exstrophy, duplication, posterior urethral valves, ectopic ureter, and ureterocele.
- List the common causes and sonographic appearance of cystitis.
- Identify the sonographic appearance of reflux, neurogenic bladder, and bladder wall abnormalities.
- Describe common mechanisms for bladder trauma and the appearance of pathologies related to trauma.
- List common causes of bladder wall thickening.
- Describe the sonographic appearance of benign and malignant bladder tumors.
- Define stress incontinence and describe sonographic techniques used in the diagnosis.
- Identify technically satisfactory and unsatisfactory sonographic examinations of the lower urinary tract.

KEY TERMS

bladder flap hematoma

cystitis

diverticula

ectopic ureter

exstrophy

neurogenic bladder

posterior urethral valves

squamous cell carcinoma

transitional cell carcinoma

urachal cyst

ureterocele

vesicoureteral reflux

GLOSSARY

cystoscopy procedure in which a scope is used to evaluate the urethra, bladder, and pelvic ureters

hematuria presence of red blood cells in the urine; hematuria can be microscopic (not visible with the naked eye) or macroscopic

trabeculated bladder thickened, irregular bladder wall frequently seen in patients with long-standing obstruction or neurogenic bladder

voiding cystourethrogram (VCUG) a procedure used to evaluate for urinary reflux in which the patient is catheterized and the bladder is filled with a contrast agent; the bladder is examined under fluoroscopy to evaluate for vesicoureteral reflux both before and during patient voiding

The lower urinary tract consists of the pelvic ureters, bladder, and urethra. Whenever a reference is made to the urinary system, the kidneys come to mind first. The ureter, bladder, and urethra are also part of the urinary system and play important roles in transporting, storing, and eliminating urine. The pelvic ureter and urethra are conduits in the process of elimination of urine. The bladder is located anatomically between these two structures and functions as a reservoir for urine storage. The primary focus of this chapter is the urinary bladder. The normal pelvic ureter and the urethra are not usually seen sonographically, but these structures may be visualized with coexisting pathologic conditions.

The urine-filled bladder is one of the most accessible abdominopelvic organs for sonography examinations. Recognition of normal bladder anatomy, including its position, size, shape, and appearance, helps the sonographer identify congenital anomalies of the bladder, pathologies, and abnormalities in the surrounding anatomy.

ANATOMY AND ORGANOGENESIS

During early embryology of the human urogenital system, three sets of kidneys develop—the pronephros (early in the 4th embryologic week), mesonephros (late in the 4th week), and the metanephros (5th week)—in three successive waves, from cranial to caudal, with the third, most inferior pair of kidneys (metanephros) becoming the permanent kidneys.[1] The caudal end of the hindgut has a dilated chamber, the cloaca. The cloacal endoderm is in close contact with the surface ectoderm, and together, they form the cloacal membrane. An extension from the cloaca into the umbilical cord is the *allantois*. The intermediate mesoderm of the gastrula bulges into the dorsal aspect of the intraembryonic coelom as a urogenital ridge on each side. This further develops into two ridges: a medial genital (gonadal) ridge and a lateral nephrogenic ridge (or cord). A mesonephric (wolffian) duct and paramesonephric (müllerian) duct form in the nephrogenic ridge or cord.[1]

In approximately the 7th gestational week, the urorectal septum between the allantois and hindgut fuses with the cloacal membrane, dividing it into the ventral (anterior) urogenital sinus and a dorsal (posterior) rectum.[2] The upper part of the urogenital sinus is the fusiform bladder. The lower pelvic and phallic parts of the urogenital sinus form the urethra and related glands and structures in each sex. The wolffian ducts give rise to the ureters; they also form the efferent tubules, duct of the epididymis, vas deferens, seminal vesicles, and ejaculatory ducts in males and the epoophoron, paroophoron, and Gartner duct in females.

The ends of the mesonephric ducts (wolffian and müllerian) and the endodermal cloaca form the urinary bladder.[1] The cloaca—the terminal, caudal, blind-ended portion of the hindgut—is the major structure that forms the lower part of the urinary and genital tract. Its primary function is to serve as the primitive receptacle into which the reproductive and excretory tracts empty.

The metanephric duct (future ureter) develops from a ureteric bud growing from the caudal end of the mesonephric duct. In a short time, the metanephric duct shifts anteriorly and makes its own connection with the cloaca/urogenital sinus/bladder.

At the 8th week of gestation, all embryos have identical primordia in the indifferent stage of urogenital development, with gonads capable of developing into testes or ovaries. In males, the paramesonephric (müllerian) ducts degenerate. The mesonephric ducts become the ductus deferens, ejaculatory ducts, and seminal vesicles. The urogenital sinus develops into the urinary bladder, prostate gland, bulbourethral glands (Cowper gland), paraurethral glands, and prostatic, membranous, and penile (spongy) urethra.[1] In females, the mesonephric (wolffian) ducts degenerate, and the paramesonephric ducts develop into the uterine tubes, uterus, and upper part of the vagina. The urogenital sinus forms the bladder, urethra, greater vestibular and paraurethral glands, vestibule, and lower part of the vagina.[1]

Initially, the bladder is contiguous with the allantois, which eventually becomes a fibrous cord, the urachus (known as the median umbilical ligament in the adult).[3] The urachus extends from the apex of the bladder to the umbilicus. In infants and children, the urinary bladder is an abdominal organ until after puberty when it becomes a true pelvic structure.[3,4]

Urinary Bladder

The bladder develops into a hollow, smooth, musculomembranous, collapsible sac that acts as a reservoir for urine. The bladder is in the retroperitoneum on the pelvic floor just posterior to the pubic symphysis.[5] Its size, position, and relationship to other organs vary according to the amount of fluid it contains.[2] The urinary bladder is lined with a mucous membrane of transitional epithelium that allows for expansion. This mucous membrane lining contains rugae or folds. When the bladder is empty, the membrane appears folded or wrinkled.[5] The mucous membrane is loosely attached to the underlying muscle coat except at the trigone region, where it is firmly attached to the muscular coat, appears smooth, and does not expand during bladder filling.

The bladder is capable of considerable distention because of the lining's elasticity and rugae and the wall's elasticity.[5] It is uniquely situated in the pelvic cavity for its function of urine storage. Bladder capacity varies greatly and depends on many factors, including the age and physical condition of the patient. The normal adult bladder is generally moderately full at 500 mL (a pint) of urine, but it may hold nearly double that if necessary.[3,5]

Normally, the bladder is a round-edged tetrahedron with a superior, a posterior, and two inferior surfaces. The superior surface has two regions: the fundus, located posteriorly, and the apex, located anteriorly. The two ureteral orifices are located in the body on the posteroinferior portion. The urethral orifice is located in the neck of the bladder and is the most inferior region.[1]

When the bladder is empty, the anterior surface lies just behind and, rarely, superior to the symphysis in both males and females.[1] The fibrous medial umbilical ligament (obliterated urachus) extends from the apex upward as a blunt cone with a solid, slender continuation in the midline of the abdominal wall and attaches to the umbilicus.[1]

Related anatomy in the pelvis varies depending on the quantity of urine and with the condition of the rectum, being pushed upward and forward when the rectum is distended.[1]

When distended with urine, the bladder can rise approximately 16 cm above the symphysis pubis. The bladder ascends into the abdominal cavity and meets with the lower anterior abdominal wall. When fully distended, it can be readily palpated or percussed. As the bladder enlarges, it loses its ovoid or spherical configuration and becomes more globular. Coils of the small intestine lie adjacent to the upper surface of the bladder and are displaced posteriorly as the bladder enlarges. With overdistention, such as acute or chronic urinary retention, the lower abdomen may visibly bulge.

When the bladder is relatively empty in the female, the fundal region of the bladder lies in contact with the anterior wall of the vagina and cervix (Fig. 13-1A). The uterus and vagina are interposed between the bladder and the rectum.[3] When the bladder is empty, the uterus rests on the bladder's superior surface. Female reproductive and pelvic muscular anatomy is greatly enhanced using the traditional full-bladder technique.

In the male, the fundus and the body of the bladder are related to the rectum, separated above by the rectovesical pouch of the peritoneum and inferolaterally on each side by a ductus deferens and seminal vesicle.[3] The prostate is a fibromuscular and glandular organ that lies just inferior to the bladder.[3] The base of the prostate is applied to the caudal surface of the bladder. The greater part of this surface is directly continuous with the bladder wall. The normal prostate encircles the prostatic urethra and prostate gland secretion enters the prostatic urethra via several ducts. The seminal vesicles lie just cephalad to the prostate under the base of the bladder. They are approximately 6 cm long and quite soft. Each vesicle joins its corresponding vas deferens to form the ejaculatory duct (Fig. 13-1B, C).

Trigone

On the floor of the bladder, a triangular region, the trigone, has no rugae and is firmly attached to the muscular coat.[6] The trigone is outlined by the three openings in the bladder: two from the ureters and one into the urethra (Figs. 13-1C and 13-2). The ureteral orifices are situated superiorly and laterally at the extremities of the crescent-shaped interureteric ridge that forms the proximal border of the trigone.[1] The urethral opening is located at its anterior, midline, lower corner at the bladder neck.

Ureters

The ureters are slender tubes that convey urine from the kidneys to the bladder.[6] Each ureter is a continuation of the renal pelvis. From there, they descend in the retroperitoneum and run obliquely through the posterior bladder wall. The average length of the ureter is 30 cm and the diameter is 6 mm.[6] The ureters are constricted in three places: (1) at the ureteropelvic junction, (2) as they cross the iliac vessels, and (3) at the junction with the bladder.

The distal ureter enters obliquely through the bladder wall by slit-like openings. This anatomic arrangement prevents the backflow of urine. As the bladder fills, the pressure increases, causing the upper and lower walls of the terminal portions of the ureter to become closely applied to each other, acting as valves to prevent regurgitation of urine from the bladder. When the bladder is distended, the openings of the ureters are about 5 cm apart; however, the distance between them is diminished by half when the bladder is empty and contracted.

Urethra

The *urethra* is a thin-walled fibromuscular tube that drains urine from the bladder and conveys it outside the body. The urethra represents the terminal portion of the urinary tract. At the bladder–urethral junction, a thickening of the detrusor smooth muscle of the bladder wall forms the *internal urethral sphincter*. This involuntary muscle keeps the urethra closed and prevents leaking between voiding. The sphincter is unique in that contraction opens it and relaxation closes it. The *external urethral sphincter* surrounds the urethra as it passes through the urogenital diaphragm. This sphincter is formed of skeletal muscle and is controlled voluntarily.[5,6]

The length and functions of the urethra differ in males and females. The female urethra is 3 to 4 cm long and functions only to convey urine from the body.[5] It lies directly posterior to the symphysis pubis and anterior to the vagina. The *external urethral orifice*—the external opening of the urethra—lies anterior to the vaginal opening and posterior to the clitoris. The opening of the urethra to the exterior is referred to as the *urinary meatus*.

The male urethra serves a double function: a conduit for eliminating urine and also as the terminal portion of the reproductive system serving as the passage for ejaculate (semen). The male urethra is approximately 20 cm long and has three regions. The *prostatic urethra*, about 2.5 cm long, runs within the prostate.[5] The *membranous urethra*, which runs through the urogenital sinus, extends about 2 cm from the prostate to the beginning of the penis. The *spongy urethra* passes through the penis and opens at its tip—the external urethral orifice.

PHYSIOLOGY

The mechanism for voiding urine (micturition) starts with involuntary and voluntary nerve impulses.[5] Even though the bladder has a greater capacity, when the volume of urine exceeds 200 to 400 mL, stretch receptors trigger transmission of impulses to the lower portion of the spinal cord, initiating the conscious desire to expel urine and a subconscious reflex, the micturition reflex.[7] The combination of voluntary relaxation of the external sphincter muscle of the bladder, reflex contraction of linear smooth muscle fibers along the urethra, and then contraction of the detrusor muscle squeezes urine out of the bladder.[5] Parasympathetic fibers transmit the impulses that cause contractions of the bladder and relaxation of the internal sphincter.[5,7,8]

Because the external sphincter is under voluntary control, we can choose to postpone bladder emptying. Voluntary contraction of the external sphincter to prevent or terminate micturition is learned and is possible only if the nerves supplying the bladder and urethra—the projection tracts of the cord and brain—and the motor area of the cerebrum are all intact.[7,8] Incontinence—involuntary emptying of the bladder—results from aging or trauma to any of these parts of the nervous system by cerebral hemorrhage or cord injury.[5–7]

Retention is an inability to empty the bladder even though the bladder contains an excessive amount of urine.[9] Catheterization may be used to relieve the discomfort accompanying

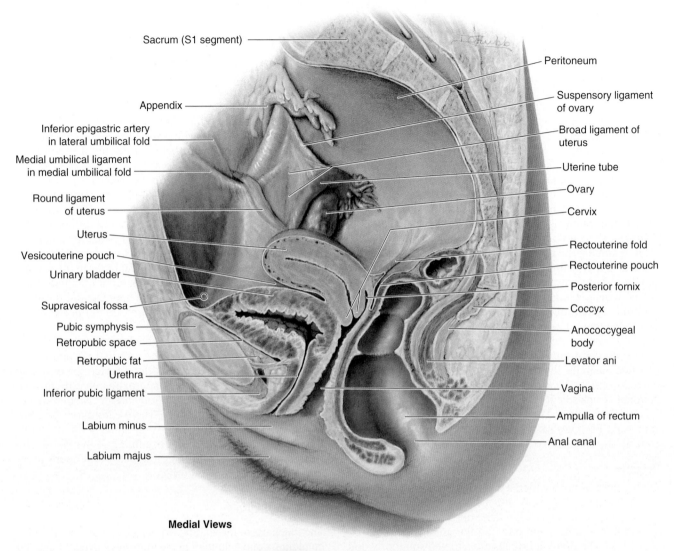

Sacrum (S1 segment)

Appendix

Inferior epigastric artery
in lateral umbilical fold

Medial umbilical ligament
in medial umbilical fold

Round ligament
of uterus

Uterus

Vesicouterine pouch

Urinary bladder

Supravesical fossa

Pubic symphysis

Retropubic space

Retropubic fat

Urethra

Inferior pubic ligament

Labium minus

Labium majus

Peritoneum

Suspensory ligament
of ovary

Broad ligament of
uterus

Uterine tube

Ovary

Cervix

Rectouterine fold

Rectouterine pouch

Posterior fornix

Coccyx

Anococcygeal
body

Levator ani

Vagina

Ampulla of rectum

Anal canal

Medial Views

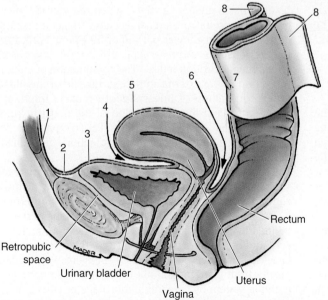

A

Retropubic
space

Urinary bladder

Vagina

Uterus

Rectum

Female:

Peritoneum passes:

- From the anterior abdominal wall (1)
- Superior to the pubic bone (2)
- On the superior surface of the urinary bladder (3)
- From the bladder to the uterus, forming the vesicouterine pouch (4)
- On the fundus and body of the uterus, posterior formix, and all of the vagina (5)
- Between the rectum and uterus, forming the rectouterine pouch (6)
- On the anterior and lateral sides of the rectum (7)
- Posteriorly to become the sigmoid mesocolon (8)

FIGURE 13-1 Normal anatomy. Coronal planes of the (**A**) female and (**B**) male pelvis show the normal anatomic relationship of the bladder with surrounding structures.

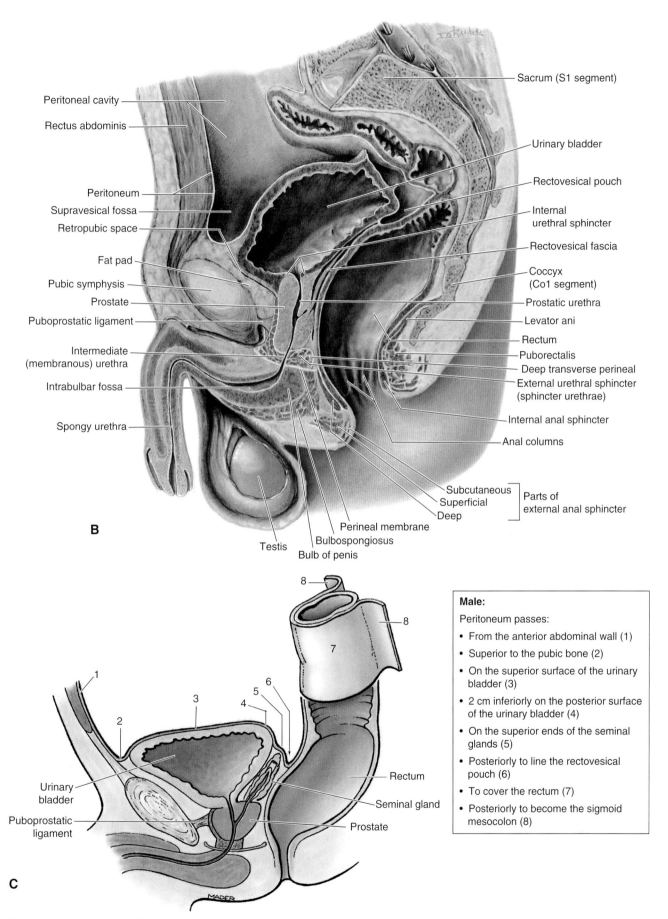

B

Peritoneal cavity
Rectus abdominis
Peritoneum
Supravesical fossa
Retropubic space
Fat pad
Pubic symphysis
Prostate
Puboprostatic ligament
Intermediate (membranous) urethra
Intrabulbar fossa
Spongy urethra

Sacrum (S1 segment)
Urinary bladder
Rectovesical pouch
Internal urethral sphincter
Rectovesical fascia
Coccyx (Co1 segment)
Prostatic urethra
Levator ani
Rectum
Puborectalis
Deep transverse perineal
External urethral sphincter (sphincter urethrae)
Internal anal sphincter
Anal columns

Subcutaneous
Superficial } Parts of external anal sphincter
Deep

Perineal membrane
Bulbospongiosus
Testis
Bulb of penis

C

Male:

Peritoneum passes:

• From the anterior abdominal wall (1)
• Superior to the pubic bone (2)
• On the superior surface of the urinary bladder (3)
• 2 cm inferiorly on the posterior surface of the urinary bladder (4)
• On the superior ends of the seminal glands (5)
• Posteriorly to line the rectovesical pouch (6)
• To cover the rectum (7)
• Posteriorly to become the sigmoid mesocolon (8)

Urinary bladder
Puboprostatic ligament
Rectum
Seminal gland
Prostate

FIGURE 13-1 (*continued*) **C:** This illustration shows the interior cutaway sections of the male urinary bladder and the prostatic urethra and a topographic anatomy of the male pelvic organs.

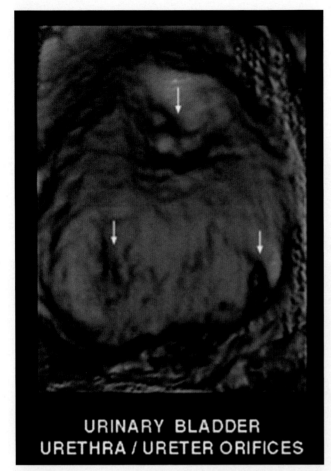

URINARY BLADDER
URETHRA / URETER ORIFICES

FIGURE 13-2 Trigone. Three-dimensional rendered image of the bladder trigone demonstrating ureteral and urethral openings (*arrows*). The three-dimensional rendered image of the inner bladder lining provides a virtual cystogram of the bladder wall. (Image courtesy of Philips Medical Systems, Bothell, WA.)

retention. 30% of patients who are catheterized routinely eventually develop a "ledge" posteriorly at the bladder neck from catheter trauma. The ledge makes voiding difficult and considerably complicates the catheterization process.

SONOGRAPHIC EXAMINATION TECHNIQUE

Patient Preparation

To visualize the bladder with the transabdominal approach, it is important that the patient prepares properly. Bladder distention is essential for optimal visualization of the bladder, bladder wall, and related anatomy. Filling the bladder can be accomplished by three methods: (1) instructing the patient to drink 16 oz of water 1 hour before the examination and not to void until the examination is completed; (2) instructing the patient not to void before the examination; or (3) catheterizing the patient and instilling fluid into the bladder through a Foley catheter. Foley catheters are not inserted routinely to fill a bladder unless it is a medical emergency. There have been many studies showing that catheter insertion may introduce infectious contaminants into the body. A Foley catheter balloon will appear as a

round cystic structure in the filled bladder and may cast shadows in areas of interest.

A fully distended bladder serves as a cystic reference in the abdominopelvic anatomy, pushes adjacent bowel and gas out of the field of view, and provides a sonographic "window" to identify pelvic anatomy. Routinely in males, the bladder, seminal vesicles, prostate, and rectum are imaged. Routinely in females, the vagina, bladder, uterus, ovaries, adnexa, and rectum are imaged. A full bladder also facilitates identification of dilated ureters. It is not necessary to restrict the diet or use catheters or enemas to reduce intestinal contents or air. Disease processes in pelvic structures can involve or mimic those of other closely related anatomy. Knowledge of pelvic anatomy, including the genitourinary tract, gastrointestinal tract, and pelvic vasculature and musculature is important.

A suitable coupling agent such as ultrasonic gel is used on the skin surface. Transducer selection should take into consideration body habitus and examination objectives. The highest-frequency transducer possible should be selected for scanning, making sure that penetration is adequate to visualize the posterior aspect of the areas of interest.

Scanning Techniques

The most widely used approach to scan the urinary bladder is the transabdominal method.[3] The patient is usually examined in the supine position. Sometimes, it is necessary to position the patient obliquely or to roll the patient into a lateral decubitus position to better demonstrate bladder wall abnormalities, the movement of debris or stones to the dependent bladder wall, or bladder tumors. The endovaginal, endorectal, and transperineal methods may also be used to a lesser extent.

The lower urinary tract should be scanned in both longitudinal and transverse planes transabdominally and may be scanned in longitudinal and coronal planes endovaginally and transperineally.[3] Using the endorectal approach, the proximal urethra can be visualized and the distal urethra is identified during penile artery evaluation.[4] Recent studies have also used translabial and transperineal approaches to evaluate female urethra and urogenital disorders such as stress incontinence.

The normal distended urinary bladder appears as an anechoic structure with visible demarcation of the echogenic smooth bladder walls.[3] The bladder wall is seen as a smooth echogenic interface and should be of uniform thickness. The thickness of the bladder wall will vary from less than 3 mm when fully distended to 5 mm when nearly empty.[3,4,10,11] A pathologically thickened bladder wall is better visualized when the bladder is fully distended.[4] If larger than 6 mm when empty or partially distended, the bladder wall should be interrogated for a pathologic process. When the bladder is scanned transabdominally, reverberation echoes are often seen anteriorly in the near field of the bladder image.[4,11] Many times, artifacts such as reverberations, grating lobes, and shadowing can be eliminated by sonography system controls and/or altering the transducer position to change the angle of the transmitted sound wave to avoid refraction from abdominal musculature[4] (Fig. 13-3A). Equipment manufacturers have added harmonics, speckle reduction, spatial compounding, and other computerized techniques

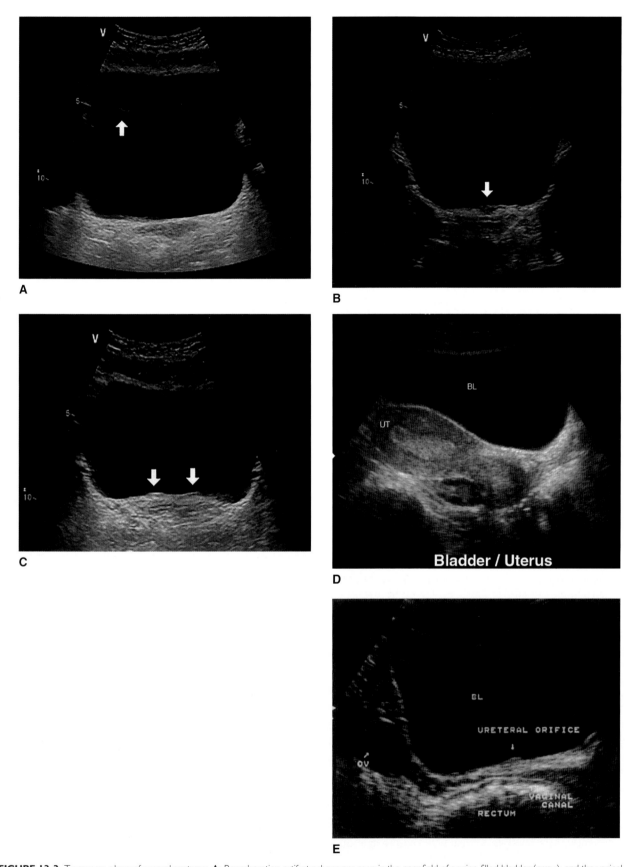

FIGURE 13-3 Transverse plane of normal anatomy. **A:** Reverberation artifact echoes are seen in the near field of a urine-filled bladder (*arrow*), and the vaginal canal is identified posterior to the bladder. **B:** The urethral orifice can be identified exiting the trigone (*arrow*). **C:** The ureteral orifices are seen as small mucosal elevations (*arrows*) as they enter the bladder. **D** and **E:** Longitudinal plane of normal anatomy. **D:** On the left, near the midline, the left ureteral orifice is seen entering the trigone. **E:** The right ureteral orifice is seen entering the trigone. *BL*, urinary bladder; *OV*, ovary; *UT*, uterus. (**E:** Image courtesy of Steven D. Hatch, Logan, UT.)

to aid in the elimination of artifact echoes. Although the normal ureters and urethra are not routinely visualized on transabdominal sonography, their location should be examined because they can be identified in some anomalies, diseases, and pathologic processes.

In females, the pelvic segment of the ureters and urethra can be evaluated with transvaginal sonography. The distal ureter can be identified by imaging in a longitudinal scan plane and moving laterally to the pelvic side wall.[12] The ureters appear as long tubular hypoechoic structures extending from the lateral aspect of the bladder base to the common iliac vessels.[13]

If the ureters are not readily seen in the sagittal scan plane, the transverse plane should be used to identify the urethral orifice. Then the probe should be slowly moved upward (anterior) to visualize the ureteral orifices near the lateral portion of the trigone.[13] Once the orifices have been identified, the transducer should be rotated to the longitudinal scan plane to lengthen out the distal ureters.

Owing to the proximity of the pelvic segments of the ureters to the common iliac vessels, color Doppler imaging may need to be used to differentiate the structures. When color Doppler imaging is applied, a ureter will not demonstrate color flow, whereas normal vessels should fill with color.

The sonographer should identify the predictable contours of the urine-filled bladder and the smooth echogenic bladder wall. If the patient has never had bladder or pelvic surgery, any deviation from the normal bladder shape, especially asymmetry, should be considered abnormal and a thorough investigation should be performed of the site of the distortion to rule out a mass. On transverse sections, the bladder should appear symmetric. Superiorly, the bladder appears rounded, but in scanning more inferiorly, it appears square owing to the parallel walls of the acetabulum (Fig.13-3B, C). On longitudinal sections, the bladder appears almost triangular, with the base of the triangle parallel with the anterior abdominal wall. In both longitudinal and transverse scans, the lateral walls appear straight or slightly indented by prominent iliopsoas muscles (Fig. 13-3D, E). As different pelvic structures are encountered, it may be necessary to angle the transducer caudad and cephalad and medial to lateral. The symphysis pubis acts as a point of reference on the body surface, where the transducer can be rocked superiorly and inferiorly on longitudinal scans to better view the superior and inferior aspects of the bladder. Transverse imaging must include tilting or a cross-plane imaging by angling the transducer from side to side while continuing to use the fluid in the bladder as a window. This produces a sharper image of the bladder wall and gives a complete sweep to interrogate the entire bladder. Longitudinal and transverse images are more easily interpreted if they are in a sequential order: right to left in the longitudinal plane with the midline image identified and inferior to superior in the transverse plane. Correct labeling must appear on all sonographic images, indicating the location of the scan, patient position, and scanning plane.

Frequently, it is possible to visualize the prostate and seminal vesicles in males using the transabdominal approach. When the transducer is angled caudad under the symphysis pubis, the prostate is seen posteroinferior to the bladder. On a longitudinal scan, the prostate appears as a heterogeneous structure at the most inferior aspect of the bladder.

On a transverse image, it appears rounded. Although newer transducers with better penetration and resolution enable sonographers to identify the prostate transabdominally in the adult male, the best way to visualize the prostate is via the endorectal approach (see Chapter 14). The seminal vesicles are seen as two small, oval, hypoechoic structures posterior to the bladder and superior to the prostate (Fig. 13-4A, B).

In patients who are catheterized, the catheter has an anechoic appearance with an echogenic margin and center. If air was used to secure the catheter's position, it may cause a shadow artifact. Sonographically, the symmetry of the catheter is identifiable as an echogenic incomplete circular structure in a urine-filled bladder (Fig. 13-5).

Routine bursts of echoes—the ureteral jet phenomenon—are seen entering the bladder from the region of the trigone.[1,3] At intervals of 5 to 20 seconds, a jet of low-intensity echoes, which lasts a few seconds, starts at the area of the ureteral orifices and flows toward the center of the bladder. Ureteral jets can occur simultaneously, but more commonly, they are separated (Fig. 13-6). Jets can be individually identified

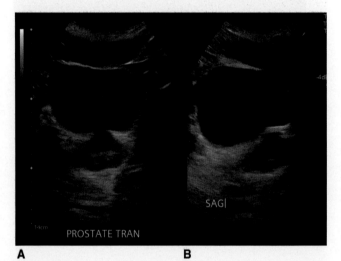

A   **B**

FIGURE 13-4 Normal male anatomy. **A:** In the transverse scan plane, the prostate is posterior to the bladder. **B:** In the sagittal scan plane, the prostate is inferior to the bladder. (Images courtesy of Susan R. Stephenson.)

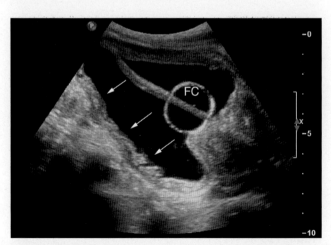

FIGURE 13-5 Foley catheter (*FC*). Longitudinal image of the urinary bladder; a *FC* can be identified within the bladder lumen. The catheter appears to be anechoic, with an echogenic exterior. Note the thickened bladder wall (*arrows*). (Image courtesy of Philips Medical Systems, Bothell, WA.)

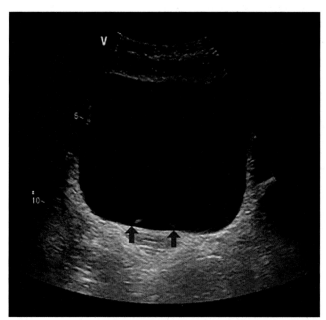

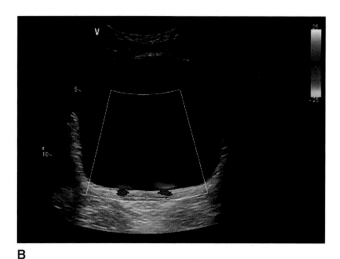

FIGURE 13-6 Transverse planes of normal ureteral jets. **A:** Simultaneous jets of low-intensity echoes (*arrows*) are visualized entering the urinary bladder. **B:** Color Doppler image demonstrates both right and left ureteral jets on the transverse image on a female patient.

on longitudinal images, but both may be seen simultaneously on a transverse image. Such jets extend up to 3 cm and broaden. After a few seconds, the low-intensity echoes become distributed in the bladder and lose intensity until they can no longer be distinguished. Color Doppler imaging is more sensitive and aids in demonstrating ureteral jets.[3] Although evaluation of ureteral jets with color Doppler imaging it cannot predict reflux, the analysis of ureteral jets with color Doppler imaging has been used successfully to determine the degree of ureteral obstruction with unilateral ureteral calculi, with either no detectable ureteral jets or continuous low-level jets on the symptomatic side.[4] In the case of bladder diverticulum, there is evidence of reversed flow of urine through the communication between the diverticulum and bladder when slight pressure is applied to the lower abdomen.

If either of the ureters is dilated, the dilated ureter can be visualized as a round, anechoic structure posterior to the bladder in the transverse plane. In the longitudinal plane, the dilated ureter can be visualized as a long, linear structure, usually posterior and to the right or left of the midline.

Bladder volume can be calculated using the formula for an ellipsoid (transverse × anteroposterior [AP] × length × 0.52).[3] The scanning equipment usually has computerized techniques to calculate volumes. The systems will calculate bladder volume once the three measurements have been entered. Bladder capacity should be noted. The capacity decreases in association with large pelvic masses, in urinary and pelvic inflammatory disease, prostatic hypertrophy, in patients receiving radiation therapy, in advanced stages of tumor infiltration, and after recent surgery.

Frequently, a postvoid residual volume calculation is also indicated.[3] To document the presence of residual urine and calculate its volume, the patient should be asked to empty the bladder. The longitudinal, AP, and transverse measurements are repeated, and another bladder volume is calculated

for comparison. Determining the amount of residual urine in patients with suspected bladder outlet obstruction has improved the treatment of these patients. Residual volume increases with age, atonic bladders, bladder neck obstruction, long-term cystitis, and advanced invasion by cancer.

The sonographer should be sure to recheck related pelvic anatomy on postvoid images. What might have appeared as a bladder might not change size postvoid, indicating an obstruction or a cystic pelvic tumor not necessarily related to the urinary system.

Three-dimensional (3D) and four-dimensional (4D) sonography has offered a whole new dimension to sonographic imaging. Obstetric and gynecologic 3D and 4D imaging are accepted as routine in the evaluation of fetal and gynecologic anatomy and pathologies. In recent years, the benefits of 3D/4D imaging of the lower urinary tract have been studied. 3D sonography has some advantages over two-dimensional (2D) imaging. An entire volume of data is stored, allowing for manipulation of the data set after the patient has left the examination room and reconstruction of images in all three scan planes. A rendered image of the interior bladder wall can provide a virtual sonographic cystoscopy examination[14] (Fig. 13-7). 3D bladder volume measurements can be obtained using a 3D technique called *virtual organ computer-aided analysis*, which also creates a 3D model of the organ.[15]

Endoluminal sonography is another imaging technique that is being investigated and is improving with revolutionary transducer technology. Initial studies using endoluminal sonography are limited by the use of high-frequency transducer (20 MHz), which allows penetration of only a few centimeters.[16] Although greater penetration is required for the upper urinary tract, the endoluminal transducer may be ideal for examining the urethra, bladder, and pelvic ureters, as researchers develop new technology for transducer construction and may find intraoperative techniques advantageous.

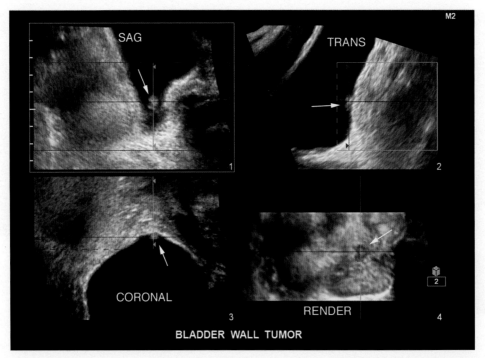

FIGURE 13-7 Three-dimensional imaging. Multiplanar reconstruction of the bladder demonstrates a small bladder tumor (*arrow*) seen simultaneously in the sagittal, transverse, and coronal planes in addition to a rendered image of the bladder lining. The intersecting lines on each image represent the same anatomic location in all three planes.

ABNORMALITIES OF THE LOWER URINARY TRACT

Duplication

Duplication of the urinary bladder is divided into three types: a peritoneal fold, which may be complete or incomplete; a septum dividing the bladder either sagittally or coronally; and a transverse band of muscle dividing the bladder into two unequal cavities.[1,4] Complete duplication of the urinary bladder is rare. One must be aware that complications may arise from variations of this anomaly. Unilateral reflux, obstruction, or infection may occur secondary to stenosis or atresia of the urethra.

Duplication of the ureters results when the embryonic ureteric bud branches prematurely and leads to partial division and separation of the related blastema.[1] Incomplete duplication includes a bifurcation of the ureter at or near the renal pelvis that unites at a variable distance between the kidney and bladder and enters the bladder as a single ureter in the normal bladder trigone.[1] Duplication is complete when there are two separate renal collecting systems and two separate ureters. The ureter from the lower renal pelvis migrates and enters the bladder in the normal ureteral orifice in the bladder trigone. The ureter from the upper pole of the kidney inserts into the bladder caudad to the ureter from the lower pole. In females, the more caudad ureter may drain ectopically into the trigone, perineum, uterus, vagina, or urethra; in males, the distal insertion can occur in the trigone, urethra, or seminal vesicles.[1,4] Duplications may be unilateral or bilateral and are more common in females than in males.

An accessory or duplicate urethra is an uncommon malformation that occurs almost exclusively in males. True duplication is associated with duplication of the bladder and usually of the genitalia.

Bladder Agenesis

An absent bladder is a rare anomaly. Most infants with bladder agenesis are stillborn, and almost all surviving infants are female.[4] During an obstetric scan, it is important to allow adequate time for the bladder to fill and empty. In cases of renal agenesis—a lethal anomaly—the bladder is not identified during an obstetric scan.

Diverticula

Diverticula of the bladder are pouch-like eversions of the wall. Bladder diverticula are produced by mucosal herniation through defects in the muscle wall arising as congenital defects or acquired lesions, usually associated with diseases resulting in bladder outlet obstruction or neurogenic conditions resulting in abnormalities in bladder function with chronically raised intravesical pressure.[3,17] One frequent form is the paraurethral (Hutch) diverticulum, which forms because the ureter is inserted at an inherently weak point in the bladder wall.[17]

Bladder diverticula are demonstrated sonographically as urine-filled outpouchings.[4,17] Careful scanning may show narrow communication between the diverticulum and the bladder, which leads to the diagnosis (Fig. 13-8A–E). Intradiverticular tumors or stones may also be identified. Because diverticula may not empty and, occasionally, actually increase in size with voiding, postvoid scans can demonstrate urine-filled diverticula.[4] Very large diverticula may be mistaken for the bladder itself, duplication of the bladder, or seminal

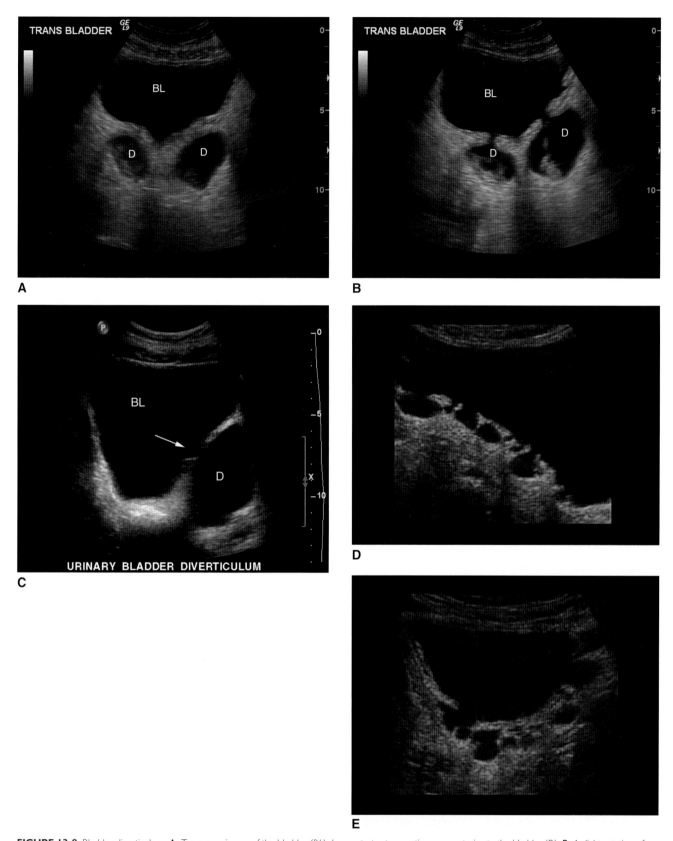

FIGURE 13-8 Bladder diverticulum. **A:** Transverse image of the bladder (*BL*) demonstrates two cystic areas posterior to the bladder (*D*). **B:** A slight rotation of the transducer reveals a connection between the cystic areas and the bladder consistent with bladder diverticula. Note the debris within the diverticula that could indicate infection. **C:** Longitudinal image of the urinary bladder shows a large diverticulum. Note the connection between the bladder and the diverticulum (*arrow*). **D:** Sagittal image of the bladder demonstrates multiple small diverticula. **E:** Transverse image of the same bladder with multiple small diverticula. (**D** and **E:** Image source: UltraSoundCases.info, the Copyright ownership: SonoSkills, the Netherlands.)

vesicle or ovarian cysts.[4] Color Doppler imaging provides a cost-benefit, rapid, and noninvasive examination for differentiating bladder diverticula from other cystic masses and fluid collections by evaluating ureteral jets. With color Doppler sonography, the diverticulum is demonstrated as a jet with alternating bidirectional flow between the bladder and the anechoic cystic diverticulum (Table 13-1).

Spontaneous rupture of bladder diverticulum is rare. Without immediate diagnosis, the condition may be mistaken for acute renal failure. Misdiagnosis and mistreatment can be fatal. Transabdominal sonography after injection of saline and air demonstrates extravasation, identifies the injury site, and is more specific than computed tomography (CT) or radiographic cystography.

Transperineal and transvaginal scanning is very effective in identifying urethral diverticula in women. The normal urethra can be routinely identified on transvaginal or transperineal scans as a hypoechoic linear structure exiting from the base of the bladder and traveling inferior to the symphysis pubis.[11] The hypoechoic to anechoic appearance of the urethral wall muscles is caused by their parallel orientation to the ultrasound beam using these techniques. Variable echogenicity depending on the relative orientation of the transducer and the structure being scanned is called *anisotropy*. Remember this whenever scanning using these techniques of the urethra so that the resulting image is not confused with anechoic urine in the urethra. Urethral diverticula appear as simple or complex collections of fluid intimately related to the urethra. These may involve both lateral aspects of the urethra or wrap around the urethra. They can contain stones or cancer. These may be differentiated from periurethral abscesses with the use of power Doppler imaging. The abscess is not vascular but, there is hypervascularity around the abscess. Clinical history is also important in the differential diagnosis if the patient is febrile.

Posterior Urethral Valves

The most common of bladder outlet obstructions results from the development of abnormal valves in the posterior urethra. The prostatic urethra is markedly dilated because of an obstruction at or just below the *verumontanum* (an elevation on the floor of the prostatic portion of the urethra where the seminal ducts enter). A posterior urethral valve usually consists of a mucosal flap originating from the verumontanum. Posterior urethral valve syndrome is the most common cause of urinary obstruction in male infants.[4] Almost 75% are discovered during the first year of life. They may present in older children but rarely occur in adults. Approximately 40% of patients have associated vesicoureteral reflux, which is usually caused by a periureteral diverticulum.[14]

The sonographic recognition of a dilated and elongated prostatic urethra helps differentiate posterior urethral valves from neurogenic bladder dysfunction. Also, with posterior urethral valves, the bladder wall appears thickened; hydroureters with dilation of the upper urinary tract may be seen (Table 13-1).

Other causes of bladder outlet obstruction include agenesis of the urethra, congenital urethral strictures, urethral tumors, and anterior urethral valves, all of which are rare.[18,19] Thickening of the bladder wall can also occur with cystitis.

Anterior urethral obstruction in males is uncommon but may be secondary to strictures, diverticula, or urethral duplication. Urethral obstruction in females is rare but may be seen in cloacal or female intersex anomalies.[19]

Exstrophy

Exstrophy of the bladder is a complete ventral defect of the urogenital sinus and the overlying skeletal system. It is frequently associated with other congenital anomalies.[20] Classically, exstrophy of the bladder represents eversion of the viscus through a defect in the anterior abdominal wall associated with separation of the pubic symphysis.[19,20] The mucosal edges of the bladder and distal ends of the ureters fuse with the skin protruding through the lower central abdominal wall, which has failed to close. Urine spurts onto the abdominal wall from the ureteral orifices. The diagnosis can be made prenatally when no bladder is visualized, a lower abdominal bulge (representing the bladder) is located and widening of the iliac crests is identified.[20]

TABLE 13-1   Bladder Abnormalities

Abnormality	Sonographic Appearance
Diverticula	Round, well-defined, thin-walled, fluid-filled masses with acoustic enhancement; variable in size. Color Doppler image demonstrates bidirectional flow between bladder and cystic diverticulum.
Posterior urethral valve	Dilated, elongated prostatic urethra (peculiar to males); subsequently, thickened bladder wall, hydroureters, or dilated upper urinary tract may develop.
Exstrophy	Eversion through anterior abdominal wall; other findings include hydronephrosis caused by ureterovesical obstruction.
Bladder neck contracture	Secondary abnormalities include vesicoureteral reflux, vesical diverticula, and large-capacity bladder.
Ectopic ureter	More common for ureter to arise from the upper moiety of a duplex kidney; 10%–20% arise from a solitary renal pelvis; may be massively dilated; may mimic multiseptate, cystic abdominal masses.
Ectopic ureterocele	Anechoic, cyst-like, thin-walled mass of variable size and shape projecting into the bladder (sometimes described as a cyst within a cyst).
Persistent urachus	Anechoic mass or diverticular outpouching between dome of the bladder and the umbilicus; cyst formation occurs if the ends seal off; adenocarcinoma or calculi may occur in a urachal cyst.

Contracture of the Bladder Neck

Narrowing of the bladder neck is a common cause of vesicoureteral reflux, vesical diverticula, large bladder capacity, and the syndrome of irritable bladder associated with enuresis. This contracture has been considered a rare phenomenon. In females, the obstruction is caused by spasm of the periurethral striated muscle, which develops secondary to distal urethral stenosis.[1]

Ectopic Ureter

The ureteric buds originate from the mesonephric duct instead of the cloaca, and this is often the embryologic basis for an ectopic insertion of the distal ureter in pelvic organs. In both sexes, the mesonephric duct migrates to a lower position on the urogenital sinus before it becomes the vas deferens in the male and disappears in the female. The ureters can be carried with it to open in ectopic locations. An ectopic ureter does not insert near the posterolateral angle of a normal trigone. Most ectopic ureters arise from the superior pelvis (upper moiety) of a duplex kidney and typically insert lower and more medially toward the base

of the bladder.[11] In males, ectopic ureters may also insert in the seminal vesicle, vas deferens, or ejaculatory duct. In females, they may insert in the bladder neck, urethra, vestibule, vagina, or uterus[1,4] (Table 13-1).

Ureterocele

The *ureterocele* is a cyst-like enlargement of the lower end of the ureter[17] (Fig.13-9A). Problems arise because (1) the ureteral opening in the wall of the sac is stenotic and, therefore, hydroureter, hydronephrosis, and infection proximal to the ureterocele are common and (2) the ureterocele sac itself may obstruct the bladder outlet or even prolapse through the urethra. An ectopic ureterocele is formed when the ectopic ureter is obstructed in the area where it enters the bladder, causing its anterior wall to balloon into the bladder.

Sonographic diagnosis of ectopic ureters and ectopic ureteroceles must include complete scanning of the kidneys. The duplex kidney may demonstrate two ureters arising from within, although frequently, they are difficult to distinguish. The ectopic ureter may be massively dilated and tortuous in the distal portion and mildly dilated proximally. Many variations have been reported.[1] These extremely large

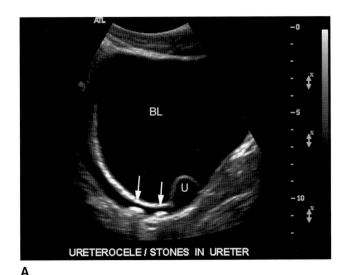

A

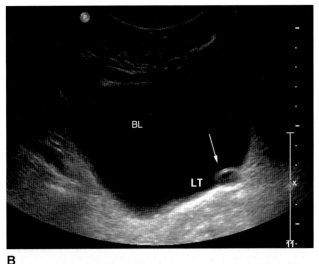

B

C

FIGURE 13-9 Ureterocele. **A:** Longitudinal image of the pelvis demonstrates a dilated ureter containing two echogenic calculi (*arrows*) and a thin-walled ureterocele (*U*) in the bladder lumen (*BL*). **B** and **C:** Transverse image of the urinary bladder shows a small thin-walled mass (*arrow*) projecting into the lumen of the bladder. Color Doppler image demonstrates the presence of a ureteral jet confirming the diagnosis of a small left ureterocele. (**A:** Image courtesy of Philips Medical Systems, Bothell, WA.)

ureters sometimes mimic multiseptate, cystic abdominal masses. Ectopic ureteroceles are dynamic structures that change shape and size according to intravesical pressure. Occasionally, a dilated ectopic ureter may indent the lower vesical wall of the bladder, simulating an ectopic ureterocele on sonography.

Simple ureteroceles are easy to see with sonography. In adults, they are usually incidental findings and are located at the expected location of the distal ureteral orifice. Sonographically, they appear as round or oval, thin-walled cystic structure on the posterior wall of a distended urinary bladder.[17,21] Real-time scanning shows these cystic areas as flexible in size as they fill and empty. Color Doppler imaging of the ureteral jets verifies the diagnosis (Fig. 13-9B, C). Pathologic processes such as stones, tumors, or recent manipulation, can cause pseudoureteroceles. Newer transducer technology makes visualization of pseudoureteroceles, which appear thicker walled, possible.

Urachal Variants

In the fetus, the bladder is located at the umbilicus and communicates with the allantoic canal, the extension of the cloacae/urogenital sinus, into the umbilical cord. The urachus is an embryonic tract formed as the bladder begins its descent into the true pelvis. As this occurs, the vertex of the bladder elongates, forming a fibromuscular appendage approximately 5 cm long surrounding the allantoic canal. This tract is normally obliterated by the time of birth. If the urachus fails to close, it creates an open channel between the bladder and the umbilicus.

There are four types of urachal anomalies[4]: (1) A patent urachus or fistula (completely patent lumen), occurs in 50% of cases. The urachus fails to close prior to birth and is usually associated with urethral obstruction. In this type, urine may drain constantly from the umbilicus. This serves as a protective mechanism to avoid an obstruction of the urinary bladder that may prevent normal fetal growth. (2) In 30% of cases, a urachal cyst develops when both ends of the urachus close off, trapping a small amount of urine in the canal. Clinically, the patient presents with a palpable mass, possible fever, and dysuria. Sonographically, a cystic structure is seen with possible internal echoes near the midline between the bladder and umbilicus. (3) A urachal sinus results, in 15% of cases, when the urachus closes at the bladder but not the umbilicus. (4) Urachal diverticulum results, in 5% of cases, when the urachus closes at the umbilicus and remains patent at the bladder.

Urachal variants are easily identified on sonography by their characteristic location adjacent to the dome of the bladder.[4] Sonographically, an anechoic mass or a diverticular outpouching between the dome of the urinary bladder and the umbilicus is identified.

Complications of a persistent urachal sinus include infection, whereas complications of a urachal cyst include adenocarcinoma, calculi formation, or both. When detected, they are easily reexamined owing to the easily assessable abdominal wall location.

A urachal remnant near the dome of the bladder can form from neoplasms. Mucinous adenocarcinoma is a leading precursor, and the remnant occurs most commonly in men aged 50 to 60 years. Stones may form in adenocarcinomas (Table 13-1).

PATHOLOGY OF THE LOWER URINARY TRACT

Cystitis

Urinary tract infections (UTIs) are extremely common, second only in prevalence to respiratory infections. UTI is a frequent cause of hospitalization in the United States and is responsible for significant morbidity and mortality.[22] Six million Americans are infected annually.[9]

Cystitis, inflammation of the bladder, always suggests predisposing risk factors, which include urethral obstruction, common rectal or vaginal fistulas, catheterization, surgical instrumentation, bladder calculi, bladder neoplasm, trauma, debilitating illness, pregnancy, sexual intercourse, renal disease, obstructive conditions, radiation therapy, diabetes mellitus, and poor hygiene.[9,22] The most common cause of all UTIs is the gram-negative intestinal bacteria *Escherichia coli*. Approximately 85% of all UTIs are caused by *E. coli*.[9,22] Cystitis is more common in females owing to the short female urethra and proximity of the urethral opening and vagina to the anal area. Most infections are *ascending*, arising from organisms in the perineal area and traveling along the *continuous mucosa* of the urinary tract, to the bladder, or possibly even further along the ureter to the kidneys, causing pyelonephritis (Fig. 13-10A–D).[9]

Cystitis usually presents as thickened bladder mucosa with hypoechoic or cystic structures along the wall.[3] Pathology Box 13-1 lists the types of cystitis, the most common etiology, and the distinctive sonographic appearance of each type based on histopathology. Diagnosis of the etiology requires correlation of the sonographic appearance with the patient's clinical signs, symptoms, and medical history.

Calculi

Bladder calculi are usually single and may be asymptomatic. They may cause inflammatory changes or acute bladder neck obstruction. Bladder neck obstruction by a calculus obstructs the flow of urine from the body. Predisposing factors to stone formation include increased concentration of salts in the urine, infection of the urinary tract, and urinary tract obstruction or stasis.[9] Stones usually appear as echogenic foci in the bladder, have an associated acoustic shadow, and shift to the dependent portion of the bladder with patient position changes (Fig. 13-11E). The anterior fluid-filled bladder provides an excellent acoustic window for the identification of bladder calculi. Stones do not have to be calcified to be identified sonographically. Sonography can distinguish uric acid stones, which have an acoustic shadow and shift position, from a bladder tumor, which appears as a fixed mass without an acoustic shadow. Intradiverticular calculi can also be identified sonographically. In a patient with diverticula, infection and stone formation are common findings owing to the stasis of residual urine remaining postvoid.

Reflux

Normally, the vesicoureteral junction allows urine to enter the bladder but prevents it from being regurgitated back into the ureter, particularly at the time of voiding. In this way, the kidney is protected from high pressure in the bladder

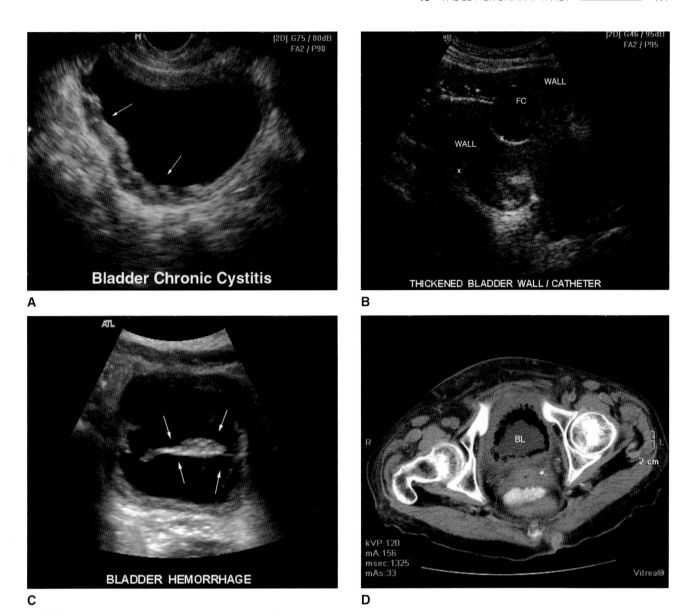

FIGURE 13-10 Cystitis. **A:** Endovaginal image of the urinary bladder shows a thickened irregular bladder wall (*arrows*) consistent with chronic cystitis. **B:** Longitudinal image of empty urinary bladder with Foley catheter (*FC*) in place. The bladder wall is extremely thickened (*between calipers*) and collapsed around the *FC*. **C:** Transverse image of the urinary bladder in a patient with hemorrhagic cystitis. A blood clot (*arrows*) is seen adhering to the thickened bladder wall. **D:** Computed tomography scan of the pelvis in a patient with emphysematous cystitis shows air within the bladder wall (*BL*). (A–C: Images courtesy of Philips Medical Systems, Bothell, WA.)

and from contamination by infected vesical urine. When this valve is incompetent, the chance for secondary development of infection in the upper urinary tract is significant.

Reflux may occur as a result of an abnormality of the trigone and secondary to anomalies such as ectopia, posterior urethral valves, paraureteric cyst, prune belly syndrome, and neurogenic bladder.[4]

Vesicoureteral reflux occurs in two distinct groups: neonatal reflux, which is seen more commonly in males; and reflux in older children, which is more common in females. Hydronephrosis, either unilateral or bilateral, can be seen on a prenatal sonography examination. There is a high incidence of contralateral renal abnormalities, including ureteropelvic junction obstruction and duplex kidney.[4] High-pressure reflux (with or without associated UTI) may be a major cause of chronic renal failure with marked scarring and atrophic changes in the kidneys (see Chapter 12).

The sonography examination is valuable in the management of children with reflux, because it is less expensive, employs nonionizing radiation, and can identify specific abnormalities. In the transverse plane, the sonographer must scan meticulously in the area where the ureters enter the bladder. Often, the ureter dilates with urine as the reflux is in progress and this may be visualized with real-time sonography.

Distal Ureteral Obstruction

Ureterovesical junction obstruction describes an obstruction at the junction of the distal ureter where it enters the bladder. To differentiate a ureterovesical junction obstruction from nonobstructive causes such as reflux, a voiding cystourethrogram (VCUG) may be necessary. The causes of distal ureteral obstruction may be congenital or acquired.

PATHOLOGY BOX 13-1
Cystitis

Type	Common Etiology	Sonographic Manifestations
Bullous	Infection	Focal bladder wall thickening in early, acute stages; small, contracted bladder in later, chronic stages
Candida albicans	Hematogenous, lymphatic, or direct inoculation from anus	Mild thickening of bladder wall; discrete, dense, fluid–fluid-debris interface shifts with changing position
Catheter induced	Irritation to bladder mucosa	Smooth, thickened, hypoechoic mucosa in early stages; redundant and polypoid in later stages
Cystic	Nonspecific inflammatory; associated with chronic cystitis or chronic catheterization	Confined to trigone; thickened, irregular mucosa with cyst-like elevations; associated intravesical mass
Emphysematous	*Escherichia coli*	Echogenic, "dirty" shadowing produced by gas collection within bladder wall
Encrusted	Urinary salts precipitate on bladder surface	Focal bladder wall thickening in early, acute stages; small, contracted bladder in later, chronic stages
Glandularis	Pelvic lipomatosis; chronic infection	Pronounced at ureterovesical junction; diffuse mucosal thickening; may have echogenic fat surrounding bladder
Hemorrhagic	Prolonged cyclophosphamide therapy	Intraluminal, echogenic debris caused by blood clots or wall thickening; focal calcification possible
Purulent	Neurogenic dysfunction and urine stasis	Pus–urine fluid level
Radiation induced	Radiation therapy	Ulceration, bladder wall sloughing, mucosal irregularity, and fistula formation in later stages
Schistosomiasis	*Schistosoma haematobium*	Polypoid bladder wall thickening; bladder wall calcifications with discrete shadowing; fibrosis and small, contracted bladder in later, chronic stages; vesicoureteral

Congenital causes include primary megaureter, primary megaureter with coexisting reflux, primary megaureter with coexisting bladder saccule, simple ureterocele, ectopic ureter, and ectopic ureterocele. Acquired causes include ureteral reimplantation procedures, infection, and stricture following the passage of stones. The sonographic findings include megaureter, hydronephrosis, and ectopic ureter, with or without ectopic ureterocele.

Neurogenic Bladder

A patient with a neurogenic bladder has lost voluntary control of voiding owing to a disturbance in the neural pathways. Depending on the nerves involved and nature of damage, the bladder becomes either overactive (spastic or hyperreflexive) or underactive (flaccid or hypotonic). *Myelodysplasia* (a neural tube defect consisting of defective development of part of the spinal cord) is the most common cause of neurogenic bladder in infants and children. Other causes include: (1) neurologic diseases (multiple sclerosis, syringomyelia, Parkinson disease), (2) congenital anomalies (partial or total absence of the sacrum or meningomyelocele), (3) systemic diseases with neurologic complications (diabetes mellitus, pernicious anemia), (4) infection (herpes zoster, poliomyelitis, spinal cord abscess), (5) trauma (vertebral fractures, operative trauma, disk herniation), (6) brain and spinal neoplasm, (7) central nervous system vascular disease, and (8) heavy metal poisoning. Neurogenic bladder is common in paraplegic patients.[7]

Individuals with overactive bladder have little to no control over voiding functions. Their bladders release urine spontaneously and frequently, although not completely. Their bladders become diminished because they are seldom filled to capacity. Because their bladders tend to retain small quantities of urine, the risk of UTI is significantly increased. Neurogenic *underactive* bladders have the opposite characteristics. Because there is damage to the neural system that informs the brain the bladder is full, the bladder continues to fill and may expand beyond the size and capacity of a normal bladder. At a certain point, the pressure of urine in the bladder will overcome the sphincter muscles' ability to retain it and urine will leak out. Like the overactive bladder, an underactive bladder fails to empty completely and retains a small amount of residual urine.

Many patients have a trabeculated bladder and spasm of the external sphincter, causing relative obstruction and narrowing of the urethra as it courses through the urogenital diaphragm. The patient may find it extremely difficult or impossible to void. Because of the obstruction, the pressure in the bladder remains constantly high, which may result in detrusor hypertrophy, the formation of saccules and diverticula, and vesicoureteral reflux[7,23] (Fig. 13-12A–C). Because the urine is chronically infected in such patients, the result may be chronic reflux pyelonephritis, the formation of struvite stones, or bladder debris.[7]

Patients with neurogenic bladder usually undergo serial excretory urography and VCUGs. Sonography is performed

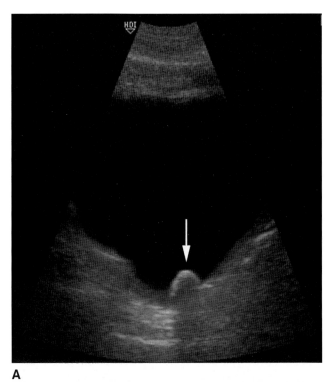

A

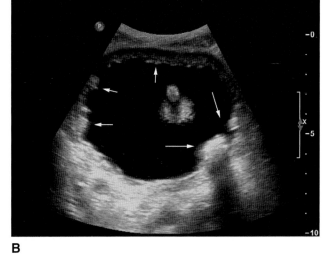

B

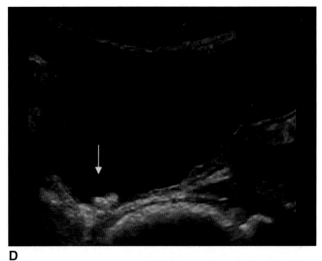

D

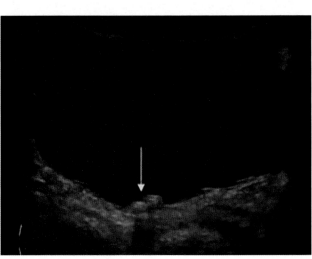

C

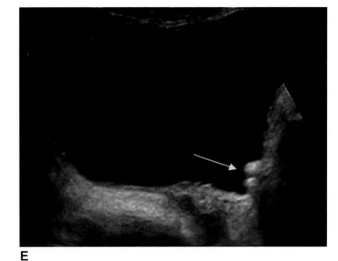

E

FIGURE 13-11 Bladder calculi. **A:** Longitudinal image of the urinary bladder shows a well-defined, hyperechoic density with an acoustic shadow along the posterior bladder wall consistent with a bladder calculus (*arrow*). **B:** Transverse image of the urinary bladder shows multiple bladder calculi (*large arrows*) and a thickened irregular bladder wall (*small arrows*). **C:** Transverse image of the urinary bladder with small hyperechoic calculi. **D:** Calculi move with change in patient position (right lateral decubitus). **E:** Calculi move with change in patient position (left lateral decubitus). (**A** and **B:** Images courtesy of Philips Medical Systems, Bothell, WA. **C–E:** UltraSoundCases.info, the Copyright ownership: SonoSkills, the Netherlands.)

to aid in the diagnosis of trabeculated bladder, ureterectasis, vesicoureteral reflux, hydronephrosis, or bladder calculi.

Bladder Wall Abnormalities

One of the most frequent sonographically observed abnormalities of the bladder is thickening of the bladder wall.

This is commonly caused by outlet obstruction. Other causes include neurogenic bladder, cystitis, edema from adjacent inflammatory processes, radiation, and primary or secondary neoplasms[10] (Pathology Box 13-2). Patients with inflammatory bladder pathology may have signs and symptoms like those of patients with urinary bladder or kidney neoplasm.[11]

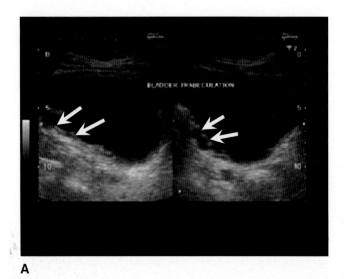

A

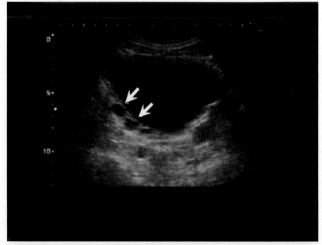

B

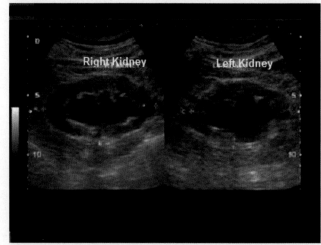

C

FIGURE 13-12 Neurogenic bladder. **A:** Longitudinal images of the urinary bladder show the presence of bladder saccules (*arrows*), a sign that bladder outlet obstruction has begun to have adverse effects on the urinary tract. **B:** A postvoid image shows a large postvoid residual within the bladder. Bladder saccules (*arrows*) are seen along the lateral wall. **C:** Longitudinal images of both kidneys show bilateral hydronephrosis.

Certain pathologic conditions are manifested with extrinsic bladder compression, invasion of the urinary bladder, or both. Endometriosis can present as an intravesical lesion by either direct extension or implantation. Regional enteritis (Crohn disease) has been reported as a loop of small bowel with thick walls and a narrowed lumen adhering to the bladder dome.[5] Focal or diffuse bladder wall thickening can occur with neurofibromatosis.[4]

TRAUMA

Rupture

Bladder rupture follows severe blunt lower abdominal or pelvic trauma or penetrating abdominal or perineal injury. If the bladder was full at the time of blunt injury, rupture is more likely to occur, spilling urine into the peritoneum. Pelvic crush injuries cause bladder rupture in 1% to 15% of cases, four-fifths being extraperitoneal. A urinoma may result from temporary sealing of a small tear. The sonographic appearance of a urinoma is of an anechoic mass with enhanced through-transmission. The mass may have irregular borders and contain septa and may compress surrounding

tissue (Fig. 13-13A, B). The best diagnostic procedure for visualizing bladder rupture is cystography.

Blood Clots

Blood clots, either from a pathologic process or from trauma, may adhere to the bladder wall, giving a sonographic appearance similar to that of a tumor (Fig. 13-14A–C). They appear as an irregularity along the mucosal surface. Most blood clots are mobile and will move freely with changes in the patient's position and will not demonstrate the presence of vascularity with color Doppler imaging.

Bladder Flap Hematoma

During a cesarean section, the surgeon incises the vesicouterine reflection of the peritoneum to obtain access to the lower uterine segment, creating a potential space between the bladder and uterus commonly known as the *bladder flap*.[24] If hemostasis is not obtained after closure of the uterine incision, a hematoma forms between the lower uterine segment and the urinary bladder (bladder flap) or

<table>
<tr><td colspan="2">

PATHOLOGY BOX 13-2
Causes of Bladder Wall Thickening

</td></tr>
</table>

Focal	Diffuse
Neoplasm	
Transitional cell carcinoma	Transitional cell carcinoma
Squamous cell carcinoma	Squamous cell carcinoma
Adenocarcinoma	Adenocarcinoma
Lymphoma	
Infectious/Inflammatory	
Tuberculosis (acute)	Cystitis
Schistosomiasis (acute); flukes living in the pulmonary venous system and its tributaries or within the veins draining the bladder; serious destruction to surrounding tissue; "swimmers itch"	Tuberculosis (chronic) Schistosomiasis (chronic)
Cystitis	
Cystitis cystica	
Cystitis glandularis	
Fistula	
Medical Diseases	
Endometriosis	Interstitial cystitis
Amyloidosis	Amyloidosis
Trauma	Neurogenic bladder
Hematoma	Detrusor hyperreflexia
Ruptured bladder	Bladder outlet
	Obstruction with muscular dystrophy

anywhere the surgical scalpel made an incision (abdominal wall, muscle).

A patient with a hematoma can present with fever, a mass, or a dropping hematocrit. An infected hematoma can manifest with the same symptoms, but the patient can additionally have leukocytosis and more pain. The fever can be caused by the infected hematoma alone or by postsurgical complications such as endometritis, septic thrombophlebitis, abscess, hematoma, or wound infection.[24]

The incidence of bladder flap hematoma is unknown. The sonographic appearances described in the literature vary significantly and include a mass as large as 15 × 12 × 9 cm (length × width × height).[22] The majority of bladder flap hematomas are complex masses with poorly defined borders that are primarily anechoic, with internal septations or debris.[24]

Because it is not possible to differentiate sonographically between a hematoma, an infected hematoma, and an abscess, the patient's clinical presentation is important.[24] A symptomatic patient with a clinical history of leukocytosis suggests an abscess; a dropping hematocrit, a hematoma; and a dropping hematocrit with leukocytosis, an infected hematoma.

If there is a suspected hematoma near the incisional site of the abdominal wall, a high-frequency (5 to 10 MHz), linear array transducer and a standoff pad may be required to examine the superficial area. If the incisional site has not healed, sterile gel and a transducer cover must be used to reduce the risk of contamination. This area may be more difficult to examine because of incisional pain and tenderness. To distinguish between a superficial wound and a subfascial hematoma, the rectus muscle must be identified. Superficial hematomas are located anterior to the rectus muscle, and subfascial hematomas are located posterior to it.[25] The typical location for a subfascial hematoma is in the prevesicular space, ventral to the bladder. Based on the sonographic appearance, a superficial hematoma or a

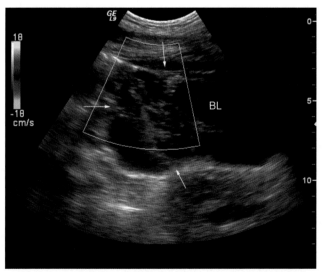

A

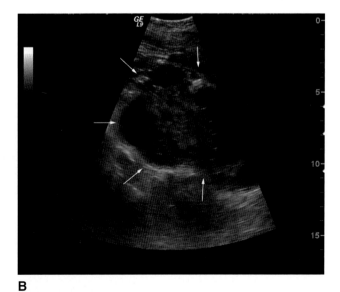

B

FIGURE 13-13 Bladder rupture. **A:** Transverse image of the pelvis in a man who experienced recent blunt pelvic trauma. A complex mass (*arrows*) is seen to the right of the urinary bladder (*BL*). This mass is consistent with a hematoma. No color flow is seen within the mass. **B:** Longitudinal image to the right of the bladder shows the complex hematoma (*arrows*).

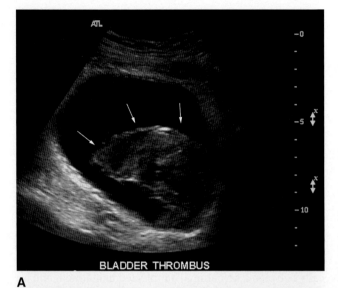

A

B

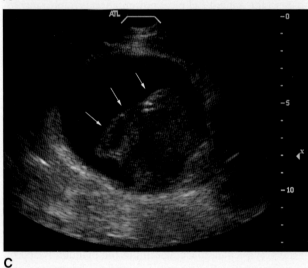

C

FIGURE 13-14 Blood clot. **A:** Longitudinal image of the urinary bladder shows a large, irregular, echogenic mass (*arrows*) along the posterior abdominal wall. This mass was diagnosed as a blood clot within the bladder. **B:** Transverse image of the urinary bladder shows a large echogenic mass (*arrows*) along the posterior bladder wall. This was diagnosed as a blood clot that developed after a renal biopsy. **C:** Longitudinal image of the urinary bladder shows a large, irregular, echogenic mass (*arrows*) along the posterior abdominal wall. This mass was also diagnosed as a blood clot within the bladder. (Images courtesy of Philips Medical, Bothell, WA.)

subfascial hematoma may appear similar to an abscess or an infected hematoma, making clinical correlation extremely important.

BLADDER NEOPLASMS

Bladder tumors are frequently found in urogenital imaging, many times in patients having renal sonography for painless hematuria. Bladder tumors are usually epithelial or uroepithelial in origin and are one of the most common tumors of the genitourinary tract. While painless hematuria is the most common symptom, other symptoms may include dysuria, urinary frequency, or urgency.[14,26] An infiltrating tumor disrupts the uniformity of the normal 3 to 5 mm bladder wall thickness (Fig. 13-15A). Hydronephrosis often occurs owing to the obstructed outflow of urine. Blood clot, benign prostatic hypertrophy, cystitis, fungal balls, stones, and bladder trabeculae can mimic bladder tumors[3,26] (Fig. 13-15B).

For initial screening of suspected bladder tumor, sonography is an excellent noninvasive, cost-effective, and nonionizing

imaging modality. Cystoscopy involves inserting a cystoscope through the urethra into the bladder. Cystoscopy with biopsy is considered the most accurate method for detecting and evaluating bladder tumors, but it is invasive and requires anesthesia.[14,26] Tumors located in the neck or dome of the bladder are difficult to detect with sonography.[3,26] The ability of sonography to detect the presence or absence of bladder tumors has varied from 33% for tumors smaller than 0.5 cm in diameter to 83% for tumors 1 to 2 cm to 95% for tumors larger than 2 cm.[3,26] Aside from the size and location of the tumor, the degree of bladder distention or obesity may affect the accuracy of tumor detection.

Endovaginal longitudinal scanning has proven effective in the diagnosis of tumors located in any part of the urinary bladder. The endovaginal approach provides good image quality, allowing the tumor to be studied in detail through the anterior wall, the neck, and the apex of the urinary bladder. Bladder tumors situated on the sidewall are harder to stage by transvaginal sonography.

Emerging research suggests that four-dimensional ultrasound (4D-US) can provide precise characterization of bladder carcinomas with image quality that is comparable to white light cystoscopy.[27]

Following the diagnosis of carcinoma of the bladder, sonography can also be helpful in staging tumors. Evidence indicates that the stage of the tumor profoundly influences curability and survival time.[28] The tumor's response to chemotherapy is the primary determinant of whether to continue therapy. Sonography is a useful adjunct to cystoscopy when serial scans of bladder tumors are performed. When sonography and cystoscopy are used together, the staging of bladder tumors is more accurate than when either study is used alone. CT is the imaging modality of choice for identifying contiguous extension of bladder neoplasms and has reduced the number of overstaging and understaging errors.[4,11,28]

Benign Neoplasms

Papilloma, a benign tumor, is a forerunner of transitional cell carcinoma (TCC). Sonographically, papillomas are usually 0.5 to 2 cm in size and have the same appearance as TCC. The most common location is along the lateral urinary bladder wall; the second most common location is the trigone.

Malignant Neoplasms

According to the National Cancer Institute, each year over 70,000 new cases of bladder cancer are diagnosed and over 14,000 will die from the disease.[29] Bladder carcinoma is the fourth most common type of cancer in men and the eighth most common in women.[29] Men, Caucasians, and smokers have up to three times

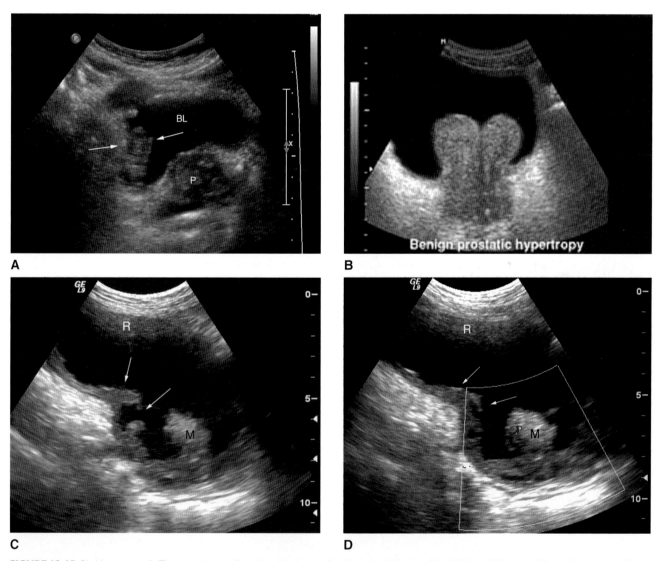

FIGURE 13-15 Bladder tumors. **A:** Transverse image of a male pelvis shows a focal irregular thickening of the right lateral bladder wall (*arrows*) consistent with bladder carcinoma. The prostate (*P*) is seen posterior to the urinary bladder (*BL*). **B:** Transverse image of a male pelvis shows a grossly enlarged prostate gland indenting the posterior wall of the bladder. An enlarged prostate gland can be mistaken for a bladder tumor. **C and D:** Longitudinal images of the urinary bladder demonstrate an irregular, echogenic mass projecting into the bladder lumen (*M*). Note the bladder wall thickening along the bladder wall (*arrows*). Reverberation is seen along the anterior bladder wall (*R*). Color Doppler image reveals flow within the mass helping to distinguish the bladder tumor from a blood clot. (**C and D:** Images courtesy of Tim S. Gibbs, Anaheim, CA.)

the risk of bladder cancer than the general population. When diagnosed and treated in a localized stage, bladder cancer is very treatable, with a 5-year cancer-specific survival rate approaching 95%.[29]

Ninety percent are TCC, a cancer that begins in the cells that normally make up the inner lining of the bladder.[26] Smoking, analgesic abuse, and industrial carcinogen exposure predispose patients to TCC cancer. Five percent are squamous cell carcinomas, the most aggressive of the malignant tumors.[24] They are associated with chronic inflammatory conditions, neurogenic bladder, stones, and patients having bladder schistosomiasis.[28] Two percent of bladder tumors are adenocarcinomas, which are associated with urachal remnants and bladder exstrophy.[11,26]

Sonographically, TCC tumors are visualized as an irregular echogenic mass, either polypoid or sessile, that projects into the lumen of the bladder; are fixed to the bladder wall; and may have associated acoustic shadowing.[3,28] Color Doppler imaging shows detectable blood flow in the malignant bladder tumor (Figs. 13-15C, D and 13-16A, B).

Whenever there is focal thickening of the bladder wall, a malignant primary urinary bladder tumor should be suspected. Sonographically, malignant masses present as echogenic structures protruding into the echo-free bladder lumen. Infiltrating tumors disrupt the normal uniformity of the bladder wall. Bladder tumors may directly invade the surrounding anatomy (Fig. 13-17A–D).

Metastatic

Metastatic urinary bladder tumors occur most commonly by direct extension from the cervix, uterus, prostate, and rectum, in that order[3] (Fig. 13-18). They may also develop from direct extension from the upper urinary system directly, or by the lymphatic or vascular system. (For a more detailed discussion, see Chapters 7, 8, and 10 and the volume *Obstetrics and Gynecology* in this series.) Prostatic cancer usually metastasizes to the seminal vesicles and perivesical connective tissue.

STRESS INCONTINENCE

The most common micturition abnormality is stress incontinence. Urinary incontinence is the most common pelvic floor dysfunction in women.[30] Forty percent of postmenopausal women are affected by incontinence.[31] The condition is caused by genuine stress incontinence, detrusor instability, voiding difficulty (overflow), fistulas, and functional or congenital disorders. It may be a temporary condition owing to UTIs. Stress incontinence is the leakage of urine from the bladder during acts that increase intra-abdominal and intravesicular pressure, such as Valsalva maneuvers, coughing, or straining.[32]

Incontinence is receiving increased attention by both the public and medical professionals. Many women suffer stress incontinence and are too embarrassed to admit it, seek help, or are unaware of available treatments. As the urogynecology surgical specialty field has emerged, the demand has increased for a more detailed understanding of normal female pelvic floor anatomy.[31–33] Sonography is being used to diagnose and treat incontinence.[32–34] Sonographic evaluation of stress incontinence requires more a detailed pelvic floor assessment. Endovaginal, endorectal, transperineal, and transabdominal methods can all be used to directly observe bladder filling and emptying.[32–34] Transvaginal sonography is sensitive and specific but cannot be used exclusively to determine urinary stress incontinence in females. The pitfalls of using the transperineal method include an overdistended bladder, poor penetration, an excessively small field of view, bowel gas, focal uterine contractions, bladder mistaken for cervix, fluid in the vaginal vault mistaken for cervix, cervical cysts, and pericervical veins.

Images obtained through 3D sonography have an important role in urogynecologic research.[32,33] A recent study utilized 3D transperineal ultrasound to assess the pelvic floor and demonstrated posterior depression of the urethra into the anterior vaginal wall, thus, indirectly suggesting lack of urethral support.[35]

Translabial ultrasound is becoming an accepted approach for urethral evaluation.[30] This technique can provide a

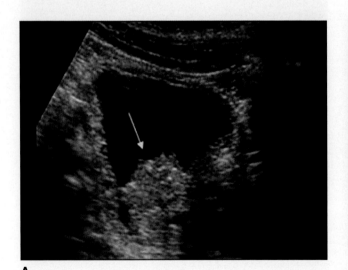

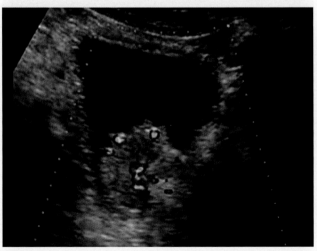

A **B**

FIGURE 13-16 Transitional cell carcinoma. **A:** Longitudinal image of a male bladder shows a large mass. **B:** Color Doppler image confirms mass vascularity. (**A** and **B:** Image source: UltraSoundCases.info. Copyright © SonoSkills, the Netherlands.)

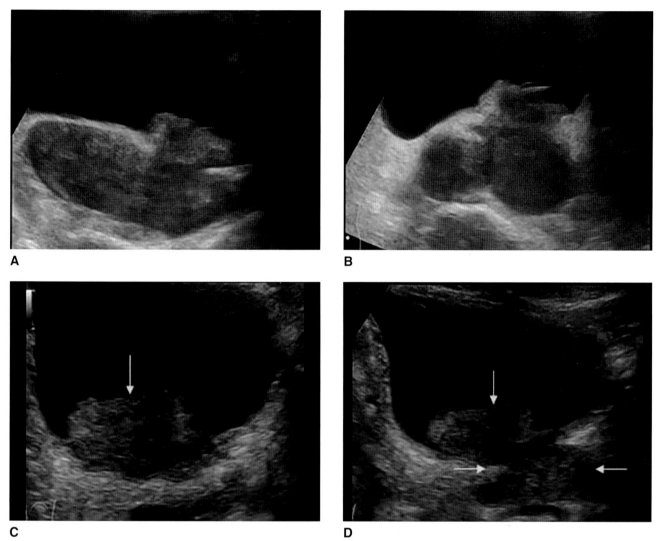

A

B

C

D

FIGURE 13-17 Direct invasion. **A:** Sagittal image of a bladder mass invading the anterior aspect of the uterus. **B:** transverse image of the same mass. **C:** Transverse image of a large bladder mass in a male patient. **D:** Transverse image of the same mass infiltrating into the prostate gland. (**A–D:** Image source: UltraSoundCases.info. Copyright © SonoSkills, the Netherlands.)

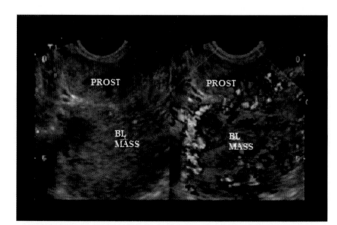

FIGURE 13-18 Metastatic invasion. Transrectal image of the prostate demonstrates a large tumor from the prostate invading the urinary bladder. Metastatic tumors of the urinary bladder can occur as a result from direct extension of prostate cancer.

dynamic assessment of urethral mobility.[36] Translabial ultrasound also allows for a better angle of insonation of the ureteral sphincter complex (USC) compared with transvaginal imaging.[37] Another advantage is the USC is not distorted by the insertion of the transducer into the vaginal canal.[37] Recent research has shown the length of the USC at rest is shorter and the mobility of the urethra increases Valsalva in patients with incontinence.[37]

Stress incontinence is caused by a poorly supported bladder neck (the section between the bladder and the urethra).[32-34] Coughing or bearing down results in the bladder neck moving inferiorly, opening the urethra opens, and pushed out urine. Depending on the extent of the findings, surgical repair can be an option. A suburethral sling and an anterior repair can be performed and consist of placing a small piece of plastic around the bladder neck to hold it in place, and at the same time, lifting the sagging bladder and stabilizing it.[31,32]

SUMMARY

This chapter discussed embryology, normal anatomy, physiology, and sonographic evaluation of the lower urinary tract. Bladder anomalies, abnormalities, and pathologies were also discussed and further summarized in the appropriate pathology boxes. Lastly, the topic of stress incontinence was described along with how sonography can be used to diagnose and treat incontinence.

REFERENCES

1. Cochard L. *Netter's Atlas of Human Embryology*. Elsevier Mosby; 2002.
2. Gray H. *Anatomy of the Human Body*. Lea & Febiger; 1918.
3. McAchran SE, Hartke DM, Nakamoto DA, et al. Sonography of the urinary bladder. *Ultrasound Clin*. 2007;2:17–26.
4. Rumack C, Wilson W, Charboneau W, Levine D. *Diagnostic Ultrasound*. 5th ed. Elsevier Mosby; 2017.
5. Marieb EN, Hoehn K. *Human Anatomy and Physiology*. 11th ed. Pearson Benjamin Cummings; 2018.
6. Scanlon VC, Sanders T. *Essentials of Anatomy and Physiology*. 8th ed. FA Davis; 2018.
7. Samson G, Cardenas DD. Neurogenic bladder in spinal cord injury. *Phys Med Rehabil Clin N Am*. 2007;18:255–274.
8. Bradley CS, Smith KE, Kreder KJ. Urodynamic evaluation of the bladder and pelvic floor. *Gastroenterol Clin North Am*. 2008;37:539–552.
9. VanMeter KC, Hubert RJ. *Gould's Pathophysiology for the Health Professions*. 6th ed. Saunders; 2017.
10. Yang JM, Huang WC. Bladder wall thickness on ultrasonographic cystourethrography: affecting factors and their implications. *J Ultrasound Med*. 2003;22:777–782.
11. Hertzberg BS, Middleton WD. *Ultrasound: The Requisites*. 3rd ed. Elsevier; 2015.
12. Bean E, Naftalin J, Jurkovic D. How to assess the ureters during pelvic ultrasound. *Ultrasound Obstet Gynecol*. 2019;53:729–733.
13. Pateman K, Mavrelos D, Hoo L, Holland T, Naftalin J, Jurkovic D. Visualization of ureters on standard gynecological transvaginal scan: a feasibility study. *Ultrasound Obstet Gynecol*. 2013;41:696–701.
14. Kocakoc E, Kiris A, Orhan I, et al. Detection of bladder tumors with 3-dimensional sonography and virtual sonographic cystoscopy. *J Ultrasound Med*. 2008;27:45–53.
15. Suwanrath C, Suntharasaj T, Sirapatanapipat H, et al. Three-dimensional ultrasonographic bladder volume measurement: reliability of the Virtual Organ Computer-aided Analysis technique using different rotation steps. *J Ultrasound Med*. 2009;28:847–854.
16. Goldberg BB, Badgley D, Liu JB, et al. Endoluminal sonography of the urinary tract: preliminary observations. *AJR Am J Roentgenol*. 1991;155:99–103.
17. Palmer LS. Pediatric urologic imaging. *Urol Clin North Am*. 2006;33:409–423.
18. Henningsen C. *Clinical Guide to Ultrasonography*. 2nd ed. Mosby; 2014.
19. Doubilet PM, Benson CB. *Atlas of Ultrasound in Obstetrics and Gynecology*. 3rd ed. Lippincott Williams and Wilkins; 2018.
20. Gearhart JP, Rink RR, Mouriquand P. The bladder exstrophy-epispadias complex. In: Gearhart JP, ed. *Pediatric Urology*. Saunders; 2010:511–546.
21. Gearhart JP, Jeffs RD. Exstrophy of the bladder, epispadias, and other bladder anomalies. In: Walsh PC, Retik AB, Stamey TA, et al, eds. *Campbell's Urology*. WB Saunders; 1998:1772–1821.
22. Drekonja DM, Johnson JR. Urinary tract infections. *Prim Care*. 2008;35:345–367.
23. Crowley L. *An Introduction to Human Disease*. 9th ed. Jones and Bartlett; 2012.
24. Winsett MZ, Fagan CJ, Bedi DG. Sonographic demonstration of bladder-flap hematoma. *J Ultrasound Med*. 1986;5:483–487.
25. Gill K. *Abdominal Ultrasound: A Practitioner's Guide*. WB Saunders; 2001.
26. Zhang J, Gerst S, Lefkowitz RA, et al. Imaging of bladder cancer. *Radiol Clin N Am*. 2007;45:183–205.
27. Jokisch F, Buchner A, Schulz GB, et al. Prospective evaluation of 4-D contrast enhanced ultrasound (CEUS) imaging in bladder tumors. *Clin Hemorheol Microcirc*. 2020;74:1–12.
28. Eisenberg R, Johnson N. *Comprehensive Radiographic Pathology*. 6th ed. Mosby; 2015.
29. U.S. National Institutes of Health. National Cancer Institute. 2010. Accessed May 26, 2017. www.cancer.gov
30. Xiao T, Chen Y, Gan Y, et al. Can stress urinary incontinence be predicted by ultrasound? *AJR Am Journal of Roentgenol*. 2019;213:1163–1169.
31. Hall R. Clinical update: pelvic floor imaging for the urogynecology patient. In: *Educators' Summit*. Seattle University; 2008–2009.
32. Unger CA, Weinstein MW, Pretorius DH. Pelvic floor imaging. *Obstet Gynecol Clin North Am*. 2011;38:23–43.
33. Mitterberger M, Pinggera GM, Mueller T, et al. Dynamic transurethral sonography and 3-dimensional reconstruction of the rhabdosphincter and urethra: initial experience in continent and incontinent women. *J Ultrasound Med*. 2006;25:315–320.
34. Oliveira F, Ramos J, Martins-Costa S. Translabial ultrasonography in the assessment of urethral diameter and intrinsic sphincter deficiency. *J Ultrasound Med*. 2006;25:1153–1158.
35. Shui W, Luo Y, Ying T, et al. Assessment of pelvic floor support to the urethra using 3D transperineal ultrasound. *Int Urogynecol J*. 2020;31:149–154.
36. Gillor M, Dietz HP. Translabial ultrasound imaging of urethral diverticula. *Ultrasound Obstet Gynecol*. 2019;54:552–556.
37. Garriga JC, Isern AP, Carballeria MR, et al. Three-dimensional translabial ultrasound assessment of urethral supports and the urethral sphincter complex in stress urinary incontinence. *Neurol Urodyn*. 2017;36:1839–1845.

CHAPTER 14

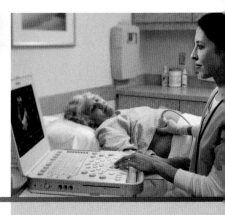

The Prostate Gland

GEORGE M. KENNEDY-ANTILLON

OBJECTIVES

- Discuss embryologic development, differentiation of structures, and hormones influencing maturation of the prostate gland.

- Identify surface, relational, and internal prostate anatomy to include differentiating the four prostate zones.

- Demonstrate routine scanning procedures to include patient preparation; patient instructions; patient position; transrectal and transabdominal scanning, biopsy techniques; technical considerations; and common scanning pitfalls.

- Describe the pathology, etiology, clinical signs, symptoms, and sonographic appearance of cysts in the male pelvis to include Müllerian duct and utricle cysts, seminal vesicle cysts, prostatic cysts (prostatic abscess), and diverticula of the ejaculatory ducts and vas deferens.

- Explain the pathology, etiology, clinical signs and symptoms, and sonographic appearance of benign prostatic hyperplasia.

- Identify the pathology, etiology, clinical signs and symptoms, and sonographic appearance of prostate calcifications.

- Categorize the pathology, etiology, clinical signs and symptoms, and sonographic appearance of prostatitis to include acute bacterial prostatitis, chronic bacterial prostatitis, chronic pelvic pain syndrome, and asymptomatic inflammatory prostatitis.

- Recognize sonographic characteristics of benign and malignant conditions of the prostate gland.

- Briefly discuss the multiparametric ultrasound (mp-US) approach of combining B-mode and Doppler ultrasound (US) with volume imaging (3D), contrast-enhanced US (CEUS) and shear wave elastography (SWE) to improve the diagnostic performance in detecting prostate cancer (PCa).

- Discuss the role of sonography in providing guidance for biopsy procedures.

- Discuss the role of sonography in evaluation of suspected male infertility.

KEY TERMS

benign prostatic hyperplasia (BPH)

digital rectal examination (DRE)

infertility

multiparametric ultrasound (mp-US)

neurovascular bundle

prostate biopsy

prostate cancer (PCa)

prostate-specific antigen (PSA)

prostatitis

transrectal ultrasound (TRUS)

transurethral resection of the prostate (TURP)

GLOSSARY

apex inferior portion of the prostate gland, located superior to the urogenital diaphragm

base superior portion of the prostate gland, located below the inferior margin of the urinary bladder

corpora amylacea calcifications commonly seen in the inner gland of the prostate

Eiffel Tower sign shadowing artifact created in the area of the urethra and verumontanum

ejaculatory duct duct that passes through the central zone and empties into the urethra; originates from the confluence of the vas deferens and the seminal vesicle

(continued)

endogenous calculi calculi formation within the substance of the prostate

exogenous calculi calculi found in the urethra

seminal vesicles paired simple tubular glands that extend from an outpouching of the vas deferens; located superior and posterior to the prostate, between the urinary bladder and rectum

surgical capsule a demarcation between the inner gland (central and transitional zones) and outer gland (peripheral zone), which is normally hypoechoic but may be echogenic if corpora amylacea or calcifications are present

vas deferens reproductive duct that extends from the epididymis to the ejaculatory duct; also known as the ductus deferens

verumontanum a longitudinal elevation or ridge of tissue on the posterior prosthetic urethral wall where the orifices of the ejaculatory ducts are located

Transrectal ultrasound (TRUS) of the prostate has improved markedly over the past several decades. Equipment technology has progressed from one of the earliest devices, a chair-type apparatus with a mechanical probe mounted in the center,[1] to current phased array, three-dimensional (3D) and high-resolution micro-ultrasound transducers (Fig. 14-1). TRUS is utilized to evaluate the prostate in the setting of malignancy, infertility, chronic pelvic pain syndrome (CPPS), and congenital abnormalities. It also plays a significant role in biopsy and treatment guidance.[1] The role of contrast agents and elastography in prostate tumor assessment is also being investigated and has shown promising results.[1-4] Additionally, studies show contrast-enhanced TRUS has a high sensitivity when detecting diffuse prostate cancers that might be missed on a baseline examination. However, current data show contrast-enhanced TRUS alone is not sufficient to confirm or exclude the presence of cancer. Combining the data acquired from individual US modalities into a mp-US approach can improve the diagnostic performance in PCa diagnosis.[4,5] Larger trials are necessary to generate more accurate estimates of the sensitivity and specificity of the individual ultrasound modalities.[5]

A sonography examination of the prostate requires a thorough understanding of the anatomy of the prostate, the sonographic characteristics of disease processes, and the unique image orientation of the transrectal transducer.

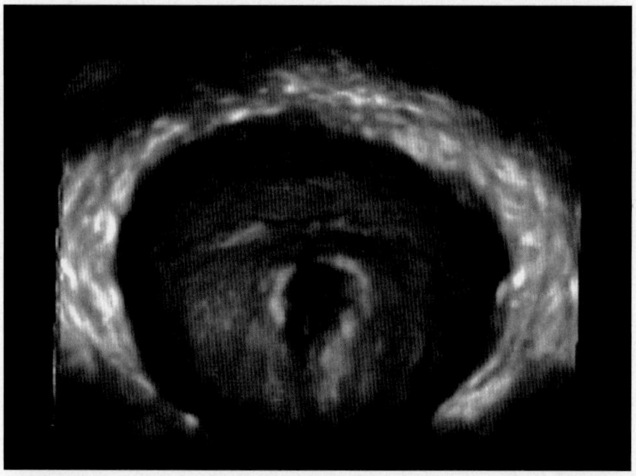

ANATOMY AND ORGANOGENESIS

During embryogenesis, all embryos start out with two paired sex ducts: the mesonephric or wolffian ducts and the paramesonephric or müllerian ducts. Each müllerian duct lies lateral to its corresponding wolffian duct.[6] This is termed the indifferent stage.[6] The mesonephric ducts are responsible for development of the male reproductive system, whereas the paramesonephric ducts will form the female reproductive system. In males, a portion of each mesonephric duct will later develop into an ejaculatory duct, vas deferens, and seminal vesicle. During the 11th gestational week, the prostate begins to form from the urogenital sinus, an endodermal derivative. It begins as multiple solid outgrowths of the prostatic portion of the urethra, which form on the posterior side of the urogenital sinus.[6] As development continues, these penetrate the surrounding mesenchyme to form the five prostatic lobes.[7] Maturation of the gland continues while testosterone levels are high. Once these levels start to decrease, the gland enters a quiescent state until puberty when testosterone levels rise again.

Gross Anatomy

The adult prostate is a funnel-shaped, exocrine gland surrounded by a fibromuscular capsule. This is not a true capsule, but rather thin, inseparable connective tissue. In the young adult, it weighs approximately 20 ± 6 g and measures on average $4 \times 3 \times 2$ cm. The prostate is composed of glandular and fibromuscular tissue and surrounds the proximal male urethra. The cephalic portion of the gland is referred to as the base and the caudal end the apex. The base is continuous with the bladder neck and the apex is adherent to the urogenital diaphragm (Fig. 14-2A). Three luminal structures traverse the prostate gland: the right and left ejaculatory ducts, and the urethra. The prostatic urethra traverses the central portion of the gland. The duct of the seminal vesicle joins the ampullae of the vas deferens to form the ejaculatory duct at the prostate base. The ejaculatory duct then extends within the central zone

FIGURE 14-1 The sonogram is a three-dimensional reconstruction of the prostate gland. (Image courtesy of Philips Medical Systems, Bothell, WA.)

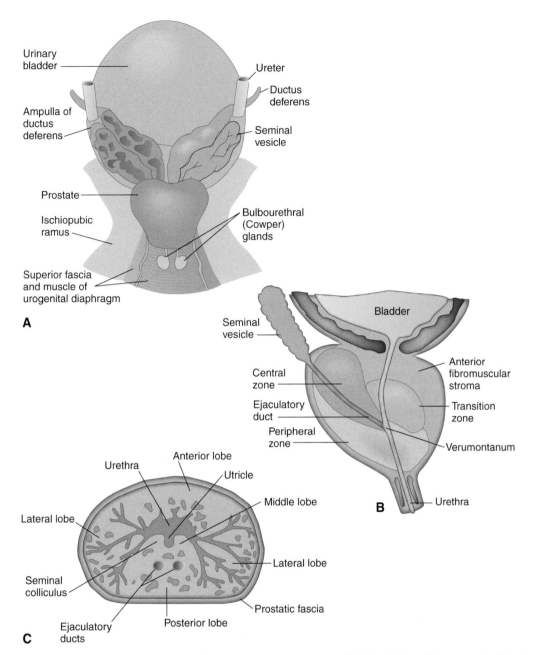

FIGURE 14-2 Male urogenital organs. **A:** Posterior view of the bladder and male accessory organs. **B:** Midsagittal view of the prostate gland showing the ejaculatory duct and urethra joining at the verumontanum. **C:** Cross section of the prostate at the utricle showing the lobes and internal prostatic structures. (Reprinted with permission from Halliday NL, Chung HM. *BRS Gross Anatomy*. 9th ed. Wolters Kluwer; 2018:187.)

of the gland to the midline where it joins the urethra at the verumontanum, a longitudinal ridge on the posterior wall of the prostatic urethra.[1,8] This structure is located at the midpoint of the prostatic urethra near the apex and is laterally flanked by the openings of the ejaculatory ducts (Fig. 14-2B). The utricle, a small epithelium-lined diverticulum at the apex of the verumontanum, is a fetal remnant of the urogenital sinus and is homologous to the female uterus[6,8,9] (Fig. 14-2C). Abnormal dilatation, cysts, or calcifications can occur at this level, and they are usually associated with urinary tract symptoms. This structure accounts for the "Eiffel Tower" appearance on transverse images of the prostate gland obtained at this level[1,10] (Fig. 14-3).

Vasculature

The prostate is supplied with blood from the internal iliac arteries via the prostaticovesical arteries.[1,11] The iliac arteries course along the medial and inferior surface of the bladder toward the prostate along the neurovascular bundle.[12] They bifurcate into the prostatic artery and inferior vesicle artery, which further branch into the urethral and capsular arteries (Fig. 14-4). The capsular vessels are arranged on the surface of the gland in five anterolateral and posterolateral groups. These capsular vessels supply approximately two-thirds of the glandular tissue.[11,12] The urethral arteries are directed inward and follow the course of the prostatic urethra, supplying the other one-third of the glandular tissue.[11,12]

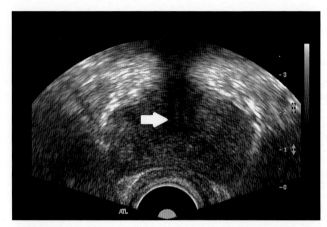

FIGURE 14-3 Verumontanum. A coronal sonogram of the normal prostate. The "Eiffel Tower" sign (*arrow*) is seen at the level of the prostatic utricle.

The venous drainage consists of a prostatic venous plexus, located between the facial layer and capsule (Fig. 14-5). These small veins drain the venous blood from the prostate gland. These vessels join the veins of the bladder and penis to ultimately drain into the internal iliac veins. The internal iliac veins then connect with the vertebral venous plexus, which is thought to be the route of bone metastasis in PCa.

Prostate Zones

The urethra is the primary anatomic reference point within the prostate, dividing the gland into an anterior fibromuscular portion and a posterior glandular portion[13] (Fig. 14-6). The glandular tissue accounts for two-thirds of the prostate and

contains four zones. Three of the zones—the peripheral zone, the transition zone, and the periurethral zone—have similar embryologic origins from the urogenital sinus, whereas the fourth zone, the central zone, is derived embryologically from the mesonephric ducts.[1,7,14] The fibromuscular structures account for one-third of the prostate.

The peripheral zone constitutes about 70% of the glandular tissue of the prostate (Table 14-1). It is located along the posterior, lateral, and apical aspects of the gland, and its ducts drain into the distal segment of the urethra between the verumontanum and the apex. The acini of the peripheral zone are small, round, and simple.[14] The peripheral zone is the most common location for carcinomas[1,15] and prostatitis to occur, with approximately 70% of prostate cancer (PCa) arising from this area. Sonographically, normal peripheral zone tissue has a homogeneous, isoechoic echotexture. It can be delineated from the central zone by a thin, hyperechoic band separating the two zones. This band, called the surgical capsule, is in the shape of a semicircle and borders the central gland laterally and posteriorly.

The central zone accounts for about 25% of the glandular tissue and is located at the base of the prostate. It is embedded in the funnel-shaped peripheral zone (Fig. 14-7). This zone narrows to an apex at the verumontanum. It surrounds the ejaculatory ducts and is located between the peripheral zone and the transition zone.[1,2] Microscopically, the central zone acini contrast strikingly in appearance with those in the peripheral zone. They are large and have irregular contours, with considerable intraluminal folds and ridges.[1,14] These morphologic differences are what set the central zone aside from the rest of the glandular tissue[16] and what presumably make it immune from most disease.[17] The stroma are composed of long, tightly arranged muscle fibers

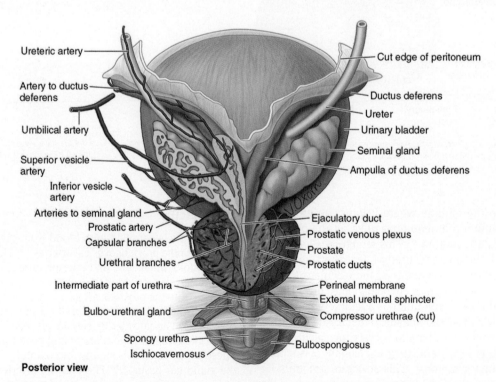

FIGURE 14-4 A drawing of the male pelvic organs, illustrating the arterial supply. The prostatic artery is shown branching into the capsular and urethral arteries. (Reprinted with permission from Dalley AF II, Agur AMR. *Moore's Clinically Oriented Anatomy*. 9th ed. Wolters Kluwer; 2022:612.)

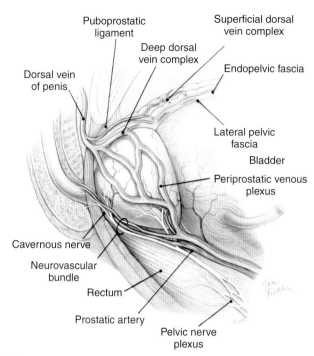

FIGURE 14-5 Parasagittal view of the prostatic venous plexus and neurovascular bundle. (Reprinted from Ohori M, Scardino PT. Localized prostate cancer. *Curr Probl Surg.* 2002;39(9):843–957. Copyright © 2002 Elsevier. With permission.)

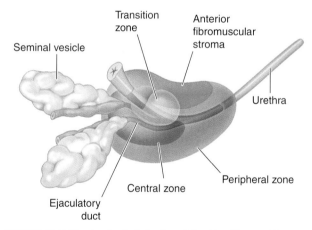

FIGURE 14-6 The drawing illustrates the relationship of the prostate zones to the urethra.

TABLE 14-1	**Prostate Zones**
Zonal Anatomy	**% of Glandular Tissue**
Peripheral zone	70
Central zone	25
Transition zone	5
Periurethral zone	<1

that sweep around the acini. Only about 5% of prostate carcinomas arise within the central zone. Sonographically, the echogenicity of the central zone is normally brighter than that of the peripheral zone.

The transition zone accounts for about 5% of the prostate gland in a young man. It consists of two small lobules found lateral to the proximal urethral segment, and is separated

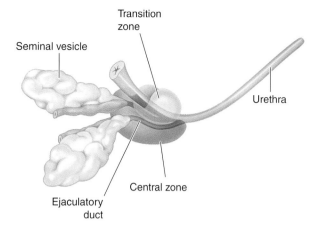

FIGURE 14-7 A drawing of the funnel-shaped central zone illustrates the ejaculatory ducts' entrance into the prostate.

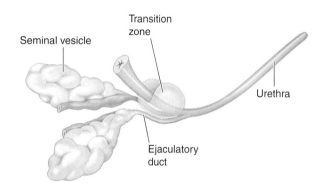

FIGURE 14-8 This drawing depicts the saddlebag-shaped transitional zone and its relationship to the urethra.

laterally and posteriorly from the outer gland by the surgical capsule (Fig. 14-8). It follows the long axis of the urethra toward the bladder neck.[17] The most caudal portion of this zone is at the verumontanum. The acini comprising the transitional zone are similar in appearance to the peripheral zone; however, the stroma is much more compact.[1] Being the most common site of involvement by benign prostatic hyperplasia (BPH), the transition zone may account for a much greater percentage of glandular tissue as men age. Also, because the transitional zone is a common location for BPH, sonographically it becomes more heterogeneous and visible. Approximately 20% of carcinomas occur in this area.[18]

The periurethral glandular tissue composes less than 1% of all prostatic glandular tissue and is embedded in the smooth muscle wall of the urethra. This region runs along most of the prostatic urethral segment.[1] The ducts of this tissue open directly into the urethral lumen. Calculi often occur in this area and are thought to be secondary to reflux of urine into these ducts.

The anterior fibromuscular stroma is a nonglandular region, composed primarily of smooth muscle. It is continuous with fibers of the bladder wall and forms the anterior portion of the prostate.[7,19]

Surrounding Structures

The seminal vesicles are paired saccular structures that lie obliquely and caudally to the prostate. The seminal vesicles are reservoirs for seminal fluid that fluctuate in size and shape secondary to levels of sexual activity. When void of seminal fluid, they appear as curvilinear, hypoechoic structures that flare out laterally. When these structures fill with seminal fluid, they become large, ovoid-shaped cystic structures. Sonographically, low-level echoes are often appreciated within the anechoic fluid.[16,20]

The ampulla of the vasa deferentia are located adjacent and medially to the seminal vesicles. In cross section, they appear as thick-walled, tubular structures. The ejaculatory ducts are formed at the junction of the ampulla of the vasa deferentia and the seminal vesicles. The prostate's posterior surface is anterior to the rectum and is separated by connective tissue called the rectovesical septum. The anterior surface is connected on either side to the pubic bone by the puboprostatic ligaments and is separated by a plexus of veins and fat. The anterior portions of the levator ani muscles cover the lateral surfaces of the prostate.

SONOGRAPHIC EXAMINATION

Indications and Contraindications

Indications for performing a sonographic evaluation of the prostate gland are numerous and continually expanding (Table 14-2). TRUS is widely used for anatomic guidance during systematic prostate biopsy. However, sonography alone is not an effective screening tool owing to a reported sensitivity and specificity of between 40% and 59% in detecting the PCa.[5,21]

TRUS is often utilized in evaluation of patients with an abnormal digital rectal examination (DRE). When a gland feels irregular, sonography is useful in identifying masses, cystic areas, or calcifications. Sonographic characteristics of a disease process may include changes in echogenicity, asymmetry, or distortion of the capsule.[22,23] Sonography may also help in identifying nonpalpable lesions. Newer technologies, such as elastography, high-resolution micro-ultrasound and contrast-enhanced ultrasound (CEUS), have been reported to improve the localization and detection

TABLE 14-2	**Clinical Role of Prostatic Evaluation**

Advantages

1. High-resolution imaging
2. Complements digital rectal examination
3. No ionizing radiation
4. Cost-effective compared with other imaging techniques
5. Dynamic imaging of blood flow

Applications

1. Biopsy guidance
2. Complementary to digital rectal examination

Indications

1. Differentiation of cystic versus solid palpable lesions
2. Abnormal prostate-specific antigen blood test
3. Evaluation of inflammatory process
4. Evaluation of male infertility
5. Guidance during biopsy or other invasive procedures
6. Evaluation of patients with a variety of clinical symptoms related to urination and/or ejaculation

of clinically significant PCa.[4,5,21,24] These modalities are widely available and desirable owing to a relatively low cost, real-time performance, and lack of ionizing radiation. This concept of mp-US, similar to multiparametric MRI, is gaining interest as a promising approach to PCa imaging.[4,5]

Other important uses of sonography include guidance during biopsy and quantification of prostate size. Ultrasound guidance assists in providing a safe and accurate method of obtaining tissue from a focal area of the gland.[25,26] It also allows for accurate biopsy device placement within a specific zone of the prostate.[7]

A patient presenting with abnormal laboratory values and a negative DRE may also undergo sonographic examination. Prostate-specific antigen (PSA) is a protein specific to the prostatic epithelium.[27] The higher the PSA value, the more likely malignancy is present, although it can be elevated in benign processes as well.[27,28] PSA is the most common blood test utilized to identify men at increased risk of prostate cancer. However, using PSA alone as a screening is not recommended and remains controversial.[28–30]

Clinical complaints of hematospermia, painful ejaculation, dysuria, and perineal pain may also warrant a prostate sonography examination.

Prostatitis is one of the most common causes of these symptoms. Sonographically, color or power Doppler imaging will show increased vascularity secondary to hyperemia when prostatitis is present. The gland may also appear enlarged and less echogenic than usual. Prostatitis may appear as a focal or diffuse process. Ultrasound is also used to detect BPH, calculi, ejaculatory duct cysts, congenital cysts, or abscesses. Sonographically, BPH will appear as an enlarged nodular inner gland. The echotexture is heterogeneous, and it can contain cystic areas. Calculi may be visualized and appear as echogenic structures that may create a shadow artifact. Cysts and abscess have a spectrum of sonographic appearances ranging from simple and anechoic to more complex collections of fluids and debris.

Infertility is another indication for TRUS. Male infertility may be related to congenital abnormalities such as agenesis or atresia of the seminal vesicles, or ejaculatory duct obstruction secondary to a cyst, mass, or calcification.[23]

A few contraindications to TRUS do exist. Significant rectal lesions such as fissures, obstructing lesions, thrombosed hemorrhoids, or prostatitis may prevent insertion of the rectal probe owing to patient discomfort.[31] Additionally, patients with these symptoms are at increased risk of bleeding or infection.

Scanning Techniques

In the early 1970s, a transabdominal approach to visualize the prostate through a full bladder was utilized (Fig. 14-9). This offered limited information owing to the limited resolution of low-frequency transducers needed to penetrate deep enough to visualize the prostate gland and owing to incomplete visualization of the entire gland. The endorectal approach provides close anatomic proximity to the pelvic organs utilizing a higher-frequency transducer, which results in improved resolution and visualization.

Before beginning a TRUS, pertinent information should be obtained including DRE and PSA results or clinical symptoms associated with infection or BPH.

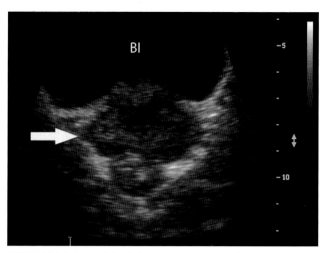

FIGURE 14-9 A transabdominal, transverse sonogram of the prostate (*arrow*). The urinary bladder (*Bl*) was used as an acoustic window to evaluate the gland. Only gross abnormalities were diagnosed using this technique.

TRUS should be performed with the patient's bladder empty to decrease discomfort. The patient is placed in a left lateral decubitus position, with the knees flexed toward the chest similar to the fetal position. The transducer is then properly prepared by placing ultrasound gel within a probe cover, which is then placed over the probe. TRUS probes can be either end-fire or side-fire, and they commonly utilize frequencies of 9 to 12 MHz or higher.[21,32] The transducer is inserted within the rectal cavity (Fig. 14-10). When a biopsy is performed, an injection of 2% lidocaine just lateral to the junction of the prostate base and seminal vesicles, at the neurovascular bundle, will significantly reduce pain.

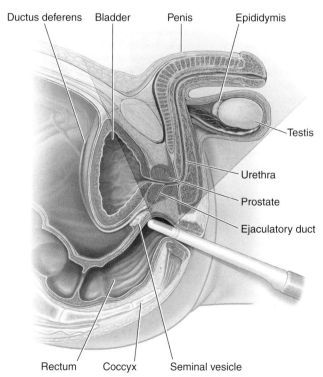

FIGURE 14-10 Scanning technique of the endorectal approach currently used to evaluate the prostate. An endorectal, end-fire transducer is used to acquire transverse and sagittal images of the prostate.

By convention, the orientation of an endorectal scan is slightly different from that of a transabdominal scan and is crucial to understand. The sonography image is inverted so that the near field is at the bottom of the image and the far field is at the top of the image. In the transverse plane, the right lobe of the gland is on the left side of the image and the left lobe of the gland is on the right side of the image. In the sagittal plane, the base of the gland is on the left side of the image and the apex of the gland is on the right side of the image. The rectal wall is in the near field and the urinary bladder is in the far field, with the prostate gland lying between these two structures.

Sonographically, the normal prostate appears as a crescent-shaped structure under the bladder base with an intact capsule. It is symmetrical and surrounds the urethra. Both the shape and echotexture of the prostate should be closely evaluated.

The capsule of the prostate should be smooth and without disruption, and the central gland should be contained within that prostatic capsule. Any disruption of this capsule deserves further exploration for pathology. The internal echo pattern is evaluated by slowly scanning through the gland beginning in a transverse plane at the base of the prostate and moving inferiorly toward the apex. If a lesion is seen within the gland, it is important to discern where the lesion is located.

Images are acquired in a transverse plane of the base, mid, and apical regions of the prostate. The base of the prostate is located superior to the verumontanum and has a half-moon shape (Fig. 14-11A). It has a homogeneous echotexture and should be isoechoic to surrounding tissue. The base of the prostate is predominately made up of the central zone. A hypoechoic arcuate line may be seen within the central portion of the base, which represents the surgical capsule. This demarcates the central gland from the peripheral gland.

The transducer is then moved slightly inferior to the level of the verumontanum, which is seen sonographically as a centrally located shadow (Fig. 14-11B). At this level, the urethra passes through the prostate and more of the central gland can be seen. The central gland appears slightly more hyperechoic than the surrounding peripheral gland. This is the level at which the prostate should be measured in both transverse and anteroposterior dimensions. In patients over age 40 years, the central gland may bulge anteriorly owing to BPH, which may change the prostate shape to an ovoid structure.

Located inferior to the verumontanum is the apex of the prostate (Fig. 14-11C). This section is typically more circular and is predominately made up of the peripheral zone. It appears slightly more heterogeneous than the homogeneous base. Because 70% of all prostate cancers occur in the peripheral zone, this is a common location for malignant lesions.

The transducer is then rotated 90 degrees to a sagittal plane. On a midline sagittal image, the urethra can be followed coursing from the bladder neck, through the prostate gland, and toward the apex (Fig. 14-12A). As the transducer is moved to the left or right, more of the central gland comes into view. At this level, the ejaculatory ducts may be visualized. As the transducer is obliqued further, the peripheral zone comes into view (Fig. 14-12B).

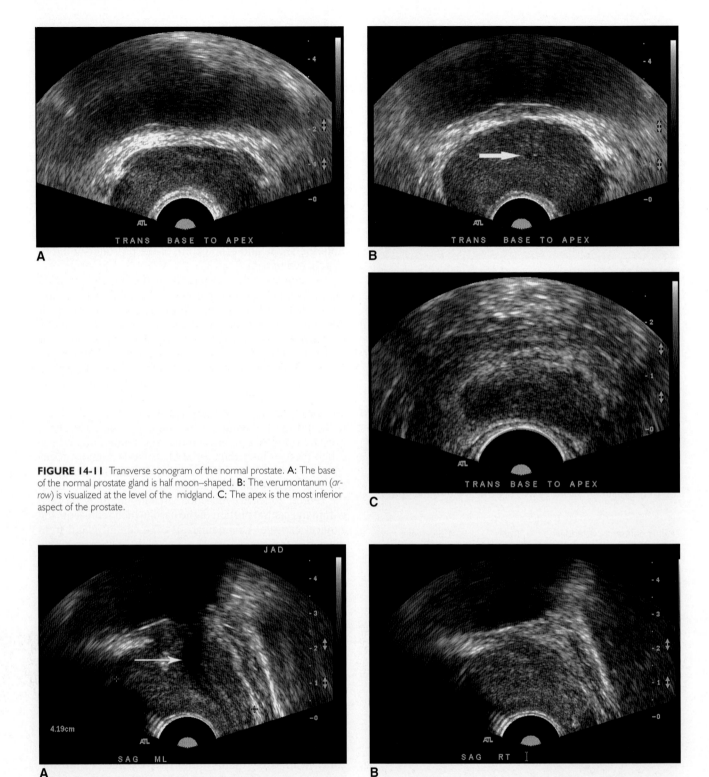

FIGURE 14-11 Transverse sonogram of the normal prostate. **A:** The base of the normal prostate gland is half moon–shaped. **B:** The verumontanum (*arrow*) is visualized at the level of the midgland. **C:** The apex is the most inferior aspect of the prostate.

FIGURE 14-12 Sagittal sonogram of the normal prostate. **A:** The midline section shows the urethra (*arrow*) coursing through the gland. **B:** The right lobe of the prostate can be identified.

The seminal vesicles and vasa deferentia should be imaged in any complete prostate evaluation. These structures are evaluated in both transverse and sagittal planes. The seminal vesicles lay laterally and superior to the base of the prostate. They should appear hypoechoic (Fig. 14-13). If the seminal vesicles appear enlarged, further investigation is required to rule out an obstructive process (Fig. 14-14A, B). The vasa deferentia are visualized in between the seminal vesicles. They are thick-walled and enter the base of the prostate (Fig. 14-15A, B). In a transverse plane, they appear as two donut-shaped structures, and in a sagittal plane, they appear as long tubular structures. The vas deferentia should be free of fluid in the normal setting.

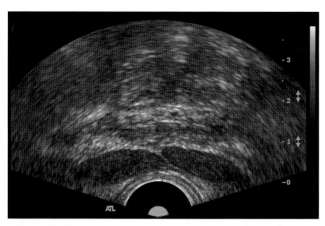

FIGURE 14-13 A transverse section demonstrates the normal seminal vesicles.

When imaging the prostate in a transverse plane, two groups of blood vessels, the periurethral and the capsular vessels, should be visualized. The periurethral vessels will be seen within the center of the prostate gland at the level of the verumontanum (Fig. 14-16). At the level of the urethra, large vessels will be seen coursing from the apex of the prostate following the urethra up toward the bladder neck. It is not unusual to see an increased amount of blood flow in this region. Color or power Doppler imaging will show capsular vessels penetrating into the parenchyma of the gland (Fig. 14-17A, B). The vessels within the gland travel in a linear progression toward the center of the gland.

Color or power Doppler imaging should also be utilized to identify signs of hyperemia either diffusely or focally within the prostate gland or increased vascularity to an identified lesion (Fig. 14-18A, B). Low flow settings and light probe pressure should be used for optimal scanning technique.

More advanced technologies such as MicroFlow Imaging (MFI) are useful in visualizing small vessels and slow blood flow signals without using contrast agents.[5]

CYSTS OF THE MALE PELVIS

Cysts arising in the male pelvis are extremely rare.[33] Patients can present with complex and perplexing clinical symptoms, ranging from urinary retention to perineal pain. There is controversy in the classification and origin of these cysts owing to the close proximity of the vasa deferentia, seminal vesicles, ejaculatory ducts, and prostate, as well as their complex embryologic development.[34]

Sonography is useful in identifying the location of a cyst and its relationship to the prostate. It also offers information about the internal characteristics of the cyst itself. Several different cystic structures may occur in the prostate, seminal vesicles, and vas deferens, including müllerian duct cysts, utricle cysts, seminal vesicle cysts, prostatic cysts, or cysts of the ejaculatory ducts or vas deferens[34] (Fig. 14-19).

Müllerian Duct and Utricle Cysts

Müllerian duct and utricle cysts are the most common type of pelvic cysts. These two cystic lesions are often discussed together because of their almost identical locations. There are, however, embryologic differences and clinical findings that suggest these lesions should be considered separately.[17,35]

Müllerian duct cysts are mesodermal in origin and arise from embryonic remnants. They occur because of failure of regression of the müllerian duct structures.[34,35] In contrast to utricle cysts, genital anomalies are not associated with true müllerian duct cysts. Unilateral renal agenesis, however, may occur. These cysts are mainly midline but may extend laterally above the base of the prostate and found between the bladder and the rectum. They are attached to the prostate

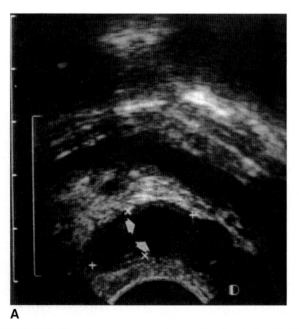
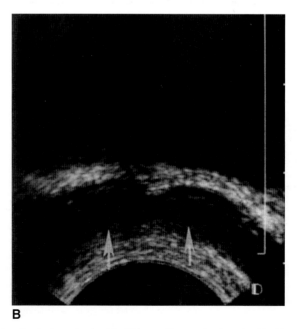

A **B**

FIGURE 14-14 **A:** The transverse sonogram shows a dilated seminal vesicle. This patient had not ejaculated for 72 hours. The saccules (*arrowheads*) of the seminal vesicle are easily appreciated when it is dilated. Distance + = 22.0 mm; distance × = 8.9 mm. **B:** On this transverse sonogram through the base of the prostate, a dilated vasa deferentia (*arrows*) is seen. (Images courtesy of Diasonics, Santa Clara, CA.)

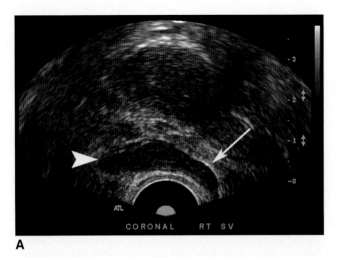

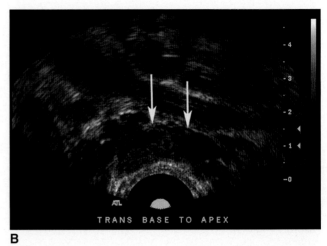

FIGURE 14-15 A transverse sonogram showing normal and abnormal vasa deferentia. **A:** A normal seminal vesicle (*arrowhead*) and a medially located vas deferens (*arrow*). **B:** On this transverse sonogram through the base of the prostate, the dilated vasa deferentia (*arrows*) are seen.

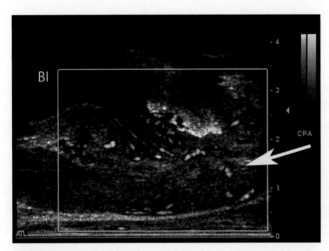

FIGURE 14-16 A sagittal, midline sonogram of the prostate gland demonstrates the periurethral vessels displayed by power Doppler image. The vessels travel along the course of the urethra through the transition zone from the bladder (*Bl*) toward the apex (*arrow*). (Image courtesy of Philips Medical Systems, Bothell, WA.)

by a stalk-like structure extending into the prostate. Patients with müllerian duct cysts will typically present with partial urinary obstruction, hematospermia, low ejaculate volume, infertility, painful ejaculation, and rectal discomfort.[34] Sonographically, these cysts appear slightly lateral from midline and superior to the base of the prostate gland (Fig. 14-20A, B). A müllerian duct cyst does not connect with the urethra or with the seminal vesicle. It is anechoic and may contain debris or calcifications. They can be very large and usually have smooth, regular borders. When aspirated, the fluid may be brownish-red and will not contain spermatozoa. This is because the müllerian system does not communicate with the wolffian duct; therefore, there is no contact between these cysts and the vasa deferentia or seminal vesicles.[34]

A utricle cyst is endodermal in origin and is usually associated with hypospadias, undescended testicles, and renal anamolies.[36] These cysts occur when the prostatic utricle is dilated. They are located directly midline and close to the verumontanum.[35] These cysts are typically smaller in size than müllerian duct cysts. Sonographically, utricle cysts appear midline and are seen at the level of the verumontanum

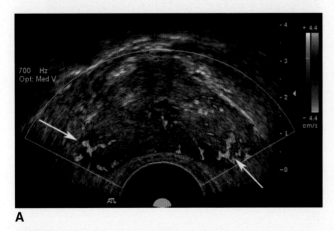

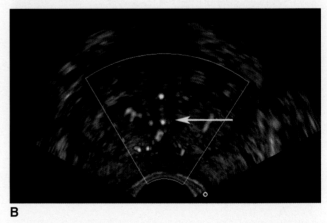

FIGURE 14-17 **A:** A transverse sonogram demonstrates the capsular vessels shown in red (*arrows*), as displayed by color Doppler image. These vessels travel throughout the capsule of the gland. **B:** On this transverse sonogram of the prostate gland, the periurethral vessel (*arrow*) is displayed by power Doppler image. (Images courtesy of Philips Medical Systems, Bothell, WA.)

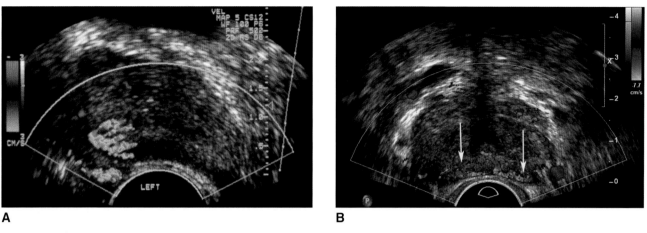

A **B**

FIGURE 14-18 **A:** A sagittal sonogram of the left prostate gland showing increased vascularity in an area of a suspicious lesion. **B:** A transverse image demonstrating abnormal peripheral zone vascularity displayed by color Doppler image (*arrows*). (Images courtesy of Philips Medical Systems, Bothell, WA.)

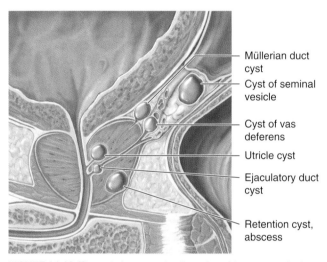

Müllerian duct cyst

Cyst of seminal vesicle

Cyst of vas deferens

Utricle cyst

Ejaculatory duct cyst

Retention cyst, abscess

FIGURE 14-19 The sagittal cross section illustration of the prostate gland shows typical locations of various cystic lesions of the prostate gland, seminal vesicle, and vas deferens.

(Fig. 14-21A, B). Utricle cysts may contain calcifications. White or brown fluid is usually aspirated and may contain spermatozoa.

Seminal Vesicle Cyst

Seminal vesicle cysts are uncommon, occurring in less than 0.005% of the male population.[37,38] Over two-thirds of reported cases are associated with ipsilateral renal agenesis.[34] This is explained embryologically by the close proximity of the abnormally developing vesicle and ureteral buds from the mesonephric duct.[39] If a seminal vesicle cyst is noted on a sonogram, both kidneys should be imaged. Sonographically, these cysts typically appear as paramedian anechoic structures (Fig. 14-22). They are smaller than müllerian duct cysts and are located more laterally. Sometimes, the functioning contralateral seminal vesicle may be enlarged.[40] When a seminal vesicle cyst is aspirated, spermatozoa are typically found, helping to differentiate it from other types of cysts.

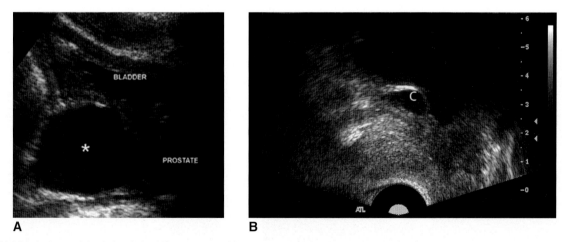

A **B**

FIGURE 14-20 **A:** A transabdominal sagittal, midline sonogram of the prostate gland demonstrates a müllerian duct cyst as a large midline cystic structure (*asterisk*) superior to the base of the prostate. **B:** This is a different patient with a müllerian duct cyst (C). The aspirated fluid of this cyst was brownish-red, but contained no spermatozoa.

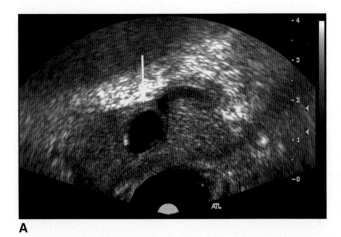

A

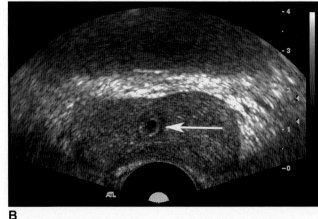

B

FIGURE 14-21 A: A transverse prostate sonogram at the level of the verumontanum shows a midline utricle cyst (*arrow*) with calcifications within the wall of the lesion. The patient presented with the characteristic postvoid dribbling. **B:** Another utricle cyst (*arrow*) is seen in this transverse prostate sonogram. This image demonstrates the characteristic location of this cyst.

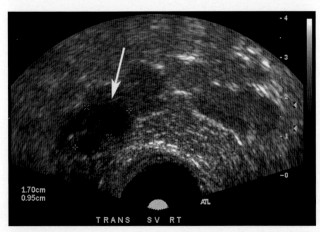

FIGURE 14-22 A transverse sonogram showing multiple seminal vesicle cysts as paramedian, anechoic structures (*arrow*).

Prostatic Cyst

There are several different types of cysts within the prostate that fall into this category. These cysts may be congenital or acquired. A retention or inclusion cyst is an acquired cyst of the prostate. It results from occlusion of a prostatic duct, causing dilatation of the glandular acini.[34] These cysts are small in size, usually 1 to 2 cm, and typically are not clinically significant. They may occur in any of the three glandular zones. Sonographically, retention cysts are simple, smooth-walled, and appear completely anechoic (Fig. 14-23A, B). They do not contain spermatozoa when aspirated.[34]

Cystic changes can be seen in the transition zone owing to BPH. These cysts are by far the most common, because BPH is a common disorder in the older male population. They occur within the hyperplastic nodules and are usually very small (Fig. 14-24). These cysts are asymptomatic, although the conditions they are seen with may cause multiple problems discussed later in this chapter.

There are other cystic lesions of the prostate that are extremely rare. Parasitic cysts, for example, result from secondary spread of echinococcus, or bilharzias, and are typically seen in males living in a region in which these parasites are endemic. Cysts may also be seen in association with carcinoma owing to a degenerative process.[34]

Prostatic Abscess

A prostatic abscess is associated with acute bacterial prostatitis, but it can also be seen in diabetic male patients. Early recognition is important, although it can be difficult to distinguish

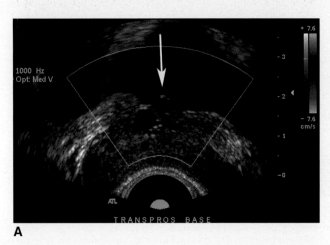

A

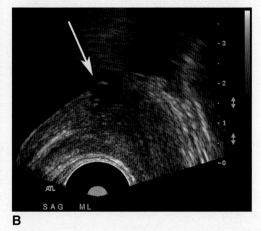

B

FIGURE 14-23 A: On a transverse sonogram of the prostate, multiple small retention cysts are seen within the base of the gland (*arrow*). **B:** A sagittal sonogram of the midline shows retention cysts (*arrow*) in the anterior section of an asymptomatic patient. This is characteristic of a retention cyst.

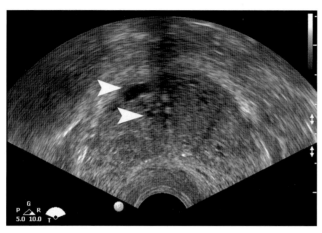

FIGURE 14-24 On a transverse sonogram, cystic changes (*arrowheads*) are seen within the hyperplastic nodules in a patient with benign prostatic hyperplasia. (Image courtesy of Philips Medical Systems, Bothell, WA.)

acute prostatitis from an abscess clinically. Symptoms are similar, including fever, chills, urinary frequency, urgency, perineal/low back pain, dysuria, and hematuria. Sonographic findings include focal or diffuse complex areas occurring in any part of the prostate gland.[2] These findings in a patient with the appropriate clinical findings are suspicious for an abscess. As mentioned previously, color or power Doppler imaging may show hyperemic blood flow. The diagnosis is confirmed by aspiration and microscopic evaluation of the fluid and is treated with antibiotics.

Diverticulum of the Ejaculatory Duct of Vas Deferens

A diverticulum or cyst of the ejaculatory duct or vas deferens can occur owing to a distal obstruction of the spermatic ductal system by a congenital abnormality or inflammation.[34] These lesions may be mistaken for seminal vesicle cysts; however, sonographic visualization of normal seminal vesicles can distinguish the two. Large ejaculatory duct diverticula are associated with perineal pain, dysuria, hematospermia, and ejaculatory pain.[20] These cystic structures are typically seen between the base of the prostate and the seminal vesicles, and they can occur along the ejaculatory duct course. If large, they may be confused with a müllerian duct or utricle cyst. Ejaculatory duct cysts can contain calculi, which can result in the seminal vesicle on the affected side becoming dilated.[20] Aspiration of these cysts will yield spermatozoa, proving that it does communicate with the spermatic system, which is typically not the case with a utricle or müllerian duct cyst.

BENIGN PROSTATIC HYPERPLASIA

BPH is the most common symptomatic tumor-like condition in the male population. It is a diffuse, nodular enlargement within the transition zone of the prostate. The cause is not well understood but is thought to be related to hormonal changes owing to the aging process. This condition is rarely seen in men under the age of 30 but is commonly seen in men over the age of 40 years and peaks around the age of 60 years.[2] BPH is exclusively a disease of the preprostatic region.[17] The nodules typically arise from the transition zone,

with some arising from the periurethral zone. Because the urethra passes through this zone, these patients typically present with urinary symptoms (Fig. 14-25). BPH acts as an obstructive process to the flow of urine. Symptoms include frequency, nocturia, dribbling, and difficulty starting a stream. On rectal examination, the prostate feels soft, boggy, and nodular. Sonographically, BPH shows enlargement of the central gland in an anteroposterior direction[7] (Fig. 14-26). This can be either symmetric or asymmetric in appearance, with the latter being more concerning for malignant changes. In contrast to a normal gland, the prostate no longer has a crescent shape but appears more rounded and can be up to four times its original size (Fig. 14-27A, B). There are three primary types of BPH:

- homogeneous stromal hyperplasia, which is sonographically hypoechoic;
- glandular hyperplasia, which may look hypoechoic or hyperechoic, depending on the cystic changes and gland size; and
- a combination of both types, resulting in a stromal and glandular hyperplasia; this form is the most common and is heterogeneous in appearance.[41]

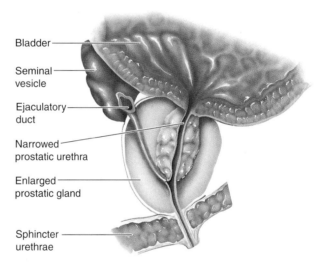

FIGURE 14-25 This illustration demonstrates the passing of the urethra through the prostate and how benign prostatic hyperplasia distorts the pathway. (Asset provided by Anatomical Chart Co., Philadelphia, PA.)

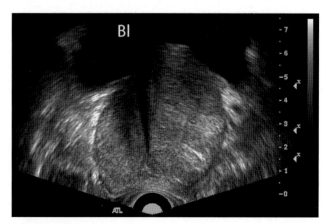

FIGURE 14-26 A transverse sonogram on a 57-year-old patient with frequency and nocturia owing to benign prostatic hyperplasia demonstrated the central gland as significantly enlarged pushing into the bladder (*Bl*).

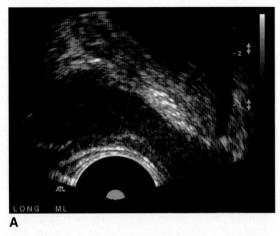
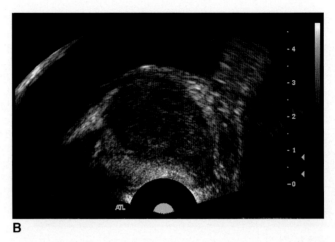

A   **B**

FIGURE 14-27 The two images demonstrate the contrast between a young, healthy prostate and a prostate affected by benign prostatic hyperplasia. Both sonograms are of the midgland. **A:** A 22-year-old patient with a normal, crescent-shaped gland. **B:** A 52-year-old with benign prostatic hyperplasia. Notice how the gland is more rounded in comparison.

As BPH develops, the peripheral gland becomes compressed, making it difficult to evaluate. When BPH is present, the central gland is often easier to visualize with sonography because as the disease develops, the glandular tissue becomes increasingly heterogeneous, thus differentiating it from the homogeneous peripheral zone.[23] This heterogeneous pattern is a result of the multiple interfaces between the stromal and glandular tissues of the hyperplastic central gland. In this setting, an increased stiffness of the gland may be appreciated on shear wave elastography (SWE).[7] BPH is commonly found when performing TRUS on men over the age of 40 years.

Transurethral resection of the prostate (TURP) is done to relieve the symptoms caused by compression of the prostatic urethra. Using a cystoscope, a surgeon removes the excess tissue, thus creating a large defect at the level of the bladder. The TURP defect, when seen sonographically, can be dramatic (Fig. 14-28).

PROSTATE CALCIFICATIONS

Prostatic calculi are frequently encountered in urologic practice and their presence is usually reported as an incidental finding. The exact incidence of these calculi is unknown because most are small, asymptomatic, and difficult to detect by DRE.[42] They are extremely common but rarely give rise to symptoms. However, the conditions they are associated with may cause symptoms. Prostate calculi can be classified into two groups: endogenous and exogenous. Endogenous calculi are found within the substance of the prostate and form from prostatic fluid. Exogenous calculi are found in the urethra and are derived primarily from urine.[43]

Endogenous calculi are the true prostatic stones. One of the most common causes of endogenous calculi is the consolidation and calcification of the corpora amylacea, which normally occurs with age. Corpora amylacea are a result of the prostatic acini progressing through their cycle of cell atrophy, degeneration, and death. This occurs most often in the posterior segment and along the surgical capsule.

Any pathologic process, such as BPH or prostatitis, can cause endogenous calculi. Inflammation of the gland can cause an imbalance of pH levels in the prostatic secretions.[44] This disrupts the calcium citrate acid balance and causes the condensation of calcium salts onto already formed small stones and corpora amylacea. As these stones get bigger, they block the ducts, causing a stasis of secretions within the ducts. This stasis results in additional stone formation, leading to the multiple calculi seen in patients with chronic prostatitis.[44] The association of calculi with BPH can also be explained by this process.[42] As nodular hyperplasia develops, the acini of the prostate may become obstructed resulting in stasis of secretions.

Sonographically, calculi are easily appreciated (Fig. 14-29). They occur within the parenchyma of the gland and range in size from very small to very large, some becoming as big as 3 cm or more.[44] They are often associated with distal acoustic shadowing and color Doppler artifact. Additionally, they may appear in clusters or alone. These stones are different in location and sonographic appearance from those that occur within the ejaculatory ducts or urethra.

Ejaculatory duct calcifications are often seen during a TRUS (Fig. 14-30). They can be an incidental finding or cause symptoms such as hematospermia or painful ejaculation. They develop for reasons similar to prostate calculi. If a cystic lesion or inflammation obstructs the ejaculatory

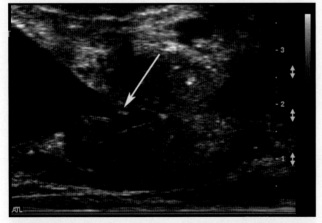

FIGURE 14-28 This 65-year-old has a transurethral resection defect. The central gland has been removed (*arrow*), distorting the typical appearance of the mid gland. (Image courtesy of Philips Medical Systems, Bothell, WA.)

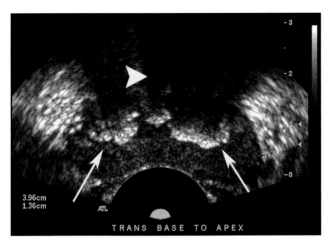

FIGURE 14-29 A transverse sonogram, numerous endogenous prostatic calculi (*arrows*) are seen along the surgical capsule of this midgland sonogram. Characteristic acoustic shadowing is present (*arrowhead*).

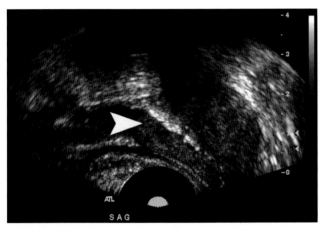

FIGURE 14-30 A sagittal sonogram with calculi (*arrowhead*) is identified lining the ejaculatory duct. These calculi provide for excellent viewing of the course of the ejaculatory duct.

ducts, stasis may occur, resulting in the concretion and calcification of fluid. Hematospermia and painful ejaculations result because of the passage of these stones. On a sonogram, these calcifications can be seen lining the ejaculatory duct. They are best appreciated in a sagittal plane and may help to visualize the sometimes difficult-to-image ejaculatory ducts. They may or may not cause an acoustic shadow.

Periurethral calcifications involve the urethra, which passes through the prostate. They are exogenous calculi and are derived primarily from urine. Periurethral calculi outline the course of the urethra and are particularly well seen on midline images.

PROSTATITIS

Prostatitis is a poorly understood condition that is difficult to diagnose both clinically and sonographically. It is a broad term used to describe inflammation of the prostate and sometimes the surrounding areas.[45,46] Many men are often diagnosed incorrectly with this condition owing to confusion in the literature regarding its pathogenesis, diagnosis, and treatment. Much of the confusion lies in the variety of organisms that may infect the prostate and the vague symptoms the patient may present with. The clinical diagnosis of prostatitis is made by an evaluation of expressed prostatic secretion (EPS) for either positive bacterial cultures or inflammatory cells. The National Institutes of Health (NIH) lists four categories of prostatitis: acute bacterial, chronic bacterial, chronic abacterial/CPPS (including inflammatory and noninflammatory disease), and asymptomatic prostatitis.[47] This classification system is based on a complex clinical and pathologic assessment[45–48] (Pathology Box 14-1).

Acute Bacterial Prostatitis

The presentation of acute bacterial prostatitis is unique, and the diagnosis is usually straightforward. Patients are typically acutely ill, with a fever, and severe lower urinary tract symptoms (LUTS). The disease is associated with large numbers of gram-negative bacteria present within the urine, which reflux into the intraprostatic ducts.[45,49] This form of prostatitis is easily diagnosed by a urine test. At the time of the DRE, the prostate will feel hard and swollen and is often very tender. Typically, a vigorous examination is contraindicated because it can precipitate bacteremia.[50] Therapy usually consists of a series of bactericidal antibiotics and palliative care.

Chronic Bacterial Prostatitis

Chronic bacterial prostatitis may be difficult to diagnose and treat owing to the wide variety of clinical presentations. The same organisms cause the acute form, yet these patients have not necessarily had an episode of acute bacterial prostatitis. Common complaints include discomfort in the penis, scrotum, and perineum, with irritative voiding symptoms such as dysuria, urgency, and frequency. This disease is characterized by relapsing urinary tract infections, even after appropriate treatment.[45,51] Quite often, physical examination will disclose no findings.

Chronic Abacterial Prostatitis/Chronic Pelvic Pain Syndrome

Chronic abacterial prostatitis/chronic pelvic pain syndrome (CP/CPPS) is an inflammation of the prostate of unknown

PATHOLOGY BOX 14-1
Classification of Prostatitis

	Perineal Pain	EPS	Leukocytes (Urine)
Acute bacterial	+	+	+
Chronic bacterial	±	+	+
Chronic abacterial/ CPPS			
Inflammatory	±	+	±
Noninflammatory	±	0	0
Asymptomatic	0	+	0

CPPS, chronic pelvic pain syndrome; EPS, expressed prostatic secretion.

etiology and has an incidence eight times higher than that of bacterial prostatitis.[50] Studies suggest the causes can include the following: a nanobacteria not detected by conventional cultures, elevated prostatic pressures, and voiding dysfunction.[45,50] The clinical symptoms are like those observed in patients with bacterial prostatitis. Patients afflicted with CP/CPPS are difficult to manage because an infectious process is not easily detected, and there is usually no history of urinary tract infections. Inflammatory and noninflammatory subtypes are differentiated by the presence or absence of inflammatory cells in EPS.

Noninflammatory CPPS is typically seen in young to middle-aged men, who experience abnormal or irritative urinary flow and lower back and perineum pain. It has been demonstrated that spasms and narrowing of the prostatic urethra owing to neuromuscular dysfunction are responsible for these symptoms.[49,52] Stress is also thought to play a primary role in the etiology of noninflammatory CPPS.

Asymptomatic Prostatitis

Patients with asymptomatic inflammatory prostatitis are, as the name implies, asymptomatic for prostatitis. However, clinically they appear to have an inflammatory disease. There is no evidence of bacterial infection or leukocytes in the EPS and the DRE is normal. Infection is usually found in cells from a prostate biopsy or during evaluation for other disorders.[45,49] Because the patient is asymptomatic, therapy is warranted only if there is an underlying problem.[50] Alternatively, interest is growing in the theory that inflammation may be a precursor to cancer, and treatment has shown to decrease PCa risks.[45]

Sonographic Findings of Prostatitis

The role of sonography is to differentiate between patients with a genuine inflammation of the gland versus patients with symptoms but no signs of inflammation. Understanding the pathogenesis of this disease helps in making a sonographic diagnosis. The prostate is infected by the ascent of organisms from the lower urethra. Once organisms gain access to the lower prostatic urethra, there is easy access to the ducts of the peripheral zone. Any increase in intraurethral pressure will encourage reflux of urine and organisms into these ducts. Typically, the central zone ducts are not invaded because their oblique entry into the urethra acts like a valve.[51] This accounts for the greater incidence of prostatitis within the peripheral zone.

The sonographic evaluation of patients with symptoms of prostatitis should include grayscale and color Doppler imaging. Grayscale findings are sometimes helpful but not always definitive. One of the most common findings is a hypoechoic halo in the periurethral area.[52] This should not be confused with the cylindrical smooth muscle of the preprostatic sphincter found at the base of the prostate. Another frequent finding is a heterogeneous echo pattern of the peripheral gland with capsular thickening and or irregularity (Fig. 14-31A, B). This pattern is most often seen in chronic cases of prostatitis. It is caused by areas of scarring and necrosis caused by previous episodes of inflammation. It is also important, when evaluating these patients, to rule out the presence of an abscess because that would require more immediate treatment. Fortunately, these lesions are rare but can occur during an acute episode or in diabetic patients.[45,49] The sonographic findings of an abscess include focal hypoechoic or anechoic lesions with a thickened wall and/or septations. The sonography examination often causes extreme discomfort for the patient, specifically when scanning the area containing the abscess.

Calculi may be visualized within the gland of a patient with chronic prostatitis. These calculi may be a result of an inflammatory reaction or part of the pathogenesis of the disease, which includes the reflux of urine, as well as organisms, into the prostatic ducts. It has been suggested in the literature that the presence of prostatic calculi may be the cause of recurrent bouts of prostatitis.[53] The calculi may harbor the bacteria that cause prostatitis, making it impossible for antibiotic therapy to be effective.

Color or power Doppler imaging may be useful in detecting a hyperemic flow pattern often associated with infection and abscess. Hyperemia may be diffuse or focal (Fig. 14-32A, B). However, it should be borne in mind that increased blood flow is not specific to inflammatory lesions.

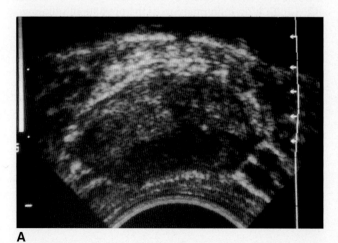
A

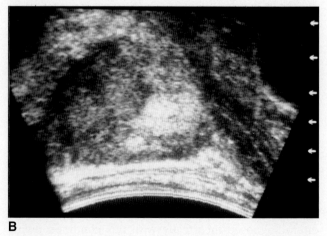
B

FIGURE 14-31 Sonograms of the midgland were obtained on patients with acute prostatitis. **A:** A transverse image showing the heterogeneous echo texture of the peripheral gland. **B:** A sagittal image of the left prostate gland on a patient with known prostatitis.

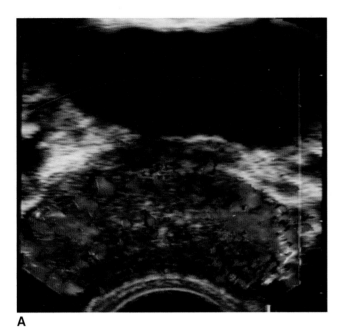 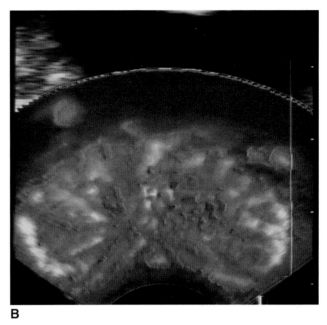

A **B**

FIGURE 14-32 Transverse sonograms of the midgland were obtained on a 32-year-old with acute prostatitis. **A:** Multiple vessels are seen in the peripheral gland, displayed by color Doppler imaging. **B:** Large parenchymal vessels are seen using power Doppler imaging.

PROSTATE CANCER

PCa is the second most common and fifth most aggressive neoplasm among men worldwide.[10,12,14,54] It is estimated that one in seven men will be diagnosed with PCa in their lifetime.[54] A few risk factors have been identified, including being of African descent, which is the most common, as well as genetics and obesity.[10,12,54] One study performed by Carter et al,[56] evaluating prostate autopsy data, found that 20% of men in the sixth decade of life and 50% of men in the eighth decade of life had histologic evidence of prostate cancer.[57] According to the NIH's Surveillance, Epidemiology, and End Results study, approximately 75% of all prostate cancers are detected by an abnormal PSA.[58] Owing to a high rate of false positives, overdiagnosis, and overtreatment, PSA testing recommendations have become more conservative.[59,60] The United States Preventive Task Force (USPSTF) recommended in 2012 against routine PSA screening for PCa in all men.[28,29] Individual screening in targeted populations at high risk for PCa and males over 50 years old who desire screening is now recommended.[61] The PSA can be reported in several different forms: total, age-adjusted, density, velocity, and free with respective charts and guidelines for each test. Typically, a value greater than 4 to 10 ng/mL is considered borderline with a 25% risk for PCa, and a value greater than 10 ng/mL is associated with a greater than 50% risk.[54] More sophisticated screening systems are currently being studied.

The usefulness of early diagnosis of PCa and achieving substantial improvements in patient morbidity and mortality rates remain to be demonstrated. That is why controversy exists in the literature regarding the utility of screening, early detection, and overtreatment of this cancer.[28,54,55] The diagnosis of early-stage PCa may cause less harm than in the past because these cancers are now commonly managed with active surveillance, and they are not thought to benefit from immediate treatment.

Most patients referred for TRUS for PCa present with either a bladder outlet obstruction, an abnormal PSA level, or an abnormal DRE. Other symptoms include bone pain, weakness, weight loss, anemia, and azotemia.[62]

DRE was previously considered the gold standard for screening of prostate cancer, but it was found to be very subjective and missed 44% to 59% of cancers.[63] PSA has become the primary test for identifying patients at increased risk of prostate cancer. However, it can be elevated in BPH and prostatitis as well.[27,63,64] Therefore, definitive diagnosis relies on sonography-guided systematic biopsy, the current gold standard.[55] In conjunction with clinical findings, TRUS can be a valuable tool and can serve as an important adjunct to the management of prostate cancer.[63-65]

Sonographic Evaluation

TRUS offers an evaluation of the zonal anatomy and sites through which extracapsular extension (ECE) can occur.[66] Eighty percent of cancers originate in the outer gland (peripheral and central zones) and 20% originate in the inner gland (periurethral and transitional zones).[31] The surgical capsule defines the plane between the inner and outer glands. PCa behaves differently in each anatomic zone and is thought to be related to its embryologic derivitative.[14] Although cancer of the prostate may have a variety of appearances, classically it presents as a hypoechoic lesion.[23,31] Adenocarcinoma is the most commonly diagnosed PCa with a vast majority arising from the peripheral zone.[67] Approximately 85% of prostate adenocarcinomas are multifocal in origin, as opposed to a solitary discrete mass.[67] Sonographically, it is not uncommon for adenocarcinoma to appear isoechoic to surrounding prostate tissue. Therefore, TRUS alone has a predictive value of only 6% for PCa diagnosis.

There are several anatomic weaknesses of this gland that result in ECE.[67] The first is within the prostatic capsule of the peripheral zone. Most tumors tend to grow along the prostatic capsule in an oblong fashion.[68] These tumors can easily extend into the subcapsular space. Another area is the trapezoid area, which is located inferior to the apex of the prostate, posterior to the urethra, and anterior to the rectal sphincter. The capsule of the apex can be very thin or absent and provides an excellent escape from the peripheral zone into the trapezoid area. Seventy-five percent of all tumors occur within 3 to 6 mm of the apex, making this a popular tumor location. The seminal vesicle "beak" sign may be visualized when an anatomic weakness occurs in the central zone (Fig. 14-33). This is a defect in the prostatic capsule that occurs where the vas deferens and seminal vesicle enter the central zone to form the ejaculatory duct. This defect provides another potential pathway for tumor extension. On a sagittal sonographic image, this defect looks like a bird's beak. The invaginated extraprostatic space is another weakness of the central zone. This is the location where the vascular-lymphatic channels invaginate the capsule and follow the ejaculatory duct to the verumontanum (Fig. 14-34). This space is in direct contact with glandular tissue of the central gland, offering another pathway for tumor spread. The final anatomic weakness of the central zone is a defect of the prostatic capsule at the bladder neck. Tumor may escape from the junction of the bladder neck and the central zone.

A sonography-guided biopsy is recommended if a lesion is seen near any of the aforementioned anatomic weaknesses. SWE has a high sensitivity and specificity compared with TRUS in tumor characterization and surgical margins. This modality displays elasticity values taken from a region of interest (ROI) and displayed in kPa or in m/sec. PCa usually appears stiffer than the surrounding tissue and can be targeted during biopsy. The capsule exhibits a soft rim artifact, which can be lost with ECE.[21,60]

Origins and Characterizations

The peripheral zone is the location of origin of 70% of prostate cancers[31] (Fig. 14-35). They can be multifocal and are typically in direct contact or close to the capsule. Most

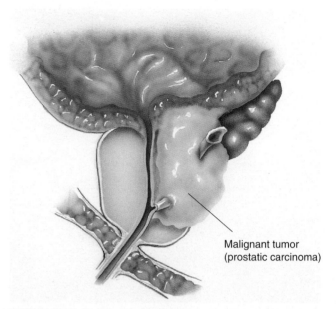

Malignant tumor
(prostatic carcinoma)

FIGURE 14-34 Prostate cancer is the second most common malignant tumor in men. This disease is complicated by the transfer of cancer cells directly to other parts of the body through a plexus of veins. (Reprinted with permission from the Anatomical Chart Company.)

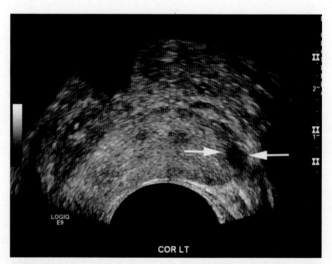

FIGURE 14-35 Prostate cancer. This image of the prostate reveals a small hypoechoic mass (between *arrows*) in the peripheral zone, which was eventually diagnosed as prostate cancer. (Reprinted with permission from Sanders RC, Hall-Terracciano B. *Clinical Sonography: A Practical Guide*. 5th ed. Wolters Kluwer; 2015: Figure 55-8.)

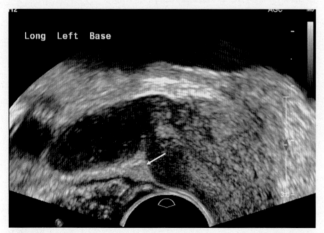

FIGURE 14-33 A sagittal sonogram of a normal prostate demonstrates the "beak" (*arrow*) where the seminal vesicle and vas deferens enter the central zone. (Reprinted with permission from Shirkhoda A. *Variants and Pitfalls in Body Imaging: Thoracic, Abdominal and Women's Imaging*. 2nd ed. Wolters Kluwer Health/Lippincott Williams & Wilkins; 2010:615.)

of these cancers involve the apex of the prostate because this is the location of the greatest portion of peripheral glandular tissue. Tumors within the peripheral zone can easily spread to the central zone because of the weak interface separating these two zones. The central zone is the site of origin for 1% to 5% of prostate cancers, likely owing to its wolffian duct origin. Cancer may spread to the ejaculatory ducts via the invaginated extraprostatic space. When the ejaculatory ducts are involved, a "halo" sign may be seen on transverse images caused by the surrounding tumor. Tumor may also cause a partial obstruction of the duct, resulting in a dilated seminal vesicle. The remaining 20% of cancers originate in the transitional zone. Cancers of the transition zone commonly arise circumferentially in proximity to the anterior fibromuscular stroma and are most often discovered during a TURP.[41] They can originate in either glandular acini or within a hyperplastic nodule. Tumors originating within the glandular acini arise medially, frequently invading the anterior fibromuscular stroma. These tumors tend to remain within the inner prostate gland until they become quite large. Tumors arising from a hyperplastic nodule tend to remain encapsulated. Localized asymmetry and a hypoechoic lesion within the transition zone are highly suspicious.[41]

Attempts have been made to categorize PCa by a specific sonographic characteristic. Most (Fig. 14-36A–C) malignant lesions contain fewer sonographically detected interfaces and thus appear hypoechoic, but they can be variable in appearance.[10,68] Most cancers undergo morphologic changes, such as increased cellular density, increased mircovascularity, and loss of glandular architecture, rendering them stiffer than the surrounding normal tissue.[21,60] However, all cancers are not stiff and all stiff lesions are not cancer.[60] If the lesion is small, it may appear isoechoic with the surrounding tissue. SWE and CEUS can be used to identify abnormal foci not visible on grayscale or Doppler imaging and represent a promising approach to PCa imaging.[4,59,60] Alternatively, large, diffuse tumors can go sonographically undetected because of total replacement of the gland. The difficulty in evaluating a diffuse lesion is that there is no normal tissue for comparison.

It is important to keep in mind that a hypoechoic lesion is not always specific for cancer. In fact, the majority of suspicious hypoechoic areas within the peripheral zone result from benign causes.[31,67,68] These include inflammation, fibrosis, infarction, smooth muscle surrounding the ejaculatory ducts, BPH, atrophy, and lymphoma. Other factors also hinder the specificity of sonography, including the location of the tumor, the presence or absence of an interface with surrounding benign tissue, and BPH. Thus, although sonography is useful in certain cases, it will not detect most cases of prostate cancer. Using a mp-US approach, beginning with B-mode TRUS and color Doppler imaging, then adding techniques like MicroFlow imaging (MFI), SWE, and CEUS can increase detection rates of clinically significant PCa compared with utilizing only a single US modality.[4] If a suspicious lesion is seen sonographically, further evaluation by biopsy is warranted (Fig. 14-37).

BIOPSY GUIDANCE PROCEDURES

Sonography is used almost universally for guidance during biopsy of the prostate gland[23] (Fig. 14-38A, B). Ultrasound guidance offers safe and accurate placement of the biopsy needle to obtain a tissue sample from the prostate whether it be a systematic biopsy or a lesion-specific biopsy.

Ultrasound-guided biopsies of the prostate were first described in the early 1980s using a transperineal approach. Currently, the endorectal approach is the method of choice and performed on an outpatient basis. Both techniques are safe, accurate, and only mildly uncomfortable when certain precautions are taken to correctly perform the examination. Periprostatic nerve block is the most common and popular method of anesthesia, as well as the use of lidocaine gel.[69]

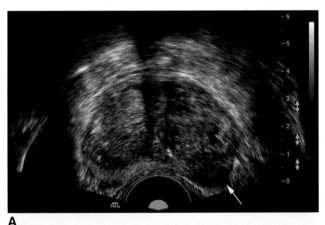

A

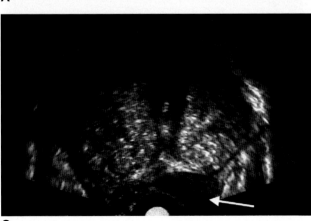

C

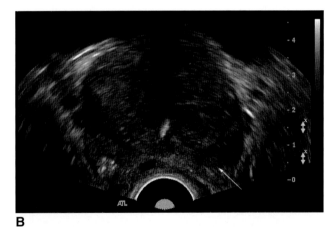

B

FIGURE 14-36 A: A transverse sonogram of the prostate gland is obtained at the level of the verumontanum. The hypoechoic lesion (*arrow*) is seen within the peripheral zone on the left side of the gland. **B:** This sonogram is of a hypoechoic malignant lesion (*arrow*) within the prostate. **C:** A classic hypoechoic malignant lesion (*arrow*) is seen on this sonogram. This was a histologically proven cancer. (**A** and **B**: Images courtesy of Philips Medical System, Bothell, WA.)

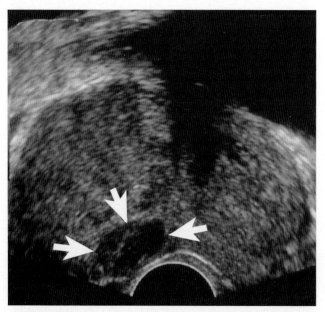

FIGURE 14-37 A hypoechoic area immediately adjacent to the rectum (*arrows*) represents a prostate carcinoma. (Reprinted with permission from Daffner RH, Hartman MS. *Clinical Radiology: The Essentials.* 4th ed. Wolters Kluwer Health/Lippincott Williams & Wilkins; 2013:304.)

There is a risk of prostate contamination by fecal material using the endorectal approach. For this reason, a cleansing enema is often given before the biopsy and antibiotics administered prophylactically to minimize the risk of sepsis. Other minor side effects reported are blood in the urine, stool, or sperm. This technique may not be appropriate when an abscess is suspected because of the risk of infection with fecal material. The transperineal approach does not require a cleansing enema or antibiotic coverage, and it is increasingly being used during magnetic resonance imaging (MRI)-guided biopsy. It does, however, require extensive use of a local anesthetic directly into the perineum.

Sonographic guidance can be utilized to localize a nonpalpable, sonographically suspicious lesion,[66,70] or as guidance for systematic biopsies of known sites of anatomic weakness, including the following: (1) the seminal vesicle beak, (2) the invaginated extraprostatic space which follows the ejaculatory ducts to the verumontanum, and (3) the trapezoid area.[41] Sonographic guidance also assists in staging PCa by obtaining tissue from areas where microscopic ECE is likely to be present. Other applications include draining fluid or sampling suspicious tissue within range of the transducer and needle.

INFERTILITY

The use of sonography in the evaluation of male infertility is limited, yet it often offers valuable information. There are several conditions of the prostate that affect fertility, including congenital abnormalities and prostatitis. Vasography, the examination for determining the reproductive tract patency, is invasive and can cause scarring of the vasa deferentia.[60] Endorectal sonography is an inexpensive and less invasive examination capable of detecting many abnormalities associated with infertility.

Ten percent of male infertility patients present with azoospermia or lack of spermatozoa within the ejaculate.[71] A minority of these patients with this condition will have an obstructive lesion within the prostate or an endocrine disorder. The remainder have an untreatable testicular defect. A clinical workup involves a DRE to rule out the presence of a mass and to confirm the presence of the accessory organs (seminal vesicles and vasa deferentia). If mature sperm are being produced, a blockage must be occurring to prevent the passage of spermatozoa through the ejaculatory ducts, which results in the absence of sperm in the ejaculate. Structural abnormalities of the male pelvis causing azoospermia include congenital or acquired cysts of the prostate or absence or atresia of the vasa deferentia.

Low ejaculate volume is different from azoospermia. In this setting, sperm may be present, but the overall amount of ejaculate is decreased. Clinically, low ejaculate volume is significant and generally treatable. It occurs in about 7% of male infertility patients. This condition may result from a blockage or congenital anomaly of the seminal vesicles. The seminal vesicles store seminal fluid, which makes up a portion of the ejaculate.[72] A partial obstruction along the ejaculatory duct may be present, allowing some sperm in the ejaculate, but an overall decrease in fluid. Finally, a

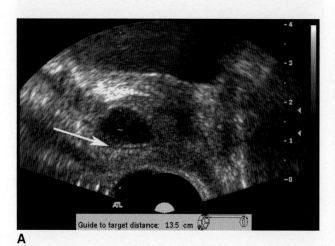

A

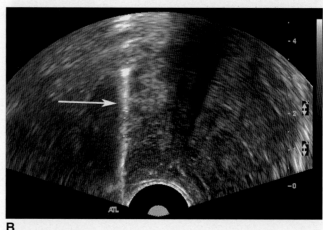

B

FIGURE 14-38 A: On a sonographically guided endorectal biopsy, the echogenic-appearing needle can provide a target distance marker. **B:** The needle is seen as an echogenic, linear structure (*arrowhead*) passing through the prostate gland. (Images courtesy of Philips Medical Systems, Bothell, WA.)

secretory dysfunction of the gland owing to prior infections may result in low ejaculate volume.

Interest has grown, recently, concerning the possible relation of infections of the prostate and male subfertility. Leukocytospermia is typically seen as a clinical sign of genital tract infection and has been associated with adverse effects on sperm number, motility, and sperm velocity.[73] An elevated number of leukocytes in prostatic secretions is typical of acute and chronic bacterial and nonbacterial prostatitis.[74] Acute inflammatory conditions of the prostate gland are often associated with transient disturbances in its secretory function and with changes in sperm quality.

Sonography is most useful in male infertility in the evaluation of the seminal vesicles and the ampullae of the vasa deferentia. Both seminal vesicles and ampullae should be present and free of abnormalities in the normal setting. Absence of the vas deferens and ampulla is a common cause of obstructive azoospermia. Absence of a seminal vesicle may result in low ejaculate volume, although spermatozoa would still be present within the ejaculate.[74] If absence of a seminal vesicle or vas deferens is suspected, the kidneys should be evaluated for associated abnormalities or atresia.[37]

Enlargement of these structures may also be indicative of an obstruction. However, unless the seminal vesicles are grossly enlarged, enlargement may also be the result of sexual abstinence or age. If, however, the seminal vesicles appear grossly enlarged and the above conditions do not apply, a distal obstruction of the ejaculatory duct must be suspected. It is important to rule out cystic structures or calculi that may be obstructing these ducts.[75] These lesions become significant in the presence of fertility issues, such as low ejaculate volume and azoospermia.

SUMMARY

- The prostate gland is retroperitoneal, anterior to the rectum, and inferior to the urinary bladder.
- The normal prostate gland should appear symmetrical with the majority of the parenchyma appearing homogeneous with medium-level echoes.
- The central and transition zones usually are not sonographically distinct.
- The peripheral zone appears homogeneous and slightly hyperechoic relative to adjacent parenchyma.
- Seminal vesicles should be ovoid structures that are symmetric in size, shape, and hypoechoic echogenicity compared with the prostate.

- If distinguished sonographically, the vas deferens is medial to the seminal vesicles with a similar echo texture and the ejaculatory ducts will appear as bright double lines.
- TRUS is the scanning approach of choice.
- Overall, sonography is a useful mechanism of assessing the prostate gland for a variety of abnormalities and for providing biopsy and treatment guidance.
- Its utility as a screening tool for malignant lesions is limited.
- Mp-US has shown to increase PCa detection rates, with more studies needed.

REFERENCES

1. Shetty S. Transrectal ultrasonography (TRUS) of the prostate. *Medscape*. Accessed July 31, 2010. http://emedicine.medscape.com/article/457757-overview
2. McAchran SE, Resnick MI. Prostate ultrasound: past, present, and future. *Ultrasound Clin*. 2006;1:43–54.
3. Frauscher F, Gradl J, Pallwein L. Prostate ultrasound—for urologist only? *Cancer Imaging*. 2005;5:S76–S82.
4. Mannaerts CK, Wildeboer RR, Remmers S, et al. Multiparametric ultrasound for prostate cancer detection and localization: correlation of B-mode, shear wave elastography and contrast enhanced ultrasound with radical prostatectomy specimens. *J Urol*. 2019;202:1166–1173.
5. Correas JM, Halpern EJ, Barr RG, et al. Advanced ultrasound in the diagnosis of prostate cancer. *World J Urol*. 2021;39(3):661–676. doi:10.1007/s00345-020-03193-0
6. Moore KL, Persaud TVN. The urogenital system. In: Moore KL, Persaud TVN, eds. *The Developing Human: Clinically Oriented Embryology*. 8th ed. Elsevier Saunders; 2008:287–328.
7. Muldoon L, Resnick MI. Results of ultrasonography of the prostate. *Urol Clin North Am*. 1989;16(4):693–702.
8. Levin TL, Han B, Little BP. Congenital anomalies of the male urethra. *Pediatr Radiol*. 2007;37:851–862.
9. Dean GE. Congenital prostatic abnormalities. *Curr Prostate Rep*. 2008;6:39–42.
10. Nghiem HT, Kellman GM, Sandberg SA, et al. Cystic lesions of the prostate. *Radiographics*. 1990;10:635–650.
11. Keener TS, Winter TC, Berger R, et al. Prostate vascular flow. *Am J Roentgenol*. 2000;175:1169–1172.
12. Neumaier CE, Martinoli C, Derchi LE, et al. Normal prostate gland: examination with color Doppler US. *Radiology*. 1995;196(2):453–457.
13. McNeal J. The prostate gland: morphology and pathobiology. *Monogr Urol*. 1988;9:36–54.
14. Laczko I, Hudson DL, Freeman A, et al. Comparison of the zones of the human prostate with the seminal vesicle: morphology, immunohistochemistry, and cell kinetics. *Prostate*. 2005;62:260–266.
15. Raja J, Ramachandran N, Munneke G, et al. Current status of transrectal ultrasound-guided prostate biopsy in the diagnosis of prostate cancer. *Clin Radiol*. 2006;61:142–153.
16. Fornage BD. Normal US anatomy of the prostate. *Ultrasound Med Biol*. 1986;12:1011–1021.
17. McNeal JE. Normal and pathologic anatomy of prostate. *Urology*. 1981;17(3):11–16.
18. Kaye K. *Prostate Ultrasound Anatomy: Normal and Pathological*. American Urological Association Annual Meeting; 1989.
19. Ishidoya S, Endoh M, Nakagawa H, et al. Novel anatomical findings of the prostatic gland and the surrounding capsular structures in the normal prostate. *Tohoku J Exp Med*. 2007;212:55–62.
20. Littrup PJ, Lee F, McLeary RD, et al. Transrectal US of the seminal vesicles and ejaculatory ducts: clinical correlation. *Radiology*. 1988;168:625–628.
21. Liau J, Goldberg D, Arif-Tiwari H. Prostate cancer detection and diagnosis: role of ultrasound with MRI correlates. *Curr Radiol Rep*. 2019;7:7.
22. Brawer M. Techniques of examination. In: Resnick M, ed. *Prostatic Ultrasonography*. B.C. Decker; 1990:25–35.
23. Rifkin MD, Dahnert W, Kurtz AB. State of the art: endorectal sonography of the prostate gland. *Am J Roentgenol*. 1990;154:691–700.

24. Laurence Klotz CM. Can high resolution micro-ultrasound replace MRI in the diagnosis of prostate cancer? *Eur Urol Focus.* 2020;6(2):419–423. doi:10.1016/j.euf.2019.11.006

25. Vincent R, Sebastien D, Panhard X, et al. The 20-core prostate biopsy protocol—a new gold standard? *J Urol.* 2008;179:504–507.

26. Loch AC, Bannowsky A, Baeurle L, et al. Technical and anatomical essentials for transrectal ultrasound of the prostate. *World J Urol.* 2007;25:361–366.

27. Hernandez J, Thompson IM. Prostate-specific antigen: a review of the validation of the most commonly used cancer biomarker. *Cancer.* 2004;101(5):894–904.

28. Kearns JT, Holt SK, Wright JL, et al. PSA screening, prostate biopsy, and treatment of prostate cancer in the years surrounding the USPSTF recommendation against prostate cancer screening. *Cancer.* 2018;124(13):2733–2739. doi:10.1002/cncr.31337

29. Fenton JJ, Weyrich MS, Durbin S, et al. Prostate-specific antigen-based screening for prostate cancer: evidence report and systematic review for the US Preventive Services Task Force. *JAMA.* 2018;319(18):1914–1931. doi:10.1001/jama.2018.3712

30. Jones JS. Prostate cancer: are we over-diagnosing or under-thinking? *Eur Urol.* 2008;53:10–12.

31. Shapiro A, Lebensart PD, Pode D, et al. The clinical utility of transrectal ultrasound and digital rectal examination in the diagnosis of prostate cancer. *Br J Radiol.* 1994;67:668–671.

32. Paul R, Korzinek C, Necknig U, et al. Influence of transrectal ultrasound probe on prostate cancer detection in transrectal ultrasound-guided sextant biopsy of prostate. *J Urol.* 2004;64(3):532–536.

33. Moukaddam HA, Haddad MC, El-Sayyed K, et al. Diagnosis and treatment of midline prostatic cysts. *Clin Imaging.* 2003;27(1):44–46.

34. Galosi AB, Montironi R, Fabiani A, et al. Cystic lesions of the prostate gland: an ultrasound classification with pathological correlation. *J Urol.* 2009;181:647–657.

35. VanPoppel H, Vereecken R, De GP, et al. Hemospermia owing to utricle cyst: embryological summary and surgical review. *J Urol.* 1983;129:608–609.

36. Elder JS, Mostwin JL. Cyst of the ejaculatory duct/urogenital sinus. *J Urol.* 1984;132:768–771.

37. Arora SS, Breiman RS, Webb EM, et al. CT and MRI of congenital anomalies of the seminal vesicles. *Am J Roentgenol.* 2007;189:130–135.

38. Labanaris AP, Zugor V, Meyer B, et al. A case of a large seminal vesicle cyst associated with ipsilateral renal agenesis. *Sci World J.* 2008;8:400–404.

39. Sheih CP, Hung CS, Wei CF, et al. Cystic dilatations within the pelvis in patients with ipsilateral renal agenesis or dysplasia. *J Urol.* 1990;144:324–327.

40. Anderson WAD. Anderson's pathology. In: Anderson WAD, Kissane J, eds. *Anderson's Pathology.* 8th ed. Mosby; 1985.

41. Lee F, Torp P-ST, Siders DB, et al. Transrectal ultrasound in the diagnosis and staging of prostatic carcinoma. *Radiology.* 1989;170(3, pt 1):609–615.

42. Narayan S, Mongha R, Kundu AK. Gross calcification within the prostate gland and its significance and treatment. *Indian J Surg.* 2008;70:203–204.

43. Suh JH, Gardner JM, Kee KH, et al. Calcifications in prostate and ejaculatory system: a study on 298 consecutive whole mount sections of prostate from radical prostatectomy or cystoprostatectomy specimens. *Ann Diagn Pathol.* 2008;12:165–170.

44. Griffiths G, Clements R, Peeling W. Inflammatory disease and calculi. In: Resnick M, ed. *Prostatic Ultrasonography.* B.C. Decker; 1990.

45. Potts J, Payne RE. Prostatitis: infection, neuromuscular disorder, or pain syndrome? Proper patient classification is key. *Cleve Clin J Med.* 2007;74(suppl 3):S63–S71. doi:10.3949/ccjm.74.suppl_3.s63

46. National Institute of Diabetes and Digestive and Kidney Disease. Prostatitis: inflammation of the prostate. Updated July 2014. Accessed January 24, 2021. https://www.niddk.nih.gov/health-information/urologic-diseases/prostate-problems/prostatitis-inflammation-prostate

47. Naber KG. Management of bacterial prostatitis: what's new? *BJU Int.* 2008;101(suppl 3):7–10.

48. Weidner W, Anderson RU. Evaluation of acute and chronic bacterial prostatitis and diagnostic management of chronic prostatitis/chronic pelvic pain syndrome with special reference to infection/inflammation. *Int J Antimicrob Agents.* 2008;31(suppl 1):S91–S95.

49. Weidner W, Wagenlehner FM, Marconi M, et al. Acute bacterial prostatitis and chronic prostatitis/chronic pelvic pain syndrome: andrological implications. *Andrologia.* 2008;40(2):105–112.

50. Schaeffer AJ. Prostatitis: US perspective. *Int J Antimicrob Agents.* 1998;10:153–159.

51. Blacklock NJ. The anatomy of the prostate: relationship with prostatic infection. *Infection.* 1991;3:S111–S114.

52. Gulek B, Evliyaoglu Y. Transrectal sonographic findings in chronic prostatitis: a comparative study with an asymptomatic control group. *J Diagn Med Sonogr.* 2008;24:88–92.

53. Shoskes DA, Lee CT, Murphy D, et al. Incidence and significance of prostatic stones in men with chronic prostatitis/chronic pelvic pain syndrome. *Urology.* 2007;70(2):235–238.

54. Barsouk A, Padala SA, Vakiti A, et al. Epidemiology, staging and management of prostate cancer. *Med Sci (Basel).* 2020;8(3):28. doi:10.3390/medsci8030028

55. Rawla P. Epidemiology of prostate cancer. *World J Oncol.* 2019;10(2):63–89. doi:10.14740/wjon1191

56. Carter HB, Piantadosi S, Isaacs JT. Clinical evidence for and implications of the *multistep* development of prostate cancer. *J Urol.* 1990;143:742–746.

57. Franks L. Latent carcinoma of the prostate. *J Pathol Bact.* 1954;68:603–616.

58. Carroll P, Coley C, McLeod D, et al. Prostate-specific antigen best practice policy. Part 1: early detection and diagnosis of prostate cancer. *Urology.* 2001;57:217–224.

59. Ji Y, Ruan L, Ren W, et al. Stiffness of prostate gland measured by transrectal real-time shear wave elastography for detection of prostate cancer: a feasibility study. *Br J Radiol.* 2019;92(1097):20180970. doi:10.1259/bjr.20180970

60. Gandhi J, Zaidi S, Shah J, Joshi G, Khan SA. The evolving role of shear wave elastography in the diagnosis and treatment of prostate cancer. *Ultrasound Q.* 2018;34(4):245–249. doi:10.1097/RUQ.0000000000000385

61. Moyer VA; U.S. Preventive Services Task Force. Screening for prostate cancer: U.S. Preventive Services Task Force recommendation statement. *Ann Intern Med.* 2012;157(2):120–134. doi:10.7326/0003-4819-157-2-201207170-00459

62. Carey BM. Imaging for prostate cancer. *Clin Oncol.* 2005;17:553–559.

63. Dogra VS, Turgut AT. Prostate carcinoma: evaluation using transrectal sonography. In: Hayat MA, ed. *Methods of Cancer Diagnosis, Therapy, and Prognosis: General Methods and Overviews, Lung Carcinoma and Prostate Carcinoma.* Springer; 2008:499–520.

64. Pallwein L, Mitterberger M, Pelzer A, et al. Ultrasound of prostate cancer: recent advances. *Eur Radiol.* 2008;18:707–715.

65. Brawer MK. The diagnosis of prostatic carcinoma. *Cancer.* 1993;71(suppl 3):899–905.

66. Matlaga BR, Eskew LA, McCullough DL. Prostate biopsy: indications and technique. *J Urol.* 2003;169:12–19.

67. Hricak H, Choyke PL, Eberhardt SC, et al. Imaging prostate cancer: a multidisciplinary perspective. *Radiology.* 2007;243:28–53.

68. Linden RA, Halpern EJ. Advances in transrectal ultrasound imaging of the prostate. *Semin Ultrasound CT MR.* 2007;28(4):249–257.

69. Mallick S, Humbert M, Braud F, et al. Local anesthesia before transrectal ultrasound guided prostate biopsy: comparison of 2 methods in a prospective, randomized clinical trial. *J Urol.* 2004;171:730–733.

70. Djavan B, Margreiter M. Biopsy standards for detection of prostate cancer. *World J Urol.* 2007;25:11–17.

71. Jarow JP. Transrectal ultrasonography of infertile men. *Fertil Steril.* 1993;60:1035–1039.

72. Simpson WL Jr, Rausch DR. Imaging of male infertility: pictorial review. *Am J Roentgenol.* 2009;192:S98–S107.

73. Barratt C, Bolton A, Cooke I. Functional significance of white blood cells in the male and female reproductive tract. *Hum Reprod.* 1990;5:639–648.

74. Purvis K, Christiansen E. Infection in the male reproductive tract. Impact, diagnosis and treatment in relation to male infertility. *Int J Androl.* 1993;16(1):1–13.

75. Jarow J. Transrectal ultrasonography in the evaluation of male infertility. In: Resnick M, ed. *Prostatic Ultrasonography.* B.C. Decker; 1990.

CHAPTER 15

The Adrenal Glands

AMBER WOOTEN

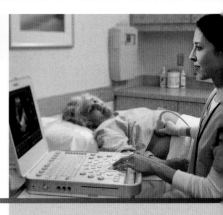

OBJECTIVES

- Identify the sonographic role in the evaluation of the adrenal glands.
- Describe the embryologic development of the adrenal glands.
- Discuss the anatomy and physiology of the adrenal cortex and medulla.
- List the hormones secreted by the adrenal cortex and medulla.
- Identify conditions caused by hyposecretion and hypersecretion of adrenal hormones.
- Identify the normal sonographic appearance of the adrenal glands.
- Describe adrenal gland scanning technique, patient positions, and scanning pitfalls.
- Discuss the differential diagnosis for solid adrenal masses.
- Discuss alternative imaging modalities used to evaluate the adrenal glands.

GLOSSARY

adrenal cortex outer parenchyma of the adrenal gland that makes up 90% of the organ's weight and secretes corticoids including cortisol and aldosterone

adrenal medulla inner portion of the adrenal gland that secretes the catecholamines epinephrine and norepinephrine

adrenocorticotropic hormone (ACTH) hormone secreted by the pituitary gland that causes the adrenal gland to produce and release corticosteroids

endoscopic ultrasound (EUS) an ultrasound transducer on a thin flexible endoscope is inserted in the mouth or anus to visualize the walls of the upper or lower digestive tract and surrounding organs

multiple endocrine neoplasia (MEN) syndrome a group of autosomal dominant disorders characterized by benign and malignant tumors of the endocrine glands

KEY TERMS

Addison disease

adenocarcinoma

adrenal adenoma

adrenal cyst

adrenal hemorrhage

Conn syndrome

Cushing syndrome

hyperadrenalism

hypoadrenalism

myelolipoma

pheochromocytoma

Waterhouse–Friderichsen syndrome

In contrast with other examinations of the abdomen, transabdominal sonographic imaging is not the first-choice imaging modality for screening adrenal glands or detecting adrenal pathology. Examination of the adrenal glands challenges the skills of novice and experienced sonographers alike and requires a working knowledge of exact adrenal anatomic locations and landmarks. However, combining planar flexibility and improved beam-resolution capabilities of modern ultrasound equipment with maneuvering the patient into multiple positions increases the likelihood of producing quality sonographic images of the adrenal glands.[1-3] In addition, since the mid-1990s, endoscopic ultrasound (EUS)

and intraoperative ultrasound (IOUS) have developed as tools for high-resolution sonography evaluation of suprarenal and retroperitoneal masses. Using a 7.5-MHz transducer positioned 1 to 2 cm from the adrenal gland, EUS and IOUS are particularly useful for detecting adrenal metastases and staging cancer.[4,5] As new technologies are introduced for transabdominal imaging, such as three-dimensional/four-dimensional (3D/4D) imaging and elastography, these tools also become available for EUS and IOUS applications.[6,7]

This chapter provides an overview of relevant anatomy, embryology, scanning techniques, functional and morphologic adrenal pathology, and the sonographic appearance of the normal gland as well as adrenal pathology. As a sonographer, it is important to develop critical-thinking and problem-solving skills for sorting out the origin and extent of abdominal masses, including those of suprarenal and retroperitoneal origin. Related techniques are discussed. In addition, EUS, IOUS, computed tomography (CT), magnetic resonance imaging (MRI), and associated nuclear medicine imaging procedures are presented as related to adrenal imaging. Owing to technical improvements in all the diagnostic imaging modalities and the increased use of these modalities, more clinically silent or unexpected masses are being detected. The general term for an unexpected mass detected during an imaging procedure being performed for unrelated disease is "incidentaloma." This term may be applied to any unexpected mass occurring anywhere in the body. Adrenal incidentaloma (AI) has become a common term in the medical literature and represents a diagnostic challenge that includes discovery of masses, which range from benign, nonfunctional lesions to malignant tumors such as pheochromocytomas, adrenocortical carcinomas, or metastases from other primary cancers.[8] Sonographers have a role both in the initial detection of AIs and in gathering diagnostic information regarding newly discovered AIs.

ANATOMY

Embryology

The adrenal gland consists of two distinct parts: the cortex and the medulla. Each develops from different embryonic tissues, forms different anatomic and functional structures, and combines within a common capsule.[9,10] The result is two endocrine glands in one organ. Most glands of the body develop from epithelial tissue. In contrast, the adrenal cortex is derived from the mesoderm of the same region that gives rise to gonadal tissue.[9,10] The central tissue or adrenal medulla is functionally part of the sympathetic nervous system developed from the neural crest cells that also give rise to postganglionic sympathetic neurons.[9-11] As a result, some adrenal medullary pathology may appear ectopically along the paths of these sympathetic neurons usually near the celiac axis, whereas ectopic adrenocortical tissue may be located inferiorly along the path of gonadal tissue migration.[9-11] In addition, extra-adrenal chromaffin cells also normally deposit near the aortic bifurcation to form the organ of Zuckerkandl.[10-12]

Cortex

During gestational weeks 5 and 6, the fetal cortex is first recognized bilaterally as a groove between the developing dorsal mesentery and gonad.[9,10] During weeks 7 and 8, the cells arrange into cords with dilated blood spaces, forming a thin capsule of connective tissue that encloses the gland[9,10] and develops an intimate relationship with the superior pole of the kidney. If the kidney does not develop normally, there will be a discoid distortion in the shape of the adrenal gland.[9,10] Initially, the fetal adrenal gland is larger than the kidney and 10 to 20 times the relative size of the adult adrenal gland.[9,10] During the remainder of fetal life, the cortical tissue is composed of two zones comprising 75% to 80% of the bulk of the gland.[10,11] By week 8, the cortex produces precursors to androgen, estriol, and corticosteroids.[9,10] After birth, the inner zone undergoes involution, whereas the thinner outer zone continues to develop into

the adult adrenal cortex, which takes on a yellow color.[9-13] By the age of 3 years, the cortex differentiates into three zones: (1) zona glomerulosa, (2) zona fasciculata, and (3) zona reticularis. Each zone develops different cellular arrangements and becomes functionally specialized, producing mineralocorticoids, glucocorticoids, and gonadocorticoids, respectively[9-12,14] (Fig. 15-1).

Medulla

Specific ectodermal cells ascend from the neural crest, migrate from their origin, and differentiate into sympathetic neurons of the autonomic nervous system.[9-11] Some of these primitive autonomic ganglia differentiate even further into endocrine cells, designated chromaffin cells, and migrate to form a mass on the medial surface of the fetal adrenal cortex.[9-11] Soon, these chromaffins, or pheochrome cells, invade the developing cortex, establishing the primordium of the adrenal medulla.[9,10] On cut section, the medulla has a red, brown, or gray color depending on the level of blood perfusion.[15] As mentioned previously, chromaffin cells also form the organ of Zuckerkandl.[10-12]

Relational Anatomy

Like the kidneys, the adrenal glands are retroperitoneal. They are generally anterior, medial, and superior to the kidneys.[9,10,13,15] The cortex and medulla are encapsulated by a thick inner layer of fatty connective tissue.[12,13] A thin, fibrous outer capsule attaches to the gland by many fibrous bands, providing the adrenals with their own fascial supports so that they do not descend if the kidneys are displaced or absent.[9,12] The glands are attached to the anteromedial aspect within renal fascia (also referred to as Gerota fascia), and abundant adipose tissue (perinephric fat) surrounds each gland, separating it from the kidneys[11,12,16] (Fig. 15-2).

Right Adrenal

The right adrenal gland is located posterior and lateral to the inferior vena cava (IVC), medial to the right lobe of

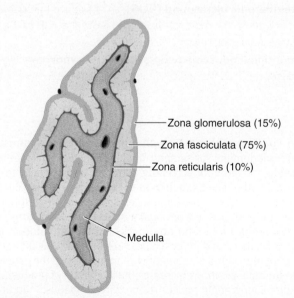

FIGURE 15-1 Adrenal gland. The anatomic sectional illustration of the adrenal gland demonstrates the medulla surrounded by three differentiated zones of the cortex.

Zona glomerulosa (15%)

Zona fasciculata (75%)

Zona reticularis (10%)

Medulla

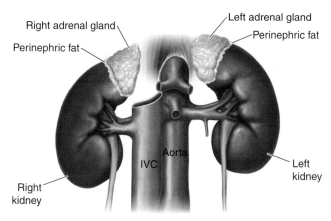

FIGURE 15-2 Relational anatomy. The illustration demonstrates the antero-medial relationship of the adrenal glands to the kidneys. *IVC*, inferior vena cava.

the liver and lateral to the crus of the diaphragm.[9,10,13,15,16] The right adrenal gland has been described as sitting like a triangular cap on the anterior, medial, and superior aspects of the superior pole of the right kidney.

The anterior surface of the right adrenal gland is shaped like a pyramid. Two areas make up the anterior surface: the medial area is narrow and lies posterolateral to the IVC and the lateral, somewhat triangular, portion is in contact with the liver.[9,10,13,15,16] The superior end of the lateral area is devoid of the peritoneum as it comes in contact with the bare area of the liver, and the inferior portion is covered by reflected peritoneum from the inferior layer of the coronary ligament[12,13,15] (Fig. 15-3).

A curved ridge separates the posterior dorsal surface into superior and inferior parts. The superior convex portion rests on the diaphragm, and the inferior concave portion

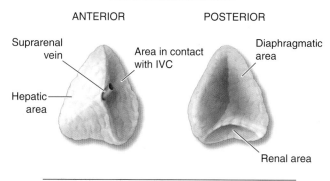

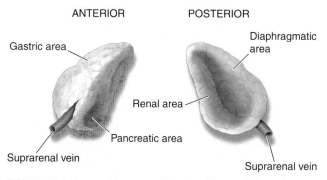

FIGURE 15-3 Topographic anatomy. There is a difference in the surface anatomy of right and left adrenal glands. *IVC*, inferior vena cava.

is in contact with the superior–anterior surface of the right kidney[15] (Fig. 15-3).

Left Adrenal

The left adrenal gland appears draped in an elongated, crescent, or semilunar shape on the medial aspect of the left kidney's superior pole.[9-13,15,16] The left gland is larger than the right, and extension to the left renal hilus is a normal variant.

The anterior portion can be separated into superior and inferior parts. The superior area is situated posterior to the peritoneal wall of the lesser sac and is covered by the peritoneum of the omental bursa, which separates the gland from the cardiac portion of the stomach.[15] The inferior area is not covered by the peritoneum and lies posterior and lateral to the pancreas[9,10,12,13,15,16] (Fig. 15-3). The splenic artery and vein course between the pancreas and the left adrenal gland.

The posterior surface is in close proximity to the splanchnic nerves.[6,15] It is divided into a medial and a lateral area by a vertical ridge. The larger lateral area rests on the kidney and the medial posterior area on the crus of the diaphragm[12,13,15] (Fig. 15-3).

Systemic and Lymphatic Vessels

Similar to other endocrine glands, the adrenals are among the most vascular organs of the body.[13,15,16] The vasculature of the adrenal gland is distinguished from other organs in that the arteries and veins do not actually course together. The abundant arterial supply may contain as many as 50 to 60 small terminal arterioles, whereas the venous blood is channeled almost completely through a single, large venous trunk.[12,13,15,16]

Arteries

Three arteries supply each gland: the superiorly located suprarenal branch of the inferior phrenic artery, the superior and medially located branch of the aorta, and the inferiorly located suprarenal branch of the renal artery[12,13,15,16] (Fig. 15-4).

These arteries are distinctively classified into three types: short capsular arterioles, intermediate cortical arteries (long branches that go through the cortex to the medulla), and the medullary sinusoids.[15]

Veins

In each adrenal gland, a central vein runs the length of the gland and exits at the hilum.[12] The right suprarenal vein empties directly into the posterior aspect of the IVC as a short (4 to 5 mm) vessel, which exits the gland on the mid-anteromedial surface.[12,15] The left suprarenal vein drains directly inferior and medial into the left renal vein.[12,15] Frequently, the left inferior phrenic vein and the left suprarenal vein join before emptying into the left renal vein[12,15] (Fig. 15-4).

Lymphatics

Lymph channels drain from the adrenal cortex and medulla to the hilar area.[15] Following the arterial pathways, larger lymphatic vessels drain into para-aortic and lumbar lymph nodes, which drain to the cisterna chyli, thoracic duct, and eventually into the subclavian vein, whereas a few lymphatic vessels drain into the posterior mediastinal lymph nodes.[12,17]

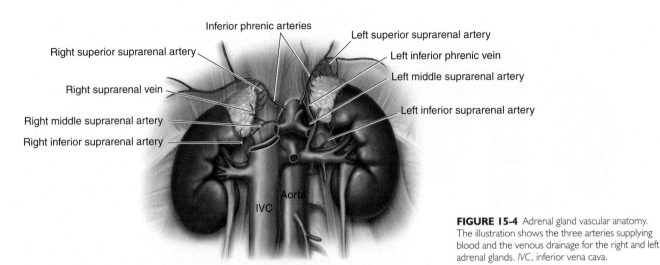

FIGURE 15-4 Adrenal gland vascular anatomy. The illustration shows the three arteries supplying blood and the venous drainage for the right and left adrenal glands. *IVC,* inferior vena cava.

PHYSIOLOGY

Just as their origin and structure are unique, the function and control of hormones differ for these two different glands in one organ. Adrenal pathology and some medications have the potential to disrupt the level of adrenal hormone secretion and associated regulatory mechanisms.[11,14,18–20] Hormones produced by the adrenal cortex, such as cortisol, are essential to life and must be replaced if both adrenal glands are removed.[11,14,18–20]

Cortex

The cortex makes up 90% of the adrenal gland. By 3 years of age, the cortex develops into three epithelial layers, each one evolving functionally into very specialized zones, producing steroid hormones consistent with their mesodermal source. The zona glomerulosa, the outer layer directly beneath the connective tissue covering, makes up 15% of the cortex and produces aldosterone, a mineralocorticoid.[9,10,13,14,16] The zona fasciculata, the middle layer, comprises 75% of the cortex and the zona reticularis, the inner layer, accounts for the remaining 10% of the cortex[9–11,13,16] (Fig. 15-1). Cortisol, a glucocorticoid, and two gonadocorticoids, estrogen and androgen, are produced by the zona fasciculata and zona reticularis.[9,10,13,14,16]

Hormone secretion is often controlled by the negative feedback mechanisms.[14] Low blood concentrations of a hormone trigger the hypothalamus to secrete the primary regulating factor, *corticotrophin-releasing hormone* (CRH), which triggers the anterior lobe of the pituitary to release adrenocorticotropic hormone (ACTH).[14] As blood concentrations of ACTH increase, adrenal hormone activity increases, producing a higher concentration of hormones, such as cortisol, in the bloodstream. This increased concentration of the adrenal hormone inhibits CRH and ACTH and, ultimately, hormone synthesis. When the blood concentration of one or more of the adrenal hormones drops to low levels, the cycle is repeated.[14,18] Adrenocortical hormone secretion, function, and regulation are summarized in Table 15-1.

Medulla

Originating from ectodermal cells, the medulla secretes catecholamine hormones, similar to the posterior pituitary and thyroid glands. The medulla's chromaffin (pheochrome) cells, the hormone-producing portion, surround large blood-filled sinuses.[9,10,13,16]

Epinephrine (adrenalin) and norepinephrine (noradrenalin) are the two principal hormones synthesized by the medulla. Epinephrine constitutes about 80% of the total secretion, and its action is more important than norepinephrine. Release of both hormones is usually stimulated through the sympathetic nervous system.[11,14]

Adrenal nerve stimulation results in prompt discharge of medullary hormones without materially influencing cortical secretion.[11,14] Hormone secretion is controlled directly by the autonomic nervous system, and innervation by the preganglionic fibers allows the gland to respond to the neural stimulus.[14] The anticipation or presence of stress or pain causes the hypothalamus to signal the sympathetic preganglionic neurons to stimulate the chromaffin cells to increase output of epinephrine and norepinephrine.[11,14] Functionally, the medulla is a large sympathetic ganglion, which triggers action via hormone release instead of through axons.[11,14] The body responds by (1) accelerating the heart rate and constricting the vessels, causing increased blood pressure; (2) accelerating the rate of respiration and dilating the respiratory passage; (3) decreasing the rate of digestion to make available more blood to the muscles, increasing the efficiency of muscle contraction; and (4) increasing the blood sugar level to provide energy, thus stimulating cellular metabolism.[11,14] This physiologic response to stress is better known as the *fight-or-flight response.*[11,14,18] Hypoglycemia, hypotension, hypoxia, hypovolemia, and exposure to temperature extremes may also stimulate medullary secretion of epinephrine and norepinephrine.[11,14] Like the glucocorticoids of the adrenal cortices, these hormones help the body resist stress; however, unlike the cortical hormones, the medullary hormones are not essential to life.[11,14]

FUNCTION TESTS

There are many different kinds of laboratory tests to evaluate adrenocortical function. They can be divided into two types: tests that determine the absolute values in serum and urine versus tests that check the interdependency of the various hormones. Table 15-2 summarizes the significance of increased and decreased variance from normal laboratory values for various serum and urine tests.

TABLE 15-1	Adrenal Hormone Secretion, Function, and Regulation[7,11,21]		
Layer	**Hormone**	**Function**	**Regulation**
Zona glomerulosa	Aldosterone is responsible for 95% of mineralocorticoid hormone activity	Regulates sodium and potassium levels, which affect fluid and electrolyte homeostasis, including extracellular fluid volumes; primary activation through the renin–angiotensin system	Complex process; release triggered by a. dehydration, sodium deficiency, hemorrhage or b. elevated potassium levels ACTH has minor role in stimulation secretion.
Zona fasciculata	Glucocorticoids, including cortisol or hydrocortisone (most abundant), cortisone, and corticosterone	Major effect on metabolism of lipids, proteins, and carbohydrates; encourages fat storage; when more energy is required, assists in gluconeogenesis, which helps resist both mental and physical stress; hormones trigger anti-inflammatory and immunosuppressive responses	High stress or low blood concentration (negative feedback mechanism)
Zona reticularis	Regardless of gender, secretes both male and female gonadocorticoids (estrogens and androgens)	Promotes normal development of bones and reproductive organs; affects secondary sex characteristics but not as much as hormones from ovaries and testes	Low blood concentration (negative feedback mechanism)

ACTH, adrenocorticotropic hormone.

TABLE 15-2	Tests of Adrenal Function[7,11,21]		
Sample Source	**Steroid**	**Variation**	**Clinical Implications and Accompanying Conditions**
Serum	Adrenocorticotropic hormone (ACTH, corticotropin)	Increase	Addison disease, ectopic ACTH syndrome, pituitary adenoma, pituitary Cushing syndrome, primary adrenal insufficiency, and stress; drugs causing elevation: amphetamine sulfate, calcium gluconate, corticosteroids, estrogens, ethanol, lithium carbonate, metyrapone, and spironolactone
		Decrease	Primary adrenocortical hyperfunction (owing to tumor or hyperplasia) and secondary hypoadrenalism; drugs causing suppression: dexamethasone
Serum/urine	Aldosterone	Increase	Adrenal tumor (adenoma), aldosteronism (primary, secondary), bilateral adrenal gland hyperplasia, cirrhosis, chronic obstructive lung disease, congestive heart failure, Conn syndrome (with decreased renin), stress, hemorrhage, hyponatremia, hypovolemia, idiopathic cyclic edema, inadequate renal perfusion causing continual activity of the renin–angiotensin system (renin level is also high), nephrosis (lower nephron), nephrotic syndrome, renovascular hypertension (with hypokalemia), low-sodium diet, and excessive licorice consumption; drugs causing elevation: corticotropin, diuretics that promote sodium excretion, fludrocortisone, and potassium
		Decrease	Addison disease, primary hypoaldosteronism, salt-wasting syndrome (high-sodium diet), septicemia, stress, diabetes mellitus, and pregnancy-induced toxemia; drugs causing suppression: fludrocortisone and methyldopa
Serum/urine	Cortisol	Increase	Pituitary tumor causing ACTH-dependent increase (Cushing disease), Cushing syndrome causing ACTH-independent increase, adrenal gland hyperplasia, pregnancy-induced hypertension, exercise, severe hepatic disease, hyperpituitarism, hypertension, hyperthyroidism, infectious disease, obesity, acute pancreatitis, pregnancy, severe renal disease, burns, shock, stress (severe heat, cold, trauma, psychological), surgery, and amenorrhea (urine); drugs causing elevation: long-term corticosteroid therapy (virilism), corticotropin, estrogens, oral contraceptives, and vasopressin
		Decrease	Addison disease from primary hypofunction of the cortex or secondary to hypofunction of the pituitary gland, iatrogenic adrenal insufficiency, adrenogenital syndrome, AIDS, chromophobe adenoma, craniopharyngioma, hyperkalemia, hypoglycemia, hyponatremia, hypophysectomy, pituitary necrosis, renal-glomerular dysfunction (urine), and Waterhouse–Friderichsen syndrome; drugs causing suppression: withdrawing corticosteroids after long-term administration, dexamethasone, dexamethasone acetate, and dexamethasone sodium phosphate
Urine	17-Ketogenic steroids (17-KS)	Increase	Adrenogenital syndrome, Cushing syndrome, adrenal carcinoma, burns, hirsutism, hyperadrenalism, infectious disease, obesity, pregnancy, surgery, and virilization; drugs causing elevation: cephalothin, corticosteroids, digoxin, meprobamate, oral contraceptives, penicillin, phenothiazine, and spironolactone
		Decrease	Addison disease, cretinism, hypoadrenalism, hypopituitarism, Simmonds disease, postovary or testicle removal, and wasting away diseases in general; drug intake includes ampicillin, dexamethasone, estrogens, glucose, morphine, phenytoin, prednisone, and prednisolone

Of the limited tests available for testing medullary function, 24-hour urine samples are typically used for catecholamines.[11,14,18,20] Metanephrines are measured in urine, whereas dopamine may be assessed via urine or blood samples.[18,20] With hypertension, pheochromocytoma, or neuroblastoma, urine levels of catecholamine, vanillylmandelic acid (VMA), or both may be elevated.[11,14,18,20]

Multiple tests are designed to determine the true functions and interdependency of the hypothalamus, pituitary, kidneys, and adrenals, including stimulation and suppression testing for ACTH, aldosterone, and cortisol.[11,14,18,19]

SONOGRAPHIC SCANNING TECHNIQUE

Preparation

Usually, patients receive no preparatory instructions for sonography of the adrenal glands, but when there is suspicion of a mass or metastases or a need to image any retroperitoneal anatomy sonographically, it is recommended that the patient fast approximately 6 to 8 hours before the examination.

Scanning Protocol

Evaluation of adrenals may be approached with the patient in supine or decubitus positions. Common protocols typically begin with transverse scanning, followed by longitudinal and/or coronal assessment. Slight or small scanning maneuvers are used to obtain desired images. One of the imaging goals for adrenal sonography is to document unilateral versus bilateral pathologic involvement. As with most sonographic examinations, width and anteroposterior measurements in transverse sections and length measurements from the longitudinal/coronal sections are required. Various breathing excursions and suspended inspiration may be used to optimize visualization of both adrenal glands.

The sonographer should select the highest-frequency transducer that will provide adequate penetration, given an adrenal depth range of 4 to 12 cm, depending on the patient's size.[21] Selection of a transducer with a small footprint will also facilitate scanning through intercostal spaces.[1,3] Magnifying the field size may improve visualization of small structures. Scanning the patient in a prone position is uncommon, although this method is useful to show the spatial relationship between a large adrenal mass and the adjacent kidney.

Right Adrenal

For imaging the right adrenal, the liver and sometimes the right kidney are useful acoustic windows (Fig. 15-5). Successful utilization of the liver as an acoustic window depends on hepatic size and attenuation characteristics (Fig. 15-6). Starting with transverse scans using an intercostal approach, the section of the IVC located medial and anterior to the upper pole of the kidney should be found.[1,2] The plane should be directed toward the lateral and posterior aspects of this portion of the IVC while also keeping the ultrasound beam perpendicular to the spine. The adrenal gland should be seen in this location anterior to the crus of the diaphragm. The entire right adrenal gland is evaluated by scanning transversely from the renal hilus and proceeding superiorly (Fig. 15-5).

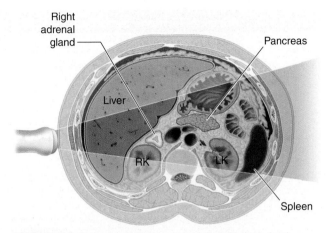

FIGURE 15-5 Right adrenal gland scan technique. With the patient in a supine position, a series of transverse images are obtained through the intercostal spaces of the right adrenal gland, using the liver and kidney as acoustic windows. *LK*, left kidney; *RK*, right kidney.

Longitudinal or coronal scanning of the right gland can be accomplished with several approaches[1,3] (Fig. 15-6). A higher success rate has been reported when utilizing the liver as an acoustic window and scanning the patient in a left lateral decubitus position.[6,22,23] From an intercostal window, the transducer is angled anterior toward the IVC and posterior toward the right kidney until the entire gland is visualized in the longitudinal or coronal plane (Fig. 15-7).

Left Adrenal

The left adrenal gland is more difficult to locate and document. Conventionally, the left adrenal has been imaged with the patient in the right decubitus position, using the spleen or left kidney as an acoustic window[21,22,24] (Fig. 15-8). Identifying the left adrenal and its alignment is first done in the transverse plane. The left adrenal should lie between the left kidney and the aorta, with the pancreatic tail and splenic vein marking the superior margin of the gland.[25]

Longitudinal or coronal scans may be easier to obtain with the patient in a right anterior oblique position using a left posterior oblique scanning plane. First, in the transverse plane, the aorta medial and anterior to the upper pole of the left kidney or the spleen should be located, until the axis of the left kidney and the position of the aorta are determined and the left adrenal gland is identified between these structures[22,23] (Fig. 15-9A). With the patient in the same position, the transducer should be rotated into the longitudinal/coronal plane. When imaging the left adrenal gland, the transducer may have to be oriented obliquely (Fig. 15-9B).

In the mid-1980s, Krebs and colleagues[21,24] introduced an alternative approach to improve localization and delineation of the left adrenal gland. The patient is placed in a 45-degree left posterior oblique position, termed the *cavasuprarenal line position*.[21,24,26] The transducer is placed on the patient's right side, allowing the acoustic beam to pass through a double vascular acoustic window, the IVC, and the aorta[21] (Fig. 15-10). The protocol starts with transverse scans until the left adrenal gland is located; longitudinal views follow. With this position, the success rate is 90%, compared with 60% in the same patient population using the conventional approach.[21,24]

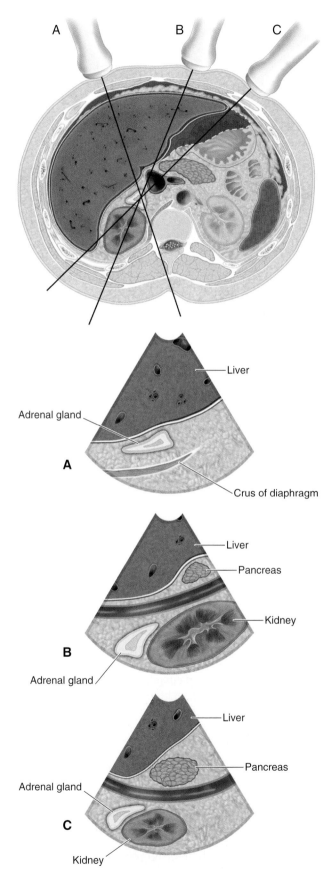

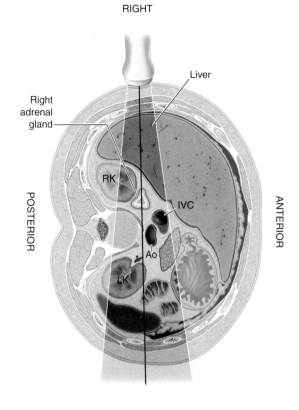

FIGURE 15-7 Left lateral decubitus technique. With the patient in a left lateral decubitus position, the right adrenal gland may be easier to visualize as the inferior vena cava (*IVC*) moves forward and the aorta (*Ao*) moves over the crus of the diaphragm. *LK*, left kidney; *RK*, right kidney.

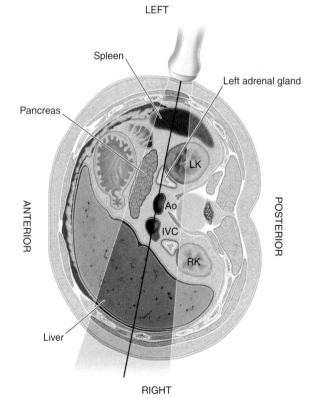

FIGURE 15-6 Transverse sectional planes of the right adrenal gland. The sectional transverse illustration demonstrates the relationship of the adrenal glands to other anatomic structures. Longitudinal images of the right adrenal gland as obtained with the patient in a supine position, using the liver as an acoustic window. (**A**) and (**B**) can be obtained on most patients, whereas (**C**) requires a prominent left liver lobe.

FIGURE 15-8 Right lateral decubitus technique. Using the spleen or the left kidney (*LK*) as an acoustic window, transverse images of the left adrenal gland can be made with the patient in a right lateral decubitus position. *Ao*, aorta; *IVC*, inferior vena cava; *RK*, right kidney.

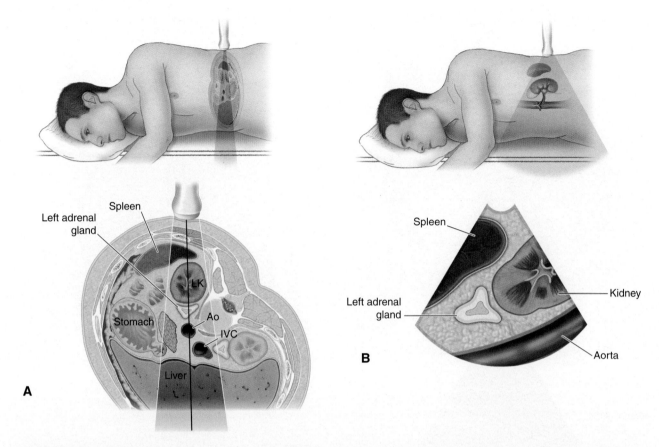

FIGURE 15-9 Right anterior oblique technique. **A:** With the patient lying in a right anterior oblique position, the left kidney (*LK*) and aorta (*Ao*) are aligned in a transverse plane until the left adrenal gland is located. **B:** After the left adrenal gland is identified in the transverse plane, longitudinal images of the entire gland are easier to obtain. *IVC*, inferior vena cava.

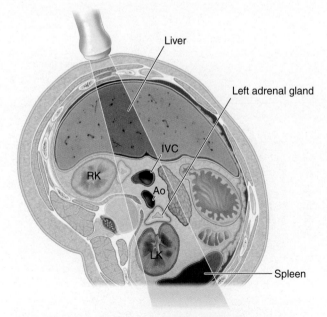

FIGURE 15-10 Cava-suprarenal line position. The cava-suprarenal line position uses the inferior vena cava (*IVC*) and aorta (*Ao*) as a double vascular acoustic window for visualizing the left adrenal gland.[35–37] *LK*, left kidney; *RK*, right kidney.

Pitfalls

The size, location, and pathology of the adrenals and of surrounding structures impose significant limitations on sonographic visualization. Cirrhosis with fatty infiltration of the liver and obesity interfere with adequate penetration. Shadowing from the ribs and narrow intercostal spaces also make this approach challenging.

The right adrenal gland may be obscured by gas and food in the second portion of the duodenum. It is important to differentiate the crus of the diaphragm as a tubular structure located medial to the right adrenal, because it can be mistaken for a normal gland.[27] The right adrenal gland is usually displaced posteriorly when the retroperitoneal fat line is displaced by liver disease.[27,28]

Structures that converge in the area of the left adrenal may mimic this gland: the esophagogastric junction, stomach, gastric diverticula, splenic vessels, portosystemic collateral vessels, tail of the pancreas, prominent hepatic lobes, medial lobulations of the spleen, superior lobulations of the kidney, or adjacent tumors.[1,3,27,29–32] A more posterolateral approach or the cava-suprarenal line position may be indicated for proper visualization of the left adrenal gland.[21,24]

NORMAL SONOGRAPHIC ANATOMY

Fetal adrenal glands are quite large, and 90% of the time at least one can be imaged after 26 to 27 weeks of gestation.[33] In adults, the adrenal glands are much smaller. The glands are generally located anterior, medial, and superior to the kidneys and vary in shape and configuration.[11,32] Their size varies from 3 to 6 cm long, 2 to 4 cm wide, and 3 to 10 mm thick; the adult adrenals weigh 4 to 14 g.[1,3,22,23,32,34] Transabdominally, the cortex and medulla are usually sonographically indistinguishable, because the normal internal texture appears homogeneous and hypoechoic.[32] The glands are usually surrounded by highly echogenic fat, and in some patients, only the echogenic fat can be identified in contrast to an anechoic adrenal gland.[32] Higher-resolution transducers such as those used for endoscopic and intraoperative applications are able to routinely detect the hyperechoic medullary echoes against the hypoechoic cortical echoes and the hyperechoic halo of fatty tissue.[4,17]

Right Adrenal

The right adrenal gland is identified superior to the kidney and lateral to the right crus of the diaphragm.[23,32] On transverse sections, the gland is described as having a triangular, trapezoid, or inverted Y or V shape, with the tail extending from the anteromedial aspect of the right kidney[3,30,32,35] (Fig. 15-11A). In a longitudinal plane scanning the medial aspect of the gland, the anteromedial ridge appears as a curvilinear or S-shaped structure and is visualized posterior to the IVC, slightly above or at the level of the portal vein.[1,22,23,32,35] Moving laterally in longitudinal planes through the right adrenal gland, the anterior and posterior wings spread open and the gland takes on an inverted Y or V shape[35] (Fig. 15-11B, C). The anterolateral portion is medial and posterior to the right lobe of the liver and posterior to the duodenum.[32] Care should be taken to differentiate the right adrenal gland from the more medial hypoechoic/anechoic tubular right crus of the diaphragm.

Left Adrenal

Lateral to the left crus of the diaphragm and lateral or slightly posterolateral to the aorta, the left adrenal gland is visualized superior and medial to the kidney.[22,32,35] This gland is described as having a triangular or semilunar appearance (Fig. 15-12A). Because the stomach lies posterior to the lesser omental sac (a potential space that is usually collapsed), the superior portion of the adrenal gland can appear directly behind the stomach.[1,35] The inferior portion of the gland lies posterior to the pancreas. The splenic artery and vein can be identified passing between the left adrenal gland and the more anterior pancreas.[32,35] On longitudinal sections posterior to the pancreas, the left adrenal has a sonographic configuration similar to that of the right gland[35] (Fig. 15-12B–D).

PATHOLOGY

In most cases of suspected adrenal disease, CT is the imaging modality of choice.[29–31,36,37] Better visualization of the adrenal areas is obtained with CT, particularly in patients with adequate

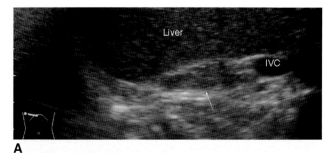

A

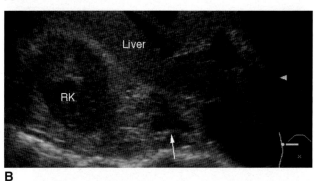

B

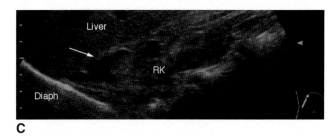

C

FIGURE 15-11 Sonographic appearance of right adrenal gland. **A:** This transverse section of the normal right adrenal gland (*arrow*) demonstrates its relationship to the liver, inferior vena cava (*IVC*), and diaphragm. **B:** This transverse section of the normal right adrenal gland (*arrow*) demonstrates its relationship to the liver and right kidney (*RK*). **C:** In longitudinal sections moving from lateral to medial, a normal V- or Y-shaped right adrenal gland (*arrow*) is seen in relation to the *RK*, liver, and diaphragm (*Diaph*). (Images courtesy of Dr. Taco Geertsma, Gelderse Vallei, Ede, The Netherlands.)

retroperitoneal fat.[37] In addition, MRI, scintigraphy, positron emission tomography (PET), and blood and urine testing are used to refine the diagnoses of adrenal pathologies. Sonography provides an alternative for screening children from families with the multiple endocrine neoplasia (MEN) syndromes, pregnant women, and poor candidates for CT who have a paucity of retroperitoneal fat.[37] Indications for sonography of the adrenals and retroperitoneum include evaluation for the presence of local or regional metastases; localized tumor invasion; origin of retroperitoneal masses; characterization of adrenal hemorrhage, cyst, or tumor for cystic and solid components; patency of local veins and IVC; hypertrophy of the gland; and follow-up on nonresected adrenal masses.

Because a mass may be encountered incidentally during routine abdominal or renal scanning, it is important to understand adrenal pathology and its clinical manifestations, to correlate laboratory values, and to identify normal and abnormal sonographic appearances. A change in the normal appearance of the gland's size and configuration is a key

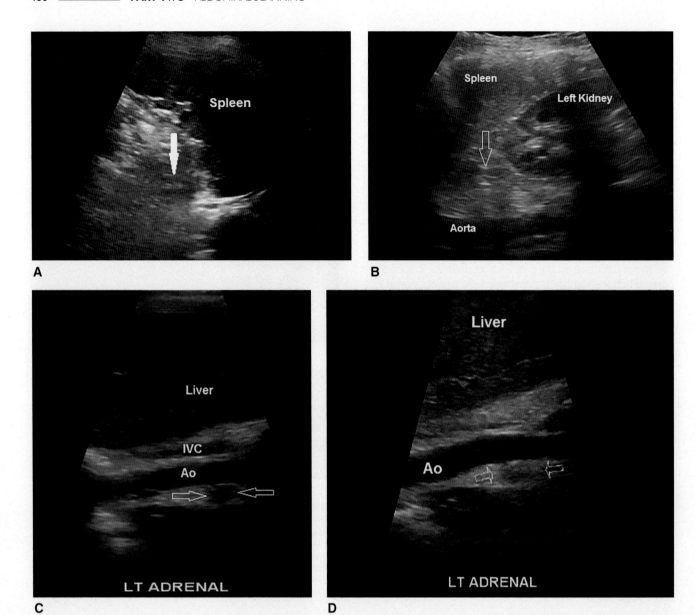

FIGURE 15-12 Sonographic appearance of the left adrenal gland. **A:** Transverse section demonstrates the triangular shape of a normal left adrenal gland. **B:** On a longitudinal section with the patient in a right posterior oblique position, the normal V or Y shape of the left adrenal gland and its relationship to the left kidney, spleen, and aorta can be identified. **C** and **D:** The normal left adrenal gland (*arrowheads*) is seen in a coronal section (medial to lateral) using the cava-suprarenal line position. The patient is tilted 45 degrees, and the beam passes through the liver, inferior vena cava (*IVC*), and aorta.

indicator for adrenal abnormalities. An increase in size can cause compression or displacement of surrounding structures. With right adrenal disease, the retroperitoneal fat line, IVC, and right renal vein may be displaced anteriorly, whereas the right kidney is displaced inferiorly or posteriorly[28] (Fig. 15-13A, B). An enlarged left adrenal gland may displace the splenic vein anteriorly and the left kidney inferiorly or posteriorly.[28] An adrenal mass should be differentiated from a renal mass by identifying the echo interface separating the mass from the upper pole of the kidney[32,35] (Fig. 15-13B, C). On rare occasions, an adrenal tumor may invade the adjacent kidney (Fig. 15-13D–G). As with other abdominal pathology, adrenal masses may present with irregular outer margins and can indent adjacent organs and vascular structures. Regardless of pathologic origin, large adrenal masses tend to outgrow their vascular supply, potentially producing irregular internal hypoechoic and hyperechoic

areas representing central necrosis, liquefaction, or hemorrhage[32] (Fig. 15-14A–F and Pathology Box 15-1).

Developmental Anomalies

See Pathology Box 15-1.

Agenesis

The most important congenital disorders are the adrenocortical hyperplasias, which cause alterations and increases in steroid synthesis. These are discussed later in the chapter with hyperadrenalism.

Congenital Hypoplasia

There are two types of congenital adrenal hypoplasia: anencephalic and cytomegalic. In both types, essential hormone production is altered.

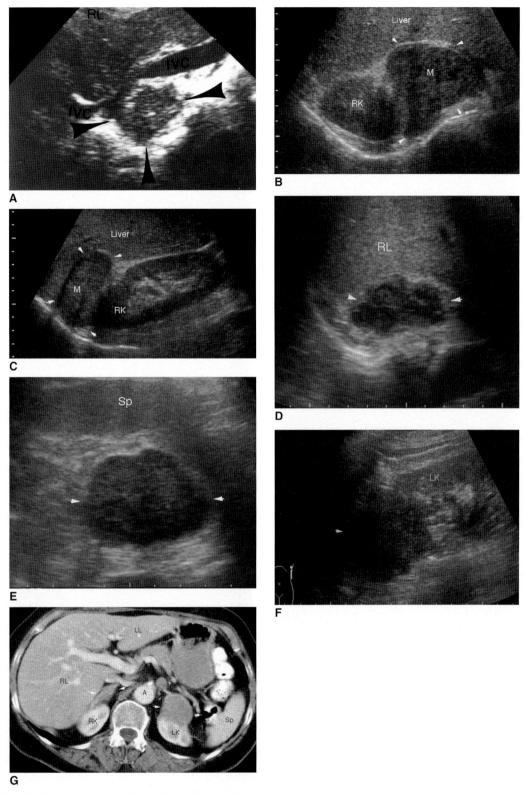

FIGURE 15-13 Adrenal metastases. **A:** On a longitudinal section, a right adrenal metastatic mass (*arrowheads*) measuring 4 cm in average diameter is seen posterior to the right liver lobe (*RL*) indenting and displacing the inferior vena cava (*IVC*). The primary site was bone cancer. **B:** On a transverse section of a patient with right adrenal metastases from lung cancer, the adrenal mass (*M, arrowheads*) displaces the liver anteriorly and right kidney (*RK*) laterally. **C:** A longitudinal section on the same patient showing the adrenal mass (*M, arrowheads*) distorting the suprarenal space. An adrenal mass should be differentiated from a renal mass by identifying the echo interface separating the mass from the upper pole of the *RK*. **D–G:** These sonograms demonstrate bilateral predominantly hypoechoic solid masses (*arrowheads*), representing metastases to right and left adrenal glands from a lung carcinoma. **D:** A transverse section of the right adrenal mass is identified posteromedial to the *RL*. **E:** A transverse section of the left adrenal mass is identified medial to the spleen (*Sp*). **F:** A longitudinal section demonstrates the left adrenal mass superior to and infiltrating the left kidney (*LK*). **G:** On the computed tomography image, the location and relational anatomy of the bilateral adrenal masses (*arrowheads*) are demonstrated. The appearance of the left adrenal mass on computed tomography gives the impression of a renal mass. *A*, aorta; *LL*, left liver lobe; *M*, mass; *RK*, right kidney, *RL*, right liver lobe; *Sp*, spleen. (Images courtesy of Dr. Taco Geertsma, Gelderse Vallei, Ede, The Netherlands.)

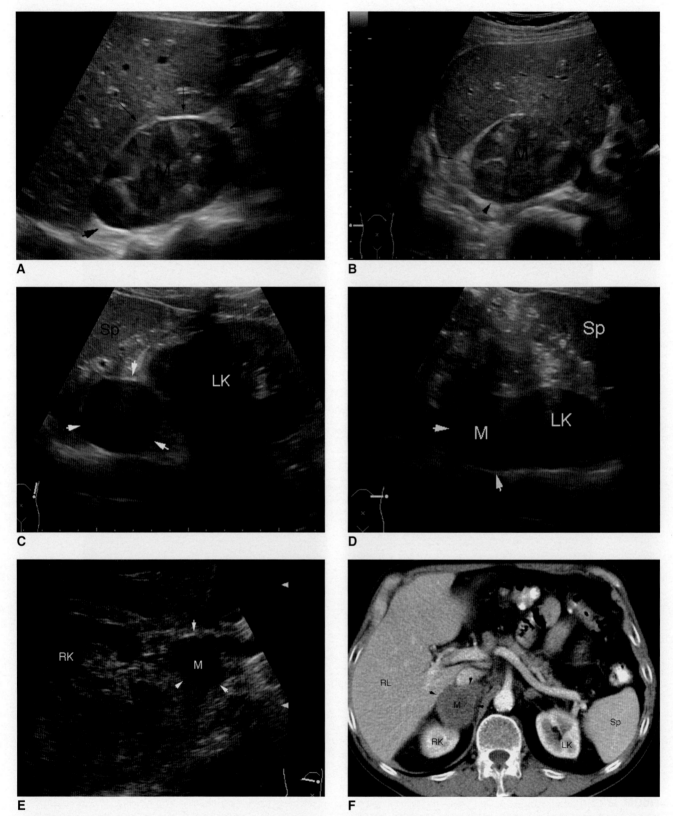

FIGURE 15-14 Solid adrenal masses. **A–D:** These sonograms demonstrate solid masses (*M, arrowheads*), representing bilateral metastases to right and left adrenal glands from a melanoma. The longitudinal (**A**) and transverse (**B**) aspects of the right adrenal mass are identified posterior to the right liver lobe, superior to the right kidney (*RK*). Images demonstrate anterior and superior distortion of the Gerota fascia and fat between the adrenal gland and right lobe of the liver (*arrows*). The longitudinal (**C**) and transverse (**D**) aspects of the left adrenal mass are identified medial to the spleen (*Sp*) and superomedial to the left kidney (*LK*). Anterior margin of mass is poorly defined on transverse image (**D**). **E** and **F:** This patient has a unilateral metastasis to the right adrenal gland. A solid right adrenal mass was identified on both ultrasound and CT images. The left adrenal gland was unremarkable. **E:** On a transverse section, the adrenal mass (*M, arrowheads*) is differentiated by the echo interface separating the mass from the upper pole of the *RK*. **F:** On the CT image, the location and relational anatomy of the right adrenal mass (*arrowheads*) are demonstrated. *A*, aorta; *RL*, right liver lobe. (Images courtesy of Dr. Taco Geertsma, Gelderse Vallei, Ede, The Netherlands.)

Pathology	Etiology	Sonographic Appearance
Metastatic disease	Develops from squamous cell carcinoma of the lung, breast, gastrointestinal tract, thyroid, pancreas, kidney, lymphoma, melanoma	Small masses (4–5 cm); usually bilateral solid, well circumscribed, encased within the adrenal; located anteromedially; may have irregular margins and can indent IVC and displace kidney; necrosis (hypoechoic) or areas of hemorrhage (hypoechoic) may occur within the mass
Developmental anomalies	Agenesis–adrenocortical hyperplasia; congenital hypoplasia: anencephalic–cerebral, pituitary, or hypothalamic; cytomegalic unknown; ectopic unknown	Location and size are not commonly identified sonographically
Cyst	Develops from hemorrhage, trauma, or idiopathic causes	Rounded, fluid-filled mass with a thin, smooth wall, unilocular or multilocular; calcifications may be present, with acoustic shadowing affecting through-transmission; ring calcification has a higher incidence of malignancy; hemorrhage with dense clot presents a thick, hyperechoic area of the pseudocyst type
Hemorrhage	Birth trauma or anoxia, systemic disease, anticoagulant therapy, metastases, adrenal trauma	Echo pattern variable, depending on age of hemorrhage; complex mass located anterosuperior to kidney may displace it; may shrink; calcifications, if present, appear as focal, hyperechoic areas, with or without acoustic shadowing
Abscess and infection	Opportunistic infections in immunocompromised patients	Both adrenal glands appear enlarged and hypoechoic; hepatosplenomegaly is usually present with lymphadenopathy in patients with HIV/AIDS

IVC, inferior vena cava.

In an anencephalic fetus, usually stillborn, the adrenal gland consists of only a provisional cortex with no fetal zone.[38] The cause of the disorder is either cerebral, pituitary, or hypothalamic.

The cause of the cytomegalic type is unknown. An unusual adrenal cortex is made up histologically of large eosinophilic cells. Usually, the gland weighs less than 1 g and is not identifiable by ultrasound. With early diagnosis, early replacement steroid therapy promotes long-term survival.[38]

Ectopy

Ectopic adrenal glands consist mainly of accessory cortical material and can occur anywhere from the diaphragm to the pelvis[9–12,38]: in the kidney, liver, retroperitoneal tissues, ovary, testis, and in the tissues accompanying the spermatic cord. The ectopia may have either cortical or cortical and medullary cellular components. On surgical resection, ectopic adrenocortical tissue is identified by its bright yellow color. Because of their location and size, ectopic adrenal glands are not commonly identified with sonography.

Cysts

Relatively infrequent and usually asymptomatic, adrenal cysts may be incidental findings. The endothelial type may be subdivided into lymphangiomatous (41%) and angiomatous (3%), pseudocysts (40%) are secondary to hemorrhage into or around the gland, and epithelial cysts (6%) result from cystic degeneration of adenomas and parasitic cysts.[3,32]

Adrenal cysts demonstrate the characteristic sonographic cystic appearance with marked through-transmission and posterior enhancement.[1,39] They appear as rounded, fluid-filled masses with thin, smooth walls.[1] They may be unilocular or multilocular, small or large[32] (Fig. 15-15A, B). Calcifications are found in 15% of cases and dense clot retraction may persist, providing a thick, hyperechoic area in the pseudocystic variety[32,35] (Fig. 15-15C). Most adrenal cysts are benign, but adrenal cysts with a "ring" calcification are more often malignant.[35] The calcified cyst wall (aka eggshell) produces a thick, hyperechoic ring that may or may not cast an acoustic shadow[3,35,37] (Pathology Box 15-1). For a purely cystic mass, percutaneous fine-needle aspiration may be indicated to examine the contents or relieve symptoms associated with pressure.[32]

Hemorrhage

Hemorrhage of the adrenal gland is seen most often in newborns, especially after a difficult delivery in which fetal oxygen is diminished or cut off for some time (see Chapter 20). Hemorrhage can also be precipitated by adrenal trauma, surgery, stress, anticoagulant therapy, adrenal vein thrombosis, adrenal neoplasms, metastases, or septicemia.[1,3,40,41] The right side is often more involved in the hemorrhagic process, which is probably associated with right adrenal venous drainage directly off the IVC. Trauma-induced hematomas usually resolve without clinical complications, unless the trauma is bilateral, because an Addisonian crisis is a risk associated with bilateral hemorrhage.[1,40]

Depending on the stage of organization, the echo pattern of adrenal hemorrhage varies. The appearance can range from an acute hyperechoic suprarenal mass to the hypoechoic-to-anechoic pattern of a resolving chronic hematoma[3,32,39,42] (Fig. 15-16A–C). With age, the mass typically shrinks, and calcifications can appear as focal, hyperechoic areas with associated acoustic shadowing[3,39,40,42] (Pathology Box 15-1).

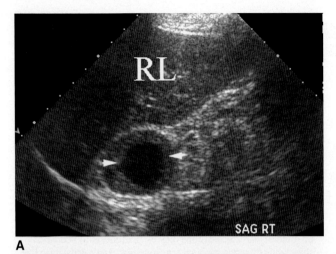

A

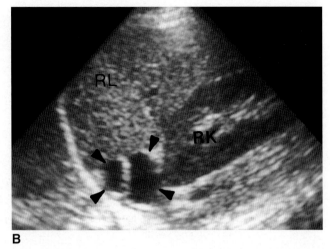

B

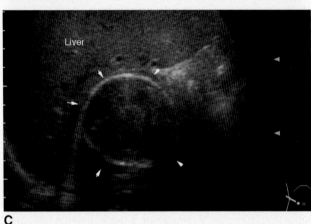

C

FIGURE 15-15 Adrenal cysts. **A:** A unilocular right adrenal gland cyst (*arrowheads*) posterior to the right liver lobe (*RL*) can be identified in this longitudinal/coronal section. This was an incidental finding. **B:** This patient presented with right upper quadrant pain. The sonographic examination imaged a bilobed, mostly anechoic mass (*arrowheads* and *cursors*) measuring 4 cm in the anteroposterior dimension. On the longitudinal section, the bilobed mass is identified superior to a normal-appearing right kidney (*RK*) and posterior to the *RL*. **C:** Calcified cyst (*arrowheads*). The transverse aspects of the right adrenal cyst are identified posterior to the *right liver lobe and* superior to the right kidney. On this patient, a radiograph demonstrated a circumferential calcification of cyst wall. (**C:** Image courtesy of Dr. Taco Geertsma, Gelderse Vallei, Ede, The Netherlands.)

Inflammation/Infection

Abscess and Infection

Adrenal abscess is extremely uncommon in adults, although less rare with neonates following traumatic delivery or septicemia (see Chapter 20). Adrenal abscess formation in adults has been associated with opportunistic infections (i.e., *Bacteroides, Escherichia coli,* histoplasmosis, *Nocardia asteroides, Proteus, Salmonella,* and tuberculosis) in immunocompromised patients (i.e., HIV/AIDS, hemophilia, or thalassemia minor), with direct contamination through an invasive procedure or trauma, as a complication to hemorrhage, and with regional contamination from appendicitis.[11,43,44] With percutaneous drainage or aspiration and proper antibiotics, patients can have a full recovery.[43,44]

In patients with HIV/AIDS, focal adrenal lesions are associated with neoplastic changes (lymphoma and/or Kaposi sarcoma) and infections (candida, cryptococcus, cytomegalovirus [CMV], herpes, mycobacterium, toxoplasmosis, and/or tuberculosis).[1,45] Complications of systemic infections including tuberculosis, fungal sources, and viruses can also lead to primary adrenal insufficiency or hypoadrenalism.[11,14,18] The appearance of Addison disease symptoms may appear gradually, as the adrenal glands are destroyed by these rampant infection processes and deficiencies occur in the production of cortical hormones.[11,14,18] However, the adrenalitis associated with CMV seldom claims more than half of the glandular tissue, so Addisonian crises rarely

strike patients with isolated CMV infections.[45] Caution is advised when co-treating CMV-infected HIV/AIDS patients with steroids, because these medications may temporarily disguise impending adrenal insufficiency.[45]

Histoplasmosis, which is disseminated through numerous body systems, requires treatment; otherwise, it can be fatal.[46] Disseminated histoplasmosis is rare but occurs at higher rates in immunocompromised patients. Both adrenal glands appear enlarged and hypoechoic.[46] Hepatosplenomegaly is usually present along with lymphadenopathy in patients with HIV/AIDS (Pathology Box 15-1). This appearance is also consistent with tuberculosis and is further discussed later.

CORTICAL PATHOLOGY

Adrenal cortex pathology can be divided into three categories: disorders that diminish steroid output, disorders that increase steroid production, and lesions that have no functional effect. The presentation of cortical disease categories contributes to an understanding of the range of sonographic appearances of adrenal diseases.

Hypoadrenalism (Hypocorticism)

Hypoadrenalism or adrenocortical hypofunction may be caused by primary disorders of the cortex or by secondary failure in the elaboration of ACTH (Pathology Box 15-2). The clinical manifestation, atrophic or necrotic destruction

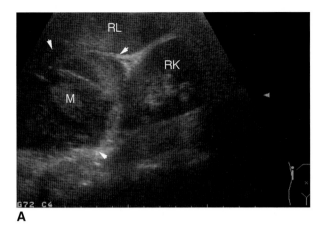

A

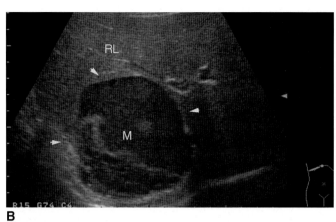

B

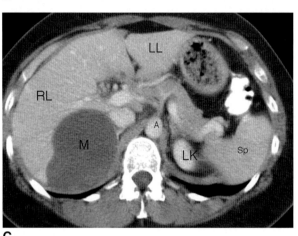

C

FIGURE 15-16 Adrenal hemorrhage. This case demonstrates an adrenal hemorrhage with septated cystic mass with internal echoes. A complex, predominantly hypoechoic mass measuring 9 cm in maximum diameter was identified in the subhepatic space. Posterior enhancement is noted on the sonograms. **A:** The longitudinal section demonstrates the mass (*M, arrowheads*) superior to the right kidney (*RK*) and inferior and posterior to the right liver lobe (*RL*). **B:** On the transverse section, the primarily hypoechoic, complex mass (*M, arrowheads*) is identified posterior and lateral to the *RL*. **C:** On the computed tomography image, the location and relational anatomy of the right adrenal hemorrhage (*M, arrowheads*) are demonstrated. *A*, aorta; *LK*, left kidney; *LL*, left liver lobe; *Sp*, spleen. (Images courtesy of Dr. Taco Geertsma, Gelderse Vallei, Ede, The Netherlands.)

PATHOLOGY BOX 15-2
Disorders of the Adrenal Cortex

Disorder	Etiology	Sonographic Appearance
Hypoadrenalism	Addison disease caused by idiopathic atrophy of the adrenal cortex	Unable to identify
	Addison disease caused by tuberculosis	Solid, enlarged, and nodular, with hyperechoic capsule; may appear complex, with areas of necrosis
	Waterhouse–Friderichsen syndrome	Hemorrhage may occur (see Pathology Box 15-1)
Aldosteronoma	Conn disease	Hypoechoic, small (1–2 cm), round masses
Hyperplasia	Cushing or Conn disease, adrenogenital disease	Normal or diffusely enlarged; solid, cystic, or complex, with or without focal zones of necrosis within the gland

---

of the cortex, is usually not detectable by ultrasound, but complications such as hemorrhage can be identified.

Chronic Primary Hypoadrenalism (Addison Disease)

The chronic form of hypoadrenalism (Addison disease) is the most common.[11,18] Insufficient secretion of adrenocortical hormones results from the insidious and profound atrophy of the adrenal glands. Addison disease is uncommon (4 cases per 100,000 population); it becomes evident only when 90% of functioning adrenocortical cells have been destroyed.[11,18] The two major causes of adrenal destruction are idiopathic atrophy (80%) and glandular destruction attributed to an autoimmune disorder, infection, or tuberculosis (20%).[11,18] Females are more often affected by the idiopathic atrophic type and males by the type caused by tuberculosis.[47]

Clinical symptoms depend on the degree of hormone deficiency. Because of adrenal atrophy, the steroid response is diminished or absent, causing an increase in the pituitary gland's production of ACTH.[10,11,14,18] Because ACTH has melanin-stimulating properties, about 98% of affected persons present with changes in skin color.[11,14,47] Other clinical manifestations include sodium and potassium retention; renal impairment; and decreases in blood volume, sugar, and lipids.[11,14,18] Symptoms can include fever; fatigue; muscle weakness; hypotension; and gastrointestinal distress such as nausea, vomiting, weight loss, and diarrhea.[11,14,18] The disease may be managed by administration of steroids, but patients are vulnerable to all forms of stress, which may trigger hypoadrenal crisis and shock.[11,14,18]

As mentioned previously, systemic infections including tuberculosis, fungal sources such as histoplasmosis, and viruses such as CMV and AIDS may lead to primary adrenal insufficiency or hypoadrenalism.[11,14,18,45] As the adrenal glands are destroyed by these infections, cortical hormonal deficiencies are revealed.[11,14,18] Sonographic appearances vary depending on the extent of gland destruction and tissue necrosis. During acute stages, there is diffuse glandular enlargement, whereas chronic infection usually leads to patterns of atrophy and calcification.[45]

When Addison disease is caused by tuberculosis, the glands are enlarged, firm, and nodular, with a thick capsule. The sonographic appearance can range from a normal echoic appearance to hyperechoic with areas of necrosis. Small, irregular, and contracted adrenal glands that usually are not identified on ultrasound occur with idiopathic Addison disease.

Chronic Secondary Hypoadrenalism

Any disorder to the hypophyseal-thalamic axis that reduces the output of ACTH causes atrophy of the adrenal cortex and decreases secretion of cortisol and androgen.[11,18] The most common cause is abrupt cessation of exogenous steroid therapy.[11,18] Other causes include metastatic cancer, infection, infarction, bilateral hemorrhage, bilateral adrenalectomy, and irradiation.[1,11,18] A syndrome of hypoadrenalism similar to Addison disease results, except that hyperpigmentation is absent with diminished ACTH.[11,18] The adrenal glands may be moderately to markedly shrunken, may appear leaf-like, and become difficult to identify in the periadrenal fat.[38]

Acute Hypoadrenalism (Waterhouse–Friderichsen Syndrome)

Massive destruction of the adrenals can occur at any age and in a variety of settings, causing acute adrenal insufficiency (Addisonian or adrenal crisis).[38] Hemorrhagic destruction of the adrenal glands occurring owing to widespread pneumococcal, meningococcal, or gram-negative septicemia is known as *Waterhouse–Friderichsen* syndrome.[11] Immediate intervention, such as the administration of glucocorticoid therapy and treatment of the underlying infection, is necessary or death will rapidly ensue.[11] Caution should be exercised to avoid treating hyponatremia too fast to prevent additional complications.[11,18]

Hyperadrenalism (Hypercorticism)

With hyperadrenalism, the three types of corticosteroids produced by the adrenal cortex result in three distinctive but sometimes overlapping clinical manifestations: Cushing syndrome, Conn syndrome or aldosteronism, and adrenogenital syndrome or congenital adrenal hyperplasia (CAH).[11,18]

Cushing Syndrome

In Cushing syndrome, excessive glucose production results from hypersecretion of cortisol from the adrenal cortex.[11,14]

The most common cause is treatment of nonendocrine disorders with long courses of potent glucocorticoid drugs such as prednisone and dexamethasone.[11,18] Three clinically similar forms of Cushing syndrome result from glucocorticoid overproduction.[11,48] Hypersecretion of ACTH by the anterior pituitary (Cushing disease, 68% to 80% of cases) and ectopic ACTH syndrome from adenocarcinoma, oat-cell carcinoma of the lung, or other malignant neoplasms (8% to 12%) are two ACTH-dependent forms.[11,48] Most patients with ACTH-dependent forms of Cushing syndrome have symmetrically enlarged glands, whereas 30% have normal-sized glands.[48–50] The third form involves ACTH-independent processes, which account for 15% to 20% of Cushing syndrome cases and always are adrenocortical neoplasms, usually hyperfunctioning adenomas, carcinomas, or a few other rare entities.[48,49] A pseudo-Cushing syndrome occurs rarely (<2%) with alcoholism or major depression. In children, tumors are the most common cause, and the child's growth ceases if treatment is not begun before the epiphyses of the child's bones have sealed.[11]

Cushing syndrome is characterized by increases in cortisol secretion, which trigger increases in gluconeogenesis and result in elevated serum glucose levels.[11,18] Eventually, the islet cells of the pancreas are no longer able to produce sufficient amounts of insulin and diabetes mellitus results.[11] Protein loss occurs almost everywhere except in the liver.[47] This loss results in weakened muscles and elastic tissue, producing a protuberant abdomen and poor wound healing.[11,14] Humoral immunity is impaired, decreasing the threshold for infection.[18] With the loss of collagen in the skin, the tissues become very thin and susceptible to tearing and bruising. Red welts and striae are seen, mostly over the abdomen and thighs.[11] Owing to the melanin-stimulating properties of ACTH, hyperpigmentation may be seen.[11,14] Osteoporosis can result, causing weakness and fractures.[11,18] Hypertension is also evident in most cases.[11,18]

Hyperaldosteronism (Conn Syndrome)

Primary hyperaldosteronism, or Conn syndrome, is the result of excessive and uncontrolled secretion of the mineralocorticoid aldosterone.[11,14,18] It is uncommon, and in 80% to 90% of patients, it results from a benign aldosterone-producing adrenal adenoma.[8,37,49] Bilateral cortical hyperplasia and rare carcinomas account for the remaining 10% to 20% of the cases. Both categories of tumors are known as aldosteronomas.[49] These lesions are difficult to detect because more than 20% are less than 1 cm in size.[49]

Secondary hyperaldosteronism is not a disease process but results from hypersecretion of aldosterone in response to stimulation of the renin–angiotensin system.[11,18] This occurs when almost any factor decreases the blood supply to the kidneys, raising the plasma renin level and increasing subsequent excessive aldosterone secretion.[11,18]

The clinical features of this disorder are a direct result of aldosterone's functions of conserving sodium and losing renal potassium.[11,14,18] Hypernatremia (excess sodium in the blood) and hypokalemia (extreme potassium depletion in the blood) are the principal clinical manifestations.[11,14,18] The condition is suspected whenever a hypertensive patient exhibits concurrent hypokalemia.[11,18] Conservation of sodium leads to water retention, increasing the volume in the extracellular and vascular compartments, causing arterial hypertension.[11,14,18] Potassium loss most commonly results in muscle cramps and weakness.[11] Because the kidneys are the primary site of sodium conservation, renal functional alterations occur.[11,14,18] The sonographic appearance of aldosteronoma is presented in Pathology Box 15-2 and is discussed in the section on Cortical Tumors.

Congenital Adrenal Hyperplasia (Adrenogenital Syndrome)

CAH encompasses at least six distinctive autosomal recessive syndromes, each characterized by a congenital deficiency of a specific enzyme involved in the biosynthesis of adrenal steroids.[11,18] Ultrasound evaluation of the fetus or neonate with CAH will demonstrate enlarged adrenal glands with a characteristic cerebriform pattern (resembling the appearance of brain gyri) (Fig. 15-17). With bilateral hyperplasia, the enzyme deficiencies may also result from postpubertal adrenal hyperplasia, adrenal adenoma, or adrenal carcinoma.[11] The effect of the deficiencies impairs synthesis of cortisol and distorts other aspects of steroidogenesis.[38] In most cases, this increases levels of ACTH, leading to adrenal hyperplasia and subsequent overstimulation of the pathways of steroid hormone production, particularly those involving the production of adrenal androgens.[11,14] All of these

syndromes are adrenogenital, representing an abnormal expression of androgen excess—the ultimate result in most cases is the same: virilization.[11,18]

Newborn girls with CAH have ambiguous external genitalia, resembling those of boys.[11,18] Reconstructive surgery, if indicated, can be performed during the first 2 years of life to reduce the size of the clitoris, separate the labia, and exteriorize the vagina.[11,18] Internal female genitalia are normal. Boys are seldom diagnosed at birth unless they have enlarged genitalia, lose salt, or manifest adrenal crisis.[11,18]

The age and sex of the affected person determine the nature and severity of the disorder when adrenogenital syndromes are caused by benign or malignant tumors. Precocious sexual development and elevated plasma 17-hydroxy-progesterone levels aid in the diagnosis.[11,18] Early diagnosis is important, because the deficiency can often be controlled, allowing normal sexual and physical development.[11,18]

Hyperfunctioning adrenal glands can appear normal or diffusely enlarged but with normal shape.[38] With nodular hyperplasia, a solid, cystic, or complex mass, with or without focal zones of necrosis, may present in the adrenal gland[29] (Fig. 15-18). Because the sonographic appearance is used to describe and characterize, and not to make tissue-specific

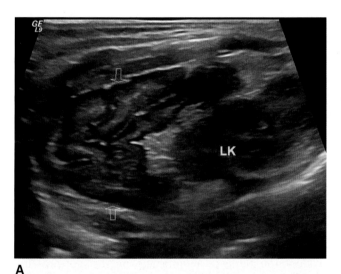

A

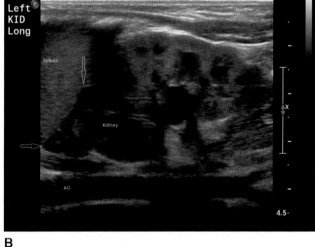

B

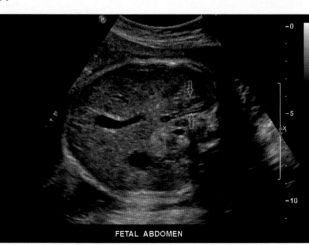

C

FIGURE 15-17 Congenital adrenal hyperplasia. **A:** Neonate born with ambiguous genitalia. Karyotype confirmed a chromosomal female.[46] The adrenal glands (*arrows*) were enlarged and demonstrated a cerebriform pattern. A pelvic ultrasound performed confirmed a normal uterus and ovaries. **B:** Normal adrenal gland (*arrows*) in a neonate. **C:** Normal adrenal gland (*arrows*) in the fetus. *LK*, left kidney. (**A:** Image courtesy of Linda S. Woolpert, Grand Rapids, MI; **B** and **C:** Images courtesy of Susan Raatz Stephenson, Salt Lake City, UT.)

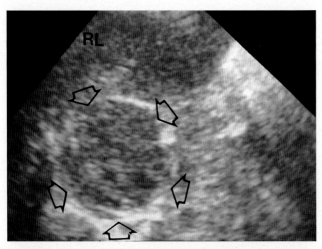

FIGURE 15-18 Hyperadrenalism. The right adrenal gland appears as a solid mass (within *arrowheads*) on the transverse section made on a 4-month-old girl displaying clinical signs and symptoms of hyperadrenalism. *RL*, right liver lobe. (Image courtesy of Helen Johnson, Salt Lake City, UT.)

diagnoses, correlation with the patient's clinical findings and laboratory values expedites interpretation of the sonographic study (Pathology Box 15-2).

Incidentaloma

The general term for an unexpected mass detected during an imaging procedure being performed for unrelated disease is "incidentaloma." This term may be applied to any unexpected mass, occurring anywhere in the body. AI has become a common term in the medical literature and represents a diagnostic challenge, which includes discovery of masses, which range from benign, nonfunctional lesions to malignant tumors such as pheochromocytomas, adrenocortical carcinomas, or metastases from other primary cancers.[8] These incidental masses are detected on 4% to 5% of CT studies.[51,52]

Diagnoses and treatments for incidentalomas vary based on two important clinical criteria: patient history of cancer and hyperfunction of the mass.[8,11,53,54] Multiple studies have revealed that in patients with a history of extra-adrenal malignancy, 45% to 73% of the incidentalomas are metastases.[34,51,55] This is not surprising because lung cancer commonly metastasizes to the adrenal glands.

In contrast, in recent studies on the general population of patients without a history of cancer, the majority of incidentalomas (60% to 94%) were nonhypersecreting adenomas, 1% to 22% were cysts, 6% to 15% were myelolipomas, 0% to 11% were pheochromocytomas, whereas 0% to 4% were adrenocortical carcinomas and 0% to 2% were metastases.[11,34,51-53,56] Subclinical Cushing syndrome was present in 5% to 20% of patients with incidentalomas, which should account for hypersecreting adenomas.[11]

Unilateral hyperfunctioning lesions (adenomas, aldosteronomas, pheochromocytomas, and adrenal hyperplasias) are usually treated surgically.[8,11,53,54] Laparoscopy is used for small tumors (1 to 2 cm).[11] Adrenalectomy is also indicated for nonfunctioning masses larger than 4 to 6 cm in size and lesions that are potentially malignant.[11,54,57] Bilateral masses require alternative or combination treatments to avoid adrenal insufficiency. Gland enlargement, change in appearance on follow-up, or atypical appearance on CT and/or MRI also justify gland removal.[11,58]

Cortical Tumors

Adenomas

Adrenal gland nodules measuring less than 3 cm are found in approximately 2% to 9% of patients on autopsy; the majority are nonfunctioning, slow-growing cortical adenomas.[31,38,59] An adenoma may also be one part of the MEN syndromes.[38] Most are benign, poorly encapsulated tumors, 1 to 5 cm in diameter, and consist of lipid-filled cells that do not secrete hormones.[38] Generally, a single-ovoid nodule larger than 1 cm is considered an adenoma; multiple or bilateral nodules located either inside or outside the capsule are considered expressions of nodular hyperplasia.[38] Adenomas greater than 2 cm in size are more likely to be functional and may cause Cushing syndrome (hypercortisolism).[49] Administration of ACTH causes adrenal adenomas to grow in the same way it stimulates adrenal hyperplasia. Adenocarcinoma, however, is independent of pituitary influence and does not respond to ACTH administration.[47]

An adenoma is sonographically difficult to detect because of its anatomic location and the presence of surrounding retroperitoneal fat. Criteria used to support the diagnosis of an incidental adrenal adenoma include a small (<5 cm) round or oval mass, clear separation of the margins from adjacent structures, and no evidence of growth on serial examinations[37] (Fig. 15-19A–E and Pathology Box 15-3). Such masses are frequently only 1.5 to 2 cm in diameter, with no calcifications or central necrosis.[48,49,53] Their homogeneous, hypoechoic sonographic appearance is similar to that of aldosteronomas, which cause Conn syndrome and generally appear sonographically as small, round, relatively anechoic masses.[1]

Myelolipomas

Adrenal myelolipoma is a rare benign tumor of the adrenal cortex. Of uncertain etiology, it is composed of mature, lipid-rich, macrosomic fatty tissue with a variable proportion of hematopoietic elements resembling bone marrow.[1,3,48,60,61] The lesion is found between the fourth and sixth decades of life, with an equal incidence in men and women.[26,31] Generally, myelolipomas are unilateral, less than 5 cm in size, hormonally inactive, and therefore asymptomatic.[1] Large or bilateral lesions may become symptomatic, causing pain or endocrine dysfunction owing to hemorrhage, necrosis, or pressure on adjacent structures.[60,61]

A combination of sonography, CT, and angiography can lead to a fairly specific preoperative diagnosis of an adrenal myelolipoma.[60,61] Sonographically, the tumor is usually a well-defined, markedly hyperechoic mass demonstrating an interrupted, posteriorly displaced hemidiaphragm resulting from a velocity artifact caused by the lipomatous content[3,60,62] (Fig. 15-20A–C and Pathology Box 15-3). The sonographic examination is useful in localizing the anatomic origin of these upper quadrant abnormalities, especially on the right side.[60] If it is detected sonographically, the differential diagnosis includes retroperitoneal lipoma, retroperitoneal liposarcoma, renal angiomyolipoma, lymphangioma, increased abdominal fat deposition, and retroperitoneal teratoma.[3,32,60,61] A more complicated appearance is created when an adenoma is imbedded within the myelolipoma or the mass is primarily myeloid tissue.[1,48]

CT examination should follow detection of a lipomatous lesion by sonography because CT is capable of identifying

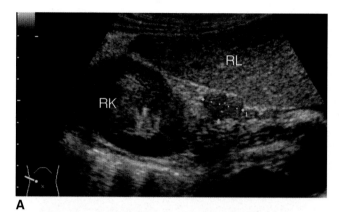

A

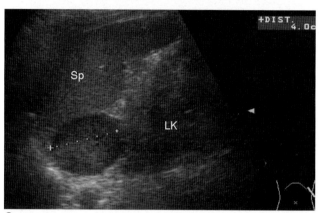

C

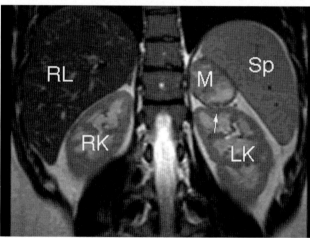

E

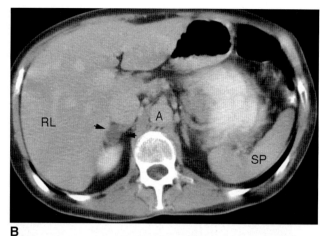

B

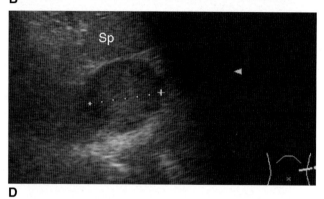

D

FIGURE 15-19 Adrenal adenomas. **A:** On a transverse section, a small right adrenal adenoma appears as an isoechoic mass (*calipers*) measuring 1.9 × 1.3 cm. **B:** On the computed tomography (CT) image of the same patient, the location and relational anatomy of the right adrenal adenoma (*arrowhead*) are demonstrated. The mass is posteromedial to the right liver lobe and superomedial to the right kidney. Differential diagnosis includes nonfunctioning adrenal adenoma. Nonfunctioning adrenal adenomas require no special treatment, but the patient should be kept under observation for tumor growth or development of hypersecretory function. Adrenal insufficiency is rarely observed unless both glands are involved. Left gland is normal (*arrow*). **C–E:** On another patient, this left adrenal adenoma appears as a hypoechoic mass measuring 4 cm in maximum diameter identified in the subsplenic space. **C:** The longitudinal section demonstrates the mass (*calipers*) superior to the left kidney (*LK*) and inferior and medial to the spleen (*Sp*). **D:** On the transverse section, the primarily hypoechoic mass (*calipers*) is identified posteromedial to the spleen (*Sp*). **E:** On coronal magnetic resonance imaging (MRI), the location and relational anatomy of the left adrenal mass (*M*) are demonstrated. No mass is identified in the region of the right adrenal gland. The tissue planes between the retroperitoneal organs are clearly delineated and show the adenoma indenting the upper pole of the left kidney on the MRI (*arrow*). *A*, aorta; *RL*, right liver lobe; *RK*, right kidney. (Images courtesy of Dr. Taco Geertsma, Gelderse Vallei, Ede, The Netherlands.)

PATHOLOGY BOX 15-3
Adrenocortical Tumors

Tumor	Sonographic Appearance
Adenomas	Hypoechoic, small (1.5–2 cm), round, encapsulated mass; clear separation of the margins from adjacent structures; may have calcifications
Myelolipomas	Hyperechoic, well-defined mass with interrupted posterior hemidiaphragm; if small, may blend with perirenal fat
Cancer	Hyperechoic, solid, larger masses; echo pattern varies with necrosis or hemorrhage; may invade vasculature and displace surrounding organs

the fatty nature of the mass.[61] On CT, a myelolipoma appears as a well-defined, fatty suprarenal mass with negative or low attenuation values compared with the high-attenuating adrenal gland tissue, other tissue types, or hemorrhage.[48,60] These masses also appear hyperintense on T1-weighted in-phase MRI and hypointense on fat-saturated MRI.[48] If present, liposarcomas are nonhomogeneous, poorly defined, and infiltrative.[63] On angiography, an adrenal myelolipoma appears as an avascular mass in the adrenal gland rather than in the kidney or liver.[60] Venography demonstrates displacement of veins around the tumor.

Cancer

Cortical cancers, such as adenocarcinomas, often produce steroids (36% to 90%) and are usually associated with one of

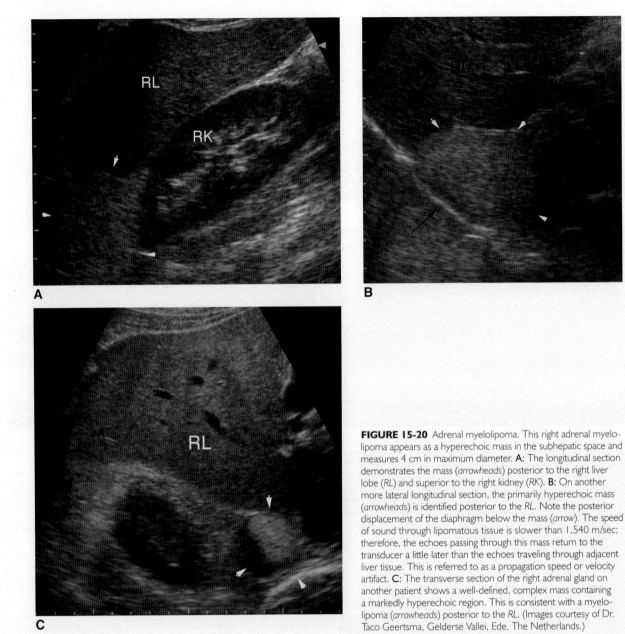

FIGURE 15-20 Adrenal myelolipoma. This right adrenal myelolipoma appears as a hyperechoic mass in the subhepatic space and measures 4 cm in maximum diameter. **A:** The longitudinal section demonstrates the mass (*arrowheads*) posterior to the right liver lobe (*RL*) and superior to the right kidney (*RK*). **B:** On another more lateral longitudinal section, the primarily hyperechoic mass (*arrowheads*) is identified posterior to the *RL*. Note the posterior displacement of the diaphragm below the mass (*arrow*). The speed of sound through lipomatous tissue is slower than 1,540 m/sec; therefore, the echoes passing through this mass return to the transducer a little later than the echoes traveling through adjacent liver tissue. This is referred to as a propagation speed or velocity artifact. **C:** The transverse section of the right adrenal gland on another patient shows a well-defined, complex mass containing a markedly hyperechoic region. This is consistent with a myelolipoma (*arrowheads*) posterior to the *RL*. (Images courtesy of Dr. Taco Geertsma, Gelderse Vallei, Ede, The Netherlands.)

the hyperadrenal syndromes—those that are nonfunctioning are highly malignant.[3,11,32,38] Adrenal carcinomas are rare, accounting for only 2% of cancers in the world.[7,11] They may appear to be encapsulated and many exceed 20 cm in diameter, producing palpable abdominal masses.[11,38] These tumors may show zones of hemorrhage and necrosis.[38] Cortical cancers tend to invade the adrenal vein, IVC, and lymph nodes and commonly metastasize to regional and periaortic nodes, with hematogenous spread to the lungs, liver, bones, and other viscera.[1,3,11,32,38] Cortical cancers are solid-looking masses larger than most adrenal masses: 3 to 6 cm for hyperfunctioning tumors and greater than 6 cm for nonfunctioning lesions.[3] The echogenic appearance varies with the presence and degree of hemorrhage and necrosis, with nonfunctioning neoplasms appearing more complex and hyperechoic, whereas hyperfunctioning masses are more likely to be uniformly hypoechoic.[3] Calcifications are seen in 19% of cases.[31] Invasion of the mass into surrounding

vasculature and displacement of normal tissue contour and location help identify the mass (Fig. 15-21A–F and Pathology Box 15-3).

MEDULLARY PATHOLOGY

Pheochromocytoma

Patients with pheochromocytomas typically present with mild-to-marked hypertension (90%), headache (80%), sweating (65%), and tachycardia (50%).[11,14,18] Additional signs and symptoms also relate to the excessive and/or intermittent catecholamine secretion from these tumors. The rule of 10 describes the incidence of many features: 10% malignant, 10% bilateral or multiple, 10% hereditary syndromes, 10% pediatric, 10% extra-adrenal locations (paragangliomas), and 10% are normotensive nonfunctioning tumors.[11,50,64] Pheochromocytomas are rare (2 to 8 per million) but occur

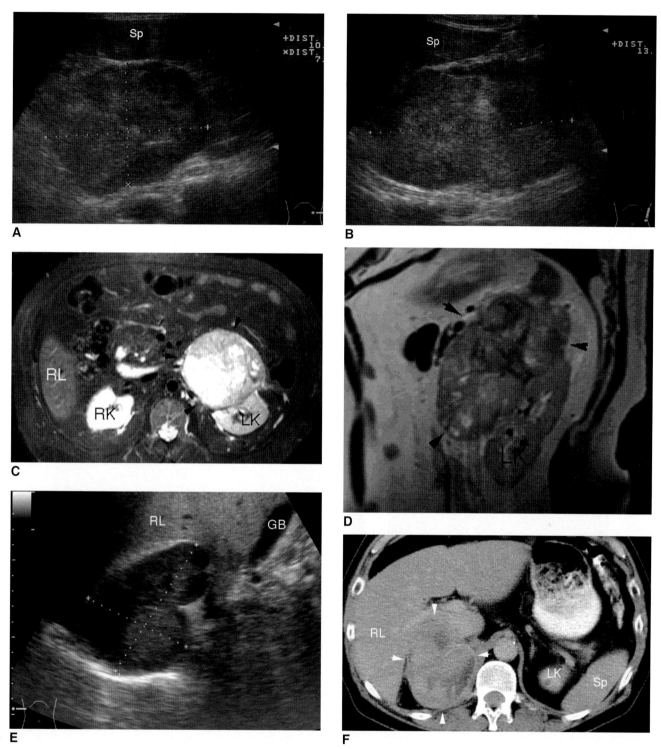

FIGURE 15-21 Adrenal carcinoma. Sonographic and magnetic resonance imaging (MRI) examinations documented a very large mass in the subsplenic region consistent with adrenocortical carcinoma. Sonographic characteristics of the mass include fairly well-defined margins with focal areas of increased and decreased echogenicity likely owing to hemorrhage and necrosis. The mass measured approximately 11 × 14 cm. The MRI did not demonstrate metastatic spread or involvement of the right adrenal gland. **A:** The transverse section demonstrates the cortical mass (*calipers*), medial to the spleen (*Sp*). **B:** On the longitudinal section, the cortical cancer (*calipers*) displaces the *Sp* anteriorly. **C:** On the transverse MRI, the location and relational anatomy of the left adrenal mass (*arrowheads*) are demonstrated. No mass is identified in the region of the right adrenal gland. **D:** On the longitudinal section MRI, the mass, spleen, and left kidney (*LK*) appear to be compressed into the left upper quadrant. Tissue variations on the MRI are consistent with the irregular echogenicity seen by ultrasound. The large dimensions and relational anatomy of the left adrenal mass (*arrowheads*) to the *LK* and diaphragm are demonstrated. **E** and **F:** Sonographic and computed tomography (CT) examinations documented a large mass in the subhepatic region consistent with adrenocortical carcinoma. Sonographic characteristics of the predominantly hypoechoic mass include fairly well-defined margins with focal areas of increased and decreased echogenicity likely owing to hemorrhage and necrosis. The mass measured approximately 10 cm. The CT images do not demonstrate metastatic spread or involvement of the left adrenal gland. **E:** On the transverse section, the primarily hypoechoic mass (*calipers*) is identified posterior to the right liver lobe (*RL*) and lateral to the gall bladder (*GB*). **F:** On the transverse CT image, the location and relational anatomy of the right adrenal mass (*arrowheads*) are demonstrated. No mass is identified in the region of the left adrenal gland. Tissue variations on the CT are consistent with the irregular echogenicity seen by ultrasound. *RK*, right kidney. (Images courtesy of Dr. Taco Geertsma, Gelderse Vallei, Ede, The Netherlands.)

at a higher frequency in patients with hypertension (1%), hereditary endocrine tumor syndromes; MEN type 2A and 2B, von Hippel–Lindau, and neurofibromatosis (NF-1), as well as neuroectodermal dysplasia syndromes; and von Recklinghausen neurofibromatosis, tuberous sclerosis, and Sturge–Weber syndrome.[11,20] These patients are routinely screened, so the masses are usually smaller when initially detected.[50] For some patients, the incidence of pheochromocytomas is dramatic at 50% to 70% for MEN 2A and 90% and bilateral for MEN 2B.[65] Patients with MEN syndromes are often treated with prophylactic cortical-sparing or complete bilateral adrenalectomies with hormone replacement.[20,36] In addition to these hereditary syndromes, which demonstrate genetic mutations that contribute to a higher risk for pheochromocytomas, there are sporadic genetic mutations, which can be passed by carriers. First-degree relatives should be screened when new cases are discovered.[20,64]

Benign and malignant pheochromocytomas have similar biochemical characteristics, such as elevated levels of urinary catecholamine, plasma-free metanephrine, and other metabolites such as VMA.[11,14,20,32,37,47] Clinical manifestations, laboratory values, and metastases to liver, lymph nodes, lungs, or bones help establish a diagnosis of malignancy. The sustained elevation of catecholamine secretion can lead to cardiomegaly, left ventricular failure, cardiomyopathy, and ultimately death owing to heart failure.[47] Generally, treatment consists of surgical removal of the gland and epinephrine and norepinephrine substitution therapy.

These tumors are usually well encapsulated, are ovoid to round, and may be palpable.[39,50] They are highly vascular masses and, if rupture occurs, massive hemorrhage can be fatal.[47] This tumor occurs in both sexes, usually between ages 25 and 50 years.[38] Pheochromocytomas are usually larger than 2 cm in size at detection and average 5 to 6 cm in size.[39] Sonographic appearance includes a broad spectrum from (1) hyperechoic, hypoechoic, or isoechoic solid tumors; (2) homogeneous or heterogeneous echogenic solid tumors; (3) complex masses; and (4) cystic masses.[65,66] This variety is attributed to the spectrum of their gross morphologic appearances.[65,66] The well-marginated mass may appear quite large, with purely solid homogeneous components or with complex heterogeneous echoes representing hemorrhage and/or necrosis[32,39,65] (Fig. 15-22A, B). Calcification may also be present in an eggshell pattern along the outer margin of the tumor.[39] Larger masses may displace surrounding organs and/or indent vasculature (Pathology Box 15-4).

CT is the imaging modality of choice for the initial detection and localization as indicated by the presence of a soft tissue mass, potential speckled calcifications, and intense contrast enhancement with nonionic contrast media.[50] When central necrosis is present, the peripheral rim of tumor retains the intense enhancement on CT.[50]

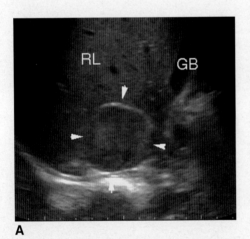
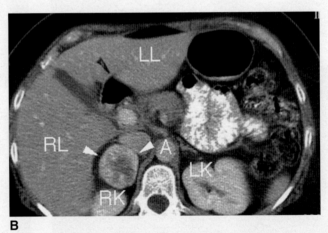

FIGURE 15-22 Pheochromocytoma. In the right adrenal gland, a pheochromocytoma (*arrows*) approximately 4 cm in maximum dimension. **A:** On the longitudinal section, the primarily isoechoic round mass with sharply marginated walls (*arrow*) is identified posterior to the right liver lobe (*RL*) and lateral to the gallbladder (*GB*). **B:** On the transverse section, the right adrenal mass (*arrow*) is demonstrated medial to the right kidney (*RK*), and posterior to the right liver lobe (*RL*). (Images courtesy of Dr. Taco Geertsma, Gelderse Vallei Hospital, The Netherlands.)

PATHOLOGY BOX 15-4
Tumors of the Adrenal Medulla

Tumor	Sonographic Appearance
Pheochromocytoma	Broad spectrum (hyperechoic, hypoechoic, echogenic, complex, cystic), marginated, or encapsulated; solid components of homogeneous or heterogeneous echoes may represent hemorrhage or necrosis; larger masses displace surrounding organs or indent vasculature; may be bilateral or external to the adrenal
Neuroblastoma	Generally affect children (see Chapter 20); hyperechoic, poorly defined borders; focal echogenic areas may be present owing to calcifications; hypoechoic areas may be present owing to necrosis; inferior and lateral displacement of kidney

MRI may also be used to characterize these tumors, which are isointense or hypointense to the liver on T1-weighted images.[65] T2 weighting reveals high intensity in areas of hemorrhage.[50,65] Unfortunately, the appearance of pheochromocytomas on MRI also overlaps with metastases and lipomatous adenomas.[50] A definite benefit of CT and MRI is concurrent detection of additional tumors associated with MEN syndromes.[50] Scintigraphy offers whole-body imaging and the ability to simultaneously detect extra-adrenal lesions and metastases.[50] Specific radionuclides used for detection of pheochromocytomas are discussed later in this chapter.

Neuroblastoma

Neuroblastoma is a highly malignant tumor of the adrenal medulla that is generally found in children (Pathology Box 15-4; see Chapter 20).

Metastatic Disease

For patients with a history of cancer, multiple imaging modalities are used for locating new lesions, staging the disease, and treatment planning. Adrenal glands are the fourth most common site of metastases after lungs, liver, and bones.[32,37] Metastases to the adrenal glands occur from squamous cell carcinoma of the lung (33%); breast carcinoma (30%); lymphoma, leukemia, and melanoma; and carcinoma of the gastrointestinal tract, thyroid, pancreas, and kidney (37%), and they tend to be bilateral.[3,32,37,39,55,59] There is a 25% incidence of adrenal involvement in non-Hodgkin lymphoma[32] (see Pathology Box 15-1).

Small adrenal metastases characteristically are hypoechoic, round, or oval, and they are located anteromedial to the upper pole of the kidney[32,35] (Fig. 15-14E, F). Larger metastases (>4 cm) tend to be irregularly shaped, heterogeneous in texture, and may show central necrosis. These masses can also indent the posterior wall of the IVC and displace the kidneys inferiorly[32,37] (Figs. 15-3A, 15-14A–D, and 15-23A–C). Hypoechoic and hyperechoic areas within these masses may represent necrosis and/or hemorrhage[32] (Figs. 15-13A–G and 15-14A–F and Pathology Box 15-4). Tumor extension into the IVC is specific for adrenocortical carcinoma.

With nonenhanced CT, the nonnecrotic rim of tissue may show high attenuation. On delayed contrast-enhanced CT, metastases enhance rapidly, but contrast washout is slow.[29,49,53] Although adrenal metastases and lymphomas are often bilateral (50%); this is not unique to the presentation of cancer[29,53] (Fig. 15-13D–G). Hyper- and hypofunctional diseases that commonly occur bilaterally include hyperplasia, infections, and hemorrhage.[53] Less frequently,

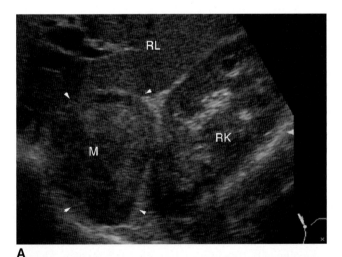

A

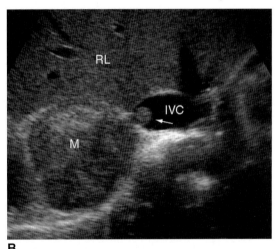

B

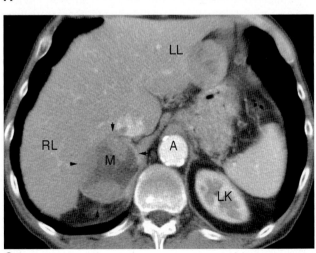

C

FIGURE 15-23 These sonograms demonstrate a predominantly solid mass (*M, arrowheads*), representing metastases to the right gland from a lung carcinoma. The longitudinal (**A**) and transverse (**B**) aspects of the right adrenal mass are identified posteromedial to the right liver lobe (*RL*) and superior to the right kidney (*RK*). The transverse sonogram also demonstrates direct tumor invasion (*arrow*) into the inferior vena cava (*IVC*). **C:** On the computed tomography image, the location and relational anatomy of the right adrenal mass (*M, arrowheads*) are demonstrated. No mass was identified in the region of the left adrenal gland. *A*, aorta; *LL*, left liver lobe; *LK*, left kidney. (Images courtesy of Dr. Taco Geertsma, Gelderse Vallei, Ede, The Netherlands.)

pheochromocytomas, myelolipomas, and masses replacing normal adrenocortical tissue (adenomas and adrenocortical carcinomas) occur bilaterally.[53] Failure to identify accompanying adrenal insufficiency is life-threatening.[11,18]

Only about half of the adrenal masses in patients with known primary tumors prove to be malignant on biopsy examination.[37] Therefore, a solitary nonfunctioning adrenal tumor should not be assumed to be metastatic disease without being correlated with other findings.[37] Percutaneous aspiration biopsy is capable of distinguishing metastases from a benign adenoma or a primary adrenal carcinoma.[37] Collision tumor describes an existing adrenal adenoma, which is secondarily infiltrated by a metastasis.[49,67] This tumor produces a mixed-signal MRI anatomically consistent with the adenoma and metastasis components.

OTHER IMAGING PROCEDURES

Radiography

With advances in tomographic and volumetric imaging technology, traditional radiographic examinations are no longer the procedure of choice for the adrenal gland; however, incidental radiographic findings may indicate adrenal gland pathology. Calcifications may be visualized on an abdominal radiograph of the kidneys, ureters, and bladder, which is the "scout study" prior to excretory urography, intravenous pyelography (IVP), or nephrotomography (tomography eliminates obscuring overlying structures). The presence of calcifications is not specific because they occur in 10% of adrenal tumors and 15% of adrenal cysts. In adrenal cysts, calcifications are usually located at the periphery and appear more curvilinear, like an eggshell.[35,37] Approximately 70% to 80% of adrenal masses can be detected by combined IVP and tomography, relying on both the delineation of the mass and demonstration of the degree to which it impinges on the kidney. Small adrenal masses, such as aldosteronomas and extra-adrenal pheochromocytomas, are difficult to demonstrate with these modalities.[37]

An angiography examination is specific in demonstrating vascular adrenal masses[60] and the vascular supply to tumors and provides useful information for the surgical team. Angiography may not be specific, though, in differentiating neoplasms from hyperplasia or delineating hypovascular lesions. Venography demonstrates the displacement of veins around the tumor. Venography with venous blood sampling of circulating hormones is 100% accurate in differentiating between a unilateral adenoma and bilateral adrenal hyperplasia.[40,49] The risks of angiography, venography, and venous sampling include intra-adrenal hemorrhage with pain, infarction, and possibly Addison disease.[40]

Computed Tomography and Magnetic Resonance Imaging

Thin-collimation CT is the first-choice imaging modality for evaluating most cases of suspected adrenal disease.[30] In comparison to sonography, CT is superior in detecting normal adrenal glands, especially in obese patients.[29,49,55,65] Several adrenal lesions have inherent tissue characteristics detectable on CT that permit a confident diagnosis based on these images alone.[29,49,53] The use of other imaging modalities

(MRI, scintigraphy, and PET) in addition to blood and urine testing contributes to refining the diagnosis in most cases.[34,49,65] MRI offers multiple techniques for evaluating adrenal masses.[58] Both T1- and T2-weighted images may be utilized to obtain a diagnosis, with adenomas producing weak signals, pheochromocytomas strong ones, and carcinomas intermediate signals.[37,58,65]

Diagnostic protocols have been developed and continue to be refined regarding the use of CT and MRI for identifying, characterizing, and treating adrenal lesions. MRI is as sensitive as CT in the identification of a variety of adrenal abnormalities. Diagnosis usually relies on multiple criteria, and even after extensive imaging, biopsy may still be required to rule out malignancy.[29] For example, with oncology patients, noncontrast CT is the first step in the diagnostic imaging process. If the attenuation rate of the tumor area is less than 10 Hounsfield units (HU), it is classified as a benign adenoma.[29,49,53] If the mass does not meet this criteria, then a delayed contrast-enhanced CT (10 minutes) or chemical shift MRI is the next step. The delayed contrast-enhanced CT provides information about the perfusion of the lesion and the rapidity of washout of the contrast media. Lesion attenuation values less than 30 HU and greater than 50% washout of contrast media at 10 minutes identify another group of benign adenomas.[29,49] Tumors that do not meet these criteria are destined for biopsy or further evaluation by MRI. Similar to CT, with the more costly contrast MRI, adenomas show rapid enhancement and rapid washout of contrast material. On chemical-shifted MRI, adenomas show signal drop-off, which is not seen with malignant lesions.

The advantages of MRI are multiple acquisition and reconstructed planes and use of nonionizing radiation, whereas limitations include cost and availability.[31,58] Chemical shift MRI or T2-weighted MRI is used for the detection of pheochromocytomas. Pheochromocytomas are often, but not always, T2 hyperintense.[65] MRI is useful for the detection of recurrence and ectopic pheochromocytomas (aka paragangliomas).[49]

MRI and CT imaging continue to improve, and differences occur in technologies and methodologies. For example, single- and multiple-row helical CT scanners produce somewhat different image features for some adrenal masses.[53] Further research data will need to be collected to determine how these changes in technology and methodology impact the image characteristics that may eventually become uniquely diagnostic for a variety of lesions evaluated by CT and MRI. When laboratory testing and imaging procedures are not conclusive, biopsy becomes necessary. CT remains the preferred method to provide needle guidance, although these percutaneous procedures are not without complication.[40,49,68]

Radionuclide Studies

Radiopharmaceuticals are used to locate and differentiate specific types of adrenal masses. The major benefits of nuclear medicine procedures are that the images are based on active tissue physiologic function and can be collected from a whole-body perspective, which is particularly useful for identifying ectopic masses and metastases.[65,69] Fusion imaging in the form of SPECT/CT and PET/CT will likely continue to increase because it offers the integration of anatomic and functional data for the diagnosis and treatment of cortical and medullary adrenal disease.[55]

Meta-iodobenzylguanidine (^{131}I-MIGB or ^{123}I-MIGB) and [111]Indium-octreotide (Somastatin analog) are radiopharmaceuticals used to locate adrenomedullary tumors such as neuroblastomas and pheochromocytomas.[49,65,69] Pheochromocytomas are visualized with both radionuclides 50% of the time, 25% of the time only with MIGB, and the other 25% of the time with only In[111].[49] Therefore, using the second radionuclide when there is nonvisualization with the first ensures localization of all adrenal and extra-adrenal pheochromocytomas and paragangliomas of similar embryonic origin when using whole-body scans.

An investigational but very successful radionuclide, [131]Iodine 6-beta-iodomethyl-19-norcholesterol (NP-59) is used to detect and differentiate aldosteronomas from adrenocortical hyperplasia. In patients with ACTH-independent Cushing syndrome, bilateral increased uptake of NP-59 indicates adrenocortical nodular hyperplasia whereas unilateral increased uptake suggests an adrenocortical adenoma. Absent or faint uptake is considered normal if there are no other signs or symptoms of adrenal disease.[55,69] Currently, NP-59 is not U.S. Food and Drug Administration (FDA)–approved and has limited availability.[49,55,59]

Using a whole-body imaging PET approach, the radiopharmaceutical fluorine-18 fluorodeoxyglucose (PET/FDG) is very good at distinguishing benign adrenal masses from malignant adrenal tumors and metastatic disease.[49,55,65,69] Increased costs and reduced availability are limitations for PET/FDG.[70]

Endoscopic Ultrasound

EUS is a useful tool for assessing the adrenal gland when this invasive procedure is already planned. There is a significant potential to gather additional information regarding the presence of adrenal masses, adjacent lymphadenopathy, and for staging lung cancers, which commonly metastasize to the adrenal glands.[5,68] Gastric and duodenal windows are used to image with 5- to 7.5-MHz radial, linear, and/or curvilinear transducers.[5,68] This technique can place the transducer as close as 1 to 2 cm from gland. As a result, the acoustic appearance of a normal adrenal gland is that of seagull-shaped hyperechoic medullary echoes against the hypoechoic cortical echoes and the hyperechoic halo of fatty tissue.[17,68]

Guidance of fine needle aspiration of adrenal lesions can also be performed using this endoscopic approach (EUS-FNA).[68,71] EUS-FNA is used to differentiate benign adrenal masses from metastases or primary adrenal malignancies. This is particularly important for preoperative staging of patients with known malignancies, because adrenal glands are common metastatic sites.[5,68,71] EUS visualization of the left adrenal from a transgastric approach reaches 98%, whereas it has been reported that imaging the right adrenal gland from a transduodenal window is only successful 30% of the time with a mechanical radial transducer.[72] Others have had improved success for visualizing and performing EUS-FNA on the right adrenal by instead using a curvilinear transducer.[68,73]

EUS is minimally invasive and has minimal complications for the patient.[5,68,71,73,74] Limitations of EUS for adrenal imaging rest with the experience and motivation of the specialists who use this technology.[5,17,68,71,73]

Intraoperative Ultrasound

High-frequency IOUS is also used with a variety of laparoscopic (LIOUS) and open surgery settings.[4,74,75] Benefits of LIOUS concurrent with laparoscopic adrenalectomies are numerous. These include improved localization and guidance of complete and partial adrenalectomies, reduced blood loss owing to improved vascular visualization, identification of adjacent tumor infiltration, metastases and lymphadenopathy, fewer complications, and shorter time to recovery.[4,57,74,75] Some drawbacks to laparoscopic adrenalectomies with LIOUS are an increase in procedure duration, steep learning curve for physicians, and an increase in patient cost for adding LIOUS.[4,57,75]

SUMMARY

- The adrenal cortex and medulla develop from different embryonic tissues and are therefore two functionally distinct endocrine glands within one organ.
- The adrenal cortex comprises 90% of the gland and produces corticoids including cortisol, aldosterone, estrogen, and androgen.
- The medulla produces the catecholamines epinephrine and norepinephrine responsible for the body's fight-or-flight response to stress.
- The adrenal glands are retroperitoneal and are located anterior, medial, and superior to the kidneys.
- The right adrenal gland is triangular in shape and is located posterior and lateral to the inferior vena cava, medial to the right lobe of the liver, and lateral to the crus of the diaphragm; the left adrenal gland is larger than the right and is more crescent or semilunar in shape.
- Adrenal cysts are infrequent and usually asymptomatic, whereas most adrenal cysts are benign, and adrenal cysts with a "ring" calcification are more often malignant.

- Hemorrhage of the adrenal gland is seen most often in newborns, especially after a difficult delivery but can also be precipitated by adrenal trauma, surgery, stress, anticoagulant therapy, adrenal vein thrombosis, adrenal neoplasms, metastases, or septicemia. The right side is involved more often than the left side.
- Addison disease is a condition caused by hyposecretion of adrenocortical hormones and is characterized by fever, fatigue, muscle weakness, hypotension, and gastrointestinal distress such as nausea, vomiting, weight loss, and diarrhea.
- Cushing syndrome is caused by hypersecretion of the adrenocortical hormone cortisol, which triggers an increase in gluconeogenesis and results in elevated serum glucose levels, protein loss, and hypertension.
- Conn syndrome is caused by hyperaldosteronism and in 80% to 90% of patients, it results from a benign aldosterone-producing adrenal adenoma.
- Adrenal adenomas are typically benign, poorly encapsulated tumors 1 to 5 cm in diameter, and consist of lipid-filled cells that do not secrete hormones. Adenomas greater

than 2 cm in size are more likely to be functional and may cause Cushing syndrome.

■ Adrenal myelolipoma is a rare benign tumor of the adrenal cortex composed of fatty tissue that sonographically appears as a well-defined and markedly hyperechoic mass.

■ Adrenal adenocarcinomas occur in the adrenal cortex, often produce steroids, and are usually associated with one of the hyperadrenal syndromes; those that are nonfunctioning are highly malignant.

■ Adenocarcinomas are solid masses larger than most adrenal masses, 3 to 6 cm for hyperfunctioning tumors and larger than 6 cm for nonfunctioning lesions with a variable echogenicity depending on the degree of hemorrhage and necrosis. Nonfunctioning neoplasms appear more complex and hyperechoic, whereas hyperfunctioning masses are more likely to be uniformly hypoechoic.

■ Benign and malignant pheochromocytomas arise from the adrenal medulla and have similar sonographic and biochemical characteristics. Patients with pheochromocytomas typically present with mild-to-marked hypertension, headache, sweating, and tachycardia, and most have a history of a hereditary endocrine tumor syndrome such as MEN or von Hippel–Lindau.

■ Pheochromocytomas are usually well encapsulated, are ovoid-to-round, and may be palpable. They are highly vascular masses, and if rupture occurs, massive hemorrhage can be fatal. They have a highly variable echogenicity ranging from cystic or complex to echogenic with calcifications.

■ Adrenal metastases occur from squamous cell carcinoma of the lung, breast carcinoma, lymphoma, leukemia, melanoma and from carcinoma of the gastrointestinal tract, thyroid, pancreas, and kidney, and they tend to be bilateral.

■ CT is the modality of choice for evaluating the adrenal glands, but MRI, radionuclide studies, endoscopic ultrasound, and IOUS are also utilized.

REFERENCES

1. Little AF. Adrenal gland and renal sonography. *World J Surg.* 2000;24:171–182.
2. Suzuki Y, Sasagawa I, Suzuki H, et al. The role of ultrasonography in the detection of adrenal masses: comparison with computed tomography and magnetic resonance imaging. *Int Urol Nephrol.* 2001;32:302–306.
3. Wan YL. Ultrasonography of the adrenal gland: a review. *J Med Ultrasound.* 2007;15(4):213–227.
4. Heniford BT, Iannitti DA, Hale J, et al. The role of intraoperative ultrasonography during laparoscopic adrenalectomy. *Surgery.* 1997;122(6):1068–1074.
5. Kann PH. Endoscopic ultrasound imaging of the adrenals. *Endoscopy.* 2005;37(3):244–253.
6. Saftoiu A, Vilman P. Endoscopic ultrasound elastography—a new imaging technique for the visualization of tissue elasticity distribution. *J Gastrointestin Liver Dis.* 2006;15(2):161–165.
7. Slapa RZ, Kasperlik-Zaluska AA, Polanski JA, et al. Three-dimensional sonography in diagnosis of retroperitoneal hemorrhage from adrenocortical carcinoma. *J Ultrasound Med.* 2004;23:1369–1373.
8. Nawar R, Aron D. Adrenal incidentalomas—a continuing management dilemma. *Endocr Relat Cancer.* 2005;12:585–598.
9. Barwick TD, Malhotra A, Webb JA. Embryology of the adrenal glands and its relevance to diagnostic imaging. *Clin Radiol.* 2005;60:953–959.
10. Mangray S, DeLellis RA. Adrenal embryology and pathology. In: Blake MA, Boland G, eds. *Adrenal Imaging.* Humana Press; 2009:1–34.
11. Brunt LM, Moley J. The pituitary and adrenal glands. In: Townsend CM, Beauchamp RD, Evers BM, et al, eds. *Sabiston's Textbook of Surgery: The Biological Basis of Modern Surgical Practice.* 17th ed. Saunders Elsevier; 2004:1023–1070.
12. Banowsky JHW. Surgical anatomy. In: Novick AC, Stewart BH, Pontes JE, eds. *Operative Urology Vol 1: The Kidneys, Adrenal Glands and Retroperitoneum.* Lippincott Williams & Wilkins; 1989.
13. Stephen AE, Haynes AB, Hodin RA. Adrenal surgery. In: Blake MA, Boland G, eds. *Adrenal Imaging.* Humana Press; 2009:77–90.
14. Genuth SM. The adrenal glands. In: Berne RM, Levy MN, Koeppen BM, et al, eds. *Physiology.* 5th ed. Mosby Elsevier; 2004:949–979.
15. Standring S, ed. *Gray's Anatomy: The Anatomical Basis of Clinical Practice.* 40th ed. Churchill Livingstone Elsevier; 2008.
16. Higham CE, Coen JJ, Boland GWL, et al. The adrenals in oncology. In: Blake MA, Boland G, eds. *Adrenal Imaging.* Humana Press; 2009:65–66.
17. Chang KJ, Erickson RA, Nguyen P. Endoscopic ultrasound (EUS) and EUS-guided fine needle aspiration of the left adrenal gland. *Gastrointest Endosc.* 1996;44(5):568–572.
18. Corbett JV. *Laboratory Tests and Diagnostic Procedures with Nursing Diagnosis.* 7th ed. Prentice-Hall; 2008.
19. Trikudanathan S, Dluhy RG. Adrenocortical dysfunction. In: Blake MA, Boland G, eds. *Adrenal Imaging.* Humana Press; 2009:35–56.
20. Young WF. Adrenal medullary dysfunction. In: Blake MA, Boland G, eds. *Adrenal Imaging.* Humana Press; 2009:57–64.
21. Krebs CA, Eisenberg RL, Ratcliff S, et al. Cava-suprarenal line: new position for sonographic imaging of the left adrenal gland. *J Clin Ultrasound.* 1986;14:535–539.
22. Weinberg K. The retroperitoneum. In: Hagen-Ansert SL, ed. *Textbook of Diagnostic Ultrasonography.* 7th ed. Elsevier; 2012:440–460.
23. Yeh HC. Sonography of the adrenal glands: normal glands and small masses. *Am J Roentgenol.* 1980;135:1167–1177.
24. Krebs CA, Eisenberg RL. Ultrasound imaging of the adrenal glands. *Radiol Technol.* 1985;56:421–423.
25. Krebs CA, Rawls K. Techniques for successful scanning: positioning strategy for optimal visualization of a left adrenal mass. *J Diagn Med Sonogr.* 1990;5:286.
26. Krebs CA, Giyanani VL, Eisenberg RL. *Ultrasound Atlas of Disease Processes.* Appleton & Lange; 1993.
27. Matthew D. Possible adrenal mass. In: Sanders RC, Hall-Terracciano B, eds. *Clinical Sonography: A Practical Guide.* 5th ed. Wolters Kluwer; 2015:500–513.
28. Weinberg K. General abdominal sonography. In: Krebs C, Odwin CS, Fleischer AC, eds. *Appleton & Lange's Review for the Ultrasonography Examination.* McGraw-Hill; 2004:187–300.
29. Al-Hawary MM, Francis IR, Korobkin M. Adrenal imaging using computed tomography: differentiation of adenomas and metastasis. In: Blake MA, Boland G, eds. *Adrenal Imaging.* Humana Press; 2009:127–140.
30. Brant WE. Adrenal glands and kidneys. In: Brant WE, Helms CA, eds. *Fundamentals of Diagnostic Radiology.* 3rd ed. Lippincott Williams & Wilkins; 2007:867–886.
31. Ahua A, Thurston W, Wilson S. The adrenal glands. In: Rumack CM, Wilson SR, Charboneau JW, eds. *Diagnostic Ultrasound.* 4th ed. Elsevier Mosby; 2011:429–445.
32. Mittelstaedt CA. Retroperitoneum. In: Mittelstaedt CA, ed. *General Ultrasound.* Churchill Livingstone; 1992:714–832.
33. Filly R. Normal fetal anatomy. In: Callen PW, ed. *Ultrasonography in Obstetrics and Gynecology.* 5th ed. WB Saunders; 2008:297–362.
34. Frilling A, Tecklenborg K, Weber F, et al. Importance of adrenal incidentaloma in patients with a history of malignancy. *Surgery.* 2004;136:1289–1296.
35. Yeh HC. Ultrasound and CT of the adrenals. *Semin Ultrasound.* 1982;3:97–113.
36. Goldman SM, Coelho RD, Freire Filho E, et al. Imaging procedures in adrenal pathology. *Arq Bras Endocrinol Metabol.* 2004;48(5):592–611.

37. Mitty HA. Adrenal disease. In: Eisenberg RL, ed. *Diagnostic Imaging: An Algorithmic Approach.* Lippincott Williams & Wilkins; 1988:373–386.

38. Robbins SL, Cotran RS. *Pathologic Basis of Diseases.* 2nd ed. WB Saunders; 1979.

39. Hall R. *The Ultrasound Handbook: Clinical, Etiologic and Pathologic Implications of Sonographic Findings.* 3rd ed. Lippincott Williams & Wilkins; 1999.

40. Lucey BC. Adrenal trauma and intervention. In: Blake MA, Boland G, eds. *Adrenal Imaging.* Humana Press; 2009:193–204.

41. Weissleder R, Wittenberg J, Harisinghani MG. *Primer of Diagnostic Imaging.* 5th ed. Mosby Elsevier; 2011:231–234.

42. Fleischer AC. Renal and urological sonography. In: Fleisher AC, Kepple DM, eds. *Diagnostic Sonography: Principles and Clinical Applications.* WB Saunders; 1995:470–557.

43. Dimofte G, Dubei L, Lozneanu L-G, Ursulescu C, Grigora Scedil M. Right adrenal abscess—an unusual complication of acute appendicitis. *Rom J Gastroenterol.* 2004;13(3):241–244.

44. Kao P, Liu C, Lee C, et al. Non-typhi Salmonella adrenal abscess in an HIV-infected patient. *Scand J Infect Dis.* 2005;37(5):370–372.

45. Uno K, Konishi M, Yoshimoto E, et al. Fatal cytomegalovirus-associated adrenal insufficiency in an AIDS patient receiving corticosteroid therapy. *Intern Med.* 2007;46(9):617–620.

46. Grover SB, Midha N, Gupta M, et al. Imaging spectrum in disseminated histoplasmosis: case report and brief review. *Australas Radiol.* 2005;49:175–178.

47. Bullock BL. *Pathophysiology: Adaptations and Alterations in Function.* 4th ed. JB Lippincott-Raven; 1996.

48. Rockall AG, Babar SA, Sohaib SA. CT and MR imaging of ACTH-independent. Cushing syndrome. *Radiographics.* 2004;24(2):435–452.

49. Mayo-Smith WW, Boland GW, Noto RB, et al. State-of-the-art adrenal imaging. *Radiographics.* 2001;21(4):995–1012.

50. Sohaib SA, Rockall AG, Reznek RH. Imaging functional adrenal disorders. *Best Pract Res Clin Endocrinol Metab.* 2005;19(2):293–310.

51. Barzon L, Sonino N, Fallo F, et al. Prevalence and natural history of adrenal incidentalomas. *Eur J Endocrinol.* 2003;149(4):273–285.

52. Song JH, Chaudhry FS, Mayo-Smith WW. The incidental adrenal mass on CT: prevalence of adrenal disease in 1049 consecutive adrenal masses in patients with no known malignancy. *Am J Roentgenol.* 2008;190(5):1163–1168.

53. Johnson PT, Horton KM, Fishman EK. Adrenal imaging with multidetector CT: evidence-based protocol optimization and interpretive practice. *Radiographics.* 2009;29(5):1319–1331.

54. Zarco-González JA, Herrera MF. Adrenal incidentaloma. *Scand J Surg.* 2004;93(4):298–301.

55. Gross MD, Avram A, Fig LM, Rubello D. Contemporary adrenal scintigraphy. *Eur J Nucl Med Mol Imaging.* 2007;34(4):547–557.

56. Kloos RT, Gross MD, Francis IR. Incidentally discovered adrenal masses. *Cancer Treat Res.* 1997;89:286–292.

57. Mansmann G, Lau J, Balk E, et al. The clinically inapparent adrenal mass: update in diagnosis and management. *Endocr Rev.* 2004;25(2):309–340.

58. Kenney PJ. MRI of the adrenal glands. In: Blake MA, Boland G, eds. *Adrenal Imaging.* Humana Press; 2009:141–156.

59. Yeh HC. Ultrasonography of the adrenal gland. In: Schwartz AE, Pertsemlidis D, Gagner M, eds. *Endocrine Surgery.* Informa Healthcare; 2003:370–377.

60. Cintron E, Quntero EC, Perez MR, et al. Computed tomography, sonographic, and radiographic findings in adrenal myelolipoma. *Urology.* 1984;23:608–610.

61. Dieckmann KP, Hamm B, Pickartz H, et al. Adrenal myelolipoma: clinical, radiologic, and histologic features. *Urology.* 1987;29(1):1–8.

62. Richman TS, Taylor JK, Kremkau FW. Propagation speed artifact in fatty tumor (myelolipoma): significance for tissue differential diagnosis. *J Ultrasound Med.* 1983;2:45–47.

63. Friedman AC, Hartman MD, Sherman J, et al. Computed tomography of abdominal fatty masses. *Radiology.* 1981;139(2):415–429.

64. Fernández-Cruz L, Puig-Domingo M, Halperin I, et al. Pheochromocytoma. *Scand J Surg.* 2004;93(4):302–309.

65. Remer EM, Miller FH. Imaging of pheochromocytomas. In: Blake MA, Boland G, eds. *Adrenal Imaging.* Humana Press; 2009:109–126.

66. Schwerk WB, Görg C, Görg K, et al. Adrenal pheochromocytomas: broad spectrum of sonographic presentation. *J Ultrasound Med.* 1994;13(7):517–521.

67. Schwartz LH, Macari H, Huvos AG, et al. Collision tumors of the adrenal gland: demonstration and characterization on MR imaging. *Radiology.* 1996;201(3):757–760.

68. Eloubeidi MA, Morgan DE, Cerfolio RJ, et al. Transduodenal EUS-guided FNA of the right adrenal gland. *Gastrointest Endosc.* 2008;67(3):522–527.

69. Scott JA, Palmer EL. Single photon imaging of the adrenal gland. In: Blake MA, Boland G, eds. *Adrenal Imaging.* Humana Press; 2009:127–162.

70. Roedl JB, Boland GWL, Blake MA. PET and PET-CT imaging of adrenal lesions. In: Blake MA, Boland G, eds. *Adrenal Imaging.* Humana Press; 2009:173–192.

71. Stelow EB, Debol SM, Stanley MW, et al. Sampling of the adrenal glands by endoscopic ultrasound-guided fine-needle aspiration. *Diagn Cytopathol.* 2005;33(1):26–30.

72. Dietrich CF, Wehrmann T, Hoffmann C, et al. Detection of the adrenal glands by endoscopic or transabdominal ultrasound. *Endoscopy.* 1997;29(9):859–864.

73. DeWitt JM. Endoscopic ultrasound-guided fine-needle aspiration of right adrenal masses. *J Ultrasound Med.* 2008;27(2):261–267.

74. Piccolboni D, Ciccone F, Settembre A, et al. The role of echolaparoscopy in abdominal surgery: five years' experience in a dedicated center. *Surg Endosc.* 2008;22(1):112–117.

75. Lucas SW, Spitz JD, Arregui ME. The use of intraoperative ultrasound in laparoscopic adrenal surgery: the Saint Vincent experience. *Surg Endosc.* 1999;13(11):1093–1098.

CHAPTER 16

The Retroperitoneum

JOIE BURNS

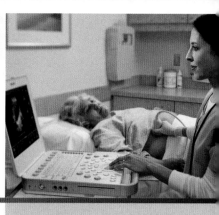

OBJECTIVES

- Identify the compartments of the retroperitoneum and the fascia that divide them.
- List the muscles, organs, and vessels normally found in each retroperitoneal compartment.
- Differentiate between the location and function of the deep abdominal (parietal) nodes and the superficial (visceral) nodes.
- List the indications for sonographic evaluation of the retroperitoneum.
- Demonstrate the scanning techniques used to image the retroperitoneum.
- Recognize the role retroperitoneal fascia play in identifying and limiting the extent of pathology.
- Describe the six scanning objectives the sonographer should employ when retroperitoneal pathology is identified.
- Differentiate the sonographic appearance of inflammatory and malignant adenopathy.
- Describe the pathology, etiology, clinical signs and symptoms, and sonographic appearance of solid lesions and fluid collection found in the retroperitoneum.
- Analyze sonographic images of the retroperitoneum for pathology.
- Identify technically satisfactory and unsatisfactory sonographic examinations of the retroperitoneum.

KEY TERMS

abscess

adenopathy

AIDS

fibroma

fibrosarcoma

hematoma

HIV

leiomyoma

leiomyosarcoma

lipoma

liposarcoma

lymphocele

retroperitoneal fibrosis

rhabdomyoma

rhabdomyosarcoma

GLOSSARY

abscess a pocket of infection typically containing pus, blood, and degenerating tissue

adenopathy also called lymphadenopathy; enlargement of lymph nodes owing to inflammation, primary neoplasia, or metastasis

extravasate fluid, such as blood, bile, or urine, which is forced out or leaks out of its normal vessel into the surrounding tissues or potential spaces

fascia a thin sheet-like tissue that separates muscles

great vessels a term used to describe the aorta and inferior vena cava together

hematoma an extravasated collection of blood localized within a potential space or tissues

HIV human immunodeficiency virus; blood-borne virus that attacks T lymphocytes resulting in their destruction or impairment, eventually leading to AIDS

mass effect distortion or displacement of normal anatomy owing to a mass, neoplasm, or fluid collection

metastasis the spread of cancer from the site at which it first arose to a distant site

orthogonal planes that are perpendicular or at 90 degrees to each other

primary neoplasm a new growth of benign or malignant origin

urinoma an extravasated urine collection owing to a tear of the urinary collecting system

Sonography plays an important role in the examination of the retroperitoneum as well as the organs and vessels located within the cavity. Although computed tomography (CT) is the preferred imaging modality for retroperitoneal neoplasms and adenopathy, the radiation dose delivered to the patient over multiple examinations must be considered. Sonography produces high-quality images without ionizing radiation, it can provide real-time biopsy guidance, and it provides safe imaging for follow-up of disease progression or resolution. The skill and creativity of the sonographer often dictates the quality of the examination produced. A thorough knowledge of anatomy, pathophysiology, and sonography physics and instrumentation is required to produce the highest quality of sonographic examination. This chapter focuses specifically on the normal anatomy and pathologies found in the retroperitoneum.

ANATOMY OF THE RETROPERITONEUM

The parietal peritoneum is the outermost of two membranes that enclose most of the intra-abdominal contents, including the intestines, liver, pancreatic head, spleen, and pelvic organs. The other membrane, the visceral peritoneum, lies in direct apposition to the parietal membrane, thus forming a potential space. The area lying behind the peritoneal membrane is referred to as the *retroperitoneum*. The retroperitoneum is a complex abdominal space located between the parietal peritoneum and anterior to the transversalis fascia.[1,2] It extends from the diaphragm superiorly to the pelvic brim inferiorly.[3–5]

Retroperitoneal Compartments

The retroperitoneum is divided into three major compartments or spaces by the anterior and posterior perirenal fascia.[6] These retroperitoneal compartments are the anterior pararenal space, the perirenal or perinephric space, and the posterior pararenal space.[1,6,7] The fascial planes are fused superiorly but remain unfused caudally. The literature frequently refers to both the anterior and posterior as Gerota fascia, although it is more correct to reference the anterior renal fascia as Gerota fascia and the posterior renal fascia as Zuckerkandl fascia.[8] The anterior renal fascia courses anterior to the great vessels, kidneys, and adrenal glands and extends across the midline to fuse with the posterior renal fascia laterally. The posterior renal fascia fuses with the anterior renal fascia laterally and tracks posterior to the kidney to blend with the anterior layer of the thoracolumbar fascia and the psoas fascial sheath medially.

An understanding of the retroperitoneal fascia is important to define the retroperitoneal compartments (Fig. 16-1A, B).

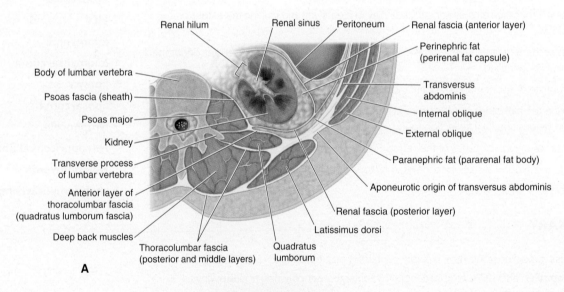

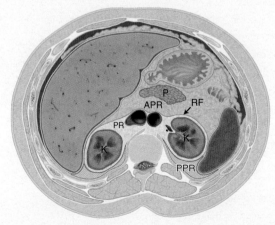

FIGURE 16-1 Retroperitoneum. **A:** A transverse sectional retroperitoneum illustration at the renal hilum level demonstrates the fascial planes and musculature relationship. **B:** The transverse drawing illustrates the three major compartments: anterior pararenal space (*APR*), perirenal space (*PR*), and posterior pararenal space (*PPR*). *K*, kidney; *P*, pancreas; *RF*, renal fascia.

Anterior Pararenal Space

The anterior pararenal space is bordered anteriorly by the posterior parietal peritoneum and posteriorly by the anterior perirenal fascia.[6] The space communicates with the opposite side around the pancreas.[1] Inferiorly, this space communicates with the extraperitoneal space of the pelvis and the posterior pararenal space.[9] The communication is important because it allows cells and fluid to travel between the two spaces. Along with a variable amount of fat, some portions of the digestive organs are embedded in this layer including the pancreas; distal common bile duct; the second, third, and fourth parts of the duodenum; and the ascending and descending colon.[10]

Perirenal or Perinephric Space

The perirenal space is bordered anteriorly by the anterior renal fascia and posteriorly by the posterior renal fascia. Superiorly, the fascias fuse and attach to the diaphragmatic crura bilaterally immediately superior to the adrenal glands. Inferiorly, the perirenal space is open at the level of the pelvic brim because the fascial perirenal sheaths remain unfused. The perirenal space encloses the kidneys, adrenal glands, perinephric fat, and the prevertebral aorta and inferior vena cava (IVC).[1,10]

Posterior Pararenal Space

The posterior pararenal space lies between the posterior renal fascia and the transversalis fascia. This space contains no organs, only fat.[10] The retrofascial space is located immediately posterior to the posterior pararenal space and it contains the psoas muscle posteromedially and the quadratus lumborum muscle posteriorly. The retrofascial space is not technically part of the retroperitoneum, but its muscles are frequently referred to in discussions of the retroperitoneal space.

Table 16-1 lists the organs and vessels contained in the retroperitoneum.

ANATOMY OF THE LYMPHATIC SYSTEM

The lymphatic system extends throughout the body with lymph vessels found immediately adjacent to normal arteries and veins.[7,11] Unlike the vascular system, the lymph vessels end in a blind-ending plexus of tubes at the vascular capillary level. The lymphatic system acts as a fluid recovery system, collecting nearly 3 L of plasma fluid that oozes from the normal vascular capillaries into the extracellular space. The lymphatic system also collects cellular debris and bacteria within the extracellular fluid, as well as absorbing and transporting dietary fat. Because the lymphatic system returns excess fluid to the bloodstream, homeostasis (internal fluid balance) is maintained.

The fluid that enters the lymphatic plexus is referred to as *lymph*. This thin, colorless, or slightly yellow fluid has a cellular composition similar to blood plasma. Lymph flows from the lymph capillary plexus toward the great vessels in the abdomen, eventually to the right and left subclavian veins in the thorax. The right lymphatic duct conducts lymph collected from the right head, neck, arm, and chest back into the venous system at the confluence of the right internal jugular and the right subclavian vein. The thoracic duct conducts lymph collected from the rest of the body back into the venous system at the confluence of the left internal jugular and the left subclavian vein. The chyle cistern is a dilated collecting area found in the midretroperitoneum that collects lymph from the lower extremities and pelvis before it ascends to the thoracic duct[7,11] (Fig. 16-2A, B).

Lymph moves through lymphatic vessels, passing through lymph nodes along the way. Each lymph node is a small mass of lymphatic tissue that filters the lymph fluid, phagocytizing foreign proteins and infectious debris, and generating and sending lymphocytes to infected tissues. Lymph nodes are described based on their location. See Table 16-2 for a list of commonly affected abdominopelvic lymph node groups and measurements that indicate abnormal size.

In the retroperitoneum, lymph nodes are generally divided into deep abdominal or parietal lymph nodes and superficial abdominal or visceral lymph nodes. Parietal nodes are those lymph nodes found in the retroperitoneum surrounding the principal blood vessels. They are grouped according to the arterial vessel with which they are associated. In the upper retroperitoneum, aggregations can be found around three unpaired vascular branches: inferior mesenteric, superior mesenteric, and celiac. Groups found in the lower retroperitoneum include the external, common, internal iliac, and epigastric.

Nodes are positioned 360 degrees around the aorta and IVC. Those that lie posterior to the great vessels (aorta and IVC) provide the most reliable indicator of lymphadenopathy because they frequently displace the aorta or IVC anteriorly (Fig. 16-3).

Visceral nodes are located within the peritoneal cavity and are generally found at the hilum of organs. The most common groups are gastric, hepatic, pancreatic, splenic, and various groups associated with branches of the colic artery.

A special type of lymph node found along the small bowel and mesentery are called *lacteals*. Lacteals take on a milky white appearance because they also absorb dietary fat.

SCANNING TECHNIQUE AND NORMAL SONOGRAPHIC APPEARANCE

Ideally, patients should be fasting for 6 to 8 hours prior to the examination. This will reduce bowel gas and fluid that may be confused with pathology; however, if needed, an examination of the retroperitoneum may be performed

TABLE 16-1	Retroperitoneal Organs and Structures	
Diaphragmatic Crura	**Aorta**
Pancreas	Inferior vena cava
Distal common bile duct	Superior mesenteric artery
Second, third, and fourth parts of duodenum	Superior mesenteric vein
Kidneys	Hepatic artery
Adrenals	Splenic artery
Lymphatic vessels and nodes	Splenic vein

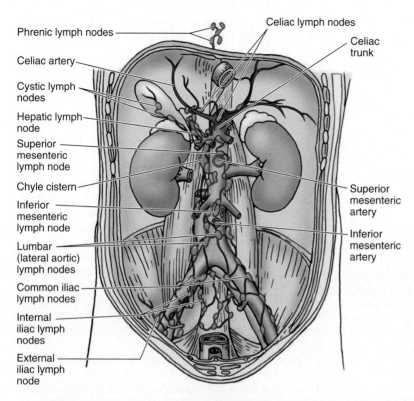

Phrenic lymph nodes

Celiac artery

Cystic lymph nodes

Hepatic lymph node

Superior mesenteric lymph node

Chyle cistern

Inferior mesenteric lymph node

Lumbar (lateral aortic) lymph nodes

Common iliac lymph nodes

Internal iliac lymph nodes

External iliac lymph node

Celiac lymph nodes

Celiac trunk

Superior mesenteric artery

Inferior mesenteric artery

FIGURE 16-2 Lymphatic system. This illustration shows the parietal node groups of the abdominopelvic cavity and their relationship to the blood vessels. (Reprinted from Moore K, Dalley A, Agur A. *Clinically Oriented Anatomy.* 6th ed. Lippincott Williams & Wilkins; 2010:316, with permission.)

TABLE 16-2   Abdominopelvic Lymph Node Groups[4,5,7,11]

	Location	Abnormal Size (mm)
Retroperitoneum		
Retrocrural	Posterior to the diaphragmatic crura	>6
Retroperitoneal	Encircling the aorta (periaortic) or inferior vena cava (pericaval) or both (interaortocaval)	>10
Mesenteric and celiac	Anterior to the abdominal aorta surrounding the origins of the celiac axis and mesenteric arteries	>10
Pelvic	Along the common, external and internal iliac (hypogastric) arteries and veins; also referred to as the *iliac chain*	>15
Intraperitoneal		
Gastrohepatic	Within the superior portion of the lesser omentum that suspends the stomach from the liver	>8
Perisplenic	At the splenic hilum	>10
Parapancreatic	Between the duodenal sweep and the pancreatic head anterior to the inferior vena cava	>10
Hepatic hilum	Surrounding the porta hepatis	>6

without any patient preparation. Owing to the retroperitoneum's deep position, a 3-to-6-MHz sector or curvilinear transducer should offer adequate penetration and a wide field of view for most adult retroperitoneal examinations. Higher-frequency transducers should be used on smaller children whereas lower-frequency transducers provide better penetration on obese patients.

The retroperitoneum may be scanned using an anterior, coronal, or posterior approach. The anterior approach frequently involves directing the sound beam through the left lobe of the liver in the epigastric region or through a fluid-filled stomach when overlying bowel gas obstructs visualization of deeper anatomy. Coronal scan planes are frequently used, directing the beam through the liver on the right and the spleen on the left, to evaluate kidneys, adrenals, and midline retroperitoneal structures that are not seen well from an anterior approach. The posterior or flank scanning approach may be employed, directing the ultrasound beam through the deep back muscles (see Fig. 16-1), when the anterior and coronal approach offer

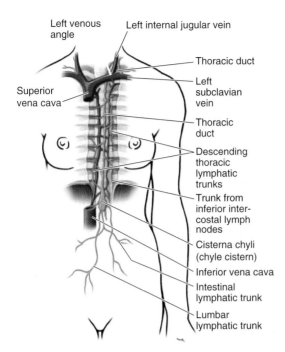

Left venous angle
Left internal jugular vein
Thoracic duct
Superior vena cava
Left subclavian vein
Thoracic duct
Descending thoracic lymphatic trunks
Trunk from inferior intercostal lymph nodes
Cisterna chyli (chyle cistern)
Inferior vena cava
Intestinal lymphatic trunk
Lumbar lymphatic trunk

FIGURE 16-3 Retroperitoneal lymph nodes. This illustration demonstrates the deep abdominal lymph vessels following the course of the major blood vessels. The chyle cistern is a dilated collecting area found in the midretroperitoneum collecting lymph from the lower extremities and pelvis before it ascends to the thoracic duct. The thoracic duct receives lymph collected from the rest of the body and returns it back into the venous system at the confluence of the left internal jugular and the left subclavian vein. (Reprinted from Moore K, Dalley A, Agur A. *Clinically Oriented Anatomy.* 6th ed. Lippincott Williams & Wilkins; 2010:316, with permission.)

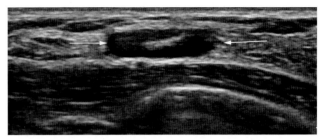

FIGURE 16-4 Lymph node. The longitudinal image displays a normal ovoid-shaped hypoechoic lymph node. Note the echogenic central fatty hilum. The arrows depict the medial and lateral edges of the lymph node. (Image courtesy of Philips Medical Systems, Bothell, WA.)

proximal aorta. Muscles identified during the retroperitoneum examination include the quadratus lumborum and psoas. Both muscles appear hypoechoic with bright linear fibers running along the length of the muscle. Care must be taken not to mistake these muscles for inflammation or fluid collections when they are well developed in very muscular patients. When there is a question, the patient may be asked to flex and extend his or her hip. The muscle can be seen to extend and contract with leg movement.

less than desirable imaging. Rolling the patient into oblique, decubitus, and prone positions using the above scanning approaches will shift air and organ position and potentially improve imaging.

The retroperitoneal examination should include assessment of the kidneys, pancreas, and vasculature for size, relationship, neoplasm, fluid collection, and mass effect. Normal lymph nodes are not seen in the retroperitoneum. Normal superficial lymph nodes may be identified as hypoechoic almond-shaped structures with a bright fat containing hilum (Fig. 16-4). Normal adult adrenal glands are rarely identified, except in extremely thin patients.

A variable amount of fat is identified in the retroperitoneal compartments depending on the patient's body fat composition. Generally, more obese patients demonstrate more pronounced amounts of fat in each space. Typically, there is a more generous amount of fat in the perirenal space than in the other retroperitoneal compartments. The anterior and posterior pararenal spaces may not be distinguishable from the perirenal space in average and thin patients. The perirenal fascial planes may be identified only occasionally. When seen, they appear as very fine echogenic lines surrounded by fat. Fat typically appears moderately echogenic and homogeneous in these spaces. In some obese patients, the perinephric fat may appear anechoic and should not be mistaken for fluid (Fig. 16-5A, B).

The diaphragmatic crura may be identified fairly routinely. As a muscular structure, the diaphragmatic crura appear as a hypoechoic linear structure surrounded by hyperechoic tissue running obliquely between the aorta and the IVC in the transverse epigastric plane and anterior to the longitudinal

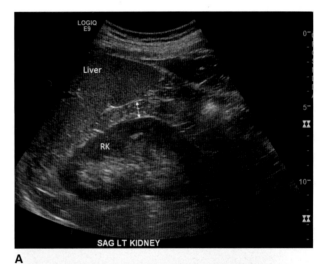

A

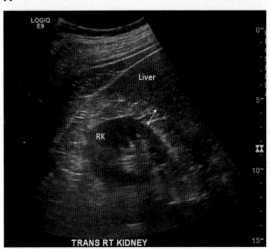

B

FIGURE 16-5 Retroperitoneal fat. The perirenal space contains more fat than the other retroperitoneal compartments. **A:** A longitudinal image of the right kidney (*RK*) and liver with echogenic fat (*arrows*) seen surrounding the kidney. **B:** The transverse image of the right kidney also displays echogenic fat (*arrows*).

PATHOLOGY OF THE RETROPERITONEUM

When a mass is identified in the retroperitoneum, the sonographer should demonstrate the following:

- The abnormality in orthogonal planes
- Measurements of the mass in three dimensions
- Mass characteristics (cystic/fluid, solid tissue, air, calcification, borders, wall thickness, septa, etc.)
- The relationship of the mass to surrounding anatomy/mass effect
- The organ or area of mass origin
- Blood flow characteristics and feeding vessel(s) using color, power, and spectral Doppler imaging

Solid Lesions

Solid masses found in the retroperitoneum are usually metastatic and most frequently involve the lymph nodes. Although primary tumors do occur in the retroperitoneum, they are rare. The role of sonography in evaluating retroperitoneal adenopathy is limited. Sonography can detect the presence of solid masses and, in cases where intestinal gas or overlying bony structures do not obscure retroperitoneal imaging, may demonstrate the relationship of these masses to normal structures. The exact histologic nature of solid masses cannot, however, be definitively ascertained by sonography alone. When solid lesions are noted, the patient should be referred for additional diagnostic testing such as CT, magnetic resonance imaging (MRI), and possibly fine-needle biopsy of the solid mass.[12]

Lymphadenopathy

Lymphadenopathy, also called *adenopathy*, describes the enlargement of lymph nodes caused by inflammation, primary neoplasia, or metastasis. The pattern of lymph node enlargement can provide important clues to the origin and type of pathology. Sonographically, enlarged lymph nodes appear as oval- to round-shaped masses with a low-to-medium-level echo pattern compared with the more hyperechoic fat of the retroperitoneum. Lymphadenitis is the enlargement of lymph nodes owing to an inflammatory process. Although lymph nodes are enlarged with lymphadenitis, they typically maintain an ovoid shape and fatty hilum. On color or power Doppler images, lymphadenitis demonstrates hyperemia within the node (Fig. 16-6A, B). Primary malignant nodes, like those seen with lymphoma, tend to become more hypoechoic to anechoic and round-shaped, with a length-to-width ratio of less than two[5] (Fig. 16-7A, B). Additional node characteristics that increase the likelihood of malignancy include asymmetric cortical widening and a loss of the normal fatty hilum, with color Doppler images demonstrating avascular areas within the node or mass effect on normal vascular tree within the node.[5] Metastatic adenopathy tends to appear more echogenic and heterogeneous[5] (Fig. 16-8A, B). Care must be taken to adjust color and power Doppler settings to levels that are sensitive to low flow levels when evaluating lymph nodes.

Enlarged nodes in the retroperitoneum may also fuse together, forming a lobulated mantle-like soft tissue mass anterior to the aorta and the IVC. Adenopathy may completely encase the abdominal great vessels, moving them away from the vertebral column. It may also demonstrate a mass effect on arterial branches, displacing them from their normal position while compressing surrounding veins (Fig. 16-9A, B).

Lymphadenopathy is a very common finding in patients with acquired immune deficiency syndrome (AIDS). Patients infected with the blood-borne virus human immunodeficiency virus (HIV) experience depression of their immune system owing to this virus' destructive effect on T lymphocytes. Without retroviral medical therapy, the

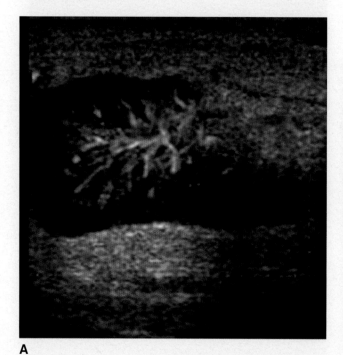

A

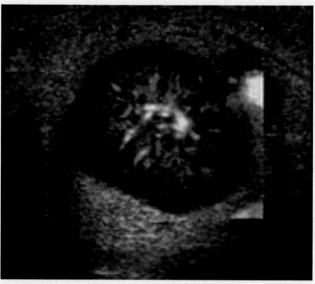

B

FIGURE 16-6 Lymphadenitis. Longitudinal (**A**) and transverse (**B**) images of an infected lymph node demonstrate hyperemia with power Doppler.

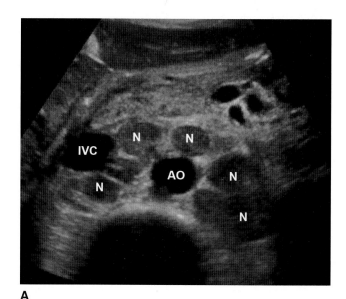

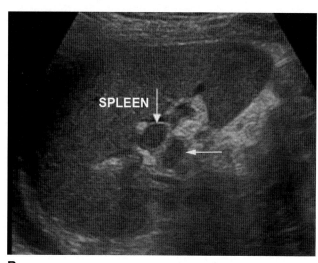

A

B

FIGURE 16-7 Lymphadenopathy. **A:** Retroperitoneal lymph nodes (*N*) are seen surrounding the aorta (*AO*) and inferior vena cava (*IVC*). The lymph nodes are more rounded in shape and a normal fatty hilum is not seen. **B:** Rounded lymph nodes (*arrows*) are seen at the splenic hilum. (**A:** Image courtesy of Philips Medical Systems, Bothell, WA. **B:** Image courtesy of Dr. Taco Geertsma, Gelderse Vallei, Ede, The Netherlands.)

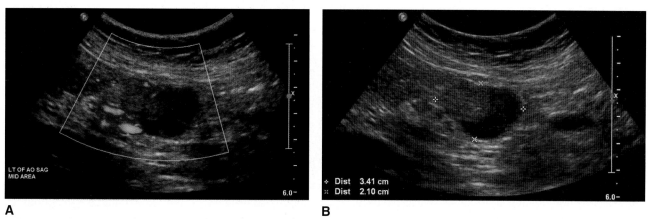

A

B

FIGURE 16-8 Mesenteric node. Longitudinal images obtained with power Doppler (**A**) and with measurements (**B**) in the area left of the aorta in a patient with hepatocellular carcinoma demonstrates metastatic changes in blood flow, appearance, and size.

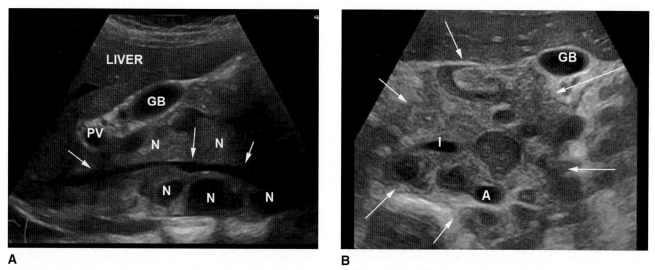

A

B

FIGURE 16-9 Midline adenopathy. **A:** Longitudinal image of the abdomen demonstrates compression of the inferior vena cava (*IVC; arrows*) by lymphadenopathy seen anterior and posterior to the vessel. **B:** Transverse midline image demonstrates an echogenic mass encompassing and compressing the aorta (*A*) and IVC (*I*). The mass is consistent with lymphadenopathy. *GB*, gallbladder; *N*, retroperitoneal lymph nodes; *PV*, portal vein. (Images courtesy of Dr. Taco Geertsma, Gelderse Vallei, Ede, The Netherlands.)

patient's immune system fails and the disease evolves into AIDS. AIDS patients experience multiple opportunistic infections and neoplasms. The more common opportunistic fungal, viral, and bacterial infections include *Mycobacterium avium* complex infection, tuberculosis, candidiasis, cytomegalovirus, and herpes. These infections frequently affect the gastrointestinal tract and are demonstrated on sonography as hypoechoic-appearing lymphadenopathy and gut wall thickening. Tuberculosis may demonstrate very low attenuating, anechoic lymph nodes owing to necrosis, and punctuate echogenicities within the kidneys. Common neoplasms associated with AIDS include Kaposi sarcoma and lymphoma. Kaposi sarcoma is associated with chest and skin neoplasms and adenopathy. The AIDS-related lymphomas are of B-cell origin and include primarily non-Hodgkin lymphoma. AIDS lymphomas tend to affect the central nervous system, gastrointestinal tract, liver, and lungs. In the abdomen, hypoechoic retroperitoneal adenopathy is frequently seen.[5] With current improvements in retroviral and prophylactic medications, AIDS is rarely seen.

CT is the imaging modality of choice to evaluate retroperitoneal adenopathy because of its ability to generate standard and reproducible views of abnormal nodes without bowel gas interference.[5] Sonography can be used to guide biopsy and assess the effects of lymphadenopathy on vascular and urinary structures of the retroperitoneum during therapy without additional radiation to the patient. Therapies related to lymph node enlargement are dependent on the cause but may include medical therapy to treat infection, chemotherapy, radiation therapy, or surgical removal with malignancies.[12]

Retroperitoneal Fibrosis

Retroperitoneal fibrosis, also called *Ormond disease* or *chronic periaortitis*, is a chronic inflammatory process that results in fibrous tissue proliferation, affecting and encasing the great vessels, ureters, and lymphatics of the retroperitoneum.[13–16] The disease affects middle-aged males twice as often as females.[5] The majority of cases of retroperitoneal fibrosis are idiopathic, thought by some to be autoimmune in nature.[16] Other causes include infiltrating neoplasia of the stomach, lung, breast, colon, prostate, and kidney; methysergide (medication prescribed to treat migraine headaches) use; and less frequently Crohn disease, sclerosing cholangitis, radiation therapy, aneurysm surgery or leakage, retroperitoneal infections, and urine leakage into the retroperitoneum.[5,16]

The ureters are frequently affected, demonstrating a characteristic medial deviation or complete stenosis, resulting in unilateral or bilateral hydronephrosis.[9,15,16] Additional symptoms include unintended weight loss, nausea, malaise, hypertension, and renal insufficiency.[9]

Although CT is the imaging modality of choice for initial diagnosis, sonography is frequently used to follow this disease process. Sonographically, retroperitoneal fibrosis appears as a hypoechoic, smoothly marginated clump or layer in the para-aortic area of the perinephric space and may be mistaken for plaque surrounding the distal aorta (Fig. 16-10A–H). Treatment includes corticosteroid therapy with ureteral stenting in cases of ureteral stenosis and medical therapy for concomitant renal insufficiency.

Primary Neoplasms

Solid retroperitoneal tumors are rare. Primary malignancies include liposarcoma, leiomyosarcoma, rhabdomyosarcoma, myxosarcoma, and fibrosarcoma. Benign retroperitoneal tumors include lipoma, leiomyoma, rhabdomyoma, myxoma, and fibroma. Malignant tumors tend to appear larger and more complex than their benign counterparts. These neoplasms tend to demonstrate mass effect on the vasculature of the retroperitoneum, compressing the IVC, ureters, urinary bladder, and extrahepatic bile ducts. The role of sonography beyond characterizing the neoplasm, evaluating the size, and demonstrating its blood flow characteristics is to demonstrate whether or not the tumor has infiltrated adjacent organs, because complete surgical resection determines prognosis.[5]

Liposarcoma is the most common primary malignancy of the retroperitoneum, representing 95% of all fatty retroperitoneal tumors.[5] This slow-growing neoplasm affects middle-aged males more frequently than females. Patient complaints include abdominal pain, unintended weight loss, anemia, and a palpable mass.[17] CT remains the imaging modality of choice; however, sonography may be employed initially owing to its noninvasive nature. Sonographically, liposarcoma demonstrates a poorly marginated, lobulated, complex mass that displaces adjacent anatomy rather than infiltrating it. One remarkable characteristic of retroperitoneal liposarcomas is the immense size some of them attain before diagnosis.[17] Tumors weighing 20 pounds or more are not rare. Liposarcomas occur more frequently anterior to the spine and psoas muscles[5] (Fig. 16-11A–D).

Leiomyosarcoma is the second most common primary retroperitoneal malignancy. This smooth muscle tumor may occur in the uterus, gastrointestinal tract, or in the retroperitoneal cavity and may originate in the wall of the IVC.[18–20] Leiomyosarcoma typically affects middle-aged females.[18] Patients complain of an abdominal mass, pain, unintended weight loss, nausea, vomiting, and abdominal distention. Leiomyosarcoma frequently demonstrates bloodborne metastases to the liver, lung, brain, and peritoneum. Approximately 40% of patients demonstrate metastases at the time of diagnosis. Sonographically, these lesions present a mixed echo texture. Internal necrosis and hemorrhage produce fluid-filled areas within a well-circumscribed mass. Erosion of adjacent visceral walls may result in the presence of gas within the mass. This complex solid tumor is indistinguishable from other retroperitoneal neoplasms such as liposarcoma, lymphoma, and adrenal malignancy. Treatment consists of complete surgical resection, chemotherapy, and radiation therapy[5,20] (Fig. 16-12).

Because solid masses cannot displace the musculoskeletal structures of the back, clinical detection may be delayed. Frequently, the tumor must grow large enough to displace intraperitoneal contents before it can be palpated anteriorly. When the mass is finally detected, it is quite large and may have been present for as long as 20 years or more. Typically, the patient presents with a large, protruding abdomen or complains of increasing abdominal girth, weight loss, or abdominal pain. If the tumor has spread to the intestinal tract, symptoms such as nausea, vomiting, anorexia, diarrhea, and altered bowel habits may develop. Involvement of the kidneys or ureters, either by direct invasion or mechanical

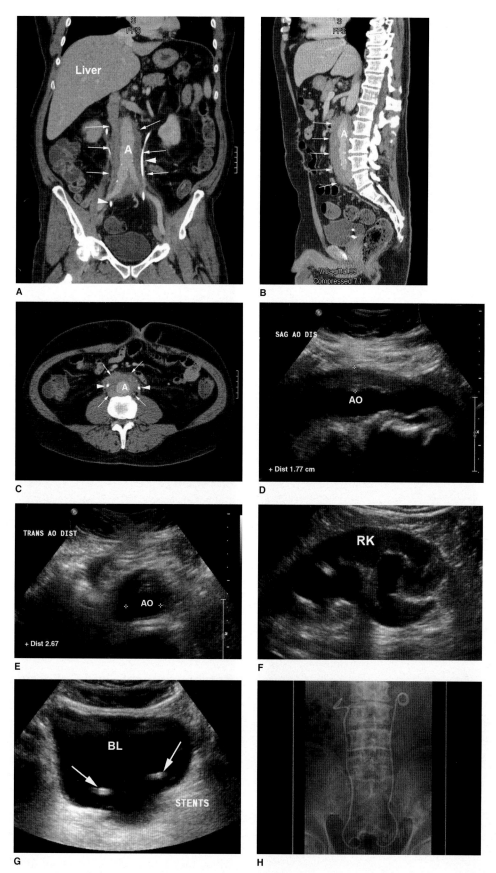

FIGURE 16-10 Retroperitoneal fibrosis. Coronal (**A**), sagittal (**B**), and computed tomography (**C**) images demonstrate retroperitoneal fibrosis (*arrows*) surrounding the aorta (*A*). Bilateral ureteral stents (*arrowheads*) are seen on the coronal and axial images. Longitudinal (**D**) and transverse (**E**) sonography images of the same patient demonstrate hypoechoic fibrosis seen surrounding the anechoic aorta (*AO*). **F:** Longitudinal image of the right kidney (*RK*) demonstrates moderate hydrone-phrosis secondary to ureteral compression by the tumor. **G:** Transverse image of the urinary bladder (*BL*) demonstrates bilateral echogenic ureteral stents (*arrows*) projecting into the bladder lumen. **H:** The abdominal radiograph demonstrates bilateral ureteral stents. (**H:** Image courtesy of Dr. Taco Geertsma, Gelderse Vallei, Ede, The Netherlands.)

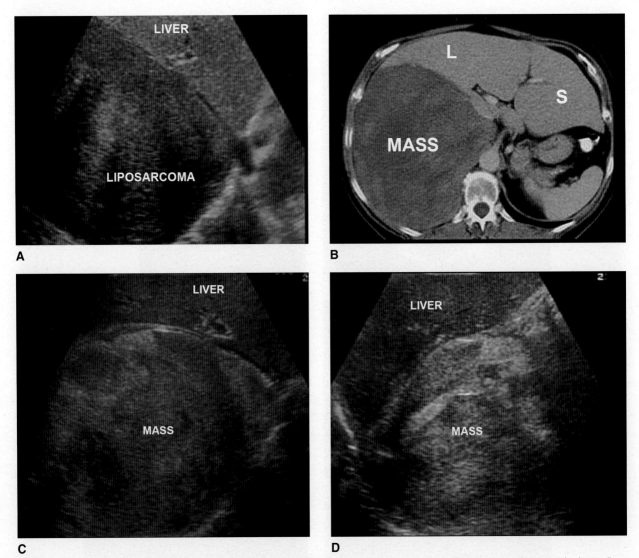

A **B**

C **D**

FIGURE 16-11 Liposarcoma. **A** and **B:** A large heterogeneous mass seen posterior to the liver on both sonography and computed tomography. It was diagnosed as a retroperitoneal liposarcoma. On this patient, the transverse (**C**) and longitudinal (**D**) images of the right upper quadrant demonstrate a large heterogeneous mass posterior to the right lobe of the liver. The mass was diagnosed as a liposarcoma. *L,* liver; *S,* spleen. (Images courtesy of Dr. Taco Geertsma, Gelderse Vallei, Ede, The Netherlands.)

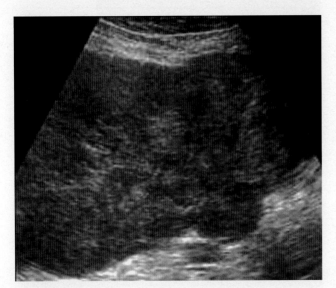

FIGURE 16-12 Leiomyosarcoma. This large, heterogeneous, well-circumscribed mass seen in the retroperitoneum was diagnosed as a leiomyosarcoma. (Image courtesy of Dr. Taco Geertsma, Gelderse Vallei, Ede, The Netherlands.)

compression, may lead to hydronephrosis and subsequent pyelonephritis and uremia.

Retroperitoneal Fluid Collections

Fluid collections of the retroperitoneum are relatively common and include abscesses, hematomas, urinomas, and lymphoceles. Because they may all have the same sonographic appearance, it is impossible to differentiate the pathologic process on the basis of sonography alone; however, correlation of sonographic findings with the patient's clinical history can frequently provide a presumptive diagnosis. Fine-needle aspiration of suspicious areas provides more specific information on the nature of the mass. Identifying the compartment in which the collection is localized may help narrow the diagnostic possibilities. Fluid collections will conform to the space in which they form, frequently demonstrating sharp corners at organ interfaces. This knowledge may also be helpful in determining the cause and nature of the fluid collection.

The anterior pararenal space is the most common site of retroperitoneal infections. Because the appendix frequently occupies a retrocecal position and lies outside the peritoneal cavity, and because portions of the duodenum and colon also border the anterior pararenal space, perforation by trauma, inflammation, or as a sequela of bowel disease can lead to retroperitoneal infection. In cases of pancreatitis, digestive enzymes are extravasated and cause an inflammatory response in the anterior pararenal space.[13,21,22] Typically, this develops into a pseudocyst. As proteolytic digestive enzymes destroy the cell walls within the pancreas, additional enzymes are released into the interstitial spaces, precipitating further destruction of pancreatic parenchyma. Necrosis of blood vessel walls may also cause hemorrhage into the anterior pararenal space, increasing the fluid content[22] (Fig. 16-13A, B). In some cases, the tissue-dissolving capabilities of the pancreatic enzymes cause further spread of the fluid into the posterior pararenal space.[21,22]

Fluid collections within the perirenal space or contained within Gerota fascia are generally associated with renal abnormalities.[9] Nephritis with subsequent abscess formation, rupture of a renal artery aneurysm, or bleeding from a renal neoplasm may all create a perinephric fluid collection. Sonographically, the fluid collection is contained within the borders of the renal fascia and does not demonstrate significant movement with alterations in patient position.

The posterior pararenal space is bounded anteriorly by the posterior renal fascia and posteriorly by the transversalis fascia. Because it does not contain any specific organs, alterations in anatomic appearance are due solely to processes that originate outside this space. Hemorrhage from trauma or ruptured vessels may dissect along the posterior pararenal space. Postoperative infections from aortic grafts may produce abscess collections, and leaking anastomoses may allow blood to collect there. The most common cause of posterior pararenal fluid collections is aortic disease.

Hematoma

Bleeding into the retroperitoneum may be the result of trauma, hemophilia, malignant invasion, surgery, or anticoagulant therapy. It may also occur spontaneously.

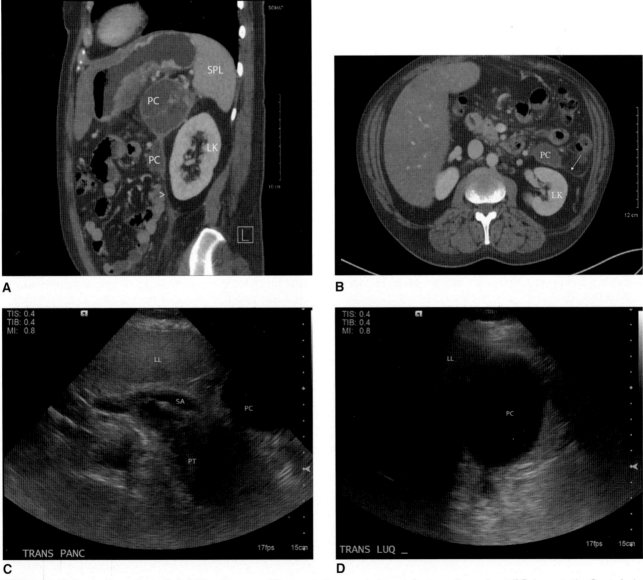

FIGURE 16-13 Pancreatic pseudocyst. Sagittal (**A**) and transverse (**B**) computed tomography images of a pancreatic pseudocyst (*PC*) demonstrating Gerota fascia (*cursor, arrow*). The fascia was not visible on the sonogram. Transverse (**C**) and (**D**) ultrasound images of a pancreatic pseudocyst (*PC*) adjacent to the pancreatic tail (*PT*) and left liver (*LL*). *LK*, left kidney; *SPL*, spleen.

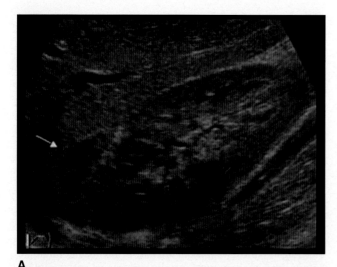

A

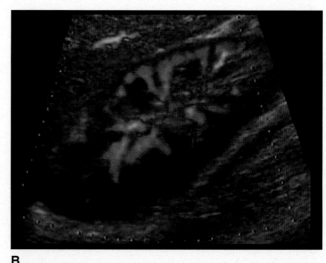

B

FIGURE 16-14 Longitudinal images (**A** and **B**) of the right kidney with a hematoma compressing the superior anterior pole (*arrow*). Note the absence of color flow in the hematoma (**B**). (Images courtesy of Dr. Taco Geertsma, Gelderse Vallei, Ede, The Netherlands.)

Spontaneous retroperitoneal hemorrhage is associated with primary renal malignant tumors (30%), benign renal neoplasms (30%), vascular diseases such as aneurysm rupture and arteriovenous malformation (25%), inflammation and infection (10%), anticoagulant therapy, hemodialysis, and primary adrenal neoplasms less frequently. The classic patient complaint is sudden onset of flank pain.[5] CT is the preferred imaging modality; however, sonography may be requested as an initial imaging modality or to follow up a known hematoma for resolution. Coagulating blood presents a variable appearance depending on the age of the bleed. Initial bleeding appears anechoic, becoming more echogenic with thrombin organization, taking on the echogenicity of splenic parenchyma. As the hematoma ages, it begins to retract and lyse, becoming more hyperechoic and complex in its appearance. Eventually, the hematoma is completely resorbed or may deposit a calcification at the hemorrhage site. Treatment is dependent on the cause of the hemorrhage. Thrombus does not contain vascularity and should not be mistaken for a neoplasm (Figs. 16-14A, B and 16-15A, B).

Lymphocele

Lymphocele is an extravasated lymphatic fluid collection within the retroperitoneum. These are typically iatrogenically induced following node dissection for cancer staging or following surgery or renal transplant where the lymph vessels are disrupted. They may also occur following trauma. Lymphoceles typically develop within 10 to 21 days following surgery, but they may develop up to 8 weeks following renal transplant.[5,9] Typically, these fluid collections are small and resolve on their own. However, if they become large, causing hydronephrosis or inducing edema, they will be treated with percutaneous drainage, surgery, or sclerosing agents.[5] Lymphoceles appear similar to a simple cyst but may appear more complex with thin septa seen on sonography.

Urinoma

Retroperitoneal urinoma is an extravasated urine owing to a tear of the urinary collecting system and continued renal function. Urinoma may occur owing to nonobstructive causes such as blunt or penetrating trauma, surgery,

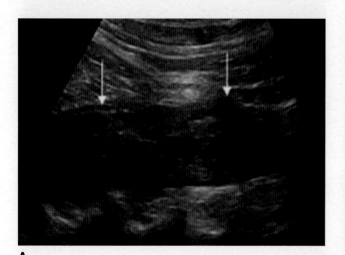

A

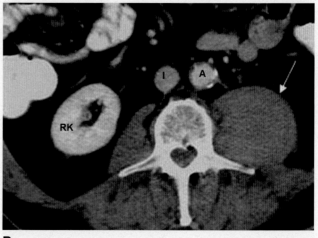

B

FIGURE 16-15 Psoas muscle hematoma. **A:** Longitudinal image of the left retroperitoneum demonstrates an ovoid complex mass (*arrows*) consistent with a psoas muscle hematoma. **B:** Computed tomography scan of the same patient demonstrates a left-sided mass (*arrow*) adjacent to the spine. The mass was diagnosed as a psoas muscle hematoma. *A*, aorta; *I*, inferior vena cava; *RK*, right kidney. (Images courtesy of UltrasoundCases.info, owner SonoSkills.)

or infection. Obstructive causes are more common and include ureteral obstruction or bladder outlet obstruction owing to neoplasm, calculi, or congenital anomaly. Common patient complaints include fever, nausea, malaise, hematuria, and a compressible tender mass. Treatment includes aspiration of the urinoma and treatment of the primary cause. On sonography, this simple fluid collection is typically confined to the perirenal space (Fig. 16-16). The sonography examination should also include a search for the primary cause. The retroperitoneum should be examined for evidence of retroperitoneal fibrosis, ureteral strictures and calculi, and renal dysplasia.[5]

Retroperitoneal Abscess

Retroperitoneal abscess may develop as an extension from an adjacent organ such as renal infection, diverticulitis, and Crohn disease or owing to an existing retroperitoneal fluid collection that has become infected. Additionally, immunosuppressed patients and those with diabetes mellitus, ureteral obstruction, recent trauma, or surgery are at an increased risk for developing retroperitoneal abscess.[5] Clinically, abscess presents with an elevated white blood cell count, malaise, and fever. The sonographic appearance of abscess is very nonspecific, ranging from infiltrated solid tissue to a complex or thick-rimmed fluid collection with debris and possibly air (Fig. 16-17). Sonography cannot differentiate a complex fluid collection from an abscess. Aspiration is required to make a definitive diagnosis and may be the primary therapy.[22] Color and spectral Doppler imaging should be used to ensure that the complex fluid collection is not an aneurysm before aspiration is performed.

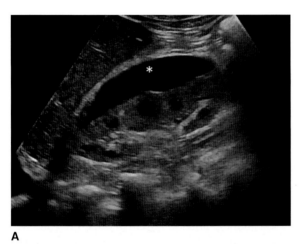

A

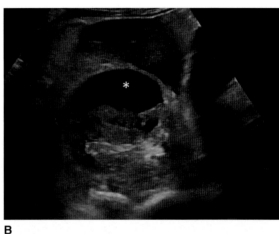

B

FIGURE 16-16 Urinoma. Longitudinal (**A**) and transverse (**B**) images of the kidney demonstrate an anechoic fluid collection (*asterisk*, *) compressing the kidney posteriorly and inferiorly within the renal capsule following percutaneous nephrolithotripsy. The fluid collection was diagnosed as a urinoma. (Image courtesy of UltrasoundCases.info, owner SonoSkills.)

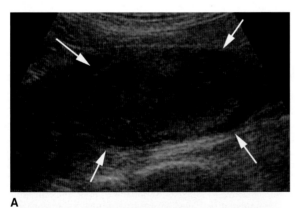

A

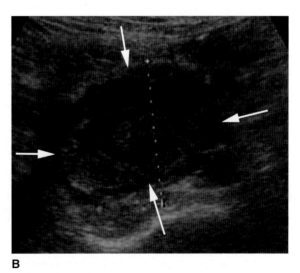

B

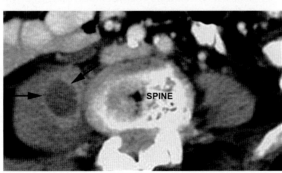

C

FIGURE 16-17 Psoas muscle abscess. Longitudinal (**A**) and transverse (**B**) images of the right retroperitoneum demonstrate a large hypoechoic mass (*arrows*) in the region of the psoas muscle. **C:** Computed tomography of the same patient demonstrates an abscess of the right psoas muscle. (Images courtesy of Dr. Taco Geertsma, Gelderse Vallei, The Netherlands.)

SUMMARY

- CT is the primary modality for evaluating the retroperitoneal cavity, but sonography can be used to evaluate the retroperitoneum, guide biopsy, or drainage procedures, and can be used for follow-up evaluations for lymphadenopathy, fluid collections, or solid masses.
- The retroperitoneum is located behind the parietal peritoneum, extends from the diaphragm superiorly to the pelvic brim inferiorly, and is divided into three major compartments by two fascial planes and the anterior and posterior renal fascia.
- The anterior pararenal space contains portions of the digestive tract, the pancreas, and the distal common bile duct.
- The perirenal space contains the kidneys, adrenal glands, perinephric fat, and the aorta and inferior vena cava.
- The posterior pararenal space lies between the posterior renal fascia and the transversalis fascia and contains no organs, only fat.
- The lymphatic system, comprised of the lymph nodes and lymphatic vessels, functions to return excess fluid from the interstitial spaces to the bloodstream, removes cellular debris and bacteria, and sends lymphocytes to infected tissues to help fight infection.
- Parietal lymph nodes are found surrounding the principal abdominal blood vessels and are grouped according to the artery with which they are associated, whereas visceral nodes are located at the hila of abdominal organs.
- When evaluating a retroperitoneal mass, the abnormality should be imaged in orthogonal planes; measurements should be obtained in three dimensions, the relationship of the mass to the surrounding anatomy, the origin of the mass, the mass characteristics, and blood flow characteristics should be documented.
- Lymphadenopathy describes the enlargement of lymph nodes caused by inflammation, primary neoplasia, or metastasis.
- Sonographically, enlarged lymph nodes typically appear as oval- to round-shaped masses with a low-to-medium-level echo pattern.
- Primary malignant nodes tend to be more hypoechoic to anechoic, more rounded than oval in shape, and have an asymmetric cortical widening and a loss of the normal fatty hilum.

- Enlarged retroperitoneal lymph nodes may fuse together to form a lobulated mantle-like soft tissue mass anterior to the great vessels or may completely encase the vessels, elevating them away from the vertebral column.
- Retroperitoneal fibrosis is typically idiopathic and may affect the ureters, resulting in unilateral or bilateral hydronephrosis.
- Although solid retroperitoneal tumors are rare, primary malignancies include liposarcoma, leiomyosarcoma, rhabdomyosarcoma, myxosarcoma, and fibrosarcoma.
- Liposarcoma is the most common primary malignancy of the retroperitoneum.
- Leiomyosarcoma is a smooth muscle tumor and is the second most common primary retroperitoneal malignancy, sonographically appearing as a large complex mass.
- Benign retroperitoneal tumors include lipoma, leiomyoma, rhabdomyoma, myxoma, and fibroma.
- Retroperitoneal fluid collections include abscess, hematoma, urinoma, and lymphocele.
- Retroperitoneal infections most commonly occur in the anterior pararenal space as a result of appendicitis, bowel inflammation, trauma, or pancreatitis.
- Fluid collections within the perirenal space are generally associated with renal abnormalities such as nephritis, ruptured renal artery aneurysm, or bleeding from a renal neoplasm.
- Fluid collections in the posterior pararenal space are most commonly associated with aortic disease and may include hemorrhage from rupture or infection from surgical procedures.
- Hematoma formation in the retroperitoneum may occur as the result of trauma, hemophilia, malignant invasion, surgery, anticoagulant therapy use, or may occur spontaneously.
- A lymphocele typically occurs following node dissection for cancer staging or following surgery such as renal transplant where the lymph vessels are disrupted.
- A urinoma occurs as a result of a tear in the urinary collecting system that may result from trauma, surgery, infection, or obstructive causes.
- Retroperitoneal abscess may develop as an extension from an adjacent organ such as renal infection, diverticulitis, and Crohn disease or owing to an existing retroperitoneal fluid collection that has become infected.

REFERENCES

1. Auckland AK. Unexplained hematocrit drop: rule out perinephric hematoma; possible perinephric mass. In: Sanders RC, Hall-Terracciano B, eds. *Clinical Sonography: A Practical Guide.* 5th ed. Wolters Kluwer Health; 2016:188–195.
2. Mirilas P, Skandalakis JE. Surgical anatomy of the retroperitoneal spaces part II: the architecture of the retroperitoneal space. *Am Surg.* 2010;76:33–42.
3. Kumar P, Mukhopadhyay S, Sandhu M, et al. Ultrasonography, computed tomography and percutaneous intervention in acute pancreatitis: a serial study. *Australas Radiol.* 1995;39:145–152.
4. Pick TP, Howden R, eds. *Gray's Anatomy: Anatomy, Descriptive and Surgical.* Random House; 1995.
5. Dähnert W. *Radiology Review Manual.* 5th ed. Lippincott Williams & Wilkins; 2003.
6. Ishikawa K, Idoguchi K, Tanaka H, et al. Classification of acute pancreatitis based on retroperitoneal extension: application of the concept of interfascial planes. *Eur J Radiol.* 2006;60:445–452.
7. Moore KL, Dalley AF, Agur AM. *Clinically Oriented Anatomy.* 7th ed. Wolters Kluwer Health; 2013.
8. Chesbrough RM, Burkhard TK, Martinez AJ, et al. Gerota versus Zuckerkandl: the renal fascia revisited. *Radiology.* 1989;173:845–846.
9. Lee SL, Ku YM, Rha SE. Comprehensive reviews of the interfascial plane of the retroperitoneum: normal anatomy and pathologic entities. *Emerg Radiol.* 2010;17:3–11.
10. Lee YJ, Oh SN, Rha SE, et al. Renal trauma. *Radiol Clin North Am.* 2007;45:581–592.
11. Moore KL, Agur AM, Dalley AF. *Essential Clinical Anatomy.* 5th ed. Wolters Kluwer Health; 2015.

12. Bertino RE, Saucier NA, Barth DJ. The retroperitoneum. In: Rumack CM, Wilson SR, Charbonneau JW, et al, eds. *Diagnostic Ultrasound.* Vol 1. 4th ed. Elsevier Mosby; 2011:447–485.

13. Paetzold S, Gary T, Hafner F, et al. Thrombosis of the inferior vena cava related to Ormond's disease. *Clin Rheumatol.* 2013;32(suppl 1):S67–S70.

14. Moussavian B, Horrow MM. Retroperitoneal fibrosis. *Ultrasound Q.* 2009;25:89–91.

15. Vaglio A, Palmisano A, Corradi D, et al. Retroperitoneal fibrosis: evolving concepts. *Rheum Dis Clin North Am.* 2007;33:803–817.

16. Sinescu I, Surcel C, Mirvald C, et al. Prognostic factors in retroperitoneal fibrosis. *J Med Life.* 2010;3:19–25.

17. Han HH, Choi KH, Kim DS, et al. Retroperitoneal giant liposarcoma. *Korean J Urol.* 2010;51:579–582.

18. Fried AM. Spleen and retroperitoneum: the essentials. *Ultrasound Q.* 2005;21:275–286.

19. Hemant D, Krantikumar R, Amita J, et al. Primary leiomyosarcoma of inferior vena cava, a rare entity: imaging features. *Australas Radiol.* 2001;45:448–451.

20. Al-Saif OH, Sengupta B, Amr S, et al. Leiomyosarcoma of the infrarenal inferior vena cava. *Am J Surg.* 2011;2:e18–e20.

21. Tchelepi H, Ralls PW. Ultrasound of acute pancreatitis. *Ultrasound Clin.* 2007;2:415–422.

22. Rivera-Sanfeliz G. Percutaneous abdominal abscess drainage: a historical perspective. *Am J Roentgenol.* 2008;191:642–643.

CHAPTER 17

The Thyroid Gland, Parathyroid Glands, and Neck

AMBREE PENROD

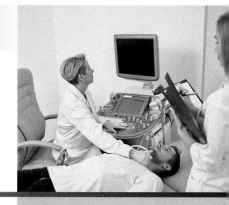

OBJECTIVES

- Describe the thyroid gland embryology, surface anatomy, anatomic variants, and the common relational landmarks.
- Discuss the physiology of the thyroid gland to include how each of the three thyroid hormones enables thyroid function.
- Correlate laboratory values and clinical indications associated with hyperthyroidism and hypothyroidism.
- Explain the sonographic evaluation of the thyroid gland to include patient preparation and protocol and demonstrate the examination procedure.
- Differentiate normal and pathologic sonographic appearances associated with thyroid gland disease or pathology.
- Describe the pathology, etiology, clinical signs and symptoms, and sonographic appearance for thyroid gland cysts, nodules, adenomas, goiters, thyrotoxicosis/hyperthyroidism, hypothyroidism, thyroiditis, thyroid disease in pregnancy, and thyroid carcinoma.
- Explain the indications and guidelines for fine-needle aspiration.
- Describe the parathyroid glands' embryology, surface anatomy, anatomic variants, and the common relational landmarks.
- Discuss the physiology of the parathyroid glands to include the importance of parathyroid hormone regulating calcium and phosphorus concentrations in extracellular fluid.
- Correlate laboratory values and clinical indications associated with hypercalcemia and hypocalcemia.
- Explain the sonographic evaluation of the parathyroid glands to include patient preparation and protocol and demonstrate the examination procedure.
- Differentiate normal and pathologic sonographic appearances associated with disease or pathology of the parathyroid glands.
- Describe the pathology, etiology, clinical signs and symptoms, and sonographic appearance for primary hyperparathyroidism to include adenomas, hyperplasia, and carcinoma.
- Differentiate the varying sonographic appearances associated with normal anatomy and disease or pathology of the neck.
- Describe the etiology, clinical signs and symptoms, and sonographic appearance of developmental cysts for the thyroglossal duct cyst, branchial cleft cyst, and cystic hygroma.

KEY TERMS

anaplastic carcinoma

calcitonin (thyrocalcitonin)

elastography

euthyroid

follicular carcinoma

Graves disease

Hashimoto thyroiditis

Hürthle cell carcinoma

hypercalcemia

hyperparathyroidism

hyperplasia

hypocalcemia

hypothyroidism

medullary carcinoma

papillary carcinoma

subacute thyroiditis (de Quervain disease or granulomatous thyroiditis)

thyroiditis

thyrotoxicosis/ hyperthyroidism

thyroxine (T_4)

triiodothyronine (T_3)

■ Identify the usefulness of diagnostic imaging to differentiate between a hematoma and deep neck space infections.

■ Describe the pathology, etiology, and important sonographic appearance and criteria to differentiate normal versus pathologic cervical lymph nodes.

GLOSSARY

adenoma parathyroid adenoma, a benign, solid tumor of the parathyroid gland that secretes parathyroid hormone, which results in elevated levels of serum calcium thyroid adenoma, a benign, solid tumor of the thyroid gland

adenopathy enlargement of the glands

anaplasia a loss of differentiation of cells, which is a characteristic of tumor tissue and occurs in most malignant tumors

cervical adenopathy enlargement of the lymph nodes

cold nodule (photon-deficient area) seen on a nuclear medicine study as region of thyroid where the radioisotope has not been taken up; the area may correspond to a palpable mass

euthyroid state in which the thyroid gland is producing the right amount of thyroid hormone

fine-needle aspiration (FNA) invasive procedure using a small gauge needle to obtain a tissue specimen from a specific lesion

goiter focal or diffuse thyroid gland enlargement often owing to iodine deficiency; multiple nodules may be present

Graves disease an autoimmune hyperthyroidism caused by antibodies that continuously activate thyroid-stimulating hormone receptors; it is characterized by enlarged thyroid, protrusion of eyeballs (exophthalmos), a rapid heartbeat, nervous excitability

Hashimoto thyroiditis (chronic lymphocytic thyroiditis or Hashimoto disease) most common inflammatory disease of the thyroid gland; usually occurs in genetically predisposed individuals, often presents in patients with other autoimmune disorders that may be associated with the formation of antibodies against normal thyroid tissue, and often accompanied by marked hyperemia

heterotopic occurring at an abnormal place or upon the wrong part of the body

hyperparathyroidism disorder associated with elevated serum calcium levels; usually caused by benign parathyroid adenoma

hyperthyroidism oversecretion of thyroid hormones

hypothyroidism underactive thyroid hormones

indolent causing little pain (indolent tumor) or slow growing (indolent lesion or tumor)

isthmus thin band of thyroid tissue connecting the right and left lobes

longus colli muscles wedge-shaped muscle posterior to the thyroid lobes

microcalcifications tiny hyperechoic foci that may or may not shadow; sometimes present within a thyroid nodule

papillary carcinoma most common form of thyroid cancer

parathyroid hormone hormone produced by the parathyroid glands that regulate serum calcium and phosphorus

sternocleidomastoid muscles large muscles located anterolateral to the thyroid

strap muscles sternohyoid and sternothyroid muscles located anterior to the thyroid

thyroglossal duct cyst developmental fluid-filled space; congenital anomaly located anterior to trachea extending from the base of the tongue to the isthmus of the thyroid

thyroid inferno increase in color Doppler vascular flow in the thyroid

thyroiditis inflammation of the thyroid

thyroid-stimulating hormone hormone secreted by the anterior pituitary gland that stimulates the thyroid gland to secrete thyroxine (T_4) and triiodothyronine (T_3)

Sonographic evaluation of the neck provides an important diagnostic screening procedure for the evaluation of both the thyroid gland and parathyroid glands, as well as the soft tissues of the neck. Using a high-resolution, high-frequency transducer, the noninvasive examination provides a fast and an accurate assessment of anatomy without patient preparation. Sonographic guidance is important during such interventional procedures as fine-needle aspiration (FNA) and alcohol ablation of adenomas of the parathyroid glands.[1]

THYROID GLAND

The thyroid gland is the site of synthesis, storage, and controlled secretion of thyroid hormones.[2] It is the largest endocrine gland in the human body and functions to control the basal metabolic rate (BMR).[3] With the development of high-resolution, high-frequency probes designed for scanning small parts, sonography has established itself as a superior modality for imaging the thyroid gland.[4] Its greatest clinical value is in confirming mass location, differentiating between cystic and solid lesions, and imaging the biopsy needle during FNA. The thyroid gland is subject to an array of maladaptations, which are presented along with their sonographic appearance in this chapter.

Embryology

Emerging between the third and fourth gestational weeks, the thyroid gland is the earliest endocrine glandular structure to appear in the human embryo.[5] The gland develops from an invagination in the floor of the primitive pharynx at the level of the first and second branchial arches, a point in the adult corresponding to the base of the tongue. This invagination is lined by cylindrical epithelial cells and can be distinguished at 16 to 17 days of gestation. These cells separate to form their pharyngeal connections by the fifth gestational week and migrate downward in front of the primitive pharynx and the developing hyoid bone. During this period of growth, the vesicle becomes a solid mass of epithelial cells and severs its connection with the pharyngeal cavity. This journey leaves behind a trace of epithelial cells known as the *thyroglossal tract* (*duct*), which normally solidifies and ultimately atrophies.[6] Dividing into two lobes connected by an isthmus at 7 weeks, the thyroid gland forms a shield over the front of the trachea and thyroid cartilage, becoming fully developed by the end of the first trimester.[6]

Anatomy

The thyroid gland is located in the anterior neck, surrounded by a fibrous capsule. It consists primarily of a right and left lobe, with a relatively thin isthmus, which unites the lobes usually over the second and third cartilaginous rings of the trachea.[7] The superior border of the lateral lobes begins at approximately the thyroid cartilage (*pomum Adami* or Adam's apple) and extends inferiorly (Fig. 17-1A, B).

The thyroid gland weighs approximately 30 g in the adult.[3,8] The size and shape of the thyroid lobes vary with age, body surface area, and gender, being slightly larger in females.[9] On longitudinal sections, the lobes appear elongated in tall individuals and appear more oval on short individuals.[10] The mean length measures 40 to 60 mm, mean anteroposterior (AP) diameter is 13 to 18 mm, and the mean isthmic thickness is 4 to 6 mm.[11] Sonography is very accurate for calculating thyroid gland volume when needed to determine treatment or evaluate response to treatment. The volume can be determined with linear measurements or mathematical formulas for each lobe,[10] and vary by gender with female volumes ranging from 10 to 15 mL and males from 12 to 18 mL.[3]

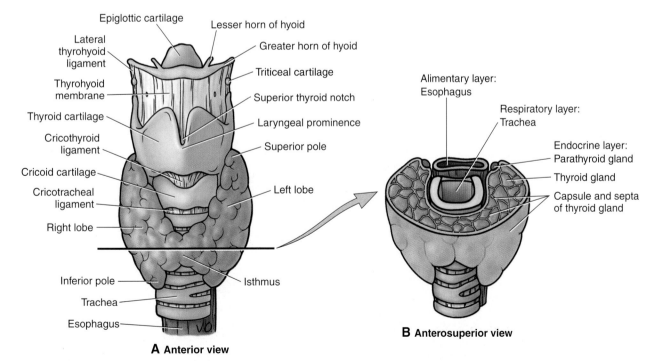

FIGURE 17-1 Thyroid gland anatomy. **A:** The illustration demonstrates the relationship of the normal thyroid gland from an anterior view and (**B**) an anterosuperior view, which includes the three layers of cervical viscera. (Reprinted with permission from Moore KL, Agur AMR, Dalley AF II. *Essential Clinical Anatomy*. 5th ed. Wolters Kluwer Health; 2015:604.)

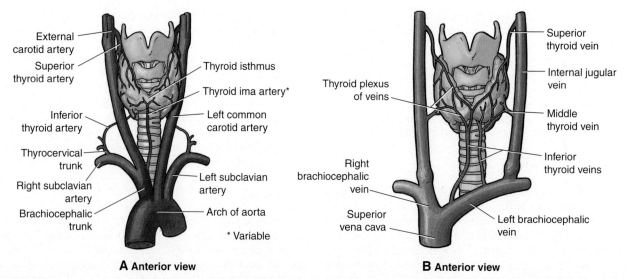

A Anterior view **B** Anterior view

FIGURE 17-2 Thyroid gland vascularity. **A:** The anterior view illustration demonstrates the arterial supply to the thyroid gland and **(B)** illustrates an anterior view of the venous drainage of the thyroid gland. (Reprinted with permission from Moore KL, Agur AMR, Dalley AF II. *Essential Clinical Anatomy.* 5th ed. Wolters Kluwer Health; 2015:607.)

Four arteries provide a rich blood supply to the thyroid gland. The upper poles of the gland receive blood from paired superior thyroid arteries that arise from the external carotids. Two inferior thyroid arteries originate at the thyrocervical trunk of the subclavian artery and supply the lower thyroid poles[12] (Fig. 17-2A). Normal peak velocities from the major thyroid arteries are 20 to 40 cm/sec and normal peak velocities from the intraparenchymal arteries are 15 to 30 cm/sec.[10] On the anterior surface, three pairs of veins normally drain the thyroid plexus.[12] The superior thyroid veins correspond to the superior thyroid artery and drain the superior lobes. The middle thyroid veins drain the middle lobes and the inferior thyroid veins drain the inferior poles. The superior and middle thyroid veins drain into the internal jugular vein and the inferior thyroid veins drain into the brachiocephalic veins[12] (Fig. 17-2B).

Anatomic Variants

Deviations during any stage of development may lead to aberrant configurations or heterotopic locations of the thyroid gland. If the thyroglossal duct fails to involute completely, its persistence is a 1 to 3 cm cystic, fluid-filled remnant located anywhere along the route of the duct.[6] The thyroglossal duct cyst is the most common congenital cyst found in the neck.[13]

The most critical abnormality is the absence of the thyroid gland (athyrosis). This rare condition is associated with cretinism or congenital hypothyroidism. Early identification and intervention with hormone replacement can stave off the physical and mental deficiencies associated with congenital hypothyroidism.

More commonly, the gland may differentiate into configurations other than an isthmus and two lateral lobes. The variation occurring most often is a pyramidal lobe, which has been identified to some degree in approximately as many as 50% of normal patients.[5] Developmentally, the pyramidal lobe arises from the caudal portion of the thyroglossal tract. Usually, this lobe is small, extending midline upward from the isthmus, but it can arise from either lobe, more often the left lobe than the right[12] (Fig. 17-3).

Other anatomic variations include the absence of an isthmus with the gland appearing as two independent lobes, the absence of one lobe with enlargement of the remaining lobe, or continuity from one lobe to the other effectively obliterating the isthmus.[5]

Thyroid gland development can occur ectopically at any point along the pathway of descent.[12] A normal gland may also rest entirely above (suprahyoid or prelaryngeal) or below the hyoid bone. Lingual thyroid, although relatively rare (1 in 100,000 cases of thyroid disease), is the most common location for functional ectopic tissue.[13] This placement is usually identified by an incidental finding of a mass at the back of the tongue.[14]

Other ectopic locations include under the tongue (sublingual), the mediastinum (substernal), and rarely the

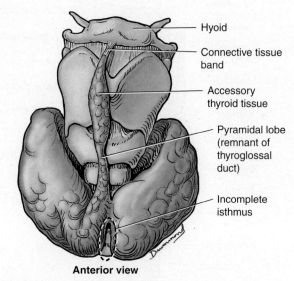

Anterior view

FIGURE 17-3 Anatomic variations. An anterior view illustration demonstrates anatomic variations, which include accessory thyroid tissue, pyramidal lobe, and incomplete isthmus. (Reprinted with permission from Moore KL, Agur AMR, Dalley AF II. *Essential Clinical Anatomy.* 5th ed. Wolters Kluwer Health; 2015:607.)

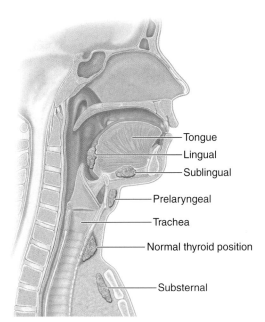

FIGURE 17-4 Ectopic thyroid gland locations. The illustration of a lateral view demonstrates the common sites for an ectopic thyroid gland.

tracheal or esophageal wall (Fig. 17-4). Small amounts of histologically functioning tissues may also be found along the internal carotid artery, the supraclavicular fossa, adjacent to the aortic arch or between the aorta and the pulmonary trunk, within the upper portion of the pericardium or mediastinum, and even within the interventricular septum.[5,6,15]

Anatomic Landmarks

Many anatomic landmarks help to define the thyroid gland on a sonogram (Fig. 17-5A). On transverse images, the common carotid artery and internal jugular vein form the posterior lateral border of the gland. The artery is located medial to the vein. These structures are distinguished from the thyroid gland by echogenic walls and anechoic centers with color or pulsed wave Doppler imaging also available to assist in clarifying the anatomy. The longus colli muscle appears as a low-level, echogenic structure defining the posterior border of the gland. The air-filled trachea forms the medial border and appears hyperechoic, with posterior shadowing. The sternothyroid, sternohyoid, and omohyoid muscles, collectively called the *strap muscles*, form the anterolateral border of the gland. The sternothyroid muscle is directly superficial to the thyroid gland and is bordered by the sternohyoid anteriorly and the omohyoid laterally. The sternocleidomastoid is located lateral and superficial to the omohyoid. The very thin platysma muscle surrounds the neck, but its superficial location and indistinct density make it difficult to image with sonography. The thyroid gland appears as a rounded structure of low- to medium-level echoes, homogeneous in texture (Fig. 17-5B).

When imaged in the longitudinal (parasagittal) planes, the jugular vein and carotid artery appear as long, tubular, anechoic structures located laterally to the thyroid gland. Moving medially from these landmarks, the longus colli muscle, located posteriorly, becomes visible as a low-level, echogenic structure (Fig. 17-5C, D). The thyroid gland again is distinguished by its low- to medium-level, homogeneous echo pattern.

Physiology

Normal physical and mental growth depends on a healthy, functioning thyroid gland. The principal responsibility of the thyroid gland is maintenance of body metabolism.[2] Protein, carbohydrate, lipid, and vitamin metabolism all rely on or are affected by thyroid hormone action. Additionally, thyroid hormones modulate oxygen consumption and enhance the rate of glucose uptake by fat tissue. Lipolysis and fatty acid mobilization from fat stores are magnified in the presence of thyroid hormone and blood serum cholesterol levels are generally lowered.[3]

The thyroid gland secretes three hormones: triiodothyronine (T_3), thyroxine (T_4), and calcitonin, also called *thyrocalcitonin*.[2] The thyroid gland's parafollicular cells, or C cells, secrete calcitonin, which lowers the plasma calcium level by inhibiting mobilization of calcium from the bone. The follicular cells of the thyroid gland chemically process iodine to secrete T_3 and T_4.[8] The synthesis of these hormones depends on the availability of iodine and the gland's ability to process it properly.[3] When comparing secretion, the thyroid gland produces 90% of the less potent T_4 and only 10% of the more potent T_3; however, T_4 is converted to the more powerful T_3, which has the greatest metabolic effect and binds more efficiently to nuclear receptors in target cells.[2]

Maintenance of circulating concentrations of T_3 and T_4 is achieved by a dynamic regulatory system involving the hypothalamus, the pituitary, and the thyroid gland.[2] Thyrotropin, secreted by the anterior pituitary (adenohypophysis) thyrotroph cells, orchestrates thyroid hormone production. The secretion of thyroid-stimulating hormone (TSH) is modulated by both the T_3 and T_4 hormones and by thyrotropin-releasing hormone (TRH) from the hypothalamus.[2] Utilizing a classic negative feedback system, a drop in circulating thyroid hormones decreases the BMR. The falling BMR stimulates TRH, which in turn provokes the release of TSH. Thus inspired, the thyroid gland liberates the necessary T_3 and T_4, thereby returning the BMR to normal and retiring the cycle. Because the effects of thyroid hormones represent a complex integration of events at both the cellular and holistic levels, disease states that interfere with this system can have serious consequences.[2]

Laboratory Tests

Thyroid hormones circulate in the blood both free and bound to thyroxine-binding globulin (TBG).[6] Thyroid gland with normal laboratory values is referred to as an *euthyroid*, which means the gland is producing the right amount of thyroid hormone. There are several tests for diagnosing thyroid disease, an example of which is given in (Table 17-1). The range of these values may vary somewhat among laboratories and in different geographic locations, and additional labs may be added to this list in different circumstances. For example, laboratory tests for calcitonin are done only for known or suspected cases of medullary carcinoma of the thyroid gland.

Diagnosing thyroid disease early is important because most are responsive to medical or surgical management.[6] These include conditions associated with excessive release of thyroid hormones (hyperthyroidism), those associated with thyroid hormone deficiency (hypothyroidism), and mass lesions of the thyroid gland.[6]

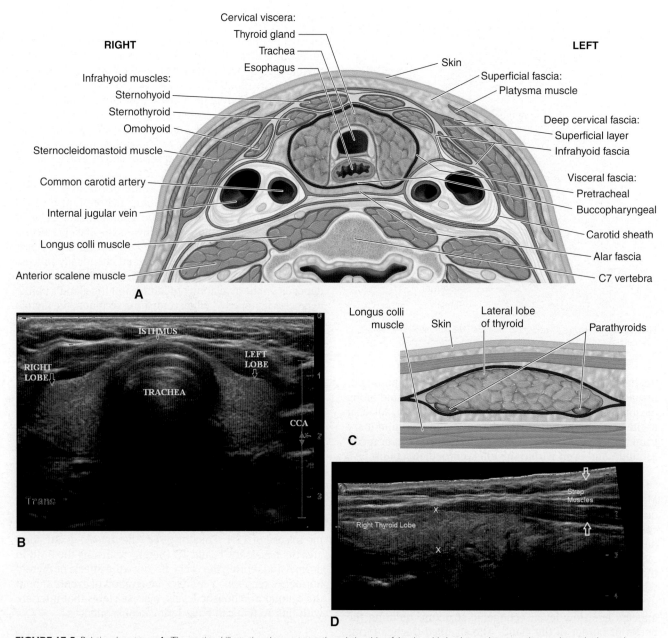

FIGURE 17-5 Relational anatomy. **A:** The sectional illustration demonstrates the relationship of the thyroid gland, vasculature, and musculature in the neck. (Reprinted with permission from Tank PW, Gest TR. *Lippincott Williams & Wilkins Atlas of Anatomy*. Wolters Kluwer Health/Lippincott Williams & Wilkins; 2009:305.) **B:** Transverse image of a normal thyroid. Note the homogeneous texture. **C:** A longitudinal section of either the right or left lobe will show the thyroid gland relationship to the distally located longus colli muscle. **D:** A longitudinal sonogram is performed with a panoramic imaging option and demonstrates a normal right lobe (*cursors*) of the thyroid gland and the strap muscles (*arrows*). *CCA*, common carotid artery.

TABLE 17-1	Thyroid Laboratory Values
T_4 free	0.8–2.4 ng/dL
T_4 total	4–11 ng/mL
Thyroxine-binding globulin (TBG)	12–30 mg/L
T_3 total	75–220 ng/dL
TSH	0.3–3.04 U/mL

T_3, triiodothyronine; T_4, thyroxine. TSH, thyroid-stimulating hormone.

Sonographic Examination Technique

Sonography proves useful in a variety of situations when examining the neck. Sonographic examination can reliably distinguish between cystic and solid masses, provide guidance for FNA sampling or treatment of lesions,[16] and establish pathology in the thyroid or neck following a normal clinical exam with nonpalpable lesions, as may be the case in patients with a history of therapeutic radiation to the head and neck. Serial sonographic examinations are also used to follow the size of suspected benign nodules on patients receiving suppressive therapy or in those patients who require continued monitoring for growth of nodules. Sonographic exams aid in the determination of when further examination through biopsy or surgery may be necessary as is the case when nodules fail to decrease in size or continue to grow over a period of time. Additionally, sonography facilitates the treatment of several benign and malignant conditions through the use of sonographically guided percutaneous ethanol injection, which has been used as an alternative to surgery in patients not suitable for surgical intervention or in patients with recurrent cysts following FNA.[16]

To begin the examination, the medical history should be reviewed from the referring physician and the pertinent information obtained from the patient. Information about symptoms, duration, current treatment, history of therapeutic radiation, and locations of any palpable masses is necessary when interpreting the final images. If the patient has had a radioisotope scan or any prior imaging exams, sonographers should attempt to access and review the images and the associated reports because this will allow them to tailor their exam to attempt to answer any questions raised by preceding tests, or to follow up on indicated areas of concern. If the patient presents with a mass, either the patient should be made to identify its location or, if the mass is palpable only to the referring physician, a description of the area of interest should be obtained.

No patient preparation is required for thyroid gland sonography, although some facilities recommend limiting food and drink 1 hour prior to the examination to reduce gastric reflux in patients subject to this problem. With the patient in a supine position, the shoulders and upper back should be elevated with a pillow or rolled towel, hyperextending the neck.[17] This will permit easier access to the thyroid gland. The sonographer should be cautious with elderly patients and other patients in whom this position may cause dizziness or neck strain and should not overextend the neck in any patient. If this position is not tolerable, the patient should be requested to elevate the chin up and back as far as possible, and, if needed, the patient's head should be turned away from the side being examined in order to gain surface area for scanning.

The highest-frequency transducer available should be selected, remaining aware that the thyroid gland is a superficial structure and that near-field resolution will be important. Most current sonography equipment offer 7.5- to 15-MHz short-focus linear transducers specifically designed for small parts scanning. The movable focal zone (if applicable) should be adjusted to the area of interest in the gland. In patients with thick necks, or occasionally in those who have had radiation therapy, a lower-MHz transducer may be needed for penetration. Resolution is diminished at this lower frequency, which compromises structural clarity but may be necessary in these situations.

Scanning protocol includes multiple transverse, longitudinal, and oblique views. The sonographer should begin superiorly at the level of the mandible and then move inferiorly in the transverse plane until the characteristic pattern of the thyroid gland is identified. The homogeneously echogenic pattern results from the numerous follicles and surrounding supportive tissue that constitutes the thyroid gland. Sonographically, it is similar in appearance to normal parenchyma in the liver and testes and hyperechoic in appearance relative to adjacent musculature.[7] The sonographer should stay alert for extra thyroid masses, such as enlarged lymph nodes or parathyroid glands,

and proceed slowly through the gland and beyond, paying particular attention to subtle textural or structural changes. The procedure should be repeated for the opposite lobe. An attempt should be made to image both lobes and the isthmus on a single image with or without the use of wide screen settings. When a single image is not possible, most equipment will allow dual-screen imaging, which displays two images side by side. This feature provides a method for presenting both thyroid lobes and the connecting isthmus simultaneously when unable to fit the entire gland on a single image. Panoramic imaging is useful when scanning enlarged glands and, in some cases, may be the only way to demonstrate the thyroid gland in its entirety. The sonographer should record as many images as necessary to document normal or abnormal structures and at least acquire representative images from the upper, middle, and lower portions of both lobes, including the isthmus. Each lobe should be measured in both the AP and transverse planes, and the isthmus should be measured in the AP plane. Imaging of the lower poles can be enhanced by asking the patient to swallow, which momentarily raises the thyroid gland in the neck.[10]

To scan the longitudinal plane, the sonographer should begin lateral to the thyroid gland, imaging the carotid artery or jugular vein and move the transducer medially, again noting both the architecture of the gland and any extraglandular structures. The gland should be measured in its longest projection, using the dual-screen, wide-screen, or panoramic function if necessary. The examination should also be extended laterally to include the region of the carotid artery and jugular vein in order to identify enlarged cervical chain lymph nodes, superiorly to visualize submandibular adenopathy, and inferiorly to define any pathologic supraclavicular nodes.[10] Color Doppler and pulsed wave Doppler imaging contribute to the thyroid gland sonography examination by revealing internal vascular detail. They are perhaps most helpful when examining ambiguous isoechoic or complex masses. The presence or absence of Doppler flow may help to differentiate among solid vascular masses, simple serous cysts with echogenic fluid, necrotic solid masses, and hemorrhagic cysts. When nodules are identified during an exam, their size should be measured as the thyroid gland was measured, in three dimensions, in longitudinal, anterior-to-posterior, and transverse planes, and their location within the gland should be documented along with any identifying characteristics of the nodule. If multiple nodules are noted, they should be numbered with their location documentation to allow for follow-up when it is required.

Pathology of the Thyroid Gland

The thyroid gland is host to benign, malignant, autoimmune, and metastatic conditions, all of which have varied and often overlapping sonographic appearances. Sonography is most useful in differentiating solid from cystic lesions and in patients in whom there is uncertainty about the origin of a neck mass. The sonography examination for thyroid gland disease should serve to amplify and clarify the clinical, laboratory, nuclear medicine, and cytopathology data obtained for a patient.

Cysts

Thyroid cysts are common in humans but the term is often used loosely to define thyroid disease.[18] The true epithelium-lined cysts in the region of the thyroid gland are uncommon and are almost always benign.[13] Two true cysts are the thyroglossal duct cyst and the branchial cleft cyst, which can be differentiated from each other by their location. Thyroglossal duct cysts tend to be midline and branchial cleft cysts tend to be lateral to the carotids. More information regarding these two cysts in presented in the section on Developmental Cysts.

Benign nodular thyroid disease is common among adults and the prevalence increases with age.[19] Sonographic evaluation indicates that 15% to 25% of these solitary thyroid nodules are either cystic or predominantly cystic and are sonographically described as either a mixed or a complex lesion.[18,19] The etiology of the cystic portion of the thyroid nodule is usually hemorrhage or is subsequent degeneration of preexisting nodules.[20] FNA cytology provides the diagnosis of benign versus malignant and cystic versus solid lesions.[18] Percutaneous ethanol injection is used to initially treat benign cystic nodules or as follow-up treatment for recurrent thyroid cysts.[19,20] The response rate to the ethanol injection ranges from 72.1% to 93.9%.[18] Malignant cystic nodules are surgically removed.[18]

Sonographically, a simple cyst will be circular or oval, with discrete margins; contain no internal echoes; and exhibit posterior enhancement (Fig. 17-6A). Comet tail artifacts can frequently be encountered in complex cystic thyroid nodules, and they are likely related to the presence of colloid substances in the cyst[21] (Fig. 17-6B). A hemorrhagic cyst may contain blood and debris and may appear as a complex mass with irregular borders and internal septa (Fig. 17-6C). When more densely echogenic fluid is gravitationally layered in the posterior portion of a cystic cavity, the likelihood of hemorrhagic debris is very high (Fig. 17-6D). Sonographically, papillary carcinomas may present with varying amounts of cystic change, may appear almost indistinguishable from benign cystic nodules, or may appear as uneven cystic structures, with finger-like pedunculated mass(es) larger than 2 cm seen projecting into the lumen[18] (Fig. 17-6E). FNA is important to distinguish these from one another and to obtain a diagnosis.

Thyroid Nodule

In the United States, the estimated prevalence of thyroid nodules found by palpation alone ranges from 4% to 7% and sonography detects nodules in 20% to 76% of the adult population.[22] They are more common in women and increase in frequency with age and with decreasing iodine intake.[22] Based on the technetium-99m (Tc-99m) radioiodine scintigraphy examination, they are classified either as "hot" (hyperfunctioning/autonomous) or as "cold" (nonfunctioning).[23] A cold nodule is one that does not absorb the radiopharmaceutical used for evaluating the gland and therefore appears as an area of decreased or absent activity on the resulting nuclear image. In contrast, a hot nodule traps an excessive amount of isotope and presents as a dense collection of activity.

Patients with a thyroid nodule palpated on physical examination, which subsequently appear as cold nodules on a nuclear medicine study, are often referred to sonography for further evaluation. Approximately 80% to 85% of thyroid nodules are cold and 10% to 15% of these are malignant.[24] About 5% to 10% of solitary thyroid nodules are hot nodules, which usually implies benignity.[23] Currently, no single sonographic criterion distinguishes benign thyroid nodules

from malignant thyroid nodules with complete reliability.[10] It is possible to make an accurate prediction of malignancy and recommend FNA when suspicious sonographic signs are seen in combination with multiple signs of thyroid malignancy.

Adenomas

A thyroid adenoma is a benign, neoplastic growth of thyroid glandular epithelium usually contained within a fibrous capsule.[6] Most adenomas are solitary but they may also develop as part of a multinodular process.[10] Although the terms *adenoma* and *nodule* are used interchangeably, an adenoma is a specific new tissue growth (neoplastic) and a nodule may include a carcinoma, a normal gland lobule, or any other focal lesion. Benign adenomas account for 5% to 10% of thyroid nodules and are seven times more common in females than in males.[10] Most adenomas are derived from follicular epithelium, and a small minority of these are toxic and cause hyperthyroidism owing to autonomous function.[13] Based on the degree of follicle formation and the colloid content of the follicles, the rare adenomas make up these histologic subtype classifications: macrofollicular (simple colloid), microfollicular (fetal), embryonal (trabecular), Hürthle cell (oxyphil, oncocytic) adenomas, atypical adenomas, and adenomas with papillae.[8] Adenomas grow slowly, remain dormant for years, and are more common in the fifth and sixth decades of life.[6] In order to be palpated on physical examination, an adenoma must reach a size of 0.5 to 1 cm. This explains why sonography has detected small nodules on a thyroid gland that was not detected on palpation. When a hyperfunctioning adenoma suppresses normal thyroid gland tissue, the normal tissue atrophies and the adenoma appears as a hot nodule against a background of minimal uptake on a radionuclide examination.[6] A toxic hyperfunctioning adenoma may provoke thyrotoxicosis. The distinction between toxic and nontoxic adenomas cannot be made with sonography. Adenomas are typically asymptomatic but can grow large enough to exert pressure or develop hemorrhage, thus, becoming problematic.

The sonographic features of adenomas are influenced by the amount of structural degeneration and vary widely, appearing cystic to complex or solid. One other sonographic feature previously thought to indicate a benign nodule often associated with an adenoma is calcification along the rim, but malignant nodules may also have this appearance[10] (Fig. 17-7A, B). The most common appearance is that of a solitary, well-circumscribed, oval or circular mass of variable size and echogenicity. Small, solid adenomas with uniformly low echogenicity can be mistaken for cysts. The distinction is made by noting the absence of through sound transmission behind a solid lesion. A peripheral hypoechoic-to-anechoic halo that completely or incompletely surrounds an adenoma is a relatively consistent finding. The halo, however, cannot be used as the only criterion and additional statistical information is necessary to establish the halo's specificity.[9] A halo in the nodule periphery may be seen with benign or malignant conditions and suggests that there is an acoustic interface that does not reflect the ultrasound across two different types of histology in the region of the benign or malignant nodule and the surrounding thyroid gland.[25] In the case of an adenoma, this halo is thought to represent the fibrous capsule and the perinodal blood vessels, which can be seen by color Doppler imaging, and mild edema

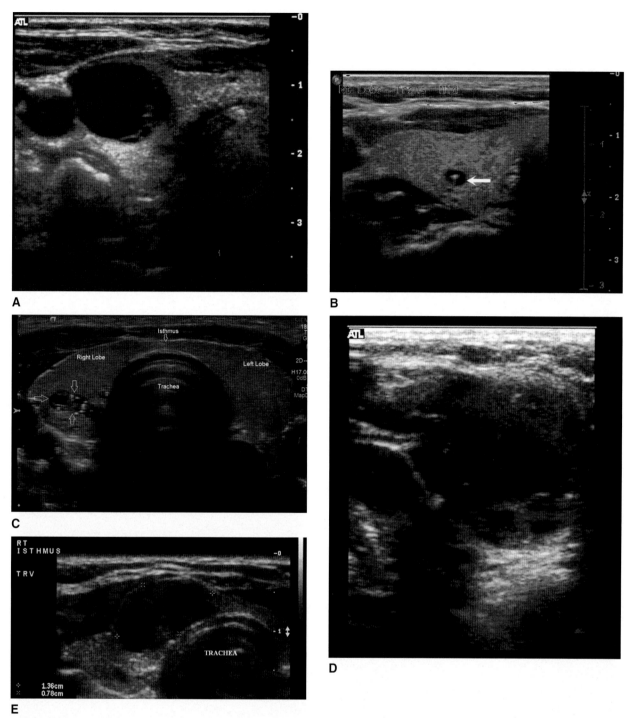

FIGURE 17-6 Thyroid cysts. **A:** A transverse image through the right thyroid midlobe region shows a well-circumscribed anechoic structure, with good through sound transmission and debris along the posterior wall representing colloid elements within the cyst. **B:** A transverse image through the right thyroid lobe shows a small central colloid cyst (*arrow*) with a "comet tail" artifact beneath the small echogenic structure within the colloid cyst. **C:** A small complex thyroid cyst is identified in the right lobe on this transverse image. (Courtesy of Siemens Medical Solutions USA, Inc.) **D:** This transverse image through the right thyroid lobe shows a complex thyroid mass, which on biopsy was identified as a degenerating cyst. **E:** On this transverse image of the right thyroid/isthmus region, the sonographic appearance is similar to Figure D; however, the cytology report from a sonography-guided biopsy on this 32-year-old woman revealed papillary carcinoma.

or compressed normal thyroid parenchyma (Fig. 17-7C). Color Doppler imaging performed on an adenoma may have a "spoke and wheel" appearance with peripheral blood vessels extending toward the center of the lesion[10] (Fig. 17-7D, E). Adenomas greater than 2.5 to 3 cm commonly display the sonographic characteristics of a complex cyst. These adenomatous cysts tend to have irregular shapes and borders with thickened walls, an incomplete capsule and are less sharply demarcated from surrounding tissue. Although imaging research is providing increased statistical probabilities to distinguish benign and malignant nodules, imaging procedures cannot be used as the only dependable criteria to distinguish adenomas from other benign or malignant nodules[21] (Fig. 17-7F–I).

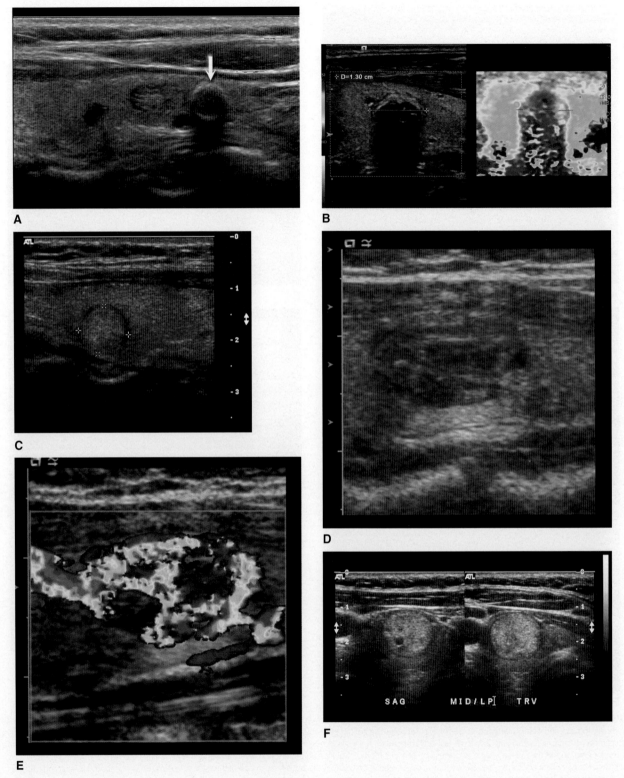

FIGURE 17-7 Sonographic appearance of adenoma. **A:** An image from a 71-year-old female of the left thyroid lobe demonstrates three different presentations of adenomatous nodules. The *open solid arrow* points to a calcified nodule. Note the highly echogenic anterior-curved wall and dense shadowing. **B:** The sonogram shows an echogenic anterior peripheral (eggshell) calcification with shadowing. The sonographic appearance of peripheral curved calcification was previously inclusive to only benign nodules but to a much lesser extent been seen with malignant nodules. (Courtesy of Siemens Medical Solutions USA, Inc.) **C:** This longitudinal image through the left thyroid lobe in a 41-year-old woman demonstrates a hypoechoic halo surrounding the nodule. Fine-needle aspiration of the area marked by *cursors* returned a diagnosis of a benign hyperplastic nodule consistent with a nodular goiter. **D, E:** On these two images on a 41-year-old woman patient, the fine-needle aspiration results described an adenoma. A longitudinal image (**D**) of the left thyroid gland shows a solitary nodule. On the color Doppler image (**E**), the circle of color is at the periphery of the nodule and the linear color signals are coursing toward the center. **E–H:** These four images represent biopsy-proven benign adenomatous cysts or degenerating adenomas. Although there are some recurrent sonographic appearances associated with benignity, imaging alone cannot definitively predict benign versus malignant biopsy outcomes. **F:** A longitudinal and transverse image through the right thyroid lobe shows a hypoechoic, round-to-oval mass surrounded by a thin halo.

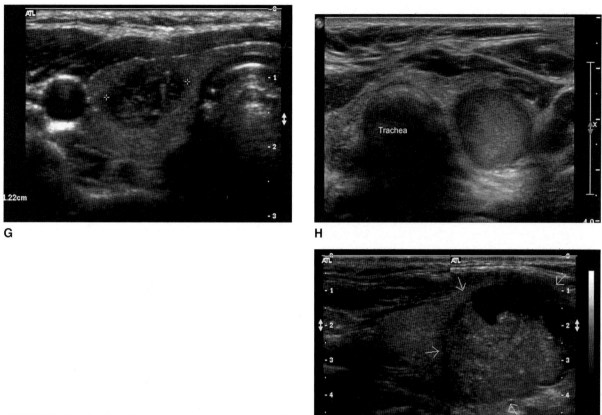

FIGURE 17-7 (*continued*) **G:** A transverse scan made through the right thyroid lobe shows a complex mass measuring 1.22 cm (*cursors*). **H:** A transverse image through the left thyroid lobe shows an oval mass. **I:** A longitudinal image through the left thyroid lobe shows a degenerating adenoma seen as an oval mass with internal cystic components (*arrows*).

Goiters

A nontoxic goiter is also termed simple, colloid, or multinodular and refers to an enlargement involving the entire gland without producing nodularity and without evidence of a functional disturbance.[6] The enlarged follicles are filled with colloid.[8] Nontoxic goiter occurs in both an endemic distribution with more than 10% of the population affected and a sporadic distribution.[8] Endemic goiter occurs in geographic areas where the soil, water, and food supply contain low levels of iodine. The decrease or lack of iodine leads to decreased synthesis of thyroid hormone and a compensatory increase in TSH. Increased TSH levels lead to follicular cell hypertrophy, hyperplasia, and goitrous enlargement.[8] *Sporadic goiter* is defined as a benign enlargement of the thyroid gland in euthyroid subjects living in an iodine-sufficient area. The sporadic goiter can be diffuse, uninodular, or multinodular.[26] The cause of sporadic goiter is usually not apparent and may be related to ingestion of substances or hereditary enzymatic defects that interfere with thyroid hormone synthesis.[8] The peak age of subjects with sporadic goiter is between 35 and 60 years and women are three times more likely than men to have the disease.[10]

Owing to recurrent episodes of hyperplasia and involution, simple goiters may convert into multinodular goiters. Nodularity of the thyroid gland can be the end stage of diffuse nontoxic goiter. As new follicles develop and outgrow their blood supply, hemorrhagic necrosis of all or part of the nodule results. Scarring then produces an inelastic network into which new follicles are squeezed, resulting in the formation of nodules.[14] Calcifications, fibrosis, degenerative cysts, and hemorrhage result in the heterogeneous sonographic appearance. Multinodular goiters may be multilobulated with an asymmetrically enlarged gland. The pattern and location of enlargement are unpredictable and may involve only one lobe or may expand growing behind the sternum and clavicles to produce the intrathoracic or plunging goiters.[8] Multinodular goiters may be nontoxic or may induce thyrotoxicosis (toxic multinodular goiters). As is the case of the simple goiter, the incidence of multinodular goiter is greater in females than in males.

The size of nontoxic goiters ranges from a doubling in size (40 g) to a massive enlargement in which the thyroid weighs a few hundred grams to more than 2,000 g.[6,8] Symptoms caused by large goiters are usually associated with compressing the esophagus (dysphasia), trachea (inspiratory stridor), neck veins (venous congestion), or laryngeal nerve (hoarseness).[6]

The sonographic appearance may be nonspecific and varies with pathogenesis of the goiter. The visualization of a dominant nodule, a tender spot, or a region of focal hardness may provide pathologic clues[25] (Fig. 17-8A, B). A second type of pathology may be suggested if one region in a goiter presents an echo pattern distinct from the rest of the goiter. It is important to note if there is a region within the goiter that displays sonographic features associated with increased risk

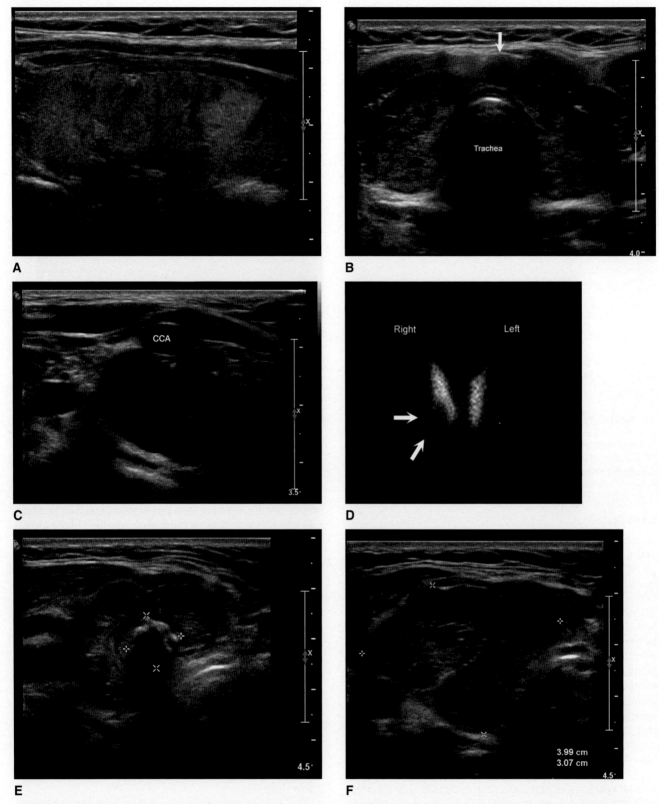

FIGURE 17-8 Goiters. **A:** This 79-year-old woman was referred to sonography following a computed tomography diagnosis of a multinodular goiter. The longitudinal image of the right thyroid lobe demonstrates diffuse enlargement and general heterogeneity. **B:** The transverse sonogram on this patient shows a diffusely enlarged, heterogeneous thyroid. There is an increased anteroposterior (*AP*) diameter of the isthmus when compared to the normal mean diameter measurement of 4 to 6 mm (*arrow*). An isthmus measuring greater than 1 cm is a reliable marker for diffuse thyroid enlargement. This patient was diagnosed with a multinodular goiter. **C, D:** A transverse sonogram (**C**) of the right lower thyroid pole in a 30-year-old woman shows a complex mass, which appears as a cold nodule on nuclear imaging. On the scintigram (**D**), one can see an irregular margin and diminished activity in the lower right pole (*arrow*). A biopsy cytology report identified a necrosing colloid nodule with associated cyst. **E, F:** These transverse images of the right thyroid lobe obtained on the same patient show diffuse heterogeneity mass with both internal cystic components and calcification. Although the presence of calcifications creates concern for a malignant process, this mass proved to be a benign adenomatoid multinodular goiter on biopsy. *CCA*, common carotid artery.

TABLE 17-2   Value of Sonographic Examination for Goitrous Patients[25]

- Differentiates thyroid gland enlargement from adipose tissue or muscle.
- Identifies large unilateral mass in distinction to an asymmetric goiter
- Confirms pattern and location of enlargement and extensions (substernal, intrathoracic, plunging)
- Provides the correct interpretation to correlate varying clinical impressions among several examiners
- Objectively documents volume changes in response to suppressive therapy with thyroid hormone
- Monitors patients undergoing long-term treatment with lithium for mental illnesses (bipolar, depression, schizophrenia)

for malignancy, which include hypoechogenicity, solidity, microcalcification, irregular margin, and a taller-than-wide shape[27] (Fig. 17-8C–F). Neoplasm and lymphomas have been demonstrated in goiters.[25] Table 17-2 lists additional usefulness of sonographic examinations in goitrous patients.

Thyrotoxicosis/Hyperthyroidism

Thyrotoxicosis is a hypermetabolic state caused by elevated levels of free T_3 and T_4.[28] The terms thyrotoxicosis and hyperthyroidism are often used interchangeably because the condition is caused most commonly by hyperfunction of the thyroid gland.[8] Hyperthyroidism is correct to use if elevated levels arise from hyperfunction, as occurs in Graves disease; thyrotoxicosis is correct to use if the increased hormone levels reflect excessive leakage of hormone out of a nonhyperactive gland.[8] Primary hyperthyroidism is a form of thyrotoxicosis in which excess thyroid hormone is synthesized and secreted by the thyroid glands.[8] Secondary hyperthyroidism is rare and is caused by TSH-secreting pituitary adenomas[28] (Pathology Box 17-1).

Pathogenesis of either thyrotoxicosis or hyperthyroidism produces common clinical manifestations (Pathology Box 17-2). Children with Graves disease often have accelerated growth spurts and advanced bone age, symptoms of emotional lability, hyperactivity, difficulty concentrating, and occasionally failure to thrive.

The underlying cause of hyperthyroidism in 50% to 80% of cases is Graves disease.[28] Graves disease is an autoimmune disease and about 75% of autoimmune diseases occur in women, most often during the childbearing years.[29] Graves

PATHOLOGY BOX 17-1
Causes of Primary and Secondary Hyperthyroidism[8,28]

Causes of Primary Hyperthyroidism

- Graves disease
- Toxic multinodular goiter
- Solitary hyperfunctioning nodules
- Follicular thyroid carcinoma (rare)
- Thyroiditis
- Ingestion of exogenous thyroid hormone administered for hypothyroidism

Causes of Secondary Hyperthyroidism

- Secretion of excessive amounts of thyroid hormone by ectopic thyroid arising in ovarian teratomas (struma ovarii)

PATHOLOGY BOX 17-2
Clinical Manifestations of Hyperthyroidism[6,8,28]

Cardiovascular system: increased cardiac output and decreased peripheral resistance; tachycardia at rest; loud heart sounds

Endocrine system: enlarged thyroid gland (goiter); hypercalcemia and decreased parathyroid hormone secretions

Gastrointestinal system: weight loss; increased peristalsis leading to diarrhea, nausea, vomiting, anorexia, abdominal pain

Integumentary system: excessive sweating, flushing, and warm skin; heat intolerance; temporary hair loss; palmar erythema

Musculoskeletal system: muscular weakness; children experience accelerated growth spurts and advanced bone age

Nervous system: nervousness; restlessness; short attention span; fatigue; fine hand tremor (particularly when outstretched); insomnia; increased appetite; emotional instability

Pulmonary system: dyspnea; reduced vital capacity

Reproductive system: oligomenorrhea or amenorrhea; erectile dysfunction and decreased libido

Sensory system (eyes): elevated upper eyelid (decreased blinking and staring feature); fine tremor of lid; variable eye changes

disease can occur at any age or gender but is most common in women of reproductive age.[30] Research indicates a multifactorial etiology where different factors come together to cause Graves disease, such as heredity, the body's immune system, age, gender, and possibly stress.[29]

Graves disease is characterized as a multisystem syndrome consisting of one or more of the following: (1) hyperthyroidism, (2) diffuse thyroid enlargement (goiter), (3) ophthalmopathy (protrusion of the globe owing to fat accumulation and inflammation with edema), and (4) Graves dermopathy (pretibial myxedema characterized by subcutaneous swelling on the anterior portions of the legs and by indurated and erythematous skin).[28]

Thyrotoxicosis has a variety of causes, and determining the cause is important because treatment and expected outcomes will vary accordingly, though it will normally focus on controlling excessive thyroid hormone production.[28] The diagnosis is based on symptoms of thyroid hormone excess and evaluating elevated serum-free T_4 and T_3 variances. TSH levels are increased in primary hyperthyroidism and decreased in secondary hyperthyroidism. Radioactive iodine uptake is a good diagnostic tool to determine the etiology of thyrotoxicosis.

Sonography for thyrotoxicosis and hyperthyroidism can assess the size of the thyroid gland to facilitate decisions regarding treatment.[25] Graves disease can present with either a normal-sized or an enlarged gland. When the gland is enlarged, the echo texture will usually be more heterogeneous compared to a diffuse goiter, which has numerous, large intraparenchymal vessels.[10] Normal-sized glands will have a more uniform pattern. Hypervascularity is observed in most patients with Graves disease and has been quantified by the number of vessels per square centimeter measured on the greatest longitudinal view.[31] The term "thyroid inferno" demonstrating multiple tiny areas of flow in the glandular tissue is often used to describe the hypervascular pattern

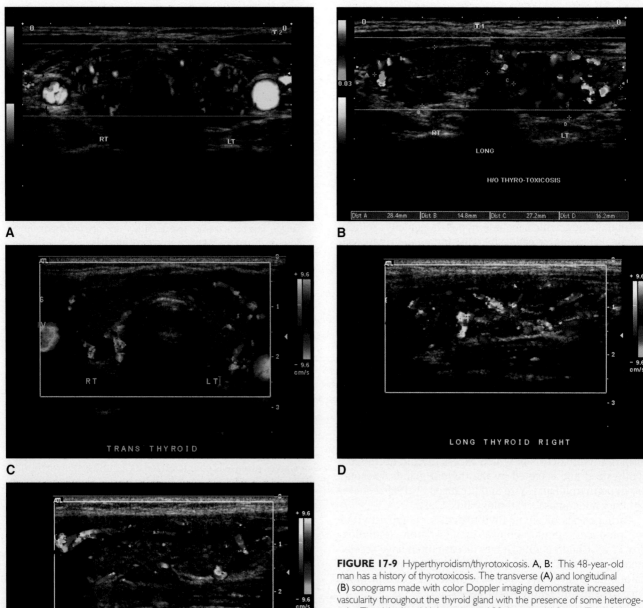

FIGURE 17-9 Hyperthyroidism/thyrotoxicosis. **A, B:** This 48-year-old man has a history of thyrotoxicosis. The transverse (**A**) and longitudinal (**B**) sonograms made with color Doppler imaging demonstrate increased vascularity throughout the thyroid gland with the presence of some heterogeneity. The right thyroid lobe measured 28.4 mm × 14.8 mm. The left thyroid lobe measured 27.2 mm × 16.2 mm. (Images complements of Thyroid. http://www.ultrasound-images.com/thyroid.htm/ http://www.ultrasound-images.com. Dr. Joe Anton, MD, India.) Graves disease. **C–E:** This 19-year-old woman presented with thyroid enlargement and a history of Graves disease. The transverse (**C**) and longitudinal sonograms of the right lobe (**D**) and left lobe (**E**) made with color Doppler imaging show markedly increased vascularity and a more heterogenic thyroid gland. (Images courtesy of LaNae Holman, Alamosa, Colorado.)

seen on color Doppler images (Fig. 17-9A–E). A bruit or thrill can often be heard over the gland. Spectral Doppler images may demonstrate peak velocities exceeding 70 cm/sec.[10]

Hypothyroidism

Hypothyroidism is the most commonly occurring thyroid function disorder and affects between 0.1% and 2% of individuals in the United States.[28] It is a clinical syndrome caused by a deficient production of thyroid hormone that results in reduced thyroid hormone action in the peripheral tissues. Hypothyroidism may be primary or secondary. There

is a greater incidence and increased number of causes of primary hypothyroidism arising from an intrinsic abnormality in the thyroid gland (Pathology Box 17-3). Secondary (central) hypothyroidism occurs less frequently than primary hypothyroidism and includes those conditions that cause either pituitary or hypothalamic disease or damage resulting in failure to stimulate normal thyroid function.[28] The conditions contributing to secondary hypothyroidism include pituitary adenoma; tumors impinging on the hypothalamus; irradiation; medication (dopamine, lithium); congenital disorders; and, rarely, Sheehan syndrome.

PATHOLOGY BOX 17-3
Causes of Primary Hypothyroidism[8,28]

Defective hormone synthesis

Autoimmune disease (Hashimoto thyroiditis most common); postpartum thyroiditis

Endemic iodine deficiency

Iodine excess

Iodinated contrast agents used in imaging; amiodarone medication; health tonics

Iatrogenic loss of thyroid tissue

Radioactive iodine treatment of Graves disease; external neck irradiation (head/neck neoplasm, breast cancer, Hodgkin disease); thyroidectomy

Inflammatory conditions, viral syndromes, or infiltrative disorders

Neoplasia; leukemia; sarcoidosis; hemochromatosis; amyloidosis; mycobacterium tuberculosis infection; *Pneumocystis carinii* infection; cystinosis

Congenital defect

Rare inborn errors of thyroid hormone synthesis

PATHOLOGY BOX 17-4
Clinical Manifestations of Hypothyroidism[6,8,28]

Cardiovascular system: reduction in stroke volume and heart rate results in lowered cardiac output; increased peripheral vascular resistance to maintain systolic blood pressure; cool skin and cold intolerance; enlarged heart; decreased intensity of heart sounds; electrocardiogram (EKG) changes

Endocrine system: increased thyroid-stimulating hormone (TSH) production in primary hypothyroidism; enlarged pituitary thyrotropes, increased serum prolactin levels with galactorrhea; decreased rate of cortisol turnover but with normal cortisol levels

Gastrointestinal system: constipation, weight gain, and fluid retention; decreased absorption of most nutrients; decreased protein metabolism; edema; decreased glucose absorption and delayed glucose uptake; elevated serum lipid values

Integumentary system: dry, flaky skin; dry, brittle head and body hair; reduced nail and hair growth; slow wound healing; myxedema; cold skin

Hematologic system: decrease in red cell mass leading to normocytic, normochromic anemia; macrocytic anemia associated with vitamin B_{12} deficiency and inadequate foliate or iron absorption in the gastrointestinal tract

Musculoskeletal system: muscle aching and stiffness; slow movement and slow tendon jerk reflexes; decreased bone formation and resorption, increased bone density; aching and stiffness in joints

Nervous system: confusion, syncope, slowed speech and thinking, memory loss; lethargy, headaches, hearing loss, night blindness; slow clumsy movements

Pulmonary system: dyspnea; myxedematous changes in respiratory muscles leading to hypoventilation and carbon dioxide retention contributes to myxedema coma

Reproductive system: in men, decreased androgen secretion; erectile dysfunction, decreased libido, and oligospermia; in women, increased estriol formation; low total hormone values but with increased amounts of unbound hormone; anovulation, decreased libido, and a high incidence of a spontaneous abortion

Urinary system: reduced renal blood flow and glomerular filtration rate; increased total body water and dilutional hyponatremia; reduced production of erythropoietin

The most common cause of primary hypothyroidism in areas of the world where iodine levels are sufficient is chronic autoimmune thyroiditis. The literature also refers to the disease as chronic lymphocytic thyroiditis, Hashimoto disease, and most commonly as in this chapter as Hashimoto thyroiditis. The name of the disease is derived from a 1912 report where Hashimoto described patients with goiters and intense lymphocytic infiltration of the thyroid gland.[8] It is estimated three-fourths of hypothyroidism cases are because of Hashimoto thyroiditis,[6] which occurs in genetically predisposed individuals and is associated with high iodine intake, selenium deficiency, smoking, and chronic hepatitis C.[28] This disorder is most prevalent between 45 and 65 years of age, has a female predominance of 10:1 to 20:1, and clusters in families with a concordance rate in monozygotic twins between 30% and 60%.[8] Patients with Hashimoto thyroiditis may also present with other autoimmune disorders such as Sjögren syndrome, lupus, rheumatoid arthritis, fibrosing mediastinitis, sclerosing cholangitis, and pernicious anemia and are at an increased risk for the development of B-cell lymphoma (non-Hodgkin).[13] The autoimmune disease can also occur in children to a much lesser extent and is a major cause of nonendemic goiter in children.

The clinical manifestations of hypothyroidism vary, depending on its cause, duration, and severity. The spectrum extends from subclinical hypothyroidism to overt hypothyroidism to myxedema coma.[28] Common signs and symptoms include weakness and fatigue, dry skin, cold intolerance, hoarseness, weight gain, constipation, menstrual irregularities, and decreased sweating (Pathology Box 17-4). The diagnosis is usually made serologically.

The sonographic appearance of Hashimoto thyroiditis changes with the duration of the disease. Over time, the normal homogeneous echo texture is replaced by a coarse and a more heterogeneous texture with multiple ill-defined hypoechoic areas separated by thickened fibrous strands.[13] The thyroid gland is usually diffusely abnormal and no normal parenchyma can be identified

(Fig. 17-10A–C). The best imaging clue is a moderately enlarged, lobular thyroid gland without calcifications or necrosis. An indication of diffuse enlargement of the thyroid gland is often best noted by determining if the isthmus measures greater than 1 cm anteroposteriorly. Often, color Doppler demonstrates hypervascularity in the early stages of Hashimoto thyroiditis (Fig. 17-10D, E). The sonographic characteristics of autoimmune diseases seen in Graves disease are also seen in Hashimoto thyroiditis and include enlargement of the thyroid gland with reduced echogenicity, heterogeneity, and hypervascularity. These sonographic features are more enhanced in Graves disease; however, the sonographic appearance without clinical history, serology reports, and, in some cases, FNA are nonspecific because the same sonographic appearance is also demonstrated in diffusely infiltrative papillary or follicular thyroid cancer.[32] Hashimoto thyroiditis can also

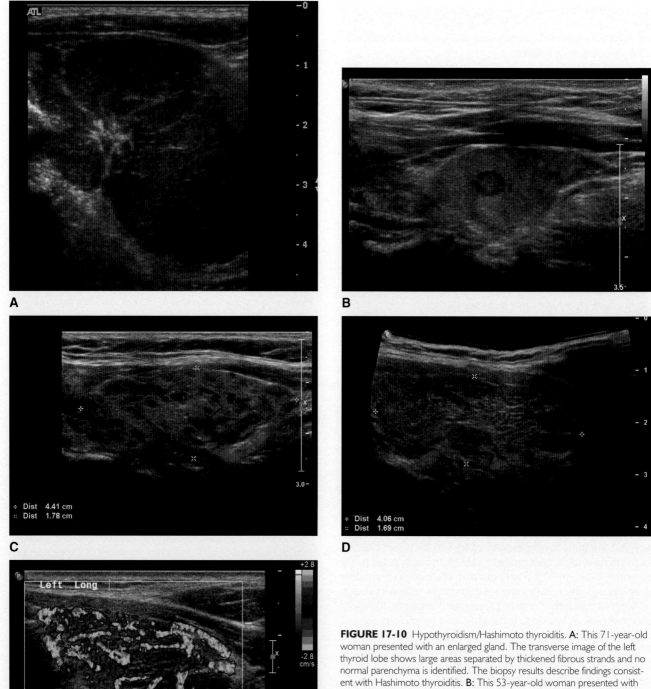

FIGURE 17-10 Hypothyroidism/Hashimoto thyroiditis. **A:** This 71-year-old woman presented with an enlarged gland. The transverse image of the left thyroid lobe shows large areas separated by thickened fibrous strands and no normal parenchyma is identified. The biopsy results describe findings consistent with Hashimoto thyroiditis. **B:** This 53-year-old woman presented with known Hashimoto thyroiditis. A patient presenting with single or multiple nodules makes the distinction between Hashimoto thyroiditis and multinodular goiter difficult to conclude from only the imaging characteristics. This representative longitudinal image of the right thyroid lobe shows an echogenic oval mass. The fine-needle aspiration results were in agreement with the patient's presenting diagnosis. **C:** This 45-year-old woman presented with a palpable thyroid nodule. The longitudinal image of the right thyroid lobe shows multiple small nodules, which give the appearance of a multinodular goiter. The fine-needle aspiration results diagnosed Hashimoto thyroiditis. **D, E:** The images of a left thyroid lobe were made without (**C**) and with (**D**) color Doppler imaging. On this patient with Hashimoto thyroiditis, the image demonstrates the hypervascularity seen in the early stages of the disease.

cause nodules, and other benign and malignant nodules can coexist with Hashimoto thyroiditis,[13] thus making it difficult to differentiate these conditions based on sonographic appearance alone. The presence of normal-appearing thyroid parenchyma amid the nodules favors a multinodular goiter, but information regarding the presence of the antithyroglobulin antibodies found in Hashimoto thyroiditis is necessary for a definitive diagnosis. In patients who do progress to end-stage Hashimoto thyroiditis, the thyroid gland becomes fibrotic, ill-defined, and heterogeneous, and it begins to atrophy.[13]

Thyroiditis

Thyroiditis encompasses a diverse group of disorders characterized by some form of thyroid gland inflammation. Generally, the clinical manifestations and symptoms for this group of disorders vary but most present with hypothyroidism or thyrotoxicosis followed by hypothyroidism (Pathology Box 17-5).

Subacute thyroiditis (de Quervain disease or granulomatous thyroiditis), along with Graves disease and Hashimoto thyroiditis, is one of the more common parenchymal diseases of the thyroid gland.[13] The disorder is most common between the ages of 30 and 50 and the female-to-male ratio is between 3:1 and 5:1.[8] Although it is a nonbacterial inflammation of the thyroid gland, it is often preceded by a viral infection because the majority of patients have a history of an upper respiratory infection just before the onset of subacute thyroiditis.[8,28] There have been reported clusters in association with coxsackievirus, mumps, measles, adenovirus, and other viral illnesses, and cases cluster seasonally peaking in the summer.[8]

The gland may be unilaterally or bilaterally enlarged and firm with an intact capsule, and it may be slightly adherent to surrounding structures.[8] The sudden or gradual onset of subacute thyroiditis is characterized by neck pain, which may radiate to the upper jaw, throat, or ears and which may be intensified when swallowing. Clinical suspicion occurs when the patient presents with fever, tenderness, fatigue, malaise, anorexia, and myalgia coexisting with inflammation of the thyroid gland.[8] The thyroid gland inflammation and hyperthyroidism are usually transient and resolve in 2 to 6 weeks, and spontaneous recovery of thyroid function usually occurs within 6 to 8 weeks.[8] Aside from some fibrosis, recovery is almost always complete.

The sonographic appearance of either acute or subacute thyroiditis is most often that of a diffusely enlarged, hypoechoic thyroid gland with normal or decreased vascularity owing to the presence of diffuse edema compressing the vessels.[13] The presence of hypoechoic and hyperechoic nodules is common, and that significantly reduces specificity of the sonographic image (Fig. 17-11).

Thyroid Disease in Pregnancy

Thyroid diseases are the second most common endocrinopathy and affect women of reproductive age and produce well-described complications in reproductive dysfunction, pregnancy, and the puerperium (the 42 days following

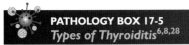

PATHOLOGY BOX 17-5
Types of Thyroiditis[6,8,28]

Acute thyroiditis (suppurative thyroiditis; infectious thyroiditis)

Rare inflammatory disease usually affecting children

Caused mainly by bacteria but may be caused by any infectious organism

Resolves after treating cause

Hashimoto thyroiditis

Autoimmune with antithyroid antibodies

Hypothyroidism is permanent

Iatrogenic hypothyroidism

Caused by radioiodine thyroid ablation (radiation induced), prescription drugs such as amiodarone, lithium, interferons, cytokines (drug-induced), or thyroidectomy

Depending on cause, hypothyroidism may be transient to permanent

Postpartum thyroiditis

Autoimmune with antithyroid antibodies

Occurs in up to 7% of all women

Spontaneous recovery in most women

Persistent hypothyroidism does occur

Subacute thyroiditis (de Quervain thyroiditis, granulomatous thyroiditis)

Possibly viral cause

Inflammation resolves usually in 2 to 8 weeks followed by spontaneous recovery of thyroid function usually in 6 to 8 weeks

Subacute thyroiditis (lymphocytic thyroiditis, painless thyroiditis, or silent thyroiditis)

Possibly inherited susceptibility

Incidence from 1% to 10% of all thyroiditis cases

Course similar to subacute thyroiditis but pathologically identical to Hashimoto thyroiditis

Thyrotoxicosis followed by hypothyroidism

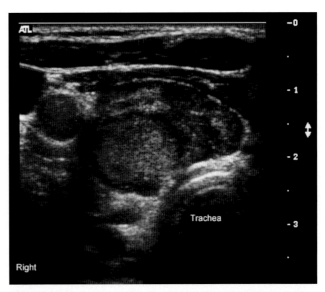

FIGURE 17-11 Acute thyroiditis. The 29-year-old woman presented with a short history of sore throat, difficulty swallowing, and tender thyroid. The laboratory data included markedly elevated thyroid-stimulating hormone and decreased free T$_4$. The transverse image of the right thyroid lobe shows a diffusely enlarged, complex echo pattern with an oval nodule. The diagnosis of acute thyroiditis was based on the patient's symptoms, clinical data, physical examination, and complex echo pattern seen on the sonographic images.

childbirth).[33] The array of thyroid diseases in pregnancy is similar to those in the nongravid population. During pregnancy, a number of physiologic adaptations and hormonal changes alter maternal, fetal, and neonatal thyroid function. Maternal physiologic changes early in pregnancy include an increase in thyroid-binding globulin (TBG), and as human chorionic gonadotropin (hCG) increases and levels peak, there is a partial inhibition of the pituitary gland that yields a transient decrease in TSH between weeks 8 and 14 of gestation.[33] Another physiologic adaptation affecting maternal thyroid function is a reduction in plasma iodine owing to fetal iodine usage and increased maternal renal clearance of iodine. The decreased plasma iodide level is associated with a noticeable increase in thyroid size in approximately 15% of women[33]; however, the increased size is not correlated with abnormal thyroid function tests. Sonographic measurement of thyroid gland in more than 600 women who did not have thyroid disease confirmed a mean increase in size of 18%, with the gland returning to normal size during the postpartum period.[33]

The most common maternal thyroid dysfunction that occurs after an abortion, miscarriage, or delivery is postpartum thyroiditis (PPT). It occurs in 7% to 10% of postpartum women, although this varies depending on iodine intake and genetic factors.[34] The classic description includes thyrotoxicosis followed by hypothyroidism, and treatment will depend on the phase of thyroiditis and degree of symptoms.

Sonographically, these cases will exhibit the nonspecific decrease in echogenicity and diffuse enlargement of the thyroid gland similar to those seen in other thyroid abnormalities. A definitive diagnosis is made with clinical data.

Thyroid Carcinoma

Thyroid nodules are very prevalent and are found by palpation in 4% to 7% of an asymptomatic population, with sonography in 13% to 67% of cases, and at autopsy in 50% of cases.[24] Most thyroid nodules are benign, and approximately 5% to 15% are malignant.[35] Of these, papillary carcinoma accounts for the vast majority of thyroid cancers followed in frequency by follicular, medullary, anaplastic, and Hürthle (subtype of follicular) cell cancer[13] (Table 17-3). Clinical criteria suggestive of a malignant neoplastic thyroid nodule include solitary nodules versus multiple nodules, nodules in younger patients versus older patients, and nodules in males versus in females. The incidence of thyroid malignancy increases in patients with a history of radiation exposure or radiation treatment to the head or neck. Although these general trends may favor a malignant diagnosis, they are of little significance without the morphologic evaluation of an FNA biopsy and histologic study of surgically resected thyroid parenchyma.[8] There is no simple noninvasive imaging criterion to diagnose a minority of patients who will prove to have malignant thyroid nodules while reassuring the majority of patients who have benign disease.[36] There are certain sonographic characteristics associated with either an increased risk or with a low risk of thyroid cancer (Table 17-4). The sonographer should be able to identify these sonographic characteristics and must realize they are of limited significance when evaluated independently; however, it is possible to make an accurate prediction when multiple signs of thyroid malignancy appear in combination.[24,32,37,38]

TABLE 17-3 Relative Frequencies of Thyroid Malignant Masses[6,8,47,49]

Type	% of Cases
Papillary carcinoma	75–85
Follicular carcinoma	10–20
Medullary carcinoma	5
Anaplastic carcinoma	<5
Hürthle cell carcinoma (subtype of follicular carcinoma)	3 to <10
Lymphoma	<5

TABLE 17-4 Sonographic Characteristics[13,25,33,36–45]

Associated with Increased Thyroid Cancer Risk	Associated with Low Thyroid Cancer Risk
• Hypoechogenicity • Entirely solid • Microcalcifications • Intrinsic hypervascularity (central part) • Incomplete or absent halo • Ill-defined margin • Shape: tall > wide • Local invasion and lymphadenopathy • Elasticity indication of increased tissue stiffness compared with normal tissue	• Hyperechoic or isoechoic • Cystic elements • Large, coarse calcifications (except medullary thyroid cancer) • Eggshell calcifications (few exceptions) • Perinodular hypervascularity (peripheral, circumference) or avascular nodule • Inspissated colloid; comet tail shadowing

Malignant nodules typically appear solid and hypoechoic compared with normal thyroid parenchyma. This finding is not particularly useful in and of itself because the majority of nodules are benign and a hypoechoic appearance is also noted in approximately 55% of benign nodules.[32] Marked hyperechoic nodules are probably benign,[25] whereas marked hypoechogenic nodules are suggestive of malignancy.[32]

The presence of calcifications within a nodule may occur in both benign and malignant disease and can be classified as microcalcifications (<2 mm) or macrocalcification (>2 mm).[38,39] Microcalcifications present sonographically as punctate hyperechoic foci without acoustic shadowing and may present a twinkling pattern. The presence of microcalcifications is one of the most specific features of thyroid malignancy and may represent calcium salts in the psammoma bodies associated with primary tumors and cervical lymph node metastases.[10] Microcalcifications are commonly found in papillary thyroid cancer (PTC) but have been described in follicular and anaplastic thyroid carcinomas as well as in benign conditions such as follicular adenoma and Hashimoto thryoidits.[32] Kim et al.[39] classified these three sonographic patterns of macrocalcifications: (1) solitary calcifications that are either linear or round hyperechoic structures greater than 2 mm sonographically presenting with or without acoustic shadowing located in the middle of the nodule or along the margin of the nodule encompassing less than 120 degrees of the circumference; (2) eggshell calcifications that are curvilinear hyperechoic structures parallel to the margin of the nodule encompassing 120 degrees or more of the circumference; and (3) all other coarse but not otherwise specified calcifications. The presence of solitary macrocalcifications and peripheral or eggshell calcifications of the thyroid nodule has been an indicator of benignity especially in the absence of other suspicious sonographic findings.[40] The clinical suspicion for malignancy increases in the presence of at least one or more of the other sonographic characteristics associated with an increased thyroid cancer risk, such as marked hypoechogenicity, irregular or microlobulated margins, and taller-than-wide shape.[39,40] Macrocalcifications are the most common type of calcifications found in medullary thyroid cancer and may coexist with microcalcifications in papillary cancers. In a person 40 years or younger, calcifications in a solitary nodule are suspicious of malignancy because the relative cancer risk is greater than in a person over 40 years of age.[25]

Color or power Doppler sonography should be used to evaluate vascular flow within a thyroid nodule. Intrinsic hypervascularity is defined as flow in the central part of the tumor that is greater than in the surrounding thyroid parenchyma and perinodular flow is defined as the presence of vascularity around at least 25% of the circumference or periphery of a nodule. Marked intrinsic hypervascularity with disorganized vascularity mostly in well-encapsulated forms is seen in 69% to 74% of PTC cases.[32] The intrinsic hypervascularity in and of itself is not specific and can also be seen in more than 50% of benign, solid thyroid nodule lesions.[41] Perinodular, circumferential, or peripheral flow is more characteristic of benign thyroid lesions but has also been found in 22% of thyroid malignancies.[32,37] A completely avascular nodule is likely benign.[37]

The halo or hypoechoic rim seen in some thyroid nodules is produced by a pseudocapsule of fibrous connective tissue, a compressed thyroid parenchyma, and chronic inflammatory infiltrates.[32] Although a complete uniform halo around a nodule is highly suggestive of benignity, an absent halo is not significantly associated with either the presence or absence of thyroid cancer because it is not identified sonographically in more than half of all benign thyroid nodules.[38] Approximately 10% to 24% of papillary thyroid carcinomas have either a complete or an incomplete halo.[32,37]

The well-defined margin is typical of benign thyroid nodules but there is an overlap with malignant nodules.[13] An ill-defined thyroid nodule margin is one in which more than 50% of the margin is not clearly demarcated. Sonographically, some papillary thyroid carcinomas have a misleadingly well-demarcated margin but are encapsulated at histologic review.[32] The sonographic appearance of minimally invasive follicular carcinoma may have some features in common with that of follicular adenoma. Without sonographically demonstrating invasion beyond the capsule, the appearance of either a well-defined or poorly defined margin without other criteria is an unreliable basis for determining malignancy or benignity.[32,38,39]

Sonographically evaluating the thyroid nodule to determine if it is taller than wide in shape (greater AP dimension than transverse dimension) may be potentially useful. The taller-than-wide shape is thought to be because of a centrifugal tendency in tumor growth, which does not necessarily occur at a uniform rate in all dimensions.[32] Kim et al.[39] reported a triple criteria for malignant sonographic features that included (1) solid thyroid nodules with the taller-than-wide shape, (2) marked hypoechogenicity (decreased echogenicity compared with the surrounding strap muscle), and (3) irregular or microlobulated margins.

Highly specific signs of thyroid malignancy include tumor invasion or lymph node metastasis. Direct tumor invasion sonographically can be identified with subtle extension of the tumor beyond the thyroid gland contours or with frank invasion of adjacent structures. Suspicion of lymph node metastases should be elevated with the sonographic appearance of a rounded bulging shape, increased size, replaced fatty hilum, irregular margins, heterogeneous texture, calcifications, cystic areas, and vascularity throughout the lymph node instead of normal central hilar vessels with Doppler instrumentation.[32] The clinical manifestations of compression and invasion include cough, dyspnea with invasion of the trachea, hoarseness with invasion of the larynx, and dysphagia with invasion of the laryngeal nerve or the esophagus.[8] The pathogenesis of anaplastic thyroid carcinoma, lymphoma, and sarcoma is aggressive local invasion.[32]

Elasticity describes a mechanical tissue characteristic that prevents displacement of stiffer tissue when placed under pressure such as with compression from an ultrasound probe.[42,43] Elastography is an imaging method used to evaluate the stiffness of soft tissues and to display new information about the internal structure of tissue.[44] With further clinical correlations, elastography may become a significant diagnostic technique to help differentiate the malignant nodule, which tends to be harder (stiffer) than normal tissue or the benign nodule. The three primary types of elasticity imaging are (1) strain imaging, (2) color elasticity, and (3) shear wave imaging. Strain imaging uses a software program with conventional sonography equipment and ultrasound probe to first receive the echo from the tissue; second, lightly compress the tissue with the ultrasound probe along the insonation axis to cause some displacement; and third, receive a second, postcompression digitized echo from the same tissue.[43] Color elasticity continues to use the push and tract displacement technique of strain image but adds a chromatic scale assigned to different levels of elasticity.[44] Shear wave elastography is based on the automatic generation and analysis of transient shear waves that are quantitative and reproducible based on the stiffness of a thyroid nodule, which sets it apart from other elasticity imaging modes[42] (Fig. 17-12). The preliminary correlation studies between the histologic pattern of thyroid nodules and shear wave elastography and the ability to quantitatively measure soft tissue stiffness are important steps in differentiating pathology. Zhang et al.[42] completed a meta-analysis with a total of 568 benign and 130 malignant nodules for a total 698 thyroid nodules in 469 patients. The conclusions of the study indicated that shear wave elastography has high sensitivity and specificity and can potentially reduce FNA.[42] As equipment technology continues to advance, comparing the sensitivity, specificity, positive predictive value, and negative predictive value for shear wave elastography, conventional sonography, and FNA biopsy may decrease the number of FNA biopsies performed.

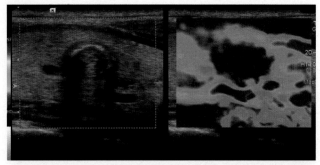

A

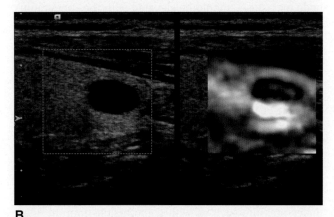

B

FIGURE 17-12 Elasticity Imaging. Comparing the mechanical tissue characteristics preventing displacement of (**A**) stiffer tissue in a solid thyroid mass with (**B**) a thyroid cyst. (Courtesy of Siemens Medical Solutions USA, Inc.)

However, one has to take into consideration that shear wave elastography can be affected by the trachea, carotid artery, and other surrounding structures.[42]

Papillary Carcinoma

Papillary carcinoma is the most common malignant tumor of the thyroid gland, accounting for 75% to 85% of all thyroid cancers. It develops in patients of any age and it occurs most frequently between 20 and 50 years of age. The female-to-male ratio is 3:1 in adults.[6] Most papillary carcinomas present as (1) a painless, palpable nodule in an otherwise normal gland; (2) a nodule with enlarged cervical lymph nodes; or (3) cervical lymphadenopathy in the absence of a palpable thyroid nodule. Like most benign nodules, a papillary carcinoma tends to move freely during swallowing.[8] More advanced disease is suspected if a patient presents with hoarseness, dysphagia, cough, or dyspnea.

There are a number of variant forms of papillary thyroid carcinomas. The most common variant is the pure papillary carcinoma, which accounts for about 55% to 66% of all well-differentiated thyroid carcinomas.[45] The second most common is the follicular variant of papillary thyroid carcinoma, which accounts for about 9% to 22.5% of all papillary thyroid carcinomas.[45] The encapsulated variant occurs in about 10% of all papillary thyroid carcinomas. The tall cell variant tends to occur in older individuals, has the poorest prognosis, and may be misdiagnosed as Hürthle cell tumors.[8]

A variety of diagnostic tests have been employed to separate benign form malignant thyroid nodules. The FNA biopsy cytology test has a higher diagnostic accuracy than the radionuclide scanning, sonography, or elastography. Treatment varies and may consist of a partial lobectomy, radical neck dissection, or both, followed by suppressive therapy.

Generally, papillary carcinoma is considered the least aggressive of the thyroid tumors. The prognosis is excellent and there is little difference in life expectancy from that of the general population for patients less than 50 years of age. The overall survival rate is 98%.[8] In children, the outlook of recovery is good even in cases with lung metastases.[6] The prognosis is more serious in patients older than 50 years of age and papillary carcinoma is more aggressive in men than in women.[6] The prognosis is also poorer in cases where the primary neoplasm is larger, more aggressive, and has a direct extension into the adjacent soft tissues.[6] The proportion of papillary and follicular elements contributes little to the prognosis, but less differentiated papillary carcinomas tend to be more aggressive. The presence of metastases to cervical nodes at the time of surgery does not change the prognosis, and less than 10% of these patients succumb to the tumor. In fatal cases of papillary carcinoma, death is caused principally by metastases to the lungs or brain or by obstruction of the trachea or esophagus.[6]

Sonographic appearance may include one or more of the following: hypoechogenicity (in 90% of the cases) owing to closely packed cell contents and minimal colloid substances; microcalcifications owing to deposition of calcium salts in psammoma bodies, which appear as tiny, punctate hyperechoic foci, hypervascularity with disorganized vessels, and if there is metastasis to the lymph nodes, tiny punctate calcifications may appear in the affected lymph nodes[10] (Fig. 17-13A–F).

Follicular Carcinoma

The second most common thyroid cancer is follicular carcinoma, and it accounts for 10% to 20% of diagnosed cases.[8] The female-to-male ratio is 3:1 and most cases affect individuals in the fourth and fifth decades of life.[6,8] There is an increased incidence in geographic areas of endemic goiter where there is a dietary iodine deficiency,[6] whereas papillary carcinomas are more common in areas of sufficient or excess iodine intake. The pathology comes to clinical attention as a slow-growing, enlarging, painless nodule.

Follicular thyroid carcinomas are subdivided into minimally invasive and widely invasive variants, which differ in histology and clinical course.[10] An accurate diagnosis can only be made histologically.[24] The minimally invasive follicular carcinoma is a well-defined, encapsulated tumor. It usually is diagnosed when the tumor extends into but not entirely through the capsule.[6] The widely invasive follicular carcinomas are not well encapsulated and invasion of the vessels and the adjacent thyroid is more easily demonstrated.[10] Unlike papillary carcinoma that has a propensity for invading lymphatics, both types of follicular carcinoma differ in that metastasis spreads hematogenously, especially to the bone, lungs, liver, and elsewhere.[1] Metastases to the neck nodes are distinctly rare with follicular cancer.[13] Distant metastases are present in 5% to 20% of the minimally invasive variant and in 20% to 40% of the widely invasive variant.[13] The prognosis depends on the size of the primary and the presence or absence of capsular and vascular invasion and, to a lesser extent, on the level of anaplasia in the lesion.[8] Minimally invasive follicular tumors have a cure rate of at

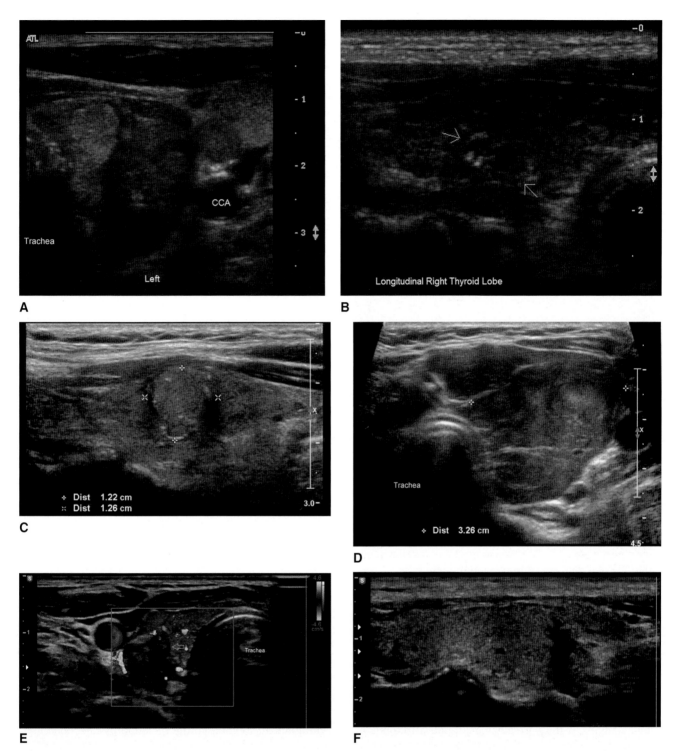

FIGURE 17-13 Papillary carcinoma in different patients diagnosed by fine-needle aspiration cytology. Note the variation in appearance, size, and texture. **A:** A transverse image through the left thyroid lobe demonstrates a hypoechoic slightly lobulated lesion with tiny hyperechoic punctate calcifications. **B:** A longitudinal image of the right thyroid lobe shows a heterogeneous but isoechoic mass (*arrows*) containing microcalcifications. **C:** A longitudinal image of the left thyroid lobe shows a hypoechoic, homogeneous oval mass with microcalcifications and an irregular thick halo. **D:** A transverse image of the left lobe demonstrates an elongated hypoechoic and heterogeneous mass. Images **E** and **F** are sonograms from the same patient. **E:** The transverse image shows a complex mass in the right lobe. **F:** A jagged edge hypoechoic mass is seen in the transverse image. The post-op report confirmed papillary carcinoma with one lesion in the right lobe measuring 0.7 mm and two lesions in the left lobe measuring 0.2 mm and 0.1 mm with extension in the lymph nodes. *CCA,* common carotid artery. (Courtesy of Susan Raatz Stephenson, Salt Lake City, UT.)

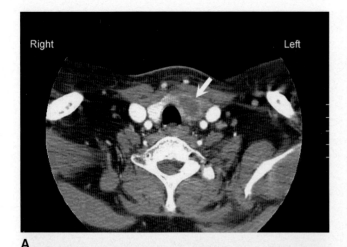

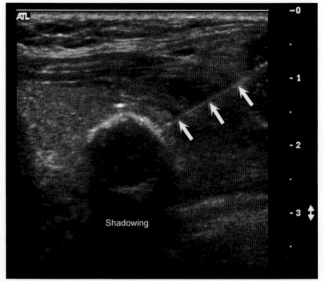

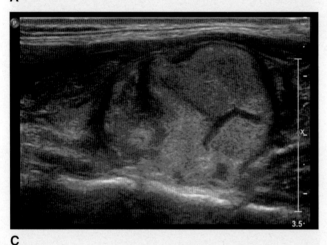

FIGURE 17-14 Follicular carcinoma. **A:** The computed tomography (*CT*) with contrast image demonstrates the sectional neck anatomy and a heterogeneous area beginning in the isthmus and extending throughout the left thyroid lobe *arrow*. **B:** On the same patient with the CT exam, the transverse sonogram of the left thyroid mass shows diagonal white line *arrows* entering the image from the right, which is the biopsy needle used during a sonography-guided fine-needle aspiration biopsy. The tissue was described as having a smooth calcified rim with difficult gritty penetration. The cytology report diagnosed follicular carcinoma. **C:** The 42-year-old woman in this case presented with a lump in the neck. The longitudinal image of the left thyroid lobe shows a hypoechoic lobular, irregular mass demonstrating some vasculature seen as anechoic vessels. The fine-needle aspiration cytology report diagnosed follicular carcinoma.

least 95% compared with a survival of about 50% for the widely invasive form.[6] The 20-year mortality for all patients with follicular cancer is approximately 25%.[13]

Follicular carcinomas are treated with lobectomy or subtotal thyroidectomy. Widely invasive tumors are treated with total thyroidectomy, which is usually followed by the administration of radioactive iodine.[8]

The sonographic features of follicular carcinoma overlap the appearance of follicular adenomas, which is explained with the cytologic and histologic similarities in the two entities.[10] The two lesions cannot be distinguished on sonography or with FNA.[13] Sonographic features that suggest follicular carcinoma are rarely seen but include irregular tumor margins, a thick irregular halo, and a tortuous or chaotic arrangement of internal blood vessels on color Doppler images[10] (Fig. 17-14A–C).

Medullary Carcinoma

Medullary thyroid carcinoma accounts for no more than 5% of all thyroid carcinoma.[6] It is a neuroendocrine neoplasm derived from the thyroid gland's parafollicular cells, which are similar to normal cells but secrete calcitonin (C cells).[8] Serum calcitonin can be used as a tumor marker.[13] The disease occurs in sporadic forms with approximately 80% of cases and in familial forms in approximately 20% of cases.[6] The mean age is 50 years for sporadic cases and 20 years for familial cases.[8] The female-to-male ratio in sporadic cases

is 1.5:1 with a slight female predominance, but in familial cases, the inheritance is autosomal dominant with an almost equal sex distribution.[6] Sporadic cases of medullary carcinoma come to medical attention most often as a mass in the neck, sometimes associated with local effects such as dysphagia or hoarseness. Patients often suffer a number of symptoms related to endocrine secretion, which includes carcinoid syndrome (serotonin) and Cushing syndrome with one-third of the patients having watery diarrhea owing to vasoactive intestinal secretions.[6,8] Patients with the familial form of medullary carcinoma are often afflicted with multiple endocrine neoplasia (MEN) type 2, which includes hyperparathyroidism, episodic hypertension, and other symptoms attributable to the secretion of catecholamines by pheochromocytoma.[8] Sporadic medullary carcinomas and those arising in patients with MEN type 2 are aggressive lesions with a propensity to metastasize hematogenously and have a 5-year survival rate of 50%.[8] They has a more aggressive behavior than the differentiated carcinomas and do not respond to either chemotherapy or radiation therapy.[13] In contrast, familial medullary carcinomas not associated with MEN are often fairly indolent lesions.[8]

The sonographic appearance of medullary carcinoma is usually similar to papillary carcinoma although local invasion and metastasis to cervical nodes occur more often in patients with medullary carcinoma.[13] The features include a hypoechoic solid mass, and microcalcifications are common.[10,13] Often, coarse calcifications are seen in the primary tumor, the lymph nodal metastases, and even in hepatic metastases.[10]

Anaplastic Carcinoma

Anaplastic thyroid carcinomas are undifferentiated tumors of the thyroid follicular epithelium.[8] This thyroid cancer accounts for less than 5% of thyroid malignancies. The female-to-male ratio is 4:1 and it occurs typically in people over 60 years with a mean age of 65 years.[6] The incidence is greater in endemic goiter areas. Of the patients diagnosed with anaplastic carcinoma, over 50% have a long-standing history of multinodular goiter; approximately 20% have a history of differentiated carcinoma; and another 20% to 30% have a concurrent differentiated thyroid tumor, which is frequently a papillary carcinoma.[6,8] The findings lead some to speculate that anaplastic carcinoma develops from more differentiated tumors as a result of one or more genetic changes.[8]

In striking contrast to the differentiated thyroid carcinomas, anaplastic carcinomas are aggressive tumors, with widespread metastases, and a dismal prognosis with less than 10% of patients surviving for 5 years.[6,8,13] The clinical course for these highly malignant tumors is a rapidly enlarging bulky neck mass that compresses and destroys local structures. Compression and invasion symptoms such as dyspnea, dysphagia, hoarseness, and cough are common.[6,8] In many cases, the disease has already spread beyond the thyroid capsule into adjacent neck structures or has already metastasized to the lungs when the patient presents for the initial examination. There is no effective therapy for anaplastic carcinoma and death results from the aggressive growth and the compromise to vital structures in the neck.[8]

Sonography may not be able to adequately examine the large size of the tumor or extent of tumor invasion and involvement. Computed tomography (CT) and magnetic resonance imaging (MRI) are better imaging modalities to accurately demonstrate the extent of the disease. Sonographically, anaplastic carcinoma usually appears as a large, solid, hypoechoic mass with demonstration of encasing or invading blood vessels and, if present, invasion of the neck muscles.[10,13]

Hürthle Cell Carcinoma

Hürthle cell cancer is frequently grouped with follicular thyroid cancers because they have some similarities. Microscopically, Hürthle cells do look different than follicular cells. The cells are also called oxyphilic cells and the cancer is referred to as oxyphil cell cancer. Hürthle cells are large thyroglobulin-producing epithelial cells and are found in both nonneoplastic and neoplastic thyroid lesions.[46] The Hürthle cell neoplasm is classified as either a benign Hürthle cell adenoma or a malignant Hürthle cell carcinoma, both of which consist of at least 75% Hürthle cells and a paucity of colloid cells.[46,47] The diagnosis of Hürthle cell carcinoma, as with follicular carcinoma, requires histologic identification of capsular or vascular invasion, or nodal and/or distant metastasis.[47] Hürthle cell carcinomas account for approximately 3% but less than 10% of differentiated thyroid malignancies. Although they are uncommon and there is some controversy regarding Hürthle cell carcinoma clinical behavior, they are more aggressive than either papillary or follicular cell carcinoma, which makes their timely diagnosis important for cancer prognosis and therapy.[46] Most studies show that advanced age, male gender, large primary tumor size, degree of invasion, and recurrence are poor prognostic indicators.[47] A total thyroidectomy is usually the treatment of choice with different follow-up therapy.

Sonography is an important tool in evaluation of the thyroid gland; however, there is a limited number of current publications regarding the appearance of either benign or malignant Hürthle cell neoplasms and are clinical descriptions of a single entity.[46] In retrospective studies, researchers concluded there is a wide spectrum of sonographic appearances.[46,47] At this time, sonography can define the size and shape of the tumor, but an accurate diagnosis is only possible with pathologic evaluation of resected tumors.

Lymphoma

Lymphoma originating in the thyroid gland is distinctly uncommon, accounting for less than 5% of all thyroid malignancies. It can occur either as a manifestation of generalized lymphoma or as a primary abnormality, and it is usually a non-Hodgkin variety.[13] Most cases arise in the clinical setting of chronic thyroiditis (Hashimoto thyroiditis) with subclinical or overt hypothyroidism and are highest in regions where this disorder is frequent. Like chronic thyroiditis, it is more common in women with a female-to-male ratio of 4:1.[6] The mean age at presentation is the seventh decade of life. The clinical presentation usually includes a rapidly growing mass and symptoms of airway obstruction with a history of long-standing thyroiditis. The treatments of choice are usually radiation therapy and chemotherapy. Surgery is often performed to diagnose the primary thyroid lymphoma. Research on the accuracy of FNA biopsy for diagnosis for subclassification of lymphoma is ongoing.[48] The 5-year survival rate ranges from nearly 90% in early-stage cases to less than 5% in advanced, disseminated disease.[10]

Sonographically, lymphoma usually appears as a large, solid, hypoechoic mass that compresses adjacent thyroid parenchyma or infiltrates the thyroid parenchyma.[13] The mass may appear lobulated and have large areas of cystic necrosis as well as encasement of adjacent neck vessels.[10] Color Doppler evaluation most likely will demonstrate a predominantly hypovascular or a chaotic blood vessel distribution and arteriovenous shunts. If the patient has chronic lymphocytic thyroiditis, the adjacent thyroid parenchyma may be heterogeneous.[10]

Metastases

Metastases to the thyroid gland are infrequent and occur late in the course of neoplastic disease; they spread most commonly by hematogenous route and less frequently by lymphatic routes.[10] When it does occur, metastases are from melanoma, breast, lung, and renal cell carcinoma. None of these lesions has a characteristic sonographic appearance; however, metastatic disease should be considered when a solid thyroid nodule is identified in a patient with a known extrathyroidal malignancy[13] (Fig. 17-15).

Fine-Needle Aspiration

Although there has been great progress and promise with shear wave elastography, conventional imaging examinations cannot definitively distinguish between benign and malignant thyroid nodules and adenopathy. FNA biopsy is the primary evaluation method of a palpable thyroid nodule.[1]

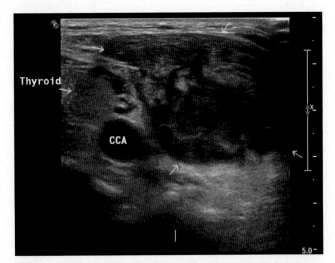

FIGURE 17-15 Metastases. The 56-year-old man is undergoing radiation treatment for throat cancer. A transverse image through the left neck adjacent to the thyroid demonstrates a mixed echoic pattern in a large mass (*arrows*) compressing thyroid gland tissue (*arrow*). The report from the fine-needle aspiration diagnosed metastatic squamous cell carcinoma. *CCA*, common carotid artery.

The actual diagnosis of thyroid cancer is made from the cytologic evaluation of the thyroid follicular epithelial cells and minute tissue fragments obtained either from an FNA biopsy or a surgical resection.

Indications and Guidelines

FNA biopsy of thyroid nodules and adenopathy is a diagnostic tool used for differentiation and patient management. FNA is essential for decision-making and is capable of providing highly accurate information by confirming benignity or suspected malignancies before the commencement of nonsurgical treatments, such as chemotherapy or radiation therapy, or by determining the nature of an indeterminate nodule.[10,24] Sonography-assisted FNA biopsy is a minimally invasive and safe procedure that can be performed on an outpatient basis.[49] Both the Society of Radiologists in Ultrasound (SRU) and the American Thyroid Association (ATA) as well as the American college of Radiology (ACR) provide useful guidelines for the management of thyroid nodules.[50,51] The physicians writing the ATA and SRU guidelines include endocrinologists and endocrine surgeons and those writing the SRU guidelines also include radiologists. Their recommendation is to strongly consider FNA when the nodule has microcalcifications 1 cm or more in size, when the nodule is solid or almost entirely solid, when the nodule has coarse calcifications, and when the nodule is 1.5 cm or greater in size. The guidelines developed by the ACR is called Thyroid Imaging and Reporting Data System (TI-RADS).[50] This system assigns point values to the *composition, echogenicity, shape, margin,* and *echogenic foci* and makes recommendations of FNA or follow-up according to the awarded scores. The points associated with these features are then added and lead to a categorization of risk ranging from benign to highly suspicious. The possible outcomes using this lexicon are TR1—benign, TR2—not suspicious, TR3—mildly suspicious, TR4—moderately suspicious, and TR5—highly suspicious. Recommendations for FNA are made according to their TI-RADS score and depending on the size of the nodules imaged. FNA is recommended in those measuring

greater than 1 cm in the three higher-risk categories and in the lower-risk categories only if the nodule measures over 2.5 cm.[50] Referencing these guidelines provides a good decision-making tool for referring physicians and sonologists to determine which patients should be recommended the FNA biopsy procedure. The benefit for the majority of patients is the assurance of benign disease and for the minority of patients is the diagnosis of malignant disease. Side effects from the FNA biopsy procedure are uncommon but may include bleeding, which is especially true in patients using anticoagulants, antiplatelet agents, or those who have a bleeding diathesis.[25] The effect of bleeding can be diminished in some patients if their condition allows discontinuing anticoagulant medication or antiplatelet agents prior to the procedure. Other effects may include hoarseness, infections, and the remote consideration of seeding the needle track with thyroid cancer.[25] In cases where FNA biopsy is to be performed on bilateral masses, the precautionary measure is to schedule separate appointments. Although rare, the development of a post-procedure hematoma could compress the trachea, which, if present bilaterally, could have catastrophic consequences for the patient.

Protocol

The outpatient procedure is performed in a sonography room using standard sterile technique. When the patient first enters the room, applying ice to the patient's neck helps anesthetize the skin as well as reduce blood flow to the area. The patient should be placed in the same position used for a standard thyroid gland examination with the patient in a supine position and the shoulders and upper back should be elevated with a pillow or rolled towel, hyperextending the neck.[17] This will permit easier access to the thyroid gland. Cautious approach is required with elderly patients and other patients in whom this position may cause dizziness or neck strain and the neck should not be overextended in any patient. If this position is not tolerable, the examiner should request the patient to elevate the chin up and back as far as possible and, if needed, turn the patient's head away from the side being examined in order to gain surface area for accessing the requested FNA site. The examiner should review any previous sonography examinations and reexamine the area to be biopsied. Prior to prepping the patient's neck, the best approach should be demonstrated and discussed with the provider performing the procedure. A 25-gauge needle is usually used, and because it is small, it can be sonographically visualized best when parallel to the transducer face (perpendicular to the beam). The advantage of performing a sonographically guided FNA biopsy is the real-time visualization of the needle because it enters the mass better and enables the provider to accurately select the intended site. Once in the mass, the provider will pull back slightly on the syringe, creating mild suction while collecting tissue by moving the needle within the area of interest. Some providers prefer to use the natural capillary action of the needle alone for this process. The sampled cells are transferred to laboratory slides and submitted for analysis (Fig. 17-16). The sonographic protocol also provides the provider with guidance for percutaneous treatment of neck pathology such as alcohol ablation of parathyroid adenomas or ethanol injection of benign cystic thyroid lesions.

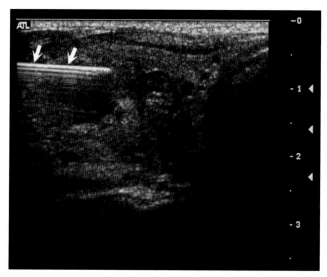

FIGURE 17-16 Fine-needle aspiration (*FNA*) biopsy. The aspiration needle (*arrows*) can be identified during FNA of a complex right thyroid nodule. Note the reverberation artifact from the needle. This needle is positioned perpendicular to the sound beam, which is parallel to the transducer, allowing for better visualization and guidance during the procedure.

Limitations

According to the American Cancer Society, the repeat rate is 2 in every 10 biopsies, a benign diagnosis is made in 7 of 10 biopsies, and a cancer diagnosis is made in 1 of every 20 biopsies.[52] The high repeat rate is because of aspiration of fluid from a cystic lesions, and it has a higher association with a FNA biopsy procedure performed by palpation versus sonography guidance.[10] Factors that will help decrease the rate of the sample inadequacy include an experienced sonographer for lesion targeting and localization, the level of experience of the individual performing the biopsy and obtaining the aspirate, and immediate on-site cytologic examination.[49] With an ample aspirate, cytologic examination is more effective for diagnosing papillary, medullary, and anaplastic carcinoma[53] but lacks specificity in diagnosing follicular carcinoma, Hürthle cell carcinoma, and lymphomas. These cases and other suspicious biopsy aspirates require surgical excision.

PARATHYROID GLANDS

Embryology

The embryonic development of the parathyroid glands is a complex process of cell differentiation and migration of the glands from the sites of origin in the pharynx and pharyngeal pouches to the usual anatomic location near the thyroid gland. The pharyngeal pouches (or branchial pouches) form on the endodermal side between the arches. The pharyngeal grooves (or clefts) form from the lateral ectodermal surface of the neck region to separate the arches.[54] The paired superior and paired inferior parathyroid glands have different embryologic origins.[5,55] Between the fifth and sixth gestational weeks, the parathyroid glands derive from the endoderm of the third and fourth pharyngeal pouches.[55]

The superior parathyroid glands arise from the dorsal wing of the fourth pharyngeal pouch.[5,56] At the seventh gestational week, the superior parathyroid glands lose connection to the pharynx and migrate caudally to attach with the posterior aspect of the mid-to-upper portion of the thyroid gland.[5] At autopsy, the final position for 80% of the superior parathyroid glands is within a 2-cm area located slightly superior to the recurrent laryngeal nerve and slightly inferior to the thyroid artery.[55]

The inferior parathyroid glands arise from the dorsal wing of the third pharyngeal pouch, along with the thymus. The ventral wing becomes the thymus.[5] During fetal development, the "parathymus glands" migrate caudally.[55] The inferior parathyroid gland loses its connections with the thymus, and the migration usually stops at the dorsal surface of the thyroid gland, outside of the fibrous capsule.[5] The final position of the inferior parathyroid glands is variable. Usually, over 60% come to rest at or just inferior to the posterior aspect of the lower pole of the thyroid gland.[55]

When migration is complete, the normal adult anatomical location of the superior and inferior parathyroid glands, which developed respectively from the fourth and third pharyngeal pouch, is now opposite of the pharyngeal rostrocaudal order.

Anatomy

Most adults have four parathyroid glands: two superior glands located posterior to the midportion of the thyroid gland and two inferior glands located in a slightly more variable position. The inferior parathyroid glands are located posterior or just inferior to the lower thyroid pole in approximately 60% of adults and are located within 4 cm of the lower thyroid pole in approximately 20% of adults[13] (Fig. 17-17). Microscopically, about three-fourths of the parathyroid glands are composed of chief cells and oxyphil cells and the remainder is composed of adipose tissue scattered throughout the parenchyma.[6] Normal parathyroid glands vary from a yellow to a reddish-brown color based on the amount of yellow parenchymal fat and chief cell content.[55] The parathyroid glands are typically somewhat flattened, oval, almond-shaped structures measuring $1 \times 3 \times 5$ mm.[13] Although enlarged, diseased, or cystic parathyroid glands may be differentiated from normal surrounding anatomy, imaging and visualizing the normal parathyroid glands is a challenge owing to their variable locations, small size, and isoechoic texture when compared to the normal thyroid gland.

Anatomic Variants

Accessory or supernumerary "fifth" parathyroid glands are found in approximately 13% of individuals at autopsy.[55] In one study, two-thirds of the supernumerary cases revealed the fifth parathyroid gland inferior to the lower pole of the thyroid gland associated with the thyrothymic ligament or the thymus and one-third had the supernumerary parathyroid gland in the vicinity of the thyroid between the orthotopic superior and inferior parathyroids.[56] Absence of parathyroid glands, defined as less than four, is noted in approximately 3% of individuals at autopsy.[5] In about 25% of cases, the inferior parathyroid glands fail to dissociate from the thymus and continue to migrate lower in the neck or into the mediastinum.[55]

Ectopic parathyroid glands occur in 15% to 20% of patients.[5] Owing to the long course of descent during

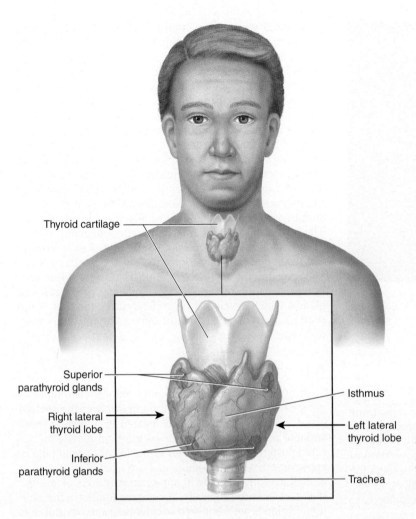

Thyroid cartilage

Superior parathyroid glands

Right lateral thyroid lobe

Inferior parathyroid glands

Isthmus

Left lateral thyroid lobe

Trachea

FIGURE 17-17 Anatomic location of the parathyroid glands. The superior and inferior thyroid glands are commonly located on the posterior surface of the thyroid gland surface. When evaluating the parathyroid glands, the scanning area should be large enough to include an investigation lateral and inferior of the thyroid.

embryologic development, the ectopic locations for the inferior parathyroid glands range from the level of the mandibular angle to the pericardium.[56] The most common ectopic location for the inferior parathyroid glands is in the anterior mediastinum and occurs in approximately 5% of ectopic cases.[56] Other common ectopic locations include the posterior mediastinum and retroesophageal and prevertebral regions.[5,55] It is interesting to note that even in their ectopic locations, the parathyroid glands are symmetrical from side to side when comparing right with left at 80% for the superior and 70% for the inferior glands.[56] The parathyroid glands have also been identified entering the thyroid gland capsule and embedding into the thyroid gland, resulting in intrathyroidal parathyroid gland(s).[5]

Physiology

The chief cells of the parathyroid glands are the primary source for the production of parathyroid hormone (PTH). PTH is the most important endocrine regulator of calcium and phosphorous concentrations in extracellular fluid, with the major target cells being in the bone and the kidney. The metabolic functions of PTH in supporting serum calcium and phosphorous levels includes activating osteoclasts, which influences the release of calcium by the bones; augmenting

the absorption of calcium in the intestinal tract; increasing renal tubular reabsorption of calcium that conserves free calcium; increasing conversion of vitamin D to its active dihydroxy form in the kidneys; and increasing urinary phosphate excretion that lowers the serum phosphate level.[8] These normal metabolic activities act in a classic feedback loop in the following ways: (1) An increase in the level of free calcium inhibits further PTH secretion. (2) When serum calcium levels are low, PTH secretion increases to act on target organs (skeletal, renal, and intestinal) and to enhance calcium absorption.

Laboratory Tests

A fasting blood PTH test is usually performed with a calcium test to monitor patients with a parathyroid condition or to help diagnose the reason for a variance in calcium levels (hypercalcemia or hypocalcemia).[57] Normal PTH values are 10 to 55 pg/mL and may vary slightly among different laboratories. Elevated values may occur with chronic renal failure, hyperparathyroidism, and vitamin D deficiency as well as other entities. Decreased values may occur with accidental removal or autoimmune destruction of the parathyroid glands, hypoparathyroidism, and metastatic bone tumors as well as other entities.

Sonographic Examination Technique

The preparation and protocol for a sonography examination of the parathyroid glands are the same as for a thyroid gland examination. For sonographic evaluation, the examiner should concentrate on the region between the posteromedial thyroid gland and the longus colli muscle.[7] The superior parathyroid glands are slightly more medial than the inferior parathyroid glands. The common ectopic locations for parathyroid glands can also be evaluated. On a transverse section, particular attention should be given to the area medial to the carotid artery, posterior to the lateral lobe of the thyroid gland, and anterior to the longus colli muscle. The parathyroid glands normally measure $1.0 \times 3.0 \times 5.0$ mm in size and are similar in echogenicity to the adjacent thyroid gland and surrounding tissues, making it difficult to distinguish sonographically.[1] If the parathyroid glands are visualized, their location, size, and number should be documented, and measurements should be made in three dimensions.[17] Minor bundles (containing the recurrent laryngeal nerve and inferior thyroid artery) may be mistaken for a parathyroid adenoma. These bundles are located posteriorly and slightly medial to the lateral thyroid lobes. The esophagus, which often appears between the left lateral thyroid lobe and the trachea may also be visualized. The posteriorly located longus colli muscle may also be mistaken for parathyroid disease. It is important that any suspected pathology can be identified, as such, in both longitudinal and transverse planes.

Pathology of the Parathyroid Glands

Evidence of parathyroid disease is often sought in patients who present with signs and symptoms of hyperparathyroidism, particularly those with hypercalcemia. Hypercalcemia occurs with excessive calcium levels, which can be caused by a number of diseases. The most common causes include hyperparathyroidism; calcium resorption with bone metastases from breast, prostate, or cervical cancer or hematologic malignancy; sarcoidosis; and excess vitamin D.[58] The clinical manifestations may include weight loss, anorexia, dyspepsia, peptic ulcer disease, pancreatitis, and nausea. Renal colic, hematuria, polyuria, and nocturia result from renal tubular dysfunction and diminished ability of the kidney to concentrate urine. Nephrolithiasis and urolithiasis, bone and joint pain, arthritis, and gout may also be present. Other presentations in patient history may include short-term memory loss, lack of energy and enthusiasm, and insomnia.

Hypocalcemia occurs with low serum calcium levels and may be either asymptomatic or life-threatening. Mild decreases in calcium can produce paresthesias around the mouth and in the digits, muscle spasms in the hands and feet (carpopedal spasm), and hyperreflexia.[58] Hyperirritability, fatigue, and anxiety are common symptoms. Severely reduced levels may induce dementia, depression, psychosis, and local or generalized seizures. Severe symptoms may include muscle spasm that can interfere with breathing and cause death.[58] Chronic hypocalcemia may affect ectoderm, producing dry skin, coarse hair, and brittle nails. Patients who have undergone partial or complete thyroidectomies may have had an inadvertent removal of all parathyroid glands and are at higher risk for developing hypoparathyroidism and consequently hypocalcemia.

In addition to the inadvertent removal of all parathyroid glands, there are a number of underlying causes of deficient PTH secretion resulting in hypoparathyroidism.[8] Other underlying causes include congenital absence of all glands, primary (idiopathic) atrophy, and familial hypoparathyroidisms.

Hyperparathyroidism is characterized by a greater than normal secretion of PTH. The two major classifications of hyperparathyroidism are primary and secondary and a less common tertiary.[8] The pathophysiologic mechanisms are somewhat different for each classification.[28] Primary hyperparathyroidism represents an autonomous, spontaneous PTH overproduction. Secondary hyperparathyroidism generally results as a secondary compensatory enlargement and hypersecretion that usually affects all parathyroid glands in patients with chronic renal insufficiency or vitamin D deficiency.[1] Tertiary hyperparathyroidism is the development of autonomous parathyroid hyperplasia, and it is often a result of an underlying disease such as parathyroid hyperplasia after long-standing hyperplasia secondary to renal failure.[6]

Primary Hyperparathyroidism

Primary hyperparathyroidism is one of the most common endocrine disorders and is characterized by inappropriate excess secretion of PTH by one or more of the parathyroid glands.[8,58] Most cases are detected with routine laboratory tests indicating elevated serum calcium levels and inappropriately high levels of PTH compared with the calcium level.[13] Primary hyperparathyroidism is usually caused by a single parathyroid adenoma in 80% to 85% of cases, by parathyroid hyperplasia in 10% to 15% of cases, and by parathyroid carcinoma in approximately 1% of cases.[58] It is usually a disease of adults and tends to affect patients between the ages of 40 and 60 years.[13] Over half of the patients with primary hyperparathyroidism are older than 50 years of age, and cases are rare before 20 years of age.[55] The female-to-male ratio is 2.5:1 with an increased incidence in women after menopause.[13,55] Although some cases of primary hyperparathyroidism are associated with prior external neck irradiation, long-term lithium therapy, or an inherited syndrome commonly related to MEN type 1 (MEN 1), most cases of primary hyperparathyroidism are sporadic and related to adenomas or hyperplasia.[55]

Surgery, considered the definitive treatment of primary hyperparathyroidism, is generally reserved for individuals with documented complications (osteoporosis, nephrolithiasis, or gastrointestinal or neuropsychiatric complications), severely elevated serum calcium levels, marked hypercalciuria, or individuals younger than 50 years of age.[28]

Adenoma

A solitary adenoma is a benign lesion and may involve any one of the four parathyroid glands with equal frequency.[55] Most adenomas are located in either the superior or inferior parathyroid glands and are adjacent to the thyroid gland.[1] Approximately 3% of cases are found in the same ectopic locations as the parathyroid glands, which includes the low neck, mediastinum, retrotracheal/retroesophageal, undescended/carotid sheath, and intrathyroidal.[1,13]

Sonographically, the parathyroid adenomas appear as hypoechoic, homogeneous solid masses. The echogenicity is usually less than the thyroid gland and may be so hypoechoic as it simulates a cyst.[13] The vast majority are homogeneously solid, and about 2% have an internal cystic components, most often owing to cystic degeneration, or less commonly, they are true simple cysts.[55] Adenomas are usually oval and less often appear as teardrop-shaped or round lesions. As the parathyroid glands enlarge, the adenoma dissects between longitudinally oriented tissue planes in the neck and acquires a characteristic oblong shape in the craniocaudal direction.[55] Most adenomas range in size from 0.8 to 1.5 cm and are usually less than 3 cm, but may reach 5 cm.[9,55] Smaller adenomas resected surgically in minimally enlarged, normal-appearing parathyroid glands have been found to be hypercellular on pathologic examination[55] (Fig. 17-18A–E). Examining enlarged parathyroid glands with color flow Doppler imaging may demonstrate a hypervascular pattern with prominent diastolic flow, or a peripheral vascular arc that may allow for differentiation from hyperplastic regional lymph nodes, which have a central hilar flow pattern.[1] Sonography may detect an enlarged extrathyroidal feeding artery supplying the adenoma, which often originates from branches of the inferior thyroidal artery.[55]

Hyperplasia

Primary hyperplasia is the enlargement of all four parathyroid glands; however, the enlargement is frequently unequal and asymmetric with apparent sparing of one or two glands.[8] Hyperplasia may occur sporadically or be associated with

MEN syndromes (MEN types 1 and 2A).[6] Approximately 75% of sporadic cases occur in women and are associated with external radiation and intake of lithium.[6] One-third of sporadic cases demonstrate monoclonality, which suggests a neoplastic basis for the proliferation of chief cells.[6] These sporadic cases have both chief cell hyperplasia and multiple small adenomas in the same gland.

Because hyperplasia usually affects more than one gland, it should be suspected when multiple nodules are identified; whereas the sonographically similar parathyroid adenomas should be suspected when a solitary nodule is identified. The sonographic appearances of hyperplasia has these potential pitfalls: (1) misinterpreting hyperplasia as a solitary adenoma; (2) missing hyperplasia when glandular enlargement is minimal; (3) difficulty distinguishing hyperplasia versus adenoma when there is sparing of one or two glands; and (4) misinterpreting normal cervical structures, such as veins adjacent to the thyroid gland, the esophagus, or the longus colli neck muscles, which may sonographically simulate a parathyroid adenoma.[1,55]

Carcinoma

Parathyroid carcinoma is a functioning tumor found in 1% of patients with primary hyperparathyroidism. These tumors occur equally in both sexes principally between 30 and 60 years of age.[8] They should be included as a diagnostic

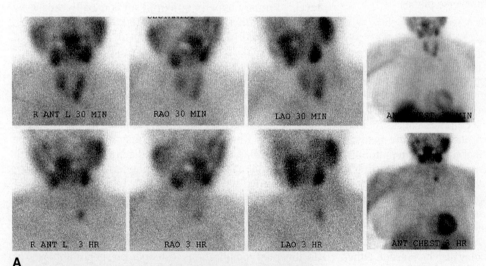

A

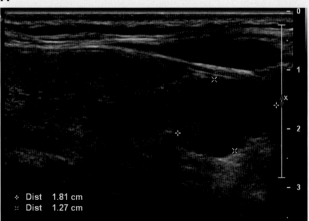

B

FIGURE 17-18 Parathyroid gland adenoma (**A, B**) and mass (**C–E**). **A, B:** The 66-year-old woman presented with elevated serum calcium levels. **A:** Images obtained from the radionuclide parathyroid study demonstrate increased focal uptake inferior to the left lower thyroid. **B:** On the same patient with the nuclear medicine exam, the longitudinal sonogram of the left inferior medial thyroid gland area shows a mass with mixed hyperechoic, hypoechoic, and cystic regions in the same left parathyroid gland region. Cursors mark the area corresponding to the focal increased uptake seen on the technetium-99m radionuclide exam. Based on the imaging appearances and the patient's history, the diagnosis was a parathyroid gland adenoma.

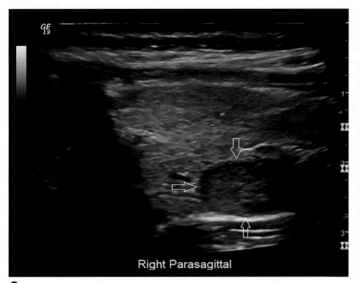

C

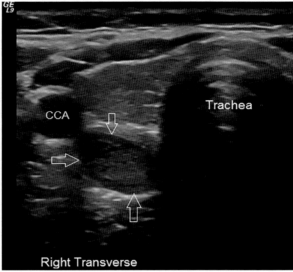

D

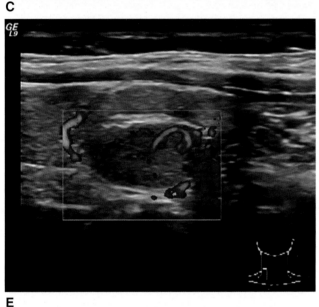

E

FIGURE 17-18 (continued) **C–E:** The right inferior parathyroid mass (arrows) was an incidental finding in an asymptomatic female with normal lab values. The mass is not causing any symptoms and has not been biopsied or diagnosed. CCA, common carotid artery. **E:** The longitudinal power Doppler sonogram shows a polar feeding vessel. (**D, E:** Courtesy of Darla Matthew, Las Cruces, NM.)

consideration for patients with primary hyperparathyroidism, particularly when the patient has a very high serum level of calcium, has had an abnormal gland excised, or has a palpable neck mass that is firm and immobile. Parathyroid carcinomas are often slow-growing, indolent masses with a lobular contour measuring more than 2 cm compared to the average 1 cm for adenomas. The mass often adheres to the surrounding soft tissues.[6] Sonographically, carcinomas frequently have a lobular contour with a heterogeneous internal architecture and internal cystic components.[55] The appearance may be similar to a large benign adenoma. A parathyroid carcinoma may demonstrate more attenuation than is normally seen with parathyroid adenomas or hyperplasia but differentiation is difficult prospectively. There is general agreement that a diagnosis of carcinoma based on cytologic detail and appearance is unreliable unless there is evidence of gross invasion to adjacent structures such as vessels or muscle.[8] If gross invasion occurs, it is an uncommon finding that is the only reliable preoperative sonographic criterion

for the diagnosis of malignancy.[55] Despite surgical removal of the tumor, local recurrence occurs in one-third of the cases, and about one-third of the cases develop metastases to regional lymph nodes, lungs, liver, and bone.[8] In fatal cases, death is most often caused by hyperparathyroidism rather than carcinomatosis.[6]

NECK

Sonography is excellent for neck anatomy evaluation and can identify intrathyroidal from extrathyroidal pathology, distinguishing between solid and cystic masses and, when needed, providing biopsy guidance.

Developmental Cysts

The more common developmental cysts that are sonographically identifiable in the neck include thyroglossal duct cysts, branchial cleft cysts, and cystic hygromas.

Thyroglossal Duct Cyst

A thyroglossal duct cyst is a congenital anomaly that develops within the remnant of the thyroglossal duct, which courses from the posterior third of the tongue to the thyroid cartilage.[59] Over half of all cases occur in the first decade of life with decreasing incidence from children to adults and rare occurrences in elderly patients, and they affect both sexes equally.[60] Cysts can form anywhere along the course of the duct; however, 65% of cysts occur at the infrahyoid level.[59] For most patients with thyroglossal duct cyst, surgical excision is curative.[6] The sonographic examination can provide the surgeon with preoperative assessment of the thyroglossal duct cyst size, location, and involvement, if any, of the surrounding musculature and may exclude the need for CT or MRI.[60]

Branchial Cleft Cyst

In early embryo development, the neck is shaped like a hollow tube with four circumferential ridges termed *arches,* which develop into the musculoskeletal and vascular components of the head and neck. During embryonic maturation, the thinner regions between the arches, termed *clefts,* are located on the lateral or skin side and the pouches are located on the medial or pharynx side.[61] The pouches develop into the middle ear, tonsils, thymus, and parathyroid glands. The first branchial cleft develops into the external auditory canal. The second, third, and fourth branchial clefts merge to form a sinus, which normally become involuted. The most widely held belief why developmental abnormalities within the branchial cleft occur is incomplete obliteration of the cervical sinus though there are other theories including incomplete obliteration of thyropharyngeal duct, cystic degeneration of cervical lymph nodes, trapped epithelium from the parotid gland, pharyngeal pouch, and branchial cleft.[62] With no communication with the inner mucosa or outer neck skin, the trapped arch remnants form a branchial cleft cyst (also known as a *lateral cervical cyst*).[62] On rare occasions, the branchial cleft fails to become involuted and a complete fistula with both external and internal openings forms between the pharynx and skin[61] (Fig. 17-19).

First branchial cleft cysts are usually identified on contrast-enhanced axial CT and are either located in the auditory canal (type I) or in the submandibular area (type II).[61] Second branchial cleft cysts account for 95% of branchial anomalies and are identified by sonography along the anterior border of the upper third of the sternocleidomastoid muscle and adjacent to the muscle. Third branchial cleft cysts are rare and extend from the same skin location as a second branchial fistula but occur deep into the sternocleidomastoid muscle and extend farther medially between the internal and external carotid arteries at the carotid artery bifurcation.[61,63] Fourth branchial cleft cysts are rare and arise from various neck locations, including the thyroid gland and mediastinum.[61]

Ahuja and colleagues identified four variable sonographic appearances for second branchial cleft cysts found in 17 adult

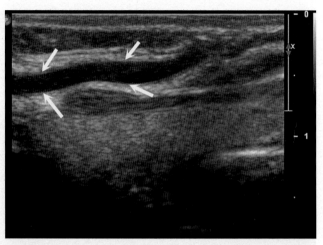

FIGURE 17-19 Branchial cleft fistula. This 1-month-old boy presented with an opening in the lateral/anterior neck. A longitudinal image shows a homogeneously hypoechoic structure with some internal debris (*arrows*). A fistula is formed when the cleft fails to involute; whereas, if no communication existed, the trapped arch remnants would form a branchial cleft cyst.

patients: anechoic (41%), homogeneously hypoechoic with internal debris (23.5%), pseudosolid (12%), and heterogeneous (23.5%).[62] Posterior enhancement was identified in 70% of cases, and in all cases, the cysts were located in their classical location posterior to the submandibular gland, superficial to the carotid artery and internal jugular vein, and closely related to the medial and anterior margin of the sternocleidomastoid muscle.[62] There are other benign cystic lateral neck masses that can mimic branchial cleft cysts and abscesses, and necrotic adenopathy can be difficult to distinguish from a branchial cleft cyst especially if it has been previously infected.[63]

Cystic Hygroma

A cystic hygroma is a congenital modification in the cervical lymphatic system. Over 60% are associated with chromosomal abnormality such as Turner syndrome but other aneuploidies are common such as trisomy 21 and trisomy 18.[13] These benign congenital masses occur at many sites but most often appear from the posterior occipital region and are most frequently visualized sonographically as large cystic masses on the lateral aspect of the neck. A cystic hygroma usually appears thin-walled and can be multilocular and multiseptated.

Pathology

Sonography is an excellent diagnostic tool used to evaluate masses in the salivary gland, hematomas, deep neck space infections, and cervical lymph node pathology.

Hematoma

Neck hematomas following trauma or surgery will appear as cystic, solid, or mixed masses, depending on the degree of coagulation. Because an abscess may present with a similar sonographic appearance, an accurate clinical history is imperative for differentiation. Patients with a hematoma may present with a history of recent surgery or other soft tissue assault, whereas patients with an abscess present clinically with elevated temperature, elevated white blood cell count, and tenderness.

Deep Neck Space Infections

Once a deep neck space infection is initiated, it may progress to either an inflammation and phlegmon or to fulminant abscess with a purulent fluid collection. The distinction is important because the treatment for these two entities is different.[64] Deep neck space infections are relatively uncommon but are a serious health problem with significant risks of morbidity and mortality.[64] Although the incidence and mortality rates have been reduced with the advancements in antibiotic medication, the diagnosis and treatment of infections in this area are difficult and potentially lethal complications may arise. Deep neck space infections are most commonly odontogenic in origin in adults, and tonsillitis is the most common etiology in children.[64] The infection can be caused by other infections, aspiration, drug use, postbiopsy or surgical procedures, and trauma. The etiology is unknown for 20% to 50% of cases.[64] The patient presents with the signs and symptoms of pain, recent dental procedures, upper respiratory tract infections, neck or oral cavity trauma including surgery or biopsy, respiratory difficulties, immunosuppression or immunocompromised status, or dysphagia. The infectious process can arise or spread to any potential space located between layers of fascia in the neck. The most common spaces that are likely to harbor an abscess are the submandibular space, the retropharyngeal space, and the parapharyngeal spaces.

The usefulness of diagnostic imaging varies and is based on the patient's age and the location of the infection. Sonography is helpful to distinguish between phlegmon and an abscess, give information about the condition of surrounding vessels, guide FNA procedures, and act as a guide to the need for further imaging with CT or MRI. CT is considered the gold standard in the evaluation of deep neck space infections and is capable of imaging infections extending into the chest.[65] MRI increases both the time and expense involved but provides excellent soft tissue resolution to help localize regional involvement.

The sonographic appearance of an abscess, although variable, is most often a partially or fully fluid-filled, thick-walled mass. In the presence of gas-forming organisms, small pockets of hyperechoic air can be seen within the collection.[66] Enlarged, hypoechoic lymph nodes may be identified surrounding the abscess.[66]

Cervical Lymph Node Pathology

Cervical lymph nodes are located along the lymphatic channels of the neck and have been classified for staging of cancers and reclassified for sonographic evaluation, allowing the adoption of a systematic protocol for examination.[67] These nodes are also common sites of pathologic involvement with metastases, lymphoma, lymphadenitis, tuberculosis, reactive hyperplasia, and other conditions of benign lymphadenitis.[67,68] Evaluating cervical lymph nodes is an important follow-up on patients with head and neck carcinoma.[69,70] CT and MRI can be used to evaluate cervical lymph nodes; however, CT is less sensitive than sonography in detecting small nodes and MRI is less sensitive than sonography in detecting calcification within lymph nodes that can be identified sonographically.[67] Sonography is sensitive in identifying lymph nodes as small as 2 mm and intranodal calcifications that are useful features to identify metastatic nodes form papillary and medullary carcinoma of the thyroid gland.[67,68]

Normal cervical lymph nodes are usually found in the submandibular, parotid, upper cervical, and posterior triangle regions, whereas the distribution of cervical lymph nodes is different in patients with metastatic head and neck carcinomas, non-Hodgkin lymphoma, and tuberculosis.[67,69]

The normal nodes appear hypoechoic when compared to adjacent soft tissue with an echogenic hilus.[69] The echogenic hilus is a hyperechoic linear structure, which is continuous with adjacent soft tissue and is usually considered as a sign of benignity[67] (Fig. 17-20A). The shape of a normal lymph node is predominantly oval, elongated, or elliptical, except for the submandibular and parotid regions where the nodes appear round.[67,69] Normal lymph nodes less than 5 mm usually appear avascular because the blood vessels are too small to be detected, whereas, approximately 90% of normal lymph nodes with a maximum diameter greater than 5 mm present with hilar vascularity.[67,69] The use of nodal size and vascular resistance has not produced a firm criterion to differentiate normal from abnormal nodes.[67,70] Finding a value as a cutoff point using a short-axis measurement of 5 mm, 8 mm, and 10 mm increases the sensitivity as nodal size increases but it decreases the specificity as nodal size decreases. Nodal size is not useful as the sole criterion in differential diagnosis; however, it is clinically very useful when the size of lymph nodes in a patient with known carcinoma increases on serial sonography examination, when metastasis is strongly suspected, and when evaluation of progressive change of nodal size is required while monitoring treatment response of the patient[69] (Fig. 17-20B).

The sonographic appearance helpful in differentiating metastatic nodes include hypoechoic nodule, except it is hyperechoic when the metastasis is from PTC carcinoma because intranodal calcification is common in this condition.[67,70] Metastatic nodes tend to be round in shape, the echogenic hilus is absent, and there is intranodal cystic necrosis, increase in size on serial examinations, and peripheral or mixed vascularity.[67,69] The metastasis may also originate from the lung, breast, gastrointestinal tract, or pancreas as well as local head and neck carcinoma (Fig. 17-20C). The differentiation of normal and abnormal cervical lymph nodes is not always possible based on sonographic features and the diagnosis is still based on histology.[68]

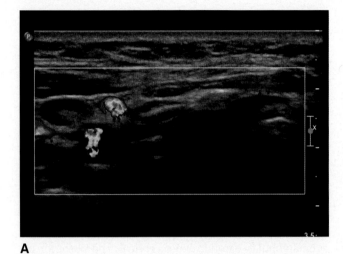

A

B

C

FIGURE 17-20 Cervical lymph nodes. **A:** The sonogram shows an example of a lymph node with a prominent fatty hilum. The blood flow into the hilum is usually seen and will confirm identification of the hilum. **B:** The *cursors* mark normal lymph nodes seen on the sonograms made in the left lateral neck on a post-thyroidectomy patient. **C:** This transverse image through the right inferior thyroid gland between the common carotid artery (*CCA*) and trachea shows an enlarged, hypoechoic lymph node without a typical fatty hilum (*arrows*). The sonography examination is on a 25-year-old woman with known thyroid papillary carcinoma. Biopsy confirmed local metastasis of the patient's thyroid cancer. Compare this lymph node with those appearing in images A and B.

SUMMARY

- The thyroid gland is located in the anterior neck usually over the second and third cartilaginous rings of the trachea.
- The thyroid gland is surrounded by a fibrous capsule and consists primarily of the right and left lobes that are united by a relatively thin isthmus.
- The thyroid gland is responsible for maintenance of body metabolism and secretes three hormones: triiodothyronine (T_3), thyroxine (T_4), and calcitonin (thyrocalcitonin).
- Sonographically, the normal thyroid gland parenchyma appears as a homogeneous gland of medium- to high-level echoes.
- The most common cause of thyroid gland disorders worldwide is iodine deficiency, which may result in goiter formation and hypothyroidism.
- Most thyroid nodules are benign and approximately 5% to 6.5% are malignant.
- Most adults have four parathyroid glands, two superior and two inferior, located on the posterior surface of the thyroid gland.
- The parathyroid glands regulates calcium and phosphorous concentration in extracellular fluid and secretes PTH.

- If normal parathyroid glands are visualized, the examiner should document the location, size, and number and make measurements in three dimensions.
- Primary hyperparathyroidism is the most common endocrine disorder.
- Developmental cysts of the neck include thyroglossal duct cyst, branchial cleft cyst, and cystic hygroma.
- Pathology of the neck includes hematomas and deep neck space infections and cervical lymphadenopathy.
- Sonography of the neck, thyroid gland, and parathyroid glands is an excellent diagnostic test for determining the internal architecture and precise location of intrusive pathology.
- The sonography examination relies on the skill, knowledge, and accuracy of the sonographer who must pay attention to the texture, outline, size, and shape of both normal and abnormal structures.
- The patient will benefit most when the sonographic appearance is correlated with patient history, clinical presentation, laboratory function tests, and other imaging modalities to compose a clinically helpful picture.

REFERENCES

1. Kuntz KM. Neck mass. In: Henningsen C, Kuntz K, Youngs D, eds. *Clinical Guide to Sonography*. 2nd ed. Elsevier; 2014:359–368.
2. Brashers VL, Huether SE. Mechanisms of hormonal regulation. In: Huether SE, McCance KL, eds. *Understanding Pathophysiology*. 6th ed. Elsevier; 2017:439–459.
3. Dighe M, Barr R, Bojunga J, et al. Thyroid ultrasound: state of the art part 1—thyroid ultrasound reporting and diffuse thyroid diseases. *Med Ultrason*. 2017;19(1):79–93. doi:10.11152/mu-980
4. Baker S. Neck mass. In: Sanders RC, Hall-Terracciano B, eds. *Clinical Sonography: A Practical Guide*. 5th ed. Wolters Kluwer; 2016:691–703.
5. Zapanta PE, Meyers AD. Embryology of the thyroid and parathyroids. *Medscape: eMedicine*. March 2016. Accessed March 10, 2017. http://emedicine.medscape.com/article/845125-overview
6. Rubin R, Rubin E. The endocrine system. In: Rubin E, Gorstein F, Rubin R, eds. *Rubin's Pathology: Clinicopathologic Foundations of Medicine*. 4th ed. Lippincott Williams & Wilkins; 2005:1125–1171.
7. DeJong MR. Thyroid scanning protocol. In: DeJong MR, ed. *Sonography Scanning: Principles and Protocols*. 5th ed. Elsevier; 2021.
8. Kumar V, Abbas AK, Aster JC, Anirban M. The endocrine system. In *Robbins & Cotran Pathologic Basis of Disease*. 10th ed. Elsevier; 2021:1065–1132.
9. Hagen-Ansert SL. The thyroid and parathyroid glands. In: Hagen-Ansert SL, ed. *Textbook of Diagnostic Ultrasonography*. Vol 1. 8th ed. Elsevier Mosby; 2017:618–641.
10. Huppert BJ, Reading C, Solbiati L, et al. The thyroid gland. In: Rumack CM, Levine D, eds. *Diagnostic Ultrasound*. Vol 1. 5th ed. Elsevier Mosby; 2017:691–758.
11. Needleman L. Thyroid and parathyroid. In: Goldberg BB, McGahan JP, eds. *Atlas of Ultrasound Measurements*. 2nd ed. Elsevier Mosby; 2006:328–332.
12. Agur AMR, Dalley AF, Moore KL, Moore KL. *Moore's Essential Clinical Anatomy*. Wolters Kluwer Health; 2019.
13. Middleton WD, Kurtz AB, Hertzberg BS. *Ultrasound: The Requisites*. 3rd ed. Elsevier Mosby; 2015.
14. Malek H, Raheleh H. A rare case of coexistence ectopic lingual thyroid and thyroglossal cyst with TC 99 & thyroid scintigraphy. *Indian J Otolaryngol Head Neck Surg*. 2021. doi:10.1007/s12070-021-02721-7
15. Lin, Q, Qilu G, Rong F, et al. Ectopic thyroid gland located on the L4 vertebral body. *Medicine*. 2021;100(2):e24042. doi:10.1097/md.0000000000024042
16. Alcântara-Jones, DM, Lucas MB, Nunes TF, et al. Percutaneous injection of ethanol for thyroid nodule treatment: a comparative study. *Arch Endocrinol Metab*. 2021;65(3):322–332. doi:10.20945/2359-3997000000363
17. AIUM–ACR–SPR–SRU practice parameter for the performance and interpretation of a diagnostic ultrasound examination of the extracranial head and neck. *J Ultrasound Med*. 2018;37:E6–E12.
18. Lin JD, Huang BY, Hsueh C. Application of ultrasonography in thyroid cysts. *J Med Ultrasound*. 2007;15:91–102.
19. Sung JY, Baek JH, Kim YS, et al. One-step ethanol ablation of viscous cystic thyroid nodules. *AJR Am J Roentgenol*. 2008;180:1730–1733.
20. Kim DW, Rho MH, Kim HJ, et al. Percutaneous ethanol injection for benign cystic thyroid nodules: is aspiration of ethanol-mixed fluid advantageous? *AJNR Am J Neuroradiol*. 2005;26:2122–2127.
21. Hoang VT, Trinh CT. A review of the pathology, diagnosis and management of colloid goitre. *Eur Endocrinol*. 2020;16:131–135.
22. Popoveniuc G, Jonklaas J. Thyroid nodule. *Med Clin North Am*: 2012;96(2): 329–349.
23. Low SCS, Sinha AK, Sundram FX. Detection of thyroid malignancy in a hot nodule by fluorine-18-fluorodeoxyglucose positron emission tomography. *Singapore Med J*. 2005;46:304–307.
24. Yeung MJ, Serpell JW. Management of the solitary thyroid nodule. *Oncologist*. 2008;13:105–112.
25. Blum M. Ultrasonography of the thyroid. *Thyroid Disease Manager*. July 2020. Accessed January 14, 2022. http://www.thyroidmanager.org
26. Samuels MH. Evaluation and treatment of sporadic nontoxic goiter—some answers and more questions. *J Clin Endocrinol Metab*. 2001;86:994–997.
27. Xiang P, Chu X, Chen G, et al. Nodules with nonspecific ultrasound pattern according to the 2015 American Thyroid Association malignancy risk stratification system: a comparison to the Thyroid Imaging Reporting and Data System (TIRADS-Na). *Medicine (Baltimore)*. 2019;98:e17657.
28. Brashers FL, Jones RE, Huether SE. Alterations of hormonal regulation. In: Huether SE, McCance KL, eds. *Understanding Pathophysiology*. 6th ed. Elsevier; 2017:460–489.
29. Office on Women's Health. Graves' disease fact sheet. November 2017. Accessed January 14, 2022. https://www.womenshealth.gov/a-z-topics/graves-disease
30. Davies TF, Andersen S, Latif R, et al. Graves' disease. *Nat Rev Dis Primers*. 2020;6:52.
31. Baldini M, Orsatti A, Bonfanti MT, et al. Relationship between the sonographic appearance of the thyroid and the clinical course and autoimmune activity of Graves' disease. *J Clin Ultrasound*. 2005;33:381–385.
32. Hoang JK, Lee WK, Lee M, et al. US features of thyroid malignancy: pearls and pitfalls. *Radiographics*. 2007;27:847–865.
33. Neale DM, Cootauco AC, Burrow G. Thyroid disease in pregnancy. *Clin Perinatol*. 2007;34:543–557.
34. Smith A, Eccles-Smith J, D'Emden M, Lust K. Thyroid disorders in pregnancy and postpartum. *Aust Prescr*. 2017;40(6):214–219. doi:10.18773/austprescr.2017.075
35. Paajanen I, Metso S, Jaatinen P, Kholová I. Thyroid FNA diagnostics in a real-life setting: experiences of the implementation of the Bethesda system in Finland. *Cytopathology*. 2018;29: 189–195.
36. Hong Y, Liu X, Li Z, et al. Real-time ultrasound elastography in the differential diagnosis of benign and malignant thyroid nodules. *J Ultrasound Med*. 2009;28:861–867.
37. Chan BK, Desser TS, McDougall IR, et al. Common and uncommon sonographic features of papillary thyroid carcinoma. *J Ultrasound Med*. 2003;22:1083–1090.
38. Frates MC, Benson CB, Doubilet PM, et al. Prevalence and distribution of carcinoma in patients with solitary and multiple thyroid nodules on sonography. *J Clin Endocrinol Metab*. 2006;91:3411–3417.
39. Kim MJ, Kim EK, Kwak JY, et al. Differentiation of thyroid nodules with macrocalcifications: role of suspicious sonographic findings. *J Ultrasound Med*. 2008;27:1179–1184.
40. Kim BM, Kim MJ, Kim EK, et al. Sonographic differentiation of thyroid nodules with eggshell calcifications. *J Ultrasound Med*. 2008;27:1425–1430.
41. Frates MC, Benson CB, Doubilet PM, et al. Can color Doppler sonography aid in the prediction of malignancy of thyroid nodules? *J Ultrasound Med*. 2003;22:127–131.
42. Zhang B, Ma X, Wu N, et al. Shear wave elastography for differentiation of benign and malignant thyroid nodules: a meta-analysis. *J Ultrasound Med*. 2013;32:2163–2169.
43. Sohn YM, Kim MJ, Kim EK, et al. Sonographic elastography combined with conventional sonography: how much is it helpful for diagnostic performance? *J Ultrasound Med*. 2009;28:413–420.
44. Pickerell DM. Elastography: imaging of tomorrow? *J Diagn Med Sonogr*. 2010;26:109–113.
45. Yoon JH, Kim EK, Hong SW, et al. Sonographic features of the follicular variant of papillary thyroid carcinoma. *J Ultrasound Med*. 2008;27:1431–1437.
46. Maizlin ZV, Wiseman SM, Vora P, et al. Hürthle cell neoplasms of the thyroid: sonographic appearance and histologic characteristics. *J Ultrasound Med*. 2008;27:751–757.
47. Lee SK, Rho BH, Woo SK. Hürthle cell neoplasm: correlation of gray-scale and power Doppler sonographic findings with gross pathology. *J Clin Ultrasound*. 2010;38:169–176.
48. Kwak JY, Kim EK, Ko KH, et al. Primary thyroid lymphoma: role of ultrasound-guided needle biopsy. *J Ultrasound Med*. 2007;26:1761–1765.
49. Kim MJ, Kim EK, Park SI, et al. US-guided fine-needle aspiration of thyroid nodules: indications, techniques, results. *Radiographics*. 2008;28:1869–1886.
50. Grant EG, Tessler FN, Hoang JK, et al. Thyroid ultrasound reporting lexicon: white paper of the ACR Thyroid Imaging, Reporting and Data System (TIRADS) Committee. *J Am Coll Radiol*. 2015;12(12 Pt A):1272–1279.
51. Haugen BR. 2015 American Thyroid Association management guidelines for adult patients with thyroid nodules and differentiated thyroid cancer: what is new and what has changed? *Cancer*. 2017;123:372–381.
52. American Cancer Society. Detailed guide: thyroid cancer. May 2020. Accessed January 14, 2022. https://www.cancer.org/cancer/thyroid-cancer/detection-diagnosis-staging/how-diagnosed.html

53. Anderson TJ, Atalay MK, Grand DJ, Baird GL, Cronan JJ, Beland MD. Management of nodules with initially nondiagnostic results of thyroid fine-needle aspiration: can we avoid repeat biopsy? *Radiology.* 2014;272(3):777–784.

54. Graham A, Okabe M, Quinlan R. The role of the endoderm in the development and evolution of the pharyngeal arches. *J Anat.* 2005;207:479–487.

55. Huppert BJ, Reading CC. The parathyroid gland. In: Rumack CM, Levine MA, eds. *Diagnostic Ultrasound.* Vol 1. 5th ed. Elsevier Mosby; 2017:732–758.

56. Fancy T, Gallagher D III, Hornig JD. Surgical anatomy of the thyroid and parathyroid glands. *Otolaryngol Clin North Am.* 2010;43:221–227.

57. American Association for Clinical Chemistry. PTH: the test. November 2021. Accessed January 14, 2022. http://www.labtestsonline .org/understanding/analytes/pth/test.html

58. Huether SE. The cellular environment: fluids and electrolytes, acids and bases. In: Huether SE, McCance KL, eds. *Understanding Pathophysiology.* 6th ed. Elsevier; 2017:114–133.

59. Patel S, Bhatt AA. Thyroglossal duct pathology and mimics. *Insights Imaging.* 2019;10:1–12.

60. El-Ayman YA, Naguib SM, Abdalla WM. Huge thyroglossal duct cyst in elderly patient: case report. *Int J Surg Case Rep.* 2018;51:415–418.

61. Branstetter BF. Branchial cleft cysts. *Medscape: eMedicine.* April 2018. Accessed January 14, 2022. http://emedicine.medscape .com/article/382803-overview

62. Gonzalez-Mourelle A, Vicente-Fernandez C, Pombo-Castro M, Vazquez-Mahia I, Lopez-Cedrun JL. Branchial cleft cysts: serie of 33 cases and review of the literature. *Ital J Anat Embryol.* 2018;123:194–198.

63. Lanham PD, Wushensky C. Second branchial cleft cyst mimic: case report. *Am J Neuroradiol.* 2005;26:1862–1864.

64. Murray AD. Deep neck infections. *Medscape: eMedicine.* April 2020. Accessed January 14, 2022. http://emedicine.medscape. com/article/837048-overview

65. Craig FW, Schunk JE. Retropharyngeal abscess in children: clinical presentation, utility of imaging, and current management. *Pediatrics.* 2003;111:1394–1398.

66. Turkington JR, Paterson A, Sweeney LE, et al. Neck masses in children. *Br J Radiol.* 2005;78:75–85.

67. Ying M, Ahuja AT. Ultrasound of neck lymph nodes: how to do it and how do they look? *Radiography.* 2006;12:105–117.

68. Ahuja AT, Ying M. Sonographic evaluation of cervical lymph nodes. *AJR Am J Roentgenol.* 2004;184:1991–1699.

69. Ying M, Ahuja A, Wong KT. Ultrasound evaluation of neck lymph nodes. *ASUM Ultrasound Bull.* 2003;6:9–17.

70. Leboulleux S, Girard E, Rose M, et al. Ultrasound criteria of malignancy for cervical lymph nodes in patients followed up for differentiated thyroid cancer. *J Clin Endocrinol Metab.* 2007;92:3590–3594.

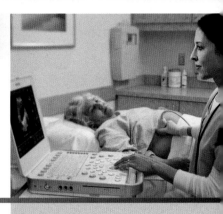

CHAPTER 18

The Breast

CATHERINE CARR-HOEFER

OBJECTIVES

- Discuss sonography's role in the evaluation of the breast.
- Explain the indications for sonography of the breast, as well as its advantages and limitations.
- Identify the role of other modalities and newer applications used in breast imaging.
- Describe normal breast anatomy and corresponding appearance of the sonographic layers/zones, as well as changes with age and hormone status.
- Demonstrate the sonographic techniques used for breast evaluation.
- Describe the methods used to annotate breast sonograms.
- Explain how patient positioning affects sonomammographic correlation.
- Discuss ACR BI-RADS categories and risk classification for breast cancer.
- List the characteristics of simple and complicated cysts, and complex cystic and solid breast masses.
- Identify common cystic lesions found in the breast.
- Describe inflammatory and traumatic conditions that can affect the breast.
- Differentiate the sonographic and mammographic characteristics of benign breast lesions from malignant lesions.
- Identify common benign and malignant solid breast masses.
- Discuss benign and malignant conditions that affect the male breast.
- Identify imaging characteristics of normal- and abnormal-appearing lymph nodes.
- List common sonography-guided interventional procedures used to diagnose or to treat diseases of the breast.
- Discuss the normal appearance and complications that can arise in the augmented breast.
- Discuss the role of elastography and emerging technologies in breast imaging.

GLOSSARY

adenopathy enlargement or changes involving the lymph nodes due to infection, inflammatory disease, or cancer

areola pigmented skin surrounding the nipple

axilla armpit, significant because it contains lymph nodes that drain the breast tissue

BI-RADS Breast Imaging Reporting and Data System; published by the American College of Radiology to promote the use of consistent terminology when characterizing and reporting imaging findings, as well as classifying findings into risk categories for cancer; provides recommendations for patient management; data collection tool

KEY TERMS

abscess

adenopathy

BI-RADS

breast augmentation

breast cyst

breast sonography

colloid carcinoma

complex cyst

complicated cyst

core needle biopsy

ductal carcinoma in situ

elastography

extracapsular rupture

fat necrosis

fibroadenoma

fibrocystic change

fine-needle aspiration

galactocele

gynecomastia

hamartoma

hematoma

inflammatory carcinoma

intraductal papilloma

invasive ductal carcinoma

intracapsular rupture

invasive lobular carcinoma

lipoma

lobular carcinoma in situ

(continued)

mammography

mastitis

medullary carcinoma

Mondor disease

Paget disease

papillary apocrine metaplasia

papillary carcinoma

postsurgical scar

sebaceous cyst

seroma

triple-negative breast cancer

tubular carcinoma

whole-breast sonography

brachytherapy radiotherapy technique involving implantation of a radiation source in the breast, at/near the lumpectomy site, to treat the tumor bed and adjacent tissues; form of accelerated partial breast irradiation

cooper ligaments thin connective tissue bands that extend through the breast to the skin and provide structural support to the breast; also referred to as suspensory ligaments of Cooper

desmoplasia fibroelastic host response; reactive fibrosis that occurs in the tissues surrounding many invasive malignant breast lesions

elastography technique used to evaluate tissue stiffness by measuring deformation of tissues following a compressional force or by pulses of an acoustic radiation force; methods include strain and shear-wave elastography

in situ (noninvasive) breast cancer carcinoma in situ; the malignant cells are confined within the boundaries of the duct and/or lobule and have not extended into adjacent tissue

invasive breast cancer malignant cells have infiltrated past the boundaries of the breast duct and/or lobule into adjacent tissue; with access to blood or lymph vessels, metastasis can occur

multicentricity coexistent cancers within different quadrants or separated by greater than 5 cm within the breast

multifocality additional malignant lesions within a breast quadrant or within 5 cm of the primary tumor, typically indicating spread of cancer via the ducts

sentinel node first node in the drainage basin of a primary cancer and at most risk for metastasis; the presence or absence of cancer cells in this node is used in staging the tumor

spiculation finger-like extensions from a mass most often seen with invasive cancer; images as straight lines that radiate from the surface of a mass

terminal ductolobular unit (TDLU) the functional unit of the breast; composed of a lobule and its draining extralobular terminal duct; has histologic importance because most benign and malignant breast diseases arise from this structure

triple-negative breast cancer invasive breast cancer that tests negative for estrogen and progesterone receptors and for overexpression of human epidermal growth factor receptor 2

Sonography is a useful complement to physical examination, mammography, as well as magnetic resonance imaging (MRI) in the assessment of breast disease. The sonography examination provides a real-time tomographic display of the breast without ionizing radiation. In addition, the relative comfort of the examination and low cost make sonography an attractive choice for breast evaluation.

Mammography is the most common imaging modality used to evaluate the breast and remains the only widely used screening tool proven effective at reducing breast cancer mortality.[1-6] High-quality mammography is capable of detecting suspicious patterns of microcalcifications, which is typically the first imaging sign of a developing malignancy.[1-7] Early cancer detection and treatment improves long-term survival by decreasing the incidence of lymph node involvement and metastasis to distant sites. Although digital mammography has improved pathology detection in certain breast types, mammography still has some diagnostic limitations. It cannot detect all breast masses. Lesions are more readily detected in a radiolucent, fatty breast and can be obscured in a radiopaque dense breast. Mammography alone does not determine whether a mass is cystic or solid because radiodensity can be similar. Localization of a mass is difficult if seen on only one radiographic view. Occasionally, superimposition of a focal area of normal breast tissues can create a pseudomass that may be difficult to differentiate from a real lesion on two-dimensional (2D) mammography. Digital breast tomosynthesis (DBT), or 3D mammography, allows breast tissues to be viewed "layer by layer," which improves mass detection and reduces false-positive findings; however, not all patients may have access to this newer technology.[4-7] In addition, radiographic features of some breast malignancies are similar to those of benign masses so the level of diagnostic confidence is reduced.

For these reasons, adjunctive imaging tests are often recommended for breast evaluation in certain patients. When used in addition to mammography or physical examination, high-resolution sonography often improves diagnostic accuracy and assists in appropriate patient management.

CLINICAL ROLE OF BREAST SONOGRAPHY[4-18]

Table 18-1 summarizes the indications and advantages of sonographic evaluation of the breast. Sonography's proven ability to differentiate between cystic and solid masses allows palpable and radiographically indeterminate lesions to be characterized before invasive tests are considered. Dense fibroglandular tissue can hinder mass detection, especially on 2D mammography. Conversely, solid lesions are more evident on a sonogram when contrasted against hyperechoic fibroglandular tissue than in a less echogenic fat-replaced breast. Sonography serves as the primary nonionizing imaging modality used to evaluate symptomatic patients who are young, pregnant, or lactating, which are patient groups often associated with increased breast density that compromises radiographic evaluation.

Because sonography allows a tomographic display of the breast without painful compression, it is useful for examining patients with breast trauma, inflammatory changes, augmentation mammoplasty, or postirradiation changes. Sonography can also help evaluate the male breast for physiologic or pathologic changes. Mammography is often difficult to perform on these patients.

Following contrast-enhanced MRI evaluation, targeted "second-look" ultrasound (US) can assess an area of suspicious enhancement, a worrisome lesion, or an abnormal lymph node, especially when not visible by mammography. Careful correlation is needed owing to the differences in patient positioning between these modalities. If sonography can detect the MRI finding and image-guided intervention is recommended, then US guidance is typically preferred to MRI to biopsy a suspicious finding.[6,9]

Sonographic guidance is highly useful during the performance of interventional and therapeutic breast procedures. High-resolution, real-time sonography can assist needle placement during aspiration or biopsy procedures, affording direct visualization of the needle tip as it approaches and enters the mass. Evacuation of cystic lesions, drainage of abscess cavities, and sampling of suspicious solid masses and lymph nodes can be observed and confirmed. Clip marker placement to identify the site of mass after tissue sampling, or in conjunction with cancer therapy planning, can be performed using sonographic guidance.

Although sonography is useful in a number of clinical settings, there are limitations that should be recognized. The diagnostic quality of a sonographic breast examination is very operator and equipment dependent. As with other imaging modalities, differentiation between some benign and malignant solid lesions is less reliable when imaging patterns are similar. Even some normal structures and imaging artifacts (e.g., costal cartilage, Copper ligament shadowing) can be mistaken for pathology by an inexperienced breast imager. Newer high-frequency broadband transducers, harmonic imaging, spatial compounding, three-dimensional (3D) multiplanar imaging, and advanced processing techniques have increased sonography's ability to assess lesion characteristics. Some manufacturers apply special processing filters to enhance the sonographic detection of microcalcifications.[19] However, the thin image planes and limitations in resolution restrict conventional sonography's ability to assess the exact size, shape, and distribution patterns of microcalcifications within the breast that are readily detectable by mammography. Limitation in detecting suspicious calcifications is one reason why sonography is not approved as a "primary" breast cancer screening tool; however, sonography and contrast-enhanced MRI are most commonly used as supplemental screening tools to detect occult cancers in certain at-risk women and those with radiographically dense breasts when the efficacy of mammography is reduced.[1-4,20-22]

Advancements in sonographic imaging such as automated whole-breast scanners, volumetric 3D and 4D imaging, image fusion technology, volume navigation, sonoelastography, contrast imaging, as well as development of computer-assisted detection (CAD) programs and lesion analysis software are some of the progressive changes to enhance sonography's role in breast pathology recognition and diagnosis.

TABLE 18-1 Breast Sonography: Clinical Role	
Indications[a]	**Advantages**
• Characterization of palpable breast mass or breast-related sign or symptom	• Noninvasive, painless
• Suspected or apparent abnormality detected on other imaging tests (e.g., mammography, MRI)	• Nonionizing examination
• Initial imaging test before age 30 (not at high risk for breast cancer) and in pregnant or lactating female	• Tomographic display
• Evaluation of clinical concern when mammography is compromised or contraindicated (e.g., dense breast, inflammation, trauma, irradiation, male breast)	• Real-time imaging and needle guidance
• Evaluation of the augmented breast	• Cyst versus solid mass differentiation
• Guidance during breast biopsy and other interventional procedures, including biopsy of abnormal lymph nodes	• Mass detection in radiographically dense breast
• Supplement to mammography to screen for occult breast cancer in certain patient populations (e.g., dense breast patient at elevated risk), or with when MRI is contraindicated or not available	• Mass characterization for BI-RADS risk assessment
• Treatment planning for radiation therapy	• Chest wall imaging
	• Implant imaging
	• Doppler, elastography capabilities
	• 3D/4D capabilities
	• Mass localization when seen on one mammographic view
	• Contrast injection not required
	• Low cost; widely available

MRI, magnetic resonance imaging.
[a]Indications adapted from American College of Radiology. *ACR Practice Parameter for the Performance of a Breast Ultrasound Examination*. American College of Radiology; 2016. Accessed December 15, 2020. http://www.acr.org

ANATOMY[4,5,8,15,23]

The breasts, or mammary glands, are paired, dome-shaped structures lying along the chest wall anterior to the level of the second to sixth ribs (Fig. 18-1). As exocrine glands, the primary function of these modified sweat glands is to produce milk to nourish maternal offspring.

The breast tissue resides within thin layers of the superficial pectoral fascia. The anterior layer of this fascia travels just beneath the skin within the superficial fat, whereas the deep fascial layer lies near the fascia covering the pectoralis muscle. A layer of loose connective tissue between the deep layer of the superficial fascia and the pectoralis fascia is called the retromammary space. This potential space allows mobility of the breast over the chest wall.

The skin, nipple, and areola comprise the external surface of the breast. The outer epidermis and underlying dermis of the skin contain hair follicles, sebaceous, and sweat glands. The nipple is a round fibromuscular papilla projecting from the center of the breast that is encircled by the pigmented areola. Small bumps on the areola mark the sites of sebaceous glands (Montgomery glands), which secrete an oily substance to lessen drying and cracking of the nipple during breastfeeding.

The female breast is primarily composed of glandular, fatty, and fibrous connective tissues that vary in proportion based on the individual's age and hormonal status.

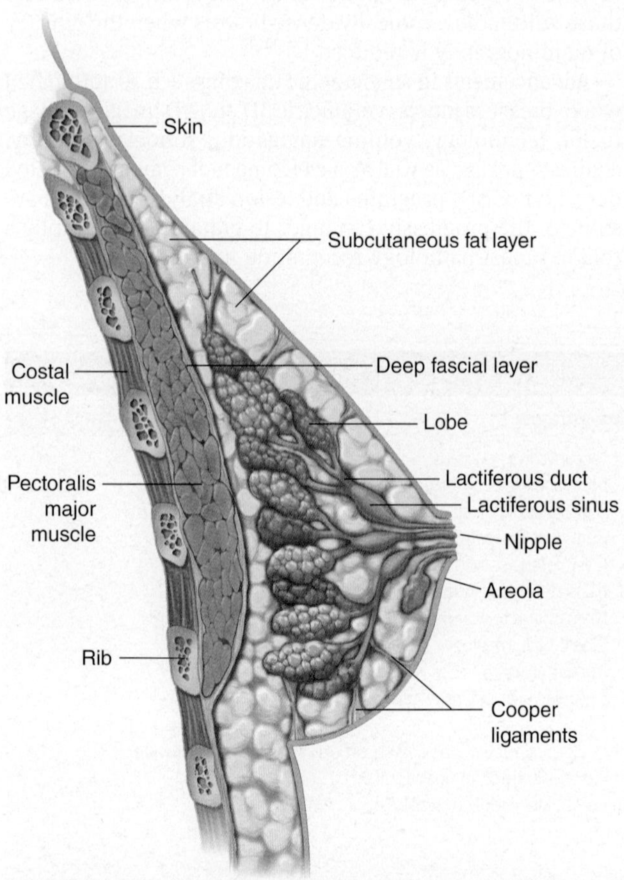

The glandular elements of the breast primarily function to produce and transport milk. The stromal elements consist of fat, fibrous connective tissues, and blood vessels, lymphatics, and nerves.

Between the skin and the chest wall, the breast is subdivided by fascial planes into three layers: the subcutaneous fat layer, the mammary (parenchymal) layer, and the retromammary fat layer. These breast layers are also referred to as the premammary, mammary, and retromammary layers or zones.

The parenchyma (fibroglandular tissue) contains the functional glandular elements of the breast and supporting connective tissues. Within this mammary layer are approximately 15 to 20 overlapping lobes arranged in a radial manner around the nipple. Each lobe contains 20 to 40 terminal ductolobular units (TDLUs), which are the functional units of the breast. A TDLU is composed of a lobule and its draining extralobular terminal duct. Each lobule contains an intralobular portion of the terminal duct that drains numerous, small terminal ductules (Fig. 18-2). During late pregnancy, these ductules transform into tiny sac-like, milk-producing glands called *acini* or *alveoli* that involute after the lactation period ceases. Each lobe has a branching network of lactiferous ducts that transport milk from the TDLUs to the nipple. Smaller subsegmental and segmental ducts join to form a main lactiferous duct that becomes progressively larger. One major lactiferous duct empties each breast lobe and extends radially toward the nipple. Beneath the areola, the main duct focally enlarges at the ampulla or lactiferous sinus, which serves as a reservoir for milk during breastfeeding. Some major ducts from the lobes may join at the sinus level before exiting as excretory ducts through tiny openings at the summit of the nipple.

The ducts are lined by an inner epithelial cell layer and an underlying myoepithelial cell layer. The myoepithelial cells contract to help transfer milk out of the TDLUs during lactation. Breast ducts are surrounded by a basement membrane that separates ductal structures from adjacent tissues.

The TDLU is of histologic importance because most benign and malignant breast diseases arise from this

FIGURE 18-1 Anatomic sectional illustration demonstrating the major anatomic components of the adult female breast and chest wall.

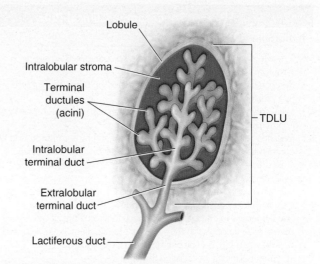

FIGURE 18-2 Terminal ductolobular unit (*TDLU*). A TDLU is composed of an extralobular terminal duct and a lobule. Each breast lobe contains numerous TDLUs.

structure. The majority of the glandular tissue lies in the upper outer quadrant (UOQ) of the breast. The TDLUs are typically confined to the mammary layer; however, a TDLU may occasionally project between a Cooper ligament into the superficial breast or retromammary layer. A portion of mammary tissue may also extend into the axilla, forming the axillary tail of Spence.

The breast stroma helps provide support to the breast. Adipose tissue (fat) is found in the premammary (subcutaneous) and retromammary layers and fills out the spaces between the lobes and the lobules. Although the breast slides easily over the pectoralis major muscle, the gland itself is firmly attached to the skin by thin connective tissue bands known as *Cooper ligaments*. These suspensory ligaments extend radially through the breast from the deep pectoral fascia to the skin, enclosing fat lobules and providing structural support. Interlobular stromal tissue and Cooper ligaments make up the dense connective tissue. Hormonally responsive, loose intralobular stroma surrounds the smaller ducts of the lobule. Loose periductal fibrous tissue surrounds the larger ducts.

Posterior to the breast and pectoral fascia are muscles that separate the breast tissue from the chest wall. The pectoralis major muscle lies beneath the upper two-thirds of the breast. The smaller pectoralis minor muscle lies beneath the major muscle. The serratus anterior muscle extends under the lateral breast. The external oblique muscle is beneath a portion of the lower outer breast and the rectus abdominis abuts part of the lower inner breast.

The primary arterial blood supply to the breast is from the internal thoracic (mammary) artery and the lateral thoracic artery. The internal thoracic artery is a branch of the subclavian artery, whereas the lateral thoracic artery arises from the axillary artery. Additional blood supply includes the thoracoacromial and intercostal arteries. Arterial anastomoses occur beneath the areola.

Venous drainage is through superficial and deep networks. Venous anastomosis occurs in a circular pattern around the base of the areola (circulus venosus). Deep veins follow the path of the arteries to drain the breast, with most drainage heading to the axillary vein. There are connections between the intercostal veins and the vertebral plexus that are potential pathways for bone and nervous system metastasis.

Lymph vessels originate in the connective tissues near the lactiferous ducts and communicate with the subareolar plexus (Sappey plexus). Lymph drainage is from deep to superficial networks. Numerous lymphatics lie under the skin. Lymph vessels drain into lymph nodes and follow venous drainage pathways out of the breast. Small intramammary lymph nodes are found within the breast, especially in the UOQ and near the axilla. The vast majority of breast lymph drains into the ipsilateral axillary lymph node chain (~75%). Lymphatic channels less often drain medially into the internal mammary (parasternal) nodes, which lie within the intercostal spaces alongside the sternum. Some lymph vessels drain to the opposite breast, toward the diaphragm, or to abdominal nodes. Axillary lymph nodes can be classified by anatomic location or by surgical level (Table 18-2). For surgical and staging purposes, the axillary nodes are subdivided by level relative to the pectoralis minor muscle.

The nerves of the breast are located along the skin and within the glandular tissue. Innervation of the breast is primarily derived from branches of the lateral and anterior cutaneous branches of the second to sixth intercostal (thoracic) nerves. The fourth intercostal nerve serves the nipple. Superficial sensory nerves join the cervical, brachial, and intercostal nerves.

SONOGRAPHIC ANATOMY[4-10,13-15,23]

The anatomic components of the breast are easily demonstrated by high-resolution sonography. The appearance of the normal female breast varies widely from patient to patient and depends on the relative amounts of fat, connective, and glandular tissue in the scanning plane. Unlike 2D mammography, sonography allows sectional evaluation of the breast, one "slice" at a time, from the skin surface to the chest wall, allowing delineation of all breast layers or zones (Fig. 18-3).

The skin layer is seen as two thin, reflective bands encasing a band of medium-level echoes representing the dermis. Scanning through an acoustic offset better delineates the skin. Normal skin thickness is usually 2 mm or less but slightly thicker near the areola and inframammary fold. The hyperechoic interface between the skin and subcutaneous fat should be intact. Changes in skin contour and thickness may indicate neoplastic, traumatic, postirradiation, or inflammatory changes at or below the skin surface.

The nipple displays a homogeneous texture of medium-level echoes. Connective tissue within the nipple and the irregular

TABLE 18-2   Classifications of Axillary Lymph Nodes

Anatomic Classification	Surgical Classification
• Anterior (pectoral) group: along lower border of pectoral minor muscle; near lateral thoracic vessels; receives most of lymphatic drainage. • Posterior (subscapular) group: along posterior lower axilla; by subscapular vessels. • Lateral (axillary vein) group: along the axillary vein at lateral wall of axilla. • Central group: lie in adipose tissue, deep to pectoralis minor muscle; medial to axillary vessels; most superficial and most easily palpated. • Apical (medial, infraclavicular) group: medial and posterior to pectoralis minor muscle at apex of axilla; near subclavian vessels; drainage path for other axillary node groups. (*Apical and infraclavicular nodes are sometimes listed as separate axillary node groups.*)	• Level I nodes: low axillary nodes lying lateral to the pectoralis minor muscle • Level II nodes: midaxillary nodes lying beneath the pectoralis minor muscle • Level III nodes: high axillary nodes lying medial to the pectoralis minor muscle *Note:* *Interpectoral (Rotter) group: located between pectoralis major and minor muscles by pectoral branch of thoracoacrominal artery; included as level II nodes.*

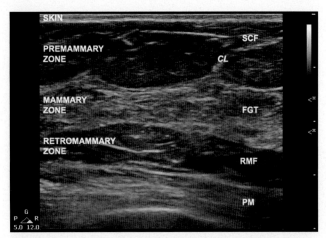

FIGURE 18-3 Normal adult female breast. Sonogram of breast zones (layers) between the skin and the chest wall: the *premammary zone* contains subcutaneous fat (*SCF*) outlining Cooper ligaments (*CL*); the *mammary zone* contains the fibroglandular tissues (*FGT*); and the *retromammary zone* contains retromammary fat (*RMF*). The mammary zone is encased within the anterior and posterior mammary fascial planes. Deep to the breast lies the pectoralis muscle (*PM*) of the chest wall. (Image courtesy of Philips Healthcare, Bothell, WA.)

contour of the nipple–areolar complex can cause acoustic shadowing. Probe compression and the use of ample scanning gel will flatten the nipple and reduce trapped air pockets to lessen shadowing. Transducer angulation beneath the nipple, the use of spatial compound imaging, or utilizing the two-handed peripheral scanning technique allows better evaluation of subareolar structures.

The premammary layer (subcutaneous fat layer) lies between the skin and the mammary layer and does not extend beneath the nipple. When equipment settings are properly set, the echogenicity of normal breast fat will be a midlevel gray shade. Blood vessels within this subcutaneous fat layer are easily compressed by transducer pressure. Cooper ligaments are best seen in the subcutaneous layer and imaged as thin, hyperechoic, curvilinear bands ascending from deep in the breast toward the

skin and encasing the fat lobules. At times, streaks of acoustic shadowing are seen at oblique interfaces from these connective tissue ligaments, caused by refraction of the sound beam.

The mammary layer lies deep to the subcutaneous fat and contains the breast parenchyma and supporting tissues. This mammary zone is enclosed between the reflective interfaces of the anterior and posterior mammary fascia.[9,10] In the adult breast, the mammary layer has the greatest variation in echo pattern depending on the distribution of glandular, fibrous, and fatty tissues. Dense stromal fibrous tissue is very hyperechoic relative to fat, whereas glandular (periductal, lobular) tissue is nearly isoechoic to fat (Fig. 18-4). Tubular fluid-filled ducts may be seen radiating from the nipple and into the breast core (Fig. 18-5). Major lactiferous ducts are best imaged with radial scans. Generally, ducts measure 2 mm or less but are often larger at the lactiferous sinus and during lactation.

The retromammary layer lies between the posterior mammary fascia and the pectoralis major muscle and contains small fat lobules and some suspensory ligaments. This retromammary fat layer appears thinner on a sonogram than the subcutaneous fat layer.

At the chest wall, the pectoralis major muscle lies immediately posterior to most of the breast. The pectoralis minor muscle lies beneath the major muscle in a more superolateral location. These muscles appear as striated hyperechoic and hypoechoic linear bands of echoes that run parallel to the chest wall. Recognition of the pectoral major muscle is important to confirm ample US penetration of the breast and to help determine whether a deep lying cancer is invading through the pectoral fascia.

Deep to the pectoral muscles are the ribs and intercostal muscle of the thoracic cage. Laterally, the bony portion of the ribs attenuates the sound beam, resulting in acoustic shadowing. Medially, the costal cartilage of the ribs appears as oval structures containing low-level echoes seen best on sagittal scans (Fig. 18-6). Care must be taken not to mistake the cartilaginous portion of the ribs for a breast mass. Rotating the transducer in orthogonal scan planes will confirm

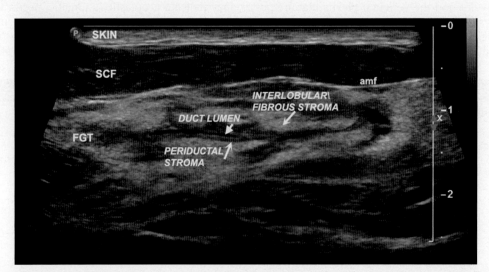

FIGURE 18-4 Fibroglandular tissue (*FGT*). The echogenicity of the periductal tissue and intralobular fibrous tissue is nearly isoechoic to fat. The dense interlobular fibrous tissue is hyperechoic to fat. Anechoic fluid is present within the duct lumen. The anterior mammary fascia (*amf*) separates the FGT in the mammary zone from the subcutaneous fat (*SCF*). (Image courtesy of Philips Healthcare, Bothell, WA.)

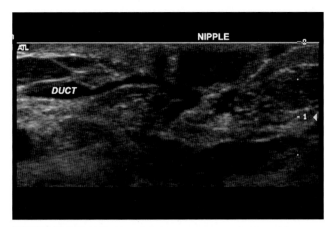

FIGURE 18-5 Fluid-filled breast ducts are seen converging toward the nipple. Radial scan planes best visualize major lactiferous ducts.

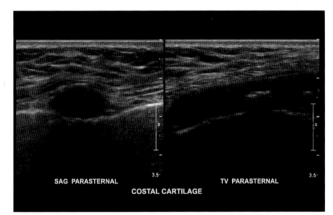

FIGURE 18-6 Costal cartilage. A cross section of the rib cartilage can be mistaken for a hypoechoic mass when scanning in the sagittal scan plane near the sternum. Rotating the transducer 90 degrees shows the linear extent of the cartilage and connection to the rib.

the cartilage is not a mass. The hyperechogenic interface beneath the chest wall demarcates total sound reflection from the lung.

Normal lymph nodes can be imaged by sonography, especially in the axilla. Normal intramammary nodes are less often detected. The size of a normal intramammary node is typically less than 1 cm, but axillary nodes can be larger. Normal nodes are oval or reniform in shape, circumscribed, and display a symmetrically thin hypoechoic outer cortex and a hyperechoic fatty hilum (Fig. 18-7). Color Doppler identifies a single feeding artery and draining vein at the hilum. Axillary nodes that contain mostly fat and have a very thin cortical rim may be difficult to delineate from adjacent structures. Enlarged lymph nodes may indicate inflammatory or neoplastic change.

VARIATIONS IN NORMAL PATTERNS

The proportionate amount of stromal and glandular tissues in the female breast depends on the patient's age, parity, and whether she is premenopausal or postmenopausal, pregnant or lactating, or obese. The prepubertal breast is small and fatty. At puberty, estrogen and progesterone stimulate breast development by promoting duct growth and lobular development. The adolescent breast becomes increasingly glandular, whereas the amount of surrounding fat diminishes.

The adult breast has the greatest range of appearances. Characteristically, the young, nulliparous female breast is densely glandular, with little internal or surrounding fat. Sonographically, the glandular tissue appears isoechoic to mildly hyperechoic compared with fat. Over time, more hyperechoic fibrous stroma is apparent within the mammary zone that can partially attenuate the sound beam. With increasing age and number of pregnancies, fatty replacement of the parenchyma begins to occur. Isolated, hypoechoic fat lobules in the mammary layer may appear "mass like" compared with the more echogenic surrounding fibroglandular

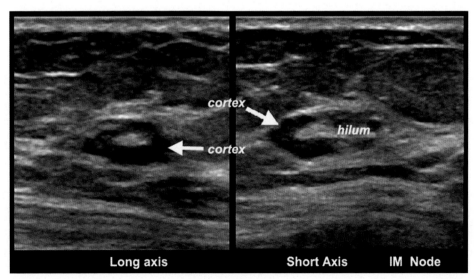

FIGURE 18-7 Normal intramammary lymph node. This small, circumscribed, oval node displays a hypoechoic cortex and hyperechoic fatty hilum. The cortex has a "C-shaped" appearance in cross section.

tissue; however, fat lobules are very compressible and often merge into other fat lobules on the orthogonal scan plane.

In the breast of the pregnant or lactating woman, glandular elements proliferate within the mammary layer, compressing the surrounding fat layers. Acini within the breast lobules develop and begin milk secretion in response to hormones that include placental lactogen, chorionic gonadotropin, and prolactin. The overall texture of this glandular parenchyma can become weakly echogenic compared with denser connective tissues within this layer. Duct dilatation may be marked during late pregnancy and lactation.

The postmenopausal breast may show complete or near-complete fatty replacement as the lobules and ducts atrophy as hormonal influences decline. Cooper ligaments are easily seen encasing the fat lobules. However, older, nulliparous women or those on hormone replacement therapy (HRT) may retain considerable amounts of glandular tissue.

DEVELOPMENTAL ANOMALIES[5,15,23,24]

In both genders, breast development begins in utero along bilateral ectodermal milk lines that extend from the axilla to the inguinal region. Although there are several points along the milk lines for breast tissue to develop, one paired set of breasts grow from mammary ridges located in the thoracic region. Rudimentary ducts arising from epithelial breast buds are present in both females and males at the time of birth. In the neonate, there may be some transient breast enlargement and milky nipple discharge because of residual circulating maternal hormones.

Developmental anomalies of the breast are uncommon. Some are associated with abnormal endocrine gland development or hormonal dysfunction and may not become apparent until puberty. Congenital nipple inversion is a normal variant. An accessory nipple (*polythelia*) is the most common congenital breast anomaly. A completely formed accessory breast (*polymastia*) is rare. These supernumerary anomalies can occur anywhere along the milk line. Accessory breast tissue in the axilla (without a nipple) is occasionally present. Underdevelopment (*hypoplasia*) or excessive growth (*hypertrophy*) of the breast tissue may affect one or both breasts. *Athelia* indicates congenital absence of the breast nipple. *Amastia* refers to absent development of the nipple, areola, and breast tissue. Poland syndrome is associated with underdevelopment or absence of the breast, nipple, and chest muscles. *Amazia* refers to absence of breast tissue development although the nipple is present. This acquired condition may be secondary to excessive chest wall radiation or inadvertent excision of premature breast tissue development in a child.

Before the age of 8 years, growth of one breast occasionally occurs before the other. By puberty, however, both breasts are usually comparable in size and development.[24] This variant, referred to as unilateral early ripening or unilateral premature thelarche, should not be mistaken for pathology and does not necessitate excision. Early developing glandular tissue images as a small, mildly hypoechoic region under the nipple corresponding to the palpable region of subareolar nodularity.

If development of both breasts occurs before 8 years of age, precocious puberty is suspected. Causes are varied. Sonographic signs of precocious puberty may include ovarian enlargement with prominent follicular cysts, the presence of a hormone-secreting ovarian tumor (e.g., granulosa–theca cell tumor), a large-for-age uterus, or an adrenal tumor.

BREAST SONOGRAPHIC EXAMINATION AND INSTRUMENTATION[4–18]

Before scanning, the indication for the examination, as well as any pertinent prior mammograms, breast sonograms, and/or other correlative imaging tests, is reviewed. The clinical history and the location of palpable masses, biopsy scars, and other changes of the skin, nipple, and breast contour are documented. Correlation of clinical and relevant imaging tests with the sonographic findings is imperative so the interpreting physician can more accurately assign a risk classification, provide a differential diagnosis, and make recommendations for patient management.

The American College of Radiology (ACR) publishes practice parameters and minimum equipment requirements for the performance of breast sonography.[16–18] Proper transducer selection, equipment setup, patient positioning, and scanning technique are essential to produce high-quality images.

Transducer Requirements

Based on 2016 ACR practice parameters, breast sonography should be performed utilizing a high-resolution, real-time, linear-array, broad-bandwidth transducer operating at a center frequency of at least 12 MHz and preferably higher.[4,16] Ultra-broadband transducers are now available that span even wider frequencies ranges, up to 15 to 18 MHz at the higher end (e.g., L17-5; eL18-4). High-frequency, broadbandwidth transducers provide better spatial and contrast resolution. Higher frequencies enhance image resolution and optimize detail of more superficial structures, whereas lower frequencies allow better penetration of attenuative tissues and deep lying structures. During the examination, the highest frequency capable of adequate sound penetration of the region of interest should be used.

Equipment and Grayscale Settings

Equipment settings must be optimized to display an image that clearly demonstrates all breast tissue from the skin line to the chest wall or for the selected region of interest. Handheld transducer footprints of 35 to 50 mm enable effective survey scanning of the breast. Important system controls include output power, time gain compensation (TGC), overall gain, dynamic range, as well as optimization of focal zones, image size, and image depth. In addition, image optimization is augmented by using harmonics, spatial compounding, speckle reduction, and speed-of-sound correction features, as applicable.

Appropriate grayscale setup is important for breast sonography. The gain settings, dynamic range, and processing curves should be set so that normal breast fat displays a medium-level gray shade. Using accepted ACR lexicon, the echogenicity of other breast structures and masses are described as being hypoechoic, isoechoic, or hyperechoic compared with normal (subcutaneous) fat.[4,6] Correct TGC settings will allow normal breast fat to be displayed with the same echogenicity within the premammary, mammary, and retromammary breast layers.

Proper sound beam focusing reduces volume-averaging artifacts and enhances detail of the area of interest. During survey of the breast, the number of focal zones should be increased to span depth of the mammary zone. When evaluating a mass, the focal zone should be placed at, or slightly below, the level of the mass to enhance resolution and posterior acoustic effects. Matrix-array transducers allow elevation plane focusing to further enhance near-field imaging.

Patient Positioning

Patient positioning during breast sonography can vary depending on breast size, mass location, or as needed for sonomammographic correlation. In general, the patient should be positioned in a manner that minimizes the thickness of the portion of the breast being examined. The patient is typically placed in a "supine-oblique" or "contralateral-oblique" position. This is accomplished by rolling the supine patient approximately 30 to 45 degrees, allowing placement of a wedge support to elevate the side of the body to be examined. The adjacent arm is extended near the head, which helps to stabilize the breast and provides access to the axillary region. The breast should appear flattened with the nipple centered. The reduction in breast thickness allows sound penetration by higher frequencies and orients major tissue planes more parallel to the face of the transducer optimizing sound beam reflection. This patient positioning can be used to scan the entire breast but is particularly useful when examining the outer breast. Steeper obliquity may be needed to scan large breasts or very lateral lesions. A straight supine position is often preferred when examining medial lesions.

Sometimes, a patient can only feel a mass while in a specific position. Scanning the patient in that position allows correlation of clinical and sonographic findings. For more accurate sonomammographic correlation of a breast mass, it may be helpful to scan certain patients in positions that simulate the mammographic views.

Scan Procedure and Technique

Based on site protocol and indication, either a targeted examination or a whole-breast sonographic examination is performed utilizing a handheld, high-resolution transducer. Targeted examinations are more common and limited to the quadrant or region of clinical concern, such as for a palpable mass, or to further characterize a mammographic or MRI finding. Some indications for a whole-breast examination include the search for satellite lesions and lymph node involvement in a patient with a known cancer or suspicious lesion to assist staging. In addition, sonography can canvas the breast to evaluate implant integrity.

As a supplement to mammography, a bilateral whole-breast US screening examination is warranted for some women with compromised mammograms due to high breast density and for women at high risk for breast cancer who are not the MRI candidates (or unable to easily access breast MRI testing). Screening US can be performed using a handheld transducer or an automated whole-breast system.

For a breast US examination, the patient is properly positioned, and a warm scanning gel is applied to the skin. The breast is methodically surveyed in overlapping orthogonal (perpendicular) scan planes with special attention paid to the areas of concern. Orthogonal scan planes include sagittal (longitudinal) and transverse, or radial and antiradial image planes (Fig. 18-8). Radial and antiradial scan planes are of particular value during breast imaging. Radial scans better follow lobar anatomy and are often best for examining major lactiferous ducts or for documenting mass location relative to the nipple. Scanning the entire volume of a solid breast mass in both radial and antiradial planes can increase detection of tumor extension coursing toward the nipple within a major duct or branching outward into smaller ducts.

The skin overlying a palpable lump can be marked before scanning or the location confirmed during the examination. *Echopalpation* (*sonopalpation*) refers to concurrent palpation of a region of interest while scanning.[10,15] For example, the sonographer secures the palpable area between two fingers while scanning directly over the lump. This allows direct correlation of clinical and sonographic findings. Alternatively, the sonographer can place a thin marker producing a shadowing artifact (e.g., opened metal paper clip) between the transducer and palpable finding. Images are taken with and without this "marker" to correlate and document the location of the palpable finding. The image should be annotated as the "palpable" area of interest.

The use of an acoustic standoff between the transducer and the breast improves delineation of the skin layer and very superficial breast masses by optimizing near-field focusing and reducing artifacts. In most cases, extra scanning gel is a sufficient standoff. When a standoff pad is used, the thickness of the acoustic offset should not exceed 1 cm so that the focal plane (elevation focus) is not shifted out of the breast.[10]

Scanning with a variety of beam angles is needed to fully evaluate the margin characteristics of a breast mass. This can be accomplished by rocking and angling the transducer (heel–toe maneuver) and by using spatial compounding.[10]

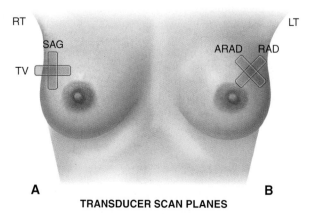

FIGURE 18-8 Orthogonal scan planes. **A:** Schematic of traditional sagittal (*SAG*) and transverse (*TV*) scan planes. **B:** Radial (*RAD*) and antiradial (*ARAD*) scan planes are particularly useful for evaluating ductal structures and mass features.

Enlarging the image to the region of interest and focusing at the level of the mass allow better inspection of mass features.

During the breast examination, applying variable amounts of transducer pressure to compress the underlying tissues is beneficial for a variety of reasons. Compression decreases breast thickness for better sound penetration by higher frequencies. Applying transducer pressure flattens Cooper ligaments to reduce critical angle shadowing. Compression will also reduce or eliminate false acoustic shadowing beneath a benign lesion or scar tissue, whereas malignant shadowing tends to persist. Alternating the application and release of transducer pressure (ballottement) helps assess the compressibility and mobility of breast masses, as well as the movement of internal echoes in complicated cysts and dilated ducts. In contrast, too much transducer pressure is detrimental during Doppler evaluation because vessel compression can reduce or ablate blood flow.

Positional changes can be advantageous when trying to shift internal debris, fluid–debris levels, or fat–fluid levels within a complicated cystic mass, or move a dependent milk-of-calcium sediment layer.

Key lesions should be documented with and without caliper measurements.[4,16] Minimally, the maximal dimensions of a mass should be recorded in at least two planes (orthogonal planes preferred). Maximal dimensions, rather than mean diameter, correlate better with mammographic measurements. Obtaining measurements in three dimensions (maximal length, height, and width) allows for more accurate comparison of lesion size, or calculation of mass volume, for follow-up imaging or after intervention. Height-to-width ratios can also be calculated when assessing benign and malignant imaging characteristics.

Obtaining a comparison scan of the opposite breast in the same region can be helpful when sorting out questionable findings and helps to contrast inflammatory or traumatic changes with the normal breast tissue. Side-to-side comparison is also helpful when assessing axillary nodes.

Based on site protocol and reason for the examination, representative images are acquired of the region of interest, or expanded to document each breast quadrant, the subareolar region, and the axilla, when indicated. Important findings are documented.

Minimum documentation of a handheld, whole-breast screening US examination that is negative for mass detection should include a representative view of each breast quadrant (at the same level) and the retroareolar region. These can be taken in a single scan plane, such as the radial plane.[10,18]

Images are appropriately labeled, interpreted, and archived. Most digital picture archiving and communication system (PACS) can archive dynamic cine clips, showing full sweeps of the breast tissue, pathologic conditions, and needle placement during interventional examinations.

Image Annotation[4,9,10,13,16]

Breast sonograms should document the facility's name and location, the examination date, the patient's name, date of birth and/or identification number, and the initials (or another notation) as to the sonographer/physician performing the examination.

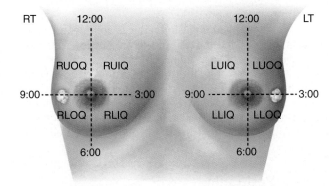

QUADRANT AND CLOCK-FACE ANNOTATION

FIGURE 18-9 Quadrant and clockface image annotation: upper outer quadrant (*UOQ*), upper inner quadrant (*UIQ*), lower inner quadrant (*LIQ*), and lower outer quadrant (*LOQ*). Using the clockface annotation, a mass lateral to the nipple in the right breast is located at 9 o'clock (RT 9:00), whereas a mass lateral to the nipple in the left breast is located at 3 o'clock (LT 3:00).

Accurate labeling of each image should include side (right or left), transducer location and scan plane, and mass location in the breast, in order to accurately document findings for the interpreting physician. Proper image annotation is also important for follow-up comparison and to relocate a mass before intervention.

Over the years, a variety of labeling methods have been used to annotate breast sonograms, including the quadrant, clockface, and 1-2-3: A-B-C methods (Figs. 18-9 and 18-10). Current ACR practice parameters state that the location of a breast lesion on the sonogram should be annotated using the clockface position, distance in centimeters from the nipple (not the areola), and the transducer orientation.[16] Many systems provide a breast body marker for additional documentation of transducer position and scan plane. One way to annotate a right breast mass located 5 cm from the nipple in the radial scan plane is "RT 9:00 5 CM FN RAD." Most breast imaging transducers have a footprint of 3.8 to 5 cm, which is helpful as a measuring guide. Using a ruler or placing a piece of tape with centimeter marks along the

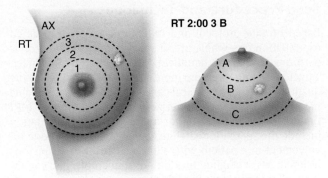

"1-2-3 A-B-C" ANNOTATION

FIGURE 18-10 1-2-3: A-B-C annotation. The breast is divided into three concentric rings from the areola to denote the relative distance of a mass from the nipple: *1*, inner third of the breast; *2*, mid third; *3*, outer third of the breast. To denote the relative distance of a mass from the skin to the chest wall, the breast is divided into thirds: *A*, anterior third; *B*, mid third; *C*, posterior third of breast. A peripheral right breast mass at the 2 o'clock position, in the mid mammary zone, can be annotated, "RT 2:00 3 B."

side the transducer helps to estimate mass–nipple distance. Some new breast transducers are now manufactured with centimeter marks embedded along the side of the transducer. On occasion, two closely positioned masses may reside in the same scan frame. In such situations, an additional measurement of the distance from the skin to the mass (mass depth) can help differentiate these lesions in the final report.

The "1-2-3: A-B-C" labeling method has been used to note the relative distance of a mass from the nipple, as well as the depth within the breast.[9,10] This method also had value when relocating a mass, especially when intervention was to be done at a different facility. Some facilities still elect to record the depth of a lesion using the A-B-C method in addition to the more current ACR annotation recommendations.

Specialty Techniques

Most current breast handheld sonography systems have split-screen capabilities, extended field-of-view (EFOV), or convex linear (trapezoidal) 2D imaging features that allow larger spans of breast anatomy and masses to be displayed and measured.

Harmonic imaging and spatial compounding are now common equipment features that improve contrast and spatial resolution during breast imaging. These techniques reduce image artifacts (e.g., speckle, noise, reverberation) and show better margin delineation, which help make subtle masses, such as small isoechoic lesions, more apparent on the sonogram. Spatial compounding creates a single real-time image from multiple scan angles and improves margin delineation. Besides reducing detrimental image artifacts, spatial compounding may also reduce demonstration of helpful attenuation artifacts. The sonographer should be aware that enhancement beneath a small cyst or subtle shadowing from a cancer may be reduced or eliminated at higher levels of spatial compounding yet be apparent on conventional imaging. Therefore, scanning a region of interest with and without spatial compounding may be necessary.

Many newer generation scanners have a system control that the sonographer can use to adjust the speed of sound, especially when imaging the fatty breast. Sound travels slower in fat than in soft tissues. Applying speed-of-sound correction can improve spatial and contrast resolution for better image quality. Improvements include better depiction of mass margins, tissue interfaces, and calcifications.

3D imaging provides surface or volume rendering of breast masses that can be further manipulated after completion of the scan. A volume data set can also be viewed in multiple static image planes (multiplanar), which is particularly helpful when assessing margin and wall characteristics of solid masses and complex cysts. 3D US shows breast masses in three orthogonal planes. Compared with conventional 2D imaging, the additional coronal plane is of particular value when analyzing the growth pattern of masses and effects on surrounding tissues. Reconstructed coronal scans better illustrate malignant features such as spiculation (Fig. 18-11) shown as a "retraction/star" pattern, compared with a "compression" pattern seen with more circumscribed benign masses.[25] Real-time 3D imaging (4D) may be of value during guidance procedures.

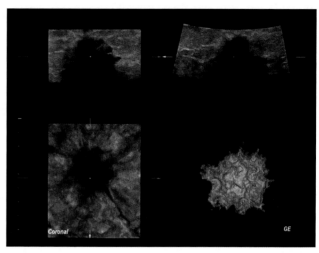

FIGURE 18-11 Three-dimensional (3D) sonogram. Malignant spiculation, displaying a "star" pattern, is best appreciated on the reconstructed coronal plane (bottom left image). A volume rendering of the mass is shown on the bottom right. (Image courtesy of GE Healthcare, Milwaukee, WI.)

SONOGRAPHIC–MAMMOGRAPHIC CORRELATION[6,7,15]

Breast sonography usually follows clinical and mammographic examinations with the hope of providing more specific diagnostic information for appropriate patient management. The breast sonographer must have at least a basic understanding of mammography in order to properly correlate sonographic with mammographic findings. Table 18-3 compares the tissue densities and echogenicities of common breast structures seen on mammography and sonography.

Mammography is performed on asymptomatic patients to screen for occult breast cancer or on symptomatic patients to diagnose a clinical concern. The standard of care has been 2D full-field digital mammography (FFDM). However, many sites also offer 3D mammography, known as digital breast tomosynthesis (DBT), which allows breast tissue to be additionally reviewed in layers besides standard screening views.

A 2D mammogram is a superimposed image of all breast tissue compressed between the X-ray image receptor and a compression plate. Images are labeled for the specific view and breast side (laterality). Standard mammographic screening projections are the craniocaudal (CC) and the mediolateral oblique (MLO) views (Fig. 18-12). Besides these standard views, additional views (e.g., spot compression, magnification, 90-degree lateral) may be obtained during a diagnostic mammogram to better assess a palpable mass or to further examine an abnormality found on the screening examination.

For the mammographic CC view, the X-ray tube is oriented vertically over the breast with the patient upright. The breast is positioned so that the X-ray beam enters the superior (cranial) breast and exits the inferior (caudal) breast. The side marker is always placed by the lateral breast. With the nipple centered, this view demonstrates the medial, central, and lateral breast.

The MLO view shows breast tissue from the axilla to the inframammary fold and includes a portion of the pectoralis muscle and lower axilla. The nipple is seen in profile. The

TABLE 18-3 **Comparison of Tissue Densities and Echogenicities**	
Mammogram Density	**Ultrasound Echogenicities**
Fat Density: (radiolucent—gray) • Fat • Fat density mass (e.g., oil cyst; lipoma; galactocele) • Fatty hilum of lymph node **Water Density:** (radiodensity greater than fat; described as low, equal to, or high density compared with equal volume of fibroglandular tissue) • Fibroglandular tissues; ducts • Blood vessels • Cooper ligaments • Cortex of lymph node • Solid and cystic masses • Pectoralis muscle **Calcium:** (appears radiopaque) Calcifications ***Other:*** ***Foreign body:*** *(radiopaque)* • *Clip marker* • *Silicone* • *Pacemaker* ***Air – VAB site:*** *(lacks density; appears black)* **Notes:** • Mass density does not differentiate solid from cystic masses. • Mass detection is best in fat-replaced breast.	**Isoechoic/Nearly Isoechoic:** (midlevel grayshade) • Fat (reference tissue) • Lipoma • Glandular (epithelial) tissue; adenosis; periductal/lobular tissue • Certain solid masses and complicated cysts **Hyperechoic:** (more echogenic than normal fat) • Interlobular stromal fibrous tissue • Cooper ligaments • Skin; fascial interfaces • Edematous fat/fibrosis • Echogenic capsule; cyst wall • Muscle: striated hyperechoic/hypoechoic bands **Hypoechoic:** (less echogenic than normal fat) • Nipple • Complicated fluid; inspissated duct secretions • Benign/malignant solid mass (some cancers are markedly hypoechoic) • Lymph node cortex (abnormal nodes may be markedly hypoechoic or nearly anechoic) **Anechoic:** (without internal echoes) • Simple cyst; certain fluid collections • Blood; duct secretions; dilated lymphatics • Saline/silicone implant

side marker is placed near the axilla at the outer breast. Depending on body habitus, the plane of the image receptor for the MLO view is approximately 45 degrees (± 15 degrees) from horizontal to be parallel with the plane of the pectoralis muscle. Unlike a true 90-degree lateral projection, the X-ray beam passes from the superomedial to the inferolateral breast for the MLO projection. For screening purposes, the MLO view shows the greatest amount of breast tissue in a single view. This projection best images the UOQ and axillary tail but may exclude some posteromedial tissue. Lower axillary lymph nodes are often visible on this projection.

Although not a screening view, a true 90-degree lateral projection shows a true profile of the breast and accurately shows the superior-to-inferior location of masses relative to

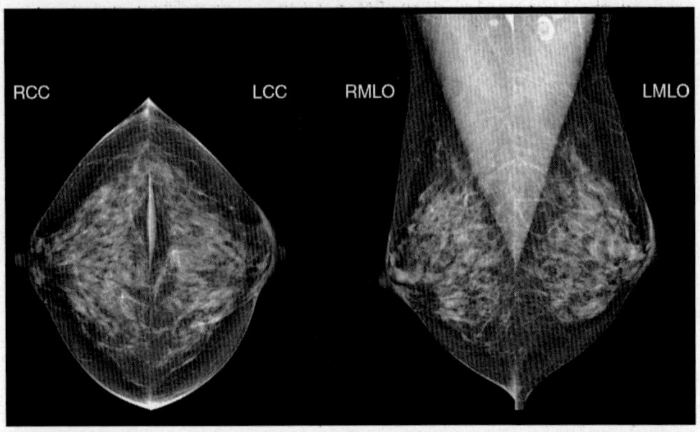

FIGURE 18-12 Mammographic standard views of both breasts. Craniocaudal (*CC*) view shows the lateral, central, and medial breast with the nipple centered. The side marker denotes the outer breast. The mediolateral oblique (*MLO*) view shows the upper to lower breast with the nipple in profile. The lower axilla and pectoralis muscle are seen on the MLO view. The side marker is always placed by the outer breast near the axilla. (Image courtesy of Hologic Inc., Marlborough, MA.)

the posterior nipple line. However, this view restricts seeing the axillary region. This mammogram view is helpful for mass localization before biopsy and for demonstration of air–fluid or fat–fluid levels or dependent milk-of-calcium sediment.

The size, shape, location, and surrounding tissue density need to be compared when correlating a breast mass on mammography and sonography.[9,10] Differences in technique, patient positioning, and direction of tissue compression between the mammogram and the sonogram can affect the relative location, orientation, and shape of a breast mass when correlating imaging findings. The margin characteristics and tissues surrounding a mass should be compared between modality images for concordance (e.g., mass surrounded by fat). During mammographic positioning, breast tissues (and masses) are pulled away from the chest wall. During sonography, structures are pushed toward the chest wall by transducer compression in an anteroposterior (AP) direction, making breast layers appear thinner. Taking this into account, a mass that abuts the anterior mammary layer on the mammogram should still correlate with that location on the sonogram. Compression can also alter the shape and orientation of some masses when correlating findings between modalities.

The radiologist can assist the sonographer when triangulating the true location of a breast mass seen on a mammogram before US scanning because patient positioning is different. The CC view shows the lateral, central, or medial location of a mass with minimal rotation and best correlates with the US location. Because of the oblique path of the X-ray beam for the MLO view, a mass may project higher or lower on the mammogram than its actual location in the breast. A medial mass can actually lie higher, whereas a lateral mass can lie lower in the breast than where it is shown on the MLO view. This is especially true for more peripheral lesions near 3:00 or 9:00. This must be taken into account when performing the US scan and may necessitate scanning a larger wedge of tissue to locate the mass. Remembering the acronym "MULD" for *medial-up* and *lateral down* will help the sonographer remember this concept during sonomammographic correlation. Generally, a more centrally located breast mass (near 12:00, subareolar, or 6:00) is more accurately shown as to its true location on standard screening mammogram views.

Real-time scanning an entire breast hemisphere is often needed to locate a mass seen on only one mammographic view. For example, a mass shown only on the CC view in the lateral breast may necessitate scanning the full outer hemisphere of the breast.

With the patient supine, it is occasionally difficult to be certain whether a mass seen by sonography is the same mass demonstrated by mammography, especially in larger breasted women. By scanning the patient in a position that simulates the radiographic projection, the sonographic location of a mass can be more accurately correlated, although breast tissues will be less compressed. To simulate the CC projection during the sonography examination, the patient can sit upright and use her opposite hand to lift the lower surface of the breast so the nipple is in profile.[14,15] This technique can be helpful to locate a mass seen only on the CC view.

SONOGRAPHIC DESCRIPTORS AND CLASSIFICATION OF FINDINGS[4–16,26]

The ACR originally developed the Breast Imaging Reporting and Data System (BI-RADS) to standardize the reporting of mammographic findings, as well as classifying findings into risk categories for cancer.[4] The BI-RAD system is now also applied to the classification of sonography and MRI findings. Recommendations for patient management follow the level of risk assessment (Table 18-4).

Breast patients are often referred for US examination based on a screening mammogram report that states the following: BI-RADS Category 0: incomplete; needs additional imaging

evaluation. In such cases, the radiologist will require "more information" before assigning a final risk category. Often, these are cases when a mass or focal asymmetry is present on the mammogram and sonography is needed to further characterize the mass as solid or cystic and to provide other diagnostic imaging features that may favor a benign versus a suspicious process.

The ACR published a "BI-RADS Breast Ultrasound Lexicon" to promote the use of more consistent terminology when describing and reporting sonographic findings (Table 18-5).[4,16] When applicable, similar terms are applied to mammographic and sonographic features. The ACR BI-RADS lexicon also includes descriptions of tissue composition to be reported with screening breast US examinations. Breast tissue composition on US can appear homogeneously fatty, or display homogeneous echogenic fibroglandular tissue with little surrounding fat, or show a more heterogeneous echo pattern.

When a mass is demonstrated by sonography, its imaging characteristics must be carefully examined, as well as any effects on surrounding tissues. A mass occupies space and must be confirmed in orthogonal US scan planes. Real-time imaging facilitates complete inspection of a mass. For lesion analysis, primary US features include mass shape, orientation in the breast relative to the skin line, margin characteristics, internal echo pattern, and posterior acoustic features. Mass features of most importance for cancer risk assessment are shape, orientation, and margin characteristics.[4,9,10,16]

Sonographic features most characteristics of a benign solid breast mass are oval shape, a parallel orientation relative to the skin (wider-than-tall, horizontally positioned), and a smoothly circumscribed margin. A circumscribed mass shows sharp demarcation from surrounding tissues along its entire margin. An oval mass is elliptical or egg shaped and may display two or three surface undulations, alternatively referred to as gentle lobulation or macrolobulation. Using the BI-RADS US lexicon, "irregular" is a descriptor of shape rather than margin. Unlike cysts, solid breast masses are less often round. An oval, parallel-oriented lesion will have a greater length than height, a feature referred to as "wider-than-tall."[9,10] Benign solid masses tend to be mildly

TABLE 18-4	American College of Radiology Ultrasound BI-RADS Assessment Categories		
Assessment Category		**Likelihood of Malignancy**	**Management**
0	Incomplete—Need additional imaging evaluation	NA	Recall for additional imaging
Final Assessment Categories			
1	Negative	Essentially 0%	Routine screening
2	Benign	Essentially 0%	Routine screening
3	Probably benign	>0% but ≤2%	Short-interval (6 months) follow-up or continued surveillance
4	Suspicious 4A—*Low suspicion* 4B—*Moderate suspicion* 4C—*High suspicion*	>2 but <95%	Tissue diagnosis
5	Highly suggestive of malignancy	≥95%	Tissue diagnosis
6	Known biopsy-proven malignancy	NA	Surgical excision when clinically appropriate

Reprinted with permission from Sickles EA, D'Orsi CJ, Bassett LW, et al. ACR BI-RADS® Mammography. In: *ACR BI-RADS® Atlas, Breast Imaging Reporting and Data System*. American College of Radiology; 2013.

TABLE 18-5 **American College of Radiology BI-RADS Ultrasound Lexicon**	
BREAST TISSUE	
Tissue composition (screening only)	• Homogeneous background echotexture—fat • Homogeneous background echotexture—fibroglandular • Heterogeneous background echotexture
FINDINGS	
Masses: Occupy space and should be seen in two different planes on 2D imaging; three planes on volumetric 3D imaging	**Shape** • Oval • Round • Irregular
	Orientation • Parallel (*wider-than-tall: horizontal*) • Not parallel (*taller-than-wide: vertical*)

	Margin
	• Circumscribed
	• Not circumscribed
	  • Indistinct
	  • Angular
	  • Microlobulated
	  • Spiculated

	Echo pattern • Anechoic • Hyperechoic • Complex cystic and solid • Hypoechoic • Isoechoic • Heterogeneous
	Posterior features • No posterior features • Enhancement • Shadowing • Combined pattern
Calcifications	• Calcifications in a mass • Calcifications outside a mass • Intraductal calcifications

Associated features	• Architectural distortion
	• Duct changes
	• Skin changes
	  • Skin thickening
	  • Skin retraction
	• Edema
	• Vascularity
	  • Absent
	  • Internal vascularity
	  • Vessels in rim
	• Elasticity assessment
	  • Soft
	  • Intermediate
	  • Hard

Special cases	• Simple cyst
	• Clustered microcysts
	• Complicated cyst
	• Mass in or on skin
	• Foreign body including implants
	• Lymph nodes—intramammary
	• Lymph nodes—axillary
	• Vascular abnormalities
	  • AVMs (arteriovenous malformation; pseudoaneurysms)
	  • Mondor disease
	• Postsurgical fluid collection
	• Fat necrosis

Based on American College of Radiology. *BI-RADS Atlas-Breast Ultrasound.* 5th ed. 2013. Refer to Atlas for full description of lexicon terms. Accessed November 20, 2020. www.acr.org.

hypoechoic or isoechoic compared with fat and show normal sound transmission (no posterior features) or mild enhancement. A purely hyperechoic lesion or focal region of hyperechoic fibrous stromal tissue in the area of clinical concern also favors a benign diagnosis.

Sonographic features most suspicious for malignancy include an irregular shape, nonparallel orientation (taller-than-wide, vertically positioned), and a margin that is not circumscribed along all, or any portion, of the mass. Round masses are also considered "not parallel" in orientation. Margins that are "not circumscribed" may be indistinct, angular, microlobulated, or spiculated. An indistinct margin is ill-defined and shows no clear demarcation between the lesion's border and surrounding tissues. The presence of a thick echogenic rim can also make margins indistinct. In addition, a cancer may show a combination of circumscribed and noncircumscribed features.

Echogenicity alone is a less specific criterion when predicting cancer because most benign and malignant solid masses are hypoechoic compared with normal subcutaneous fat. However, a markedly hypoechoic mass is a suspicious finding, especially when combined with other worrisome imaging features.

Masses attenuate sound differently. Shadowing is a suspicious posterior feature of a solid mass and can, in part, reflect fibrotic changes within and around the lesion (e.g., desmoplasia), but may also occur with certain benign processes. In addition, higher grade, more cellular breast cancers can show sound enhancement.

A heterogeneous echo pattern shows as mixture of internal echogenicities and has less validity in predicting cancer.[4] A complex cystic and solid mass displays both anechoic (cystic or fluid) and echogenic (solid) components and can be worrisome in the absence of known infection or trauma.

When detected by US, breast calcifications are reported as calcifications in a mass, calcifications outside a mass, or intraductal calcifications. Calcifications can be benign or malignant and are better detected and characterized as to size and distribution by mammography. Because of their tiny size (<0.5 mm), microcalcifications do not shadow on US because of smaller than the sound beam width and are typically best seen within a hypoechoic breast mass. A breast mass with microcalcifications is suspicious for cancer. However, newer high-resolution transducers and equipment processing features have made microcalcifications more discernible with US imaging. Macrocalcifications are typically benign.

Associated features are listed in the ACR lexicon. These include changes in adjacent tissues or structures owing to the presence of a breast mass or abnormality. Associated changes in the skin, tissues planes, Cooper ligaments, ductal structures, and vascularity provide additional clues when differentiating benign from malignant growth patterns. Sometimes, a focal area of architectural distortion or tissue disruption is evident without a focal mass. A benign mass typically compresses, rather than disrupts, adjacent tissues. Suspicious findings include straightening or thickening of Cooper ligaments, obliteration of tissue planes, or aberrations in ductal patterns. The presence of intraductal extension from a tumor should be sought because it impacts surgical management.[7,10]

Duct changes that occur in the breast include cystic dilatation, irregular caliber and/or arborization, ductal distortion by a mass, ductal extension to or from a suspicious mass, or an intraductal mass, thrombus, or debris. Skin changes can manifest as areas of thickening or retraction can indicate underlying malignancy, inflammatory cancer, or be related to benign inflammation, prior trauma, or radiation. Breast edema produces increased echogenicity of affected tissues and may have a reticulated appearance from dilated lymphatics and interstitial fluid. Tissue edema can have benign causes (e.g., mastitis, congestive heart failure, irradiation) but could also manifest with malignancy (e.g., inflammatory carcinoma, lymphoma).[4,14]

Elasticity assessment of breast masses is a recent addition to the lexicon, although not available at all US facilities. Elastography evaluates the stiffness of breast lesions relative to adjacent tissues. Similar to clinical palpation, benign masses tend to be soft or compressible, whereas malignant masses tend to be hard or stiff when assessed by elastography methods. Using the ACR lexicon, stiffness characteristics are reported as *soft, intermediate,* or *hard.*[4] Elastography is performed in conjunction with 2D US imaging. Greater reliance is given to the morphologic features seen on 2D imaging for equivocal findings.

Breast cancers typically show several suspicious imaging findings, but not always. Some cancers resemble a benign mass, whereas some benign masses and inflammatory and traumatic changes mimic cancer, so close correlation with clinical history and related imaging examinations is important. Because mass characterization is also affected by technical factors, adherence to proper scanning technique and equipment setup is critical, as well as recognition of diagnostic pitfalls.

Special cases are listed in the ACR BI-RADS US lexicon that include conditions with a unique diagnosis or display specific findings, including *simple cyst, clustered microcysts, complicated cysts, mass in or on the skin, foreign body including implants, lymph nodes, vascular abnormalities, postsurgical fluid collections,* and *fat necrosis.*[4] These are discussed later in this chapter, along with further discussion on solid breast mass assessment and elastography.

BREAST DISEASE AND TISSUE VARIATIONS

A variety of physiologic and pathologic changes affect the breast, many of which have features detectable by imaging techniques. Many of these conditions are reviewed in this chapter.

Sonographic Assessment of Cystic Breast Masses[4–15,27]

During the sonographic examination of a breast mass, the first step is to determine whether the mass is cystic or solid. Cystic breast masses can be described as simple cysts, clustered microcysts, complicated cysts, or complex cystic and solid masses based on imaging findings. Classifying a simple breast cyst is easy when diagnostic criteria are met but can be confusing when cyst fluid is complicated by cellular debris, hemorrhage, or infection. Cystic masses that contain solid elements add to diagnostic uncertainty and require additional workup to determine their benign or, possibly, malignant nature. Clinical history and correlative imaging factor into making a differential diagnosis.

Simple Cyst

True cysts are epithelial-lined, fluid-filled masses. Most breast cysts are related to fibrocystic change (FCC) and develop over time from progressive dilatation of small ducts within an obstructed TDLU. Cysts are the most common cause of breast lumps in women aged 35 to 50 years. They can be single or multiple in number and range from millimeters to several centimeters in size. Ductal secretions and fluid reabsorption contribute to variability in cyst size. With time, most cysts regress or involute. Cysts are uncommon in young or elderly women. However, in postmenopausal women receiving HRT, a cyst may develop, persist, or enlarge.

Signs and Symptoms

Small and flaccid cysts are often asymptomatic. Tense or enlarging cysts are usually palpable and may be tender. Palpable cysts are typically round or oval, smooth, and freely mobile. Most cysts are compressible unless tense.

Mammographic Features

On a mammogram, cysts appear as round or oval, smoothly marginated water density masses that are often equal in density to the surrounding parenchyma. These circumscribed masses compress adjacent tissues and are encircled by a thin radiolucent rim, referred to as the *halo sign* (Fig. 18-13A). Although findings appear benign, mammography alone cannot tell whether a circumscribed water density lesion is cystic or solid, so a sonography examination is recommended for mass characterization.

Sonographic Features of a Simple Cyst

The accurate diagnosis of a simple breast cyst is a key role of sonography and is important for subsequent patient management. Diagnostic criteria for a simple cyst are summarized in Table 18-6. Diagnostic US findings include a round or oval shape, a thin-walled circumscribed wall, absent internal echoes (anechoic), and posterior enhancement. Thin refractive edge shadowing is often apparent unless scanning with spatial compounding. In addition, transducer pressure can show the compressibility and mobility of a cyst. No color Doppler signal will be generated by the fluid-filled mass. When strict criteria are met, the diagnosis of a simple cyst can be made with a high level of confidence, allowing for a

TABLE 18-6 **Sonographic Features: Benign Simple Cyst**	
Primary Findings	**Additional Findings**
• Round or oval shape • Smooth, thin, circumscribed margin • Absent internal echoes (anechoic) • Posterior sound enhancement	• Absent Doppler flow signal • Compressibility with transducer pressure (unless tense cyst) • Mobility with transducer pressure

Note: Spatial compounding can reduce edge shadowing and the degree of distal sound enhancement.

BI-RADS 2 (benign) ACR classification (Fig. 18-13B). In such cases, no intervention or follow-up is required unless the cyst is symptomatic or enlarges, or if the presence of multiple cysts reduces mammographic efficacy for cancer screening.

Technical Considerations

Appropriate equipment settings and scanning technique are critical to ensure diagnostic accuracy. Angulation of the sound beam allows all walls to be visualized, helping to exclude wall thickening or an intracystic mass. Proper focusing and the use of spatial compounding and/or harmonic imaging enhance margin delineation and help reduce internal artifacts. A true simple cyst should be echo free at normal gain settings and retain a crisp back wall at low gain. Sound enhancement may diminish when a cyst is small, viscous, lies deep near the muscle, or can be related to technical factors (e.g., poor focusing, use of spatial compounding).

Clustered Microcysts[4]

Clustered microcysts describes a grouping of tiny cysts (each <2 to 3 mm) separated by thin (<0.5 mm) intervening septations or walls. This finding represents cystic dilatation of the tiny ductules (acini) within an enlarged breast lobule. At times, the surface may appear microlobulated, somewhat like a cluster of grapes, yet the margin remains distinct. Occasionally, tiny, dependent, hyperechoic foci may be evident, reflecting *milk of calcium*. Microcyst clusters with thin septations, and no solid components, are typically benign[4,5] (Fig. 18-14). The presence of thick isoechoic septations or solid components increases the risk of an intracystic papilloma or malignancy.

Complicated Cysts versus Complex Cystic and Solid Masses

Some cystic breast masses contain internal echoes or wall changes that are evident with high-resolution sonographic systems. These masses do not meet "simple cyst" criteria and are, instead, classified as complicated cysts or complex cystic and solid masses. A "nonsimple" breast cyst should be evaluated for signs of acute inflammation or infection and for more worrisome signs of neoplastic change. Possible causes of real echoes within a cystic breast mass are listed in Table 18-7.[9,10]

Circumscribed, thin-walled, complicated cysts are typically benign and often related to FCCs. These are frequently nonpalpable incidental findings and often coexist with simple cysts. Only rarely is a true intracystic tumor present, which may be benign or malignant.

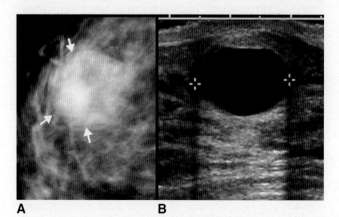

FIGURE 18-13 Simple cyst. **A:** Mammogram shows a rounded, circumscribed, water density mass with a radiolucent halo (*arrows*). **B:** Conventional sonogram demonstrates a rounded, circumscribed, thin-walled, anechoic mass with posterior enhancement and refractive edge shadowing.

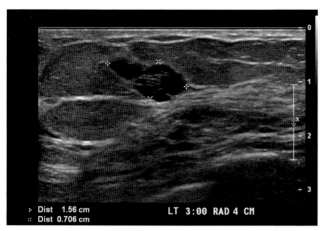

FIGURE 18-14 Cyst cluster. Sonogram showing a cluster of cystically dilated acini (ductules) within an enlarged lobule with thin intervening septations. Microcyst or macrocyst clusters are possible depending on the degree of ductule dilatation.

TABLE 18-7   Causes of Real Echoes within Nonsimple Cysts[9,10]

- Cellular debris
- Cholesterol crystals
- Epithelial cells; apocrine cells (floating, papillary)
- Protein globules; foam cells; fat globules
- Blood; pus
- Fibrous intervening walls of cyst cluster
- Intramural neoplasm (rare)

TABLE 18-8   Sonographic Features of Nonsimple Cysts

Complicated Cysts	Complex Cystic and Solid Mass (Suspicious Findings)
Thin-walled cyst containing • Homogeneous low-level internal echoes • Mobile internal echoes • Fluid–debris level • Fat–fluid level	• Thick wall (≥0.5 mm) • Thick septations (≥0.5 mm) • Intracystic mass (intramural nodule) • Mixed solid/cystic components

Sonographic Features

Sonography of a nonsimple cystic mass involves assessment of the cyst wall, internal echo pattern, movement of internal echoes, and surrounding tissues (Table 18-8). Color- or power-mode Doppler assesses for vascularity of the cyst wall and internal contents.

Complicated cysts represent breast cysts with internal debris without a discrete solid component.[4,9,10,27] Otherwise, these cysts maintain a thin, circumscribed wall and typically show distal acoustic enhancement. Echoes within complicated breast cysts can present as a fluid–debris level, a fat–fluid level, or homogeneous low-level internal echoes (Fig. 18-15 A–C). The mobility of the internal echoes and fat–fluid levels can be assessed by changing the patient's position or applying and releasing transducer pressure over the mass. Increasing the system's transmit power or applying Doppler can induce lightweight echoes within a cyst (e.g., cholesterol crystals) to move or "stream" away from the transducer.[9,10] The internal echoes may appear to scintillate. A color flash generated by these moving particles is termed "color streaking" when applying color- or power-mode Doppler to the cyst contents. The nondependent echogenic layer of a fat–fluid level can take 5 minutes or longer to shift with positional changes.[9,10]

Circumscribed, thin-walled, complicated cysts, especially when coexist with other simple cysts, or bilateral cysts, favor a benign diagnosis, such as that with FCC.

An "acorn cyst" describes a cyst that displays a nondependent echogenic layer. A cyst with a fat–fluid level can have this appearance when the echogenic lipid layer floats anteriorly. Showing movement of this fat layer helps to differentiate this finding from a crescent-like layer of echogenic papillary apocrine metaplasia (PAM) that is fixed to the wall. When using power Doppler fremitus, a true papillary lesion within a cyst will vibrate and transmit the fremitus artifact, whereas a nonattached fat layer will not.[9,10]

Homogeneous internal echoes within a complicated cyst can mimic a solid mass. Inspissated foam or gel cysts are often filled with diffuse low-level internal echoes. Sources of these internal echoes include proteinaceous or fatty material, or PAM.[9,10] Compressibility and lack of internal Doppler vascularity can help differentiate a "solid-appearing" complicated cyst from a true solid mass. Sonoelastography can sometimes

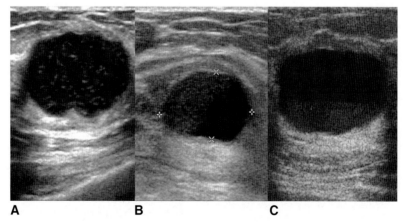

FIGURE 18-15 Complicated cyst examples with **(A)** floating internal echoes, **(B)** a partially shifted fat–fluid level, and **(C)** a fluid–debris level. The cyst walls are thin and circumscribed, and posterior enhancement is present.

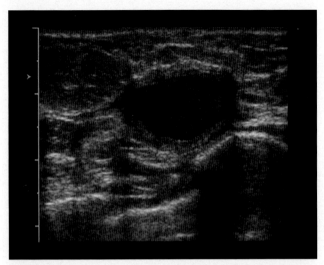

FIGURE 18-16 Infected cyst. Uniform isoechoic wall thickening and low-level internal echoes are features of this inflamed cyst. Color Doppler (not shown) showed blood flow along cyst wall.

these include galactocele, fat necrosis, phyllodes tumor with prominent cystic elements, hematoma, and abscess. Because suspicious findings necessitate intervention, correlation with clinical history and mammographic findings is important if biopsy is deferred.

Technical Considerations

Before characterizing a cyst as complicated or complex, technical factors and sound beam focusing must be optimized to eliminate as many "false echoes" from artifacts as possible. Common detrimental artifacts include reverberation, slice thickness artifacts, and clutter. The gain settings should be set high enough to visualize true echoes within cyst fluid without introducing false echoes. Harmonics and spatial compounding can help reduce troublesome artifacts.

Assessment and Treatment

Patient history and other imaging findings are helpful when considering a differential diagnosis for a complicated or complex cystic mass. In most cases, well-circumscribed, thin-walled complicated cysts are benign and part of the spectrum of FCCs.

Classification of complicated/complex cysts into BI-RADS categories is reported in the literature.[4,5,10] A benign (BI-RADS 2) classification can be appropriate for asymptomatic, thin-walled, circumscribed, complicated cysts with mobile internal echoes or fluid–debris levels, especially in the setting of bilateral multiple breast cysts. When discovered on a baseline sonography examination or as an incidental finding, asymptomatic complicated cysts with homogeneous internal echoes and clustered microcysts are generally classified as "probably benign." In such cases, the patient may be offered short-interval follow-up.

Aspiration of a benign simple cyst is not needed unless the patient is symptomatic (e.g., discomfort, tense palpable cyst), or when numerous cysts compromise mammographic quality. Benign-appearing aspirates that are green, yellow, clear, or black can be discarded.[9] Aspiration or core biopsy may be needed to differentiate an echo-filled complicated cyst from a solid mass. Cysts filled with PAM may not aspirate.[9] Aspiration is warranted for symptomatic complicated cysts. A bloody aspirate should undergo cytologic analysis to exclude malignant cells. Cysts that recur after aspiration or cannot be completely aspirated may require excision. Aspiration can be diagnostic and therapeutic for cysts suspected to be acutely inflamed or infected. Purulent fluid aspirated from a symptomatic cyst should be sent for Gram stain and culture to determine whether the cyst is infected or just inflamed.[9,10]

With suspicious complex cystic and solid lesions (BI-RADS 4), large core or sonography-directed vacuum-assisted biopsy (VAB) is preferred to cyst aspiration because the cyst wall and solid components are of histologic importance. Placement of a marker clip serves as a landmark should excision be required.

Benign Cystic Masses and Related Conditions[4-15]

Fibrocystic Change

FCC is the most common benign diffuse breast condition. Women are typically most symptomatic during late reproductive life (35 to 55 years). FCC is not considered a

be useful in this clinical setting. Aspiration may be warranted to differentiate some complicated cysts from a solid mass.

Cysts complicated by inflammation or infection affect the cyst wall and internal contents. Sonographic features worrisome for acute inflammation or infection include uniform isoechoic wall thickening, hyperemia of the cyst wall, and, possibly, internal fluid–debris level (Fig. 18-16).[9,10] Heavier white blood cells (WBCs) or tumefactive sludge tend to settle dependently within an infected cyst and can take longer to shift with positional changes. Color- or power-mode Doppler can display blood vessels coursing along the wall of a hyperemic inflamed cyst, as opposed to tumoral vessels coursing across the cyst wall. Supportive clinical features of inflammation include focal pain, tenderness, and, possibly, redness and thickening of the overlying skin. Fibrotic cyst wall thickening from prior inflammation typically lacks hyperemic change.

Older hemorrhagic, infected, or oil cysts may develop thin-walled (eggshell) calcification, causing acoustic shadowing that may obscure all or a portion of the cyst contents.

Complex *cystic and solid mass*, rather than complex cyst, is the preferred ACR BI-RADS term used to describe a mass that displays both anechoic (cystic or fluid) and discrete echogenic (solid) components.[4] Although most lesions are benign, such findings increase suspicion for neoplastic change. Worrisome sonographic findings include wall thickening (≥0.5 mm), thick internal septations (≥0.5 mm), intracystic mural nodule, or a mixed cystic/solid mass. Both the outer wall and any solid intracystic component should be evaluated for suspicious imaging features (e.g., noncircumscribed margins, duct extension, or invasion past the cyst wall).[10] Echoes from benign proliferative changes along the cyst wall or from an intramural tumor will not shift with positional changes. Doppler confirmation of blood flow within an eccentrically thickened wall or a fibrovascular stalk suggests neoplastic growth rather than PAM. A true intramural neoplasm, such as an intracystic papilloma or carcinoma, is rare. Ductal carcinoma in situ (DCIS) and necrotic neoplasms can also present as complex cystic and solid lesion by sonography.

Certain benign masses and fluid collections can image as complex cystic and solid masses. Besides papillary lesions, "disease" but rather signifies several changes considered to be aberrations of normal development and involution. With aging, female estrogen levels can predominate as menstrual cycles become irregular and ovulatory patterns change. This hormonal imbalance helps induce changes that primarily affect the ducts, lobules, and connective tissues of the TDLUs. Key features of FCC include epithelial hyperplasia, adenosis, stromal fibrosis, and cyst formation. Most FCC findings are nonproliferative and do not increase breast cancer risk.

Signs and Symptoms

At least half of adult women develop some symptoms related to FCC, including breast tenderness or pain, fullness, and nodularity. Symptoms are usually bilateral and often increase before menses. Nipple discharge, if present, can be from more than one duct orifice and involve both breasts and is often yellow or green in color. Symptoms diminish after menopause unless, but may persist if, a woman is on HRT.

Mammographic Features

Common features of FCC include the presence of bilateral, rounded, circumscribed water density masses, and benign scattered round/punctate parenchymal calcifications. In some patients, milk-of-calcium sediment within microcysts appears as "teacup-shaped" calcifications. Multiple enlarged lobules (adenosis) can give the parenchyma a "snowflake" appearance. Increased radiodensity of the breast parenchyma can hinder detection of some cysts and lobular changes. Certain benign FCC alterations such as sclerosing adenosis, radial scars, and focal fibrosis can occasionally produce suspicious imaging findings.

Sonographic Features

The most common sonographic finding is the presence of multiple cysts of varying sizes in both breasts (Fig. 18-17). Some complicated and septated cysts fall within the spectrum of FCC. When seen, clustered microcysts may show tiny hyperechoic foci, reflecting milk of calcium. Stromal fibrosis can increase parenchymal echogenicity and sound attenuation. The fibroglandular tissue may have a basket-weave appearance with ductal prominence. High-resolution sonography may detect small solid nodules related to FCC. Enlarged lobules (adenosis) can measure up to 7 mm and appear as isoechoic

or hypoechoic solid nodules. Nodular adenosis may appear as a circumscribed mass. Sclerosing adenosis may display an irregular shape, microlobulation, or microcalcifications, making differentiation from cancer difficult.

Galactocele

A galactocele is a milky cyst caused by obstruction of a lactiferous duct in the pregnant or lactating woman. This retention cyst tends to develop after abrupt cessation or suppression of lactation and contains fat, proteins, and lactose. A subareolar location is common, but galactoceles also occur in a peripheral TDLU. A galactocele may persist past the lactation period, undergo oily transformation, and become a lipid (oil) cyst. Rupture of an infected galactocele can lead to mastitis and subsequent abscess formation.

Signs and Symptoms

A galactocele is the most common benign mass to develop in a lactating patient. The presenting mass is usually firm but mobile. Tenderness or mastitis can accompany an infected galactocele.

Mammographic Features

A galactocele appears as a circumscribed mass containing radiolucent (fat density) material, which is a benign feature. Radiolucency varies with the fat and protein content. Increased parenchymal density of the lactating breast can hinder mammographic detection of some masses. A thin rim of wall calcification may occur with older lesions.

Sonographic Features

This round or oval, circumscribed mass can be unilocular or multilocular in appearance. Although galactoceles can be anechoic, variable amounts of internal echoes reflect from milk-laden contents (Fig. 18-18), often presenting as a complicated cyst. A fluid–fat level can be present and slowly shifts with positional changes. Doppler confirms the absence of internal blood flow. Posterior enhancement may be less than that seen with a simple cyst. Rim calcification, if present, can impede sound transmission. Associated

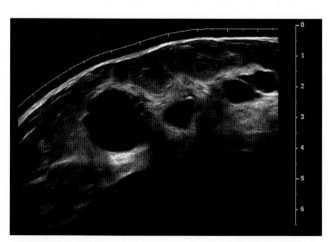

FIGURE 18-17 Fibrocystic change showing multiple breast cysts on this extended field-of-view high-resolution scan. (Image courtesy of Philips Healthcare, Bothell, WA.)

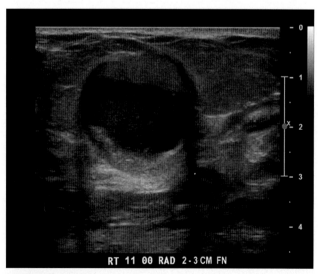

FIGURE 18-18 Galactocele. Sonogram shows a unilocular cystic mass of mixed echogenicity due to milky-fatty contents. An echogenic nondependent fat layer is present in this mass. (Reprinted with permission from Carr-Hoefer C. *Breast Ultrasound: A Comprehensive Sonographer's Guide.* Pegasus Lectures; 2007.)

findings in the lactating patient are prominent glandular tissue and dilated ducts.

Differential Diagnosis

Oil cysts and other complicated cysts can have similar sonographic appearances. If mastitis is present, an infected cyst or localized abscess is considered. A tender mass with a thick hyperemic wall can indicate an infected galactocele.

Treatment

Resolution of the galactocele is usually spontaneous, but aspiration using a low-gauge needle is often curative.

Sebaceous Cyst and Epidermal Inclusion Cyst

Sebaceous and epidermal cysts are small, benign, skin appendage masses that result from obstructed sebaceous glands or hair follicles and contain sebum or keratin. The superficial location is a clue to their origin, residing within or just beneath the dermal layer of the skin. Sebaceous cysts are often located at the inferior or medial margins of the breast or near the axilla. Occasionally, epidermal cysts form after breast trauma (e.g., needle biopsy, reduction mammoplasty). Retention cysts can also develop within the Montgomery glands of the areola. Infected or ruptured sebaceous cysts can lead to abscess formation.

Signs and Symptoms

Nodules are palpable because of their superficial location. The skin pore overlying the obstructed gland may be darkened. Skin reddening and tenderness overlying the cyst can indicate infection.

Sonographic Features

Sebaceous and epidermal cysts are round or oval in shape with smooth, thin-walled, circumscribed margins. The cyst can be completely or partially located within the dermis or project beneath the skin into the subcutaneous fat (Fig. 18-19). Focal skin thickening usually accompanies the cyst. When a cyst projects into the subcutaneous fat, the surrounding dermis can have a "claw-like" appearance. Although these cysts can be anechoic, the greasy or waxy contents often generate low- to medium-level internal echoes, fluid–fat

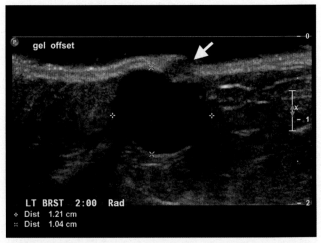
FIGURE 18-20 Sebaceous cyst with tract to skin (*arrow*). Extra scan gel and near-field focusing optimize imaging of this superficial mass.

levels, or produce a multilaminated appearance. Posterior acoustic enhancement is typically preserved. Slight angulation of the sound beam can improve detection of a narrow, hypoechoic, excretory duct or inflamed hair follicle that extends from the cyst to the skin surface (Fig. 18-20). Color Doppler reveals no internal blood flow. Cysts of skin origin can be classified as BI-RADS 2 benign lesions.[4]

Signs of cyst infection or abscess formation are sought when tenderness and skin reddening are present. Over time, sebaceous cysts may develop wall calcification with associated acoustic shadowing.

Technical Considerations

These superficial lesions are best delineated utilizing a very high-frequency transducer, an acoustic offset (such as extra scan gel), and proper near-field focusing. A small footprint (hockey stick) linear transducer can optimize imaging small superficial cysts.

Benign Inflammatory Conditions[4–15]

Mastitis

Mastitis, or inflammation of the breast, presents most often during pregnancy and lactation but can affect women at any stage of life. Causes are varied. Nonlactational forms of mastitis may result from an infected or ruptured cyst, a ruptured ectatic duct, postsurgical infection, periductal inflammation, or due to granulomatous conditions.

Puerperal mastitis represents breast inflammation related to lactation. It is the most frequent cause of acute mastitis. Bacteria, typically *Staphylococcus aureus*, can enter the ducts through a skin abrasion or cracked nipple or ascend via the ducts. Obstructed lactiferous ducts are susceptible to infection. Dilated infected ducts can show thick isoechoic walls and internal echoes from inspissated milk. With puerperal mastitis, infection can begin centrally within a lactiferous duct or develop more peripherally in a galactocele. Without appropriate treatment, an abscess may develop. Infection may potentially spread by way of the blood and lymph vessels to other parts of the breast.

Mammography is compromised in the woman with acute mastitis due to increased breast density from edema and

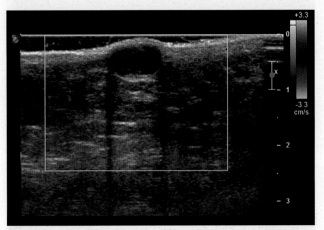
FIGURE 18-19 Sebaceous cyst. Oval circumscribed cystic mass located within the dermal layer of the skin and partially extending into the superficial fat. Internal echoes reflecting greasy contents. Doppler confirms absence of internal blood flow in this cyst extending from the skin into the superficial fat.

also from glandular proliferation related to lactation. Breast tenderness can further limit adequate tissue compression. Depending on the patient's age and clinical history, sonography is often the initial imaging examination for patients presenting with mastitis to search for complications such as abscess formation.

Mammary duct ectasia and periductal (plasma cell) mastitis primarily affects subareolar structures. This uncommon, chronic, nonlactational form of mastitis presents closer to menopause, although younger women with congenital nipple inversion are also at risk. Symptoms can include subareolar nodularity, a thick sticky nipple discharge, nipple retraction, and discomfort. Clinical features can mimic cancer; however, the ductal ectasia–periductal mastitis complex is usually bilateral in presentation. Subareolar ducts become distended with thick secretions and debris. Irritation and damage to the duct wall can allow secretions to leak into surrounding tissues, inciting periductal inflammation. Periductal fibrosis may follow and eventually shorten the ducts, resulting in nipple retraction. Mammogram features include an increase in subareolar density from dilated ducts or from a possible abscess. Calcification can develop both within and around the affected ducts.

In patients with periductal mastitis, sonography is primarily used to determine whether the cause of subareolar nodularity is from duct ectasia, abscess, or due to a mass. Dilated mammary ducts converging toward the nipple may display thick walls and contain echogenic, inspissated secretions. Color Doppler may show increased blood flow along the duct wall. Rupture of a duct can incite formation of a subareolar or periareolar abscess that may develop fistula tracts. Over time, there can be fibrous obliteration of the duct lumen.

Abscess

Abscesses are localized areas of pus and necrotic tissue that develop in a small percentage of patients with breast infection. Most often, abscesses form beneath the nipple (subareolar), or they may develop under the skin (subcutaneous), within the gland (intramammary), or deep to the gland in front of the pectoral muscles (retromammary).

Signs and Symptoms

Acute mastitis presents with varying degrees of fever, pain, skin reddening and thickening, and a purulent discharge. An elevated WBC count supports infection. In this setting, a palpable mass can indicate an abscess. Axillary nodes may be enlarged and tender.

Sonographic Features

The sonographic appearance varies with the stage and distribution of the inflammatory process. The inflamed, thickened skin prompts a search for an underlying infected duct or fluid collection. Swollen edematous breast tissues scatter and attenuate the sound beam, requiring lower frequencies to adequately penetrate the tissues. Edema can increase the echogenicity of the subcutaneous fat, which reduces delineation of the Cooper ligaments and other tissue planes. Dilated subdermal lymphatic channels or interstitial fluid may be seen. Comparison of the inflamed breast to a similar region in the normal contralateral breast allows the sonologist to appreciate the degree of inflammatory change.

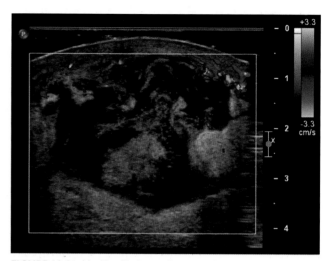

FIGURE 18-21 Mastitis with abscess. Sonogram shows a large complex-appearing fluid collection in a lactating patient with fever, breast swelling, and skin reddening. Associated skin thickening and hyperechogenicity of adjacent tissues is present. Color Doppler shows an increase in blood flow in tissues adjacent to the abscess.

An organized abscess can display varying amounts of liquefaction and tissue necrosis. An abscess appears as a complicated or complex fluid collection often with thick, irregular, or indistinct walls (Fig. 18-21). Nonuniform internal echoes, debris levels, and septations are common. Air within an abscess cavity is rare and can cause ring-down artifact. Distal sound enhancement varies with the fluid composition. An abscess can tract to various parts of the breast or peak anteriorly through the superficial fascia, forming fistula tracts to the skin. As an abscess matures, it becomes more encapsulated and well defined. Color or power Doppler documents hyperemic flow to inflamed tissues and the absence of blood flow within the abscess cavity.

Differential Diagnosis

Depending on the stage of the process, inflammatory change can mimic a hematoma, seroma, infected cyst, degenerating tumor, or even cancer.

Both inflammatory carcinoma and acute mastitis can have similar clinical findings and must be differentiated by diagnostic methods if suspicious findings are detected. Cancer can grow rapidly and disseminate diffusely when hormones are elevated in the pregnant or lactating breast.

Skin thickening and/or breast edema can also be caused by other conditions, such as direct trauma, congestive heart failure, nephrotic syndrome, lymphoma, and lymphedema. A skin burn or direct radiation exposure can inflame local tissues.

Skin retraction, architectural distortion, fat necrosis, scarring, and fibrosis may indicate residual change from a serious abscess. Clinical correlation is important.

Treatment

Most inflammatory processes resolve with proper antibiotic therapy. Aspiration of purulent fluid is diagnostic of an abscess when a fluid collection is present. Microbiology studies should include culture and Gram stain. Needle or catheter drainage with irrigation and instillation of antibiotics into the abscess cavity may augment medical treatment. In some cases, biopsy or excision may be needed to exclude an underlying malignancy if a treated abscess does not fully involute.

Mondor Disease

Mondor disease is a vascular abnormality and represents acute thrombophlebitis of the superficial veins of the chest wall and breast. The lateral thoracic, thoracoepigastric, and superior epigastric veins are most often involved. Risk factors for this rare vascular condition include breast injury, surgery, infection, hypercoagulable state, pregnancy, dehydration, and cancer. The presence of a central venous catheter may initiate clot formation and affect the internal mammary vein. Both males and females are affected.

Signs and Symptoms

Clinically, a thrombosed vein can present as a tender, palpable, cord-like superficial mass. The skin overlying the thrombosed vein can be thick and reddened, signifying focal inflammation.

Sonographic Findings

The dilated, tubular, superficial vein may have a somewhat beaded appearance and displays internal echoes from clotted blood (Fig. 18-22). Thrombus is confirmed by showing incomplete compressibility of the vein when applying transducer pressure. Doppler shows absent blood flow in the obstructed vein segment. Edema increases the thickness and echogenicity of overlying skin and the fat surrounding an acutely thrombosed vein. A partially recanalized vein may show fibrous bands within the vessel lumen. Chronic clot may eventually calcify.

The location of the thrombosed vein within the superficial fat layer helps to differentiate the tubular structure from a breast duct located in the mammary zone. Once a thrombosed breast vein is identified, the course of the clot should be traced to its draining vein to exclude extension of clot into the axillary, subclavian, or internal mammary veins.

Treatment

Symptoms often resolve over a period of several weeks without intervention. Some cases require anticoagulatory therapy. Recurrence is possible.

Benign Trauma–Related Masses[4–15]

The main causes of breast injury include blunt trauma, percutaneous interventional procedures, and surgery. Patient history is very important when establishing a differential diagnosis in a patient following trauma or infection because some residual changes can create clinical and imaging features that simulate cancer.

Hematoma

Hematomas are blood-filled breast masses that usually result from vessel damage following breast injury. Nontraumatic hematomas may develop in patients with a history of blood disorders or anticoagulant treatment.

Signs and Symptoms

Bruising and skin thickening are external signs of hemorrhage. Tenderness is present in varying degrees. A palpable mass following biopsy or trauma suggests a hematoma.

Mammographic Features

The mammographic appearance of hemorrhage varies from mild changes of increased density and skin thickening to an opaque, hemorrhagic cyst or a more sclerotic, retractive mass.

Sonographic Features

Sonography is usually the preferred imaging modality because it is less painful than mammography and can identify a fluid collection separate from other traumatized tissues. Imaging patterns of hemorrhage depend on the extent, duration, and organization of the bleed. Initially, mild skin thickening and altered echogenicity of subcutaneous fat or other affected tissues may be present. The sonographic appearance of an organizing hematoma is variable and depends on the amount of liquefaction and clotted blood present (Fig. 18-23). A hematoma can appear round, oval, or irregular in shape. Clotted blood along the periphery of the hematoma forms a fibrous wall that helps contain the blood collection. The encapsulated blood may be anechoic, but more often displays diffuse internal echoes, echogenic clot, septations, or fibrous bands. Distal acoustic enhancement is variable.

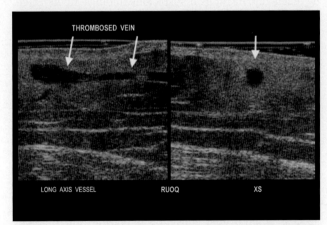

FIGURE 18-22 Mondor disease. A noncompressible thrombosed superficial breast vein (*arrows*) shows internal echoes. Edema causes an increase in echogenicity of the fat surrounding the occluded vessel. Doppler confirmed absent blood flow. (Reprinted with permission from Carr-Hoefer C. *Breast Ultrasound: A Comprehensive Sonographer's Guide*. Pegasus Lectures; 2007.)

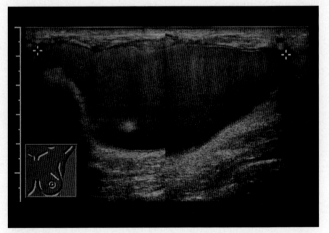

FIGURE 18-23 Hematoma. Split-screen imaging documents an 8-cm echogenic fluid collection that resulted from a seat belt injury. A small area of hyperechoic clotted blood is present. Skin thickening accompanies the area of bruising. (Reprinted with permission from Carr-Hoefer C. *Breast Ultrasound: A Comprehensive Sonographer's Guide*. Pegasus Lectures; 2007.)

Color Doppler confirms the absence of internal blood flow within a nonvascularized hematoma.

Treatment

Hematomas will typically regress over time. Residual changes can be minimal or leave signs of architectural distortion, fat necrosis, or scarring that might mimic cancer. Therefore, clinical correlation is needed on subsequent imaging.

Pseudoaneurysm

A pseudoaneurysm is a rare complication of acute breast trauma, such as with percutaneous interventional procedures, that can result from arterial vessel damage, causing spontaneous, localized hemorrhage. Instead of being contained by an arterial wall, the leaking blood jets into a false aneurysmal sac and contained by clotted blood elements.

Some predisposing factors for this vascular abnormality are anticoagulant therapy, advanced age, or other factors that cause increase breast vascularization (e.g., pregnancy, malignant invasion). To potentially reduce risk of a pseudoaneurysm, color Doppler is used to help avoid prominent blood vessels when selecting a needle path to a mass during large core breast biopsy.

Signs and Symptoms

After an interventional procedure, an enlarging mass at or near the interventional site prompts concern for a hematoma or pseudoaneurysm formation. Skin bruising may be apparent.

Sonographic Features

Grayscale imaging reveals a fluid-containing mass at the trauma site, which may be anechoic or contain variable internal echoes. Areas of echogenic clotted blood may be evident within and along the fluid cavity. Doppler plays a key role in differentiating a postbiopsy hematoma from blood flow jetting into a pseudoaneurysm. Color Doppler reveals swirling internal blood flow with a characteristic "to-and-fro" pattern ("yin–yang" sign) (Fig. 18-24).[28–30] During spectral Doppler analysis, the sample gate should be placed at the neck of the pseudoaneurysm to better document the high-velocity antegrade and retrograde blood flow pattern between the feeding vessel and the pseudosac. This Doppler pattern helps to differentiate a postbiopsy pseudoaneurysm from a rarer arteriovenous fistula that would show a high systolic velocity and low-resistive flow signal.[31]

Treatment

Treatment options vary and depend on the size of the fluid collection and the amount of blood jetting within the pseudoaneurysm. The application of external compression for a time period can help facilitate clotting. When conservative measures do not work, other treatment options include thrombin injection, angioembolization with coils, or surgical repair.

Seroma

A seroma is an accumulation of serous fluid that collects within a surgical cavity or at a biopsy site. A seroma at a lumpectomy site can help reduce contour deformity by allowing breast tissues to reshape as the fluid collection regresses. Drains are more often placed at mastectomy sites to lessen the accumulation of fluids. Seromas help identify the treatment cavity site for brachytherapy patients undergoing accelerated partial breast irradiation (APBI). Axillary seromas can follow lymph node dissections.

Signs and Symptoms

A seroma is suspected in an afebrile patient with a palpable mass at a surgical site. Larger seromas can cause pain and stretch the overlying skin.

Sonographic Features

A seroma typically conforms to the shape of the surgical cavity. The fluid may appear anechoic or display low-level internal echoes or septations (Fig. 18-25). Distal sound enhancement is evident. Doppler confirms the absence of internal vascularity.

Differential Diagnosis

Clinical findings and lab values help differentiate postsurgical fluid collections when imaging features are similar and aspiration is not desired. In the axilla, a lymphocele can mimic a seroma.

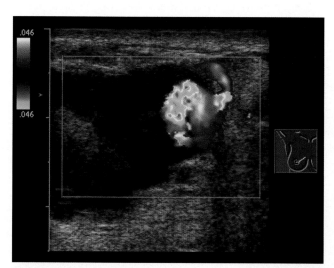

FIGURE 18-24 Pseudoaneurysm. Color-flow Doppler reveals blood flow within the neck of this postbiopsy pseudoaneurysm. (Reprinted with permission from Carr-Hoefer C. *Ultrasound for the Sonomammographer.* Sound Imaging Consulting, LLC.)

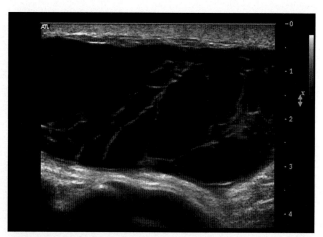

FIGURE 18-25 Seroma. Breast fluid collection with internal septations at the surgical site. (Image courtesy of Philips Healthcare, Bothell, WA.)

Treatment

Seromas gradually resolve with time; however, therapeutic aspiration is warranted if a seroma is large, persists for a long time, or becomes infected.

Fat Necrosis

Fat necrosis is an uncommon inflammatory and ischemic process that is a consequence of blunt breast trauma (e.g., seat belt injury), surgery (e.g., reduction mammoplasty), radiotherapy, or inflammation. Trauma can disrupt blood supply, causing hemorrhage and liquefaction of a focal area of breast fat, resulting in necrosis and some foreign-body reaction. Subsequently, the traumatized fat may transform into a lipid-filled (oil) cyst or evolve into a fibrous sclerotic mass. Older obese women with large fatty breasts are more prone to fat necrosis, especially within the subcutaneous fat. Large surgical excisions followed by radiation increase risk for ischemic changes. Spontaneous development has been reported in diabetic patients.

Signs and Symptoms

Palpable findings range from a smooth, mildly compressible lump to a firm, fixed, irregular mass in the region of prior breast injury. There may be associated skin thickening, dimpling, or nipple retraction. Findings are usually painless. Clinical history is important because many of these clinical features mimic signs of cancer. Not all patients recall a history of breast trauma or infection, making clinical correlation difficult. Unlike cancer, symptoms typically diminish with time. Some patients are asymptomatic, with fat necrosis being initially discovered on an imaging examination.

Mammographic Features

Findings are variable. An oil cyst appears as a round or oval, radiolucent, or mixed fat/water density mass with a radiodense fibrous capsule (Fig. 18-26A). Thin rim (eggshell) calcification may encompass an oil cyst. When a fat density mass is apparent by mammography, sonography is not needed to make a benign diagnosis. Fibrotic changes mimic cancer and include architectural distortion or a spiculated mass with or without calcifications (Fig. 18-27A).

Sonographic Features

Fat necrosis also has a range of sonographic appearances. Initially, there may be increased echogenicity of the traumatized fat in which an anechoic or hypoechoic area develops. Changes can progress into an oil cyst encompassed by a thin or thick wall. Internally, a discrete oil cyst may be anechoic, show a fat–fluid level, and display a complex cystic and solid pattern, including a mural nodule (fat globule) (Fig. 18-26B). Enhancement is variable. If rim calcification is present, acoustic shadowing may obscure portions of the cyst, complicating the diagnosis. Fat necrosis can evolve into a more solid appearance with suspicious features related to fibrosis and granuloma formation. Fibrotic fat necrosis can appear as an irregular, spiculated, hypoechoic, shadowing mass (Fig. 18-27B). Doppler flow shows no associated blood flow as tissues become avascular with fibrotic scarring.

Differential Diagnosis[4,5,8]

An appropriate differential diagnosis factors in the patient's history, the location, and imaging appearance of the mass. Fat necrosis appearing as a fibrotic or granulomatous mass can overlap imaging features of a postsurgical scar, focal fibrosis, radial scar, invasive ductal carcinoma (IDC), tubular carcinoma, or recurrent tumor. Doppler flow at the site would favor tumor growth. The presence of radiolucent fat within a mass on a mammogram can indicate an oil cyst and should be differentiated from other fat-containing masses.

Patients with Weber–Christian disease can develop multiple oil cysts in the breast, as well as fat necrosis in other parts of the body. Steatocystoma multiplex is a rare familial disorder manifested by multiple, bilateral, small keratin-filled oily cysts in the axillae, the anterior chest wall, extremities, and even the skin layer. This condition can also be seen in males.

Postsurgical Scar

A scar forms as connective tissue proliferates at the site of an injury. Postsurgical scarring can affect many tissue layers along the incision site. Scar tissue can also form following involution of a hematoma, seroma, or an abscess.

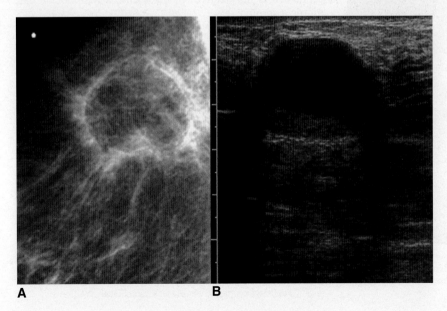

A   **B**

FIGURE 18-26 Fat necrosis: oil cyst presentation. **A:** Mammogram shows a fat density, radiolucent, rounded mass with a radiodense capsule at an old trauma site. **B:** Sonogram shows a complicated cyst with mixed echoes from fatty contents that moved with positional changes.

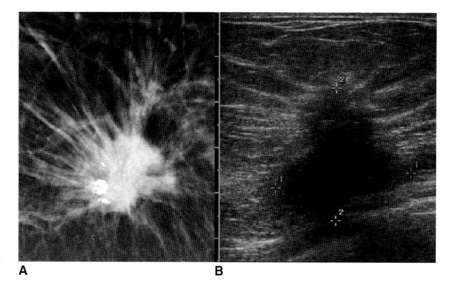

FIGURE 18-27 Fat necrosis: fibrotic presentation. **A:** Mammogram shows a radiodense spiculated mass with calcification in a fatty breast at the site of prior lumpectomy. **B:** Sonogram shows a poorly circumscribed, spiculated, hypoechoic mass with some acoustic shadowing.

Fat necrosis may complicate scarring. It may take a year for scar tissue to diminish following a benign biopsy. Radiation therapy following lumpectomy can induce significant scarring, which persists longer and potentially obscures early detection of a recurring tumor.

Signs and Symptoms

Some scars produce minimal, if any, palpable changes. Exuberant scarring at the incision site can cause thickening, firmness, and some retraction of the skin. Deeper scar tissue can present as a breast lump, which may be difficult to differentiate from recurrent tumor in some patients following breast-conservation surgery.

Mammographic Features

A radiodense scar is often better seen on one mammographic view and changes in appearance on a different projection. Patterns include architectural distortion, focal asymmetry, or a spiculated density often with dystrophic calcifications. Compression views show absence of a central mass. Skin changes include thickening, retraction, and fibrous stranding into the underlying fat. Over time, scar tissue tends to diminish in size and density on sequential mammograms.

Sonographic Features

A postsurgical scar can appear as an irregular hypoechoic area with acoustic shadowing or as architectural distortion at the surgical site. Tissue planes typically show disruption. Associated skin thickening and retraction is common. Unlike a true mass, the linear dimensions and appearance of a scar will change when scanned in orthogonal planes along the incision site (Fig. 18-28). Applying transducer pressure flattens out the connective tissue fibers, which reduces or eliminates the shadowing effect of the scar. In contrast, malignant shadowing will not significantly change with transducer pressure. No Doppler blood flow signal should be detected within scar tissue by 6 months following surgery, helping to differentiate it from a recurrent tumor.[10] The effects of a scar typically diminish over time on serial examinations.

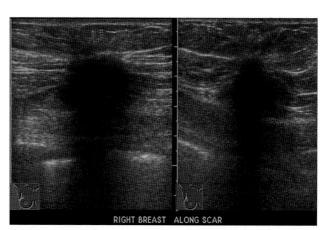

RIGHT BREAST ALONG SCAR

FIGURE 18-28 Postsurgical scar. Orthogonal scans along the incision site reveal a shadowing, spiculated area and straightening of the Copper ligaments. Note the change in dimension of the scar tissue after the transducer is rotated perpendicular to the long axis of the incision.

Sonographic Assessment of Solid Breast Masses[4–15,32]

Sonography typically follows clinical examination and mammography and provides additional diagnostic information for risk assessment. In early years, the main role of sonography was to characterize masses as cystic or solid. As the quality of sonography systems have improved, so has sonography's ability to detect more of the morphologic features of masses that correlate with benign or malignant processes. It is reported that about 80% of breast biopsies return benign results. Research studies have shown that sonography can help differentiate benign from malignant solid masses when strict imaging criteria are met.[4,5,9,10] This can impact patient care by allowing certain patients the option of short-interval follow-up imaging when findings correlate with a very high probability of being benign, while expediting biopsy of lesions with suspicious features. However, the development of a new solid mass in a postmenopausal woman, or in a patient with high-risk factors (e.g., BRCA carrier), or one that is large or fast growing is treated with suspicion, even when it displays benign imaging features.[21,22]

In 1995, Dr. A.T. Stavros and colleagues reported an algorithm for the sonographic characterization of solid breast nodules based on large-scale research studies.[10,32] Following strict criteria, solid nodules were assigned to ACR BI-RADS risk categories based on the presence or absence of specific suspicious and benign sonographic findings. Over the years, terminology regarding these US findings has been updated, as reflected in the ACR US lexicon.[4]

Using Dr. Stavros' approach, benign and suspicious features are listed in Tables 18-9 and 18-10, respectively. Based on this landmark research, the recommended approach for examining solid breast masses is to first search for the presence of suspicious sonographic findings. If one or more suspicious findings are present, the mass is minimally assigned a BI-RADS 4 (suspicious abnormality) classification and biopsy is indicated. If no suspicious findings are detected, the mass is further assessed for the presence of specific benign findings. If benign findings are present, the nodule can be classified as either BI-RADS 3 (probably benign) or BI-RADS 2 (benign). If benign findings are not present, the nodule is classified as indeterminate with low suspicion of malignancy, BI-RADS 4A, and biopsy is recommended.[10,32] The use of such an algorithm relies on the performance of a high-resolution breast sonography examination by knowledgeable and experienced sonographers and sonologists.

For the sake of comparison, benign features are discussed first. At times, the cause of a palpable lump or an asymmetric mammographic density represents a focal island of interlobular stromal fibrous tissue rather than a true mass. This is considered a benign finding if the tissue is purely hyperechoic without any gray areas larger-than-normal ducts or lobules (Fig. 18-29).[9,10,32] Certain benign masses can present as hyperechoic lesions (e.g., lipoma, angiolipoma, hemangioma, fat necrosis) and should be correlated with mammography and clinical history.[4–6] Carcinomas that are purely hyperechoic are very rare.[10] It is important to fully scan through a hyperechoic lesion to be sure it is purely echogenic because a small cancer with a tiny hypoechoic nidus and a thick echogenic rim (halo) could mimic this benign feature in certain scan planes.

TABLE 18-10 Sonographic Characterization of a Solid Mass[9,10]

Individual Findings of Malignancy	
Spiculation	Straight lines that radiate perpendicular from the surface of the mass into surrounding tissue
Thick echogenic rim	A cause of indistinct margins; can represent unresolved spiculation
Angular margins	Sharp corners that may form acute angles (occur in regions of low resistance to invasion)
Microlobulation	Small 1- to 2-mm surface lobulations that vary in number and distribution; short cycle undulations (ACR)
Nonparallel orientation (taller-than-wide)	Long axis of mass is not parallel to skin Vertically oriented; AP dimension > either horizontal dimension
Hypoechogenicity	Mass or central part of mass is markedly hypoechoic as compared with fat
Posterior shadowing	Central, partial, or complete decrease in retrotumoral echoes (often related to the degree of desmoplasia)
Microcalcifications	Tiny, hyperechoic, nonshadowing foci (best seen within mass)
Duct extension	Tumor projection from a mass into a single duct directed toward the nipple
Branch pattern	Tumor projection into multiple small ducts away from the nipple

The presence of one or more suspicious finding can place mass in either a BI-RADS 4 or BI-RADS 5 category.

Characteristically, a benign solid breast mass displaces, rather than invades, adjacent tissues as it grows and displays well-circumscribed margins that are sharply demarcated from surrounding tissues. The mass develops an oval, ellipsoid shape as it slowly grows within normal tissue planes and assumes a parallel orientation relative to the skin or

TABLE 18-9 Sonographic Characterization of a Solid Mass[9,10]

Benign Presentations	
Hyperechogenicity	Area of pure and intensely hyperechoic tissue causing a palpable or mammographic abnormality (e.g., *normal interlobular stromal fibrous tissue, echogenic fat*)

Circumscribed Solid Mass Benign Features	
Oval	Elliptical or egg shaped
Macrolobulation	Margin with three or fewer smooth gentle lobulations (when present)
Parallel orientation (wider-than-tall)	Long axis of mass is parallel to skin Horizontal dimension > AP dimension
Thin echogenic capsule	Circumscribed rim of compressed breast tissue encompassing the mass

Additionally, no suspicious findings are present.

AP, anteroposterior.

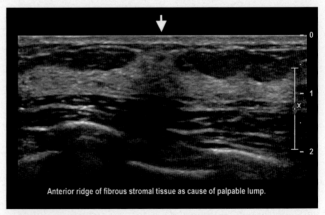

Anterior ridge of fibrous stromal tissue as cause of palpable lump.

FIGURE 18-29 Benign fibrous stromal tissue. A focal ridge of hyperechoic fibroglandular tissue (*arrow*) is seen extending anteriorly near the skin. This correlated to the patient's palpable lump during echopalpation.

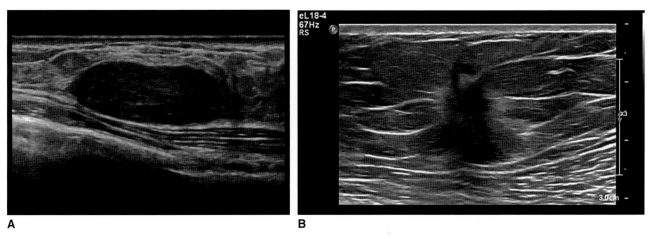

FIGURE 18-30 Sonographic characteristics. **A:** Benign features of a solid breast mass (fibroadenoma) include oval shape and thinly encapsulated circumscribed margins. The mass is wider-than-tall with orientation parallel to the skin. No suspicious associated features are seen. **B:** Malignant features of this heterogeneous mass include irregular shape, indistinct margin with thick echogenic rim, and spiculation. There are regions of marked hypoechogenicity. The mass extends through tissue planes appearing taller-than-wide (not parallel in orientation). Cooper ligaments appear straightened. (Image courtesy of Philips Healthcare, Bothell, WA.)

chest wall, appearing "wider-than-tall" (Fig. 18-30A). Two or three gentle surface macrolobulations may be present. A thin, echogenic (pseudo)capsule encompasses the entire mass that results from compression of adjacent breast tissue. If no suspicious features are present, a circumscribed solid mass with these features meets criteria for a BI-RADS 3 (probably benign) classification. Short-interval follow-up imaging (at 6 months intervals for up to 2 years) may be offered as an option to biopsy depending on patient factors. A benign (BI-RADS 2) classification can be rendered after stability of findings is established.[4,9,10,32]

Several individual sonographic findings increase suspicion for cancer during solid mass evaluation (Fig. 18-30B; Table 18-10). Cancers vary by histologic type, cellularity, vascularity, growth rate, and effect on surrounding tissues, which influence imaging appearance. Certain findings are more often associated with invasion, whereas others reflect intraductal (DCIS) components of a tumor, or other associated features. The presence of even one suspicious finding is enough to classify a solid nodule as a suspicious abnormality, although most cancers show multiple findings. Close inspection of a lesion is necessary because worrisome features might affect only a small portion of the mass.

Suspicious sonographic findings include demonstration of an irregular, heterogeneous mass with indistinct, spiculated, angular, or microlobulated margins. Spiculation is seen as hyperechoic/hypoechoic lines radiating out from the tumor and can be coarse or fine. Echogenic spiculation is best seen around fat-surrounded lesions. An indistinct, echogenic rim (halo) surrounding a mass can represent unresolved spiculation. Angular margins occur at points where there is less resistance to tumor growth, such as in fat or at the base of a Cooper ligament. Microlobulation can indicate fingers of invasive tumor or DCIS distended ducts or lobules. Cancers are often markedly hypoechoic compared with fat, especially when imaged using harmonics and spatial compounding. Occasionally, intratumoral microcalcifications are detected with high-resolution scanners. Attenuation shadowing is a worrisome finding and may be central, partial, or complete. The degree of retrotumoral shadowing often correlates with the amount

of fibrous tissue within and around the tumor. Malignant shadowing does not disappear with transducer pressure. A mass oriented within the breast that is not parallel to the skin is considered suspicious and may appear "taller-than-wide" (height-to-width ratio > 1). This feature can represent a small cancer growing within a vertically oriented TDLU or indicate cancer growth across tissue planes. Careful inspection of a mass includes the search for associated features, which includes changes to ductal patterns. Radial and antiradial scans optimize the detection of ductal extension of a tumor into a lactiferous duct leading toward the nipple, or branching into smaller peripheral ducts. These ductal changes are some of the associated features of cancer. *Additional images illustrating suspicious findings and associated features are discussed in "Malignant Breast Masses" section of this chapter.*

Benign Solid Masses[4–15,23-26,32]

This section covers many of the benign solid masses encountered during breast sonography.

Fibroadenoma

Fibroadenoma is the most common benign solid tumor of the female breast. Incidence rate is higher in patients aged 15 to 35 years. Tumors often develop before age 25. This estrogen-induced tumor represents overgrowth of the connective and glandular tissues within a breast lobule. Fibroadenomas may be single or multiple, involving one or both breasts. Large and multiple tumors occur more frequently in young black females. Older fibroadenomas may undergo involution, hyalinization, and calcification.

Fibroadenomas usually grow slowly until reaching a stable size. Most tumors measure less than 3 cm, but some grow larger. Accelerated growth can be hormonally stimulated during pregnancy, after initiation of HRT, or during immunosuppression therapy. Rapid growth can lead to infarction.

Signs and Symptoms

A palpable fibroadenoma presents as a nontender, smooth or lobular, firm or rubbery, movable mass.

Mammographic Features

Fibroadenoma appears as a water density circumscribed, oval, or round mass that may be indistinguishable from a cyst. A thin radiolucent halo supports a benign diagnosis (Fig. 18-31A). Tumors have typically equal density to fibroglandular tissue and can show a distinctive notch. Benign, coarse, "popcorn"-type calcifications are occasionally seen and help distinguish an older fibroadenoma from a cyst or a circumscribed cancer (Fig. 18-32A).

Sonographic Features

Typically, a fibroadenoma appears as an oval, circumscribed, homogeneous solid mass that may be gently lobulated (Fig. 18-31B). The wider-than-tall mass is oriented parallel to the skin. The internal echo pattern is usually isoechoic or mildly hypoechoic compared with fat. On occasion, a thin, echogenic, fibrous septation may be seen traversing the mass. Normal sound transmission is common, although some enhancement or mild shadowing is possible depending on mass composition. Color Doppler often shows some vascularity unless the mass is small.

Assessment and Treatment

When classic benign sonographic features of a fibroadenoma are present, without any suspicious imaging findings, a circumscribed solid mass is typically assigned an ACR BI-RADS 3 (probably benign) risk assessment with recommendation for short-interval follow-up imaging to assess stability, in lieu of a core biopsy.[4,5,9,10] A long-term follow-up study reported that tumor growth of more than 20% in all three dimensions over a 6-month period should prompt biopsy to exclude malignancy.[33]

A biopsy-proven fibroadenomas may not need surgical excision unless the tumor is symptomatic and large or shows atypical features.[34] Large core, percutaneous VAB has been used to excise smaller fibroadenomas as an option to surgical removal.[9,10,33,34] Other minimally invasive techniques have been used for fibroadenoma treatment, including percutaneous cryoablation, laser and radio-frequency ablation, and US-guided high-intensity–focused US ablation.[34]

Variants and Differential Diagnosis

Fibroadenomas account for most circumscribed solid breast masses. Occasionally, internal areas of cystic degeneration,

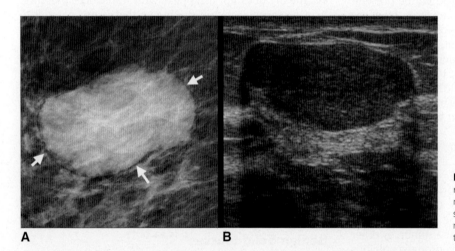

FIGURE 18-31 Fibroadenoma. **A:** Mammogram reveals a well-circumscribed, oval, water density mass with a radiolucent rim (*arrows*). **B:** Sonogram shows an oval, gently lobulated, circumscribed solid mass with a thin echogenic capsule. The wider-than-tall mass is oriented parallel to the skin.

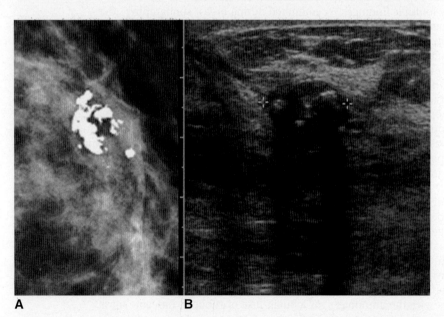

FIGURE 18-32 Calcified fibroadenoma. **A:** Mammogram reveals benign "popcorn"-type calcifications consistent with a benign degenerating fibroadenoma. **B:** Sonogram shows hyperechoic areas with acoustic shadowing from macrocalcification within the solid mass.

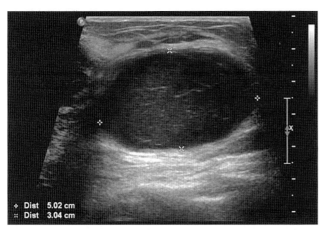

FIGURE 18-33 Juvenile fibroadenoma. Convex linear sonogram of a rapidly enlarging 5-cm palpable mass in an adolescent female. The well-circumscribed, oval, homogeneous, hypoechoic mass is oriented parallel to the skin. The cellular lesion shows some distal enhancement.

hyalinization, or calcification can cause textural inhomogeneity and alter attenuation effects. Acoustic shadowing from macrocalcifications can obscure portions of the mass (Fig. 18-32B). Findings should be correlated with the mammogram to eliminate confusion with malignant shadowing.

"Complex fibroadenomas" represent a small subset of tumors that contain proliferative changes (cysts >3 mm, epithelial calcifications, sclerosing adenosis, PAM). These complex lesions show a slight increase in relative risk for breast cancer. Because imaging features are not classic of a typical fibroadenoma, biopsy may be recommended.

Juvenile-type fibroadenomas grow rapidly during adolescence and account for up to 10% of fibroadenomas in females under age 20. Tumors can attain a large size and are usually solitary. Histologically, these uncommon tumors display a highly cellular stroma. These circumscribed tumors are usually homogeneous and can demonstrate prominent vascularity and posterior enhancement (Fig. 18-33).

Giant fibroadenomas describe tumors that measure over 5 cm in size.

A differential diagnosis for circumscribed breast tumors measuring greater than 3 cm is listed in Table 18-11 and refined based on clinical and imaging features. Biopsy or excision is advocated for large (>3 cm) and fast-growing lesions even when benign-appearing on imaging tests, so as to not miss the diagnosis of a phyllodes tumor or a circumscribed cancer (e.g., malignant phyllodes, high-grade IDC, medullary carcinoma).[6,11]

TABLE 18-11 Differential Diagnosis of Large Circumscribed Solid Breast Masses

Benign	Malignant
Fibroadenoma >3 cm	High-grade invasive ductal
Juvenile/giant fibroadenoma	carcinoma
Phyllodes tumor	Malignant phyllodes/sarcoma
Pseudoangiomatous stromal	Medullary carcinoma
hyperplasia	Primary lymphoma
Secretory adenoma	BRCA-associated breast cancer
Hamartoma	(TNBC)

Clinical history is taken into account when listing a differential for a mass >3 cm.

Adenoma and Secretory Adenoma

Adenomas are less common than fibroadenomas and are primarily composed of glandular elements. Slowly growing tubular adenomas can occur in young patients. Secretory (lactating) adenomas present during pregnancy or the lactation period in response to elevated hormones. It is questioned whether a secretory adenoma is a new lesion or represents accelerated growth of an existing fibroadenoma or tubular adenoma during pregnancy.

Signs and Symptoms

A new palpable, mobile, enlarging mass in a pregnant or lactating patient can indicate a secretory adenoma and should be differentiated from a galactocele.

Sonographic Features

Sonography is chosen over mammography to evaluate the pregnant or lactating breast. A secretory adenoma is typically an oval, circumscribed, parallel-oriented solid mass. Internal areas of increased echogenicity and some fluid-filled slits are likely related to milky secretory products (Fig. 18-34). Prominent vascularity is often a Doppler feature. Lesions can grow large and tend to regress in size after lactation ceases. Tubular adenomas are well-circumscribed, isoechoic to hypoechoic, oval, homogeneous breast masses with normal to enhanced sound transmission.

Phyllodes (Phylloides) Tumor

A phyllodes tumor is a rare fibroepithelial neoplasm with a "leaf-shaped" growth pattern. The tumor resembles fibroadenoma but has more stromal cellularity and contains narrow, cyst-like clefts of mucinous, hemorrhagic, or cystic fluid. The median age at presentation for phyllodes is during the late fourth decade, which is later than is typical for a fibroadenoma. The tumor is usually unilateral and can grow to a huge size, sometimes suddenly. Phyllodes represent 1.0% or less of all breast tumors but are the most common breast sarcomas. A woman with the inherited condition, Li–Fraumeni syndrome, is at increased risk for phyllodes. Although usually benign, a borderline tumor can undergo malignant transformation and has the potential to metastasize. This occurs in about 25%

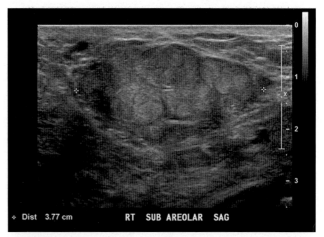

FIGURE 18-34 Secretory adenoma. A lactating woman noticed a rapidly enlarging breast mass. Sonography displays a large, lobulated, circumscribed, parallel-oriented mass with isoechoic and hyperechoic internal echoes. The mass diminished in size after cessation of breastfeeding.

of tumors.[8] Malignant phyllodes more often metastasize via the blood to the lungs, bones, and liver rather than involving the lymph nodes. Chest wall invasion is possible. Treatment includes wide local excision or mastectomy. Recurrence is possible if excision is not complete.

Signs and Symptoms

The palpable mass is discrete, nontender, and mobile. A large mass may bulge and stretch the skin, causing pressure and edema. The axilla is usually clinically normal.

Sonographic Features

Imaging features are often similar to those of fibroadenoma. However, demonstration of cystic spaces, especially within a large, discrete, solid lesion, suggests the diagnosis of a phyllodes tumor (Fig. 18-35). Calcification is not typical. Malignant phyllodes tumors tend to be more lobulated, grow larger, and double in size faster than benign lesions.

Pseudoangiomatous Stromal Hyperplasia

Pseudoangiomatous stromal hyperplasia (PASH) is a benign, solid, mesenchymal tumor that contains extensive slit-like spaces that resemble vascular channels. This often large, hormonally stimulated mass can grow quickly and is more prevalent in reproductive-aged women and those on HRT. Imaging patterns vary, but features can mimic fibroadenoma or phyllodes tumor on US examination.

Hamartoma

A hamartoma is an unusual benign mass made up of varying amounts of normal or dysplastic fibrous, epithelial, and fatty breast tissues. Alternative names include fibroadenolipoma, lipofibroadenoma, and adenolipofibroma based on predominating tissue components. This pseudotumor is located within the mammary zone and represents a focal malformation of breast development. FCCs, PASH, and, rarely, cancer may develop within tissues of a hamartoma.

A patient with Cowden disease (multiple hamartoma syndrome), a rare genetic disorder, shows increase risk for developing cancer, including breast cancer.

Signs and Symptoms

Hamartomas are usually unilateral and often measure over 3 cm when diagnosed. Palpable masses are painless, often with a soft, rubbery consistency, and smooth or lobulated surface. Compressibility varies with the tissue makeup.

Mammographic Features

A hamartoma appears as a smooth or lobulated encapsulated lesion, containing mixed radiolucent and radiodense areas. This "breast within a breast" pattern has been described as resembling a "piece of cut sausage." Benign calcifications are occasionally present. Mammography is better than sonography at differentiating fat within the lesion, which typically indicates a benign mass.

Sonographic Features

The circumscribed oval mass displays a mixed echo pattern, with isoechoic, hyperechoic, and hypoechoic elements reflecting the mixture of tissue makeup (Fig. 18-36). When fatty or fibrous components predominate, hamartomas may sonographically resemble a heterogeneous lipoma or fibroadenoma.

Lipoma

A true lipoma is a common benign nodule composed of mature adipose tissue surrounded by a thin connective tissue capsule. Lipomas can arise in many areas of the body, including the axilla, breast, and chest wall, and typically reside within subcutaneous tissues. Palpable nodules are slow growing, usually unilateral, and generally range from 2 to 10 cm in size. Large lipomas are susceptible to internal fat necrosis.

Signs and Symptom

When palpable, the painless fatty mass is typically smoothly circumscribed, movable, soft, and compressible.

Mammographic Features

Delineation of a small lipoma is difficult in the fatty breast. Larger masses displace surrounding tissues. A lipoma

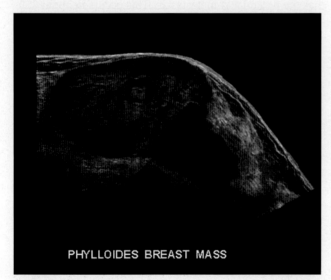

PHYLLOIDES BREAST MASS

FIGURE 18-35 Phyllodes tumor. This fast-growing, lobulated, circumscribed solid mass shows internal cystic areas. (Image courtesy of Philips Healthcare, Bothell, WA.)

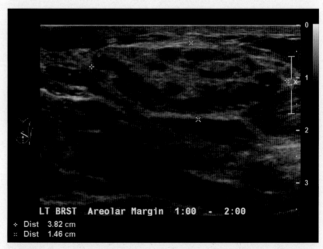

LT BRST   Areolar Margin 1:00 - 2:00
+ Dist 3.82 cm
:: Dist 1.46 cm

FIGURE 18-36 Hamartoma. Sonogram shows a mass within the mammary zone that displays a mixture of echogenicities representing a combination of fibroglandular tissues and fat.

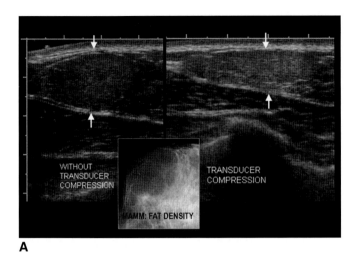

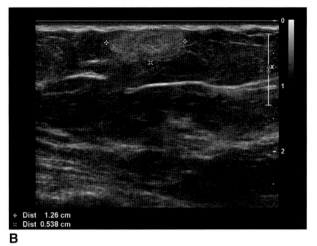

FIGURE 18-37 Lipoma. **A:** Transducer pressure confirms compressibility of a soft, palpable, mildly echogenic, circumscribed mass. Mammogram (*inset*) confirms a radiolucent fatty mass. **B:** Hyperechoic lipoma is present within the subcutaneous fat. (Reprinted with permission from Carr-Hoefer C. *Breast Ultrasound: A Comprehensive Sonographer's Guide*. Pegasus Lectures; 2007.)

appears as a round or oval, circumscribed, purely radiolucent mass surrounded by a thin radiopaque fibrous capsule (Fig. 18-37A). A pure fat density mass is a benign finding (BI-RADS 2) and does not require sonography for further risk assessment. However, sonography can help differentiate a lipoma from a fat-containing cyst.[4,5]

Sonographic Features

On a sonogram, a lipoma is smooth-walled, thinly encapsulated nodule with an echogenicity that is isoechoic or mildly hyperechoic compared with the adjacent normal fat. Lipomas can be homogeneous or may contain multiple fine linear echoes. There may be mild posterior enhancement.

Recognition of a lipoma may be difficult in the isoechoic fatty breast. A lipoma may also be missed if it is larger than the field of view of the linear-array transducer. Split-screen or EFOV imaging will better display the spatial extent of a large lipoma. Echopalpation allows direct correlation of real-time imaging findings with the clinical findings. A lipoma is soft and usually compresses by at least 30% with overlying transducer pressure and does not indent the pectoralis muscle. This can be documented using dual-screen imaging or with cine clips (Fig. 18-37A).

A small hyperechoic lipoma in the subcutaneous fat is readily discernable (Fig. 18-37B). A differential diagnosis for a hyperechoic subcutaneous lesion may include focal fat edema, fat necrosis, fibrous change, or hemangioma depending on the patient's history.

Benign Papillary Lesions

Benign papillary breast masses have various US presentations, including an intraductal mass, a solid mass, or a complex cystic and solid mass.

An *intraductal (large duct) papilloma* is a common duct neoplasm that most often occurs during late reproductive years. This benign proliferative mass develops from focal overgrowth of duct epithelial and myoepithelial cells and is supported by a fibrovascular stalk. A papilloma typically develops centrally, beneath, or close to the areola within a major lactiferous duct, rather than in a TDLU. A central intraductal papilloma is often solitary and can be too small

to palpate. However, some papillomas grow to several centimeters and can extend into duct branches. Malignant degeneration is rare, although the presence of a papilloma slightly increases the risk for developing breast cancer.

An ingrowing papilloma can obstruct the duct, causing a cyst to form that envelops the solid lesion. This type is termed *intracystic papilloma*. Torsion or infarction of the fibrovascular stalk can cause bleeding into the cyst.

Peripheral papillomatosis is a form of epithelial hyperplasia, causing the formation of multiple small papillary growths in the small ducts of a TDLU. The occurrence is much less common than large duct papillomas. Papillomatosis can be bilateral and affect multiple lobules in any breast quadrant. This proliferative condition can be associated with radial scars, sclerosing adenosis, atypical ductal hyperplasia, and ductal carcinoma. Papillomatosis carries higher risk for developing breast cancer than a central papilloma.

Juvenile papillomatosis can afflict teens and young women, many of which have a family history of breast cancer. The juvenile form shows papillomatosis with possible severe atypia, extensive cyst formation, and sclerosing adenosis. This uncommon condition also serves as a marker for increased breast cancer risk.

Signs and Symptoms of Intraductal Papilloma

The patient may be asymptomatic. A bloody or watery (serous) nipple discharge may be the first clinical sign of a developing lesion. A benign papilloma is the leading cause of spontaneous bloody nipple discharge from a single breast duct (Table 18-12). Occasionally, masses are palpable.

Mammographic Features

Standard mammography can miss a central papilloma with suspicion raised only by the presence of an asymmetrically dilated subareolar duct. Contrast ductography (galactography) better delineates the intraductal filling defect. A solitary papilloma can appear as a subareolar soft-tissue nodule that may have a "raspberry-like" microlobulated appearance. Clusters of soft-tissue isodense masses may indicate multiple papillomas. Occasionally, microcalcifications are present.

TABLE 18-12 **Nipple Discharge**	
Physiologic Discharge	**Pathologic Discharge**
• Bilateral • Nonspontaneous (expressed only) • Green, milky, yellow, brown, black • Involves multiple ducts	• Unilateral • Spontaneous • Bloody; clear or serous • Involves single duct • Possible association with mass skin/nipple changes
Associations: • Fibrocystic change • Breast feeding; galactorrhea • Mammary duct ectasia • Infection • Hormonal changes • Certain medications	**Associations (of most concern):** • Benign intraductal papilloma (most common cause of bloody nipple discharge from a single duct) • Cancer

With an intracystic papilloma, standard mammography does not differentiate between the solid and cystic components of this round or oval radiodense lesion. Before the widespread use of sonography, pneumocystography was used to evaluate the cyst cavity by injecting air into the cyst following fluid aspiration.

Sonographic Features of Intraductal Papilloma

A very small papilloma may escape detection. The only clue to its presence may be localized dilatation of a solitary duct. Occasionally, the duct dilates enough to allow visualization of the indwelling soft-tissue mass (Fig. 18-38). The mass may extend for a distance within the duct and into duct branches. Color Doppler demonstrates blood flow within the fibrovascular stalk of the lesion, allowing differentiation from echogenic blood or inspissated material within the dilated duct. A papilloma without associated ductal fluid appears as a circumscribed, round or oval, isoechoic to hypoechoic solid mass in the subareolar or periareolar region of the breast. Margins may show microlobulation. The presence of calcifications can raise suspicion level.

Radial scans align the transducer along the long axis of a major duct, which allows better detection of intraductal lesions. Performing "two-handed peripheral compression" can also help evaluate dilated subareolar ducts (Fig. 18-39A).[9,10]

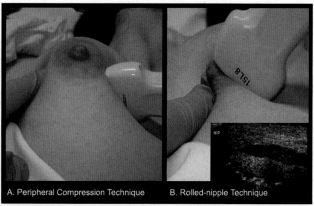

A. Peripheral Compression Technique   B. Rolled-nipple Technique

FIGURE 18-39 A: Peripheral compression technique for subareolar duct evaluation. The transducer is oriented in a radial plane along the long axis of the duct to be examined. The nonscanning hand is placed on the opposite side of breast to provide counter pressure. This maneuver brings the subareolar duct into a scan plane more parallel to the transducer. **B:** Rolled-nipple technique. The transducer is placed alongside the nipple parallel to the long axis of the excretory and subareolar duct. The index finger of the nonscanning hand is placed on the opposite side of the nipple. Light transducer pressure is applied to roll the nipple over the index finger. This maneuver allows a subareolar duct to be imaged as it passes through the nipple. The sonogram shows a nipple adenoma within a dilated excretory duct using the rolled-nipple technique (*insert*). (Reprinted with permission from Carr-Hoefer C. *Breast Ultrasound for the Sonomammographer*. Sound Imaging Consulting, LLC; 2007.)

The "rolled-nipple technique" allows a subareolar intraductal lesion to be followed into the nipple and can also identify a nipple mass, such as an adenoma (Fig. 18-39B).[10,14] Pressing over a dilated duct with the transducer may trigger nipple discharge that correlates with clinical findings.

Sonography cannot definitively differentiate benign from malignant papillary lesions, so biopsy or excision is typically warranted. As an alternative to surgical excision in certain cases, removal of a papilloma may be accomplished utilizing a VAB device.[6,35] Removal also alleviates clinical symptoms.

Sonographic Features of Intracystic Papilloma

Unlike mammography, sonography delineates both the solid and cystic components of the lesion (Fig. 18-40). A portion of the papilloma is sometimes seen extending past

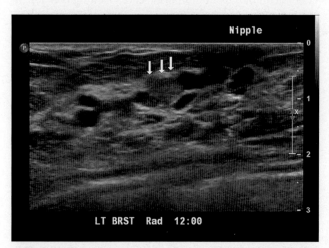

FIGURE 18-38 Intraductal papilloma. Fluid within a dilated subareolar duct outlines the small indwelling solid soft-tissue mass (*arrows*) in a patient with spontaneous nipple discharge from a single duct.

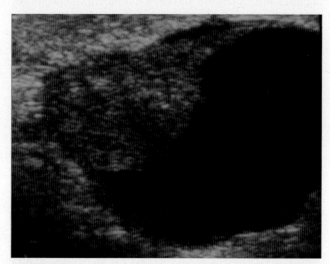

FIGURE 18-40 Intracystic papilloma. Sonogram documents a solid papillary lesion projecting into a cyst. The cyst is caused by obstruction of the duct by the indwelling mass.

the cyst wall into the duct. Doppler flow within the solid component of this complex lesion differentiates an intracystic papillary tumor from a hemorrhagic cyst with clot or from PAM. Both the cyst walls and the solid intramural nodule should be evaluated for suspicious imaging findings. This complex cystic and solid mass qualifies for a BI-RADS 4 classification. Biopsy or excision is recommended to exclude intracystic papillary carcinoma or necrotic tumor because imaging features can overlap. VAB facilitates removal of both the cyst fluids and provides tissue cores for cytologic and histologic analysis.

Sonographic Features of Juvenile Papillomatosis

In young females, a focal, ill-defined, heterogeneous mass containing several small peripheral cysts may indicate juvenile papillomatosis. Multiple small cystic areas within the stroma can give the affected lobe a "swiss cheese" appearance.

Malignant Breast Masses[4–14,26,32,36–43]

Excluding skin cancer, breast cancer is the most common malignancy affecting women in the United States. Breast carcinoma ranks second to lung cancer as the leading cause of cancer-related deaths in women over age 50. Approximately one in eight American women develop breast cancer during a lifetime.[36,37] Rates vary with race or ethnicity. The prevalence of breast cancer is highest in Caucasian women. However, African American women are more likely to die from the disease, often presenting with high-grade lesions. Breast cancer is rare in males.[36,37]

Risk factors for developing breast cancer are well documented, with many discussed here (Table 18-13).[2,3,36–44] The majority of breast cancers occur in women over the age of 50 when most are postmenopausal. Occurrence in women under age 40 is less than 5%. Besides gender and increasing age, two major risk factors are a personal or family history of breast cancer and a personal history of biopsy-proven high-risk lesion (e.g., atypical ductal/lobular hyperplasia, lobular carcinoma in situ [LCIS]/lobular neoplasia).[6] Hormonal influences include early onset of menses, nulliparity or late pregnancy, late menopause, use of combined HRT, and postmenopausal obesity. Only about 5% to 10% of breast cancers are genetically linked. *BRCA1* and *BRCA2* gene mutations significantly increase the risk for developing breast cancer. These gene mutations are also linked to ovarian, pancreas, and colon cancers. Genetically linked breast cancer tends to occur at an earlier age in both females and males and also well documented in those of Ashkenazi Jewish heritage. *BRCA* mutations pose higher risk for more aggressive breast tumors, triple-negative breast cancer (TNBC), and cancer in both breasts. Men with a BRCA2 mutation are also at higher risk for prostate cancer. The genetic condition, Li–Fraumeni syndrome, also shows an increased association of breast cancer and phyllodes tumors. High breast tissue density, as shown with mammography, is another important indicator of increased relative risk for developing cancer within the breast.[4–6]

Cancers are traditionally classified by histologic type and grade. Breast cancers are usually adenocarcinomas that arise from epithelial cells that line the breast ducts. Most cancers likely originate in a TDLU at the junction of the extralobular terminal with the lobule.[10] Malignant cells can further extend along the path of the duct into the lobule and/or migrate into larger ducts and potentially spread within the ductal system to other TDLUs within a breast lobe. Breast cancer has the highest chance ($\sim 50\%$) of developing in the UOQ where there is the greatest amount of glandular-epithelial tissue. Rarer types of malignancies include sarcomas that arise from connective tissues, primary lymphoma, leukemia, and metastases.

Certain cancers are more likely to be *multifocal* or *multicentric*, or even bilateral, which affects prognosis, surgical management, and treatment and increases recurrence rates. Multifocality describes the presence of additional malignant lesions within a breast quadrant or within 5 cm of the primary tumor, indicating spread of cancer via the ducts. Multicentricity describes coexistent cancers within different quadrants or separated by 5 cm or more within the breast. Multicentric lesions may be of the same or different histologic types.

This section discusses the pathologic, clinical, and common imaging features of many types of breast malignancies.

Noninvasive Cancer

Noninvasive breast cancer is called carcinoma in situ. The abnormal cells are confined within the boundaries of the duct and/or lobule and have not extended past the basement membrane into adjacent tissue, thus virtually eliminating the risk of metastasis.

Lobular Carcinoma In Situ

LCIS is not considered a malignancy, so it is not assigned a cancer stage.[38] However, this *lobular neoplasia* is a high-risk proliferative disease that serves as a marker for increased future risk of developing cancer (ductal or lobular) in either breast. The abnormal cells arise in the small ducts of the breast lobule, may be multifocal or multicentric, and can develop in both breasts. LCIS typically does not present with specific clinical, mammographic, or sonographic features to aid detection. Diagnosis is typically made as an incidental finding from histologic analysis of breast tissue from a biopsy or surgical specimen. LCIS has a tendency to affect premenopausal patients.

Ductal Carcinoma In Situ

DCIS is also called "intraductal carcinoma." It is the most common noninvasive cancer and typically diagnosed by screening mammography. The mean age at the time of

TABLE 18-13 **Female Breast Cancer Risk Factors**	
• Advanced age	• High breast density
• Personal and/or family history of breast cancer	• Exogenous estrogen use
• Personal history atypical ductal hyperplasia, LCIS/lobular neoplasia	• Postmenopausal obesity
• Genetic predisposition (e.g., BRCA1, BRCA2 mutation; genetic syndrome; Ashkenazi Jewish heritage)	• Alcohol consumption (>1 drink/day)
• Early menarche; late menopause	• High-dose chest radiation at young age
• Nulliparity; late age for first pregnancy	• Environmental factors

detection in women is about 50 years. This early, node-negative cancer is classified as stage 0 disease. The 5-year survival rate approaches 99% to 100% in treated patients.[36] Atypical ductal hyperplasia is a precursor to developing DCIS. Like invasive disease, DCIS can be classified by histologic grade, which helps to predict the aggressiveness of the disease and the recurrence risk. Left untreated, high-nuclear grade (comedo) DCIS is more likely, and more quickly, to progress to invasive cancer than is low nuclear grade (noncomedo) DCIS. High-grade DCIS is also more likely to recur as invasive cancer. High-grade lesions typically distend the duct with malignant cells that usually undergo extensive central necrosis and calcification. The necrotic tumor cells plug the duct with white-to-yellowish paste-like debris.

Signs and Symptoms

Such early disease is typically asymptomatic, although some patients may present with nipple discharge. Nipple discharge that is spontaneous, unilateral, bloody, or serous is worrisome. A palpable mass is uncommon.

Mammographic Features

DCIS is the earliest form of breast cancer detected by imaging techniques and best detected by mammography. DCIS represents approximately 25% of cancers detected by screening mammography. Incidence is higher in women younger than 50 years. DCIS most often presents only as suspicious calcifications, rather than a mass, on mammography. Most breast calcifications are benign, but certain patterns raise suspicion for malignancy. Suspicious microcalcifications can be irregular in size and shape. Amorphous (indistinct), coarse heterogeneous, pleomorphic, or fine linear or branching calcifications are considered more suspicious for malignancy.[4-6] Microcalcifications may also be tightly grouped (clustered) (Fig. 18-41). In other cases, sonography may be useful to exclude any related mass effect that might be missed in the radiographic dense breast before intervention.

MRI has a high sensitivity for detecting DCIS but is not used as a primary screening tool.

Sonographic Features

Sonographic features of DCIS vary. This early cancer can go undiagnosed by sonography, especially because microcalcifications can be unresolved owing to volume averaging and blend in with adjacent echogenic tissue. Suspicious calcifications are more easily identified within a distended duct or a hypoechoic mass (Fig. 18-42A, B). Microcalcifications are best seen with newer high-resolution transducers and by optimizing technical factors. Lower grade DCIS may not grossly distend the duct or TDLU. Calcifications are more evident with higher grade lesions.

The presence of intraluminal echoes and/or tiny hyperechoic foci (calcifications) within a duct is worrisome, especially when correlate with a suspicious area on mammography. The duct may appear microlobulated or show a branch pattern. Fluid within a duct helps outline intraluminal changes and duct irregularity. Alternatively, DCIS may appear as a hypoechoic nonshadowing mass that may appear microlobulated or have an irregular shape. Intracystic papillary DCIS can appear as a complex solid and cystic lesion. A microcyst cluster with thick intervening walls or solid components can also suggest early cancer. Color or power Doppler helps differentiate an intraductal neoplasm from inspissated secretions and confirms a solid mural nodule with a cystic mass. However, DCIS may not elicit a Doppler signal. 3D sonograms reconstructed in the coronal plane may help show ductal changes associated with a branch pattern.

Suspicious calcifications are typically biopsied with mammographic guidance utilizing a VAB device, followed by postbiopsy clip placement and specimen radiography to confirm adequate sampling. On occasion, sonographic guidance is elected when suspicious calcifications are well seen.

Paget Disease

Paget disease is a rare cancer involving the epidermis of the nipple and areola, often initiated by underlying DCIS within a main subareolar duct.[5] The diagnosis is often suspected clinically based on findings of redness, ulceration, and eczema-like crusting of the nipple and areola, along with nipple discharge and itching. A biopsy of the affected tissues and cytologic analysis of the nipple discharge can

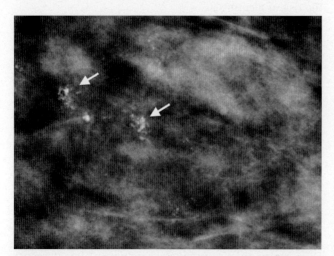

FIGURE 18-41 Ductal carcinoma in situ (*DCIS*). Mammogram shows suspicious microcalcifications (*arrows*) extending in a linear and grouped pattern in a woman with intermediate- to high-grade DCIS.

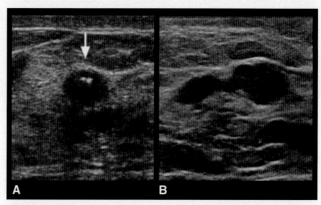

FIGURE 18-42 Ductal carcinoma in situ. **A:** Cross section of a dilated duct containing hypoechoic internal echoes and tiny, nonshadowing, hyperechoic microcalcifications (*arrow*). **B:** Tubular dilatation of a duct with internal echoes with a lobulated contour. The duct wall is intact.

yield the diagnosis. Sonography is generally not needed unless to characterize a subareolar mass.

Invasive Cancer

Invasive cancer describes cases when malignant cells breach the basement membrane of the duct and/or lobule and extend into adjacent tissues. Cancer cells can then penetrate nearby blood vessels and lymphatic channels, both pathways for metastatic seeding.

Invasive Ductal Carcinoma[4–15,25,32,36–43]

IDC is the most common breast cancer. Histologically, this cancer is also referred to as infiltrating or invasive ductal carcinoma of no special type (IDC NST) or invasive ductal carcinoma, not otherwise specified (IDC NOS). This designation is used because the cancer cells lack specific histologic features to better classify the tumor. IDC accounts for about 65% to 80% of all breast cancers and is the leading invasive malignancy. The prognosis for IDC NOS patients is usually poorer than for other invasive tumors, especially for high-grade lesions.

IDC typically incites a desmoplasia (fibroelastic) as tumor cells infiltrate neighboring tissues. Tumors often present as hard, fixed, stellate lesions (scirrhous features). Slow-growing IDCs allow more time for reactive fibrosis to occur, which helps to confine the tumor. Slow-growing lesions are often of lower grade, and the fibrous reaction can account for a large percentage of the tumor's makeup. Reactive fibrosis contributes to thickening and straightening of the Cooper ligaments that may lead to skin retraction. In contrast, fast-growing cancers lack time for much reactive fibrosis to occur, and instead, often incite an inflammatory response, causing peritumoral edema. Such tumors are often of higher grade, show expansile growth, and tend to display more circumscribed margins. High-grade lesions typically contain abundant tumor cells, plasma cells, and lymphocytes and show prominent vascularity. High-grade cancers and those with extensive intraductal (DCIS) components and ductal extension are more likely to develop satellite lesions, resulting in multifocal disease.

Signs and Symptoms

When palpable, the carcinoma is usually hard, fixed, and painless. The most common location is the UOQ. Lesions with reactive fibrosis can feel larger on palpation than their actual size. Unilateral bloody or serosanguineous nipple discharge is a worrisome finding but relatively uncommon. Secondary skin dimpling or nipple retraction or breast contour changes may be visible with advanced disease.

Mammographic Features

The principal sign of invasive cancer is an asymmetric, irregular, radiodense mass with spiculated margins (Fig. 18-43A). Associated suspicious calcifications are common, indicating DCIS component of the tumor. Surrounding architectural distortion is often noted, including thickening and straightening of the Cooper ligaments. A spiculated lesion is classified as BI-RADS 5 being highly suspicious for malignancy with a recommendation for tissue sampling. Sonography is not required to further characterize the mass unless to better assess tumor extent and to search for satellite lesions or adenopathy. However, IDC can display more indeterminate features on mammography, and sonographic evaluation is recommended before assigning a final risk classification.

Sonographic Features

As previously discussed, the presence of certain sonographic features allows classification of a mass as "suspicious for malignancy" in the absence of prior site infection or trauma (Table 18-10).[9,10,32] The vast majority of breast cancers detected with sonography will prove to be IDC. IDC often displays a variety of sonographic appearances because tumors can have a combination of invasive and DCIS components and affect the surrounding tissues as they grow. Tumors also differ in histologic makeup, grade, vascularity, and biologic behaviors.

Suspicious findings for a solid breast mass include irregular shape; noncircumscribed margins (indistinct, spiculated, angular, microlobulated); nonparallel orientation within the breast (taller-than-wide); hypoechogenicity, especially when marked; calcifications; posterior shadowing beneath

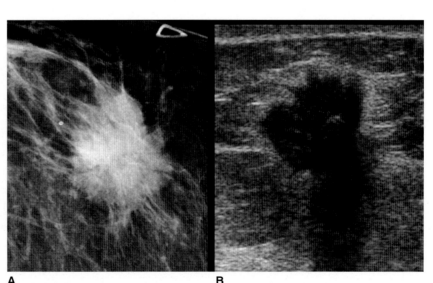

FIGURE 18-43 Invasive ductal carcinoma. **A:** Mammogram shows a spiculated, radiodense mass. Skin marker denotes the mass is palpable. **B:** Sonogram of the heterogeneous solid mass shows multiple malignant features, including irregular shape with angular margins, spiculation, thick echogenic halo, nonparallel orientation, hypoechogenicity, and partial acoustic shadowing. (Reprinted with permission from Carr-Hoefer C. *Breast Ultrasound: A Comprehensive Sonographer's Guide.* Pegasus Lectures; 2007.)

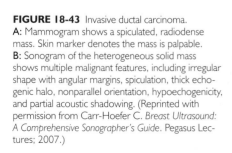

A   B

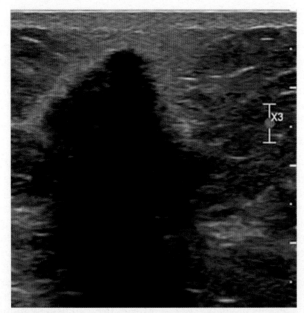

FIGURE 18-44 Invasive ductal carcinoma. Intense complete acoustic shadowing is a key suspicious feature of this carcinoma. Note indistinct margins with increased echogenicity of the mass border and adjacent tissues. (Image courtesy of Philips Healthcare, Bothell, WA.)

all or a portion of the mass; and associated ductal changes, including duct extension and/or branch pattern (Figs. 18-43B to 18-48). Some IDCs show multiple suspicious findings, whereas others do not. Some mimic a benign mass, but careful inspection will typically reveal at least one worrisome feature.

Higher grade IDC lesions can be relatively circumscribed, oval or rounded, and often markedly hypoechoic. These tumors show prominent cellularity and vascularity, resulting in increased sound transmission (Fig. 18-49) rather than shadowing. Rapid growth can incite an echogenic border of peritumoral edema rather than an indistinct rim from spiculation. The presence of other suspicious features will lessen confusion with a benign mass. Higher grade tumors may show prominent microlobulation. Tumor extension into the ducts increases the potential for satellite lesions.

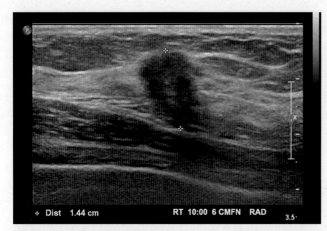

FIGURE 18-45 Malignant features. A taller-than-wide (not parallel orientation) can be a feature of a smaller cancer growing within a vertically oriented terminal ductolobular unit. This invasive ductal carcinoma also shows indistinct margins.

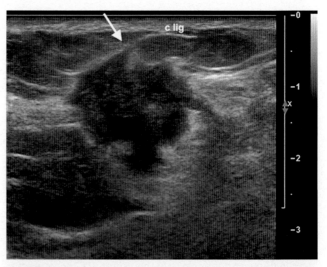

FIGURE 18-46 Malignant features. This heterogeneous invasive ductal carcinoma shows an irregular shape. Angular margins are best seen at the junction of the mass with a Cooper ligament (*arrow*). This mass also displays indistinct margins with some spiculation and straightening of Cooper ligaments. Mass orientation is not parallel to the skin. (Image courtesy of Philips Healthcare, Bothell, WA.)

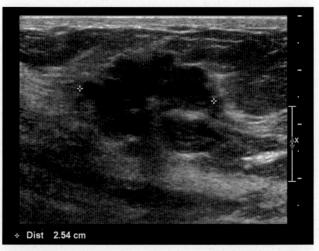

FIGURE 18-47 Malignant features. Prominent microlobulation and marked hypoechogenicity are key features of higher grade invasive breast carcinoma with intraductal components.

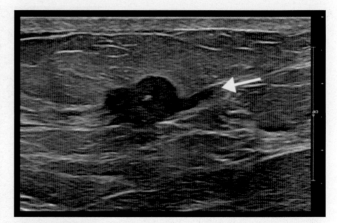

FIGURE 18-48 Malignant features. A radial scan showing duct extension (*arrow*) with tumor growing into a single duct, leading toward the nipple. Tumor involving smaller branching ducts extend away from then nipple. A calcification is noted within the mass. (Image courtesy of Philips Healthcare, Bothell, WA.)

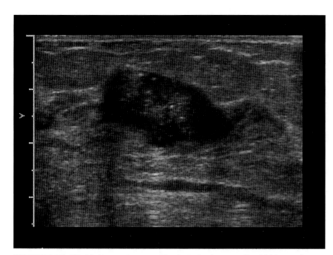

FIGURE 18-49 Malignant features. A relatively circumscribed high-grade invasive ductal carcinoma showing a heterogeneous echo pattern, near-parallel orientation, and some distal sound enhancement. Tiny, hyperechoic foci represent microcalcifications within intraductal components of the malignant tumor.

Associated signs of invasion include architectural distortion affecting any level of the breast. Cooper ligaments may appear thickened, straightened, or retracted. The skin may become thickened, flattened, retracted, or bulged. Nipple inversion is possible. Interruption of the fascial planes separating fat, glandular, and muscular structures suggests invasion. Tumors breeching the superficial or retromammary fat layers may eventually penetrate and become fixed to the skin or pectoral fascia. Secondary nodal involvement is possible.

Differential Diagnosis

Clinical correlation is important, because several benign conditions can display architectural distortion, poorly circumscribed margins, attenuation shadowing, or other sonographic features that simulate cancer (Table 18-14). A necrotic IDC may appear as a complex cystic and solid mass.

Invasive Lobular Carcinoma

Invasive lobular carcinoma (ILC) is the second most common invasive breast malignancy, representing about 10% of all breast cancer cases. This cancer often shows a diffuse infiltrative growth pattern and has higher rates of being multifocal, multicentric, and bilateral than IDC. Tumor cells

TABLE 18-14	**Solid Breast Mass: Diagnostic Pitfall**
Benign Solid Masses or Conditions Mimicking Cancer	**Circumscribed Cancers Mimicking Benign Mass**
• Fat necrosis	• High-grade invasive ductal carcinoma
• Sclerosing adenosis	
• Radial scar	• Medullary carcinoma
• Postsurgical scar	• Colloid carcinoma
• Degenerating fibroadenoma	• Papillary carcinoma
• Focal fibrosis; diabetic mastopathy	• Phylloides
	• Intracystic carcinoma
• Granular cell tumor	• Lymphoma
• Inflammatory changes	• Metastasis
• Cooper ligament shadowing	• Triple-negative breast cancer

tend to line up in "single files" and infiltrate the stroma in a diffuse manner and less often form a solitary discrete mass. Desmoplasia is not a dominant feature with ILC.

Signs and Symptoms

ILC may present as a hard fixed palpable mass. However, this cancer may, instead, feel like an area of nonspecific parenchymal thickening, making clinical diagnosis difficult. With advanced disease, the affected tissues can retract, causing a "shrinking breast."

Mammographic Features

Mammography can underestimate and even miss ILC, especially in early stages or in the radiographically dense breast. The diffuse infiltrative nature of the disease may have a radiodensity equal to or less than surrounding parenchyma. Suspicious calcifications are uncommon. ILC may present as a region of architectural distortion or asymmetric density. Findings might be better appreciated on only one mammographic view. At times, ILCs present an ill-defined mass with spiculated or obscured margins.

Sonographic Features

Sonography is helpful at confirming abnormal tissue patterns at the region of clinical or mammographic concern. Sonographic patterns are variable, but ILC often appears as an irregular, ill-defined, hypoechoic solid mass with acoustic shadowing (Fig. 18-50A, B). Subtle findings can include architectural distortion.

When ILC is suspected or confirmed by biopsy, bilateral whole-breast sonography may be indicated to search for multifocal, multicentric disease (especially if MRI examination is unavailable to evaluate the extent of disease and nodal changes). Both MRI and breast-specific gamma imaging (BSGI) show high sensitivity to detecting ILC.[40]

Special-Type Invasive Ductal Carcinomas

Tubular, medullary, colloid, and papillary carcinomas represent a small subgroup of IDCs that have morphologic and histologic features allowing specific classification. Except for tubular cancer, these special-type IDCs are usually highly cellular lesions that tend to display relatively well-circumscribed margins. Compared with IDC NOS lesions, these special-type cancers occur infrequently and usually have better prognoses with lower rates of nodal metastases.

Tubular Carcinoma

Pure tubular carcinoma accounts for about 2% of all breast cancers. However, mammographic detection has increased detection rates. This extremely well-differentiated invasive cancer is typically small, slow growing, and incites prominent reactive fibrosis. Pure tumors rarely exceed 2 cm in size and have an excellent prognosis with a low incidence of axillary lymph node metastasis. Tumors often develop within TDLUs in the peripheral breast and can arise from a radial scar. The median age of women diagnosed with tubular carcinoma is 50 years. At biopsy, tubular carcinomas are often classified as low-grade IDC NOS depending on the percentage of tubular features present. Multicentric and bilateral lesions are often coupled with LCIS in adjacent tissues. Studies suggest that a radial scar may be a precursor to tubular carcinoma.[8]

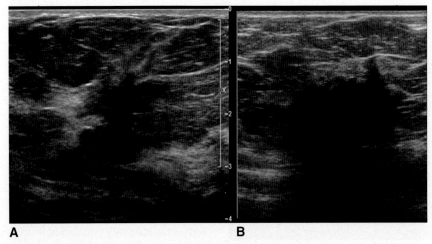

FIGURE 18-50 Invasive lobular carcinoma (*ILC*). **A:** Sonogram shows an irregular, hypoechoic area within the breast with indistinct margins. **B:** This ILC appears as a markedly hypoechoic, irregular mass, showing partial acoustic shadowing.

Signs and Symptoms

Palpable lesions tend to be fixed and may cause skin dimpling.

Mammographic Features

A pure tubular lesion can appear as a small, irregular, centrally radiodense mass often with long spicules (white-star appearance) or as an area of architectural distortion.

Sonographic Features

Tubular cancer is often a small, irregular, nonparallel, centrally hypoechoic mass with frank spiculation or surrounded by a thick, indistinct, echogenic rim (Fig.18-51). Acoustic shadowing accompanies reactive fibrosis. Adjacent Cooper ligaments can become thick and straight and potentially cause retraction of the overlying skin.

Medullary Carcinoma

Medullary carcinoma is a well-marginated cellular tumor that contains prominent lymphocytes and plasma cells. Pure tumors have been termed "circumscribed carcinoma." This uncommon tumor accounts for 5% of breast malignancies. Medullary tumors tend to develop earlier than other breast cancers, with most occurring before age 50, and represents 10% of invasive cancers in women under age 35. This cancer also shows strong association with the *BRCA1* gene mutation. Tumors can occasionally be multiple or bilateral. Medullary cancers show pushing expansile growth and compress peripheral tissues as they grow, typically eliciting little or no reactive fibrosis. Central necrosis is common in larger lesions. Calcification is uncommon. Enlarged axillary nodes may be present that are either reactive or contain metastases. The prognosis is favorable, especially for typical tumors smaller than 3 cm with negative nodes.

Signs and Symptoms

The discrete, rounded, somewhat soft and mobile palpable mass may simulate a benign mass. A large or rapidly growing mass poses concern with tumors often 2 to 3 cm at the time of diagnosis. Most are located in the UOQ.

Mammographic Features

The round or lobulated radiodense mass is usually circumscribed or partially circumscribed. Patterns may mimic a benign-appearing lesion (Fig. 18-52A). Calcification is not a typical feature.

Sonographic Features

Medullary cancer can appear as a round or oval, circumscribed solid mass that can be markedly hypoechoic and often shows distal enhancement. Close inspection of the mass will usually reveal some suspicious finding to warrant biopsy (e.g., microlobulation, multilobulation) (Fig. 18-52B). A thick echogenic halo around the mass from peritumoral edema can make margins less distinct. Central necrosis is relatively common, yielding a complex sonographic appearance. Color Doppler may reveal prominent vascularity, which helps differentiate a very hypoechoic lesion from a cystic mass.

Colloid Carcinoma

Colloid (mucinous) carcinoma is uncommon. Pure tumors account for about 2% of breast malignancies. This circumscribed gelatinous lesion contains tumor cells dispersed in pools of mucin. Pure mucinous tumors more often develop in

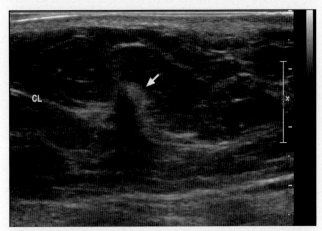

FIGURE 18-51 Tubular carcinoma. This small, peripheral, taller-than-wide, hypoechoic lesion displays a thick echogenic halo from subtle spiculation (*arrow*) and acoustic shadowing. Cooper ligament (*CL*) straightening is noted.

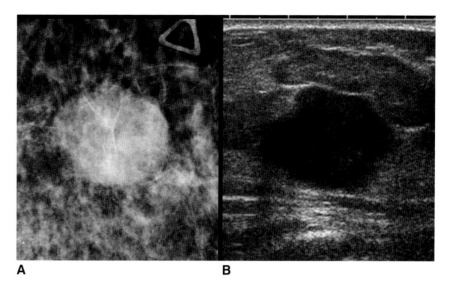

FIGURE 18-52 Medullary carcinoma. **A:** Mammogram demonstrates a rounded circumscribed mass. **B:** Sonogram shows a circumscribed, hypoechoic mass with several margin lobulations, along with some distal sound enhancement. (Reprinted with permission from Carr-Hoefer C. *Breast Ultrasound: A Comprehensive Sonographer's Guide.* Pegasus Lectures; 2007.)

A **B**

elderly women. Although slow growing, a colloid carcinoma can attain a large size. Unlike medullary cancer, internal hemorrhage is uncommon. Mixed lesions can display more invasive features.

Signs and Symptoms

When palpable, the mass can have a soft consistency or feel like an area of thickening. A large lesion may be fixed to the skin or chest wall.

Mammographic Features

Pure colloid carcinoma can appear as a lower density circumscribed mass that is round, oval, or lobulated that lacks calcifications. Mixed tumors show higher density more suspicious features.

Sonographic Features

Colloid carcinoma can image as a round or oval, circumscribed mass with possible lobulation or microlobulation (Fig. 18-53). Internal echogenicity is often isoechoic or

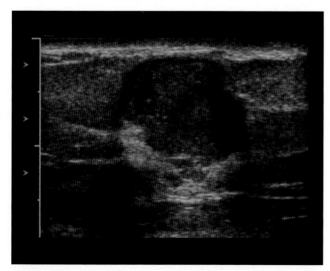

FIGURE 18-53 Colloid carcinoma. This circumscribed cancer is mildly hypoechoic compared with fat and shows distal sound enhancement.

hypoechoic compared with fat, with a homogeneous or mildly heterogeneous echo pattern. At times, internal fluid-filled spaces may be resolved. Sound transmission is normal or enhanced. A colloid cancer may occasionally mimic a fat lobule or lipoma; however, the mucinous tumor will not be compressible.

Papillary Carcinoma

Solid papillary and intracystic papillary carcinomas tend to occur in older postmenopausal women and account for 1% to 2% of invasive breast malignancies. The incidence is slightly higher in men. Papillary carcinoma can occur centrally within the breast from malignant transformation of a large duct papilloma or develop within a peripheral TDLU. Lesions can be focal or multifocal within the breast ducts. Tumor growth is usually slow. Papillary cancers are more often in situ lesions. An absence of myoepithelial cells indicates invasion; however, invasive tumors tend to be low grade. Intracystic variants frequently contain bloody fluid. Clinical and imaging features of intraductal and intracystic papillary carcinomas may not differ significantly from their benign counterparts, so histologic evaluation is important.

Signs and Symptoms

Of concern is bloody nipple discharge from a single duct, which may be associated with a relatively soft centrally located mass.

Sonographic Features

Some in situ lesions may be too small to image. The new development of a circumscribed solid or complex cystic mass in an older patient remains worrisome because imaging features of benign and invasive tumors overlap. Duct dilatation is not always present to outline a papillary lesion. Solid tumors are evaluated for suspicious findings (e.g., microlobulation, duct extension, branch pattern, calcification). Malignant intraductal papillary lesions tend to be larger, extend a greater distance within a duct, branch more extensively into adjacent ducts, and potentially disrupt the duct wall. Radial and antiradial scans better assess ductal patterns. Color Doppler can demonstrate prominent blood

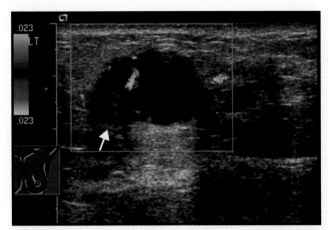

FIGURE 18-54 Intracystic papillary carcinoma. This complex cystic and solid lesion shows an intramural solid nodule (*arrow*) within a septated cystic mass. Color Doppler reveals blood flow along some of the internal septations and along the wall.

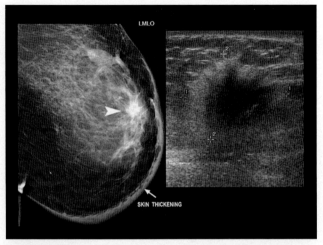

FIGURE 18-55 Inflammatory carcinoma. Postmenopausal woman with a swollen, warm breast that had a peau d'orange appearance. The mammogram shows marked skin thickening (*arrow*) primarily involving the mid to lower breast, as well as an anterior suspicious radiodense lesion (*arrowhead*). The sonogram showed an irregular, spiculated, hypoechoic mass with a thick echogenic rim (*calipers*). Biopsy of the mass and the skin confirmed invasive ductal carcinoma with tumor emboli in the subdermal lymphatics.

flow within the vascular stalk of a papillary cancer, which may show multiple feeding vessels.

An intracystic papillary carcinoma is a complex lesion with cystic and solid components or mural nodule (Fig. 18-54). There may be echoes from bleeding into the cyst fluid. Any loss of wall definition, wall thickening, or extension of the tumor beyond the cyst and duct wall suggests malignant change.

Inflammatory Carcinoma

Diffuse or inflammatory carcinoma occurs when a highly invasive cancer infiltrates the lymphatics of the skin. These are often higher grade IDCs that can disseminate within the breast. This aggressive malignancy accounts for about 1% to 5% of breast cancers. Biopsy of the skin, a suspicious breast mass, and axillary nodes help differentiate inflammatory carcinoma from benign inflammation.

Signs and Symptoms

The skin can rapidly become red, warm, and edematous and develop an orange peel (peau d'orange) appearance. These symptoms typically involve over one-third of the breast. The breast is often painful and hard. Axillary lymph nodes are usually palpable.

Mammographic Features

Patient discomfort and breast swelling limit adequate breast compression. Skin thickening is evident (Fig. 18-55). Parenchymal edema further increases breast density, making delineation of a primary tumor difficult in many patients.

Sonographic Features

A whole-breast examination is warranted to search for underlying suspicious lesions (Fig. 18-55). The inflamed skin appears thick and echogenic. Lymph vessels and veins are often dilated. Doppler reveals hypervascularity of the affected tissues. In some cases, a malignant lesion may interrupt the fat–dermal interface and directly invade the skin. Significant breast edema scatters the sound beam and degrades image detail and sound penetration, thereby allowing primary and satellite lesions to be

missed. Scanning at lower frequencies improves sound transmission but reduces resolution. Comparison imaging of the opposite breast helps to document architectural variation. Expanding imaging to the nodal regions may show adenopathy in the axillary and, possibly, the internal mammary regions.

The long-term prognosis for inflammatory carcinoma is often poor but has improved in recent years. Some high-grade cancers are initially treated with neoadjuvant chemotherapy in an effort to shrink the cancer before surgical resection. In such cases, a clip can be placed with imaging guidance to mark the tumor site. Sonography or MRI can follow the tumor's response to therapy, often showing a marked reduction in skin changes, breast edema, tumor, and nodal size.[47,48]

Clinical and imaging features of inflammatory carcinoma can mimic acute mastitis. In pregnant and lactating women, breast cancer can grow and disseminate rapidly and should prompt the search for suspicious lesions in these women presenting with breast inflammation.

The Male Breast[5–15,44]

The normal male breast consists mainly of fatty tissue, a small amount of fibrous connective tissue, and some rudimentary subareolar ducts. The skin is thicker, and the muscles are larger than those usually seen in the female breast.

Males with breast enlargement, nipple discharge, tenderness, or a palpable mass are the candidates for sonography. Mammography is often technically difficult, and magnification views are recommended for adequate evaluation of smaller breasts. Males can develop many of the types of breast masses seen in women (e.g., lipoma, fat necrosis, epidermal inclusion cyst). However, because males typically do not develop breast lobules, masses such as fibroadenomas and lobular carcinomas are rare. The most significant disorders afflicting the male breast are gynecomastia and cancer.

Gynecomastia

Gynecomastia refers to benign male breast enlargement characterized by an abnormal proliferation of ductal and stromal tissues. This is the most common male breast abnormality and is associated with an increased estrogen-to-testosterone ratio. Hormonal imbalances can be linked to physiologic, pharmacologic, or pathologic causes (Table 18-15). Depending on the underlying cause, this condition can be unilateral or bilateral, transient or persist for a long time. Physiologic gynecomastia occurs in the neonate, pubertal boys, and older men at times of their lives when estrogen levels are elevated or when testosterone levels decline.

Pseudogynecomastia refers to male breast enlargement caused by excessive fat deposition without subareolar ductal proliferation. This bilateral condition is a normal variant and common in obese males.

Signs and Symptoms

Gynecomastia usually presents as a soft-to-moderately firm, mildly tender, area of fullness or nodularity centered beneath the areola. The abnormality is typically greater than 2 cm in dimension and relatively mobile. Tenderness can subside with chronic forms.

Mammographic Features

The early "nodular" form appears as a fan-shaped, subareolar density, representing glandular tissue that gradually tapers into the surrounding fat. The flame-shaped "dendritic" form develops later and radiates deeper into the breast with possible extension into the UOQ (Fig. 18-56). There is more fibrous proliferation with this phase. The "diffuse glandular" pattern results from greater estrogen stimulation and resembles a heterogeneously dense female breast. This diffuse pattern may also be seen in transgender patients on hormone therapy.

Sonographic Features

Sonography is helpful at determining whether the cause of a subareolar density is due to a mass or gynecomastia

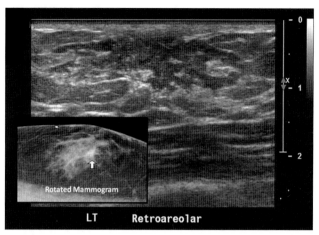

FIGURE 18-56 Gynecomastia. A middle-aged male on steroids noted breast enlargement with nodularity beneath the nipple. Sonography shows hypoechoic, subareolar, mass-like tissue with extensions into the breast core, which corresponded to fibroglandular tissue seen on the mammogram (*inset*).

(Fig. 18-56). Sonographic patterns of gynecomastia correlate well with mammography. Early changes often show a hypoechoic nodular or triangular region beneath the areola with a somewhat lobulated base. Increased vascularity on Doppler is commonly seen in this early phase of gynecomastia. The more dendritic form shows hypoechoic finger-like extensions, radiating further into the breast core surrounded by echogenic fibrous tissue. Diffuse gynecomastia can appear similar to the female fibroglandular tissue and occupy more of the mammary zone. Extra breast fat may be present.

Some patients with gynecomastia undergo sonography-guided liposuction as part of their treatment plan.

Male Breast Cancer

Breast cancer is rare in men, accounting for about 1% of all breast cancer cases. Most men affected are close to 60 years or older, which is much later than in women. Breast cancer can be genetically linked in males and shows a strong association with Klinefelter syndrome (47,XXY), BRCA, and

TABLE 18-15 **Male Breast Disease Risk Factors**	
Gynecomastia	**Breast Cancer**
Hormonal/Endocrine Imbalance	• Advanced age
• Physiologic (young age, pubertal, elderly)	• Family history breast cancer
• Hypogonadism, Klinefelter syndrome	• Inherited gene mutation: BRCA2 > BRCA1
• Testicular trauma, mumps orchitis	• Klinefelter syndrome
Neoplasm	• Liver cirrhosis
• Testicular tumor	• Testicular conditions (e.g., undescended testes, mumps
• Adrenal, renal, lung	orchitis; orchiectomy)
• Hepatoma	• Estrogen therapy (e.g., prostate cancer; transsexual treatment)
• Pituitary	• Obesity
Drug Related (examples)	• Excess alcohol consumption
• Cimetidine, digitalis, spironolactone	• Radiation therapy, especially to chest
• Marijuana, anabolic steroids	• Excessive exposure to high heat environments, certain
• Estrogen treatment for prostate cancer	occupations
Systemic Diseases / Disorders	
• Cirrhosis, chronic renal failure	
• Emphysema, tuberculosis, COPD	
• Hyperthyroidism	
• Obesity, malnutrition	
Idiopathic	

certain other gene mutations. As with gynecomastia, an elevated estrogen-to-androgen ratio increases cancer risk (Table 18-14). Because men do not undergo breast screening, cancer is usually invasive by the time of diagnosis, with IDC being the most common primary tumor. The relative incidence of intraductal and intracystic papillary carcinomas is higher in men than in women.

Primary male breast cancer is typically located beneath the areola, usually just eccentric to the nipple, with peripheral lesions presenting less often. Advanced cancer can result in skin ulceration, chest wall invasion, lymph node metastasis, and distant disease.

Signs and Symptoms

Clinically, cancer often presents as a unilateral, often painless, hard, fixed subareolar, or periareolar mass. Additional suspicious findings include bloody nipple discharge, retraction or ulceration of the nipple or skin, or palpable axillary nodes.

Mammographic Features

A lesion that is eccentric to the areola increases suspicion when trying to differentiate cancer from gynecomastia. Radiodense lesions can be round, oval, or irregular. Suspicious mammographic findings are similar to those in females, although calcifications are less often present. The close proximity of the mass to the nipple can cause skin and nipple changes. Enlarged low axillary nodes may be seen.

Sonographic Features

Some male cancers are fairly well circumscribed or may have a complex appearance (e.g., intracystic papillary carcinoma, necrotic neoplasm), whereas other lesions display definite suspicious features (e.g., irregular shape, spiculation, microlobulation, shadowing) (Fig. 18-57). Feeding vessels may be seen extending into the lesion on Doppler examination. Associated features include skin thickening and nipple retraction that are best seen when using an acoustic offset.

Other Male Breast Malignancies

Paget disease of the nipple can afflict men more than women. Other forms of cancer affecting the male breast are rare and include malignant phyllodes, lymphoma, liposarcoma, leukemia, and metastases. Nonmammary primary cancers that can metastasize to the male breast include prostate (most common), melanoma, renal, and lung cancer. Estrogen therapy for prostate cancer increases risk for male breast cancer as well as for gynecomastia.

Doppler Evaluation of the Breast[5-14]

Current sonography systems have improved Doppler sensitivity, allowing better detection of blood flow in both benign and malignant masses. Doppler, alone, has questionable efficacy differentiating benign from malignant solid masses because of overlaps in findings. Power-mode Doppler is more sensitive at blood flow detection than color Doppler. Practical uses for Doppler during a breast sonography examination are listed in Table 18-16 (Fig. 18-58).

When performing a Doppler examination, equipment settings should be optimized for low-velocity states. Too much transducer pressure will lessen or ablate blood flow, so very light touch is needed. Not all solid masses display blood flow using Doppler techniques, which can limit its utility. Microbubble contrast agents can augment Doppler flow detection within breast masses by enhancing the conspicuity of blood vessels.[9,11]

Neovascularity is a feature of cancer. In general, malignant masses tend to display more Doppler vascularity compared with benign lesions, but findings overlap. Doppler patterns reported to favor a cancer include an increased number of peripheral and penetrating (central) vessels and vessel tortuosity. Arteriovenous shunting may occur.[11] Benign masses more commonly show vessels that stretch around the periphery of the mass with fewer straight penetrating vessels. 3D Doppler may enhance detection of lesion vascularity. Cutoff values for resistive index (RI), pulsatility index (PI), and peak-systolic velocities (PSVs) have not been proved reliable enough to differentiate benign from malignant masses because of overlap between values, although some research has shown PSVs, PI, and RI values tend to be higher centrally than along the periphery in malignant lesions.[9-11]

Doppler is being used at some facilities to assess the aggressiveness of a malignant tumor and to monitor the response to therapy. Higher grade lesions tend to show increased vascularity and inflammatory hyperemia, both signs of a more aggressive tumor. A decrease in blood flow can precede tumor shrinkage following neoadjuvant chemotherapy.

Vocal fremitus is a technique using color Doppler or power-mode Doppler, in which the patient is asked to vocalize (e.g., hum "eee") during real-time imaging of an area of interest. Vibrations from the chest wall will transmit through normal breast tissues, creating flashes of color artifact. Certain abnormal tissues and masses will tend to show a "void" of color during vocal fremitus (Fig. 18-59). This vibratory defect can occur with many benign and malignant solid masses, as well as cystic masses. Although not effective at differentiating benign from malignant lesions, there are some situations when Doppler vocal fremitus is helpful.[9,10] These most often include differentiating an isoechoic solid mass from isoechoic fat lobule, differentiating malignant shadowing from benign artifactual shadowing, delineating an indistinctly marginated mass

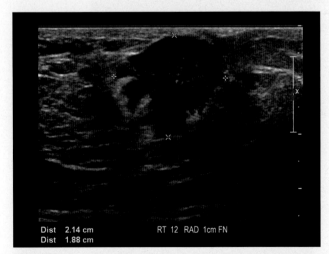

Dist 2.14 cm   RT 12 RAD 1cm FN
Dist 1.88 cm

FIGURE 18-57 Male breast carcinoma. An elderly male has a family history of breast cancer. The palpable periareolar mass corresponds to an irregular, heterogeneous, nonshadowing mass. A portion of the mass shows microlobulation and an echogenic halo.

TABLE 18-16 Doppler During Sonographic Breast Evaluation

Practical Uses

- Assess vascularity of solid mass, complex lesion, lymph node
  - (ACR lexicon) Absent vascularity, internal vascularity, vessels in rim
- Document blood flow within solid tissue to differentiate:
  - solid tumor from an echo-filled complicated cyst
  - mural nodule from an echogenic lipid layer or debris layer within a complicated cyst
  - markedly hypoechoic solid mass or abnormal lymph node from a cystic mass
- Confirm lack of blood flow within cyst, complicated cyst, fluid collection
- Document vascular stalk within intraductal or intracystic papillary mass
- Induce movement (streaming) of lightweight particles within complicated cyst fluid
- Differentiate hyperemic and inflamed tissues from normal tissues
- Differentiate blood flow in a recurrent tumor from a scar
- Differentiate a blood vessel from a fluid-filled duct
- Confirm clot within a thrombosed breast vein
- Assess flow pattern of vascular abnormality (pseudoaneurysm, AVM)
- Assess tissue response during vocal fremitus to differentiate normal from abnormal tissue

Solid Mass Assessment[a]

- Power mode more sensitive than Color Doppler for blood flow detection
- System sensitivity varies, optimize Doppler settings, use light transducer pressure
- Overlap in blood flow patterns limits Doppler's ability to differentiate benign from malignant breast masses; however, certain flow patterns are reported:
  - cancers tend to show more detectable blood flow, more peripheral and penetrating vessels (especially higher grade tumors)
  - cancers tend to show higher PSV and RIs centrally than along the mass periphery
  - benign masses tend to show rounder systolic peaks, lower PSV and RIs, peripherally and centrally
- Not all solid masses show detectable blood flow by Doppler
- Metastatic lymph nodes and primary tumors of same histologic type tend to show similar spectral waveforms
- When monitoring tumor response to neoadjuvant therapy, a decrease in Doppler blood flow can precede reduction in tumor size
- Microbubble contrast agents enhance blood flow assessment

[a]Hashmi A, Ackerman S, Irshad A. Color Doppler sonography: characterizing breast lesions. *Imaging Med.* 2010:2(2):151–163.

from adjacent tissues, and determining whether intracystic echoes are attached to the cyst wall to better differentiate a mural nodule or PAM from clotted blood or a fat–fluid level. Technical factors, such as excessive Doppler gain, transducer pressure, and focal zone placement, can alter the degree of fremitus artifact and hinder demonstration of a vibratory defect. Doppler information should be correlated with the clinical history and other imaging findings before a diagnosis is rendered.

BREAST CANCER STAGING AND PROGNOSTIC FACTORS[5,9–11,36–43,45–47]

The prognosis of breast cancer is greatly affected by the stage and extent of the disease at the time of diagnosis. Genetic testing, such as that for BRCA1 or BRCA2, provides valuable information of a person's risk for developing cancer.

Breast cancer prognosis is affected by histologic type, grade, tumor size (T), regional nodal status (N), evidence of distant

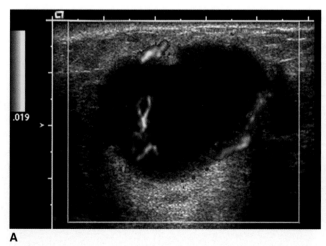

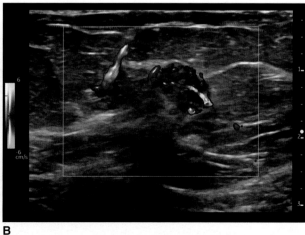

A **B**

FIGURE 18-58 Doppler. **A:** Power-mode Doppler shows sensitivity to detect blood flow within this complex cystic and solid mass and along the wall. The mass appeared internally cystic on grayscale imaging; however, internal vascularity confirmed solid internal components. **B:** Color Doppler reveals blood flow within and around a solid breast mass. (Image courtesy of GE Healthcare, Milwaukee, WI.)

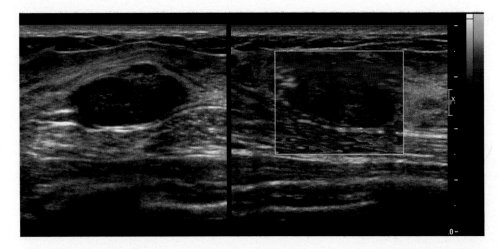

FIGURE 18-59 Fremitus. Power Doppler fremitus image shows a vibratory artifact defect (*color void*) corresponding to the solid lesion, whereas the surrounding normal tissues transmit the Doppler artifact. (Image courtesy of Philips Healthcare, Bothell, WA.)

metastasis (M), and other factors such as biologic markers and molecular subtypes. The TNM system is a classification system used to stage malignant tumors, which assists in patient management and treatment planning.[38] Regional lymph node status is a key predictor of breast cancer survival. Because metastatic disease is not curable, the goal of screening is to detect breast cancers early when tumors are small and node status is negative, thus improving long-term survival.

Using the TNM staging system, breast cancers are placed into five categories with further subcategorization to better stage the extent of involvement. Stage 0 is assigned to noninvasive cancer, such as DCIS. Stages I through IV apply to invasive carcinoma. Stage IA indicates early-stage invasive disease when tumors are small (≤2 cm) and show no nodal involvement or metastatic disease. Stage V is advanced disease with metastatic spread of cancer cells to distant sites in the body. Five-year survival rates for stage IV disease are estimated to be about 20%, compared with 98% or better for stage I.[38]

Once breast cancer has been diagnosed, typically after image-guided core needle biopsy (CNB) or VAB, additional imaging is commonly performed to help determine the extent of the disease. This can involve additional workup to search for satellite lesions in the affected breast (multifocal versus multicentric disease) and regional adenopathy and to check for involvement in the other breast. Contrast-enhanced MRI is often utilized to stage operative breast cancer because of its high sensitivity.[1-5] However, for some patients, MRI is not accessible or is contraindicated. US can provide helpful staging information in these patients regarding primary tumor size, intraductal extension, focality (Fig. 18-60), skin or chest wall involvement, bilateral involvement, and presence of abnormal-appearing nodes within the breast, as well as in the regional nodal basin.[9,11] ACR practice parameters include whole-breast US for staging purposes, when indicated.[18]

A variety of imaging modalities (CT, positron emission tomography [PET]-CT, MRI, nuclear medicine [NM], US) are utilized when metastatic disease is suspected in other parts of the body.

BRCA-Associated Breast Cancer[36,37,39,43]

Carriers of a BRCA gene mutation are at much higher risk of developing cancer over their lifetime. At least 80% of BRCA-associated breast cancers are IDC. ILC accounts for 2%

to 8%. Close to 20% of BRCA1 carriers with a malignancy are diagnosed with medullary carcinoma. Breast cancers associated with the *BRCA1* gene mutation are most often TNBCs on biologic profiling. BRCA patients with breast cancer are at significant future risk for developing a second primary in the contralateral breast. Although male breast cancer is rare, a BRCA2 gene mutation, in particular, raises cancer risk.

Breast Cancer Biomarkers[38,42,45–48]

Breast cancer is not one disease, but represents a heterogeneous array of tumor types and presentations down to the molecular level. Treatment strategies for breast cancer involve a multidisciplinary approach, typically relying on some form of surgery, radiation, and/or chemotherapy, hormonal therapy, or other targeted therapies. Besides determining histologic type and stage, additional forms of testing allow a better understanding of a cancer's biology and behavior, which impacts treatment options, tumor response, and outcomes.

Important biologic markers for breast cancer are estrogen and progesterone receptor status and overexpression of human epidermal growth factor receptor 2 (HER2). Breast cancer

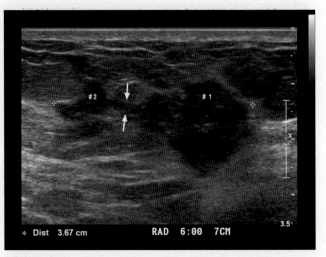

FIGURE 18-60 Multifocal invasive carcinoma. This high-grade primary tumor (*#1*) shows tumor extending into a major duct (*arrows*) that leads to a smaller satellite lesion (*#2*). Biopsy confirmed multifocal disease.

cells have hormone receptors proteins that receive signals from estrogen or progesterone to stimulate cell growth. The majority of breast cancers are estrogen-receptor positive (ER⁺) and progesterone-receptor positive (PR⁺). Treatment strategies and prognosis are quite different for a cancer that is hormone receptor positive versus one that is not. Overall, ER+ tumors have a better prognosis and tend to respond well to systemic antiestrogenic hormone therapy, rather than from chemotherapy. HER2 is another cell protein that fuels cancer growth. Overexpression of HER2 is detected in around 15% to 20% of invasive breast cancers. HER2-positive disease has a poorer prognosis with higher recurrence rates and metastatic risk than HER2-negative tumors. To limit adverse outcomes, targeted therapies have been developed to help combat HER2-positive disease in addition to chemotherapy.

The TNM system describes the anatomic stage of a cancer, whereas tumor grade, hormone receptor status, and HER2 expression describe the biologic type of the disease.[38] Knowing more about a cancer's biologic and molecular profile can lead to more personalized, and hopefully more effective, treatment strategies that can affect a patient's long-term survival.

Triple-negative breast cancer (TNBC) is the term used when hormone receptor status is negative (ER⁻/PR⁻) and the tumor lacks HER2 protein amplification (HER2⁻). The TNBC subtype accounts for about 10% to 20% of all breast cancers. Tumors tend to develop at a younger age (<50 years).[36] A higher association is noted in black and Hispanic women, as well as in BRCA mutation carriers. Most invasive breast cancers in BRCA carriers show a TNBC receptor status, especially those with a BRCA1 mutation. Tumors are typically larger, more aggressive, higher grade, and often node positive at the time of diagnosis, so effective treatment can be challenging. Distant metastasis also occurs earlier than with hormone-receptor–positive tumors. Hormonal treatment is not effective for TNBC. Rather, neoadjuvant chemotherapy is often initially offered in order to downstage the disease before surgery or radiation.

Research studies have investigated correlation between US findings and a breast cancer's tumor receptor status. Although US features vary, TNBCs tend to be rounder, hypoechoic, and display fairly circumscribed margins that may show lobulation. Some distal sound enhancement is common, rather than shadowing, as well as prominent vascularity on Doppler. Calcifications are uncommon.[11] Adjacent Cooper ligaments are often displaced rather than disrupted. Survey of the axilla may show suspicious nodes. Because some TNBCs can mimic a benign mass on initial imaging, knowledge of the patient's clinical and genetic history can expedite the decision to biopsy, rather than performing short-interval follow-up imaging. Lower grade, slower growing, non-TNBC tumors more often display suspicious US findings (e.g., irregular shape, spiculated margin, shadowing) and associated architectural distortion.

Metastatic Carcinoma and Lymph Node Assessment[4–11,36–41,48–51]

The sonographic appearance of metastatic breast disease is variable. Routes for metastasis are via the lymph channels, the blood, or by direct extension. Metastatic disease yields a poorer prognosis and alters patient management based on the extent of disease. MRI and PET-CT have become particularly helpful in assessing the extent of metastatic changes.

Besides providing anatomic images, PET-CT assesses abnormal metabolic activity of cancer utilizing a radioactive ¹⁸F-fluorodeoxglucose (¹⁸F-FDG) tracer.

Spread of Cancer from a Breast Primary

The first site of metastatic disease from a primary breast cancer is usually to the ipsilateral axillary lymph nodes, which receive most of the lymph drainage from the breast. The ipsilateral axillary, infraclavicular, and supraclavicular nodes, as well as the internal mammary (parasternal) nodes, are considered regional lymph nodes for breast cancer staging.

For surgical and staging purposes, the axillary nodes are classified as follows[5,10,11,38] (Table 18-2):
- Level I nodes: low axillary nodes lying lateral to the pectoralis minor muscle
- Level II nodes: midaxillary nodes lying beneath the pectoralis minor muscle
- Level III nodes: high axillary nodes lying medial to the pectoralis minor muscle

Interpectoral [Rotter] nodes are also grouped as level II. Malignant cells can also involve intramammary lymph nodes.

Regional lymph node involvement is a strong predictor of patient survival and impacts treatment strategies. The *sentinel lymph node* (SLN) is the first node in the drainage basin and is at most risk for metastasis. This is typically a low axillary node (level I). In past years, patients commonly underwent complete axillary lymph node dissection (ALND) after an invasive breast cancer diagnosis. Unfortunately, patients often developed significant complications, including arm lymphedema, nerve damage, and functional impairment of the arm or shoulder. More recently, SLN biopsy procedures have been used to stage the axilla, allowing surgeons to remove fewer nodes when the sentinel node is cancer free. This significantly reduces the morbid associated with complete ALND. NM *lymphoscintigraphy* is used to identify the sentinel node. A radioisotope (99m technetium-labeled filtered sulfur colloid), with or without a blue dye, is injected into the breast to map lymphatic drainage to the sentinel node. If ordered, NM images are obtained to show the uptake in the sentinel node. In the operating room, the surgeon uses a gamma probe to identify and harvest the radioactive sentinel node for microscopic analysis.[14,40]

Primary breast cancer can also metastasize to distant organs via the bloodstream. More common sites are the bone (most frequent), lung, brain, and liver.[5,13]

Sonographic Lymph Node Assessment[9–11]

Sonographically, normal lymph nodes are oval or reniform in shape, circumscribed, oriented parallel to the skin, and display a thin, symmetric, hypoechoic outer cortex and a hyperechoic fatty hilum (see Fig. 18-7). Color Doppler primarily reveals blood flow at the hilum. An axillary node with a very thin cortex and a prominent echogenic hilum may be difficult to delineate from adjacent structures. Intramammary nodes are typically small (≤1 cm), whereas normal axillary nodes are often longer. On short-axis scans, a node has a C-shaped appearance. In general, normal nodes typically have a minimum diameter of 1 cm or less.

Adenopathy can result from benign and malignant causes. Benign reactive lymphadenopathy may be due to an autoimmune disorder (e.g., arthritis, lupus), local infection

TABLE 18-17	**Sonographic Features of Lymph Nodes**
Benign Features	**Worrisome Features**
• Oval, reniform (kidney) shape • Circumscribed, smooth margins • Symmetrically thin hypoechoic outer cortex • Hyperechoic fatty hilum • Doppler flow at hilum	• Rounded, lobulated, irregular shape • Enlarged diameter • Cortical thickening >3 mm; eccentric cortical thickening • Displaced, indented, or absent echogenic fatty hilum • Markedly hypoechoic cortex • Heterogeneous cortex • Indistinct cortical wall • Transcapsular blood flow on Doppler • Side asymmetry

or inflammatory conditions, granulomatous lymphadenitis, or other etiology. Systemic conditions are more often cause bilateral adenopathy. There are also reported cases of unilateral axillary adenopathy following vaccinations, including that for COVID-19.[52] On US, reactive nodes may be enlarged and show a concentrically thickened cortex. Patients may describe associated discomfort. In some cases, reactive lymphadenopathy mimics malignant change, so correlation with clinical history is needed.

Malignant involvement of axillary nodes can result from primary breast cancer (most common), non-breast metastatic disease, and lymphoma. Metastasis can alter the size, shape, and echogenicity of lymph nodes.

Suspicious sonographic features for lymph node metastasis include nodal enlargement; rounded shape; cortical thickening (concentric, eccentric, irregular); compression, displacement, or loss of echogenic hilar echoes; markedly hypoechoic or heterogeneous cortex; or indistinct margins (Table 18-17; Fig. 18-61). Cortical thickening greater than 3 mm, especially when eccentric, is of particular concern.[9,11] A metastatic implant that focally protrudes into the echogenic hilum can have a "rat-bite" appearance.[9] Peripheral transcapsular blood flow on color-flow Doppler and side-to-side asymmetry of lymph nodes are additional

worrisome findings. Sonography has diagnostic limitations, because normal-appearing lymph nodes may still harbor malignant cells.

Sonography is often used to assess axillary disease when a suspicious mass or biopsy-proven breast cancer is present. However, some facilities do not routinely perform preoperative axillary US if findings do not change surgical management of the axilla (sentinel node biopsy versus complete ALND).[9,10,40,51]

Sonography can guide biopsy (fine-needle aspiration [FNA] or CNB) of a suspicious lymph node. A clip marker placed at the time of biopsy will mark the site for potential localization and excision, or before neoadjuvant therapy. US guidance can also be used as part of the SLN biopsy procedure.

Spread of Cancer to the Breast

Spread of cancer to the breast from another part of the body is very uncommon. Cancer cells can reach the breast via blood or lymphatic routes. Outside of the contralateral breast, the most common sources of breast metastases are melanoma and lymphoma/leukemia. Clinical history of a non-breast primary or systemic hematologic or lymphoproliferative disease allows for a broader differential diagnosis for breast masses because imaging features can overlap more common causes of breast pathology.

The most common source of metastases to the breast is from a primary cancer in the contralateral breast. Spread to the opposite breast is primarily by way of the lymphatic system and often produces diffuse architectural change without a focal mass similar to inflammatory carcinoma.

Breast metastases from extramammary malignancies are fairly rare, with cancer cells reaching the breast via the blood. Melanoma is most common distant source in females.[5] Other sources include the lung, ovary, stomach, neuroendocrine tumors, and the uterus. Prostate carcinoma is the most common source in men. Metastatic lesions most often develop in the UOQ in the superficial breast. Tumors can be single or multiple in one or both breasts. These solid lesions tend to be oval or round and hypoechoic, display relatively circumscribed margins, and typically lack calcification, spiculation, or posterior shadowing.

In rare cases, systemic diseases such as lymphoma and leukemia can also seed to the breast. Secondary disease is more common than primary non-Hodgkin breast lymphoma. On sonograms, primary lymphoma can present as solitary or multiple circumscribed or ill-defined, hypoechoic masses, often with distal sound enhancement. Enlarged, lymphomatous nodes can appear pseudocystic with absent or compressed hilar fat. Doppler reveals abundant blood flow. Infiltrative or metastatic lymphoma may show diffuse involvement of the breast and have clinical and imaging pattern similar to inflammatory carcinoma.[10] Breast changes associated with leukemia can have similar imaging patterns.

Breast Irradiation and Tumor Recurrence

Radiotherapy treatment options have broadened over the years. Standard treatment involves whole-breast external beam irradiation delivered over several weeks, which may be followed by more focused therapy called a "boost." External

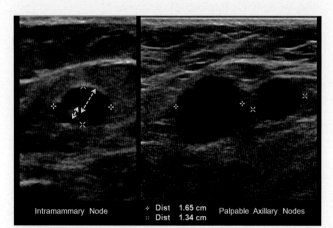

FIGURE 18-61 Metastatic lymphadenopathy. Intramammary node shows an increase in width of the cortical thickness compared with the echogenic fatty hilum. Rounded axillary nodes show marked hypoechogenicity of the cortex (nearly pseudocystic) and absent hilar echoes.

beam radiation can be delivered to both mastectomy and lumpectomy patients. Radiotherapy techniques have evolved over recent years and now include internal forms of APBI.

Sonographic Features of the Irradiated Breast

Sonography can detect changes in the irradiated breast that are not seen in the normal breast. Alterations depend on the extent of surgery, duration of radiation, and time interval since treatment. Initially, skin thickening can be marked. The subcutaneous fat layer may be altered, showing increased echogenicity, interstitial fluid, and dilated lymphatic channels. Cooper ligaments may be thickened, and the parenchyma may appear distorted, highly echogenic, and attenuative secondary to postirradiation fibrosis or from surgical scarring.[5,10] History helps to differentiate imaging patterns from other inflammatory conditions or underlying malignancy. Residual effects in these radiotherapy cancer patients take longer to diminish than postsurgical changes following a benign biopsy. Fat necrosis can develop. Pronounced residual scarring can potentially obscure detection of early tumor recurrence.

Brachytherapy[53–55]

Brachytherapy is a form of APBI and an option for certain women with early breast cancer and node-negative disease that need effective radiotherapy after a lumpectomy. In contrast to traditional whole-breast external beam irradiation, brachytherapy involves implanting a radiation source (radioactive pellets) in the breast at the lumpectomy site to treat the tumor bed and adjacent tissues. This localized form of high-dose radiation treatment is commonly delivered across 5 to 7 days, rather than 3 to 6 weeks with external beam whole-breast irradiation. Some brachytherapy protocols are as short as 2 days.[55] Because the radiation is delivered internally, brachytherapy spares more healthy tissues and organs from radiation side effects, often resulting in a better cosmetic outcome. Radiation delivery methods include insertion of multiple interstitial catheters threaded through the breast and lumpectomy bed or single insertion of an intracavitary device into the lumpectomy cavity. Different intracavitary devices are available (balloon type, multicatheter applicator).[54,55]

Although CT is widely used during planning and insertion of brachytherapy devices, US can be used to document a seroma, identifying the lumpectomy cavity; measure the distance between the skin and the seroma or balloon device for safe spacing; and guide temporary implantation of multiple interstitial catheters or the insertion of an intracavitary device for radiation delivery (Figs. 18-62 and 18-63).

Tumor Recurrence

Tumor recurrence is suspected when there is an increase in the size of the tumor bed scar or development of a new mass at the surgical site after there has been documented stability of the scar by imaging tests. Additional signs of tumor recurrence can include the interval development of microcalcifications on the mammogram or Doppler blood flow on the sonogram.[7,10,41,42]

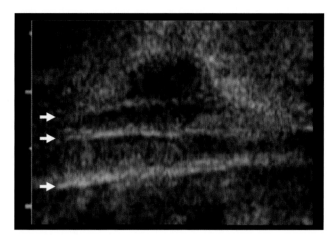

FIGURE 18-62 Brachytherapy. Linear bands of echoes (*arrows*) represent multiple interstitial brachytherapy catheters that are threaded across a seroma-filled lumpectomy bed.

Contrast-enhanced MRI is reported to be more sensitive than mammography or sonography at differentiating recurrent cancer from scar tissue 18 months or older following breast conserving surgery by detecting early tumor enhancement.[5,56]

SONOGRAPHY-GUIDED BREAST INTERVENTIONAL TECHNIQUES[6–17,57–61]

Percutaneous breast interventional procedures are both diagnostic and therapeutic and have expanded over the years. The ACR has published parameters for the performance of US-guided interventional procedures.[17] Common indications include cyst aspiration, drainage of a fluid collection such as abscess, biopsy of a suspicious solid mass or complex lesion, lymph node sampling, and presurgical localization of a nonpalpable mass. Sonography can guide placement of a marker clip following percutaneous biopsy or to document a cancer's location or extent before neoadjuvant chemotherapy or breast-conservation therapy.

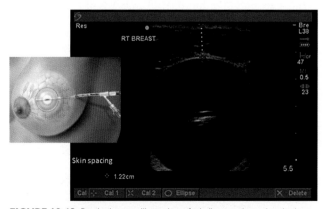

FIGURE 18-63 Brachytherapy. Illustration of a balloon catheter brachytherapy device (*inset*). Saline is infused through the catheter lumen to distend the balloon placed within the lumpectomy bed. Radioactive material is inserted through the catheter for delivery of targeted radiotherapy to the lumpectomy site and surrounding tissues. Sonogram shows a skin-to-balloon spacing distance of 1.22 cm in this patient. (Image courtesy of Hologic, Inc., Marlborough, MA.)

Less common applications for US guidance are reported, including needle placement into a subareolar duct for saline or contrast ductography when nipple cannulation is difficult.[10] Sonography can provide guidance during SLN biopsy,[51] cyrotherapy,[58] laser or radio-frequency tumor ablation,[51,60] foreign-body removal,[9] and brachytherapy procedures.[9] US also provides guidance during the removal of certain benign breast masses (e.g., fibroadenoma, papilloma) utilizing a large core VAB device.[60]

Mammographic stereotactic or tomosynthesis-guided biopsy using a VAB device is typically preferred for suspicious microcalcifications, especially those not associated with a mass, as well as for focal architectural distortion. However, with today's high-resolution transducers, sonographic visualization of calcifications has improved, allowing certain suspicious calcifications to be sampled using US guidance.[9] Calcification removal is confirmed with specimen radiography.

The advantages of sonography often make it the first choice as a guidance tool, being widely available and requiring no radiation. US procedures are often faster and offer more flexibility in patient positioning than mammographic or MRI techniques. Real-time sonography allows direct visualization of the needle tip as it approaches and enters a mass, helping to confirm accurate and adequate sampling or aspiration. Masses near the chest wall and those seen on only one mammographic view can be sampled or localized by sonography. Color Doppler capabilities allow blood flow to be quickly assessed before tumor sampling to help limit hematoma formation during a CNB or VAB procedure. Procedures are typically performed on an outpatient basis and are generally well tolerated. After sampling, the histologic or cytologic diagnosis should be compared with imaging findings to assess concordance. Discordance between US and pathology results can lead to rebiopsy or excision.

Patient Preparation

For a breast interventional procedure, the patient is fully informed of the procedure, possible complications, and alternative procedures, and then signs a consent form. Complications are uncommon but can include pain, infection, hematoma, and possible vasovagal reaction. The patient may be asked to refrain from certain blood-thinning agents (e.g., warfarin) for a limited time period before a core biopsy procedure (especially large-gauge VAB) to reduce bleeding risk. However, stopping anticoagulants is often not needed before US intervention because significant hematoma formation is uncommon.[61] Pneumothorax is a rare biopsy complication if the pleura is punctured during needle advancement.

Proper time-out with side and site verification is performed in accordance with The Joint Commission National Patient Safety Goals.

The patient is placed in a supine or oblique position so as to maximize access to the mass during US guidance. Very lateral masses can require a greater degree of patient obliquity.

Special attention is paid to the setup of sterile trays and supplies so as to maintain sterility during the procedure for infection control. A sterile transducer sleeve can be used to cover the transducer. Local anesthesia provides pain management. After CNB or VAB, manual pressure is applied over the site for 5 to 10 minutes to reduce bleeding. After covering the biopsy site with a sterile dressing, a cold pack can be applied to limit pain and swelling. Aftercare instructions should be provided.

Guidance Techniques

Most radiologists prefer the "free-handed" technique rather than employing an attachable biopsy guide for US needle guidance. The needle approach to the mass is based on the procedure type and the location of the mass within the breast. Various methods are illustrated in Figures 18-64 to 18-66.

For preoperative wire localization, surgeons often prefer to dissect the shortest distance of tissue to the mass. A near-vertical needle approach typically provides the shortest path for dye or hook-wire placement (Fig. 18-64). However, this angle of approach makes it difficult to visualize the needle shaft and tip in relation to the mass during real-time US scanning. This method should also be avoided when performing spring-loaded CNB for fear of puncturing the chest wall or when sampling a mass anterior to a breast implant.

When an oblique needle insertion path is chosen, better echo reflection from the needle may be achieved by tilting the transducer, using trapezoidal imaging, spatial compounding, or beam steering, depending on equipment features (Fig. 18-65).

The preferred method for needle biopsy is to advance the needle or biopsy probe parallel to the long axis of the transducer face and chest wall at a depth necessary to intercept the mass (Fig. 18-66). With the sound beam directed perpendicular to the needle, the needle shaft and tip are optimally seen during advancement and sampling of the mass. During spring-loaded CNB, this "parallel approach" or "long-axis" approach reduces the risk of pneumothorax or for implant puncture.[9,10]

Biopsy Procedures

Because most breast biopsies yield a benign diagnosis, minimally invasive percutaneous biopsy is preferred to open surgical biopsy for an initial diagnosis. Techniques include fine-needle aspiration (FNA) biopsy, large CNB, and directional VAB or mammotomy.

FNA is the fastest, lowest cost, and least traumatic biopsy method. This procedure is considered to biopsy certain a palpable mass, lymph node, or a mass that would be unsafe to biopsy by large core techniques (e.g., mass near an implant wall). An FNA biopsy is performed using a small-gauge (22 to 25 g) needle attached to a syringe. Multiple back-and-forth needle passes are obtained in different sections of the mass, whereas suction is applied to extract cellular material for cytologic analysis. Undersampling and false-negative rates are higher with this cytologic technique, so additional tissue sampling may be required for a definitive diagnosis. Results are also reliant on the expertise of the cytopathologist at the facility.

Minimally invasive percutaneous CNB and VAB provide multiple tissue cores for histologic analysis, allowing for more accurate diagnosis of benign versus malignant disease, and for differentiation of invasive from in situ carcinoma. Sufficient tissue cores obtained from these biopsy procedures allow for initial biologic testing (e.g., ER, PR, HER2 status) of breast cancer.[45]

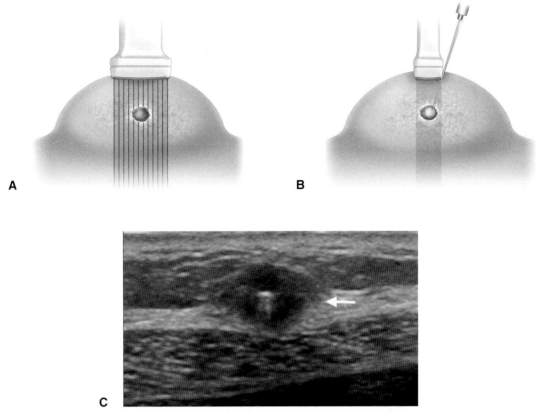

FIGURE 18-64 Method 1: sonographic needle guidance. **A:** Linear-array transducer positioned over the center of the mass. **B:** Side view showing the needle adjacent to the center of the transducer, with a slightly angled insertion path to the mass. **C:** Sonogram showing a cross section of the needle (*arrow*) within a solid mass. This approach provides the shortest path to the mass, but visualization of the needle shaft and tip is limited owing to the steep angle of insertion.

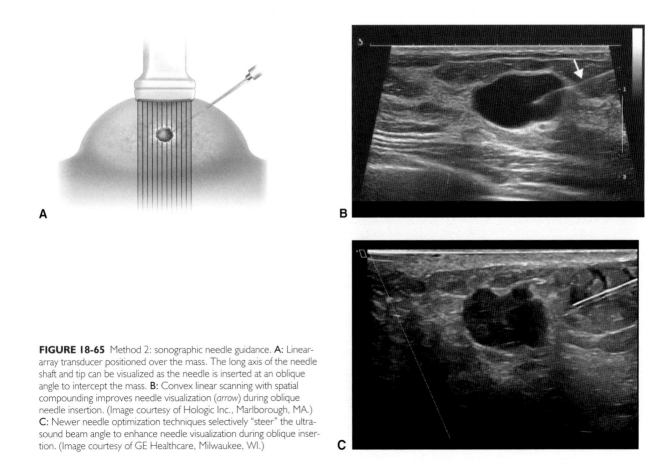

FIGURE 18-65 Method 2: sonographic needle guidance. **A:** Linear-array transducer positioned over the mass. The long axis of the needle shaft and tip can be visualized as the needle is inserted at an oblique angle to intercept the mass. **B:** Convex linear scanning with spatial compounding improves needle visualization (*arrow*) during oblique needle insertion. (Image courtesy of Hologic Inc., Marlborough, MA.) **C:** Newer needle optimization techniques selectively "steer" the ultrasound beam angle to enhance needle visualization during oblique insertion. (Image courtesy of GE Healthcare, Milwaukee, WI.)

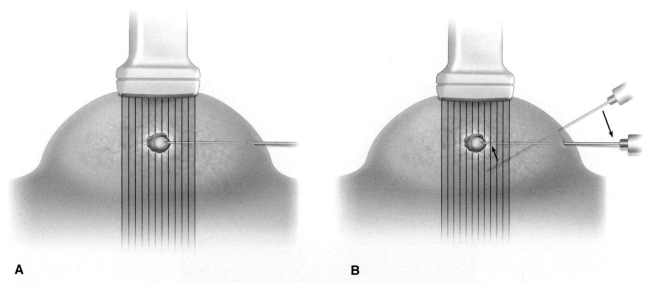

A   **B**

FIGURE 18-66 Method 3: sonographic needle guidance. **A:** The long axis of the needle is inserted parallel to the transducer or chest wall. This optimizes visualization of the needle shaft and tip and avoids needle puncture through the chest wall. **B:** Alternate method is to insert the needle obliquely and then push the needle hub down to a more parallel path. This alternate method allows needle insertion closer to the mass.

Handheld automated CNB needle devices generally vary between 14- and 18-gauge in size and have different needle and notch lengths. Spring-loaded devices are often utilized and have a throw of up to 2 cm. Advancing the needle parallel to the chest wall limits potential complications during firing (e.g., pneumothorax), especially for deep lesions, and enhances needle visualization. Unless a coaxial technique is employed, the biopsy needle needs to be withdrawn after each tissue core is obtained and then reinserted to obtain the next specimen. Using a coaxial technique, an introducer needle is advanced to the mass along the intended biopsy path. The stylet is removed to allow repeated placement of the biopsy needle for lesion sampling. This allows multiple tissue cores to be acquired without additional passes of the biopsy needle through the breast tissue. Image documentation should include labeled "pre-fire" and "post-fire" images during CNB procedures (Fig. 18-67).[17]

VAB devices allow rapid acquisition of multiple tissue cores through a single needle insertion site. The handheld biopsy probe may be connected to a separate console containing the vacuum source. Untethered handheld VAB devices are also available and affordable. Common biopsy probe sizes are 8- or 11-gauge, allowing removal of larger, more cohesive tissue cores as compared with spring-loaded CNB devices. US-guided VAB is preferred for sampling small suspicious solid lesions (<1.5 cm), visible suspicious calcifications, intraductal papillary lesions, and complex cystic and solid lesions. Because of the larger tissue core size for histologic analysis, there are lower rates of upgrading a cancerous lesion at subsequent surgical excision.

Unlike a spring-loaded core biopsy, the VAB probe is typically advanced directly under the mass. The needle aperture is opened, producing an air "ring-down" artifact that serves as a positioning landmark (Fig. 18-68). Once the aperture is properly positioned, vacuum suction is applied to pull the mass into the hollow needle through the aperture. A rotating cutter then slides across the aperture to obtain the specimen core. The vacuum pulls the specimen into a collection chamber without removal of the probe. Multiple consecutive cores are quickly acquired.

For CNB and VAB procedures, the tissue cores are placed in formalin and sent for histologic analysis. Generally, a

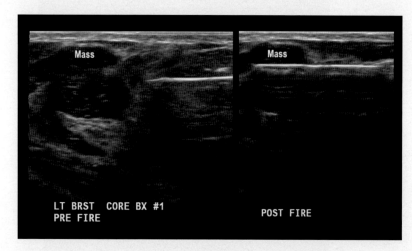

FIGURE 18-67 Large core breast biopsy. A 14-gauge, spring-loaded automated biopsy needle is inserted parallel to the transducer. The hyperechoic needle shaft and tip are well seen. The "pre-fire" image shows the needle in line with the mass. The "post-fire" image documents the biopsy site after real-time tissue sampling.

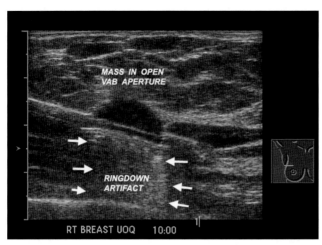

FIGURE 18-68 Vacuum-assisted breast biopsy. The biopsy probe is positioned under the mass. The posterior portion of a solid mass is seen within the needle probe aperture. Ring-down artifact (*arrows*) emanates beneath the site of the opened aperture.

minimum of three to six tissue cores are obtained depending on biopsy device and needle gauge.[17] Specimen radiography is used to document calcifications within a tissue sample.

Following CNB or VAB, a marker clip should be deployed to document the biopsy site (Fig. 18-69), which is important if surgical excision becomes necessary after a pathologic diagnosis of cancer or high-risk lesion (e.g., atypical ductal hyperplasia [ADH]), and to document the site of a benign lesion on subsequent imaging. Postbiopsy mammography further documents marker clip location relative to the intended site. Placement of markers with different shapes is advantageous when multiple lesions are biopsied or localized. Tissue markers can also be placed within a high-grade cancer in a patient receiving neoadjuvant chemotherapy to mark its location if tumor detection becomes difficult after treatment.

Sonography can also be used in the operating room to verify complete surgical excision of a localized breast mass or SLN. As an alternative to specimen radiography for some cases, the specimen can be placed in a sterile wrap or in a saline solution and scanned with US to confirm complete removal of the lesion.

Presurgical Localization

Real-time sonography is a quick, easy, and effective guidance tool for localization of nonpalpable breast masses or nodes before surgical excision. Traditionally, mass localization has been accomplished by insertion of a spring hook-wire and/or injection of methylene blue dye. Such methods have drawbacks. If only dye is used, surgery must be performed soon after localization before the dye diffuses in the parenchyma. Disadvantages of wire localization include wire extension from the patient's skin after placement, discomfort, possible wire migration or transection, and the need to coordinate same day scheduling of wire placement and subsequent surgery. Wire placement along the shortest path to the mass allows less normal tissue to be transecting as the surgeon follows the wire to the mass. However, during US guidance, a longer path may be needed to enhance wire visualization when advancing the needle/wire nearly parallel to the transducer.

Several nonwire localization techniques are now available that do not share these drawbacks.[57,61,62] Instead of a wire, these newer methods involve percutaneous insertion of radioactive or magnetic seeds, nonradioactive radar reflectors (Fig. 18-70), or radio-frequency identification (RFID) tags to localize tumors, nodes, or to bracket the extent of malignant disease before surgery. An introducer needle system houses the small (5 to 12 mm) localization device for deployment at the target site. Image-guided insertion is similar to postbiopsy clip placement. During US guidance, the radiologist can select a tissue path that enhances needle detection and device placement because it has no bearing on the surgeon's incision site. During surgery, a specialized handheld probe is moved over the skin to locate the signal activated or emitted from the localization device in the breast. A companion tabletop console emits an audio signal or shows a numeric display to accurately guide the surgeon to the mass/device location (e.g., distance to lesion). Nonwire breast localization is effective and often better tolerated by patients. Depending on the nonwire device, placement can be performed days or up to a month before surgery, allowing greater flexibility and efficiency when scheduling image-guided placement and surgery. Because the surgeon can choose an incision site close to the lesion, less normal tissue may potentially be removed, which may improve cosmetic outcome.

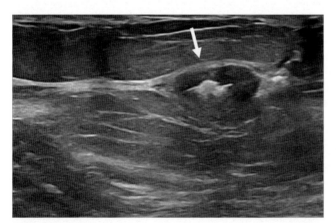

FIGURE 18-69 Tissue marker clip. Sonogram documenting postbiopsy insertion of a clip marker (*arrow*). (Trumark clip: Image courtesy of Hologic Inc., Marlborough, MA.)

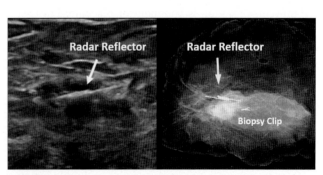

FIGURE 18-70 Nonwire localization. Sonogram and post-lumpectomy specimen radiograph of a radar reflector within a breast mass. (Images courtesy of Merit Medical, South Jordan, UT.)

THE AUGMENTED BREAST[6–11,63–68]

Although MRI is considered the most accurate imaging tool for assessing implant integrity, sonography is of much lower cost and quite useful when examining women who have undergone augmentation or reconstructive mammoplasty. In patients with breast implants, sonography allows evaluation of overlying breast tissues for pathology, as well as for changes within and around the prosthesis. Mammography may be suboptimal and more technically difficult in these patients.

Breast Implants

Over the years, there have been numerous types of implants developed for cosmetic breast augmentation and postmastectomy reconstruction, with saline and silicone being the most common. Silicone gel implants better simulate the natural feel and look of the breast compared with traditional saline implants; features often preferred by women. In 1992, the U.S. Food and Drug Administration (FDA) restricted the use of silicone implants for breast augmentation owing to safety concerns related to leakage. After that, saline implants were more widely used. However, in 2006, the FDA approved the use of certain newer generation, form-stable, silicone cohesive gel (aka gummy bear) implants with conditions for device monitoring. Since then, silicone implants have regained popularity.

More recently, a uniquely designed saline breast implant (Ideal Implant, Inc., Dallas, TX, USA) has been marketed that contains a series of implant shells nestled together and two separate saline chambers. Compared with standard saline implants, this "structured" implant better holds its shape, reduces wrinkling and folding, and gives a more natural feel to the breast, providing an alternative to silicone prostheses.

When examining the augmented breast, sonographers should understand the imaging differences between common implant types, placement sites, and related complications.

Placement Sites

For cosmetic breast enlargement, the implants are often placed beneath the glandular tissue in front of the pectoralis muscle (subglandular or prepectoral location). Women with subglandular implants require special mammographic "pushback" (Eklund) views to better visualize the overlying breast tissue. Alternatively, the implants can be inserted beneath the pectoralis major muscle (submuscular or retropectoral location), which may help reduce capsular contracture. A submuscular location is common for placement of tissue expanders and implants following mastectomy. Implants are less often inserted beneath the pectoralis minor muscle.

Normal Implant Appearance

Standard saline implants have a single anechoic lumen and an anterior filling port to allow fluid expansion to the desired size (Fig. 18-71). The fill valve may occasionally be the cause of a palpable lump near the areola. Gradual filling of a tissue expander allows the skin to stretch before placement of a permanent prosthesis.

Silicone gel implants can have single or double lumens. Single-lumen silicone gel implants are more common and come in prefilled sizes and are generally anechoic. Double-lumen

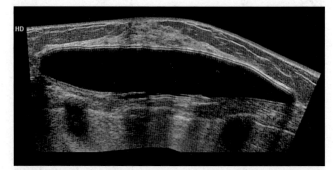

FIGURE 18-71 Saline breast implant. Extended field-of-view image of an anechoic subglandular breast implant. (Image courtesy of Philips Healthcare, Bothell, WA.).

implants have separate silicone and saline chambers. An echogenic membrane separates the chambers. A filling port extends to the expandable saline chamber. Although newer cohesive silicone gel implants are available, some women may still have older generation silicone implants. Regardless of the filler material, all breast implants have an outer silicone elastomer shell, which can be either smooth or textured.

A "fibrous capsule" naturally forms around an implant, which is an expected response to a foreign body. This fibrous reaction is more pronounced with silicone gel implants. Texturing of the implant shell can reduce the degree of capsular contracture. The inner and outer layers of an implant shell appear as two smooth, thin, parallel, hyperechoic lines when the sound beam is directed perpendicular to implant surface (Fig.18-72). An intact implant lays adjacent to the fibrous capsule. High-frequency sonography can often delineate three closely spaced echogenic lines, with the outer third line representing the fibrous capsule abutting the implant shell. This has been termed the "capsule–shell–echo" complex and is best seen with nontextured implants using a high-frequency transducer. A textured implant shell may have a thicker or fuzzier sonographic appearance.

A common implant finding is a linear infolding of the implant shell, or *radial fold*, which may extend for a variable distance from the implant margin (Fig. 18-73). Long, wavy folds may mimic a double lumen or intracapsular rupture (ICR). Some lobulation of the contour of an intact

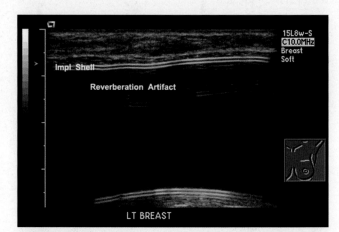

FIGURE 18-72 Saline implant. The outer and inner margins of the smooth implant shell are seen as closely spaced parallel lines abutting the fibrous capsule. The implant lumen is anechoic, although reverberation artifact is seen within the anterior implant.

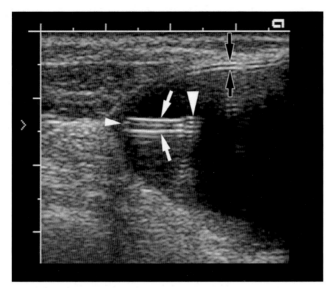

FIGURE 18-73 Radial fold. An infolding of the implant shell is seen extending a short distance into the implant lumen (*white arrows*). The abnormal fold (*white arrowheads*) is twice the thickness of single shell layer (*black arrows*). (Reprinted with permission from Middleton MS, McNamara MP Jr. *Breast Implant Imaging*. Lippincott Williams & Wilkins; 2003.)

implant, or "wrinkling" of the implant shell, is occasionally seen. An anterior wrinkle can bulge enough to be palpable in certain positions.

Reverberation artifacts are commonly present and create a band of false echoes across the anterior lumen of the implant (see Fig. 18-72). Harmonic imaging and spatial compounding help reduce imaging artifacts, thereby improving evaluation of the implant shell and reducing error when assessing implant integrity. Lighter transducer pressure can also reduce the amount of near-field reverberation within the implant.

Sound travels much slower though silicone ($\sim$ 1,000 m/s) than through saline or soft tissue (1,540 m/s). This creates a propagation speed artifact (or translation effect), whereby the posterior wall of the implant and distal structures falsely appear to extend deeper into the chest than adjacent tissues. Scanning along the edge of a subglandular silicone implant will show a "step-off" or discontinuity of the chest wall deep to the implant, which is not seen beneath saline (Fig. 18-74). This artifact is useful when trying to differentiate

a silicone from a saline implant in a patient with poor history and when a mammogram is not available for comparison.

A small amount of reactive fluid may be seen between the implant shell and fibrous capsule, termed *peri-implant effusion*. This normal finding is more common with textured implants and is not to be confused with implant rupture.

Implant Complications

Sonography can evaluate many of the complications associated with breast augmentation. Changes in implant shape, contour, and size may occur with fibrous or calcific contracture, herniation, rupture, and deflation. Capsular contracture is more often a problem with silicone implants, causing thickening and hardening of the fibrous capsule around the implant shell. This causes the implant to become rounded, hard, and immobile. Sonography will demonstrate a thickened capsule–shell complex and poor compressibility of the implant with transducer pressure. A crack in the fibrous capsule can allow focal herniation of the implant through the defect, which may present as a palpable lump. Peri-implant seroma, abscess, or hematoma may result from implant surgery, infection, or trauma. An implant may migrate in position or cause an animation deformity. Implants can also rupture due to aging, trauma, or other factors.

In 2011, the FDA reported the first possible link between breast implants and a type of non-Hodgkin lymphoma.[63] This breast implant–associated anaplastic large cell lymphoma (BIA-ALCL) was shown to develop in the scar tissue (fibrous capsule) and/or the fluid surrounding the implant. The risk appeared to be higher with certain textured implants, rather than with the filler material. Most reported cases were tracked to a certain manufacturer, and those implant types were voluntarily recalled in 2019. Signs and symptoms raising concern for BIA-ALCL include a persistent swelling, pain, lump, or hardening adjacent to the implant, which may indicate seroma formation or capsular contracture.[64] Symptoms can appear years after implant placement. Aspiration of peri-implant fluid and sampling of the fibrous capsule can be sent for specific cytologic and histologic analysis.[63] Although the chance of developing BIA-ALCL is low, there is potential risk for the spread throughout the body and even death, so knowledge of this condition is important. Women with confirmed BIA-ALCL should have both the implant and fibrous capsule removed.

FIGURE 18-74 Implant differentiation. Saline implant: There is continuity of the pectoralis muscle (*PM*) beneath the saline implant. A small amount of reactive peri-implant fluid is present (*arrowhead*). Silicone implant: In contrast, there is discontinuity of the PM and pleural reflection (*large arrows*) beneath the silicone prosthesis (step-off sign, translation effect). The slower speed of sound through silicone causes structures beneath the implant to falsely appear deeper in the body than in reality. (Reprinted with permission from Middleton MS, McNamara MP Jr. *Breast Implant Imaging*. Lippincott Williams & Wilkins; 2003.)

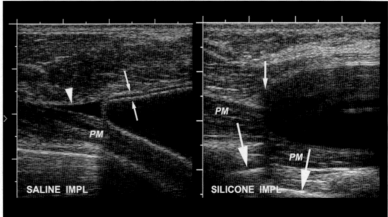

Evaluation of Implant Integrity

Saline implants are reported to more easily rupture from trauma than silicone implants. Collapse and deflation of a saline implant can be easily determined by clinical examination and mammography, without reliance on sonography. Unlike silicone, the salty fluid is reabsorbed by the body after implant rupture.

When a silicone implant ruptures, it does not quickly deflate and often goes unnoticed. The incidence of silicone implant rupture increases with the age of the prosthesis and degeneration over time. Causes of rupture vary and include damage during original insertion, direct trauma, cracks from wrinkling, and even from tight compression during mammography. An old practice of closed capsulotomy to break down fibrous contracture could also damage the underlying implant.

Noncontrast MRI and sonography are more sensitive than mammography when evaluating silicone implant integrity. Unlike saline, silicone blocks the penetration of X-rays, thereby obscuring the implant lumen and underlying tissue. This restricts detection of implant rupture on a mammogram. Sonography is not effective at determining a "gel bleed," which is microscopic passage of silicone fluid from an intact implant due to shell permeability and does not imply rupture.

When scanning the augmented breast for implant failure, it is important to closely inspect the implant lumen, the shell membrane and its proximity to the fibrous capsule, and the surrounding tissues and the axilla. High-frequency transducers are utilized to evaluate implants and overlying tissues. However, lower frequencies may be needed to penetrate the deepest portion of the prosthesis and distal structures or to penetrate significant capsular or calcific fibrosis. EFOV imaging shows a greater extent of the implant. Split-screen imaging allows side-by-side documentation of similar areas in both implants to compare implant integrity or contour changes.

Silicone implant failure is classified as ICR or extracapsular rupture (ECR). Published studies vary on the time period for implant failure of traditional silicone implants. This delayed complication most often occurs 10 to 15 years after placement.

Intracapsular Rupture

ICR describes when silicone migrates outside the implant through a breach in the implant shell but is contained by the intact fibrous capsule. This type of rupture is most common. Collapse of the implant shell may be minimal, partial, or complete. A very early sign of uncollapsed rupture is silicone trapped within radial folds. On MRI, this early feature is called the *inverted teardrop, noose,* or *keyhole sign* and is occasionally detected by US. The classic sonographic appearance of ICR is demonstration of the *stepladder sign* or *parallel-line sign* seen as multiple, parallel, echogenic curvilinear lines layered within the silicone gel contained by the fibrous capsule (Fig. 18-75).[67] This finding is usually associated with significant rupture. The stepladder sign represents sound reflecting off of overlapping layers of the collapsed implant shell suspended within the encapsulated silicone and corresponds to the *linguine sign* seen on MRI scans. The use of spatial compounding or 3D imaging may

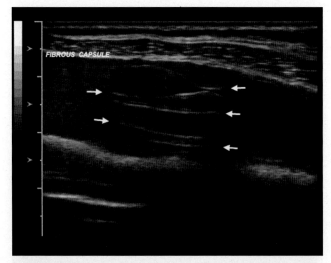

FIGURE 18-75 Intracapsular rupture. Silicone implant demonstrates multiple overlapping layers of a collapsed implant shell (*arrows*) suspended in silicone contained by the intact fibrous capsule (*parallel-line sign*). There is increased echogenicity of some of the extruded silicone.

better display the continuity of the curved edges of the collapsed implant shell.

It is uncommon for newer generation silicone implants to suffer total collapse because they have a stronger implant shell and contain more cohesive silicone gel.

A diagnostic pitfall is to confuse other band-like echoes within an intact implant with ICR, such as near-field reverberation artifacts, redundant radial folds, or double-lumen membrane interfaces. Anterior reverberation artifact can obscure detection of a minimally collapsed implant shell that might only show a slight separation from the fibrous capsule. Overall, noncontrast MRI is more reliable than sonography at diagnosing ICR, especially in patients with double-lumen implants.

A less reliable sign of ICR is the presence of low- to medium-level echoes within the extravasated silicone between the implant shell and fibrous capsule. ICR may allow the influx of body fluids, proteins, or organic salts to mix with the silicone, which can increase the echogenicity of the extravasated gel. Other materials injected into the implant to reduce contracture and infection and to promote symmetry can also cause alterations in the echo pattern of silicone and limit the efficacy of this finding.

Extracapsular Rupture

ECR indicates silicone leakage into the surrounding tissues through a breach in both the implant shell and the fibrous capsule. The presence of silicone in soft tissues can incite an inflammatory response and granuloma formation. The most specific sonographic finding of ECR is demonstration of the *echogenic noise sign*, which describes a discrete region of intense hyperechogenicity with dirty distal shadowing emanating from tissue containing free silicone (Fig. 18-76). This distinctive appearance is also termed the *snowstorm sign* and may result from marked scattering and attenuation of the sound waves when passing through tissues containing microglobules of free silicone. Although usually near the edge of the implant, free silicone can migrate along the chest wall, to the axilla, to the lymph nodes, and even travel to extramammary sites (Fig. 18-77).

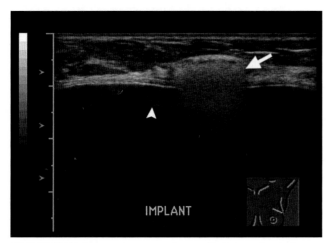

FIGURE 18-76 Extracapsular rupture. Sonographic "echogenic noise" (*arrow*) from a siliconoma near the fibrous capsule in a woman with silicone implant failure. The implant shell (*arrowhead*) is separated from the fibrous capsule.

With ECR, macroglobules of extruded silicone can appear as anechoic, hypoechoic, or complex cystic masses that may be associated with areas of echogenic noise. Because of the propagation speed variance, the back wall of a silicone gel cyst will falsely appear deeper than its true location. This elongated AP dimension helps to differentiate a silicone globule from a true cyst.

Retained silicone may be detected inside or outside the residual fibrous capsule after explantation of a silicone implant, so clinical correlation is needed. Some facilities use sonographic guidance to remove residual silicone granulomas.

Autogenous Breast Reconstruction[6,9,12,15,68]

A patient's own tissues can be used to help reconstruct the shape of the breast following mastectomy. In some patients, an implant is placed in conjunction with a tissue transfer. Some of the more common autogenous breast reconstruction procedures involve transferring muscles, fat, and skin from the abdomen or the back to rebuild the breast mound while preserving the vascular supply to the tissues, including the transverse rectus abdominis myocutaneous (TRAM) flap, the deep inferior epigastric perforator (DEIP) flap, and the latissimus dorsi myocutaneous flap procedures. Autologous tissue transfers can undergo postoperative complications; of most concern is vascular compromise that may lead to possible skin or tissue necrosis.

Autologous fat grafting can be used to improve contour deformities after lumpectomy, excisional biopsy, or implant placement, as well as for cosmetic augmentation. Fat cells are removed by liposuction from the body (e.g., abdomen, thigh, buttocks), then processed and purified before being injected back into the breast. A type of fat grafting procedure incorporates the use of a special bra device that is worn for several weeks before and after fat transfer. This devise acts as a tissue expander putting suction on the breast to create a better matrix for the fat to reside and helps maintain volume after fat transfer for a longer time period. Fat necrosis can occur after a fat transfer procedure. Common imaging findings include the formation oil cysts and dystrophic calcifications.

TECHNOLOGIC ADVANCEMENTS IN BREAST IMAGING

In recent years, there has been a variety of equipment and software improvements that aide in the detection of breast disease. Recent mammography advancements include 3D mammography (tomosynthesis) and contrast-enhanced mammography.[69] With standard digital 2D mammography, the superimposition of normal breast tissues is a common cause of false-positive examinations, resulting in patient callbacks for additional views and/or unnecessary biopsies. 3D mammography, known as digital breast tomosynthesis (DBT), acquires images in an arc-like movement of the X-ray tube, which not only obtains standard mammography views but also provides a 3D data set of the breast. This allows the radiologist to view the breast tissue "layer by layer" to better determine whether a questionable mass is real, to better define calcification and lesion characteristics, and to aide detection of lesions in women with dense breast tissue (Fig. 18-78). Compared with 2D mammography, 3D

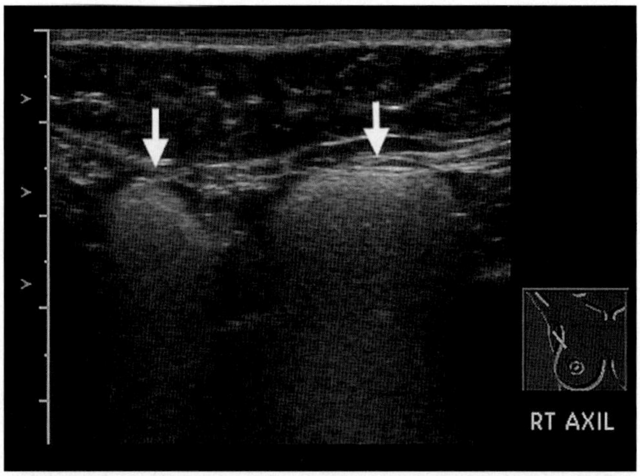

FIGURE 18-77 Silicone adenopathy. Axillary nodes display "echogenic noise" from silicone uptake (*arrows*). (Reprinted with permission from Carr-Hoefer C. *Breast Ultrasound: A Comprehensive Sonographer's Guide.* Pegasus Lectures; 2007.)

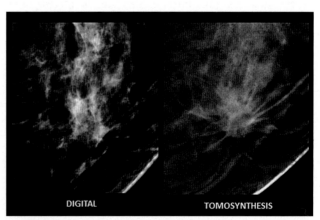

FIGURE 18-78 2D and 3D mammography. Digital 2D mammogram shows a suspicious breast mass; however, mass delineation, spiculation, and Cooper ligament straightening are better resolved on the 3D digital breast tomosynthesis slice. (Image courtesy of Hologic, Inc., Marlborough, MA.)

DBT shows greater accuracy, which reduces the number of false-positive examinations. Less patients are recalled unnecessarily for additional mammographic views. In addition, DBT detects more invasive cancers, even in dense breasts, which allows for earlier detection and treatment.

Technologic advancements continue for breast US, including 3D/4D imaging, contrast-enhanced Doppler, and elastography. Automated breast US systems have gained acceptance in many imaging centers as a way to more efficiently perform whole-breast examinations, especially during supplemental breast screening in women with dense breast. Newer tools include fusion or navigation techniques that allow side-by-side correlation of a mass seen during real-time US with the image data set from another modality (CT, MRI). CAD systems for breast US are being refined that use pattern recognition to analyze the sonographic features of breast masses for BI-RADS classification and reporting.

Emerging technologies, such as quantitative transmission (QT) US imaging, and optoacoustic (OA) imaging, have recently gained FDA approval and show promise in improving diagnostic confidence in the detection and diagnosis of breast disease, and are briefly described in this section.

Elastography[9,10,70–73]

Sonoelastography is a noninvasive technique that depicts the relative hardness or "stiffness" of tissues and masses. Breast elastography is performed in conjunction with 2D grayscale US imaging and more recently has been applied to 3D imaging. The grayscale image shows the morphologic features of a mass, whereas the elastogram depicts lesion stiffness. Images are compared side by side. The elasticity of a tissue is related to how much deformation (strain) occurs after a compressional force (stress) is applied. In the breast, "high-strain" tissues are soft and easy to compress, such as fat. Whereas "low-strain" tissues are hard (stiff) and resist deformation. The elastic features of tissues can change with disease processes. As noted with clinical palpation, cancers tend to be harder than normal breast tissues or benign masses. Two main types of elastography methods are currently used for breast evaluation: strain and shear wave.

With strain elastography, a compression force is applied to the breast tissues. This is accomplished by applying gentle transducer pressure over the region of interest, or by respiratory movements or cardiac pulsation from within the patient. Another method is to use an acoustic radiation force impulse as the source of displacement. Strain elastography typically provides qualitative information about the stiffness of a breast mass relative to the surrounding tissues. On the elastogram image, variations in tissue stiffness are depicted in either shades of gray or over a range of colors depending on the elasticity map chosen. With the current lack of color map standardization, some manufacturers denote "soft" tissue as "red" and "hard" tissue as "blue," or vice versa. Therefore, the sonographer must check the color bar designation before assessing elasticity features. In general, invasive cancers are typically stiffer and tend to measure larger on the strain elastogram than on the 2D image (Fig. 18-79). Benign masses tend to show soft-to-intermediate stiffness and can measure smaller on the elastogram. Commonly, a cyst will show a "bull's-eye" artifact on a grayscale elastogram or a trilayered (blue/green/red) pattern on a color

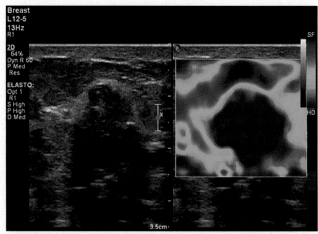

FIGURE 18-79 Strain elastogram. Dual image shows a 2D sonogram of an indistinct, nonparallel, shadowing mass. The corresponding strain elastogram shows the lesion is hard (stiff) based on the color bar. This system uses "blue" for "soft" (*SF*) and "red" for "hard" (*HD*). The lesion also appears larger on the elastogram. Findings are suspicious for cancer. (Image courtesy of Philips Healthcare, Bothell, WA.)

strain elastogram (Fig. 18-80). Performing a fat-to-lesion strain ratio and size ratios or utilizing a five-point elasticity scoring system helps provide semiquantitative information when analyzing breast lesions.

Shear-wave elastography (SWE) provides quantitative data about tissue stiffness and is more reproducible and less operator dependent. With this technique, the transducer emits a focused pulse of acoustic energy to the region of the mass, which induces the formation of shear waves that travel perpendicular to the main acoustic pulse. The propagation speed of the shear waves is directly related to tissue elasticity, traveling faster in stiff tissue than in soft tissue. The US system can differentiate the shear waves to calculate tissue stiffness in kilopascals (kPa) or in meters per second (m/s). These values are assigned to a color map on the SWE image. Lower kPa values are displayed in blue and indicate soft tissues (Fig. 18-81A). High kPa values are displayed in red and indicate stiff tissue or masses, which is concerning for malignancy (Fig. 18-81B). A "stiff rim" is another feature of some cancerous lesions. A kPa value of zero is black and a feature of a cyst.

In addition to B-mode and Doppler findings, lesion stiffness is another characteristic that may help better differentiate

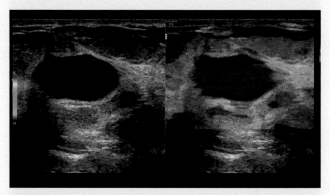

FIGURE 18-80 Strain elastogram. 2D B-mode sonogram shows a simple cyst. The color-coded strain elastogram shows a trilayer appearance typical of a cyst. The color bar indicates "red" for "soft" (S) and "blue" for "hard" (H). (Image courtesy of GE Healthcare, Milwaukee, WI.)

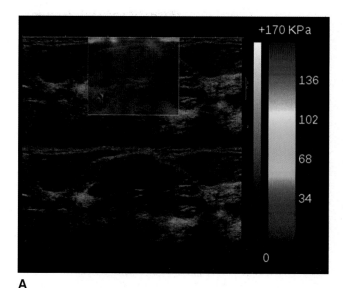
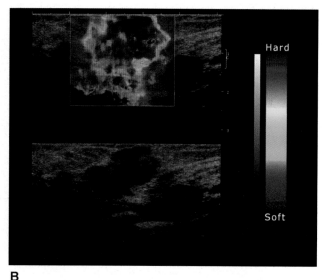

A   **B**

FIGURE 18-81 Shear-wave elastograms. **A:** 2D image shows an oval, mildly lobulated, parallel-oriented, circumscribed solid mass. Based on the low kPa value (assigned as a blue color), the mass shows soft elastic features, which is a benign pattern common with fibroadenoma. **B:** This multilobulated solid lesion displays hard (stiff) elastic features (assigned as red on the color bar), typical of a malignant mass. (Images courtesy of Supersonic Imagine; Hologic Inc., Marlborough, MA.)

benign from malignant masses. Data suggest elasticity findings may improve specificity of the US assessment of some BI-RADS 3 and BI-RADS 4a lesions, including complicated cysts. This can reduce unnecessary biopsy in some patients.[10]

Automated Breast Ultrasound Scanners and Supplemental Breast Screening[1,18,74–77]

High breast density is associated with an increased cancer risk and compromises cancer detection on standard screening mammography. Studies show that the relative risk in women with extremely dense breasts by mammography is four to six times that of a woman without dense breasts. Most states have initiated "Breast Density Notification" laws that require women to be notified if dense breast tissue was found on their mammogram. These women are encouraged to discuss with their physicians whether they might benefit from supplemental screening, such as with MRI or US.

In 2019, the ACR published practice parameters for the performance of whole-breast US for screening and staging.[18] Adjunctive screening indications for whole-breast US include women with a high lifetime breast cancer risk (≥20%) who are not the candidates for, or who cannot easily access, breast MRI and women with heterogeneously or extremely dense breasts for whom supplemental screening options have been suggested. In addition, whole-breast US is indicated for cancer staging, such as in a woman with a new diagnosis of breast cancer who is not a breast MRI candidate or cannot easily access that technology.

Supplemental whole-breast US screening examinations can be performed using handheld high-resolution transducers or with dedicated automated breast US scanners. Dedicated whole-breast US systems have been developed to reduce reliance on the operator during image acquisition by automating the scanning process and reducing scan time. Equipment design varies by company. Both supine and prone

systems are manufactured. One company utilizes a scanner assembly that houses a 15-cm reversed-curved transducer that is placed over a mesh membrane that compresses and stabilizes the breast during image acquisition. In general, the automated systems rapidly acquire image data sets of the entire breast in a preset manner and display standard image planes and reconstructed 3D coronal views (Fig. 18-82). The distance of a mass from the nipple and depth of the lesion can be quickly ascertained. Additional handheld targeted sonography devices can be directed to areas of concern as needed. The volume data set is digitally stored and retrievable on a computer workstation for radiologist review and image manipulation.

Another type of automated whole-breast US uses a standard high-frequency linear-array transducer that is mounted on a motorized arm that traverses the entire breast from superior to inferior acquiring overlapping images that include the axilla. The images are reviewed in a movie format.

With US breast screening, there needs to be a balance between acceptable recall rates and cancer detection. Studies show that the addition of a single US screening examination in women with dense breast tissue at mammography will yield an additional 2.3 to 4.6 occult cancers per 1,000 women.[10] High false-positive predictive rates associated with whole-breast US are reported to have diminished with continuing experience with this screening modality.[18]

Quantitative Transmission Ultrasound Imaging

QT US technology is an innovative advancement in automated breast imaging. This noninvasive technique provides detailed whole-breast US images without the use of radiation or contrast agents. The QT US system creates a 3D scan from volume data sets that correspond to the speed-of-sound transmission, attenuation, and reflection characteristics of breast tissues and masses.[78–80]

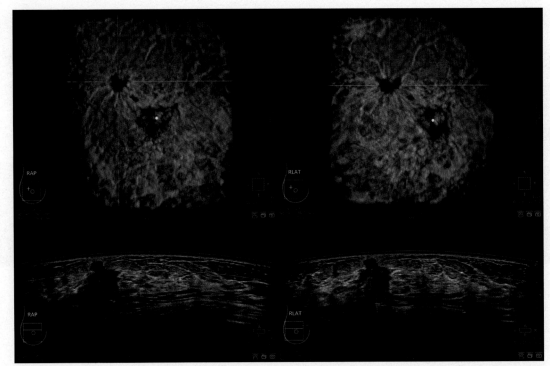

FIGURE 18-82 Automated whole-breast sonography of a breast cancer. This automated breast ultrasound system (*ABUS*) acquires 2D slices of the breast utilizing a reversed-curved 15-cm transducer. 3D data sets can produce coronal planes to more fully evaluate the characteristics of a breast lesion. The nipple location is referenced for location. (Image courtesy of GE Healthcare, Milwaukee, WI.)

The QTscan ultrasound system (QT Imaging, Inc., Novato, CA, USA) is approved by the FDA as an adjunct to mammography for breast imaging. The patient lies comfortably in a prone position on the QT scan table. The breast is placed through an opening in the table and suspended in a warm water bath. The water bath houses transducer arrays positioned around the breast that can operate in sound transmission and reflection modes. Whole-breast images are created through 3D acquisition and reconstruction, showing detailed US images of breast anatomy and pathology, which are viewable in many scan planes (Fig.18-83).

Women with dense breast tissue are at higher risk for breast cancer. Mammographic detection of cancer is compromised in such women. Besides creating detailed volumetric images of the breast, research shows promise utilizing transmission US to quantify breast density, without the need for radiation or breast compression, and to detect suspicious lesions within dense breast tissue. Clinical trials are ongoing.

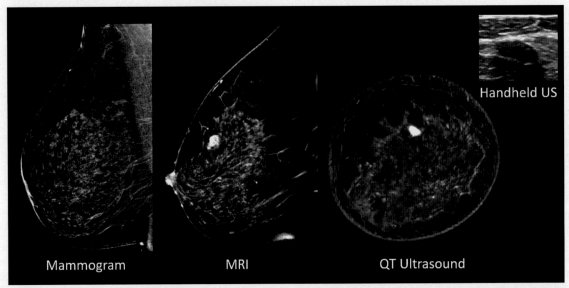

FIGURE 18-83 Quantitative transmission ultrasound (*US*) imaging. Suspicious mass across imaging modalities. Dense breast tissue on mammogram obscures optimal detection of the breast mass. Contrast-enhanced magnetic resonance imaging (*MRI*) better reveals the presence of the small lesion. QT ultrasound provides high-contrast imaging of the mass and surrounding tissues without radiation or need for contrast agents. (Images courtesy of QT Imaging, Novato, CA.)

Optoacoustic Imaging

Recent research on the use of OA imaging shows promise to better differentiate benign from malignant lesions, in hope of increasing specificity and reducing false-positive cases at biopsy. This fusion technique combines conventional breast US imaging with laser light technology to provide both anatomic and functional information about breast lesions and adjacent tissues (Fig. 18-84). The 2D grayscale image shows tumor morphology, whereas the OA component of this technology provides information about the level of hemoglobin (Hgb) oxygenation within tumors (Fig. 18-85).[81]

This technology centers on the concept that cancers are more metabolically active than normal breast tissue or benign masses. The growth and progression of breast cancer is augmented by increased vascularization and the formation new, chaotic, blood vessels (neoangiogenesis). Thus, malignant tumors tend to be more vascular and more quickly deplete oxygen from the blood as they grow. This is particularly true of higher grade invasive cancers. The OA component of the system can detect changes in breast and tumor vasculature and can differentiate normally oxygenated from more suspicious deoxygenated (hypoxic) tumors.

The OA/US image is composed of colorized maps corresponding to Hgb oxygenation within and around a lesion (green = oxygenated Hgb; red = deoxygenated Hgb) that is superimposed over the grayscale US image, or viewed side by side. Ongoing research suggests OA/US imaging can improve diagnostic confidence. For example, certain masses initially classified as BI-RADS 4A at US could be downgraded to BI-RADS 3 or BI-RADS 2. This can potentially reduce the number of unnecessary biopsies and recommendations for follow-up imaging.[81,82]

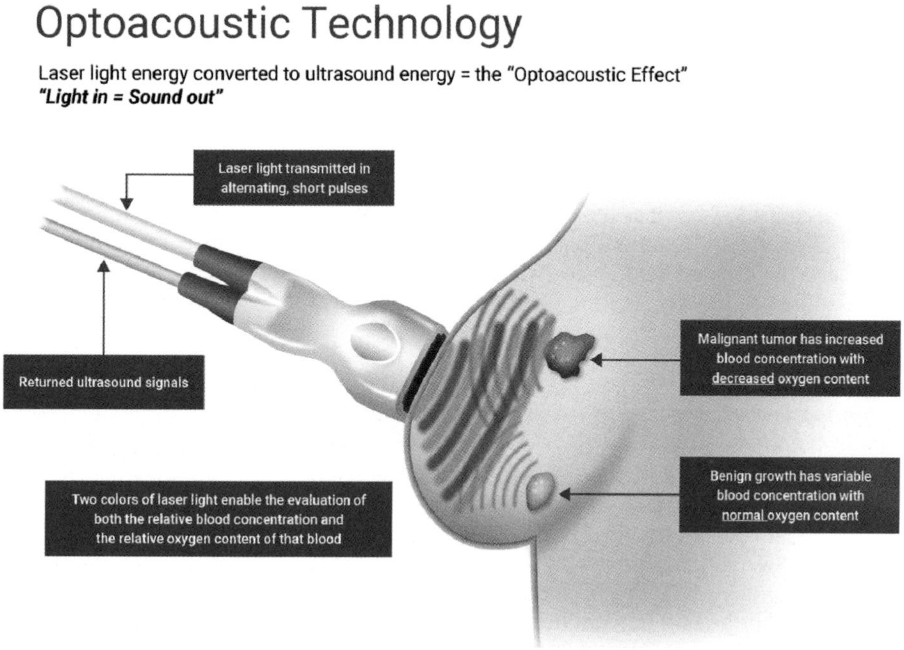

Optoacoustic Technology

Laser light energy converted to ultrasound energy = the "Optoacoustic Effect"
"Light in = Sound out"

Laser light transmitted in alternating, short pulses

Returned ultrasound signals

Two colors of laser light enable the evaluation of both the relative blood concentration and the relative oxygen content of that blood

Malignant tumor has increased blood concentration with decreased oxygen content

Benign growth has variable blood concentration with normal oxygen content

FIGURE 18-84 Optoacoustic (*OA*) technology. Illustration shows the OA/ultrasound (*US*) duplex probe that can operate in conventional 2D US imaging mode and transmit laser light at two different wavelengths into a breast mass. Hemoglobin in the blood absorbs the laser light, warms and briefly expands, and produces a pressure wave received by the transducer. The system can differentiate the relative degrees of blood concentration and oxygen content of hemoglobin in the blood. Malignant tumors tend to have increased blood concentration with decreased oxygenation, whereas benign masses have more variable blood concentration and normal oxygen content. (Images courtesy of Seno Medical, San Antonio, TX.)

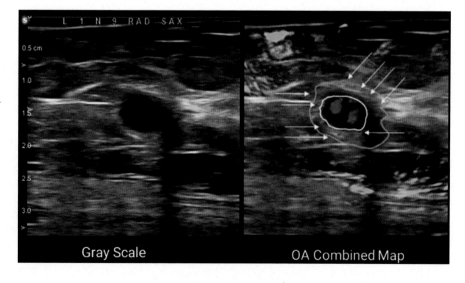

FIGURE 18-85 Optoacoustic/ultrasound (*OA/US*) duplex image. This small triple-negative breast cancer (*TNBC*) IDC could be mistaken for a probably benign mass on initial imaging. However, the OA component shows suspicious findings that upgraded classification to a BI-RADS 4. Deoxygenated vessels, shown as *red*, predominate the internal zone of the lesion (outlined by *white*). There are also multiple tortuous vessels within the boundary zone (outlined by *blue line*). Arrows point to "whisker vessels." These are suspicious findings. Most of the suspicious OA features of TNBC are within the internal and boundary zones, rather than in the peripheral zone. *IDC*, invasive ductal carcinoma. (Image courtesy of Seno Medical, San Antonio, TX.)

Gray Scale

OA Combined Map

BREAST MAGNETIC RESONANCE IMAGING[1,2,56,48,83,84]

Although mammography is the standard screening test for cancer, there are subgroups of patients with dense breast tissue for whom diagnostic efficacy is reduced. Contrast-enhanced MRI is reported to have greater sensitivity at detecting breast cancer than mammography or sonography, although false-positive findings occur from overlaps in benign and malignant breast patterns. Patients lie prone with the breast suspended in dedicated breast coils. Contrast-enhanced MRI is very effective at evaluating the morphologic features of a mass and dynamic blood flow patterns. A paramagnetic contrast agent (gadolinium) is given via intravenous (IV) injection. The neovascularity of invasive cancers, in particular, contributes to rapid, moderate-to-marked tumor enhancement and quick contrast washout on MRI images following contrast injection (Fig. 18-86). Both breasts and adjacent nodal beds can be evaluated with this nonionizing technique. The American Cancer Society published guidelines recommending contrast-enhanced MRI be used as an adjunct to mammography to screen for cancer in high-risk patients with a 20% to 25% or greater lifetime risk for the disease. MRI can look for tumor enhancement in regions of DCIS that are often associated with suspicious calcifications on the mammogram. MRI can detect multifocal, multicentric, and bilateral cancers, as well as lymph node changes, which can affect surgical and treatment planning. Suspicious masses only seen by MRI can be biopsied with this technique. MRI can also be used to assess tumor response to neoadjuvant

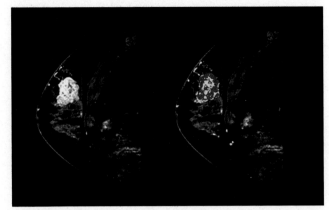

FIGURE 18-86 Contrast-enhanced magnetic resonance image. 3-Telsa sagittal scan through the breast shows marked uptake of the paramagnetic contrast. Static imaging findings and dynamic angiomap pattern indicate malignancy. (Image courtesy of GE Healthcare, Milwaukee, WI.)

chemotherapy before surgery and differentiate recurrent tumor from scar in the postsurgical patient. Noncontrast MRI is considered the best imaging tool for assessing implant integrity. Cost, limited availability, examination length, lower specificity, and the need for contrast for most examinations are some disadvantages of this technique. Abbreviated MRI imaging protocols have been introduced that significantly decrease examination time while still providing diagnostic accuracy, with the hope of increasing patient accessibility to this important test.

SUMMARY

- Mammography is still the principal technique chosen to localize and biopsy suspicious microcalcifications and remains the only widely used screening tool proven effective at reducing breast cancer mortality; however, when mammography has limited efficacy, as in a dense breast, other imaging modalities, including sonography, can be utilized to detect and localize suspicious masses.
- When used in conjunction, the strengths of sonography offset the weaknesses of mammography, providing greater diagnostic confidence.
- Sonographic evaluation of the breast is useful in young, pregnant, or lactating women; helps to differentiate between cystic and solid masses; allows palpable and mammographic or MRI indeterminate lesions to be characterized; is better tolerated in patients with breast trauma, inflammatory changes, augmentation mammoplasty, or postirradiation changes; and provides real-time guidance for interventional and therapeutic breast procedures.
- High-resolution breast sonography plays a supplemental role to mammography as a screening tool to detect occult cancer in certain women with radiographically dense breasts.
- The female breast is primarily composed of glandular, fatty, and fibrous connective tissues that vary in proportion based on the individual's age and hormonal status; the glandular elements of the breast primarily function to produce and transport milk; the stromal elements consist of fat, fibrous connective tissues, as well as blood vessels, lymphatics, and nerves.
- The breast is subdivided by fascial planes into three layers or zones: the premammary layer, the mammary (parenchymal) layer, and the retromammary layer.
- A high-frequency, broadband, linear transducer with a center frequency of 12 MHz or higher is suitable for breast sonography (ACR, 2016).
- Breast sonography systems need to provide excellent spatial and contrast resolution and the output power; TGC, overall gain, dynamic range, focal zone placement, image size, and depth must be optimized for each patient.
- Based on site protocol and indication, either a targeted examination or a whole-breast sonography examination is performed. A targeted study is limited to the quadrant or region of clinical concern, such as for a palpable mass, or to further characterize a mammographic or MRI finding. Some indications for a whole-breast examination include the search for satellite lesions and lymph node involvement in a patient with a known cancer or suspicious lesion, to screen a high-risk patient with radiographically dense breasts as adjunct to mammography, or to evaluate implant integrity.
- Images can be taken in sagittal and transverse planes, as well as in radial and antiradial orthogonal scan planes.
- Typically, annotations include the side being evaluated, the clockface position, the distance from the nipple, and the scan plane.

- The ACR BI-RADS Breast Ultrasound Lexicon is utilized in an effort to promote the use of more consistent terminology when characterizing and reporting sonographic findings.
- Most breast cysts are related to FCC; symptoms of FCC include breast tenderness or pain, fullness, and nodularity.
- Cystic breast lesions may be simple, complicated, or complex with cystic and solid components.
- Mastitis, inflammation of the breast, presents most often during pregnancy and lactation but can affect women at any stage of life. Abscess formation is a complication of mastitis. Other breast conditions related to pregnancy include galactocele and secretory adenoma.
- Hematoma, seroma, and fat necrosis are related to breast trauma and can be evaluated with breast sonography.
- Characteristically, a benign mass displaces, rather than invades, adjacent tissues as it grows and displays an oval shape and well-circumscribed margins that are sharply demarcated from surrounding tissues. Gentle lobulation may be present. Benign lesions are typically wider-than-tall with parallel orientation relative to the skin.
- Characteristics that make a mass suspicious for malignancy include irregular shape; indistinct, angular, microlobulated, or spiculated margins; an orientation not parallel to the skin (taller-than-wide); hypoechogenicity; microcalcifications; posterior shadowing; and duct changes such as duct extension or branching pattern.
- Associated features of cancer include architectural distortion with Cooper ligament straightening or thickening, skin thickening, skin or nipple retraction, and edema.
- Fibroadenoma is the most common benign solid tumor of the female breast, with a higher incidence in patients aged 15 to 35 years; sonographically, a fibroadenoma typically appears as a smooth, well-circumscribed, oval, parallel-oriented (wider-than-tall), homogeneous, solid mass that may be gently lobulated.
- Excluding skin cancer, breast cancer is the most common malignancy affecting women in the United States and ranks second to lung cancer as the leading cause of cancer-related deaths in women over age 50.
- Approximately one in eight American women develop breast cancer during a lifetime, and early cancer detection and treatment improve long-term survival by decreasing the incidence of lymph node involvement and metastasis to distant sites.
- Breast cancers are usually adenocarcinomas that originate in a TDLU; the majority of cancers develop in the UOQ where there is the greatest amount of glandular-epithelial tissue.
- Carcinoma in situ is noninvasive disease. DCIS is the most common noninvasive cancer and is stage 0 disease. LCIS is a high-risk lesion rather than a malignancy; this form of lobular neoplasia is a marker for an increased risk for developing future breast cancer.
- DCIS frequently presents only as suspicious calcifications on mammography.
- Invasive cancer describes cases when malignant cells breach the basement membrane of the duct and/or lobule and extend into adjacent tissues; cancer cells can then penetrate nearby blood vessels and lymphatic channels, both pathways for metastatic seeding.
- IDC NOS (IDC NST) is the most common breast cancer, and ILC is the second most common invasive breast cancer.
- Diffuse or inflammatory carcinoma occurs when a highly invasive cancer infiltrates the lymphatics of the skin; frequently, the result of higher grade IDCs that may disseminate within the breast.
- With inflammatory carcinoma, the skin becomes red, warm, and edematous with an orange peel (peau d'orange) appearance. The breast is often painful and hard.
- The first site of metastatic spread from a primary breast cancer is usually to the ipsilateral axillary lymph nodes, which receive most of the lymph drainage from the breast; but breast cancer can also metastasize other parts of the body, including the bone, liver, lung, and brain.
- The SLN is the first node in the lymphatic drainage basin of a breast cancer and is at most risk for metastasis.
- Gynecomastia refers to benign male breast enlargement characterized by an abnormal proliferation of ductal and stromal tissues and is associated with an increased estrogen-to-testosterone ratio. Gynecomastia usually presents as a soft, mildly tender, area of fullness or nodularity centered beneath the areola.
- Male breast cancer is rare and typically located in the retroareolar region, eccentric to the nipple.
- Common sonography-guided procedures include cyst aspiration, drainage of a fluid collection such as an abscess, biopsy of a suspicious solid mass, lymph node sampling, and preoperative localization of a nonpalpable mass.
- Sonography can be used to evaluate the integrity of saline and silicone implants and complications such as ICR or ECR.
- On elastography, malignant masses tend to be stiffer and often measure larger on the elastogram than on the 2D image.

REFERENCES

1. American College of Radiology. *ACR Appropriateness Criteria: Breast Cancer Screening.* American College of Radiology; 2016. Accessed January 12, 2021. http://www.acr.org
2. American Cancer Society. Recommendations for screening early detection of breast cancer. Accessed May 3, 2022. https://www.cancer.org/cancer/breast-cancer/screening-tests-and-early-detection/american-cancer-society-recommendations-for-the-early-detection-of-breast-cancer.html
3. National Cancer Institute. Breast cancer screening. Accessed January 12, 2021. https://www.cancer.gov/types/breast/patient/breast-screening-pdq
4. D'Orsi CJ, Sickles EA, Mendelson EB, Morris EA. *ACR BI-RADS® Atlas, Breast Imaging Reporting and Data System.* American College of Radiology; 2013.
5. Berg WA, Birdwell RL, Gombos EC, et al. *Diagnostic Imaging: Breast.* Amirsys; 2006.
6. Ikeda DM, Miyake KK. *Breast Imaging: The Requisites.* 3rd ed. Elsevier; 2017.
7. Harvey J, March DE. *Making the Diagnosis: A Practical Guide to Breast Imaging.* Saunders; 2013.
8. Mettler FA. Breast. In: Mettler FA, ed. *Essentials of Radiology.* 4th ed. Elsevier; 2019.
9. Phillips J, Mehta RJ, Stavros AT. The breast. In: Rumack CM, Levine D, eds. *Diagnostic Ultrasound.* 5th ed. Elsevier; 2017.
10. Stavros AT. *Breast Ultrasound.* Lippincott Williams & Wilkins; 2004.
11. James JJ, Evans AJ. Breast. In: Allan P, ed. *Clinical Ultrasound.* 3rd ed. Elsevier; 2014.
12. Hooley, RJ, Scoutt LM, Philpotts LE. Breast ultrasonography. State of the art. *Radiology.* 2013;268(3):642–659.

13. Hagen-Ansert SL, Salsgiver TL, Glenn ME. The breast. In: Hagen-Ansert SL, ed. *Textbook of Diagnostic Ultrasonography*. Vol 1. 2nd ed. Mosby Elsevier; 2006.

14. Carr-Hoefer C. The breast. In: Kawamura D, Lunsford B, eds. *Diagnostic Medical Sonography: Abdomen and Superficial Structures*. 3rd ed. Lippincott Williams & Wilkins; 2012.

15. Carr-Hoefer C. Breast Ultrasound: *A Comprehensive Sonographer's Guide*. 2nd ed. Miele Enterprises LLC.; 2008.

16. American College of Radiology. ACR Practice Parameter for the Performance of a Breast Ultrasound Examination. American College of Radiology; 2016. Accessed December 15, 2020. http://www.acr.org

17. American College of Radiology. ACR Practice Parameter for the Performance of Ultrasound-guided Percutaneous Breast Interventional Procedures. American College of Radiology; 2016. Accessed December 15, 2020. http://www.acr.org

18. American College of Radiology. ACR Practice Parameter for the Performance of Whole-Breast Ultrasound for Screening and Staging. American College of Radiology; 2019. Accessed December 15, 2020. http://www.acr.org

19. Anufrieva S, Blinov A, Kuznetsov A. *MicroPure-A New Technology in Clinical Breast Care*. Toshiba Medical Systems Corporation; 2014.

20. American Cancer Society. Breast cancer screening guidelines. Accessed March 17, 2021. https://www.cancer.org

21. American College of Radiology. Breast Cancer Screening for Average Risk Women: Recommendations from the ACR Commission on Breast Imaging. American College of Radiology; 2017. Accessed January 05, 2021. https://acr.org

22. American College of Radiology. Breast Cancer Screening in Women at Higher-Than-Average Risk: Recommendations from the ACR. American College of Radiology; 2018. Accessed January 05, 2021. https://acr.org

23. Kaneda HJ, Mack J, Kasales CJ, et al. Pediatric and adolescent breast masses: a review of pathophysiology, imaging, diagnosis, and treatment. *AJR Am J Roentgenol*. 2013;200(2):200–212.

24. Bock K, Duda VF, Hadji P, et al. Pathologic breast conditions in childhood and adolescence: evaluation by sonographic diagnosis. *J Ultrasound Med*. 2005;24:1347–1354.

25. Weismann C, Mayr C, Egger H, Auer A. Breast sonography—2D, 3D, 4D ultrasound or elastography? *Breast Care (Basel)*. 2011;6(2):98–103.

26. Rao AA, Feneis J, LaLonde C, et al. A pictorial review of changes in the BI-RADS fifth edition. *Radiographics*. 2016;36(3):623–639.

27. Berg WA, Sechtin AG, Marques H, Zhang Z. Cystic breast masses and the ACRIN 6666 experience. *Radiol Clin N Am*. 2010;48(5):931–987.

28. Adler K, Samreen N, Glazebrook KN, Bhatt AA. Imaging features and treatment options for breast pseudoaneurysms after biopsy: a case-based pictorial review. *J Ultrasound Med*. 2020;39(1):181–190.

29. Pesce K, Chico MA, Binder F. Breast pseudoaneurysm after core needle biopsy in a pregnant patient. *Radiol Case Rep*. 2021;16(1):35–39.

30. Sohn Y, Kim MJ, Kim E-K, et al. Pseudoaneurysm of the breast during vacuum-assisted removal. *J Ultrasound Med*. 2009;28(7):967–971.

31. Gregg A, Leddy R, Lewis M, et al. Acquired arteriovenous fistula of the breast following ultrasound guided biopsy of invasive ductal carcinoma. *J Clin Sci*. 2013;3(3):1–3.

32. Stavros AT, Thickman D, Rapp CL, et al. Solid breast nodules: use of sonography to distinguish between benign and malignant lesions. *Radiology*. 1995;196:123–134.

33. Gordon PB, Gagnon FA, Lanzkowsky L, Solid breast masses diagnosed as fibroadenoma at fine-needle aspiration biopsy: acceptable rates of growth at long-term follow-up. *Radiology*. 2003;229(1):233–238.

34. Klinger K, Bhimani C, Shames J, et al. Fibroadenoma: from imaging evaluation to treatment. *J Am Osteopath Coll Radiol*. 2019;8(2):17–30.

35. Wang ZL, Liu G, He Y, et al. Ultrasound-guided 7-gauge vacuum-assisted core biopsy: could it be sufficient for the diagnosis and treatment of intraductal papilloma? *Breast J*. 2019;25(5):807–812.

36. American Cancer Society. Breast cancer facts & figures: 2019–2020. Accessed June 5, 2021. https://www.cancer.org/content/dam/cancer-org/research/cancer-facts-and-statistics/breast-cancer-facts-and-figures/breast-cancer-facts-and-figures-2019-2020.pdf

37. National Cancer Institute. Cancer statistics. Accessed March 20, 2021. https://www.cancer.gov/about-cancer/understanding/statistics

38. American Joint Commission on Cancer. *Breast Cancer Staging*. 8th ed. Accessed March 1, 2021. http://cancerstaging.org

39. Monticciolo DL, Newell MS, Moy L, et al. Breast cancer screening in women at higher-than-average risk: recommendations from the ACR. *J Am Coll Radiol*. 2018;15:408–414.

40. Harisinghani MG. *Primer of Diagnostic Imaging*. 6th ed. Elsevier; 2019.

41. Harvey JA. The evolving role of breast radiologists. *J Breast Imaging*. 2020;2(1):1.

42. Cho N. Molecular subtypes and imaging phenotypes of breast cancer. *Ultrasonography*. 2016;35(4):281–288.

43. Lee MV, Katabathina VS, Bowerson ML, et al., BRCA-associated cancers: role of imaging in screening, diagnosis, and management. *Radiographics*. 2017;37(4):1005–1023.

44. Nguyen C, Kettler MD, Swirsky ME, et al. Male breast disease: pictorial review with radiologic-pathologic correlation. *Radiographics*. 2013;33(3):763–779.

45. Meattini I, Bicchierai G, Saieva C, et al. Impact of molecular subtypes classification concordance between preoperative core needle biopsy and surgical specimen on early breast cancer: a systematic review and meta-analysis. *Diagn Med Sonogr*. 2021;37(1):47–57.

46. Gity M, Borhani A, Mokri M, et al. Sonographic features of estrogen-negative breast cancers: A correlation with human epidermal growth factor type II overexpression. *J Diagn Med Sonogr*. 2018;34(6):484–488.

47. Kim, MY, Choi, N. Mammographic and ultrasonographic features of triple-negative breast cancer: a comparison with other breast cancer subtypes. *Acta Radiol*. 2013;54(8):889–894.

48. Sistani SS, Parooie F. Breast ultrasound versus MRI in prediction of pathologic complete response to neoadjuvant chemotherapy for breast cancer: a systematic review and meta-analysis. *J Diagn Med Sonogr*. 2021;37(1):47–57.

49. Kim S, Plemmons J, Hoang K, et al. Breast-specific gamma imaging versus MRI: Comparing the diagnostic performance in assessing treatment response after neoadjuvant chemotherapy in patients with breast cancer. *AJR Am J Roentgenol*. 2019;212(3):696–705.

50. Daugherty MW, Niell BL. Utility of routine axillary ultrasound surveillance in breast cancer survivors with previously diagnoses metastatic axillary adenopathy. *J Breast Imaging*. 2019;1(1):25–31.

51. Sun SX, Moseley TY, Kuerer HM, et al. Imaging-based approach to axillary lymph node staging and sentinel lymph node biopsy in patients with breast cancer. *Am J Roentgenol*. 2020;214(2):249–258.

52. Brown A, Shah S, Dluzewski S, et al. Unilateral axillary adenopathy following COVID-19 vaccination: a multimodality pictorial illustration and review of current guidelines. *Clin Radiol*. 2021;76(8):553–558.

53. Shaw C, Vicini F, Wazer DE, Arthur D, Patel RR. The American Brachytherapy Society consensus statement for accelerated partial breast irradiation. *Brachytherapy*. 2013;12(4):267–277.

54. HOLOGIC®. Mammosite—Breast brachytherapy. Accessed January 21, 2021. http://www.hologic.com

55. Merit Medical®. Savi Brachy: easing the burden of breast cancer treatment. Accessed January 22, 2021. http://www.merit.com

56. Molleran VM, Mahoney MC. *Breast MRI*. Saunders; 2014.

57. Hayes MK. Update on preoperative breast localization. *Radiol Clin N Am*. 2017;55(3):591–603.

58. Ward RC, Lourenco AP, Mainiera MB. Ultrasound-guided breast cancer cryoablation. *AJR Am J Roentgenol*. 2019;213(3):716–722.

59. Fornage BD, Hwang RF. Current status of imaging-guided percutaneous ablation of breast cancer. *Am J Roentgenol*. 2014;203(2):442–448.

60. Brenin DR, Patrie J, Nguyen J, et al. Treatment of breast fibroadenoma with ultrasound-guided high-intensity focused ultrasound ablation: a feasibility study. *J Breast Imaging*. 2019;1(4):316–323.

61. Somerville P, Seifert P, Destounis S, et al. Anticoagulation and bleeding risk after core needle biopsy. *Am J Roentgenol*. 2008;191(4):1194–1197.

62. Kapoor MM, Patel MM, Scoggins ME. The wire and beyond: Recent advances in breast imaging preoperative needle localization. *Radiographics*. 2019;39(7):1886–1906.

63. U.S. Food & Drug Administration. Questions and answers about breast implant-associated anaplastic large cell lymphoma (BIA-ALCL). Accessed January 14, 2021. https://www.fda.gov/medical-devices/breast-implants/questions-and-answers-about-breast-implant-associated-anaplastic-large-cell-lymphoma-bia-alcl

64. Mitry MA, Sogani J, Sutton E, et al. Rare cancer on the rise: an educational review of breast implant-associated anaplastic large cell lymphoma. *J Breast Imaging*. 2020;2(4):398–407.

65. Seiler SJ, Sharma PB, Hayes JC, et al. Multimodality imaging-based evaluation of single-lumen silicone breast implants for rupture. *Radiographics.* 2017;37(2):366–382.

66. Roller R, Chetlen A, Kasales C. Imaging of breast implants and their associated complications. *J Am Osteopath Coll Radiol.* 2014;3(1):2–9.

67. Middleton MS, McNamara MP. *Breast Implant Imaging.* Lippincott Williams & Wilkins; 2002.

68. Alvarez A. Natural breast augmentation of fat transfer: the mammographic and sonographic correlation. *J Diagn Med Sonogr.* 2012;28(1):26–32.

69. Ghaderi KF, Phillips J, Perry H, et al., Contrast-enhanced mammography: current applications and future directions. *Radiographics.* 2019;39(7):1907–1920.

70. Barr RG, Nakashima N, Amy D, et al. WFUMB guidelines and recommendations for clinical use of ultrasound elastography: part 2: breast. *Ultrasound Med Biol.* 2015;41(5):1148–1160.

71. Berg WA, Cosgrove DO, Doré CJ, et al. Shear-wave elastography improves the specificity of breast US: the BE1 multinational study of 939 masses. *Radiology.* 2012;262(2):435–449.

72. Youk JH, Gweon HM, Son EJ, Shear-wave elastography in breast ultrasonography: the state of the art. *Ultrasonography.* 2017;36: 300–309.

73. Zhou J, Zhan W, Chang C, et al. Breast lesions: evaluation with shear wave elastography, with special emphasis on the "stiff rim" sign. *Radiology.* 2014;272(1):63–72.

74. Aripoli A, Fountain K, Winblad O, et al. Supplemental screening with automated breast ultrasound in women with dense breasts: comparing notifications methods and screening behaviors. *Am J Roentgenol.* 2018;210(1):22–28.

75. Berg WA, Vourtsis A. Screening breast ultrasound using handheld or automated technique in women with dense breasts. *J Breast Imaging.* 2019;1(4):283–296.

76. Durand MA, Hooley RJ. Implementation of whole-breast screening ultrasonography. *Radiol Clin N Am.* 2017;55(3):527–539.

77. Chen L, Chen Y, Diao X-H, et al. Comparative study of automated breast 3-D ultrasound and handheld B-mode ultrasound for differentiation of benign and malignant breast masses. *Ultrasound Med Biol.* 2013;39(10):1735–1742.

78. Malik B, Klock J, Wiskin J, Lenox M. Objective breast tissue image classification using Quantitative transmission ultrasound tomography. *Sci Rep.* 2016;9(6):38857.

79. Wiskin J, Malik B, Lenox M. Quantitative assessment of breast density using transmission ultrasound tomography. *Med Phys.* 2019;46(6):2610–2620.

80. Natesan R, Wiskin J, Lee S, et al. Quantitative assessment of breast density: Transmission ultrasound is comparable to mammography with tomosynthesis. *Cancer Prev Res.* 2019;12:871–876.

81. Butler R, Lavin PT, Tucker FL, et al. Optoacoustic breast imaging: Imaging-pathology correlation of optoacoustics features in benign and malignant breast masses. *AJR Am J Roentgenol.* 2018;211(5):1155–1170.

82. Menezes GL, Pijnappel RM, Meeuwis C, et al. Downgrading of breast masses suspicious for cancer by using optoacoustic breast imaging. *Radiology.* 2018;288(2):355–365.

83. Santiago L, Candelaria RP, Huang ML. MR imaging-guided breast interventions. *Magn Reson Imaging Clin N Am.* 2018;26(2):235–246.

84. Chhor CM, Mercado CL. Abbreviated MRI protocols: wave of the future for breast cancer screening. *Am J Roentgenol.* 2017;208(2):284–289.

CHAPTER 19

The Scrotum and Penis

WAYNE C. LEONHARDT AND AARON M. CHANDLER

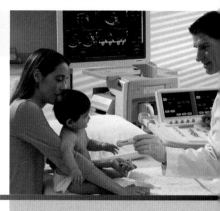

OBJECTIVES

- Illustrate the normal gross and sectional anatomy of the scrotum and penis, including the vascular anatomy.
- Describe the sonographic appearance of the normal scrotal and penile anatomy.
- Explain the technique and protocol for sonographic evaluation of the scrotum and penis.
- State the indications for a sonographic examination of the scrotum and penis.
- Identify the common pathologic conditions that can result in an acute painful scrotum and penis.
- Differentiate common extratesticular abnormalities from intratesticular abnormalities.
- Describe the sonographic characteristics and laboratory values associated with scrotal masses.
- Describe the sonographic characteristics associated with penile abnormalities.

GLOSSARY

AFP alpha-fetoprotein levels are measured during pregnancy to detect certain fetal anomalies; blood levels may also be elevated with hepatocellular carcinoma and certain testicular cancers

beta-hCG human chorionic gonadotropin is produced during pregnancy and is also secreted by some malignant tumors, including certain testicular cancers

corpora cavernosa two cylindrical columns of spongy tissue running parallel dorsally that serve as the main erectile structures in the penis

corpus spongiosum single column of spongy tissue that contains the urethra and expands distally to form the glans penis; this tissue expands slightly during an erection but not to the extent of the cavernosa

cryptorchidism undescended testicle—occurs when one or more of the testis fails to descend into the scrotum before birth

hydrocelectomy surgical procedure to remove a hydrocele

hyperemia an increase in blood flow to the tissue

infarction tissue death that occurs owing to a lack of blood flow

inguinal canal passage in the anterior abdominal wall in both females and males that transmits structures from the pelvis to the perineum

orchiopexy a surgical procedure done to fasten an undescended testicle into the scrotum or to repair an acute testicular torsion

pampiniform plexus a network of veins that drain the epididymis and testis; it is located in the spermatic cord and empties into the right and left testicular veins

KEY TERMS

choriocarcinoma

embryonal cell carcinoma

epidermoid cyst

epididymal cyst

epididymitis

epididymo-orchitis

erectile dysfunction

hematocele

hematoma

hydrocele

Leydig cell tumor

microlithiasis

Peyronie disease

priapism

scrotal hernia

seminoma

Sertoli cell tumor

sperm granulomas

spermatoceles

squamous cell carcinoma

teratoma

testicular torsion

tunica albuginea cyst

undescended testis

varicocele

(continued)

Peyronie disease (penile fibromatosis) characterized by fibrotic thickening of the tunica albuginea, resulting in the formation of fibrous plaques, which can lead to severe curvature of the penis and difficulty in achieving an erection

priapism defined as a painful and prolonged penile erection, with or without stimulation

resistive index a sonographic indicator of an organ to perfusion; it is calculated from the peak systolic velocity and the end diastolic velocity of blood flow

scrotal pearl scrotoliths or scrotal pearls are benign extra testicular macrocalcifications located within the scrotum, between the layers of the tunica vaginalis

spermatogenesis process in which spermatozoa are produced

tunica albuginea dense fibrous sheath that encapsulates and provides structure and support to the testicles and corpora of the penis

Valsalva maneuver consists of forced expiration against a closed glottis after a full inspiration; the Valsalva maneuver increases the intra-abdominal pressure and is helpful in diagnosing a varicocele and scrotal hernia

vasectomy surgical procedure in which the vas deferens is cut, tied, cauterized, or otherwise interrupted; the semen no longer contains sperm, preventing conception

yolk sac a membranous sac attached to an embryo formed by cells adjacent to the embryonic disk

High-frequency grayscale sonography with spectral, color, and power Doppler is the imaging modality of choice and the gold standard for evaluating patients with acute scrotal pain, a scrotal mass, or to assess testicular perfusion when testicular torsion is suspected.[1-3] Compared with other imaging modalities, sonography provides expedient and accurate differentiation of many causes of scrotal pain.[3-5] The diagnosis of scrotal disease is based on many factors, including a thorough clinical history, physical examination, and sonographic findings.[3,6,7] When patients present with scrotal pain or abnormality, clinical evaluation alone is difficult, and the cause of the patient's symptoms frequently remains unanswered. Sonography is used to determine whether a palpable mass is cystic or solid and differentiate between intratesticular and extratesticular abnormalities.[1,3,7] The distinction between an intratesticular lesion and an extratesticular lesion is an important one considering most intratesticular solid masses are considered malignant until proven otherwise.[8,9] Conversely, extratesticular masses tend to be benign regardless of their cystic or solid nature.[1,8,10] High-resolution grayscale sonography has been shown to be nearly 100% accurate in its ability to characterize the intrascrotal anatomy and distinguish intratesticular and extratesticular abnormalities.[3,7,14]

Sonography is also useful in the follow-up examination of infection and trauma. Incidentally, 10% to 15% of testicular tumors are identified after an episode of scrotal trauma.[11,12] Owing to its speed and efficacy, color Doppler sonography is the most useful imaging technique to establish the diagnosis of testicular torsion in addition to differentiating torsion from epididymo-orchitis.[9,13,15] With an accuracy approaching 100%, sonography is considered the primary imaging modality to assess intratesticular arterial perfusion.[13-16] Nuclear medicine and sonography are comparable in the detection of reduced or absent intratesticular flow.[15]

When a patient presents with an undescended testis, the evaluation begins with sonography to explore the inguinal canal. In 80% of cases, the undescended testis is located in the inguinal canal.[14,15] Magnetic resonance imaging (MRI) is recommended to locate intra-abdominal testes when sonography fails to locate an undescended testis within the inguinal canal. MRI is 90% to 95% sensitive for identifying intra-abdominal testes.[15]

SONOGRAPHIC IMAGING TECHNIQUE

Optimal imaging of the scrotum is achieved using a high-frequency, 12 to 18 MHz, transducer with spectral, color, and power Doppler capabilities.[3] In patients with severe scrotal swelling, a high-frequency curved linear-array transducer increases the field of view (FOV) and is useful for evaluating large segments of intrascrotal anatomy[11] (Fig. 19-1). Extended FOV imaging is extremely helpful

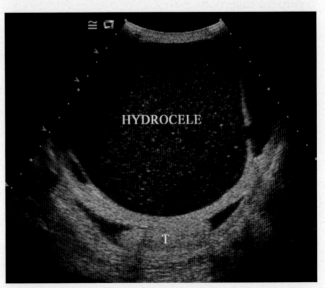

FIGURE 19-1 Convex transducer. Transverse image of enlarged scrotum best seen with a convex probe. Note the large echogenic hydrocele compressing and displacing the testis (T).

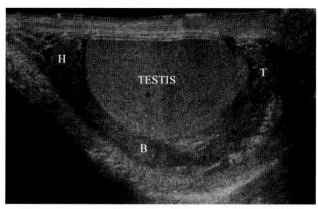

FIGURE 19-2 Extended field of view (*FOV*). Longitudinal extended *FOV* image of the scrotum, including the testis and the epididymal head (*H*), body (*B*), and tail (*T*).

when evaluating large anatomic segments with inflammatory processes and fluid collections because a wider FOV provides a greater understanding of anatomical relationships[10] (Fig. 19-2).

Using high-resolution grayscale imaging with a transducer frequency greater than 10 MHz simplifies correlating a palpable mass with real-time imaging.[11] High-frequency transducers have excellent spatial resolution and can resolve anatomic structures as small as 0.5 mm.[7,10] Imaging techniques such as harmonics, compound imaging, and multifocal zones are essential to optimizing image quality.[6] Adjusting color Doppler parameters by utilizing a low pulse repetition frequency (PRF), with a low wall filter, and a relatively high color gain output can improve the display of the intratesticular arteries.[6,10,17]

Technical Considerations

When evaluating patients for acute scrotal pain (torsion, inflammatory processes) immediately, perform a transverse image of both testes comparing echogenicity and arterial perfusion. Optimize the color and power Doppler settings.[3]

- Obtain power, color, and spectral Doppler tracings to confirm the presence or absence of intratesticular arterial and venous flow.
- Grayscale images are often nonspecific for evaluating testicular torsion and often appear normal when torsion is acute.[16]
- Spectral Doppler findings suggestive of partial torsion include asymmetry in resistive indices with decreased diastolic flow or diastolic flow reversal.[16]
- In the clinical setting of epididymo-orchitis, when focal hypoechoic areas are detected within the testis, ultrasound follow-up is recommended after antibiotic treatment is completed to confirm the diagnosis and observe resolution, so that tumor and or infarction can be ruled out.[7]
- Large hydroceles, hematomas, marked scrotal edema, and epididymo-orchitis are scrotal conditions that decrease intratesticular perfusion, mimicking testicular torsion.
- In patients presenting with acute epididymo-orchitis, spectral Doppler demonstrates decreased vascular resistance (resistive index [RI] < 0.5) compared with the normal contralateral testis and epididymis.[11]
- Reversal of the spectral diastolic component of the intratesticular arterial flow in patients with acute epididymo-orchitis suggests venous infarction.[18]

- Use color and power Doppler to differentiate epididymitis from an enlarged, noninflammatory epididymis status postvasectomy.
- Because primary varicoceles may decompress when the patient is supine, perform the Valsalva maneuver or scan the patient in the upright position to increase venous blood flow.
- Large varicoceles can extend posteriorly, lateral, and inferiorly to the testis, mimicking epididymitis.
- The inguinal canal and abdomen are imaged when hernia, secondary varicocele, undescended testis, and or postsurgical complications are suspected.
- Evaluate the spermatic cord to detect abnormalities such as solid masses, hematomas, abscess, torsion, hernias, and hydroceles.
- Use a gel standoff pad to evaluate anterior and/or superficial lesions, such as those in the tunica vaginalis.

Protocol for Real-Time Sonography

Before scanning the scrotum, review previous studies and obtain a thorough clinical history, including the patient's chief complaint, useful laboratory data, and any pertinent surgical history such as vasectomy, hernia repair, orchiopexy, and hydrocelectomy. Have the patient locate the area of pain, swelling, or palpable mass, and ask if the patient is currently being treated with antibiotics.[6,10] Once the history is obtained and documented on the anatomy worksheet, explain the procedure to the patient. The scrotal exam is performed with the patient in the supine position. The scrotum is supported on a rolled towel placed between the thighs to isolate and immobilize the anatomy for scanning.[6,11,16] The penis is positioned over the suprapubic region and covered with a second towel.[11] Generous amounts of warm gel should be applied to the scrotal skin as a coupling.[7]

Procedure for Real-Time Sonography Overview

Sonographic evaluation of the scrotum begins with a side-by-side, large-FOV image including both testes using grayscale and color Doppler imaging, comparing their echogenicity and arterial perfusion[3,10,14,19] (Fig. 19-3A, B). This is paramount in the setting of acute scrotal pain with suspected testicular torsion. Longitudinal images of each testis (lateral to medial, include cine-clips) are obtained. Oblique scanning planes are useful for demonstrating the intratesticular arteries.[20] In mid testes, document the intratesticular arterial and venous waveforms with color and color with spectral Doppler. Obtain transverse images (superior, mid, inferior, include cine-clips). Document a color Doppler image mid-testis. The relevant extratesticular structures (e.g., spermatic cord, epididymis) and skin thickness are evaluated in both longitudinal and transverse image planes[7,10] (Figs. 19-4 and 19-5). Include the body and tail of the epididymis when scanning the middle and lower portions of the testis, in the longitudinal plane.[7,11,21]

Documented Longitudinal Images

1. Longitudinal midline testis grayscale: Measure the length, and anteroposterior (AP) diameter. Midline testis: assess arterial and venous flow with color and/ or power Doppler and color with spectral Doppler. Obtain an RI measurement of arterial flow.

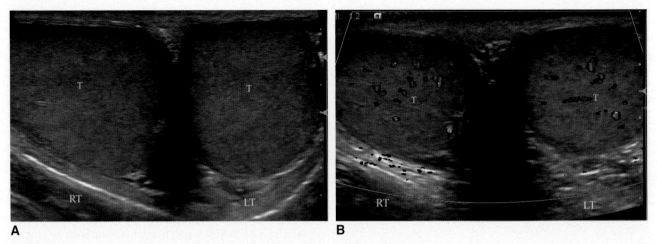

FIGURE 19-3 Comparison. **A:** Transverse image of normal bilateral right (*RT*) and left (*LT*) testes (*T*) demonstrating similar homogeneous echogenicity. **B:** Transverse image of normal bilateral right (*RT*) and left (*LT*) testes (*T*) demonstrating normal flow bilaterally.

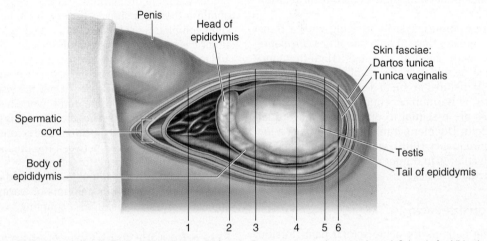

FIGURE 19-4 Schematic illustration of longitudinal scrotal anatomy and relevant adjacent structures. *1*, spermatic cord; *2*, head of epididymis; *3*, testis superior; *4*, testis—mid; *5*, testis—inferior; *6*, tail of epididymis. Note that the body of the epididymis is seen in sections 3, 4, and 5.

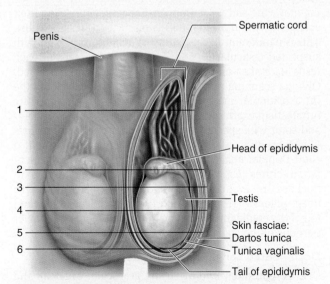

FIGURE 19-5 Schematic illustration of transverse scrotal anatomy and relevant adjacent structures. *1*, spermatic cord; *2*, head of epididymis; *3*, testis—superior; *4*, testis—mid; *5*, testis—inferior; *6*, tail of epididymis. The body of the epididymis is seen in sections 3, 4, and 5.

2. Measure the AP diameter of the scrotal wall. Subsequent images should include the lateral and medial portions of the testis.
3. Longitudinal "cine-clip" of testis lateral to medial.
4. Longitudinal epididymal head grayscale: Measure the AP diameter and length.
5. Longitudinal epididymal head with color and/or power Doppler to assess vascular perfusion.
6. Longitudinal epididymal body: The normal narrow body of the epididymis lies adjacent to the posterolateral margin of the testis. Measure the AP diameter. Perform color and/or power Doppler imaging to assess vascular perfusion.
7. Longitudinal inferior testis and epididymal tail: Measure the superior to inferior diameter of the epididymal tail. Use color and/or power Doppler to assess vascular perfusion.
8. Longitudinal spermatic cord grayscale at rest and with the Valsalva maneuver and with color and/or power Doppler, to assess venous reflux and increased flow: Measure the AP diameter of the largest vein(s) on the grayscale image.

Documented Transverse Images

1. Transverse superior testis with epididymal head in grayscale and color to assess vascularity of epididymis compared with the testis.
2. Transverse mid-testis: Obtain transverse measurement in grayscale, and document with color Doppler. Subsequent images should include inferior testis and inferior testis with epididymal tail. Obtain grayscale and color Doppler to assess the vascularity of the epididymis compared with the testis.
3. Measure the AP diameter of the scrotal wall.
4. Transverse "cine-clip" testis superior to inferior.
5. Transverse spermatic cord grayscale at rest and with the Valsalva maneuver, and with color and/or power Doppler: Measure the AP diameter of the largest vein on the grayscale image.

NORMAL ANATOMY AND SONOGRAPHIC APPEARANCE

A clear understanding of normal scrotal anatomy and vascular perfusion is paramount. Without a clear concept of normal anatomy, pathologic processes may be missed or a normal variant may be mistaken for disease.

Three major structures are contained in the scrotum: the spermatic cord; the epididymis (head, body, and tail); and the testes. The scrotum is a fibromuscular sac composed of several layers of fascia and muscle, which includes the tunica dartos, external spermatic fascia, middle spermatic fascia, cremasteric muscle, internal spermatic fascia, and tunica vaginalis.[2,3,8,14,19] The normal scrotal wall thickness is approximately 2 to 8 mm, depending on the state of contraction of the cremasteric muscle.[2,8,14,21] The normal sonographic appearance of the scrotal wall is homogeneous, and slightly echogenic, compared with the testis[7] (Fig. 19-6). The scrotum is divided into two compartments by a midline septum, the median raphe, a fibrous band of tissue that runs ventral to the undersurface of the penis and dorsal along the middle of the perineum to the anus.[2,8,10,21]

Spermatic Cord and Ductus (Vas) Deferens

The spermatic cords are paired and pass from the abdominal cavity through the inguinal canal down into the scrotum.[19]

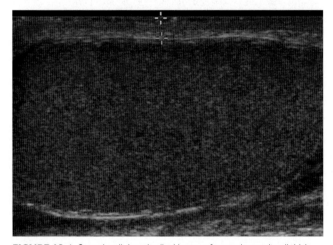

FIGURE 19-6 Scrotal wall. Longitudinal image of normal scrotal wall thickness (*calipers*).

Each spermatic cord lies above and parallel to the inguinal ligament and suspends the testis in the scrotum. The spermatic cord is composed of arteries (the testicular, cremasteric, and deferential), veins of the pampiniform plexus, nerves, lymphatics, vas deferens, and connective tissue.[2,7,8,15,22]

The ductus (vas) deferens are thick paired muscular ducts about 45 cm in length. Each duct runs in the spermatic cord, through the scrotum, inguinal canal, and into the abdomen. It is a major component of the male reproduction system. The ductus (vas) deferens is a continuation of the epididymis, (tail) and transports spermatozoa from the epididymis to the ejaculatory ducts. It is divided into three segments: (1) scrotal, inferior; (2) suprascrotal, mid; and (3) prepubic, superior.[2]

The sonographic appearance of a normal spermatic cord in the longitudinal scan is comprised of numerous hypoechoic, slightly tortuous, linear structures measuring up to 2 mm in diameter[7,15,19] (Fig. 19-7A). In the transverse plane, the sonographic appearance of the normal spermatic cord comprises of numerous hypoechoic ovoid structures with echogenic borders representing vascular walls and connective tissue[2,7,15] (Fig. 19-7B).

Normal veins of the pampiniform plexus measure less than 2 mm in diameter.[15,21] With color Doppler, the normal spermatic cord shows minimal flow within the arteries and veins of the pampiniform plexus at rest (Fig. 19-7C, D). In a normal patient, performing the Valsalva maneuver slightly increases the venous flow[7] (Fig. 19-7E, F).

The sonographic appearance of the normal ductus (vas) deferens is a linear hypoechoic structure superior to the epididymis. The cross section view shows an ovoid structure, representing a "target" or "doughnut." The ductus (vas) deferens is noncompressible and avascular. The normal thickness (AP) of the duct measures between 1.5 and 2.7 mm. The ductus (vas) deferens in the transverse dimension measures less than 0.5 mm^2 (Fig. 19-8 A, B). The scrotal, inferior portion of the ductus (vas) deferens close to the tail of the epididymis demonstrates a convoluted tortuous appearance that is hypoechoic (Fig. 19-8C).

Epididymis

The epididymides store small quantities of sperm prior to ejaculation. Additionally, they act as a conduit for sperm originating in the testis and expressed via the seminal vesicles and secrete a small portion of the seminal fluid.[7,23] The epididymis is divided anatomically into the head, body, and tail.[7] The head of the epididymis, the globus major, is located superolaterally to the testis and measures 10 to 12 mm in AP diameter, and 5 to 12 mm in length.[2,9,19] The body of the epididymis, the corpus, lies adjacent to the posterolateral margin of the testis and measures 2 to 4 mm in AP diameter.[2,14,24,25] The tail of the epididymis, or globus minor, lies on the inferolateral surface of the testis and measures 2 to 5 mm in superior to inferior diameter.[2,4,14,21,24,25] The latter continues on to become the vas deferens[2,7] (Fig. 19-9).

The normal sonographic appearance of the epididymal head is homogeneous and largely isoechoic to or slightly more echogenic than the testis.[2,9,11,16,21,24,25] The epididymal head is best evaluated in the longitudinal scan plane appearing as a triangle-, crescent-, or teardrop-shaped structure superior to the testis[2,7–9,15,21] (Fig. 19-10A). The echogenicity of the normal body and tail is isoechoic to hypoechoic compared

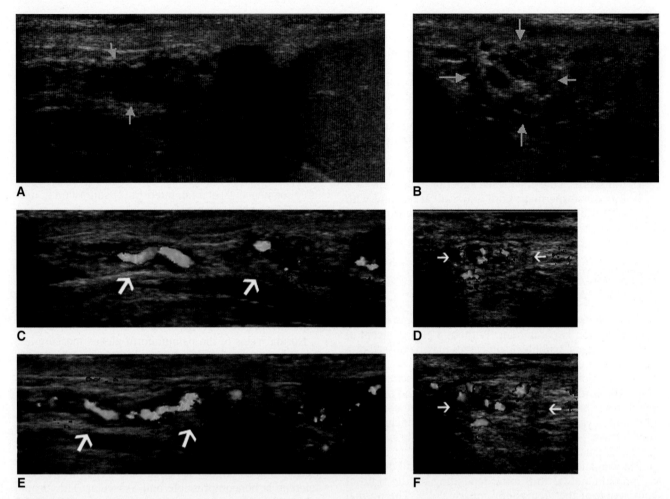

FIGURE 19-7 Spermatic cord. **A:** Longitudinal image of the normal spermatic cord (*arrows*). **B:** Transverse image of the normal spermatic cord (*arrows*) with sonolucent ducts and vessels. **C:** Longitudinal and transverse (**D**) images of the normal spermatic cord (*arrows*) with color flow at rest. Longitudinal (**E**) and transverse (**F**) images of the normal spermatic cord (*arrows*) with slightly increased venous flow during the Valsalva maneuver.

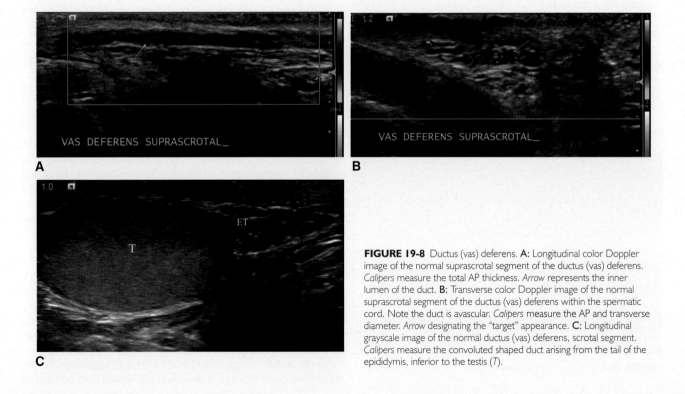

FIGURE 19-8 Ductus (vas) deferens. **A:** Longitudinal color Doppler image of the normal suprascrotal segment of the ductus (vas) deferens. *Calipers* measure the total AP thickness. *Arrow* represents the inner lumen of the duct. **B:** Transverse color Doppler image of the normal suprascrotal segment of the ductus (vas) deferens within the spermatic cord. Note the duct is avascular. *Calipers* measure the AP and transverse diameter. *Arrow* designating the "target" appearance. **C:** Longitudinal grayscale image of the normal ductus (vas) deferens, scrotal segment. *Calipers* measure the convoluted shaped duct arising from the tail of the epididymis, inferior to the testis (*T*).

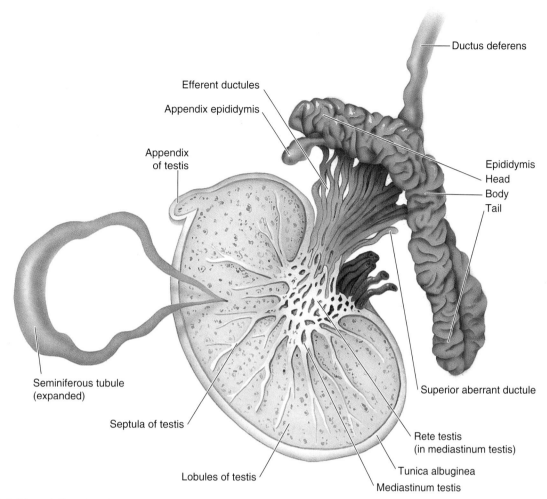

Ductus deferens

Efferent ductules

Appendix epididymis

Appendix
of testis

Epididymis
Head
Body
Tail

Seminiferous tubule
(expanded)

Superior aberrant ductule

Septula of testis

Rete testis
(in mediastinum testis)

Lobules of testis

Tunica albuginea

Mediastinum testis

FIGURE 19-9 Schematic illustration of the sagittal anatomic section of normal scrotum.

with the testis.[2,9,24,25] The narrow body and curved tail are smaller, more variable in position, usually posterior and inferior to the testis, and best evaluated in the longitudinal scan plane[2,4,15,21,24,25] (Fig. 19-10B, C). Color flow imaging of the normal epididymis demonstrates speckled intraepididymal arterial flow[7] (Fig. 19-10D).

Postvasectomy Changes in the Epididymis

When obtaining a patient history, it is important to know whether the patient has had a vasectomy. Patients with an undiscovered history of vasectomy could be misdiagnosed owing to a potential altered sonographic appearance of the epididymis. Epididymal changes occur in 40% of vasectomy patients and include enlargement of the epididymis, inhomogeneity, spermatoceles, dilatation of the rete testis, and sperm granulomas[7,8,24,25] (Fig. 19-11A–G).

Patients presenting with scrotal pain several years after vasectomy may be suspected for "postvasectomy pain syndrome," resulting from the obstruction of the efferent epididymal duct system with concomitant ductal dilatation, interstitial fibrosis, and chronic perineural inflammation.[8]

The sonographic appearance of the postvasectomy epididymis may mimic epididymitis. Clinical history and the use of color Doppler imaging differentiates between the two entities.[7]

Testis

The primary function of the testes is the production of sperm and testosterone. Spermatogenesis takes place within the seminiferous tubules.[2,23] Testosterone, secreted by the cells of Leydig, stimulates the production of sperm and is the primary sex hormone responsible for the development of male reproductive tissues and maintenance of male secondary sex characteristics.[7]

Embryologically, the testes develop between the posterior abdominal wall and the peritoneum. The testes begin to pass through the inguinal ring during the seventh month of gestation and lie in the scrotum by the eighth month. During testicular descent, in the inguinal region, the caudal genital ligament is continuous with a band of mesenchyme that connects the fetal testis to the developing scrotum.[7,26,27] This mesenchyme band is known as the *gubernaculum testis*. The gubernaculum is present only during the development of the urinary and reproductive organs and attaches to the caudal end of the testis.[7] This anchors the fetal testis to the inguinal region to prevent upward movement.[7] In the adult, this gubernaculum testis atrophies and its remnant, the scrotal ligament, extends from the inferior pole of the testis and tail of the epididymis to the skin of the scrotal wall.[7] It secures the testis, tethering it in place and limiting the degree to which the testis can move within the

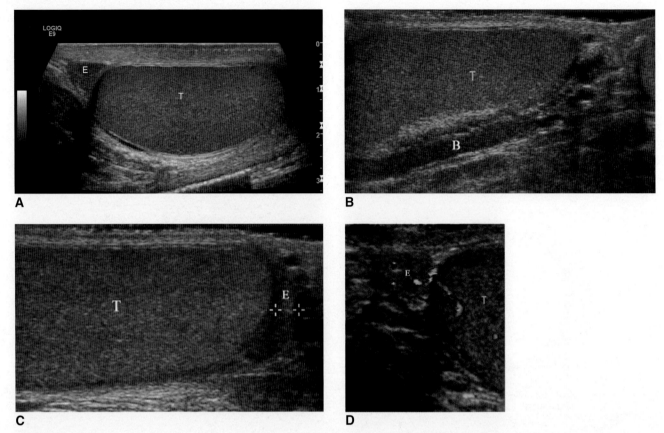

FIGURE 19-10 Epididymis. **A:** Longitudinal image of normal testis (*T*) and epididymal head (*E*). **B:** Longitudinal image of normal testis (*T*) with the body of epididymis (*B*). **C:** Longitudinal image of normal testis (*T*) and tail of epididymis (*E*). **D:** Longitudinal color image of testis (*T*) with normal flow in the epididymis (*E*).

scrotum.[7] The scrotal ligament can be seen in the presence of a hydrocele. The sonographic appearance of the scrotal ligament is an echogenic band extending from the caudal end of the testis to the scrotal wall[7] (Fig. 19-12).

As the testes descend into the scrotum, a peritoneal lining, the processus vaginalis, fuses around the testis to form the tunica vaginalis, whose communication with the peritoneal cavity obliterates after birth.[7,21] The tunica vaginalis is a peritoneal sac, composed of two layers, the visceral and parietal layers, that cover and surround the testis and epididymis except for a small posterior area.[7,15,21] The visceral layer is a serous membrane that produces secretions and covers the testis and epididymis.[6,7,15] The parietal layer is the inner lining of the scrotal wall[6,7,14,15,21] (see Fig. 19-9). The parietal layer contains lymphatics for fluid absorption.[26] Both visceral and parietal layers are separated by a potential space that normally contains a few milliliters of fluid.[6,10,15,21] Bowel (scrotal hernia) and large amounts of serous fluid (hydrocele) or blood (hematocele) can accumulate in the potential space.[7,19] In the normal scrotum, visualizing a small amount of fluid adjacent to the head of the epididymis is common.[7,12,21] This normal amount of fluid should not be misinterpreted as a hydrocele.[14,21]

The tunica albuginea is a fibrous sheath that covers the testis and is seen as a thin echogenic line[12,16,19] (Fig. 19-13). It invaginates the posterior aspect of the testis at the hilum to become the mediastinum testis.[7,9,12,16] Sonographically, the mediastinum testis is seen as an echogenic band running in a cephalocaudal orientation within the testis in the longitudinal plane[5,10,15] (Fig. 19-14A). In the transverse plane, it is

seen as an ovoid echogenic structure in the 3- or 9-o'clock position[13] (Fig. 19-14B). The mediastinum testis functions as a supporting system for arteries, veins, lymphatics, and seminiferous tubules.[9] Numerous fibrous septa extend radially from the mediastinum into the testis, dividing it into 250 to 400 pyramid-shaped compartments called *lobuli testis*.[7,10,14,16] Each lobule contains one to three seminiferous tubules. At the apex of each lobule, the tubules join the tubuli recti, which connect the seminiferous tubules to the rete testis.[10,11,14] The rete testis is a network of epithelial-lined channels embedded within the fibrous stroma of the mediastinum testis. They drain into the epididymis through 10 to 15 efferent ductules[10,14,16] (see Fig. 19-9).

High-frequency sonography can identify the normal rete testis in approximately 18% of patients. Sonographically, the normal rete testis can be seen as a hypoechoic area with striations, located adjacent to or within the mediastinum testis[10,14,15] (Fig. 19-15). Dilatation of the seminiferous tubules is referred to as *tubular ectasia* of the rete testis. This is often seen bilaterally and is associated with epididymal cysts and spermatoceles.[26]

The appendix testis and appendix epididymis are embryologic remnants (Fig. 19-16A). They are not routinely visualized by sonography unless a hydrocele is present. The appendix testis is an ovoid or elongated protuberance about 5 mm in length and is attached to the upper pole of the testis, in the groove between the testis and the epididymis[7,10,11] (Fig. 19-16B, C). The appendix testis has been identified in 92% of testes unilaterally and 69% bilaterally in postmortem studies. The appendix epididymis

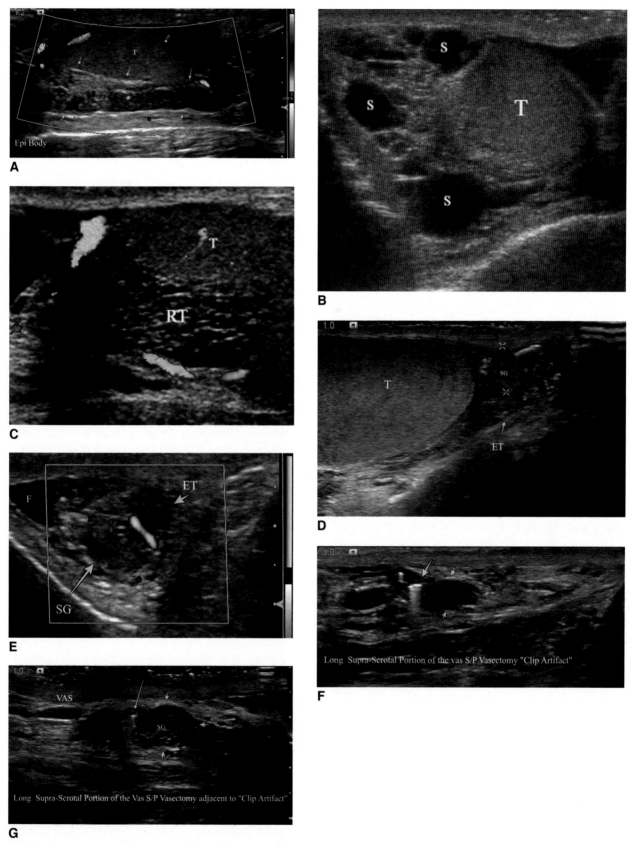

FIGURE 19-11 Postvasectomy changes. **A:** Longitudinal color Doppler image of enlarged avascular heterogeneous epididymal body (*EB*) (*arrows*) in a postvasectomy patient. Normal testis (*T*). **B:** Longitudinal image of scrotum demonstrating multiple large spermatoceles (*S*) of the head and body of epididymis. **C:** Longitudinal image of testis showing cystic changes of dilated rete testis (*RT*). **D:** Longitudinal image of diffusely enlarged hypoechoic epididymis with sperm granulomas (*SG*). Normal testis (*T*). **E:** Transverse power Doppler image of a sperm granuloma (*arrows*) with intravascular flow, within the tail of the epididymis (*ET*) postvasectomy. **F:** Longitudinal image of an enlarged "painful" ductus (vas) deferens (*arrows*) suprascrotal segment, with an echogenic "Clip Artifact" (*large arrow*) postvasectomy. **G:** Longitudinal image of a sperm granuloma (*SG*), adjacent to the "Clip Artifact" (*long arrow*) within the suprascrotal segment of the ductus (vas) deferens postvasectomy.

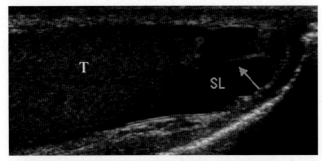

FIGURE 19-12 Scrotal ligaments. Longitudinal image of scrotal ligaments (*SL, arrow*) best seen in the presence of a hydrocele. Normal testis (*T*).

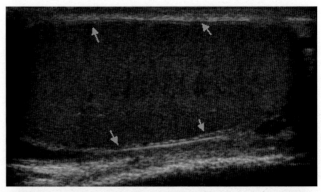

FIGURE 19-13 Tunica albuginea. Longitudinal image of testis demonstrating normal tunica albuginea (*arrows*).

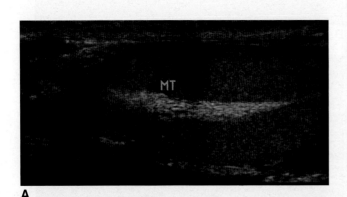

A

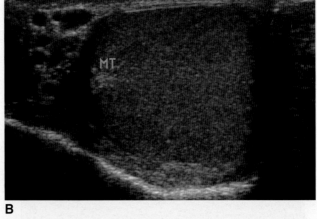

B

FIGURE 19-14 Mediastinum testis. **A:** Longitudinal image of mediastinum testis (*MT*) seen as a bright, echogenic band of fibrofatty tissue across testis. **B:** Transverse image through mediastinum testis (*MT*) seen as a bright, echogenic area in testis at the 9-o'clock position.

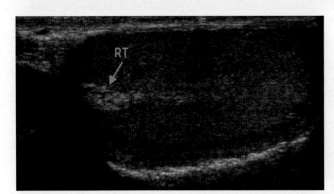

FIGURE 19-15 Rete testis. Longitudinal image of normal testis showing echogenic stroma (*arrow*) with tubules of rete testis (*RT*).

has been identified unilaterally in 34% and bilaterally in 12% in postmortem studies.[10,14] The appendix epididymis is approximately the same size as the appendix testis.[10,11] The shape of the appendix epididymis is more of a stalk-like structure.[10,11] Appendages of the testis and epididymis are visualized sonographically as isoechoic to echogenic protuberances superior to the testis and epididymis.[7,10,11,14] Occasionally, the appendix epididymis may swell or distend, forming a cyst-like structure, not to be confused with an epididymal cyst[10] (Fig. 19-16D).

The testes are bilateral, symmetrical, ovoid glands located within the scrotum. They attain their maximum size around puberty. The normal adult testis measures 3 to 5 cm in length and 2 to 3 cm in the transverse and anteroposterior diameters[2,7,14–16] (Fig. 19-17A, B). The size of both the testis and epididymis decreases with increasing age.[7,9] Sonographically, a normal adult testis appears homogeneous with medium-level echoes similar to the thyroid gland, with a smooth contour.[2,7,9,11,15]

In infants and children, the echogenicity of the testis is hypoechoic compared with that of an adult. At birth, the testes measure 1.5 cm in length and 1.0 cm in transverse diameter. Testicular size increases to 2.0 cm in length and 1.2 cm in transverse diameter by the time the infant is 3 months old.[7,15,26] During puberty, between 9 and 16 years of age, there is a significant increase in testicular echogenicity owing to the growth of seminiferous tubules.[7,26]

Arterial and Venous Anatomy of the Scrotum

Scrotal blood flow is supplied by the bilateral testicular, cremasteric, and deferential arteries.[2,6,7,9] Testicular arteries provide the major blood supply to the testis. They arise from the anterior aspect of the aorta just below the level of the renal arteries and enter the spermatic cord at the internal inguinal ring with the other cord structures.[2,7,9,10,28] In the spermatic cord, the testicular artery is joined by the deferential artery (a branch of the vesicular artery) and

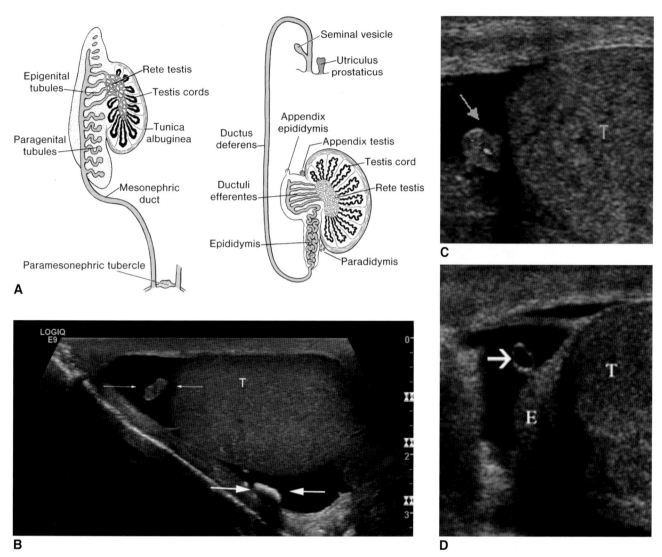

FIGURE 19-16 Appendix testis and appendix epididymis. **A:** Schematic illustration of appendix testis and appendix epididymis. **B:** Longitudinal image of testis (*T*) shows hydrocele and appendix testis (*small arrows*). Scrotal pearl is also seen (*large arrows*). **C:** Longitudinal image of normal testis (*T*) with appendix testis (*arrow*). Normal color flow is seen in the appendix. A small hydrocele is present. **D:** Longitudinal image of testis (*T*) with a cyst-like appendix epididymis (*arrow*) arising from the head of the epididymis (*E*).

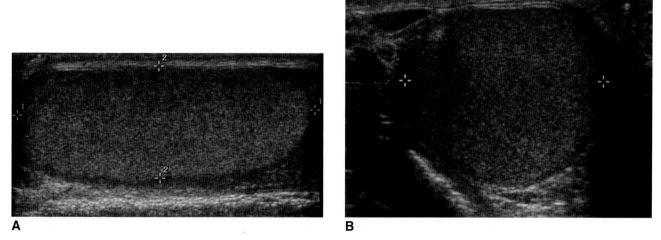

FIGURE 19-17 Testis. **A:** On the longitudinal of the normal testis, the calipers were used to measure length (1) and the width (2). **B:** Transverse image of normal testis.

the cremasteric artery (a branch of the inferior epigastric artery).[2,6,9,28] The deferential artery supplies the epididymis and vas deferens.[2,6,7,9,11,28] Major blood supply to the epididymis, however, is via the superior epididymal artery, a branch of the testicular artery.[6,11] The cremasteric artery supplies the peritesticular tissues (Fig. 19-18A, B). Both the deferential and cremasteric arteries also contribute a variable amount of blood to the testis via anastomoses with the testicular artery.[2,7,9,28]

The venous drainage from the scrotum—inclusive of the mediastinum, epididymis, and scrotal wall—is via the pampiniform plexus, which empties into the testicular veins.

The right testicular vein drains into the inferior vena cava whereas the left testicular vein drains into the left renal vein[2,7,9,28] (Fig. 19-18C).

The anatomy of intratesticular arteries is illustrated in Figure 19-18B. At the posterior superior aspect of the testis, the testicular artery pierces the tunica albuginea to form capsular arteries that run along the periphery of the testis in a layer known as the *tunica vasculosa*. Capsular arteries have centripetal branches that enter the testicular parenchyma and run toward the mediastinum testis. At the mediastinum, centripetal arteries arborize into recurrent rami arteries that course away from the mediastinum testis.

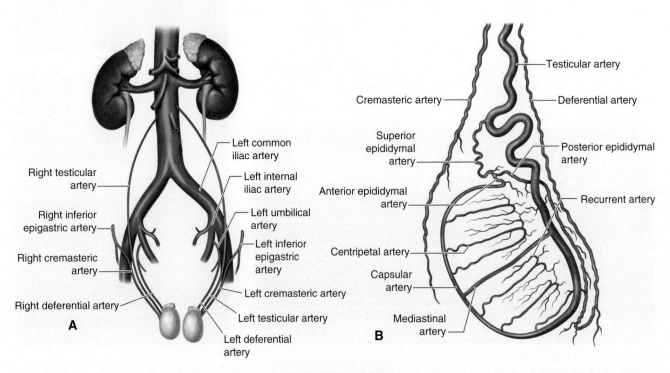

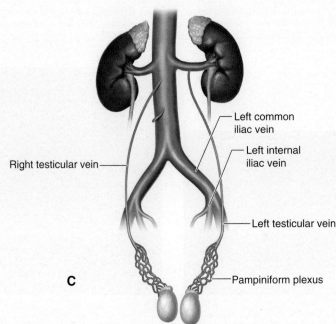

FIGURE 19-18 Vascular anatomy. Schematic illustration of normal arterial supply to the scrotum (**A**), intrascrotal arterial supply (**B**), and venous drainage form the scrotum (**C**).

In approximately 50% of normal testes, a transmediastinal arterial branch of the testicular artery enters the mediastinum and courses through the testicular parenchyma in a direction opposite to that of the centripetal arteries to supply the capsular artery. A transmediastinal vein usually accompanies the artery.[5,7,9–11,28,29] The grayscale sonographic appearance of the transmediastinal artery is a prominent hypoechoic band traversing the testis[5,9] (Fig. 19-19A). With color Doppler, the transmediastinal artery is seen as a prominent arterial branch traversing the mediastinum, demonstrating flow toward the periphery of the testis to supply the capsular arteries[5,7,10,38] (Fig. 19-19B). Flow in the transmediastinal artery courses in the opposite direction relative to the centripetal arteries.[5,6,28]

Spectral and Color Doppler Sonography of the Intrascrotal Arteries

The testis has low vascular resistance similar to that found in the brain and kidney.[7] The spectral waveform of the testicular artery, and its intratesticular branches, characteristically has a low-resistance, high-flow pattern, with a mean RI of 0.62 (range: 0.48 to 0.075)[10,11,17,28] (Fig. 19-20A). The normal spectral waveform of the epididymal artery is similar to that of the testicular artery, which is a low-resistance, high-flow waveform, with an RI ranging from 0.46 to 0.68[8,10,11,15,17] (Fig. 19-20B). Cremasteric and deferential arteries have a high-resistance, low-flow pattern with a mean RI greater than 0.75.[17,28] Supratesticular arteries (testicular, cremasteric, and deferential) within the spermatic cord demonstrate either low- or high-resistance flow patterns, depending on which artery is insonated[7,28] (Fig. 19-20C). With color Doppler, intratesticular arterial blood flow corresponds well with the described anatomic morphology.

Intratesticular arteries are oriented in vascular planes that intersect the mediastinum.

Longitudinal oblique views of the testis best demonstrate capsular and intratesticular arteries[7,28] (Fig. 19-20D).

SONOGRAPHY OF SCROTAL DISEASE

Sonography is used to evaluate the scrotum when patients present with common symptoms such as acute painful scrotum, scrotal mass, and scrotal enlargement. Scrotal pathologies by anatomic region are shown in Table 19-1.

Decrease in Size of the Testis

Decrease in the size of a testis may be a cause of infertility or an indication of a pituitary or hypothalamus gland abnormality, such as hypogonadotropic hypogonadism. Hypogonadotropic hypogonadism results from the absence of gonadal-stimulating pituitary hormones, causing underdeveloped testicles.[7,26] Other causes of testicular atrophy include cryptorchidism, "missed torsion" (ischemic damage owing to compromised blood flow), postsurgical procedures (i.e., inguinal hernioplasty, varicocelectomy), epididymo-orchitis owing to severe inflammation of the spermatic cord, and trauma.[15] The sonographic appearance of testicular atrophy is a small or shrunken heterogeneous testis displaying increased echogenicity owing to fibrosis. A uniform hypoechoic testis may be seen with associated concurrent ischemia.[7,15]

Undescended Testis

The testicles of the fetus lie in the peritoneal cavity near the inguinal canal. Most boys' testes are descended at birth but occasionally they descend later. The unilateral absence of a testis in the scrotum is an important finding because the incidence of malignant degeneration in the undescended testis is 48 to 50 times more likely than in the normally descended testis.[7,9,14] The incidence of seminoma is 2.5 to 8 times higher in patients with undescended testis than in the general population.[10,14,17] The contralateral intrascrotal testis has up to a 20% increased risk of malignancy.[26] An undescended testis is also associated with infertility because sperm are exposed to abnormally high temperatures within the abdomen and/or inguinal canal.[8,21,26] When the undescended testis is relocated and orchiopexy is performed before the age of 2, fertility is preserved.[15] Undescended testes are at increased risk for torsion and commonly associated with malignant degeneration.[26] Torsion becomes more frequent after puberty because the testis is larger than its mesentery. Sixty-four percent of patients with torsion of an intra-abdominal testis are reported to have associated testicular cancer.[26] Congenital inguinal hernia is also associated with undescended testis.[28] Failure to close the processus vaginalis, which forms the scrotal sac, increases the chance of bowel herniating into the scrotum. Approximately, 90% of patients with undescended testes have herniated sacs.[26]

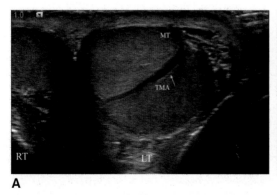
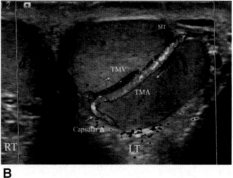

A   **B**

FIGURE 19-19 Intrascrotal arteries. **A:** Transverse image of the testis showing the transmediastinal artery (*TMA, arrow*), entering the mediastinum testis (*MT*), traversing the testis to supply the capsular artery. **B:** Transverse color image of transmediastinal artery (*TMA*) entering the mediastinum testis (*MT*), supplying capsular artery (*CA*); (*arrow*) the transmediastinal vein (*TMV*) accompanies the artery, with color flow seen in the opposite direction (*arrow*).

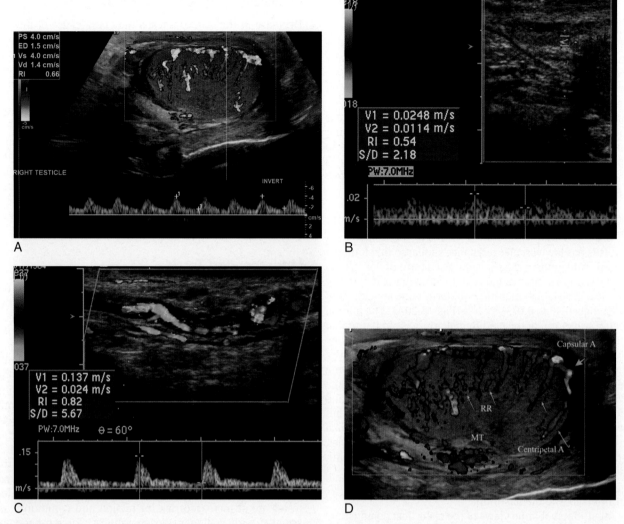

FIGURE 19-20 Spectral and color Doppler images of intrascrotal arteries. **A:** Normal spectral waveform of an intratesticular artery demonstrating low-resistance flow. **B:** Normal spectral waveform of the epididymal artery with low-resistance flow. **C:** Normal spectral waveform of the spermatic cord with high-resistance flow from either the cremasteric or deferential arteries. **D:** Longitudinal oblique images demonstrating normal intratesticular arteries. Color Doppler shows blood flow away from the Mediastinum Testis (MT). The RR are the Recurrent Rami intratesticular arteries which are demonstrated with the arrows. The Mediastinum Testis is a network of fibrous connective tissue that supports the ducts and vessels as they pass into and out of the testicular parenchyma.

TABLE 19-1	**Sonographic Appearance of Common Scrotal Lesion**	
Structure	**Lesion**	**Sonographic Appearance**
Spermatic cord	Varicocele	Dilated serpiginous veins of the pampiniform plexus (superior, lateral, and posterior) measuring >2 mm with the patient supine (Valsalva maneuver) or when the veins measure >2.5 mm with the patient standing. Color Doppler enhances dilatation and reflux.
	Hematoma/hematocele	Thickening of spermatic cord. Variable echogenicity, depending on duration. Initially hyperechoic; with age, the hematoma appears hypoechoic or complex.
	Sperm granuloma	Focal hypoechoic-to-heterogeneous solid mass. Intravascular flow present with acute inflammation.
	Hydrocele	Loculated anechoic fluid collection anterior or posterior to the spermatic cord.
	Abscess	Spermatic cord thickening with areas of increased or decreased echogenicity representing pus and microabscess. Associated spermatic cord hyperemia. Color void centrally with peripheral flow associated with focal abscess.
	Torsion	Enlarged cord with variable echogenicity, hypoechoic to hyperechoic with a "knot" or "whirlpool" mass appearance, representing venous congestion, hemorrhage, and arterial occlusion. Color Doppler reveals no flow or partial flow depending on the duration and degree of torsion.

TABLE 19-1	Sonographic Appearance of Common Scrotal Lesion (*continued*)	
Structure	**Lesion**	**Sonographic Appearance**
	Hernia	Complex mass with echogenic and anechoic areas representing omentum, air- and fluid-filled segments of bowel. Characteristic haustral appearance and peristalsis (classic appearance). Color Doppler shows blood flow within viable bowel.
	Benign neoplasms	
	Lipoma	Solid avascular echogenic mass (typical) to uniformly hypoechoic. Variable echogenicity may likely reflect the number of interstices.
	Adenomatoid tumor	Solid mass, variable echogenicity, equal to or greater than the testis. Minimal flow by color Doppler within and in the periphery of the tumor.
	Hemangioma, cholesteatoma, leiomyoma	Solid mass, variable echogenicity, hyperechoic to hypoechoic. Minimal flow by color Doppler within the tumor (specifically leiomyoma).
	Malignant neoplasms from the mesenchyme Fibrosarcoma, liposarcoma, rhabdomyosarcoma	Solid ill-defined, inhomogeneous echo texture with echogenic areas and focal anechoic areas representing necrosis.
Epididymis	Epididymitis	Enlargement of the epididymis with variable echogenicity depending on the stage of the disease. The testis is normal. A reactive hydrocele/pyocele is often seen with scrotal wall thickening.
	Acute bacterial	Enlarged hypoechoic epididymis owing to edema, with areas of hyperechogenicity, secondary to hemorrhage and infection with hypervascularity.
	Chronic	Epididymis enlarged, focal, or diffuse heterogeneity; tunica is thickened; shadowing from calcifications may be seen.
	Traumatic	Enlarged heterogeneous epididymis, hypervascularity, small hematomas, hematocele.
	Spermatocele	Cystic avascular mass with well-defined walls and few internal echoes secondary to spermatozoa and/or debris in the region of the epididymis, most often located in the head of the epididymis; may be unilocular or multilocular and displaces the epididymal head anteriorly.
	Epididymal cyst	Anechoic avascular mass with well-defined walls occurring anywhere along the epididymis.
	TB	Enlarged heterogeneous and nodular epididymis with scanty vascularity seen within or in the periphery of the nodules.
	Sarcoidosis	Enlarged heterogeneous epididymis with hypoechoic nodules.
	Sperm granuloma	Solid avascular hypoechoic or heterogeneous well-circumscribed mass, located throughout the epididymis.
	Abscess	Hypoechoic mass with irregular walls, low-level internal echoes, and peripheral hyperemia.
	Torsion	Enlarged heterogeneous epididymal body with only few vascular signals and a highly vascular epididymal head. The testis is normal on grayscale and color Doppler images.
	Adenomatoid/leiomyoma tumors	Solid well-circumscribed mass, variable echogenicity, equal to or greater than the testis. Minimal flow by color Doppler imaging within and on the periphery of the tumor.
Tunica vaginalis	Acute hydrocele	Anechoic fluid collection anterolateral to the testis, with strong sound transmission.
	Chronic hydrocele	Low-level fluid collection anterolateral to the testis with mobile echoes—that is, cholesterol crystals, fibrin bodies, inflammatory debris, septations secondary to infection and/or trauma, scrotal calcifications, and diffuse scrotal wall thickening. Power Doppler demonstrates the movement of internal debris.
	Scrotal calcifications/pearls	Highly echogenic spherical focus or foci with associated acoustic shadowing moving freely within the hydrocele.
	Acute hematocele	Complex echogenic fluid collection between the parietal and visceral layers of the tunica vaginalis.
	Chronic hematocele	Complex echogenic fluid collection with thick internal septa, scrotal wall thickening, calcifications, indistinguishable from chronic hydrocele or pyocele.
	Pyocele	Thick hemiscrotal wall; echogenic fluid collection with septations and occasionally focal mural calcifications; similar to chronic hydroceles and hematoceles.

(continued)

TABLE 19-1	**Sonographic Appearance of Common Scrotal Lesion (*continued*)**	
Structure	**Lesion**	**Sonographic Appearance**
	Hematoma	Appearance of hematoma varies with age; acutely, the scrotal wall is thickened; after 2–3 days, hypoechoic areas are seen (liquefaction); extratesticular hematomas can be solid or septated cystic masses.
	Abscess	Complex intrascrotal mass with focal hypoechoic low-level echoes or mixed areas, with irregular and hypervascular borders.
	Tunica albuginea cyst	Defined anechoic area(s) with posterior enhancement. Meets criteria for a simple cyst.
Testicular focal–benign	Hematoma/trauma	Appearance of hematoma varies with age; focal hyperechoic avascular areas are seen in the acute stage and hypoechoic to complex focal areas develop as the hemorrhage ages.
	Abscess	Focal complex mass with low-level areas, irregular and hypervascular borders.
	Focal orchitis	Ill-defined hypoechoic mass with increased blood flow.
	Liquefactive necrosis (seen in subacute torsion)	Focal anechoic areas; avascular
	Focal ischemic infarction (following infection and torsion)	Focal hypoechoic avascular mass.
	Adenomatoid tumor	Solid well-circumscribed mass, variable echogenicity, equal to or greater than the testis. Minimal flow by color Doppler imaging within and on the periphery of the tumor.
	Sarcoidosis	Solid, focal hyperechoic mass.
	Sperm granuloma	Hypoechoic-to-heterogeneous solid mass. Intravascular flow present with acute inflammation.
	Benign gonadal stromal tumors (Leydig, Sertoli)	Focal, variable echogenicity, usually hypoechoic with prominent peripheral flow by color Doppler imaging.
	Epidermoid cysts	Well-circumscribed avascular mass with variable echogenicity (hypoechoic to hyperechoic) with an echogenic or anechoic rim. Alternatively, it can contain alternating hypoechoic and hyperechoic concentric rings demonstrating an "onion appearance."
	Dermoid cyst	May simulate simple cyst or may have echogenic areas along the periphery; occasionally, the cyst itself is echogenic.
	Cystadenoma	Multiseptate cystic mass.
Testicular diffuse–benign	Orchitis	Enlarged, diffusely hypoechoic testis with hypervascularity.
	Infarcts (after trauma, infection, and torsion)	Acutely (within 24 hours), enlarged with normal or decreased echogenicity. After 24 hours, heterogeneous with hypoechoic areas representing necrosis, hemorrhage, and infarction. Absent intratesticular flow by color Doppler imaging.
	Granulomatous disease	Enlarged, irregular, heterogeneous testis; may have calcifications.
	Sarcoidosis	Enlarged heterogeneous testis with hypoechoic nodules.
	Microlithiasis	Multiple small 1–3 mm echogenic foci disseminated throughout the testis without posterior shadowing. The pattern of microliths can vary with cluster calcifications centrally and in the periphery. Bilateral involvement is common.
	Acquired atrophy	Small, hypoechoic testis.
Testicular focal–malignant	Seminoma	Uniformly hypoechoic mass; well defined (without tunica albuginea invasion), may have scattered hyperechoic areas. Color/power Doppler imaging demonstrates hypervascularity in tumors >1.6 cm.
	Embryonal cell	Predominantly hypoechoic mass, poorly marginated, texture is heterogeneous with areas of hemorrhagic necrosis or cystic change. The tumor often invades the tunica albuginea.
	Choriocarcinoma	Heterogeneous mass with extensive hemorrhagic necrosis in the central portion, with a mixed cystic and solid appearance.
	Teratoma	Large complex mass with multiple cystic areas representing bone, cartilage, smooth muscle, and other tissues.
	Yolk sac tumor	Nonspecific and inhomogeneous and may contain echogenic foci secondary to hemorrhage or hypoechoic areas owing to necrosis.

TABLE 19-1	Sonographic Appearance of Common Scrotal Lesion (*continued*)	
Structure	**Lesion**	**Sonographic Appearance**
	Lymphoma	Enlarged testis, hypoechoic lesions of various sizes with increased vascularity.
	Leukemia	Enlarged testis, hypoechoic mass with increased vascularity.
	Metastases	Multiple hypoechoic (less often echogenic) masses; rarely, both are seen together.
Testicular diffuse–malignant	Leukemia	Enlarged, hypoechoic testis with hypervascularity similar to orchitis.
	Lymphoma	Enlarged, hypoechoic testis with hypervascularity similar to leukemia.
	Diffuse embryonal cell	Enlarged, hypoechoic testis with heterogeneous echotexture, irregular margins, and focal echogenic areas owing to hemorrhage or necrosis. Tunica albuginea invasion.
	Diffuse seminoma	Enlarged, hypoechoic testis with heterogeneous echotexture, lobular or multinodular with hypervascularity similar to diffuse orchitis. The tumor is confined within the tunica albuginea.

TB, tuberculosis.

Undescended testes are bilateral in about 10% of cases.[15] Approximately 80% of undescended testes are located within the inguinal canal, and the remaining 20% are intra-abdominal (from the renal hilum to the inguinal canal).[7,17,21,23] The incidence of undescended testis has been reported in 0.28% of adult men and its incidence at birth has been reported to be 30.3% for premature infants and 3.4% for full-term infants.[7,27]

The sonographic appearance of an undescended testis is an oval or elongated well-circumscribed hypoechoic homogeneous soft tissue structure, smaller than the normal descended intrascrotal testis (Fig. 19-21). Identification of the mediastinum testis helps confirm the presence of the undescended testicle.[7,9,10,15,17,21] Because sonography is relatively inexpensive, delivers no ionizing radiation, and does not require sedation, it should be the initial imaging method for undescended testis, with adjunctive computed tomography or MRI when sonography cannot definitively localize the testis.[26]

Acute Painful Scrotum

Acute scrotal pain is a common clinical problem in both children and adults, and it often presents a diagnostic challenge for referring clinicians. Epididymitis and epididymo-orchitis are the most common causes of acute scrotal pain.[1,7,9,11,14,24,28] Differentiating patients with epididymitis from those with suspected torsion is critical. Grayscale sonography combined with color, power, and spectral

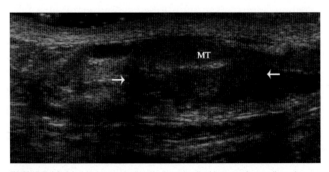

FIGURE 19-21 Undescended testis. Longitudinal image of a small, undescended testis (*arrows*) located in the inguinal canal. *MT*, mediastinum testis.

Doppler increases the diagnostic efficacy in distinguishing inflammatory from ischemic processes.[6,12,18,32] With prompt diagnosis, conditions such as ischemic necrosis and abscess can be surgically corrected to preserve testicular viability and function.[9,20,23,30]

The major causes of acute scrotal pain include epididymitis, epididymo-orchitis, focal orchitis, testicular torsion, abscess, trauma, torsion of the testicular appendices, scrotal wall inflammation, and incarcerated inguinal hernia.[7] With complete testicular torsion, arterial flow is occluded and only surgical restoration of blood flow can prevent loss of the testicle.[19] Abscess is also a surgical emergency because drainage of an abscess can prevent loss of the testicle. Epididymitis is painful, but antibiotic treatment usually resolves the symptoms fairly rapidly.[7] Left untreated, epididymitis may progress to abscess formation, testicular infarction, and necrotizing fasciitis (Fournier gangrene).[7,8,10,31]

Testicular Torsion

Testicular (spermatic cord) torsion represents 20% of scrotal disease in postpubertal males.[7] Torsion occurs most commonly during adolescence, between 12 and 18 years of age, with a peak incidence occurring at 14 years.[7,16,26] Torsion is caused by a developmental weakness of the mesenteric attachment of the spermatic cord to the testis and epididymis. This faulty development allows the testis to fall forward within the scrotum and rotate freely within the tunica vaginalis, much like a clapper inside a bell.[7,9,16,26] The severity of testicular torsion ranges from 180 to 720 degrees or greater.[5,9,11,14,16,32] Twisting of the spermatic cord results in venous congestion. Initially, this prevents venous drainage and progresses to arterial occlusion, scrotal edema, hemorrhage, and infarction.[5,12,13,16] Sonographic detection of a spermatic cord "torsion knot" has been described as a whirlpool pattern, manifested by concentric layers with increased and decreased echogenicity at the external inguinal canal above the testis and epididymis. Visualization of the torsion knot is the most specific and sensitive sign of either complete or incomplete testicular torsion[7,11,16,30] (Fig. 19-22). Pulsed Doppler should always be used in conjunction with

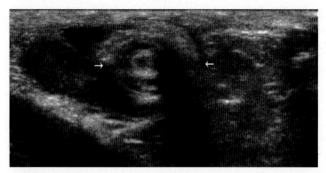

FIGURE 19-22 Testicular torsion. Longitudinal image of spermatic cord demonstrating "the knot" or "whirlpool" pattern (*arrows*) seen in testicular torsion. (Image courtesy of Dr. Vijayaraghavan S. Boopathy.)

color or power Doppler to confirm the presence of arterial and venous flow within the testis because color Doppler can be subject to motion artifacts.[13]

Early diagnosis of testicular torsion is important because it requires orchiopexy, a surgical procedure, to preserve viability and function.[7,9,11,16,26] When surgery is performed within 6 hours after the onset of pain, the salvage rate is between 80% and 100%, as opposed to 70% and 76% when performed within 6 to 12 hours.[5,14,15] After 12 hours, the salvageability drops to 20%.[6,7,14,15,26] Surgery performed after 24 hours almost never results in successful salvage of the testis and is considered a missed torsion.[5,6,11,26]

There are two types of testicular torsion: intravaginal and extravaginal[7,9,12,15,16,30] (Fig. 19-23A, B). In the intravaginal type, the testis rotates freely within the tunica vaginalis by a long stalk of mesorchium. Intravaginal torsion is the most frequent type of testicular torsion and is seen in 80% of cases.[9,11,16] Extravaginal testicular torsion occurs exclusively in newborns.[7,9,11,15,16,26] This type of torsion occurs outside the tunica vaginalis when the testes and gubernacula are not fixed and are able to freely rotate.[11,14,16]

Clinical signs of testicular torsion include a sudden onset of pain, followed by nausea, vomiting, and a low-grade fever.[32] In 50% of cases, the symptoms mimic epididymitis.[26]

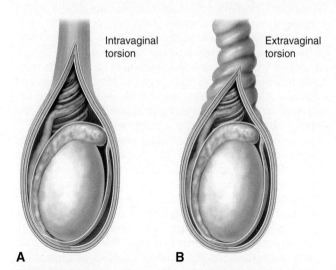

| Intravaginal torsion | Extravaginal torsion |

A   **B**

FIGURE 19-23 Types of testicular torsion. **A:** Schematic illustration of intravaginal testicular torsion. **B:** Schematic illustration of extravaginal testicular torsion.

The cremasteric reflex is usually absent, and pain cannot be relieved by elevating the scrotum.[32] When the spermatic cord twists, the affected testis maintains a higher and horizontal position in the scrotum.[16] After 24 to 48 hours, the pain usually disappears, generally indicating that the testicle is dead. In newborns, testicular torsion may present with only painless swelling and redness.[26]

Torsion can be divided into three phases: (1) acute (within 24 hours), (2) subacute (1 to 10 days), and (3) chronic (more than 10 days).[13,23] Sonographic findings in testicular torsion depend on the duration and degree of spermatic cord rotation.[7,11,15,16]

Grayscale sonographic findings alone of testicular torsion are nonspecific. Differentiation between inflammation and ischemia requires color, power, and spectral Doppler.[9,11,15,13,23,33] Within 1 to 6 hours, the affected testis maybe slightly enlarged, with normal or decreased echogenicity[7,9,11,16,23,26] (Fig. 19-24A). Epididymal enlargement (Fig. 19-24B) is common and is frequently accompanied by the "torsion knot" or "whirlpool" pattern seen in the spermatic cord (see Fig. 19-22), scrotal skin thickening, and a reactive hydrocele (Fig. 19-23C).[9,11,15,16,26] Because grayscale sonography findings are often normal in the early or acute phase of torsion, the absence of intratesticular arterial flow by color and power Doppler is diagnostic for ischemia[4] (Fig. 19-24A).

At 24 hours to 10 days—during the subacute to missed torsion phases—the testis, epididymis, and spermatic cord are enlarged with varying echogenicity.[26] The sonographic findings include a heterogeneous testis and epididymis with diffuse or focal hypoechoic changes representing necrosis, hemorrhage, and infarction[7,11,15,16,23,26] (Fig. 19-24F). Extratesticular hemorrhage within the spermatic cord is caused by congestion and blockage of venous drainage and arterial occlusion.[9,11,14–16]

With color and power Doppler sonography, patients with missed torsion or a non-salvageable testis will have absent intratesticular flow and increased peritesticular flow[7,9,15,16] (Fig. 19-24G, H).

After 10 days, classified as chronic torsion, the sonographic findings are similar to the those for the subacute phase. In time, ischemic testes become small and hypoechoic. In cases of hemorrhage infarction, the testis appears heterogeneous and fibrotic (Fig. 19-24I). The epididymis is enlarged and echogenic, representing hemorrhage and necrosis.[7,15,26]

Torsion–Detorsion and Partial Torsion of the Testis

Acute and intermittent sharp testicular pain and scrotal swelling, interspersed with long asymptomatic intervals, are characteristic of torsion–detorsion.[16] In spontaneous detorsion, there is increased perfusion, manifested by hypervascularity with a low-resistance flow pattern of the testis.[11,15,16]

The testis may be enlarged, and focal infarcts may or may not be present. Cases of partial or transient torsion can present a diagnostic challenge. There are no studies to date that validate the role of spectral Doppler sonography in partial torsion. However, there are few published case reports that suggest its usefulness. Asymmetry of the resistive indices with decreased diastolic flow or diastolic flow reversal may be seen.[11,15,16]

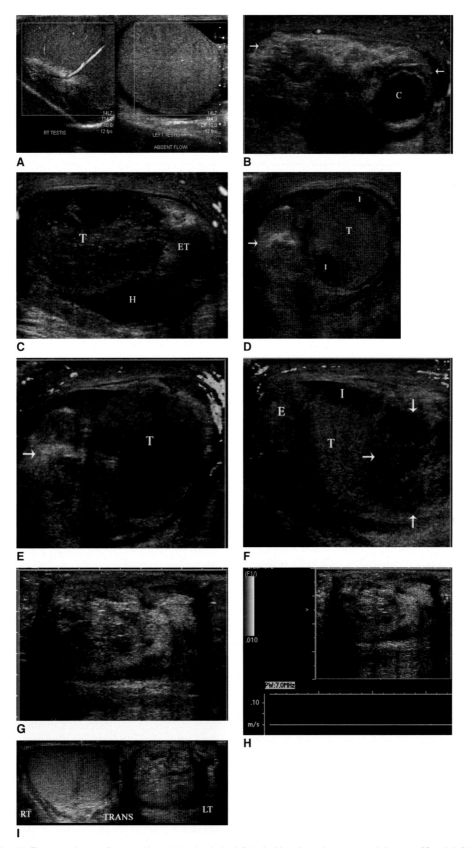

FIGURE 19-24 Torsion. **A:** Transverse image of testes with acute torsion in the left testis. Note the enlargement and absence of flow in left testis, whereas the echogenicity remains normal. **B:** Transverse image of enlarged, echogenic, torsed epididymis with hemorrhage (*arrows*). Note the absence of flow and cyst (*C*) in the epididymis. **C:** Longitudinal power Doppler image of heterogeneous, infarcted testis (*T*), with absent flow, enlarged epididymal tail (*ET*), and reactive hydrocele (*H*). **D:** Transverse image of testis (*T*) with hypoechoic focal infarcts (*I*) and epididymal hemorrhage (*arrow*) in missed torsion. **E:** Transverse color image of heterogeneous testis (*T*) with diffuse hypoechoic changes and hemorrhage in the epididymis (*arrow*). Absent flow in both the testis and epididymis is consistent with missed torsion. **F:** Longitudinal color Doppler image of testis (*T*) with diffuse hypoechoic changes (*arrows*) representing hemorrhage and infarct (*I*). Absent flow is consistent with missed torsion. Epididymal head (*E*). **G:** Longitudinal power Doppler image of a nonsalvageable testis. Note the absent intratesticular flow and increased peritesticular flow consistent with missed torsion. **H:** Longitudinal spectral Doppler image of a nonsalvageable testis with missed torsion. Note the absence of intratesticular flow. **I:** Transverse image of both testes demonstrating a missed torsion with fibrotic changes in the left testis and a normal right testis.

Torsion of the Appendages

Torsion of the appendix testis and appendix epididymis can cause acute scrotal pain mimicking testicular torsion.[2] More than 90% of torsed appendages involve the appendix testis.[11,14,16] Torsion of the appendix testis accounts for 20% to 40% of cases of acute scrotum in pubescent and adolescent males.[16] The peak incidence is between the ages of 7 and 14 years.[11,15,16] With appendiceal torsion, the testis appears normal in color duplex sonography.[5,11] The sonographic appearance of a torsed appendage varies; it may appear as a large circular hyperechoic mass with a central hypoechoic area or an enlarged circular heterogeneous mass adjacent to a normal testis and epididymis.[11,15,16] Color Doppler of appendiceal torsion shows increased periappendiceal blood flow and absent central appendiceal flow.[11] A testicular appendage larger than 5.6 mm with increased periappendiceal color flow is suggestive of torsion.[7,11,16] An associated reactive hydrocele and skin thickening are common in these cases.[2,16] Torsed appendages may ultimately atrophy and calcify.[5]

Testicular Rupture

Testicular rupture is rare.[7] It occurs when the capsule, the tunica albuginea, is torn by trauma.[12,19] Testicular rupture is associated with athletic injuries and industrial and motor vehicle accidents.[11,12,19] Early diagnosis is critical because the surgical testicular salvage rate diminishes from approximately 90% to 45% after 72 hours of onset.[7,15,19] Surgical treatment requires repair of the tunica albuginea or orchiectomy.[7,11] Failure to repair the testis may result in the loss of spermatogenesis and hormonal function, chronic scrotal pain, and secondary anaerobic infection (scrotal gangrene).[7]

Sonographic findings in testicular rupture include a contour abnormality owing to an irregular fibrous tunica albuginea, extrusion of the testicular contents into the scrotal sac, hematocele between the tunica vaginalis and parietalis, intratesticular hematoma, and infarction. The latter appears as hypoechoic or hyperechoic focal abnormalities within the testis.[11,12,15,19] The sonographic appearance of intratesticular hematomas varies with size and duration. Acute hematomas present as avascular echogenic or hypoechoic areas.[7,11,12,19] With time, liquefaction or lysis of the hematoma results in a septated fluid collection containing fine echoes.[7,34]

Disruption of the testicular echogenicity, with focal hyperechoic and hypoechoic areas in the testicle, along with an ill-defined tunica albuginea, must be considered suggestive of testicular rupture. Rupture of the tunica albuginea usually results in hemorrhage, which may occlude or decrease intratesticular arterial flow.[34] Color Doppler imaging is helpful in assessing intratesticular flow and can be used to determine surgical management.[26]

Epididymitis and Epididymo-Orchitis

Epididymitis (inflammation of the epididymis) represents 75% to 80% of all acute inflammatory processes in the scrotum.[7,9,11] Men between the ages of 20 and 30 years are most often affected.[6] In adolescents and young men, epididymitis often is secondary to sexually transmitted organisms such as *Chlamydia trachomatis* and *Neisseria gonorrhoeae*. In prepubertal boys and men over 35 years of age, the disease is most frequently caused by *Escherichia coli* and *Proteus mirabilis*.[11,19,24] The infection occurs from direct retrograde extension of pathogens, via the vas deferens, from a lower urinary tract source, such as urethritis, prostatitis, cystitis, and possibly following instrumentation such as catheterization.[8,9,11,15,24] In patients with suppressed immune systems—such as those with HIV or those receiving immunosuppression treatment for transplantation or undergoing chemotherapy—there has been a general increase in opportunistic infections of the epididymis.[24] COVID-19 causes massive endothelial inflammation throughout the body, boosting "Inflammatory Cytokines". It infiltrates multiple organ systems, including the kidney, bladder, and testicular cells. Recent studies have reported cases of acute inflammation of the testis and epididymis. Epididymitis and epididymo-orchitis were common findings in 22.5% of hospitalized patients with severe COVID-19. The sonographic appearance was similar to the classic findings of epididymo-orchitis, including enlargement, hypoechoic heterogeneous echo texture, hypervascularity, and reactive hydrocele. Thickening of the tunica albuginea and abscesses within the tail of the epididymis were also reported.[32] Less frequently, traumatic epididymitis may occur after scrotal trauma or iatrogenic injury to the epididymis during scrotal surgery.[5,12,24] The sonographic findings are similar to those for infectious epididymitis, including enlargement and hyperemia. Following trauma, the epididymis may also reveal the presence of small hematomas, resulting in enlargement and inflammatory response[12] (Fig. 19-25A, B). Differentiation between the two entities should be based on the history of trauma because the management of traumatic epididymitis does not require antibiotics.[24]

Epididymitis can affect the head, body, or tail of the epididymis; however, the entire epididymis is affected in 50% of cases.[7,35] Inflammation usually begins in the tail.[5,7,9,11,15,24] Early in the course of the disease, physical examination may demonstrate an inflamed, tense, and swollen epididymis, which may present as an enlarged tender cord separate from the testis.[24] Epididymitis is usually unilateral, but sometimes it can be bilateral.[13] If epididymitis is left untreated, it can progress to involve the spermatic cord and testis, resulting in a spermatic cord abscess or epididymo-orchitis (inflammation of both the epididymis and testicle).[7] Coexistent orchitis develops in 20% to 40% of patients owing to direct spread of infection.[5,7,9,11,15,24] Other complications include pyocele, testicular abscess, infarction, infertility, atrophy, and soft tissue necrosis (Fournier gangrene).[5,9,11,15]

Epididymo-orchitis represents approximately 25% of acute inflammatory processes of the scrotum. Untreated, acute epididymo-orchitis can progress to abscess, gangrene, infarct, pyocele infertility, and atrophy.[11,14,15] Clinical indications include fever, tenderness, and enlargement of the epididymis, testis, and hemiscrotum.[7,24]

Grayscale sonographic findings of acute epididymitis, epididymo-orchitis, and orchitis include enlargement and variable echogenicity of the affected structure. The epididymis and/or testis are usually hypoechoic owing to edema, with areas of hyperechogenicity, secondary to hemorrhage and infection[24] (Fig. 19-26A–C). Scrotal wall thickening and reactive hydrocele are common associated findings.[14,24] The hallmark of scrotal inflammatory disease is color Doppler hypervascularity of the affected structures.[28,35] The sensitivity

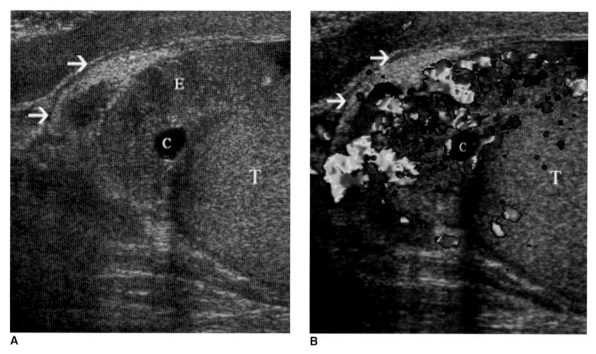

FIGURE 19-25 Traumatic epididymitis. **A:** Longitudinal image of epididymis (*E*) with hematoma (*arrows*) and cyst (*C*) in a patient with traumatic epididymitis. Normal testis (*T*). **B:** Longitudinal color Doppler image in the same patient demonstrating hypervascularity in the epididymis. *C*, cyst; *T*, testis.

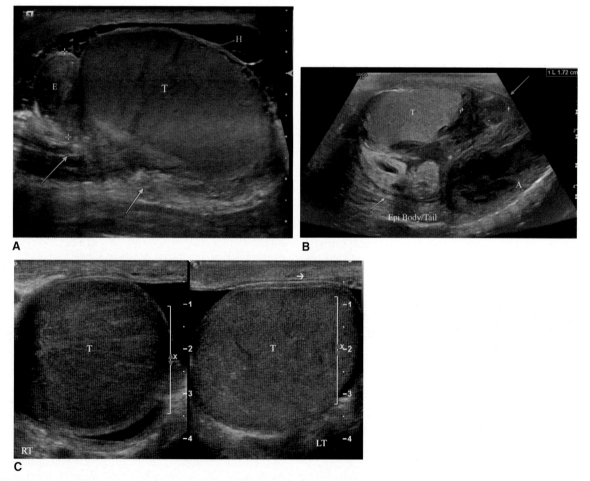

FIGURE 19-26 Acute epididymitis and epididymo-orchitis. **A:** Longitudinal image of testis (*T*) with enlarged heterogeneous epididymis (*E*) (*arrows*) in acute epididymo-orchitis. Note secondary reactive hydrocele (*H*) with septations. **B:** Longitudinal image of enlarged heterogeneous body and tail of the epididymis (*arrows* and *calipers*) in a patient with severe acute epididymo-orchitis, and concomitant scrotal abscess (*A*) inferior to the testis (*T*). **C:** Transverse image of bilateral testes (*T*) shows hypoechoic right testis with orchitis.

of color Doppler sonography for the evaluation of scrotal inflammatory disease is close to 100%.[14] In 20% of patients with epididymitis and 40% of patients with orchitis, grayscale findings are normal, and hyperemia may be the only finding.[24] Focal epididymitis occurs in approximately 25% of cases and isolated focal orchitis occurs in 10% of cases.[7,11]

In patients with epididymitis, epididymo-orchitis, and isolated orchitis, color Doppler will show increased hypervascularity within the affected areas[11,24,35] (Fig. 19-27A–G). With focal epididymitis and orchitis, there may be focal hypoechoic and hypervascular areas involving the epididymis and testis[7,11] (Fig. 19-28A, B). Conversely, isolated epididymitis usually demonstrates a sonographically normal testicle.[11] Inflammation of the spermatic cord represents secondary changes associated with epididymitis.[7,15] The grayscale sonographic image of an infected spermatic cord appears as an enlargement with areas of increased and decreased echogenicity representing edema and infection[7,24] (Fig. 19-29A). Color Doppler imaging of an infected spermatic cord will show hyperemia of both the pampiniform plexus and the supratesticular arteries[7] (Fig. 19-29B). When inflammation is severe, focal or diffuse testicular infarction may be seen.[7,11,14] Focal testicular infarcts appear sonographically as focal avascular masses[7,11,15] (Fig. 19-30). Diffuse testicular infarction shows variable echogenicity depending on the time of the ischemic event.[13,16] Color Doppler imaging of infarction will show absent flow in the affected parenchyma. With chronicity, the testis may appear small and hypoechoic.[7,15,26] Isolated orchitis is a rare phenomenon and is caused mostly by mumps or AIDS. Sonographically, the testis is enlarged and shows diffuse, focal, or multiple hypoechoic lesions.[11] Color Doppler reveals increased blood flow. Focal orchitis may be difficult to distinguish from testicular tumor.[6]

Severe untreated epididymo-orchitis resulting in scrotal, testicular, and/or epididymal abscess appears as a focal hypoechoic or mixed area, with irregular walls, hypervascular margins, and marked scrotal wall thickening with a reactive hydrocele[6,7,11] (Fig. 19-31A, B). If the abscess involves the entire scrotum, the epididymis and testis may be replaced by a complex mass and be indistinguishable.[11]

Chronic epididymitis has been classified based on its different etiologies: inflammatory, infectious, and obstructive.[8,24] Patients may also present with a history of recurrent urinary tract infections.[8] Chronic epididymitis is characterized by persistent pain lasting for at least 3 months in the scrotum, testicle, or epididymis. On clinical examination, the epididymis is moderately tender and can be differentiated from the testis.[24] In chronic epididymitis and epididymo-orchitis, the epididymis and testis are enlarged with a heterogeneous echo texture secondary to infection and hemorrhage. Calcifications and epididymal fibrosis are associated findings. The tunica albuginea also becomes thickened[8,24] (Fig. 19-32A, B). Sperm granulomas and calcifications are associated findings in patients with a history of granulomatous disease or obstruction postvasectomy.[7,8]

Scrotal and Testicular Masses

A scrotal or testicular mass can be an ominous sign. Both benign and malignant disease processes can have similar clinical findings such as pain, swelling, or presence of a palpable mass.[7,10,11] Testicular cancer accounts for approximately

1% of all cancers in men, and most often, it presents as a painless lump or swelling of the testis.[10] Testicular cancer can present with pain because of associated hemorrhage or infection.[9–11] Benign intratesticular masses that can mimic malignancy include hematomas, focal orchitis, infarction, and granuloma.[11,14] Intratesticular solid masses must be considered malignant until proven otherwise.[23] Extratesticular masses are mostly benign, with the prevalence of malignancy being approximately 3%.[8] With an accuracy approaching 100% in differentiating intratesticular from extratesticular masses, sonography is especially effective in the evaluation of scrotal masses.

Benign Scrotal Masses

Benign scrotal masses include hydrocele, spermatocele, epididymal cysts, tubular ectasia, varicocele, scrotal hernia, scrotal abscess, hematoma, hematocele, pyocele, granulomatous disease, tunica albuginea cyst, simple testicular cyst, sperm granuloma, and epidermoid cyst.

Hydrocele

A hydrocele is an abnormal accumulation of serous fluid in the potential space between the visceral and parietal layers of the tunica vaginalis, which surround the testis.[7,9,15,21] Hydroceles are the most common cause of painless scrotal swelling and may be congenital or acquired.[7,9,15] Congenital hydroceles are communicating hydroceles that occur owing to failure of the process vaginalis to close, allowing serous fluid to communicate between the abdominal cavity and the scrotum.[8] Congenital hydroceles are present in 6% of male infants at delivery, but they are present in less than 1% of adults—because most hydroceles resolve within 18 months of age.[7,8]

Acquired or reactive hydroceles are noncommunicating hydroceles that result from impaired fluid reabsorption.[7,8,15] Acquired hydroceles are often associated with infection (epididymitis and epididymo-orchitis) and torsion and are seen with 10% of malignant testicular neoplasms.[7,9,11,15,16] Up to 50% of acquired hydroceles may be secondary to trauma.[7,9,15] Rarely, large hydroceles may impede testicular venous drainage, increasing vascular resistance within the intratesticular arteries and resulting in a decrease or absence of intratesticular arterial diastolic flow[17,21] (Fig. 19-33A).

The clinical sign of hydrocele is a scrotal mass, which may or may not be painful. The classic sonographic appearance of an acute hydrocele is an anechoic fluid collection with enhanced sound transmission, surrounding the anterolateral aspects of the testis[7,9,15,21] (Fig. 19-33B). In patients with acute hydroceles, the testis is usually displaced posteromedially.[15] Chronic hydroceles may contain calcifications that produce acoustic shadowing. These calcifications, known as *scrotal pearls* or *scrotoliths*, may result from inflammatory deposits on the tunica vaginalis that have separated from the lining and/or from calcified missed appendiceal torsion[7,8,15] (Fig. 19-33C). Scrotal calcifications may be singular or multiple, filling the potential space between the layers of the tunica vaginalis testis.[7,8,15] In chronic inflammatory hydroceles, the sonographic findings may include diffuse scrotal wall thickening and echogenic septations resulting from old hemorrhage or infection[7,15,26] (Fig. 19-33D). Fine snowflake-like echoes are occasionally seen moving within

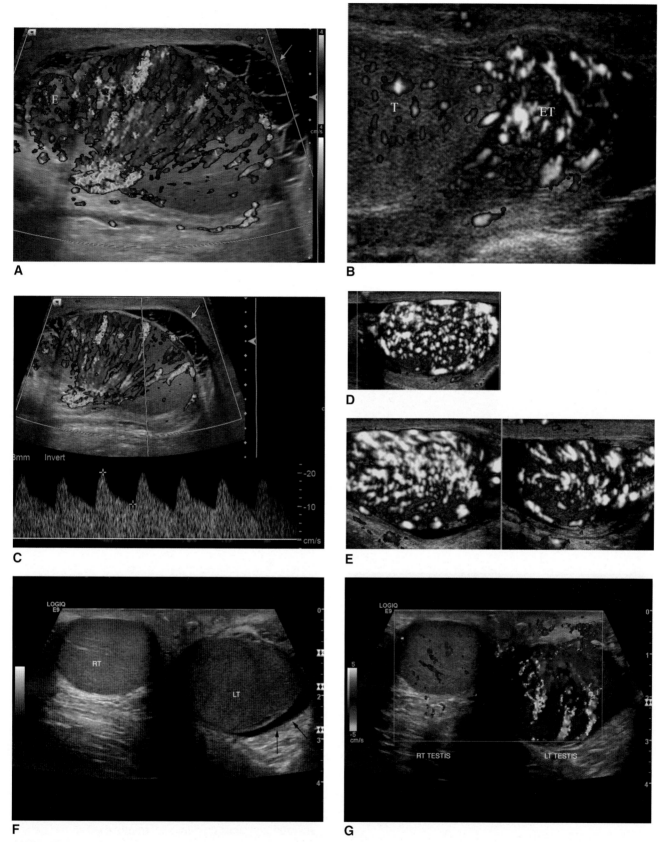

FIGURE 19-27 Color Doppler imaging. **A:** Epididymo-orchitis. Longitudinal color Doppler image of testis (*T*) and epididymal head (*E*) with diffuse hypervascularity in both testes and epididymis with septated reactive hydrocele (*arrow*). **B:** Epididymitis. Longitudinal power Doppler image of testis (*T*) showing increased vascularity in epididymal tail (*ET*). **C:** Epididymo-orchitis. Longitudinal color with spectral Doppler image of testis (*T*) showing hypervascularity with increased diastolic flow and reactive hydrocele with septations (*arrow*). **D:** Orchitis. Longitudinal power Doppler image of testis with hyperemia. **E:** Orchitis. Transverse power Doppler image of bilateral testes with orchitis shows diffuse hyperemia. **F:** Orchitis. Transverse image of both testes demonstrates a normal right testis (*RT*) and an enlarged, hypoechoic left testis (*LT*). Note small reactive hydrocele (*arrows*). **G:** Orchitis. Color Doppler image of the same patient demonstrates hypervascularity in the left testis (*LT*) consistent with orchitis.

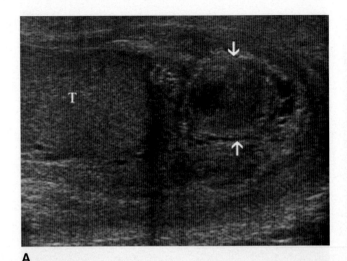

A

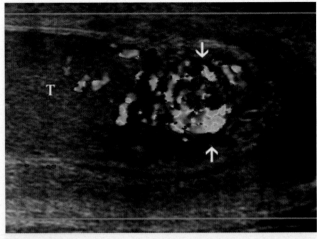

B

FIGURE 19-28 Focal epididymitis. **A:** Longitudinal image of testis (*T*) shows focal hypoechoic mass (*arrows*) in epididymal tail. **B:** Longitudinal color image of the same patient shows hypervascularity in focal hypoechoic mass (*arrows*) located in epididymal tail.

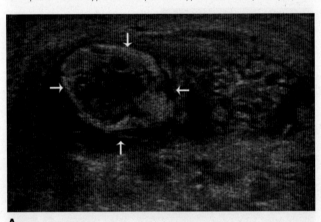

A

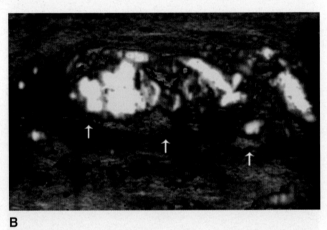

B

FIGURE 19-29 Inflammation of spermatic cord. **A:** Transverse image of enlarged spermatic cord (*arrows*) with increased echogenicity secondary to infection and hemorrhage. **B:** On the same patient, the transverse power Doppler image shows enlargement of the spermatic cord and increased flow which is referred to as "Hyperemia" and is demonstrated by the arrows.

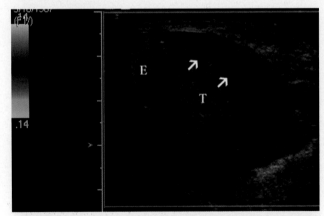

FIGURE 19-30 Intratesticular infarct. Transverse color Doppler image of testis (*T*) with focal, avascular, hypoechoic, intratesticular infarct (*arrows*). Epididymis (*E*).

the hydrocele, representing fibrin bodies or cholesterol crystals[7,9,21] (Fig. 19-33E). In addition, a large chronic hydrocele can compress the testis, causing a contour deformity and atrophy[7,26] (Fig. 19-33F).

Spermatoceles and Epididymal Cysts

Spermatoceles and epididymal cysts are the most common epididymal lesions. They have been reported in 20% to 40% of asymptomatic patients.[7,19,23] Usually presenting as painless scrotal masses, these lesions vary in size from 0.2 to 9 cm.[7,25,32] Both spermatoceles and epididymal cysts are thought to occur as a result of dilatation of the epididymal tubules, whether secondary to vasectomy, scrotal surgery, trauma, or epididymitis.[8,23,26] The most common location for spermatoceles is in the head of the epididymis, whereas epididymal cysts arise throughout the epididymis[23,26,32,34] (Fig. 19-34A). Spermatoceles usually displace the testis anteriorly, distinguishing them from a hydrocele (Fig. 19-34B), the latter of which surrounds the testis.[7,15] They are usually unilocular but can be multilocular also[9,24] (Fig. 19-34A–C).

Epididymal cysts are frequently multiple and may contain loculations similar to spermatoceles.[7,8,26] Spermatoceles generally contain nonviable spermatozoa, cellular debris, and lymphocytes, whereas epididymal cysts are lined with epithelium and contain only serous fluid.[24,32]

Sonographically, a spermatocele is a thin-walled hypoechoic mass located in the epididymal head[24] (Fig. 19-33D). Spermatoceles characteristically contain low-level echoes, owing

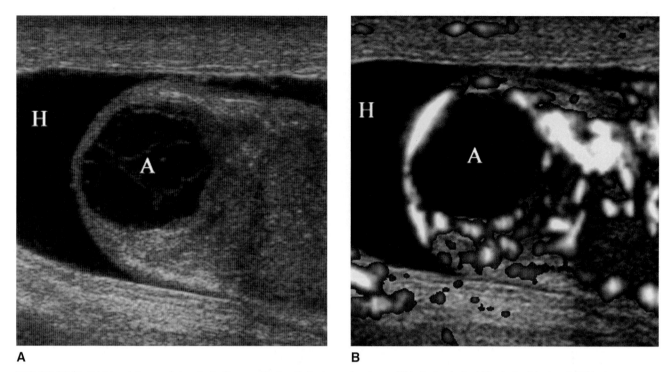

A   **B**

FIGURE 19-31 Epididymal abscess. **A:** Longitudinal image of testis with focal complex abscess (*A*) in the head of epididymis. Small hydrocele (*H*) is also present. **B:** Longitudinal power Doppler image of testis with focal complex abscess (*A*) in the head of epididymis. Small hydrocele (*H*) is also present.

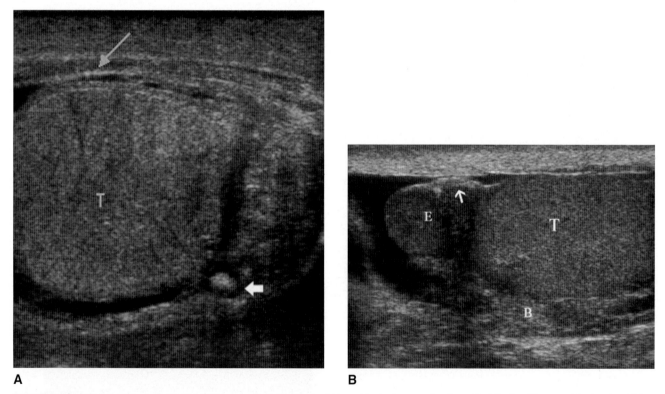

A   **B**

FIGURE 19-32 Chronic changes. **A:** Longitudinal image of testis (*T*) showing thickened tunica (*long arrow*) and scrotal calcification (*short arrow*) in chronic epididymitis. **B:** Longitudinal image of testis (*T*); epididymal head (*E*); and an enlarged, heterogeneous epididymal body (*B*) characteristic of chronic epididymitis. Thickened tunica albuginea (*arrow*) and hydrocele are also present.

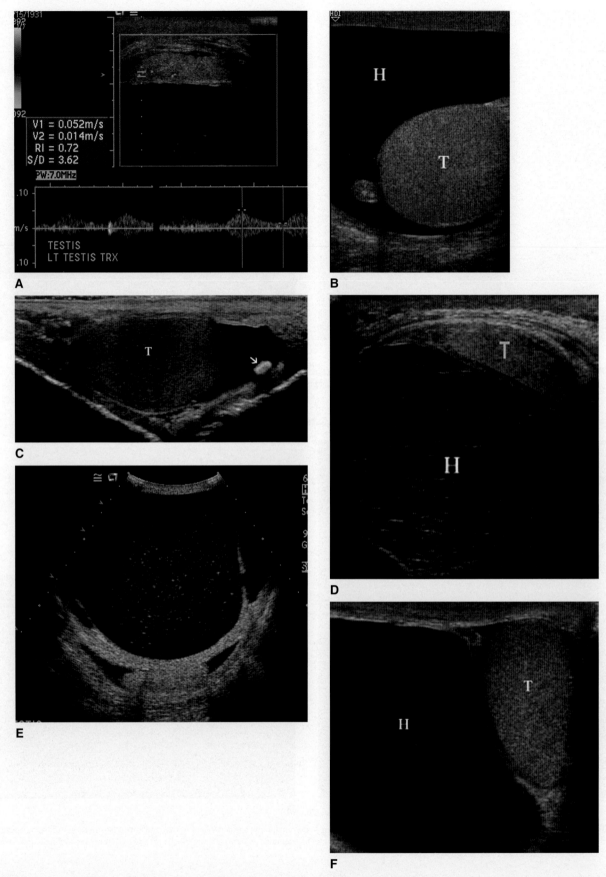

FIGURE 19-33 Hydrocele. **A:** Longitudinal duplex image of scrotum shows large hydrocele compressing testis (*T*) causing increased flow resistance. **B:** Longitudinal image of testis (*T*) with large hydrocele (*H*) surrounding the anterolateral aspect of testis. **C:** Longitudinal image of testis (*T*) with small hydrocele and scrotal pearl (*arrow*). **D:** Longitudinal image of scrotum demonstrating large, septated, chronic inflammatory hydrocele (*H*) displacing the testis (*T*). **E:** Transverse image of scrotum shows echogenic cholesterol crystals floating within a large hydrocele. **F:** Transverse image of scrotum shows large hydrocele (*H*) compressing and deforming the testis (*T*).

to the proteinaceous fluid and spermatozoa, and demonstrate posterior acoustic enhancement.[24] The sonographic appearance of an epididymal cyst is typically a well-defined, thin-walled, anechoic mass with good posterior acoustic enhancement and no internal echoes[24,25] (Fig. 19-34E, F).

Differentiating spermatoceles from epididymal cysts may be difficult if located in the head of the epididymis.[24] Color and power Doppler are useful in improving the diagnostic accuracy of a spermatocele by recognition of the "falling snow" sign[7] (Fig. 19-34G). This sign is defined as the movement of internal echoes representing solid particles, within a superficial cystic mass away from the transducer with the application of power or color Doppler imaging. This phenomenon of acoustic streaming or movement of internal echoes helps differentiate echogenic cysts from solid masses.[7,25,35]

Tubular Ectasia of the Rete Testis

Dilatation of the efferent ductules is referred to as tubular ectasia of the rete testis. Tubular ectasia is commonly

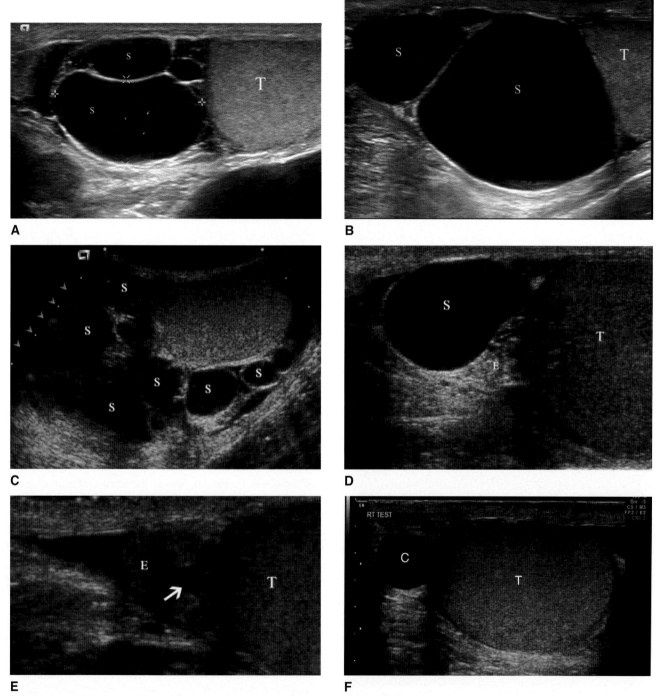

FIGURE 19-34 Spermatocele and epididymal cyst. **A:** Longitudinal image of testis (*T*) with multiple spermatoceles (*S*) in the epididymal head. Note cellular debris within the fluid (*tiny arrows*). **B:** Longitudinal image of testis (*T*) shows large spermatoceles (*S*) displacing the testis anteriorly. **C:** Longitudinal image of the testis with multiple spermatoceles (*S*) in the head and body of the epididymis. **D:** Longitudinal image of testis (*T*) shows large thin-walled spermatoceles (*S*) in the head of the epididymis (*E*). **E:** Longitudinal image of testis (*T*) shows small cyst (*arrow*) in the epididymal head (*E*). **F:** Longitudinal image of testis (*T*) shows cyst (*C*) in the epididymal head.

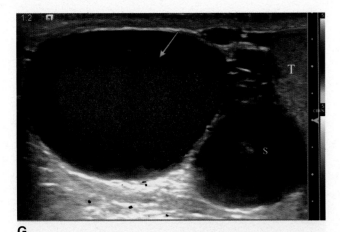

G

FIGURE 19-34 *(continued)* **G:** Longitudinal color Doppler image of large spermatoceles within the head of the epididymis (*S* and *arrow*) superior to the testis (*T*). Note color Doppler "falling snow" sign within the largest spermatocele.

seen in men older than 50 years.[24,25] It is often bilateral and associated with epididymal cysts and spermatoceles, resulting from partial or complete obliteration of the efferent ductules owing to inflammation, surgery, or trauma.[24] Tubular ectasia of the epididymis has been described in postvasectomy patients.[7,24,25] Tubular ectasia of the rete testis manifests sonographically as multiple tiny cystic tubules located within or adjacent to the mediastinum testis.[7,19,24] With color Doppler, dilated tubules are avascular and fluid filled[15] (Fig. 19-35).

Varicocele

A varicocele is formed by dilatation of the pampiniform plexus veins to a width greater than 2 mm.[3,7,9,16] Other references in the literature define a varicocele as dilatation of the pampiniform venous plexus to a width greater than 2 to 3 mm.[3,18] Currently, there is no consensus on the threshold values used to define varicocele by the maximum venous diameter. A diameter of at least 3 mm

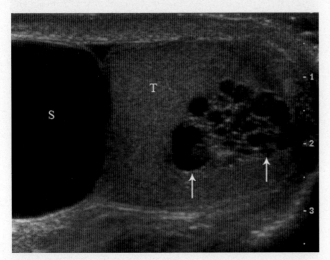

FIGURE 19-35 Tubular ectasia of the rete testis. Transverse image of testis (*T*) shows multiple, small cystic areas in rete testes (*arrows*) characteristic of tubular ectasia. Note the presence of large cystic mass, consistent with a spermatocele (*S*) adjacent to testis.

is commonly considered diagnostic for varicoceles.[18] The dilated and tortuous veins are located superior and posterior to the testis and are caused by incompetent valves in the testicular vein.[3,7,9,11] Large varicoceles can extend inferior to the testis.[7] There are two types of varicoceles: primary (idiopathic) and secondary.[7,14,15,21] Idiopathic varicoceles are present in approximately 15% of adult men, occur on the left side in 98% of cases, and are usually detected in men aged 15 to 25 years.[5,7,9,11,21] Left-sided predominance has been postulated owing to the length and angulation of the left testicular vein at the entry of the left renal vein, resulting in increased pressure and reflux. The right testicular vein drains directly into the vena cava.[3,7] Bilateral involvement is seen in 30% of men.[11] Idiopathic varicoceles normally distend when the patient is in a standing position and when the Valsalva maneuver is performed. When the patient is supine, the varices may decompress; therefore, the patient should be scanned at rest and with the Valsalva maneuver.[7] Varicoceles are the most common correctable cause of infertility, occurring in 21% to 39% of men attending infertility clinics.[7,9,21]

Secondary varicoceles result from increased pressure on the testicular vein or tributaries, which is caused by compression by an abdominal cavity or retroperitoneal mass such as a renal cell carcinoma, tumor thrombus in the left renal vein, cirrhosis, and hydronephrosis[7,9,10,15,16,21] (Fig. 19-36A, B). The appearance of secondary varicoceles is not affected by the patient's position.[21] In this situation, the abdomen and pelvis should be scanned carefully to exclude a mass compressing the testicular vein on the involved side.[7,9,11,15] Secondary varicocele and thrombosis of the pampiniform plexus may also occur in the "nutcracker syndrome," in which the superior mesenteric artery and aorta compress the left renal vein, resulting in stasis and thrombosis[8,9,11] (Fig. 19-36C, D).

Intratesticular varicocele is a rare phenomenon characterized by the dilatation of intratesticular veins, located adjacent to or within the mediastinum testis, and extending to the periphery of the testis (Fig. 19-37A, B). Ectasia of the rete testis resembles intratesticular varicocele. The Valsalva maneuver should be performed with color Doppler to differentiate between dilatation of the rete testis and varices. Most cases are associated with an ipsilateral extratesticular varicocele (predominately left side), suggesting a common pathogenesis. Testicular pain is the most common clinical presentation. The sonographic findings are similar to those of a pampiniform plexus varicocele.[7,9,11]

Clinical signs of varicocele, in addition to the scrotal mass, may include infertility and an abnormally warm scrotum. Sonographically, the varicoceles appear as multiple hypoechoic, serpiginous, tubular structures measuring greater than 3 mm in diameter with the patient supine or standing when performing the Valsalva maneuver[18] (Fig. 19-38A–C). Occasionally, low-level internal echoes can be detected in the varices secondary to slow flow.[7] Color flow Doppler defines the anatomic and physiologic aspect of varicoceles in real time, demonstrating venous enlargement and retrograde flow.[18] It is highly sensitive and specific for the detection of varicoceles, with rates approaching 100%. Color Doppler confirms the presence of varices, when increased flow is visualized within these prominent veins during the Valsalva maneuver.[7,9,11,14,15,21]

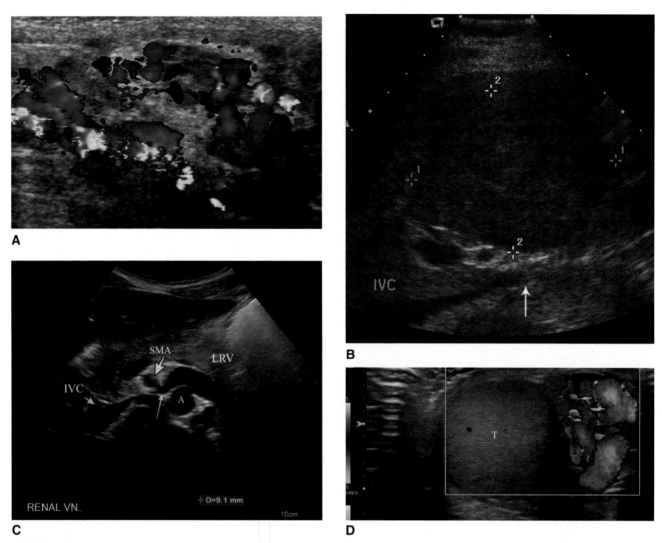

FIGURE 19-36 Secondary varicocele. **A:** Longitudinal color Doppler image of the spermatic cord with secondary varicocele resulting from abdominal mass. **B:** Longitudinal image of right upper abdomen with hypoechoic hepatocellular carcinoma (*calipers* 1, 2) compressing the inferior vena cava (*arrow*) resulting in a secondary varicocele. **C:** Transverse image demonstrating the "nutcracker syndrome" in which the superior mesenteric artery (*large arrow*) and aorta (A) compress the left renal vein (*LRV*) (*long arrow*), Note that the *LRV* is dilated owing to compression. Superior mesentric artery (SMA); Internal vena cava (IVC). (Image courtesy of Ted Whitten, Ultrasound Practitioner, Elliot Hospital, Manchester, NH) **D:** Transverse color Doppler image of the left testis (*T*) and adjacent varicocele resulting from the "nutcracker syndrome." (Courtesy of Ted Whitten, Ultrasound Practitioner, Elliot Hospital, Manchester, NH.)

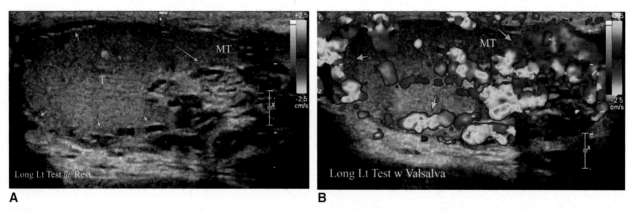

FIGURE 19-37 Intratesticular varicocele. **A:** Longitudinal color Doppler image of the left testis at rest (*T*), with dilated anechoic structures within the rete testis (*arrow*) located in the hilum of the mediastinum testis (*MT*) and in the periphery of the testis (*arrows*). **B:** Longitudinal color Doppler image of the left testis with the Valsalva maneuver. Note the increased color "bloom" within the anechoic structures (*arrows*) as described in (**A**), confirming the presence of an intratesticular varicocele (*arrows*) within the mediastinum testis (*MT*) and in the periphery of the testis (*arrows*).

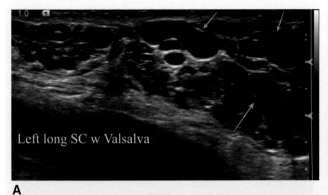

A

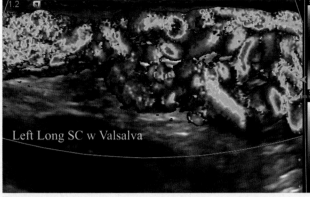

B

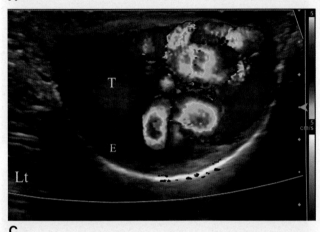

C

FIGURE 19-38 Varicocele. **A:** Longitudinal image of left scrotal varices, showing multiple, dilated, hypoechoic tubular structures (*arrows*) along the spermatic cord demonstrated with the Valsalva maneuver. **B:** Longitudinal color Doppler image of a large varicocele in the left spermatic cord demonstrated with the Valsalva maneuver. Note the dramatic increase of color within the dilated veins. **C:** Transverse color Doppler image of the inferior testis (*T*) with a varicocele adjacent to epididymal tail (*E*).

Scrotal Hernia

Scrotal hernias are inguinal hernias that descend into the scrotum. An inguinal hernia is a protrusion of peritoneal contents, usually containing omentum or bowel, through a patent processus vaginalis, the canal that connects the peritoneal cavity to the tunica vaginalis.[5,11,14,21,23] There are two types of inguinal hernias, direct and indirect, which are classified by their relationship to the inferior epigastric artery (IEA).[5,7,8,14] Direct inguinal hernias are located medial to the IEA, are more common in adults, and occur when the abdominal contents herniate through a weak point in the fascia of the abdominal wall and extend into the inguinal canal.[5,8] Indirect inguinal hernias are located lateral to the IEA and are more common in children. The latter is associated with a patent processus vaginalis, which allows abdominal contents to exit through the internal inguinal ring, extending into the inguinal canal and scrotum.[5,7,8]

Clinical examination can diagnose most scrotal hernias. The clinical sign of scrotal hernia is a persistent or intermittent scrotal mass; the patient may have abdominal pain, and there may be blood in the stool. In some cases, a hernia may present as a hard, nonreducible mass, indistinguishable from a primary scrotal mass.[8]

The sonographic appearance of an inguinal hernia depends on the contents. Hernias containing bowel are easier to diagnose than those containing only omentum.[8] Fluid- or air-filled loops of bowel with peristalsis in the scrotum or inguinal canal are diagnostic of a bowel hernia[5,7,8] (Fig. 19-39A, B). Herniated omentum is seen as a diffusely echogenic paratesticular mass that corresponds to omental fat[5,8,11] (Fig. 19-39C). Strangulated bowel, which

is more common with indirect hernias, appears as fluid- or air-filled loops of bowel within the herniated sac without peristalsis.[11] Hyperemia of the scrotal soft tissue and bowel wall are associated findings.[5,11] Extratesticular masses such as multiloculated hydrocele and hematocele with fibrous septations may mimic fluid-filled segments of bowel.

Scrotal Abscess

A scrotal abscess is most often a complication of untreated epididymo-orchitis. Less frequently, a scrotal abscess develops in patients with debilitating underlying disease such as diabetes, human immunodeficiency virus infection, cancer, or alcoholism.[8,31] The clinical presentation is usually a painful, swollen scrotum. There is an association with Fournier gangrene, also known as idiopathic gangrene of the scrotum, which is a potentially life-threatening necrotizing infection occurring in men over 50 years of age. Fournier gangrene is caused by mixed bacterial infections, most commonly *E. coli*, streptococci, proteus, and enterococci, which spread along well-defined fascial planes.[28] Sonographically, a scrotal abscess appears as a complex fluid collection with irregular borders and hyperemia around the periphery (Fig. 19-40A, B). Gas may be present, causing echogenic shadowing with ring-down artifact[8,31] (Fig. 19-40C). Scrotal wall thickening with hyperemia, in conjunction with a history of immunosuppressive conditions, warrants consideration for the diagnosis of Fournier gangrene[11,31] (Fig. 19-40D).

Scrotal Hematoma

Scrotal hematomas may be intratesticular or involve the extratesticular soft tissues such as the scrotal wall, tunica

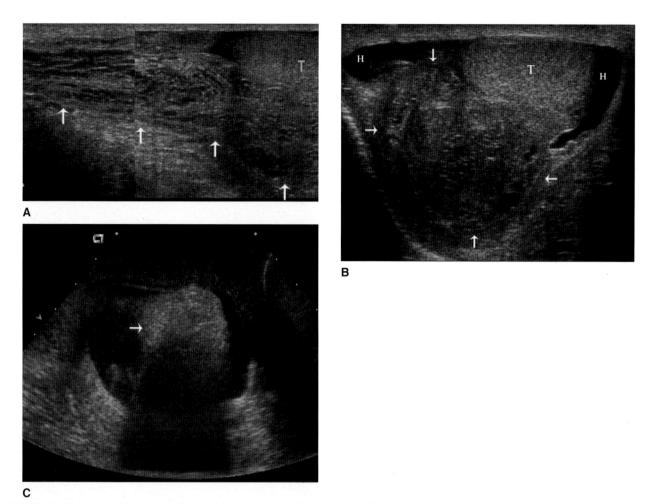

FIGURE 19-39 Scrotal hernia. **A:** Longitudinal image of the inguinal canal shows herniated bowel (*arrows*) extending into the scrotal sac. Testis (*T*). **B:** Transverse image of testis (*T*) shows herniated bowel (*arrows*) in the scrotal sac. Hydrocele (*H*). **C:** Transverse image of herniated omentum (*arrow*) in the scrotal sac with shadowing from air. Note the presence of small hydrocele in the scrotum.

vaginalis, and epididymis. Both are usually associated with a history of trauma.[11,19] Hematomas are usually focal but may also be multiple or diffuse. In extratesticular hematoma, blood collects beneath the tunica dartos and tunica vaginalis.[26] In intratesticular hematoma, the blood is contained within the scrotum itself. In both conditions, the scrotum is swollen, painful, and sometimes discolored.

The sonographic appearance of scrotal hematomas varies with size and duration. Acute hematomas present as avascular hyperechoic areas compared with adjacent testicular parenchyma. As the hemorrhage ages, the hematoma appears hypoechoic or complex with cystic components.[11,12,19] Hematomas of the scrotal wall may appear as focal thickening of the wall or as fluid collections within the wall.[11,19]

Intratesticular hematomas are less common than extratesticular hematomas and may be associated with testicular rupture. Disease processes that can mimic intratesticular hematoma include focal orchitis, testicular infarct, and testicular neoplasm.[11] With focal intratesticular and extratesticular hematomas, color Doppler will show normal perfusion to the testis and peritesticular tissues, with focal areas of absent vascularity.[11]

Hematocele

A hematocele is an accumulation of blood between the parietal and visceral layers of the tunica vaginalis and is generally the result of trauma, surgery, tumor, or torsion.[8,19] A hematocele may be either acute or chronic.[7,8,12,19] The sonographic appearance of a hematocele is a complex heterogeneous collection within the tunica vaginalis[11,12,15,19] (Fig. 19-41A). Acute hematoceles are usually more echogenic.[11,12] Sonography of chronic hematoceles demonstrates a complex heterogeneous collection with thick septations, debris, scrotal wall thickening, and occasionally focal mural calcifications[8,11] (Fig. 19-41B). Hematoceles, like hydroceles, often exert a mass effect, distorting the contour of the testis.[8] Chronic hematoceles may be difficult to distinguish from chronic hydroceles and pyoceles.[11]

Pyocele

The clinical signs of pyoceles may mimic those of infection and inflammation, with hemiscrotal swelling and pain.[7] Following trauma, iatrogenic contamination, or rupture of a testicular abscess, pus fills the potential space between the parietal and visceral layers of the tunica vaginalis.[26] The sonographic findings of a pyocele include a thick hemiscrotal wall, echogenic fluid collections with septations, and occasionally focal mural calcifications.[7,14,26]

Granulomatous Disease

Granulomatous disease of the testis and epididymis results from retrograde spread of tuberculosis (TB) from the prostate,

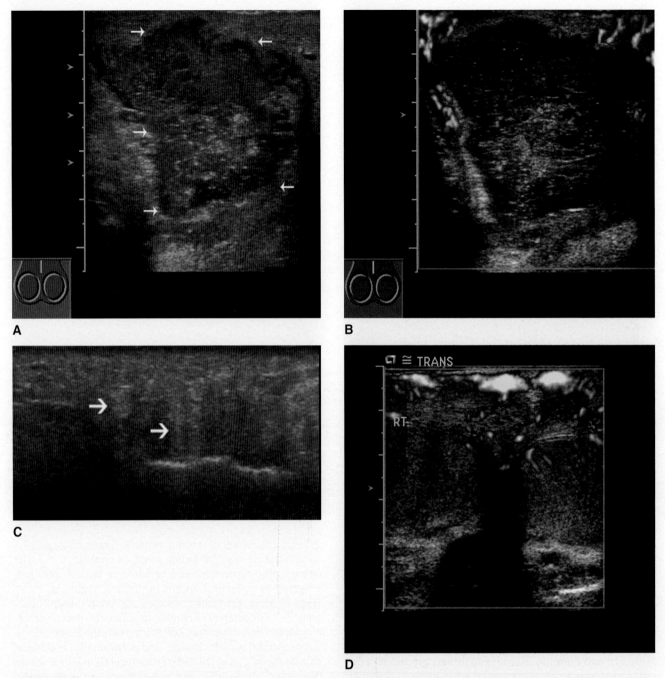

FIGURE 19-40 Scrotal abscess. **A:** Longitudinal image of the suprapubic region shows large heterogeneous wall abscess (*arrows*). **B:** Longitudinal color Doppler image of the suprapubic region shows a large heterogeneous wall abscess with hypervascular borders. **C:** Longitudinal image of scrotal wall abscess demonstrates ring-down artifact (*arrows*) from air within the abscess. **D:** Transverse image of the scrotum shows scrotal wall thickening and hyperemia.

seminal vesicles, and kidneys or from hematogenous spread. TB infection of the scrotum is rare and occurs in 7% of patients infected with the disease.[22,24] The prevalence of TB has been increasing over the past decade, owing to the number of people with HIV and the development of drug-resistant strains of *Mycobacterium tuberculosis*.[22] The genitourinary system is the most common affected extrapulmonary site for TB.[22] The peak incidence of granulomatous disease in the scrotum occurs in men aged 20 to 50 years.[24] The affected patients present with painful or painless swelling of the scrotum.[24] The epididymis is affected first, causing isolated epididymitis, which in later stages can then spread to the adjacent testes. Isolated testicular infection is rare.[24]

Tuberculous epididymo-orchitis involvement maybe either unilateral or bilateral.[7,20]

Sonographically, the epididymis is either diffusely enlarged or nodular and enlarged.[22,24] The grayscale sonographic appearance of nontuberculous epididymitis is more likely to be homogeneous, whereas tuberculous epididymitis is usually heterogeneous or nodular[22] (Fig. 19-42A). Hypervascularity is present with acute bacterial epididymitis, whereas focal linear or spotty blood flow signals may be seen in the peripheral zone of tuberculous epididymitis[24] (Fig. 19-42B). Sonographic findings in tuberculous orchitis are similar to those in tuberculous epididymitis.[24] Other associated sonographic findings include scrotal wall thickening, hydrocele,

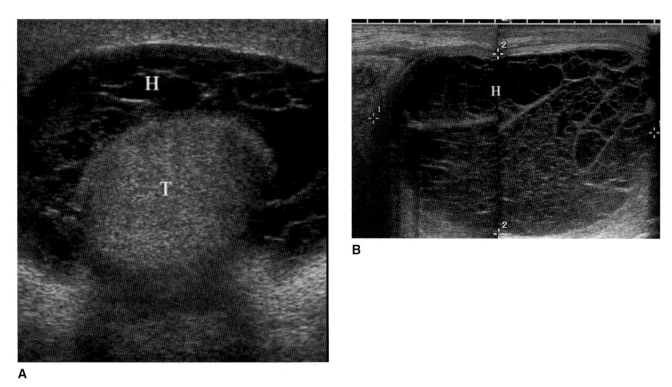

FIGURE 19-41 Hematocele. **A:** Transverse image of the scrotum with septated posttraumatic hematocele (*H*). Testis (*T*). **B:** Transverse image of the scrotum shows large hematocele (*H*) containing multiple septations. Calipers 1 and 2 were used to obtain measurements.

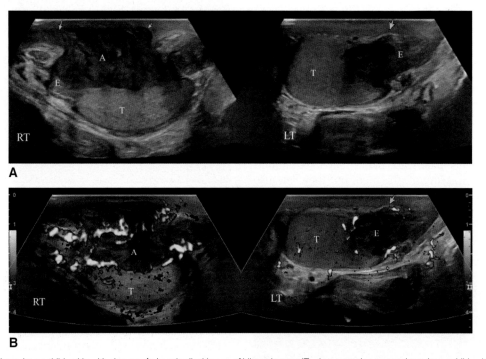

FIGURE 19-42 Tuberculous epididymitis with abscess. **A:** Longitudinal image of bilateral testes (*T*), demonstrating acute tuberculous epididymitis resulting in abscess formation (*A*) within the right testis anterior to the head of the epididymis (*E* and *arrows*). Note the heterogeneous echo texture. The left testis shows an enlarged heterogeneous epididymal tail (*E*) with a nodular contour (*arrow*). **B:** Longitudinal power Doppler image of bilateral testes (*T*), demonstrating increased peripheral vascularity associated with abscess formation (*A*), right testis, and epididymal abscess within the tail of the epididymis (*E*) on the left testis (*arrow*).

intrascrotal extratesticular calcifications, and scrotal abscess.[8,22,24] Focal lesions in granulomatous disease of the testis may mimic a primary testicular mass.[22,24]

Sarcoidosis is a noninfectious, chronic granulomatous disease that affects the genital tract. Intrascrotal sarcoidosis is rare and has been reported in the testes and epididymis.

The epididymis is more commonly affected.[8,24] Epididymal sarcoidosis occurs more often in African Americans. It is often asymptomatic, but as the epididymis becomes enlarged, patients may present with a scrotal mass or pain. Testicular granulomas may also be present.[8] The sonographic appearance of intrascrotal sarcoidosis is an enlarged heterogeneous epididymis, with hypoechoic nodules in the epididymis and/or testis.[8,24]

Tunica Albuginea Cyst

Cysts of the tunica albuginea are uncommon.[36] The etiology of tunica albuginea cysts is unknown, but these cysts are believed to be mesothelial in origin. Clinically, tunica albuginea cysts may present as a painless scrotal lump. Tunica cysts are generally seen in men in the fifth and sixth decades.[5,7,36,37]

Sonographically, tunica albuginea cysts appear as well-circumscribed anechoic areas measuring 2 to 5 mm in size, which meets all the characteristics of a simple cyst[12,15] (Fig. 19-43). The cysts are small and may be single, multiple, unilocular, multilocular, or septate.[9,36] They are generally located in the anterior and lateral aspects of the testis.[8,37] Tunica albuginea cysts can invaginate into the testicular parenchyma and simulate an intratesticular cystic lesion.[36]

Simple Intratesticular Cysts

A simple testicular cyst is an incidental finding during routine sonography examination. They appear in approximately 10% of the male population over the age of 40.[7,9,14,15,19,22] Simple testicular cysts are asymptomatic and sonographically appear as well-circumscribed anechoic areas in the testis with smooth walls and posterior acoustic enhancement[9,14,15] (Fig. 19-44). Testicular cysts range in size from 2 mm to 2 cm.[7,21] They can be located anywhere within the testis but are commonly located adjacent to the mediastinum testis.[7,15,21] Suspected causes include trauma, surgery, and prior inflammation.[14] Simple intratesticular cysts are commonly associated with extratesticular spermatoceles.[15]

Sperm Granuloma

Following trauma, vasectomy, or infection, sperm may extravasate into the surrounding tissues and produce necrosis, resulting in granulomatous formation.[24] Sperm granulomas occur in up to 40% of patients postvasectomy, but only 3% of these patients experience pain.[24] Such granulomas are often found in asymptomatic men, but they can also present as painful nodules. Sonographically, these lesions

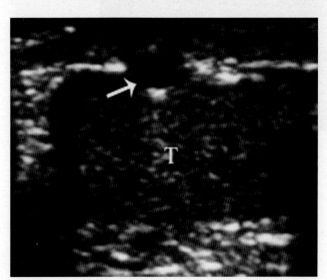

FIGURE 19-43 Tunica albuginea cyst. Longitudinal image of testis (T) shows anechoic tunica albuginea cyst (arrow).

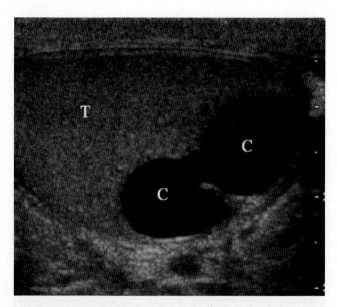

FIGURE 19-44 Intratesticular cyst. Longitudinal image of testis (T) containing anechoic intratesticular cysts (C).

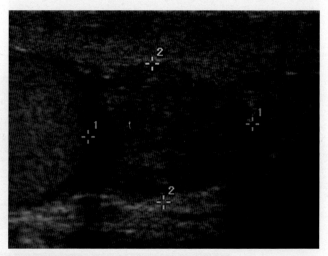

FIGURE 19-45 Sperm granuloma. Longitudinal image of enlarged epididymal tail (calipers 1 and 2) demonstrates well-defined heterogeneous mass (sperm granuloma) in a postvasectomy patient.

appear as well-defined solid hypoechoic or heterogeneous masses located anywhere in the ductal system (Fig. 19-45). Color flow Doppler shows intravascular flow with acute inflammation.[7] They most commonly occur at the cut ends of the vas deferens and can be multiple.[8,9] With improved resolution, echogenic foci noted in sperm granulomas are felt to be secondary to sperm mobility or motion of debris caused by sound waves.[24] Chronic sperm granulomas may contain calcification.[9]

NEOPLASMS OF THE SCROTUM

Extratesticular Neoplasms

Extratesticular scrotal neoplasms are rare and usually involve the epididymis. The vast majority of these masses are benign.[9,25] Only 3% of solid extratesticular masses are malignant.[8]

Benign Neoplasms

The most common extratesticular neoplasm is the benign adenomatoid tumor. It represents 30% of all extratesticular benign lesions.[8,9,25,38] These tumors are generally located within the epididymal tail, but they can occur throughout the epididymis, testis, testicular tunica, and spermatic cord.[8,9,25,38] Adenomatoid tumors usually present as a painless mass or incidental finding. They can occur at any age but are most commonly found in patients aged 20 to 50 years.[9,38]

Sonography of an adenomatoid tumor demonstrates a well-circumscribed solid mass with variable echogenicity compared with the adjacent testis[8,24,25] (Fig. 19-46). With color Doppler, there is minimal flow within and on the periphery of the tumor.[15,25] Their appearance is indistinguishable from other benign tumors such as spermatic granulomas, leiomyomas, fibromas, and lipomas of the spermatic cord.[7,25,38]

Leiomyomas are the second most common primary benign neoplasm of the epididymis. They represent 6% of epididymal tumors reported in a review of the American literature.[24] Generally, asymptomatic, leiomyomas are small, slow-growing painless, firm, intrascrotal extratesticular masses ranging in size from 1 to 4 cm, which commonly manifest in the fifth decade. Leiomyomas frequently involve the tail of the epididymis and are usually unilateral.[24] An associated hydrocele is seen in 50% of cases.

Sonographically, an epididymal leiomyoma appears as a well-circumscribed, homogeneous, solid mass with variable echogenicity with or without cystic spaces.[15,24] On color Doppler evaluation, there is minimal flow within the mass.[26,27]

Lipomas are the most common extratesticular neoplasm that involve the spermatic cord.[15] The sonographic appearance of a lipoma is a circumscribed, homogeneous, hypoechoic-to-hyperechoic structure that alters its shape with transducer compression.[8,26] The echogenicity of lipomas varies depending on the ratio of fat cells to interstitial tissue.[26]

Malignant Neoplasms

Among the malignant tumors involving the epididymis and spermatic cord, rhabdomyosarcomas are the most common, representing 6% of all non–germ cell intrascrotal tumors.[7,26] They occur predominantly in children and adolescents. Other mesenchymal sarcomas arising in the paratesticular soft tissues include leiomyosarcoma, liposarcomas, fibrosarcoma, and malignant mesenchymoma. These malignant tumors most commonly occur in the spermatic cord and in patients more than 40 years of age.[26] Of note, 30% of spermatic cord tumors are malignant.

The sonographic appearance of a leiomyosarcoma, fibrosarcoma, or liposarcoma is a solid, ill-defined, inhomogeneous, disorganized mass with echogenic and anechoic areas representing necrosis.[26] Sonographically, a rhabdomyosarcoma appears as a circumscribed, unilateral, hypoechoic lesion without a capsule measuring 1 to 2 cm in size.[7,26]

Poorly defined borders characterize invasive malignant tumors of the epididymis. With advancing tumor growth, the epididymis and testicular parenchyma may be distorted with loss of border delineation.[26]

Intratesticular Neoplasms

The vast majority of testicular neoplasms are of germ cell origin.[6,10,17,21] As a general rule, all intratesticular masses should be considered malignant until proven otherwise.[7,9,23]

Benign Neoplasms

Approximately 4% of testicular tumors are non–germ cell tumors.[14] Leydig cell tumors, also referred to as *gonadal stromal tumors*, are the most common non–germ cell neoplasm of the testis.[9,14] Although considered in the benign group, 10% to 15% of Leydig cell tumors are in fact malignant.[9,10,39] Leydig cell tumors comprise between 1% and 3% of all testicular neoplasms.[10,15] They generally occur in men between the ages of 20 and 50 years.[9,10,39] Clinical features of Leydig cell tumors may include endocrine imbalance, impotence, decreased libido, and gynecomastia.[9,10,26,40]

Sertoli cell mesenchymal tumors account for less than 1% of all testicular tumors.[9,15] The most common clinical presentation is a painless testicular mass. Feminization with gynecomastia may occur, especially with malignant Sertoli cell tumors or those with the large cell calcifying variant type.[9] Sertoli cell tumors may occur in undescended testes and in patients with feminization, Klinefelter syndrome, and Peutz–Jeghers syndrome.[9,40]

The benign Leydig and Sertoli cell tumors are usually small, less than 1 cm, well-circumscribed masses.[10] Leydig cell tumors demonstrate prominent peripheral flow by color and power Doppler.[10] The malignant forms of these neoplasms are larger (>5 cm) and have less well-defined borders.[10,15,26] Sonographically, these lesions appear as a solid testicular mass. The echogenicity of the mass varies, but it is usually hypoechoic relative to normal parenchyma.[9,10]

An epidermoid cyst is a benign teratoma with only ectodermal components and squamous metaplasia of the surface mesothelium of the testis.[15] Epidermoid cysts are rare and only account for 1% to 2% of all testicular neoplasms; they generally develop between the ages of 20 and 40 years.[10,41] Reported cases have only occurred in Caucasian and Asian individuals. There is a slightly higher prevalence in the right testis.[41] Epidermoid cysts are usually asymptomatic and present as a painless scrotal mass. Sonographically, these lesions appear as a sharply circumscribed encapsulated

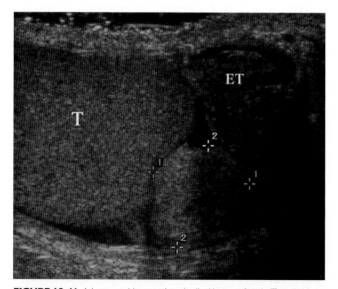

FIGURE 19-46 Adenomatoid tumor. Longitudinal image of testis (*T*) and epididymal tail (*ET*) demonstrates a well-circumscribed, hyperechoic solid mass in the tail of the epididymis characteristic of an adenomatoid tumor (*calipers 1 and 2*).

mass with variable echogenicity.[15] The lesion can contain a hypoechogenic concentric ring surrounding an echogenic center, with or without a hyperechogenic rim, commonly called a "bull's-eye" or "target" appearance. Alternatively, it can contain alternating hypoechoic and hyperechoic concentric rings demonstrating an "onion ring" appearance.[15,41] Epidermoid cysts are avascular masses.[10,15]

Adenomatoid tumors and leiomyomas are rare benign intratesticular tumors.[7,9,38] Their sonographic appearance is identical to their extratesticular manifestations.

Testicular microlithiasis (TM), also referred to as intratubular testicular calcification, is rare. The condition has been associated with a number of other diseases including infertility, cryptorchidism, male pseudohermaphroditism, Down syndrome, testicular torsion, Klinefelter syndrome, intratubular germ cell neoplasia, and granulomatous disease.[9,14,15,40,42] TM is an uncommon condition seen in 1% to 2% of patients referred for scrotal sonography.[9] It is postulated that TM is caused by defective Sertoli cell phagocytosis of degenerating tubular cells, which calcify within the seminiferous tubules.[9,42] TM is defined as multiple intratubular calcifications, within a multilayered envelope containing organelles and vesicles surrounded by stratified collagen diffusely scattered throughout the testicular parenchyma.[15] Bilateral involvement is common. Microlithiasis may be classified as limited if the presence is less than five echogenic foci per transducer field.[42] TM has been associated with testicular neoplasms in 18% to 75% of cases, with the largest series reporting a frequency of 40%.[10,14,40] One recent study showed a 21.6-fold increased relative risk for carcinoma in patients who have TM.[10,40] Because of these high associations and risks, annual follow-up sonography exams are recommended for several years after diagnosis.[10,14,42]

The sonographic findings are multiple 1 to 3 mm hyperechoic foci without posterior shadowing, disseminated throughout the testis[7,10,41] (Fig. 19-47A, B). Patterns of microlithiasis can vary, with cluster calcifications in the center and in the periphery. Color and power Doppler are useful to evaluate if concomitant masses are present.[7,14]

Malignant Neoplasms

Approximately 65% to 94% of patients with testicular neoplasms present with a painless unilateral scrotal mass, hardness of the testis, or diffuse testicular enlargement.[9] Ten percent of patients with testicular cancer present with acute pain and fever, usually initially diagnosed as epididymoorchitis, whereas 10% are detected incidentally following trauma.[7,10,15,21,40] Seminomas and testicular lymphomas may cause orchitis secondary to obstruction of the seminiferous tubules.[10]

Malignant germ cell tumors constitute 90% to 95% of intratesticular primary neoplasms.[7,9,15,21,23,40] Germ cell tumors are divided into seminomas and nonseminomatous tumors. Nonseminomatous tumors include embryonal cell carcinoma, choriocarcinoma, teratoma, yolk sac tumor, and mixed germ cell tumors.[9,10,21,40] Mixed germ cell tumors constitute approximately 40% to 60% of all nonseminomatous germ cell tumors.[10] The most common mixed germ cell neoplasm is a teratocarcinoma. These lesions contain both teratoma and embryonal cells and represent the most frequent tumor after seminoma.[10,21]

Testicular cancer accounts for 1% to 2% of all malignant neoplasms in men.[7,10,39] Testicular cancer is the fifth most frequent cause of death in men aged 15 to 34 years.[7,9,10,15] Primary cancer of the testis is 4.5 times more common in Caucasians than African Americans.[10] Patients with cryptorchidism have a 2.5 to 8 times increased risk for developing testicular cancer. TM is another risk factor for developing testicular cancer.[7,10,14]

Malignant testicular tumors are predominantly hypoechoic (92%) compared with the normal testicular parenchyma.[3,7,21] Less often, neoplasms can appear as focal hyperechoic masses, diffuse infiltration of the testicular parenchyma, or mixed lesions containing focal anechoic areas with echogenic foci. If the tumor is confined to the tunica albuginea, the testis usually retains its oval shape. Invasion of the testis and epididymis distorts the smooth contour of the testis, making it irregular and lumpy.[7,26] Sonography is sensitive in detecting malignant testicular masses, but it cannot distinguish the cell type of malignancies[7,26] (Fig. 19-48A). Color and power Doppler imaging demonstrate increased vascularity in the vast majority of malignant tumors of size greater than 1.6 cm and hypovascularity in 86% of those smaller than 1.6 cm. The presence of hypervascularity is not specific for the diagnosis of malignancy.[7,10,11,15] Infiltrating or diffuse malignancies, such as leukemia and lymphoma,

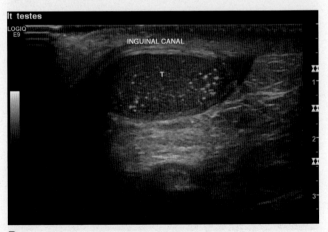

A   **B**

FIGURE 19-47 Microlithiasis. **A:** Longitudinal image of testis containing multiple, nonshadowing, hyperechoic foci. **B:** Longitudinal image of an undescended testis located within the inguinal canal. The testis contains multiple, nonshadowing, hyperechoic foci consistent with microlithiasis.

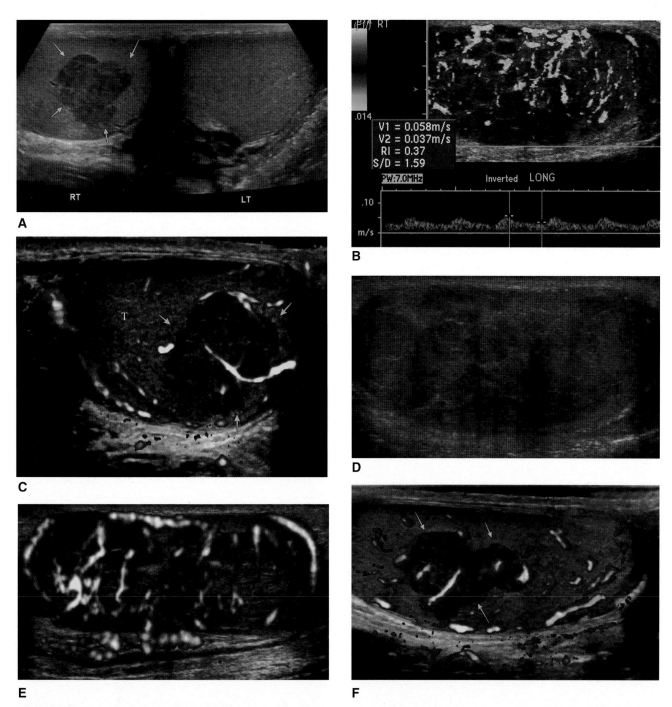

FIGURE 19-48 Malignant testicular tumors. **A:** Transverse image of bilateral tests shows a lobulated hypoechoic mass (*arrows*) within the right testis. **B:** Longitudinal spectral Doppler image of testis containing diffuse infiltrative seminoma demonstrates hypervascularity and low resistive index (*RI*). **C:** Longitudinal power Doppler image of testis (*T*) shows a focal, hypoechoic mass (*arrows*) with increased intravascular flow, consistent with a seminoma. **D:** Longitudinal image of testis shows hypoechoic, multinodular, infiltrative seminoma. **E:** Longitudinal power Doppler image of testis demonstrates hypervascularity with infiltrative seminoma. **F:** Longitudinal power Doppler image of the testis with a lobulated hypoechoic mass (*arrows*), with increased intravascular flow, proved to be a seminoma.

exhibit increased vascularity similar to diffuse orchitis, making differentiation difficult[7,10,11,15] (Fig. 19-48B). In the latter situation, clinical history is extremely important.

Other processes that may mimic testicular neoplasms include abscess, hematoma, focal orchitis, testicular infarcts, and torsion.[7,10,11] Features that tend to distinguish neoplasms from inflammatory processes are the scrotal wall thickness, the character of the epididymis, the margination of the

lesions, and the surrounding testicular parenchyma.[26] In general, with malignancy, the thickness of the scrotal wall is normal as is the epididymis, except in rare cases when the neoplasm invades the epididymis.[26] Inflammatory processes usually show thickening of the scrotal wall and fluid.[22] In 5% to 10% of patients with a testicular neoplasm, there is concurrent epididymitis or epididymo-orchitis; reactive hydroceles accompany 10% of testicular neoplasms.[26]

Seminoma

Seminoma is the most common pure germ cell tumor and accounts for 40% to 50% of primary testicular neoplasms.[7,9,10,15,21,40] Seminoma occurs most often in the fourth and fifth decades of life with an average patient age of 40.5 years.[1,17] Approximately 8% to 30% of patients with seminoma have a history of undescended testis.[7,9,14,15] The alpha-fetoprotein (AFP) level is always normal in patients with pure seminomas.[10] If a patient has an elevated AFP with seminoma histology, the tumor is treated as a nonseminomatous lesion.[10]

The sonographic appearance of seminoma is characteristically described as a well-defined homogeneous hypoechoic mass without calcification or tunica invasion[6,9,10,15] (Fig. 19-48C). Ten percent of seminomas present with small cystic areas, which correspond to dilated rete testis caused by tumor-related occlusion and liquefaction necrosis. A diffuse echotexture change may be seen secondary to seminomatous infiltration[10,40] (Fig. 19-48D, E). Color and power Doppler are useful in demonstrating hypervascularity in tumors of size greater than 1.6 cm[10,15] (Fig. 19-48F).

Embryonal Cell Carcinoma

Embryonal cell carcinoma occurs primarily in men between ages 25 and 35 and is the second most common histologic type of testicular tumor after seminoma.[9,10,40] Often invading the tunica albuginea and distorting the testicular contour, embryonal cell carcinoma is the most aggressive of the primary scrotal malignancies.[10,15,40] The AFP and beta-human chorionic gonadotropin (beta-hCG) levels are elevated in approximately 70% of patients.[10] The sonographic appearance of embryonal cell carcinoma is a hypoechoic mass, more heterogeneous than seminoma, with poorly defined borders[10] (Fig. 19-49A, B). Cystic components are seen in one-third of tumors, and calcifications or echogenic foci are not uncommon.[9,10]

Choriocarcinoma

Choriocarcinoma is a rare germ cell tumor that is seen in less than 1% patients and usually occurs in men between the ages of 20 and 30.[7,10,40] All patients with choriocarcinoma have elevated levels of beta-hCG.[3] Choriocarcinoma has the worst prognosis of any of the germ cell tumors, with death occurring within 1 year of diagnosis.[10] Sonographically, choriocarcinomas are heterogeneous and show extensive hemorrhagic necrosis in the central portion of the tumor with a mixed echo pattern.[9,10,15,40]

Teratoma

Teratoma is the second most common testicular neoplasm in children, usually occurring in children less than 4 years of age. Pure teratomas are rare in adults, but teratomatous components occur in more than 50% of all adult cases of mixed germ cell tumors. Serum AFP (38%) and beta-hCG levels are sometimes elevated.[10] Teratomas contain multiple tissue elements such as bone, soft tissue, skin, and cartilage.[9,10] Sonographically, teratomas tend to be very large and markedly inhomogeneous masses. Cystic components are common. Echogenic foci may or may not shadow, which may represent calcification, cartilage, immature bone, and fibrous tissue.[9,10,40]

Yolk Sac Tumor

Yolk sac tumors account for 80% of childhood testicular tumors, with most cases occurring before 2 years of age. They exclusively produce AFP in more than 90% of cases. Pure yolk sac tumors are rare in adults, and the presence of any yolk sac tumor element in an adult mixed cell tumor indicates a poor prognosis.[10,40] The sonographic appearance of a yolk sac tumor is nonspecific. These tumors are usually inhomogeneous and may contain echogenic foci secondary to hemorrhage or hypoechoic areas owing to necrosis.[10]

Mixed Neoplasms

Mixed germ cell tumors constitute about 40% to 60% of all germ cell tumors.[9,10] Teratocarcinoma is the most common mixed germ cell neoplasm. It contains both teratoma and embryonal carcinoma cells.[10] Teratocarcinomas are aggressive and the largest of all testicular tumors.[10] Sonographically, teratocarcinoma appears as a heterogeneous mass with

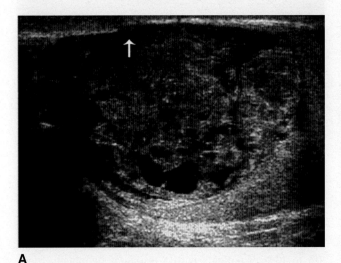

A

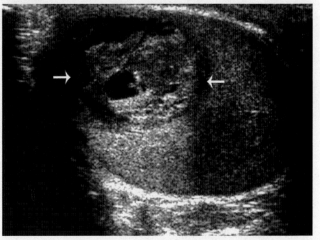

B

FIGURE 19-49 Embryonal cell carcinoma. **A:** Longitudinal image of testis containing large, heterogeneous mass with cystic areas diagnosed as an embryonal cell carcinoma. Note the presence of irregular margins with tunica albuginea invasion (*arrow*). **B:** Longitudinal image of testis demonstrates well-defined heterogeneous mass (*arrows*) with cystic areas characteristic of embryonal cell carcinoma.

echogenic foci and cystic areas secondary to hemorrhage and calcifications.

Metastases to the Testis

Metastasis to the testes is rare, with an incidence of 0.68%.[10] The most common primary tumors to metastasize to the testis are prostate (35%), lung (19%), malignant melanoma (9%), colon (9%), and kidney (7%).[10] Metastases are more common than germ cell tumors in patients over 50 years of age and are often multiple and bilateral.[26]

Lymphoma

Lymphoma accounts for 5% of all testicular neoplasms and is the most common bilateral testicular tumor. Testicular lymphoma occurs in less than 1% of patients who have lymphoma and typically occurs in older patients. Lymphoma is the most common testicular neoplasm in men over 60 years of age.[7,9,10] Testicular lymphoma is aggressive and infiltrates the epididymis and spermatic cord in 50% of cases.[10] The scrotal skin is rarely involved. Sonographically, it appears as a diffuse enlargement with hypoechogenicity or multifocal hypoechoic masses of various sizes[26] (Fig. 19-50A, B). One or both testes may be enlarged. lymphomatous tissue replaces normal testicular tissue.[7,9,10] Testicular enlargement is bilateral in 50% of cases and is commonly associated with scrotal discoloration.[22] Color Doppler imaging shows increased vascularity regardless of the tumor size. Hypervascularity seen with diffuse infiltration may resemble inflammation[7,9,10] (Fig. 19-50C, D).

Leukemia

Primary testicular leukemia is rare. The testes may be a sanctuary organ for hematologic malignancies such as leukemia and lymphoma. The blood–testis barrier prevents the accumulation of chemotherapeutic drugs within the testes.[7,10]

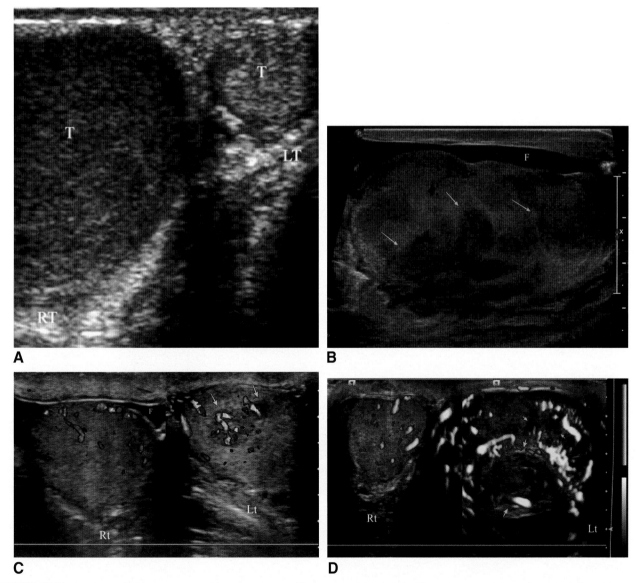

FIGURE 19-50 Lymphoma. **A:** Transverse image of the scrotum shows diffusely enlarged, hypoechoic right testis with lymphomatous invasion. Left testis is normal. **B:** Longitudinal image of the testis with multiple focal hypoechoic masses (*arrows*) proved to be lymphoma. Note the presence of fluid (*F*) anterior to the testis. (A and B: Courtesy of Ted Whitten, Ultrasound Practitioner, Elliot Hospital, Manchester, NH.) **C:** Transverse color Doppler image of the previous image (**B**) focal hypervascular masses (*arrows*) consistent with lymphoma. Note the presence of fluid (*F*) within the right hemiscrotum. **D:** Transverse power Doppler image of bilateral testes showing an enlarged hypervascular left testis. Note the multiple hypoechoic masses (*arrows*). This was a proven metastatic lymphoma involving the left testis.

Leukemic infiltration of the testis has been found in 40% to 65% of acute leukemia patients at autopsy and in 20% to 35% of patients with chronic leukemia.[7,10,14] Leukemia diffusely infiltrates the testis, resulting in hypoechoic enlargement.[3] Unilateral enlargement of the testis with normal echogenicity can also be seen. Focal, sharply defined, anechoic masses with through transmission and occasional low-level internal echoes have been described in patients with chronic lymphocytic leukemia.[9,10] Color Doppler imaging of leukemic infiltration demonstrates hypervascularity within the affected testis, similar to lymphoma.[7,9,10]

PENIS

The penis is the external male organ that serves as a conduit for the excretion of both semen and urine. Earlier, penile imaging was largely performed under plain film X-ray, urethrography, cavernosography, computed tomography, and magnetic resonance imaging. With improved high-resolution ultrasound technology, detailed sonography and Doppler evaluation of penile structure and vasculature have been utilized to image the penis.[43] In the 1990s, color Doppler ultrasound became an essential tool for the identification and classification of the causes of erectile dysfunction (ED). However, the introduction of effective oral medication has greatly reduced the demand for ultrasound in patients with impotence. Although the use of penile ultrasound has decreased, there is still a need to evaluate other

pathologies such as priapism, Peyronie disease, neoplasm, trauma, and patients who do not respond well to erectile oral medication.[44,45]

Normal Anatomy

The penis is comprised of three cylindrical columns of spongy tissue. They are composed of many sinusoidal spaces lined with smooth muscle and serve as the main erectile structures of the penis. Two corpora cavernosa run parallel along the dorsal aspect and a single corpus spongiosum, which contains the urethra, between them ventrally. The corpus spongiosum continues distally where it expands to form the glans penis, sitting over the blunt ends of the corpora cavernosa. A thick fascial sheath called the tunica albuginea binds and separates the three corpora. The tunica albuginea is comprised of two layers of thick crisscrossing fibers that encapsulate the sinusoidal tissue of the corpora and provide structure and support during an erection. The two layers are composed of an outer longitudinal layer and an inner circular layer.[45] The septum that divides the corpora contains many fenestrations that connect the sinusoidal spaces of each cavernosum. These sinusoidal spaces fill and engorge with blood during an erection. The tunica albuginea is encased by a thick fibrous envelope called Buck fascia and is then ultimately covered by a loose layer of skin (Fig. 19-51A, B). The corpus spongiosum expands slightly but adds little to the erectile state of the penis.[2,43–46]

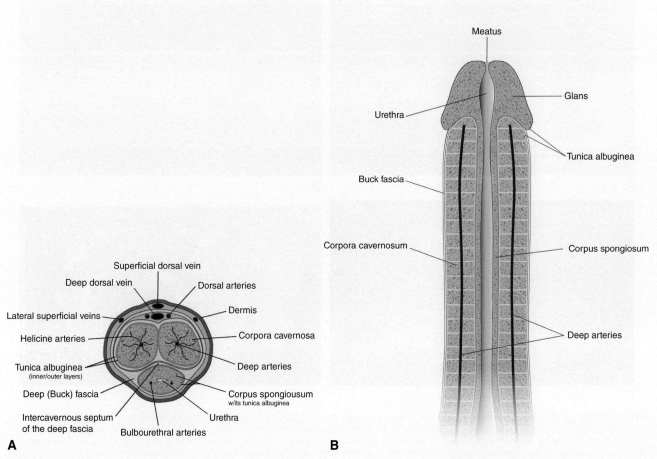

A

Superficial dorsal vein
Deep dorsal vein
Dorsal arteries
Lateral superficial veins
Helicine arteries
Tunica albuginea (inner/outer layers)
Deep (Buck) fascia
Intercavernous septum of the deep fascia
Dermis
Corpora cavernosa
Deep arteries
Corpus spongiousum w/its tunica albuginea
Urethra
Bulbourethral arteries

B

Meatus
Glans
Urethra
Tunica albuginea
Buck fascia
Corpora cavernosum
Corpus spongiosum
Deep arteries

FIGURE 19-51 Schematic illustration of transverse (**A**) and longitudinal (**B**) sections of penile anatomy. (Illustration created courtesy of David Brix.)

Vascular Anatomy

The arterial blood supply to the penis originates from the internal iliac arteries, which give rise to the internal pudendal arteries and then branch into the common penile arteries. The common penile artery divides into three branches: cavernous, bulbourethral, and dorsal arteries. The cavernous artery travels centrally and feeds the corpora cavernosa sinusoids via multiple branches called helicine arteries, which radiate out from the cavernous artery. The bulbourethral artery supplies the corpus spongiosum that contains the urethra. The dorsal artery travels dorsolateral to the midline dorsal vein and supplies the glans penis and some non-erectile tissues. It generally has little to no branches before it reaches the glans penis.[45–49]

The main venous outflow in the penis are the superficial and deep dorsal veins. The superficial dorsal vein is located outside of Buck fascia and the deep dorsal vein lies beneath Buck fascia. Drainage from corporal bodies into the deep dorsal vein originates from venules below the tunica albuginea that penetrate the tunica via emissary veins. Dorsally, the circumflex and deep dorsal veins drain into the internal iliac vein or internal pudendal vein. The superficial and deep dorsal veins connect with the pudendal venous plexus via the internal pudendal vein. During an erection, as the corpora cavernosa are expanded, the small draining veins are compressed and occluded as the fibrous tunica albuginea is stretched. This prevents blood from leaving the dilated sinusoids. The erection is reversed when muscles in the penis contract, stopping the inflow of blood and opening venous drainage channels.[45–49]

Sonographic Appearance and Imaging Techniques

Sonographic evaluation of the penis is performed with high-frequency (8 to 18 MHz) linear transducers. Many current ultrasound systems have specialized "hockey stick" probes with small linear footprints ideal for superficial vascular or small part imaging. The penis should examined with the patient in supine position and the penis in the normal anatomical orientation lying on the anterior abdominal wall. In some instances, the penis should be positioned on a towel or on the scrotum with a lateral or dorsal scanning approach.[44,47] A sufficient amount of warm sonographic acoustic gel should be used on the surface of the penis to obtain good-quality images. Excessive pressure can cause unwanted compression by the transducer, especially when the penis is in the flaccid state. The examination should be performed in transverse and longitudinal planes and from the glans to the base of the penis. A transperineal approach may be used to assess the base of the penis when appropriate.[2,44,45]

Sonographically, the midline elliptical corpus spongiosum is seen in the transverse plane with a homogeneous echotexture of medium-level echoes.[2,44,45,48,49] The spongiosum is often compressed and may be difficult to visualize optimally from the ventral approach. The paired corpora cavernosa are round or oval, lie posterior to the spongiosum in this ventral approach, which appear as symmetrical homogeneous hypoechoic cylindrical structures.[2,43,44,45,49] The corpora cavernosa and corpus spongiosum are covered by

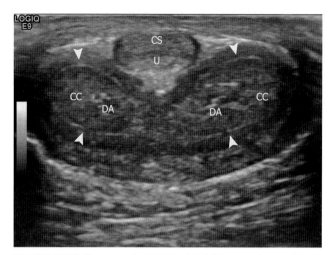

FIGURE 19-52 Transverse view of normal penis from ventral aspect. The corpus spongiosum (*CS*) with the collapsed urethra (*U*) noted within. The corpora cavernosa (*CC*) are shown with the deep artery (*DA*) located centrally. The thin hyperechoic line delineates the tunica albuginea (*arrowheads*).

the hyperechoic and linear tunica albuginea (Fig. 19-52). In the longitudinal plane, the corpora cavernosa remain homogenous with the hyperechoic tunica albuginea seen above and below the cylindrical structures.[45,49] Buck fascia is superficial to the tunica albuginea and covers all of the structures described above but is inseparable and indistinguishable from the tunica albuginea.[44,45,48] The septum penis that divides the corpora cavernosa is an extension of the tunica albuginea. The septum appears as an echogenic structure with attenuation, which can limit the evaluation of the dorsal aspect of the penis and tunica albuginea.[2,44,45,48]

PENILE PATHOLOGY

Priapism

Priapism is a persistent painful erection or tumescence of the penis that is unrelated to sexual stimulation.[44,45,48,49] Color Doppler ultrasound is the imaging modality of choice for the assessment of priapism, because it is noninvasive, widely available, and highly sensitive. Interpreting the color flow characteristics by ultrasound makes it possible to diagnose priapism and to differentiate between its low- and high-flow forms.[45,48,49]

Ischemic Priapism

The most common form of priapism is known as venous, low-flow, or ischemic priapism and is caused by decreased or absent venous drainage. The corpora cavernosa consist of multiple sinusoids lined with the smooth muscle. An erection begins with the relaxation of the smooth muscles and, consequentially, a fivefold to tenfold increase in cavernosal artery inflow. As the sinusoids expand with increase in the blood flow, the draining venules below the tunica albuginea are compressed, increasing the intracorporal pressure and rigidity. A failure along the complex neurochemical pathway preventing smooth muscle contraction and penile detumescence results in prolonged occlusion of the draining venules and trapped blood in the sinusoids. The stagnant blood flow not only occludes the venous plexus but also affects the cavernosal artery. The prolonged decrease or absence of blood flow in the deep artery will cause hypoxia of the surrounding tissues and if left untreated will result in cavernosal scarring, fibrosis, ED, ischemia, necrosis, or gangrene.[44,45] On color and spectral Doppler, the cavernosal artery presents with a complete lack of blood flow or diminished velocities with a very high-resistance flow pattern. Cavernosal sinusoids will be engorged with mixed echogenicity depending on the completeness of thrombosis[50,51] (Fig. 19-53A–D). This type of priapism is usually the result of the side effects of ED medications or the use/misuse of substances like trazodone, clozapine, thorazine, heparin, cocaine, and alcohol.[44,47,49] Other hypercoagulable risk factors include sickle cell anemia (35% to 42% will get priapism, most common in children), leukemia, thalassemia, multiple myeloma, venomous insect bites, spinal cord injury, or pelvic neoplasms.[44,45] Low-flow priapism represents a true compartment syndrome and is a urologic emergency because time is critical to prevent permanent tissue damage. The most common treatment involves

aspiration and irrigation of blood of the cavernosal bodies to prevent fibrotic activity and secure erectile function. A transient distal penile corporoglanular shunt is a simple and safe procedure often used to redirect blood from the cavernosa to the glans penis to allow absorption of blood through the corpus spongiosum.[52] The corporoglanular shunt effectively treats over 70% of patients with early stages of priapism.[52] In cases of more delayed episodes, more than 8 hours to days, patients will require more aggressive blood evacuation throughout each corpus cavernosum, using either a snake shunt or T shunt tunneling.[52,53]

Arterial Priapism

Arterial or high-flow priapism is caused by uncontrolled, increased arterial inflow to the penis.[48] Most commonly, the condition is related to blunt trauma of the penis or perineum. The surrounding erectile tissues and the tunica albuginea protect the cavernous artery, but an injury with enough force

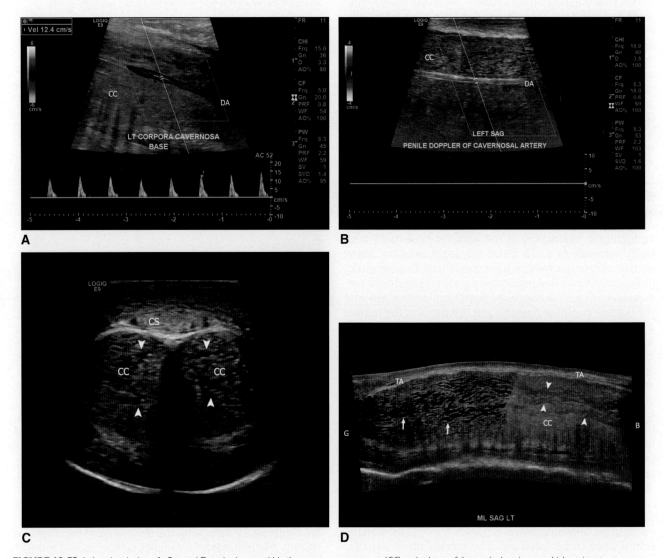

FIGURE 19-53 Ischemic priapism. **A:** Spectral Doppler image within the corpora cavernosum (*CC*) at the base of the penis showing very high-resistant, low-velocity arterial flow in the deep artery (*DA*) of a patient with ischemic priapism. **B:** Spectral Doppler image within the corpora cavernosum (*CC*) toward the glans penis, showing absent arterial flow in the deep artery (*DA*) in the same patient. **C:** Transverse view showing the spongiosum (*CS*) and the dilated sinusoids (*arrowheads*) within the corpora cavernosa (*CC*). **D:** Longitudinal image of penis with ischemic priapism. Note the echogenicity change within the corpora cavernosa (*CC*). The sinusoids (*arrowheads*) near the base (*B*) have isoechoic and hypoechoic echoes, indicating they have occlusive thrombus to mid-shaft. The sinusoids (*arrows*) near the glans penis (*G*) are more anechoic, with low-level echoes indicating fresher blood products. This patient had a corporoglanular shunt in place that partially drained the distal portion of the penis and allowed fresh blood to occupy the sinusoids. The tunica albuginea (*TA*) is well defined along the top of the cavernosum.

can create an arterial rupture that results in intercavernosal arteriovenous shunting, causing the uncontrolled fistulous flow.[54] High-flow priapism bypasses the helicine arteries and directly extends flow into cavernous sinusoidal tissue. This appears as an anechoic or hypoechoic lesion and on color Doppler as a classic blush of turbulent color fill similar to a pseudoaneurysm.[45] Spectral Doppler shows increased low-resistant flow in the cavernous arteries. The sinusoids are partially engorged as the free-flowing blood actively pools in the surrounding tissues (Fig. 19-54A, B). Despite the higher unregulated arterial inflow, this does not result in rigid and painful erections as seen in low-flow ischemic priapism because the venous channels are still competent. Because blood circulation into and out of the corpora cavernosa is not impeded, the prognosis is excellent if it is treated properly.[52,53] High-flow priapism is not considered a medical emergency because patients are at a lower risk of developing permanent tissue damage.[44,53]

Peyronie Disease

Peyronie disease is a psychologically and physically devastating disorder that manifests in middle-aged men.[55] Characterized by fibrotic thickening of the tunica albuginea, Peyronie disease is a benign, acquired, penile deformity resulting from plaque formation.[44,45,55] Although the exact cause in not fully understood, the most widely accepted hypothesis is that Peyronie is initiated by microtraumas to the erect penis with subsequent wound healing, fibrin deposition, and scar formation.[43,55] The fibrous, inelastic plaque formation leads to progressive curvature and shortening of the penile shaft along the involved area.[55] The patient may present with palpable nodules, painful erections, and/or dyspareunia.[43,45] In the flaccid state, there is no appreciable deformity.[55]

Peyronie disease is associated with other fibromatous disorders such as Ledderhose disease and Dupuytren contractures of the hands. Dupuytren disease is a fibro-proliferative condition of the palmar fascia in the hand, typically resulting in progressive contracture of one or more fingers.[56,57] Gene expression analysis indicates that an overlapping genetic predisposition to fibrotic conditions contributes to both Dupuytren and Peyronie disease.[56,57]

The fibrotic changes usually involve the dorsum of the penis but can sometimes involve the septum penis, ventral, or lateral aspects as well.[43,55] In the early stages of the disease, plaque consistency may feel soft and fleshy, whereas firm, calcified, or even ossified nodules form as the disease progresses. The detection of calcifications within the plaque suggests stabilization of the disease and provides information about appropriate treatment.[44] Often during the acute phase of the disease, there may be penile pain even when flaccid and there can be dynamic changes to the penile malformation.[44,55] During the chronic phase, the pain resolves and the deformity becomes stable in its characteristics.[55]

Grayscale ultrasound can show focal hyperechoic thickening of the tunica albuginea. Fibrosis and its associated calcifications demonstrate distal acoustic shadowing.[44] Ultrasound has 100% sensitivity in detecting calcified plaques, whereas focal isoechoic nodules or thickening in the acute phase may be more subtle and difficult to isolate, especially in the flaccid state.[55] Focal tunica thickening without posterior shadowing, isoechoic or hypoechoic lesions with posterior attenuation, and a focal break in the continuity of the tunica are all less common findings attributed to earlier stages of the disease[45,55] (Fig. 19-55A, B). Color Doppler evaluation with increased vascularity around the plaques suggests inflammatory activity, and the absence of flow can suggest stability.[43,44,55] With the recent addition of elastography, ultrasound is proving itself useful in differentiating and detecting noncalcified fibrous lesions when B-mode ultrasonography has failed to demonstrate a plaque.[58]

The normal tunica albuginea appears as a thin hyperechoic line covering the corpora cavernosa.[2] The echoes from the tunica albuginea are specular reflections and are, therefore, best demonstrated when the ultrasound beam is perpendicular to the corpora.[55] Perpendicular insonation is of particular importance when evaluating the echogenicity of plaques. Echogenic plaques might falsely appear hypoechoic owing to incorrect insonation, penile septum artifacts, or extensive fibrotic changes of the tunica.[57] Understanding the relationship of the plaque to the surrounding structures is helpful in determining the treatments and conditions with ED.[43,44,55] Intralesional plaque injections may be ineffective

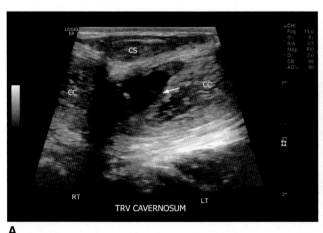

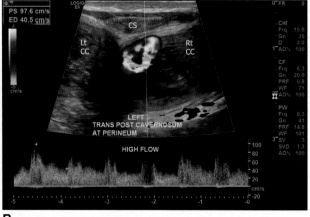

A   **B**

FIGURE 19-54 A: High-flow priapism. Transverse view of the penis in a patient with high-flow priapism. An arterial jet is noted (*arrow*) filling an anechoic vascular lesion where the cavernosal artery was ruptured. The sinusoids (*arrowheads*) are partially distended within the corpora cavernosa (*CC*). The corpus spongiosum is seen at the top of the image (*CS*). **B:** Spectral Doppler image of the turbulent vascular flow in the left corpora cavernosum (*CC*). Note the increased peak systolic velocity (*PSV*) and end diastolic velocity (*EDV*), and low-resistance arterial flow. *CS*, corpus spongiosum.

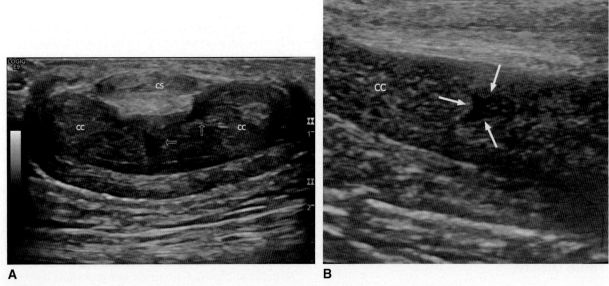

FIGURE 19-55 Peyronie disease. **A:** Transverse view of hypoechoic palpable fibrotic nodules (*arrows*) detected abutting the cavernosum (*CC*) on a patient with Dupuytren contracture of his hand. Hypoechoic nodules are typically detected in the acute inflammatory phase of the disease. Spongiosum (*CS*). **B:** Longitudinal view of a hypoechoic nodule (*arrows*) within the corpora cavernosum (*CC*) in the same patient with Dupuytren contracture.

for patients with extensive calcifications or curvature greater than 90 degrees.[55] Furthermore, plaque excision or grafting procedures on patients with marginal erectile function may worsen the erectile function or render them impotent.[55] Individuals with Peyronie disease can present with calcified nodules along the tunica of the cavernosum, resulting in veno-occlusive erectile dysfunction, owing to insufficient drainage at the site of the plaque[44,55] (Fig. 19-56A–D). Calcifications may also invade the cavernosum and occlude the cavernosal artery, resulting in arterio-occlusive impotence.[43,55] In general, penile deformities, emotional distress, and pain all contribute to ED.[47]

Erectile Dysfunction

ED is the inability to get and maintain an erection firm enough for sexual intercourse, a common problem in the aging population. Male sexual arousal is a complex process that involves the brain, hormones, emotions, nerves, muscles, and blood vessels, with ED resulting from a problem with any of these.[49] ED is classified as psychogenic (anxiety, depression, schizophrenia, stress), organic (neurogenic, hormonal, vasculogenic, drug-induced), and mixed.[44,58] Mixed ED is the most common and involves both psychogenic and organic components.[45,59]

Using color Doppler ultrasound, we can classify the organic component of ED into arterial and venous types. Patients may have arterial insufficiency or venous incompetence, or both. The physiologic process of an erection requires an increase in arterial inflow along with an increase in venous resistance. A series of coordinated events requires the presence of a normal vascular system. Although many causes of ED have been reported, approximately 80% of ED is attributed to vascular disease.[43,44,59] Penile ultrasound plays an important role in the detection of silent coronary artery disease owing to the fact ED is recognized as one of the earliest manifestations of endothelial dysfunction and peripheral vascular disease.[59]

Arteriogenic ED involves arterial insufficiency from an atherosclerotic stenosis or occlusion in arteries that feed the penile artery. Arterial causes of ED are more common in patients with diabetes, hypertension, hypercholesterolemia, and smoking history.[46,47,59] Patients with mild-to-moderate arterial insufficiency in the absence of venous incompetence are often successfully treated with oral pharmacologic therapy.[44,47,48] Patients with more severe arterial insufficiency usually require a penile implant to restore sexual function.[48,59]

In contrast, an impaired veno-occlusive mechanism causes a venous leak resulting in venogenic ED.[43] Venous incompetence results from the failure of occlusion in the draining veins despite adequate filling of the cavernosal sinusoids.[43,59] Patients may experience partial erections but rigidity cannot be fully achieved or maintained.[59] Venous competence can only be assessed if the arterial function is normal.[43] Patients with arterial insufficiency would have very little arterial inflow to expand the sinusoids enough to occlude the draining veins. Therefore, these patients can have persistent venous flow regardless of whether the veins are intrinsically competent.[43,47,48,59]

Testing for ED with ultrasound has decreased over the past few decades with the introduction of oral therapies.[43,59] For those patients who do not respond to oral medications, more involved testing may be required. The initial scan of the penis should identify any possible tumors, fibrotic plaques, calcifications, or hematomas, in addition to evaluating the appearance and tortuosity of the cavernous arteries.[44,47,59] During examination, the grayscale images of the corpora cavernosa and corpus spongiosum in transverse and longitudinal planes should be recorded. The echogenicity of the tissues and measure the transverse diameter of the cavernosal arteries should be noted.[47,59] The spectral waveforms of both cavernosal arteries should be saved and the peak systolic velocity (PSV) and end diastolic velocity (EDV) of each vessel should be recorded.

Although the anatomical and structural changes on ultrasound are informative, the functional characteristics

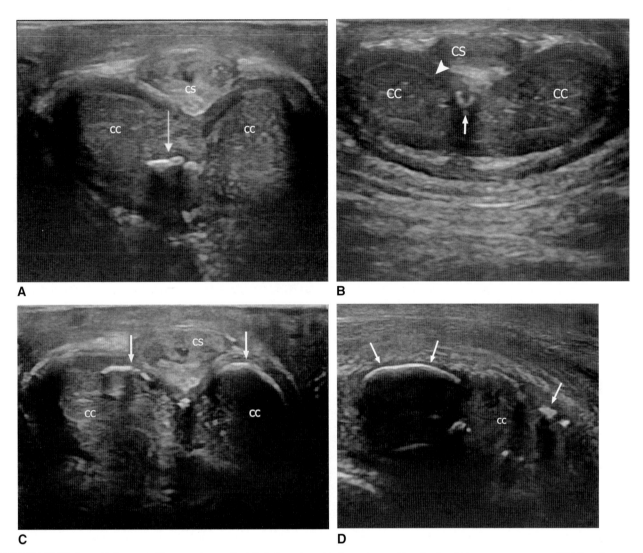

FIGURE 19-56 Peyronie disease. **A:** Transverse image of calcified plaque (*arrow*) in the septum and invading the right corpora cavernosum (*CC*). Spongiosum (*CS*). (Image courtesy of ultrasoundcases.info, © Sonoskills.) **B:** Transverse image of calcified plaque (*arrow*) in the septum abutting the tunica albuginea (*arrowhead*). **C:** Transverse view of more severe calcifications around the corpora cavernosa (*CC*) and along the tunica albuginea (*arrows*). Spongiosum (*CS*). (Image courtesy of ultrasoundcases.info, © Sonoskills.) **D:** Longitudinal image of severe calcifications (*arrows*) along the corpora cavernosum (*CC*) in a patient with Peyronie disease. (Image courtesy of ultrasoundcases.info, © Sonoskills.)

after an erection are more important.[43,59] In an office setting, patients will need a cavernosal injection to facilitate an erection to better evaluate physiologic vascular changes. Once the physician injects the vasodilator in one cavernosum, the patient should manipulate the penis to create an erection because the medication will transverse the septum to the other side.[47,48,59] If venous leakage is suspected, wrap a tourniquet or penile pressure cuff around the base of the penis to compress the dorsal vein. Remove the cuff or tourniquet after 3 minutes postinjection.[47] Measure the transverse diameter of the cavernosal arteries postinjection as well as spectral waveforms, documenting the PSV and EDV for comparison with the preinjection state.[47,59] Arterial insufficiency is diagnosed when the peak systolic velocity PSV of the cavernosal artery is less than 25 cm/s during an erection, with 92% accuracy.[43–45,47,48,59] An arterial diameter increase less than 75% postinjection in the cavernosal arteries indicates inadequate vessel compliance.[43,44,47,48,59]

Veno-occlusive ED shows a persistent cavernosal artery EDV over 5 cm/s during all phases of erection as well as visible Doppler flow in the deep dorsal vein.[43,44,46,48,59] Diagnosis based on Doppler ultrasound can only be made if the arterial inflow is normal. Persistent antegrade EDV flow rate greater than 5 cm/s when the arterial function is greater than 25 cm/s is suggestive of venous leak.[43,44,47,48,59] Other factors that need to be considered include the correlation with resistance index (RI) and dorsal vein velocity. An RI less than 0.75 is associated with venous leak in 95% of patients, and RI greater than 0.9 is associated with normal results in 90% of patients 20 minutes postinjection.[43,48,59] The dorsal vein velocity is usually less than 3 cm/s at this time; so, it is helpful to document the vein velocity. Velocities between 10 and 20 cm/s are considered moderate, whereas velocities greater than 20 cm/s are considered very high.[47,48,59] Further evaluation can be made using angiography, cavernosometry, or cavernosography with a 80% sensitivity and 100% specificity for venous leakage.[43,47,59]

The classification of disease should be determined according to department diagnostic criteria.

Penile Carcinoma

Penile carcinoma is rare and accounts for only 1,400 cases annually in the United States.[60,61] Although it accounts for 10% to 20% of all malignancies in males in Asia, Africa, and South America, it has a prevalence of only 1% in Western countries.[60] Uncircumcised men are most likely to be affected. Almost all tumors of the penis are painless, of epithelial origin, and usually involve the distal portion of the penis where they are hidden in the nonretractable foreskin.[60,61] Approximately 95% of penile cancers are squamous cell carcinomas.[60]

Penile cancers usually present in the sixth and seventh decades of life are thought to be caused by chronic irritation.[60,61] The presence of foreskin, poor hygiene, and phimosis, a condition when the foreskin is too tight to retract, are associated with the development of penile cancers through the accumulation of smegma and other irritants.[43,60] In fact, neonatal circumcision can virtually eliminate the risk of penile cancer.[60] The same strains of human papilloma virus (HPV) found to cause cervical cancers in women also have a relationship to the development of penile cancers in men.[60] Delays in seeking medical attention result in more advanced disease, and if left untreated, penile cancer has a 2-year mortality rate.[60]

Ultrasound is not the first modality of choice to determine the extent of soft tissue involvement. Most often, physicians will order an MRI because it is the most accurate owing to its superior soft tissue and spatial resolution.[43,60,62] Computed tomography does not accurately define the local extension of the primary cancer. However, it is useful in assessing metastases and postoperative complications.[60,62] On ultrasound, penile tumors can present as either hypoechoic or hyperechoic solid masses, with ill-defined borders[43,60,61] (Fig. 19-57). Dedicated ultrasound for the detection of cancer in the glans penis is not reliable in differentiating between

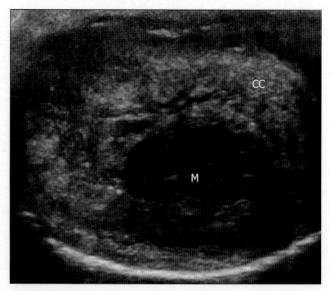

FIGURE 19-57 Penile carcinoma. Transverse view of a hypoechoic penile mass (*M*) with irregular ill-defined borders within the corpora cavernosa (*CC*). (Image courtesy of ultrasoundcases.info, © Sonoskills.)

an invasion of the subepithelial tissue and the corpora spongiosum.[60,61] Despite this, invasion into the tunica albuginea of the corpus cavernosum can clearly be demonstrated on ultrasound.[60,61] Ultrasound is utilized to evaluate inguinal lymph nodes for metastatic disease because they are usually the first site affected and to assist in ultrasound-guided lymph node biopsies.[43,60,61] Secondary or metastatic tumors of the penis have also been reported. In approximately 70% of the known cases, the primary tumor was located in the urogenital tract[60] (Fig. 19-58A, B).

The most common treatment for penile carcinoma is a partial penectomy.[60] Because the most common location is the glans penis (48%),[60] most men have enough penile length to necessitate a partial penectomy, which needs to include a 2 cm margin of tumor-free tissue necessary for amputation.[43,60] Bulky tumors or masses in the more proximal

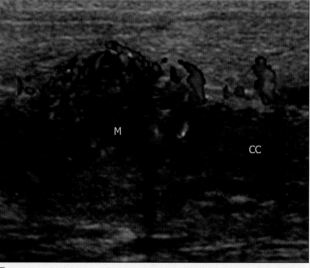

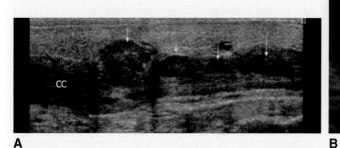

A   **B**

FIGURE 19-58 Metastatic disease. **A:** Longitudinal view of multiple hypoechoic metastatic masses (*arrows*) along the corpora cavernosum (*CC*) in a patient with prostate cancer. (Image courtesy of ultrasoundcases.info, © Sonoskills.) **B:** Color Doppler image of a metastatic lesion (*M*) within the cavernosum (*CC*) showing irregular hyperemic vascularity around the mass. (Image courtesy of ultrasoundcases.info, © Sonoskills.)

penis are treated with total penectomy and perineal urethrostomy.[60] Radiation is not frequently used because penile cancers tend to be resistant to the treatment. Approximately 30% to 50% of patients who undergo radiation will need a subsequent penectomy.[60] Chemotherapy is often limited to the treatment of metastatic lymphadenopathy.[60]

Trauma

Penile trauma can result from a blunt or penetrating injury. Imaging modalities are rarely utilized to investigate a penetrating trauma because most cases require immediate surgical exploration.[43,44] In the erect penis, trauma results from strain and increased pressure on an already thinned and stretched tunica albuginea.[43,44,63] The normal thickness of the tunica in a flaccid penis is about 2 mm, whereas during an erection, the tunica is thinned to 0.5 mm or less.[45,63,64] When an external force is applied to the erect penis, the increased intracorporeal pressure can result in a segmental rupture of one or both of the corpora cavernosa, constituting a penile fracture.[44,63] The most common cause of penile fracture is rigorous sexual intercourse as the penis hits the pubis symphysis or perineum and bends with enough force to rupture the tunica.[63,64] A blunt trauma to the flaccid penis does not lead to penile rupture and usually causes extratunical or cavernosal hematomas.[63]

Penile fractures are rare urologic emergencies. Most patients report hearing a cracking or popping sound with a sharp pain followed by rapid detumescence, swelling, discoloration, and deformity of the penis.[63,64] Fracture of the penis should be suspected on ultrasound if any loss of continuity or interruption of the tunica albuginea and disruption of the corpora cavernosa is detected.[46,63,64] Small, moderate, or broad hypoechoic hematomas surround and demonstrate the extent of that discontinuity[44,64] (Fig. 19-59A, B). Intracavernous hematomas, with or without the presence of a tunica albuginea tear, can be seen just below the tunica or in the surrounding sinusoidal spaces.[64] Penile fractures

are often associated with urethral tears, and blood products can be observed in the urethral meatus.

Although the findings may be clinically obvious, sonography can be helpful for vascular evaluation. Blunt trauma can create arterial fistulas in the sinusoidal spaces as described in high-flow priapism.[43,54,63,64] Intracavernosal hematomas are usually bilateral and result from injury to the cavernosal tissue when the base of the penis is crushed against the pelvic bones, commonly called a straddle injury.[64] Hematomas may be purely intracavernosal or extend to the perineum, scrotum, or even the thighs.[63,64] Sonographic appearance of a hematoma varies with the age of the lesion. Hematomas appear as hypoechoic, hyperechoic, or complex masses in the acute phase, eventually becoming more cystic with septations[43,63,64] (Fig. 19-60). Sonography is ideal for evaluating patients with penile trauma because it can show the integrity of the tunica albuginea as well as the extent and location of a tunica tear.[63,64] Color and spectral Doppler can also demonstrate the associated vascular injuries. The extent of the fracture, rupture, or hematoma can be limited on ultrasound but MRI can facilitate the diagnosis.[62]

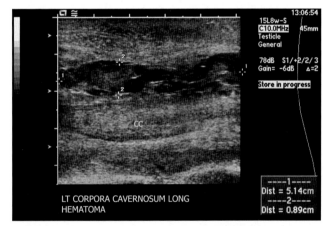

FIGURE 19-60 Trauma. Longitudinal view of a complex hematoma (*calipers*) over the corpora cavernosum in a patient with penile fracture.

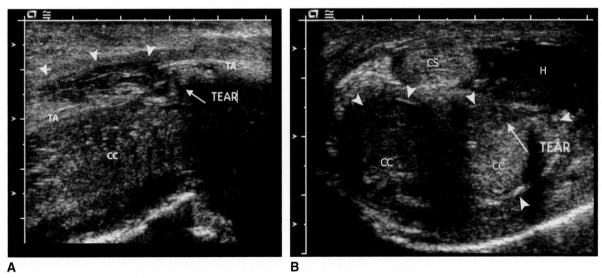

A   **B**

FIGURE 19-59 Trauma. **A:** Sagittal view demonstrates appreciable defect (*arrow* "*TEAR*") in the tunica albuginea (*TA*) of the cavernosum (*CC*) with a hypoechoic hematoma (*arrowheads*) emanating from the tear in a patient with a penile fracture. **B:** Transverse view of the hemorrhagic rupture of the left corpora cavernosum (*CC*). The defect (*arrow* "*TEAR*") shows discontinuity of the tunica albuginea (*arrowheads*), which is otherwise intact. The resulting hypoechoic hematoma (*H*) is seen in a patient presenting with a penile fracture. *CS*, spongiosum.

Penile trauma may result from foreign bodies inserted into the urethra. Urethral foreign-body insertions are rare but the behavior is commonly recurrent and driven by sexual stimulation, erectile enhancement, or attention-seeking behavior.[65] Urethral trauma related to foreign-body insertion is associated with significant risk of infection, abscess, and urethral injury with long-term tissue damage and strictures.[65] The presenting symptoms included dysuria, gross hematuria, urinary retention, urinary tract infection, and penile discharge.[65] Patients have reported a wide variety of items used for urethral insertion such as plastic, pieces of metal, paper, writing utensils, and wires. Foreign bodies on ultrasound appear as hyperechoic structures with artifacts and attenuation within the corpus spongiosum along the path of the urethra[43,65] (Fig. 19-61A, B).

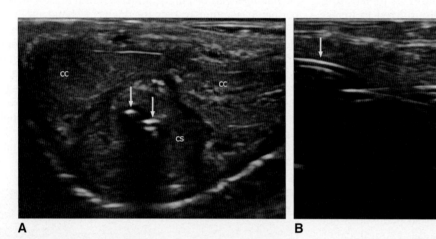

FIGURE 19-61 Foreign body. **A:** Transverse view showing a hyperechoic foreign body (*arrows*) centrally within the corpus spongiosum (*CS*). The corpora cavernosa (*CC*) are seen at the top of the image from this dorsal approach. (Image courtesy of ultrasoundcases.info, © Sonoskills.) **B:** Sagittal view of the penis with a foreign body (*arrows*) coursing through the corpus spongiosum (*CS*). Patient had inserted an electrical wire into his urethra. (Image courtesy of ultrasoundcases.info, © Sonoskills.)

SUMMARY

- Grayscale sonography with color, power, and spectral Doppler is the imaging modality of choice for evaluating patients with acute scrotal pain, undescended testis, or a scrotal mass.
- Sonographic evaluation begins with a side-by-side, large FOV image of both testes simultaneously, to compare their size, echogenicity, and vascular perfusion.
- The scrotal sac contains the testis, epididymis (head, body, and tail), and scrotal portion of the spermatic cord.
- The head of the epididymis lies superolaterally to the testes and measures 10 to 12 mm in anteroposterior diameter, and 5 to 12 mm in length.
- The tunica vaginalis is a peritoneal sac composed of two layers that surround the testis and epididymis. Serous fluid can accumulate between the layers to form a hydrocele.
- The adult testis is homogeneous with medium-level echoes and measures 3 to 5 cm in length and 2 to 3 cm in the transverse and anteroposterior diameters.
- Undescended testes are located within the inguinal canal in 80% of cases. Scrotal malignancy, torsion, and infertility are all associated with undiagnosed undescended testes.
- Causes of acute painful scrotum include epididymitis, epididymo-orchitis, orchitis, testicular torsion, trauma, torsion of the testicular appendices, scrotal wall inflammation, and incarcerated inguinal hernia.
- Color, power, and spectral Doppler are used to distinguish infectious processes from testicular torsion.
- The majority of extratesticular masses are benign, whereas intratesticular masses are considered malignant until proven otherwise.
- Varicoceles are dilated veins (≥3 mm) of the pampiniform plexus located superior and posterior to the testis. They usually occur on the left side and are associated with infertility.
- Leydig cell and Sertoli cell tumors are typically benign intrascrotal tumors and are rare.
- Testicular microlithiasis is diagnosed sonographically when more than five echogenic, nonshadowing foci are seen per transducer field. Microlithiasis is associated with an increased risk of scrotal malignancy.
- Malignant germ cell tumors constitute 90% to 95% of primary intratesticular malignancies and are divided into seminomas and nonseminomatous tumors.
- Seminomas are the most common primary testicular cancer.
- Nonseminomatous germ cell tumors include embryonal cell carcinoma, choriocarcinoma, teratoma, yolk sac tumor, and mixed germ cell tumors.
- Knowledge of normal and abnormal scrotal anatomy, consistent use of a methodical protocol, and application of the appropriate imaging parameters are essential for reliable diagnosis of scrotal disease.
- The penis consists of three cylindrical columns of spongy tissue: two corpora cavernosa and one corpus spongiosum. The spongiosum adds little to the rigidity of an erection.
- The hyperechoic fascial line that encapsulates the three columns of spongy tissue and provides structure and

support is the tunica albuginea. Another thick fibrous sheath called Buck fascia covers the tunica.

- Color Doppler is useful in determining the difference between low- and high-flow priapism. Understanding the sonographic appearances of each is crucial to deliver prompt treatment because one is a urologic emergency and the other is not.
- Penile fibromatosis or Peyronie disease is a physical and psychologically devastating disease characterized by plaque formation that can lead to deformities of the penis, painful erections, and erectile dysfunction (ED).
- ED can be a combination of many factors. Doppler ultrasound is useful in determining if a vascular etiology is responsible. ED could be caused by arterial sufficiency or venous incompetence.

- Penile carcinomas are rare and account for only 1% of all cancers in the Western world in contrast to occurring in 10% to 20% of all carcinomas in Asia, Africa, and South America. Neonatal circumcision can potentially eliminate the risk for carcinomas.
- A focal break or discontinuity of the tunica albuginea with associated hematoma is suggestive of penile fracture. Diagnosis should include a thorough correlation with patient clinical history.
- Ultrasound is a useful method, both for its availability and efficacy in penile evaluation. A knowledge of how to differentiate between normal and pathologic aspects of the penis is important for accurate diagnosis and prompt patient management.

ACKNOWLEDGMENTS

The authors extend their sincere thanks to David Brix RDMS, RVT for his assistance in creating illustrations and editing images. They would also like to thank Eric Hirshik RDMS, RVT, for his help in editing this chapter.

REFERENCES

1. Thinyu S, Muttarak M. Role of sonography in diagnosis of scrotal disorders: a review of 110 cases. *Biomed Imaging Interv J*. 2009;5:1–10.
2. Chandler AM, Leonhardt WC. Scrotal and penile sonography. In: Curry RA, Prince M, eds. *Sonography: Introduction to Normal Structure and Function*. 5th ed. Elsevier; 2021:501–516.
3. Kuhn AL, Scortegagna E, Nowitzki KM, et al. Ultrasonography of the scrotum in adults. *Ultrasonography*. 2016;35:180–197.
4. Kim W, Rosen MA, Langer JE, et al. US MR imaging correlation in pathologic conditions of the scrotum. *Radiographics*. 2007;27:1239–1253.
5. Chen P, John S. Ultrasound of the acute scrotum. *Appl Radiol*. 2006;8–17.
6. Owen CA, Winter T. Color Doppler imaging of the scrotum. *J Diagn Med Sonogr*. 2006;22:221–230.
7. Leonhardt WC, Lalani, ZH. Scrotum. In: Kawamura DM, Lunsford, BM, eds. *Diagnostic Medical Sonography*. 3rd ed. Lippincott Williams & Wilkins; 2012:529–270.
8. Woodward PJ, Schwab CM, Sesterhenn IA. Extratesticular scrotal masses: radiologic-pathologic correlation. *Radiographics*. 2003;23:215–240.
9. Gorman B. The scrotum. In: Rumack CM, Wilson S, Charboneau JW, et al., eds. *Diagnostic Ultrasound*. 4th ed. Elsevier Mosby; 2011:840–877.
10. Kocakoc E, Bhatt S, Dogra VS. Ultrasound evaluation of testicular neoplasms. *Ultrasound Clin*. 2007;2:27–44.
11. Turgut AT, Bhatt S, Dogra VS. Acute painful scrotum. *Ultrasound Clin*. 2008;3:93–107.
12. Bhatt S, Ghazale H, Dogra VS. Sonographic evaluation of scrotal and penile trauma. *Ultrasound Clin*. 2007;2:45–56.
13. Townsend RR, Cheeawai RA, Lee RS. Color evaluation of testicular torsion with subsequent blood flow after immediate manual detorsion. *J Diagn Med Sonogr*. 1999;15:197–202.
14. Dogra VS, Bhatt S, Rubens DJ. Sonographic evaluation of testicular torsion. *Ultrasound Clin*. 2006;1:55–66.
15. Paunipagar BK. Scrotal sonography. In: Ahuja AT, ed. *Diagnostic Imaging Ultrasound*. Amirsys; 2007:1020–1044.
16. Dogra VS, Gottlieb RH, Oka M, et al. Sonography of the scrotum. *Radiology*. 2003;227:18–36.
17. Mihmanli I, Kantarci F. Sonography of scrotal abnormalities in adults: an update. *Diagn Interv Radiol*. 2009;15(1):64–73.
18. Bertolotto M, Freeman S, Richenberg J, et al. Ultrasound evaluation of varicoceles: systematic literature review and rationale of the ESUR-SPIWG guidelines and recommendations. *J Ultrasound*. 2020;23:487–507.
19. Deurdulian C, Mittelstaedt CA, Chong WK, et al. US of acute scrotal trauma: optimal technique, imaging findings, and management. *Radiographics*. 2007;27:357–369.
20. Horstman WG, Middleton WD, Melson GL. Scrotal inflammatory disease: color Doppler US findings. *Radiology*. 1991;179:55–59.
21. Pearl MS, Hill MC. Ultrasound of the scrotum. *Semin Ultrasound CT MR*. 2007;28:225–248.
22. Muttarak M, ChiangMai WN, Lojanapiwat B. Tuberculosis of the genitourinary tract: imaging features with pathological correlation. *Singapore Med J*. 2005;46:568–575.
23. Futterer JJ, Heijmink S, Spermon JR, et al. Imaging the male reproductive tract: current trends and future directions. *Radiol Clin North Am*. 2008;46:133–147.
24. Lee JC, Bhatt S, Dogra VS. Imaging of the epididymis. *Ultrasound Q*. 2008;24:3–16.
25. Smart JM, Jackson EK, Redman SL, et al. Ultrasound findings of masses of the paratesticular space. *Clin Radiol*. 2008;63:929–938.
26. Hricak H, Hamm B, Kim B, eds. *Imaging of the Scrotum*. Raven Press; 1995.
27. Feld R, Middleton WD. Recent advances in sonography of the testes and scrotum. *Radiol Clin North Am*. 1992;30:1033–1049.
28. Horstman WG, Middleton WD, Melson GL, et al. Color Doppler US of the scrotum. *Radiographics*. 1991;11:941–957.
29. Middleton WD, Bell MW. Analysis of intratesticular arterial anatomy with emphasis on transmediastinal arteries. *Radiology*. 1993;189:157–160.
30. Vijayaraghavan SB. Sonographic differential diagnosis of acute scrotum: real-time Whirlpool Sign, a key sign of torsion. *J Ultrasound Med*. 2006;25:563–574.
31. Stengel JW, Remer EM. Sonography of the scrotum: case based review. *AJR Am J Roentgenol*. 2008;190:S35–S41.
32. Chen L, Huang X, YI Z, et al. Ultrasound imaging findings of acute testicular infection in patients with coronavirus disease 2019. *J Ultrasound Med*. 2020;9999:1–8.
33. Safriel Y, Cohen HL, Torrisi J. Ultrasound imaging of scrotal wall thickening and its significance in the diagnosis of Fournier's Gangrene in older men. *J Diagn Med Sonogr*. 2000;16:29–33.
34. Ledwidge ME, Lee DK, Winter,TC, et al. Sonographic diagnosis of superior hemispheric testicular infarction. *AJR Am J Roentgenol*. 2002;179:775–776.
35. Sista AK, Filly RA. Color sonography in evaluation of spermatoceles. *J Ultrasound Med*. 2008;27:141–143.
36. Martinez-Berganza MT, Sarria L, Cozcolluela R, et al. Cysts of the tunica albuginea: sonographic appearance. *AJR Am J Roentgenol*. 1998;170:183–185.
37. Burks DD, Markey BJ, Burkhard TK, et al. Suspected testicular torsion and ischemia: evaluation with color Doppler sonography. *Radiology*. 1990;175:815–821.

38. Leonhardt WC, Gooding GAW. Sonography of intrascrotal adeno-matoid tumor. *Urology.* 1992;39:90–92.

39. Singh V, Srivastava H. Leydig cell tumor of the testis—a case report. *Indian J Urol.* 2004;20:166.

40. Woodward PF, Sohaey R, O'Donoghue MF, et al. Tumors and tumor-like lesions of the testis: radiologic-pathologic correlation. *Radiographics.* 2002;22:189–216.

41. Loya AG, Said JW, Grant EG. Epidermoid cyst of the testis: radio-logic-pathologic correlation. *Radiographics.* 2004;24:S243–S246.

42. Cast JEI, Nelson WM, Early AS, et al. Testicular microlithiasis: prevalence and tumor risk in a population referred for scrotal sonography. *AJR Am J Roentgenol.* 2000;175:1703–1706.

43. King B. The penis. In: Rumack C, Wilson S, Charboneau J. *Diagnostic Ultrasound, Volume One.* Mosby-Year Book, Inc.; 1991:591–607.

44. Fernandes MA, Ferreira de Souza L, Cartafina L. Ultrasound evalu-ation of the penis. *Radiol Bras.* 2018;51(4):257–261.

45. Jung DC, Park SY, Lee JY. Penile Doppler ultrasonography revisited. *Ultrasonography.* 2018;37(1):16–24.

46. Netter F. *Atlas of Human Anatomy.* 4th ed. Saunders Elsevier, Inc.; 2006:381–382.

47. Size G, Lozanski L, Russo T. Penile testing. In: French-Sherry E, Skelly CL, eds. *Inside Ultrasound Vascular Reference Guide.* 1st ed. Inside Ultrasound, Inc.; 2018:202–207.

48. Benson CB. Duplex ultrasound evaluation of the male genitalia. In: Polak JF, Pellerito JS, eds. *Introduction to Vascular Ultrasonography.* 6th ed. Elsevier Saunders; 2012:559–578.

49. Gatz VM, Erpelding SG, Shubham G. Evaluation of penile blood flow. In: Kupinski AM, ed. *The Vascular System.* 2nd ed. Wolters Kluwer Health; 2017:427–433.

50. Halls JE, Patel DV, Walkden M, et al. Priapism: pathophysiology and the role of the radiologist. *Br J Radiol.* 2012;85:S79–S85.

51. Van Der Horst C, Stuebinger H, Seif C, et al. Priapism-etiology, patho-physiology and management. *Int Braz J Urol.* 2003;29(5):391–400.

52. Canguven O, Cetinel C, Horuz R, et al. Transient distal penile corporoglanular shunt as an adjunct to aspiration and irrigation procedures in the treatment of early ischemic priapism. *Korean J Urol.* 2013;54(6):394–398.

53. Bertolotto M, Serafini G, Savoca G, et al. Color Doppler US of the postoperative penis: anatomy and surgical complications. *Radio-graphics.* 2005;25:731–748.

54. Wu AK, Lue TF. Commentary on high flow, non-ischemic, priapism. *Transl Androl Urol.* 2012;1(2):109–112.

55. Kalokairinou K, Konstantinidis C, Domazou M, et al. US imaging in Peyronie's disease. *J Clin Imaging Sci.* 2012;2:63.

56. Nugteren HM, Nijman JM, de Jong IJ, et al. The association between Peyronie's and Dupuytren's disease. *Int J Imp Res.* 2011;23:142–145.

57. Shindel A, Sweet G, Thieu W, et al. Prevalence of Peyronie's disease-like symptoms in men presenting with Dupuytren con-tractures. *Sex Med.* 2017;5(3):135–141.

58. Richards G, Goldenberg E, Pek H, et al. Penile Sonoelestography for the localization of a non-palpable, non-sonographically visualized lesion in a patient with penile curvature from Peyronie's disease. *J Sex Med.* 2014;11(2):516–520.

59. Golijanin D, Singer E, Davis R, et al. Doppler evaluation of erectile dysfunction-part 1 & part 2. *Int J Impot Res.* 2007;19:37–42.

60. Singh AK, Saokar A, Hahn PF, et al. Imaging of penile neoplasms. *RadioGraphics.* 2005;25:1629–1638.

61. Horenblas S, Kroger R, Gallee MP, et al. Ultrasound in squamous cell carcinoma of the penis; a useful addition to clinical stag-ing? A comparison of ultrasound with histopathology. *Urology.* 1994;43(5):702–707.

62. Parker RA, Menias CO, Quazi R, et al. MR imaging of the penis and scrotum. *RadioGraphics.* 2015;35:1033–1050.

63. Kachewar SG, Kulkarni DS. Ultrasound evaluation of penile frac-tures. *Biomed Imaging Interv J.* 2011;7(4):e27.

64. Bhatt S, Kocakoc E, Rubens DJ, et al. Sonographic evaluation of penile trauma. American Institute of Ultrasound in Medicine. *J Ultrasound Med.* 2005;24:993–1000.

65. Palmer CJ, Houlihan M, Psutka SP, et al. Urethral foreign bodies: clinical presentation and management. *Urology.* 2016;97:257–260.

CHAPTER 20

The Pediatric Abdomen

TARA K. CIELMA AND ANJUM N. BANDARKAR

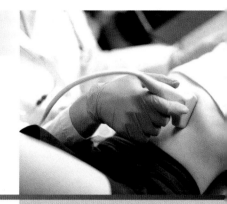

OBJECTIVES

- Demonstrate the sonographic scanning techniques, technical considerations, and routine examination for the neonatal and pediatric abdomen to include the prevertebral vessel (aorta and inferior vena cava) evaluation, liver, gallbladder and biliary system, pancreas, gastrointestinal tract, and retroperitoneum.

- Describe the pathology, etiology, and clinical signs and symptoms for anomalies and pathology of the aorta and inferior vena cava, liver, gallbladder and biliary system, pancreas, gastrointestinal tract, and retroperitoneum in the neonate and pediatric patient.

- Differentiate between the sonographic appearance of the normal prevertebral vasculature and the sonographic appearance for congenital anomalies and acquired pathology of the prevertebral vessels, liver, gallbladder and biliary system, pancreas, gastrointestinal tract, and retroperitoneum in the neonate and pediatric patient.

- Identify technically satisfactory and unsatisfactory sonographic examinations of the abdomen on the neonatal and pediatric patient.

- List the indications for the sonographic evaluation of urinary system and adrenal glands in the pediatric patient.

- Explain the protocol process for sonographic evaluation of the urinary system and adrenal glands in the pediatric patient.

- Identify the normal sonographic appearance of the urinary system and the adrenal glands in the pediatric patient.

- Describe the pathology, etiology, clinical signs and symptoms, and sonographic appearance of common congenital abnormalities, tumors, and acquired pathology in the upper and lower urinary system in the pediatric patient.

- Discuss three criteria for sonographic documentation of tumors on pediatric patients to include (1) origin of the mass, (2) extent of the mass, and (3) metastases.

- Describe the pathology, etiology, clinical signs and symptoms, and sonographic appearance of congenital abnormalities, tumors, hemorrhage, cysts, and abscesses of the adrenal glands in the pediatric patient.

- Identify technically satisfactory and unsatisfactory sonographic examinations of the urinary system and adrenal glands on the neonatal and pediatric patient.

KEY TERMS

adrenal hemorrhage

adrenocortical carcinoma

angiomyolipoma

appendicitis

biliary atresia

Budd–Chiari syndrome

Caroli disease

cavernous hemangioma

cholecystitis

choledochal cyst

cholelithiasis

cirrhosis

congenital adrenal hyperplasia

Crohn disease

cystic fibrosis

cystitis

duplicated collecting system

echinococcal cyst

glomerular cystic disease

hemangioendothelioma

hepatic fibrosis

hepatitis

hepatoblastoma

hepatocellular carcinoma

hepatoma

(continued)

GLOSSARY

AFP alpha-fetoprotein; a tumor marker frequently elevated in cases of hepatocellular carcinoma, hepatoblastoma, and certain testicular cancers

biloma a walled-off collection of bile caused by a disruption of the biliary tree, frequently caused by trauma or surgical procedures

coarctation a narrowing or constriction

enuresis involuntary discharge of urine

hemobilia hemorrhage or blood in the bile caused by bleeding into the biliary tree

hemoperitoneum blood in the peritoneal cavity

hyperalimentation the administration of nutrients through intravenous feeding

hyponatremia an electrolyte imbalance; low sodium levels in the blood

ileus failure of the normal propulsion of the digestive tract

jaundice yellowish pigmentation of the skin and whites of the eyes caused by increased levels of bilirubin in the blood

reflux occurs when valves at the junction of the ureter and bladder work incorrectly and allow urine from the bladder to back up into the ureter and kidney

ureteropelvic junction area where the renal pelvis connects to the ureter

Sonography is the noninvasive modality of choice to evaluate the neonatal and pediatric abdomen owing to the lack of ionizing radiation, the portability of the equipment, and excellent visualization of the abdominal anatomy in this age group. Critically ill patients who are sensitive to stress (i.e., transport, temperature changes) can easily and safely be examined at the bedside. Pediatric sonography presents many opportunities as well as challenges. Childhood obesity is a serious health care problem, and obese children may be as challenging to examine sonographically as adults. Obese children may also present with some disease processes previously seen only in adults, so the sonographer must have an in-depth knowledge of both pediatric and adult pathology.

SONOGRAPHIC EXAMINATION TECHNIQUES[1–3]

Scanning the pediatric age group will require sonographic equipment with a wide range of probe frequencies. Depending on the area or organ of interest, a high-frequency (7 to 10 MHz) curved or (8 to 11 MHz) micro-convex or (8 to 15 MHz) linear-array transducer is utilized. Scanning infants and small children requires the sonographer to be adept at assessing the anatomy and acquiring images quickly. Distraction techniques are used for this age group rather than sedation. Children with high level of pain, anxiety, or autism spectrum disorder with comorbid developmental delay may or may not be able to cooperate fully during the sonogram, so distractions such as headphones, development-appropriate movies, or other resources can be used to ensure the sonographer can complete the examination accurately and in a timely manner. Many health care facilities now employ Certified Child Life Specialists; these professionals may be utilized to assist with therapeutic play and assist with coping skills to manage stressful experiences.

A parent or legal guardian will most likely be present for the examination. The sonographer must be prepared to professionally interact with the parent and elicit their assistance with the examination, as needed. The sonographer should always explain the examination to the patient using age-appropriate terms, provide realistic expectations, and should answer the parent's questions about the examination in accordance with department policies and procedures. Special precautions should be taken to keep infants warm by placing blankets over all but the scanning surface. Warm gel should always be used on children. Single packets of gel for infection control must be used for neonates and critical care patients. Sterile gel packets should be used whenever a sterile area must be maintained or in cases where infection is of high concern. The sonographer must always follow infection control standards when scanning, and this can be even more important when examining pediatric patients.

A pediatric abdominal sonogram should include an assessment of all the organs, structures, and vessels of the abdomen. This chapter discusses the abdominal vessels as well as the liver, gallbladder/biliary system, pancreas, gastrointestinal (GI) tract, retroperitoneum, urinary system, and adrenal glands. The sonographer should have as much information as possible regarding the reason for the sonogram, incorporate prior diagnostic imaging, and be prepared to adapt the examination to the patient's condition and any sonographic findings.

Patient Preparation

Patient preparation will vary based on the age of the patient and the area or organ of interest. Ideally, the liver and biliary tree are best viewed with the patient in a fasting state. As infants are fed every 3 to 4 hours, the examination should be performed just before a feeding. Children aged 1 to 3 years are best examined 4 hours after fasting and older children 6 hours after fasting. Children with gastronomy (G) or gastronomy–jejunostomy (GJ) tubes are typically fasted between 4 and 6 hours before the procedure. Diabetic patients may require prioritization according to their insulin schedule and may be permitted clear liquids.

PREVERTEBRAL VESSEL EVALUATION

Sonographic Examination Technique

Patient Preparation

Although anatomically they are similar to adults, neonates and children require a different scanning approach. Using multiple planes on the neonate, the full length of the great vessels can easily be evaluated from the level of the diaphragm to the bifurcation without any particular patient preparation.

Depending on which great vessel is to be evaluated, it may be necessary to turn the patient to the appropriate side. Patients in the neonatal intensive care unit are often intubated, so if it is necessary to turn the patient onto one side or the other, it is advisable to seek the aid of the bedside nurse.

Scan Technique

In the neonate, coronal scanning is often most effective in demonstrating the aorta and inferior vena cava (IVC). Scanning from a right coronal approach is more optimal for evaluating the IVC because the vessel is closer to the transducer placed on the right lateral abdomen. Similarly, a left coronal approach on the left lateral abdomen is used to visualize the aorta.

The sonographic examination of the abdominal vessels should include assessment of the vessels in multiple scan planes and the use of color and spectral Doppler to assess blood flow. The sonographer should acquire documentary images that clearly demonstrate the aorta and IVC from proximal to distal (bifurcation), including sonographically visible branches and tributaries. Split-screen color Doppler and grayscale imaging can be used to demonstrate the vessels when grayscale alone is insufficient, or pathology is present. Color and spectral Doppler should also be used to evaluate flow in the aorta, IVC, right and left iliac arteries and veins, and right and left renal arteries and veins. Correct presentation of the abdominal aorta and IVC must be documented so that the correct location and course of these vessels are confirmed.

When present in the neonate, an indwelling catheter in the aorta and its relationship to the renal arteries should be demonstrated. Although an umbilical arterial catheter (UAC) is visible on a radiograph, the location relative to the origin of the renal arteries cannot be reliably determined. Proper location of the tip of the UAC is in the aorta well above the level of the renal arteries. Umbilical venous catheter (UVC) may also be present in the umbilicus next to a UAC (or by itself). The UVC should course through the liver via the umbilical vein and the left hepatic vein. The tip should be in the proximal IVC near the junction of the right atrium. Sonographically, the UAC and UVC are visualized as hyperechoic parallel lines with an anechoic center. Shadowing from the walls of the line may be noted when the beam is perpendicular to the catheter. It is important not to confuse this for intrahepatic calcifications, which may result as a complication from improper UVC placement.

Normal Anatomy

The sonographic appearance of the abdominal vessels in the pediatric patient is the same as in an adult (Fig. 20-1A, B). The vessels should have anechoic lumens with hyperechoic walls. The walls of the abdominal aorta may appear more echogenic than the walls of the IVC. The normal spectral Doppler of the aorta shows a pulsatile vessel with a high-resistance flow pattern (rapid upstroke, sharp systolic peak, and low-flow velocity with a small amount of reversed flow possible during diastole). The normal spectral Doppler flow pattern of the IVC is monophasic.

Congenital Anomalies

Coarctation of the Abdominal Aorta[4,5]

Hypoplasia or coarctation of the abdominal aorta is a rare congenital defect. The proximal descending thoracic aorta is affected in 98% of coarctations, only 2% of them actually affect the abdominal aorta (Fig. 20-2A, B). Renal artery stenosis occurs in more than half of abdominal coarctations. Congenital abdominal coarctation can occur at any time in embryonic development. The earlier it occurs, the more obvious the manifestations. Acquired coarctation of the abdominal aorta

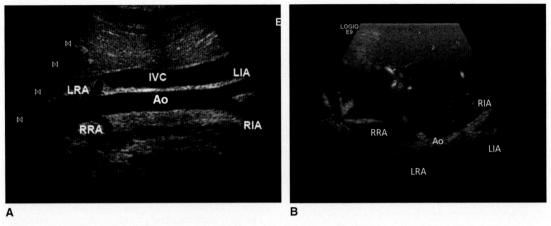

FIGURE 20-1 Abdominal vessels. The aorta (*Ao*), right and left renal arteries (*RRA* and *LRA*), right and left iliac arteries (*RIA* and *LIA*), and inferior vena cava (*IVC*) are seen in this longitudinal, coronal grayscale, and B-flow (**B**) image. (Image **A**: Courtesy of GE Healthcare, Wauwatosa, WI.)

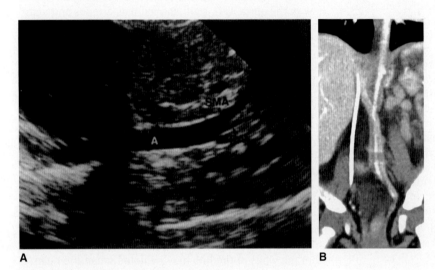

FIGURE 20-2 Coarctation of the abdominal aorta. **A:** Coarctation of the abdominal aorta (*Ao*) is demonstrated on this longitudinal section with the interruption of the abdominal aorta and collateral circulation of the superior mesenteric artery (*SMA*) and renal artery (*RA*). **B:** There is hypoplasia of the inferior abdominal aorta with hypertrophied collateral artery, which courses anterior to the midline.

has been associated with hypercalcemia, neurofibromatosis, tuberous sclerosis, rubella, and Turner syndrome. Children present with severe hypertension, headaches, and fatigue, whereas infants exhibit failure to thrive. An interrupted abdominal aorta produces vascular compromise with symptoms such as cyanotic, mottled, and discolored limbs with decreased femoral pulses. The extreme consequences of untreated severe hypertension can be fatal by the age of 30 years.

Inferior Vena Cava

When scanning the IVC and the aorta, the sonographer must note both the position and relationship of the two vessels. In the normal relationship, the IVC is located on the right side, receiving the hepatic veins as it enters the right atrium. An IVC on the patient's left side is diagnostic of situs inversus. Besides an abnormal relationship of the IVC and aorta, the IVC can also be interrupted, in which case it drains via an azygous continuation, which may lie on either the left or the right of the spine. The hemiazygous continuation lies more posterior than the aorta (Fig. 20-3A, B). Another abnormal vessel that may be imaged in the long-axis plane is an anomalous venous connection associated with total anomalous pulmonary venous return, which connects to the ductus venosus. It crosses between the aorta and IVC. Displacement or distortion of the IVC or the aorta should alert the sonographer that other anomalies may be present. Sonographers must be cognizant of the fact that unusual presentations of the aorta or IVC

and anomalous vessels in the lower abdomen may indicate complex congenital heart disease.

Acquired Pathologies[6,7]

Abdominal Aortic Thrombosis in the Neonate

The most common reason for evaluating the aorta in the neonate is for aortic thrombus, a well-recognized complication of indwelling UACs. Clinical signs of aortic thrombus include absent femoral pulses, hematuria, cyanosis, hypertension, blanching of the lower extremities, and necrotizing enterocolitis (NEC). An overly distended urinary bladder may cause some of the abovementioned symptoms.

Suspected aortic thrombus should be evaluated by a thorough scan of the entire aorta and both kidneys in multiple planes. Thrombus typically appears sonographically as echogenic material within the aortic lumen, which may totally or partially fill the vessel. The clot may be long and thick and is termed *extensive* if it fills 40% of the aorta in a sectional plane, goes to the level of the renal artery or iliac artery, or causes proximal dilatation. As the sonographic appearance of thrombus changes over time, the vessel may appear to contain thin linear structures. Color Doppler should be used to demonstrate any blood flow around the thrombus, normal flow reversal, and the presence of any collateral vessels. Grayscale and color Doppler should be used to follow the progression and/or resolution of the thrombus (Fig. 20-4A–D).

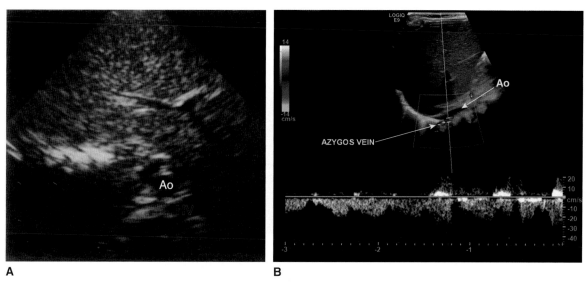

FIGURE 20-3 Interruption of the inferior vena cava. **A:** In this transverse scan low in the abdomen, the aorta (*Ao*) is demonstrated to the right of the draining venous structure. The interrupted inferior vena cava is not seen but drains through a hemiazygous vein (*azy*) with continuation seen posterior to the Ao. **B:** The pulsed Doppler spontaneous waveform of the posterior azygous vein demonstrated posterior to the proximal Ao. (Image **B:** Courtesy of Primary Children's Hospital, Salt Lake City, UT.)

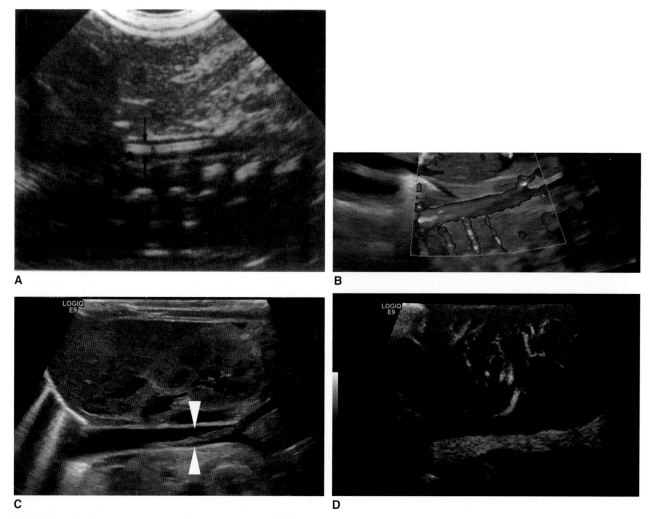

FIGURE 20-4 Umbilical arterial catheter (*UAC*). **A:** An indwelling UAC is visualized as two parallel lines (*arrow*), with an anechoic center representing the catheter lumen on this longitudinal section of the abdominal aorta (*A*). **B:** Patent vasculature is appreciated. **C:** A linear echogenic structure (*arrowheads*) extending from the mid-aorta through the aortic bifurcation into the right common iliac artery, compatible with nonobstructive thrombus in an ex-31-week neonate with DiGeorge syndrome on extracorporeal membranous oxygenation secondary to complex cardiac disease. **D:** Follow-up ultrasound demonstrates continued resolution of nonocclusive thrombus in the infrarenal aorta, seen on B-flow.

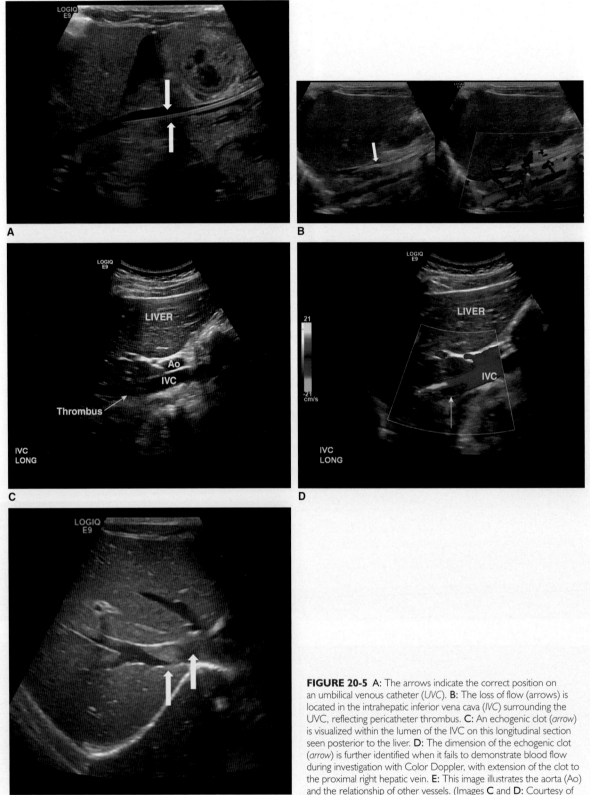

FIGURE 20-5 A: The arrows indicate the correct position on an umbilical venous catheter (*UVC*). **B:** The loss of flow (*arrows*) is located in the intrahepatic inferior vena cava (*IVC*) surrounding the UVC, reflecting pericatheter thrombus. **C:** An echogenic clot (*arrow*) is visualized within the lumen of the IVC on this longitudinal section seen posterior to the liver. **D:** The dimension of the echogenic clot (*arrow*) is further identified when it fails to demonstrate blood flow during investigation with Color Doppler, with extension of the clot to the proximal right hepatic vein. **E:** This image illustrates the aorta (*Ao*) and the relationship of other vessels. (Images **C** and **D:** Courtesy of Primary Children's Hospital, Salt Lake City, UT.)

Inferior Vena Cava Thrombosis[8]

The IVC can be a site of thrombus or calcifications in neonates. IVC thrombosis can also occur secondary to indwelling catheters (such as UVC), clotting disorders, dehydration, sepsis, nephrotic syndrome, and extension of renal and/or pelvic vein thrombosis (Fig. 20-5A, B).

Inferior Vena Cava Tumor Invasion[8]

Children can have tumor invasion into the IVC, from Wilms tumor (Fig. 20-5C–E). Tumor extension can occur from the kidney, adrenal gland (neuroblastoma), retroperitoneum (sarcoma), and from hepatocellular carcinoma (HCC), teratoma, and lymphoma. It is important to evaluate the extension of the tumor into the hepatic veins or right atrium and to seek evidence of tumor invasion into the wall of the IVC. Tumor extension appears similar to the solid texture of the tumor itself. The differential diagnosis includes simple thrombus. Computed tomography (CT) is the modality of choice for evaluating IVC wall invasion; however, sonography is the best modality for evaluating cephalad extension of IVC tumor invasion.

LIVER[9]

When imaging the neonatal or pediatric liver, it is important to image the same landmarks as in an adult examination. Special attention should be paid to the liver parenchyma, the position and size of the gallbladder, portal vein, portal vein bifurcation, hepatic artery, common bile duct, and hepatic veins.

Sonographic Examination and Technique

Scan Technique

Establishing a protocol of longitudinal, coronal, and transverse planes is important to ensure consistency from one patient to the next; however, special attention must be paid to differences, such as position of anatomy, pathology, and size. The sonographic examination of the pediatric liver should include assessment of the liver parenchyma, vessels and ligaments in multiple scan planes, and the use of color and/or spectral Doppler to assess blood flow. Patients are most commonly scanned in the supine position, but it is beneficial to utilize a left posterior oblique (LPO) position in older children and/or those with a larger body habitus. After sweeping through the entire liver, the sonographer should acquire representative images that clearly demonstrate the lobes and segments of the liver, including vascular and ligament landmarks. The sonographer should be careful to assess and document the periphery of the liver as well as the bulk of the liver; longitudinal and transverse sweeps should extend past the lateral, superior, and inferior borders of the liver. Normal measurement parameters for the liver have been reported and show correlation with age, height, and weight. Longitudinal images demonstrating the lower pole of the right kidney in relationship to the inferior margin of the liver can be helpful.

Normal Anatomy

The normal liver appears as a smooth-outlined, homogeneous organ, usually situated in the right upper quadrant of the abdomen (Fig. 20-6A). The neonatal liver may appear mildly hyperechoic. The liver is divided into a large right lobe in the right side of the abdomen, a smaller left lobe extending across the midline, a caudate lobe situated on the posterior

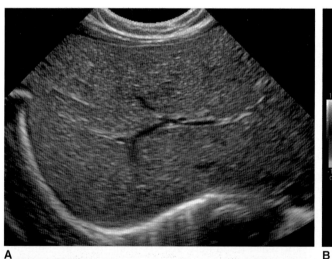

A

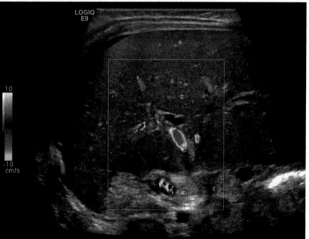

B

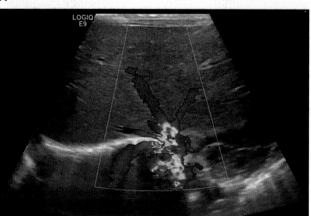

C

FIGURE 20-6 Neonatal liver. **A:** Transverse image of the liver in a neonatal patient demonstrates the normal homogeneous echo texture of liver and anechoic vasculature. (Image courtesy of Philips Medical Systems, Bothell, WA.) **B:** Transverse image of the liver in a neonatal patient demonstrating flow in the portal vein and hepatic veins. (Image courtesy of GE Healthcare, Wauwatosa, WI.) **C:** A high-frequency linear transducer is used to image the patient.

superior surface of the right lobe, and a quadrate lobe on the posteroinferior surface of the right lobe. The falciform ligament divides the right and left lobes. The liver receives a dual blood supply. The liver receives oxygenated blood from the hepatic artery, a branch of the celiac artery. Additional blood from the digestive system is carried to the liver via the portal vein, formed by the convergence of the superior mesenteric vein (SMV) and the splenic vein. The portal vein enters the liver at the porta hepatis, where it quickly branches into the right and left portal veins. The hepatic artery also enters the liver at the porta hepatis (Fig. 20-6B). The major vessels of the liver provide important visual and anatomic landmarks (Fig. 20-6C).

Applicable laboratory tests include the standard liver function tests and alpha-fetoprotein (AFP), which, if elevated, may indicate the presence of a hepatoblastoma or other malignant tumor.

Congenital Anomalies and Benign Tumors

Hemangiomas

Biliary atresia is a congenital anomaly that intricately involves the liver and is discussed in "Gallbladder and Biliary System" section. Other congenital anomalies of the liver are primarily composed of benign tumors.

Hemangiomas of the liver are congenital anomalies arising from an arteriovenous malformation, forming blood-filled spaces. They are the most common vascular liver tumor in infancy and are either cavernous (blood-filled spaces lined with a single layer of endothelial cells) or hemangioendotheliomas (the lining or endothelium is multilayered or hypertrophic, with primitive or infantile cells).

Infantile Hepatic Hemangioma[10–12]

Infantile hepatic hemangiomas usually affect infants less than 6 months of age, are typically multiple, and are associated with cutaneous hemangiomas. Patients are typically symptomatic and present clinically with hepatomegaly, congestive heart failure, and hemoperitoneum from rupture. Sonographically, the lesions can appear hypoechoic, isoechoic, or hyperechoic to adjacent liver tissue, homogeneous or complex, and may contain echogenic foci (Fig. 20-7A–F).

Depending on the composition, variable acoustic enhancement may be present.

Cavernous Hemangioma[10,13]

Hemangiomas are three times more common in girls than in boys. They may or may not be present at birth but usually become evident at about 2 months of age, or they may be found incidentally. Large hemangiomas may cause hepatomegaly, with or without accompanying abdominal distention. Hemangiomas cease to grow and then undergo spontaneous involution.

After the tumor enlarges but before regressing, the infant may experience a number of complications, including fatal rupture of the hemangioma, Kasabach–Merritt syndrome due to platelet trapping, hepatic dysfunction due to portal hypertension, intravascular coagulation, intestinal bleeding, bowel obstruction, obstructive jaundice, and irreversible congestive heart failure, as well as respiratory insufficiency caused by the mass effect.

Typical sonographic findings are of a well-defined, hyperechoic area within the liver (Fig. 20-8A). The hyperechoic appearance of hemangioma results from the multiple interfaces between the walls of the blood-filled sinuses. Less frequently, the mass is hypoechoic and may mimic a collection of simple cysts. It can also appear complex, demonstrating irregular walls and hypoechoic to anechoic areas, possibly due to necrosis (Fig. 20-8B, C). Contrast-enhanced ultrasound may be used to delineate perfusion patterns (Fig. 20-8D).

The presence of calcifications or fibrotic changes within the mass produces a hyperechoic pattern with posterior acoustic shadowing. Doppler interrogation may reveal high flow within the lesion. An enlarged hepatic artery, as well as a small distal aorta due to the increased hepatic flow, can also be seen.

Needle biopsy for confirmation of hemangiomas is a dangerous procedure that can result in fatal hemorrhage, so it is usually used as a last resort when a diagnosis cannot be reached by other means. The cytologic diagnostic criteria include the presence of benign epithelial cells, fresh blood from the mass, and no malignant cells.

The treatment of hemangioma varies with the size of the mass. Most hemangiomas undergo spontaneous involution and regression, but when a large hemangioma threatens the patient's health, aggressive procedures are instigated. A lobectomy or resection of the tumor is sometimes performed, but if the patient is experiencing congestive heart failure, hepatic artery ligation or embolization can be performed. In many cases, the lesion is responsive to steroid therapy and radiation therapy.

The differential diagnosis includes angiomatous tumors, hepatoblastoma, hepatoma and metastatic neuroblastoma, cysts, abscesses, and focal nodular hyperplasia.

Mesenchymal Hamartoma[10,14]

Mesenchymal or fibrous hamartoma is a rare congenital anomaly that arises from the connective tissue or mesenchyme of the portal tracts. It is considered to be the second most common benign hepatic mass seen in children and is more common in males.

The lesion usually presents within the first 2 years of life, with painless abdominal swelling and anorexia as the first clinical symptoms. Congestive heart failure has also been noted in patients with mesenchymal hamartoma due to arteriovenous shunting within the tumor. Patients can experience respiratory distress from the large, fluid-filled lesion if fluid accumulation has been rapid. Liver function tests are usually normal.

Sonographically, mesenchymal hamartoma is sometimes mistaken for hemangioma; however, although it frequently reveals internal septations demonstrating a complex appearance, it is avascular. These septations are strands of hepatocytes, bile duct elements, or mesenchyme separating multiple cysts. The hamartoma is usually situated in the right lobe.

The prognosis of mesenchymal hamartoma is excellent. Resection is usually all that is required, although in patients with respiratory distress, percutaneous drainage of the mass is performed before surgery.

The differential diagnosis of mesenchymal hamartoma includes mesenchymoma, hemangioma, parasitic or congenital cyst, teratoma, biliary cystadenoma, and choledochal cyst.

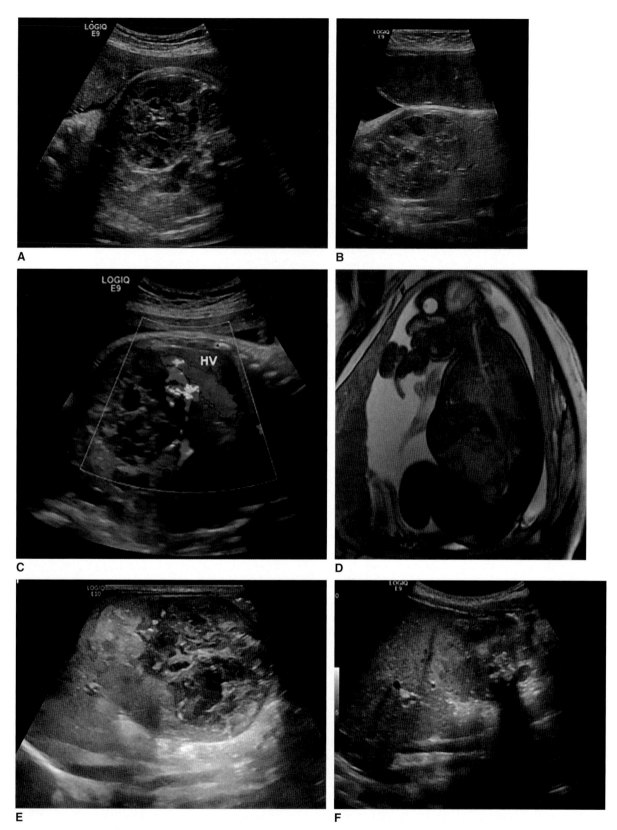

FIGURE 20-7 Infantile hepatic hemangioma. A 29-year-old primiparous woman referred at 37 weeks' gestation for evaluation of a large abdominal mass. **A:** There is a heterogeneous cystic and solid mass at the inferior aspect of the right lobe of the liver anterior and separate from the kidney and adrenal gland seen on axial and coronal (**B**) ultrasound. **C:** There is vascularity at the periphery with large portal vein, hepatic artery, and draining right hepatic vein (*HV*). **D:** Fetal magnetic resonance imaging T2- and T1-weighted sequences allow tissue characterization. T2-weighted sagittal image of a giant hepatic hemangioma. **E:** Postnatal imaging demonstrates a well-circumscribed lesion with mixed echotexture on initial examination after birth with interval decrease in size and development of shadowing calcification at 1-year follow-up (**F**) consistent with infantile hepatic hemangioma.

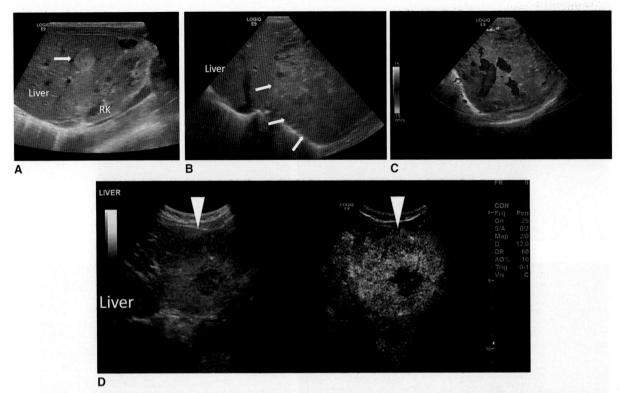

FIGURE 20-8 Hemangioma. **A:** Echogenic lesion in the right hepatic lobe, consistent with cavernous hemangioma (*arrow*). **B:** This 1-day-old male presents with abdominal distension (*arrows*). There is a well-circumscribed, solid-appearing mass in the left lobe of liver segment 3 arising exophytically along the inferior aspect. The mass has a hypoechoic to isoechoic solid-appearing periphery with a very dense echogenic apparently calcified ring-like appearance internally with the central portion difficult to characterize owing to the posterior acoustic shadowing by the calcification. **C:** On color Doppler evaluation, there is intense vascularity with large channels. **D:** Dual-screen contrast-enhanced ultrasound of an atypical hemangioma in an 8-year-old female. Following contrast administration, there is prompt peripheral nodular enhancement during the early arterial phase that progresses from peripherally to centrally according to a spoke-wheel pattern. Enhancement progresses during the late arterial and portal venous phases and becomes homogenous, with the exception of nonenhancement of the central scar and central coarse calcifications. During the delayed phase, lesion enhancement is persistently greater than the background liver, consistent with hemangioma.

Rare benign lesions include focal nodular hyperplasia, hepatic adenoma, nodular regenerative hyperplasia, and fatty tumors; all of these tumors have the same clinical presentation, sonographic appearance, and complications in adults and children.

Cysts[15]

Congenital liver cysts are relatively rare. They range in size from small to large. Polycystic disease of the liver is seen with polycystic kidney disease and von Hippel–Lindau disease. Acquired cysts include hydatid cysts and traumatic cysts caused by blunt trauma. Hemobilia can be detected if there is communication with the biliary tree. The patient is generally asymptomatic unless the lesion is large enough to impair function and cause abdominal distension. The cyst may be palpated on physical examination or found incidentally on an imaging examination.

Sonographically, simple congenital liver cysts appear as smooth-walled, anechoic lesions demonstrating good posterior enhancement. They may be completely intrahepatic, partly intrahepatic, or completely extrahepatic and attached by a stalk.

Hydatid echinococcal cysts or parasitic cysts are usually associated with exposure to livestock, farming, and dogs. After the eggs have been ingested, the gastric juices dissolve the covering of the embryo, allowing the organism to move

spontaneously and attach itself to the intestinal wall. From there, it travels through the portal system to the liver, where it lodges and creates a cyst. The sonographic appearances include simple cyst, complex cysts (daughter cysts, echogenic septa, echogenic debris, or floating membranes), and simple or complex cysts with calcifications (Fig. 20-9A–D). The peak incidence occurs in patients aged 5 to 15 years. In this population, 25% are asymptomatic and 60% present with symptoms, including urticaria, right upper quadrant pain, and abdominal swelling due to hepatomegaly. As the lung is the second most common site affected, the right more often than the left, patients with pulmonary hydatid cyst present with pain on the affected side, coughing, high fever, and dyspnea. Forty percent develop complications including rupture into the peritoneal and pleural spaces, resulting in anaphylactic shock and pneumonia. Sometimes, the organism passes through the liver and lodges in the lungs, brain, kidneys, or elsewhere. Depending on the size and location of the lesions, the patient may experience infection, impaired liver function due to biliary obstruction, or other complications due to obstruction or compression of abdominal vasculature.

Treatment usually consists of aspiration, capitonnage, omentopexy, or a combination of two or more surgical procedures.

Differential diagnosis of extrahepatic cysts includes ovarian or mesenteric cysts, whereas the differential diagnosis

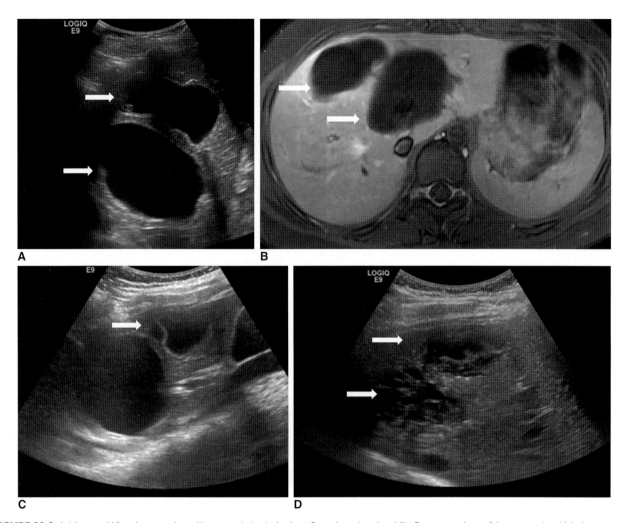

FIGURE 20-9 A 14-year-old female presenting with severe abdominal pain × 2 weeks and eosinophilia. Recent travel out of the country, in which she consumed raw meat of unknown animal origin and frequent consumption of raw/undercooked meat. **A:** Two dominant cystic lesions within the liver parenchyma representing echinococcal cysts on ultrasound and magnetic resonance imaging (**B**). **C:** The second lesion has suggestion of a water lily or floating membrane sign with split wall (*arrow*). **D:** s/p PAIR procedure (this therapeutic percutaneous technique involves puncture, aspiration, instillation, and reaspiration of a scolicidal agent). Two cystic lesions are again noted within the right lobe of the liver, cysts have decreased slightly in size and are more complex in appearance (*arrows*). Appearance is consistent with involution of daughter cysts and decreased cystic fluid.

of an intrahepatic cyst includes teratoma, mesenchymoma, and tuberculin hepatic granuloma. It is important to distinguish an intrahepatic cyst from a choledochal cyst, which involves the bile duct and is discussed in "Gallbladder and Biliary System" section.

Hepatic Trauma[15]

The most commonly injured abdominal organ in blunt abdominal trauma in children is the liver, with the right lobe involved more often than the left lobe. The types of injuries to the liver include subcapsular and parenchymal hematomas, lacerations, and fractures. Hemoperitoneum is often noted in liver trauma injuries (Fig. 20-10A–D).

Hematomas of the liver demonstrate a change in echogenicity over time, progressing from anechoic, to complex, to anechoic with possible development of calcification. Gas or air secondary to tissue ischemia and necrosis may be noted. Biloma (walled-off collections of bile) and pseudoaneurysms may be later complications of liver trauma.

Infectious and Inflammatory Disease

Hepatitis[16]

Hepatitis is a diffuse infection of the liver characterized by inflammation and hepatic cell necrosis. Nearly all cases are viral in origin (hepatitis A, B, C, D, or E; cytomegalovirus, herpes, and Epstein–Barr). Noninfectious causes include toxin exposure, drugs, sclerosing cholangitis, and autoimmune disease. Type A is transmitted by a fecal–oral route of contaminated material. Children and young adults are most often infected by the hepatitis A virus. The extent of liver damage ranges from mild involvement to widespread necrosis and hepatic failure.

The clinical symptoms vary depending on the stage of the disease. The patient can experience abdominal swelling (hepatomegaly) with pain, nausea, fever, chills, jaundice, fatigue, or loss of appetite.

Depending on the stage of the disease, the sonographic appearance of the liver can range from hypoechoic to increasingly hyperechoic. In acute hepatitis, hepatomegaly

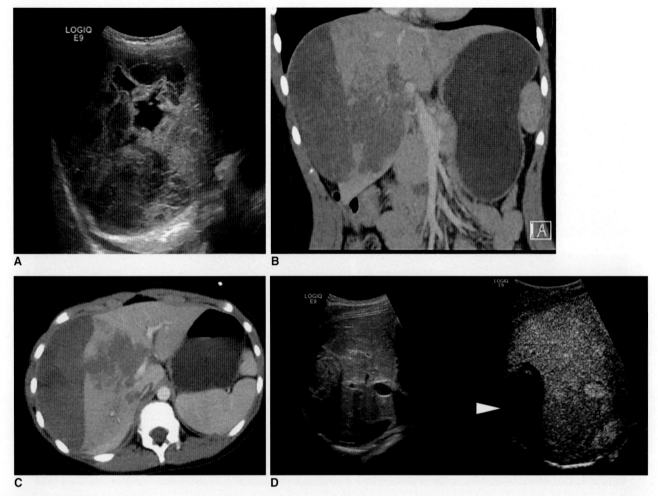

FIGURE 20-10 Hepatic trauma. Blunt abdominal trauma in an 11-year-old female kicked by a horse. **A:** Ultrasound shows a very large heterogeneous complex fluid collection centered in the right upper quadrant in keeping with known large hepatic hematoma. **B:** Coronal and axial **(C)** computed tomography demonstrate grade 4 liver laceration with a large subcapsular hematoma and intraparenchymal hematoma. **D:** Contrast-enhanced ultrasound, performed 2 years later, demonstrates chronic changes in the liver with the laceration cavity occupied largely by a chronic hematoma (*arrowhead*).

with decreased parenchymal echogenicity and increased echogenicity of the portal walls may be present. As the patient recovers, the size and echogenicity of the liver return to normal; however, with chronic hepatitis, the size of the liver may decrease but echogenicity and attenuation increase because normal liver tissue is destroyed and replaced by fibrosis and nodular regeneration. Chronic hepatitis may lead to cirrhosis, liver damage, and cancer. Therefore, routine screening sonogram is recommended in these patients. Sonography utilizing shear-wave elastography may be used to monitor the stiffness of the liver. Thickening of the gallbladder wall, small gallbladder filled with sludge, and enlarged nodes in the porta hepatitis can be found in cases of severe hepatitis (Fig. 20-11A–C).

Abscess[17,18]

The etiology of abscess is related to the source of the infection and can be introduced to the liver by various routes, including trauma, direct invasion of adjacent structures, the hepatic artery, the portal vein, umbilical vein, or the bile ducts.

Laboratory values vary. The liver enzyme levels may be normal or elevated. Patients are not usually jaundiced. Blood cultures are generally negative. Leukocytosis is common but varies among patients. In neonatal abscesses, the organism is usually Gram negative rather than Gram positive.

Intrahepatic abscesses in infants present sonographically as in older patients and vary from discretely marginated hypoechoic structures with good sound transmission to complex hyperechoic masses with poorly defined margins. Lesions that contain gas (air) are hyperechoic with acoustic shadowing and reverberation artifacts. The mass may also present with a bull's-eye appearance (a central hyperechoic area surrounded by a more anechoic one). In transplacental infection with calcifications, a bright, hyperechoic lesion with posterior shadowing can be seen (Fig. 20-12A–C).

Pyogenic Liver Abscess[17,18]

Pyogenic liver abscess (PLA) is rare in children and can be fatal. Pyogenic abscess in children is secondary to generalized infections from the bowel (appendicitis or inflammatory

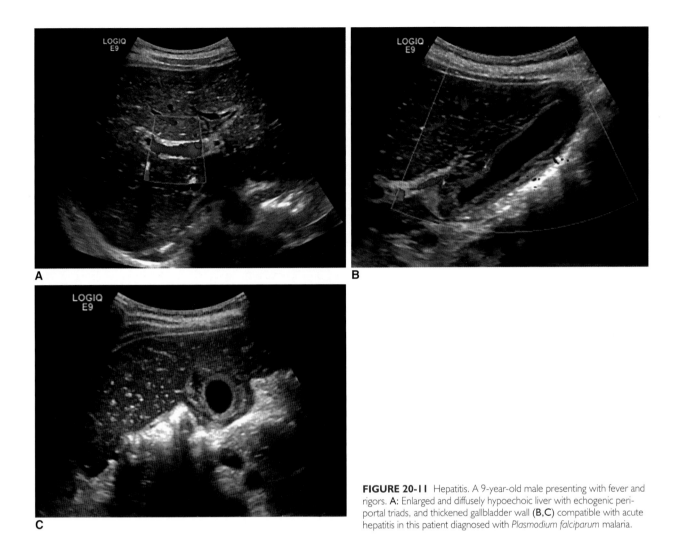

FIGURE 20-11 Hepatitis. A 9-year-old male presenting with fever and rigors. **A:** Enlarged and diffusely hypoechoic liver with echogenic periportal triads, and thickened gallbladder wall (**B,C**) compatible with acute hepatitis in this patient diagnosed with *Plasmodium falciparum* malaria.

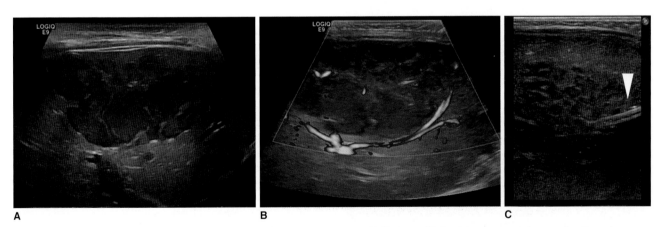

FIGURE 20-12 Liver abscess. A 9-month-old female with multifocal pneumonia and methicillin-susceptible *Staphylococcus aureus* bacteremia with tender, distended abdomen. **A:** Multiloculated septated liver abscess within the right hepatic lobe, measuring up to 6.5 cm, with mixed internal echoes. **B:** Doppler color shows no internal blood flow, with the exception of a couple of internal septations (*arrowhead*). There is hyperemia of the surrounding tissues. **C:** Image-guided aspiration of pus from the hepatic abscesses (*arrowhead*).

bowel disease), trauma, or surgery. Immunosuppression is an important predisposing condition. The most common causative agents are *Escherichia coli* and *Klebsiella pneumoniae*. PLA can also be seen in Crohn disease, chronic granulomatous disease, intestinal infection or bacteremia of any source, cholecystitis, biliary atresia, polycythemia, perforated viscus, *Candida* organisms, and hematopoietic malignancies.

Fungal Abscess[17,18]

Fungal abscess occurs most often in the immunocompromised patient and is usually due to *Candida albicans*. This type of abscess is most commonly seen as multiple small lesions with irregular walls throughout the liver and may also be seen in the spleen and kidneys. Sonographically, the lesions can appear round and hypoechoic, or hyperechoic, or have a target or wheel-within-wheel appearance (Fig. 20-13).

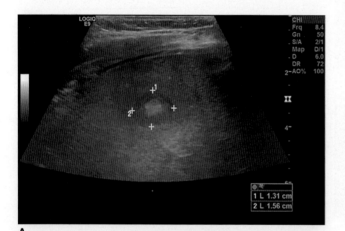

A

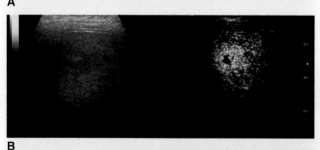

B

C

FIGURE 20-13 Fungal abscess. A 2-year-old female with acute myeloid leukemia with extended-spectrum beta-lactamases bacteremia and neutropenia. **A:** Transverse image of the liver shows a round-shaped lesion measuring 1.3 cm × 1.5 cm that presents a slightly irregular hypoechogenic ring and a hyperechogenic center. **B:** Following contrast administration, the lesion showed early enhancement of the rim of the hypoechogenic ring, without enhancement of the center, also demonstrated on delayed images (**C**).

Amebic Abscess[17,18]

Amebic liver abscess, although an adult disease, also affects children in areas, where drinking water is contaminated and sanitation is poor. Hepatic abscess is the main complication of the organism *Entamoeba histolytica*, forming in 1% of the population who is infected.

E. histolytica enters the liver from the colon via the portal system and forms a cavity that becomes the abscess. The organism resides in the wall of the abscess, and the right lobe is more commonly affected. Sonographically, the abscess can be readily identified as a hypoechoic, spherical lesion. After treatment, it can be followed with serial sonography.

Diffuse Liver Disease

Diffuse parenchymal diseases include fatty infiltration, hepatic fibrosis, cirrhosis, hemosiderosis, and metabolic diseases.

Fatty Infiltration[19–22]

Fatty infiltration of the liver is caused by chronic hepatic injury and results from an accumulation of abnormal amounts of triglycerides and lipids in the hepatocytes. Fatty infiltration may be diffuse or focal, and in children, it can be related to a variety of conditions, including malignancies, metabolic diseases, cystic fibrosis, and exposure to liver toxins. However, as childhood obesity has emerged as a significant health problem worldwide, the prevalence of fatty infiltration of the liver has increased in children. Fatty infiltration is being seen at a younger age and without the presence of other underlying risk factors.

Diffuse fatty infiltration results in hepatomegaly and sonographic findings of increased parenchymal echogenicity and attenuation of the sound beam. The resulting sonographic appearance is similar to that of older patients, including a large echogenic liver with decreased visualization of the intrahepatic vessels, posterior portions of the liver, and the diaphragm. Less common patterns of fat deposition include focal, multifocal, perivascular, and subcapsular deposition.

Metabolic Liver Disease

Metabolic liver disease is a group of disorders affecting the liver. Inborn errors of metabolism are usually due to a defect in an enzyme or transport protein that causes abnormalities in the synthesis or catabolism of proteins, carbohydrates, or fats. This is not the same as metabolic disease (or syndrome) in the adult.

These diseases may directly damage the liver, resulting in cirrhosis or liver failure. Or they may be due to a metabolic defect in the liver, causing damage to other organ systems. Metabolic disorders of the liver include glycogen storage disease (type I von Gierke disease is the most common), lipodystrophy, cystic fibrosis, Gaucher disease, and Wilson disease, all of which have the sonographic appearance of fatty infiltration of the liver (Fig. 20-14A–C).

Cirrhosis[19,21]

Cirrhosis is parenchymal destruction, scarring, fibrosis, and nodular regeneration of the liver (Fig. 20-15A–C). In infants and children, it is due to biliary atresia, cystic fibrosis, chronic hepatitis, metabolic disease (Wilson disease, glycogen storage disease, tyrosinemia, galactosemia, and

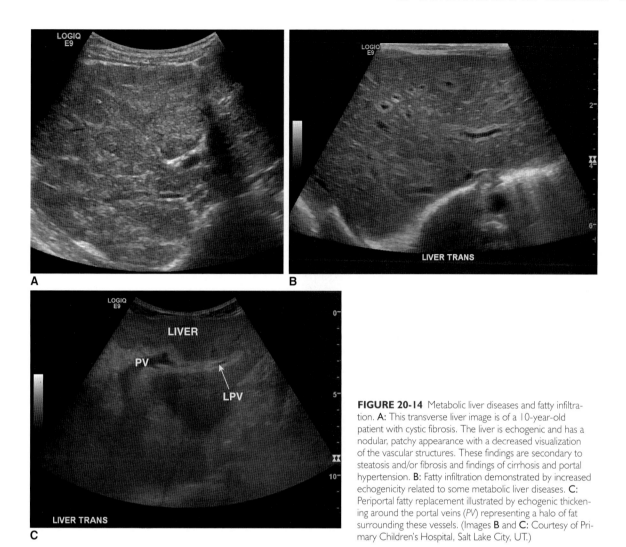

FIGURE 20-14 Metabolic liver diseases and fatty infiltration. **A:** This transverse liver image is of a 10-year-old patient with cystic fibrosis. The liver is echogenic and has a nodular, patchy appearance with a decreased visualization of the vascular structures. These findings are secondary to steatosis and/or fibrosis and findings of cirrhosis and portal hypertension. **B:** Fatty infiltration demonstrated by increased echogenicity related to some metabolic liver diseases. **C:** Periportal fatty replacement illustrated by echogenic thickening around the portal veins (*PV*) representing a halo of fat surrounding these vessels. (Images **B** and **C:** Courtesy of Primary Children's Hospital, Salt Lake City, UT.)

alpha₁-antitrypsin deficiency), prolonged parenteral nutrition, Budd–Chiari syndrome, and medications. The clinical, laboratory, and sonographic presentation is the same as in adults. Secondary signs of ascites, splenomegaly, and portal hypertension may be present.

Hepatic Fibrosis[23]

Hepatic fibrosis occurs in the absence of cirrhosis and has been associated with metabolic disorders, cystic fibrosis, biliary atresia, liver transplantation, severe congenital heart disease, cardiac transplantation, and autosomal recessive polycystic disease. Hepatomegaly and portal hypertension are common symptoms. Sonographically, the liver demonstrates increased echogenicity and biliary dilatation because of the presence of dense fibrous bands surrounding the liver lobules.

Increased echogenicity of the kidneys may also be noted.

Hemochromatosis[9,24]

Hemochromatosis occurs when an excessive amount of iron is stored within the liver. Hemochromatosis may be genetic, secondary, or transfusional. Hemosiderosis is iron storage in the liver resulting from repeated blood transfusions. The liver may demonstrate a decrease in echogenicity (Fig. 20-16). Magnetic resonance imaging (MRI) is the best imaging test for detecting hemosiderosis.

Malignant Neoplasms[10,11,25]

Primary malignant tumors of the liver are more common in children than in adults, and two-thirds of all pediatric hepatic tumors are malignant. These tumors include hepatoblastoma, HCC (hepatoma), mesenchymal (embryonal) sarcoma, and congenital neuroblastoma. Other rare liver tumors include rhabdomyosarcoma, angiosarcoma, germ cell tumors, and undifferentiated sarcomas. Primary liver tumors account for 2% to 5% of all malignant pediatric tumors. The AFP level is usually elevated in the presence of malignant hepatic tumors, and invasion of surrounding vessels is commonly noted. Because vascular invasion can impact the treatment decisions of hepatic malignancies, sonography is of vital importance to identify extension of the tumor into major blood vessels and differentiate this from thrombus formation.

Sonographically, malignancies usually demonstrate as a solitary, solid, homogeneous, hyperechoic mass and less frequently as multiple hyperechoic lesions. In some cases, a hypoechoic halo or rim may be seen, and infrequently, the malignancy may be isoechoic to normal liver tissue.

Hepatoblastoma[10,11,25,26]

Hepatoblastoma is the most common pediatric liver mass, occurring most commonly in boys younger than 5 years of age.

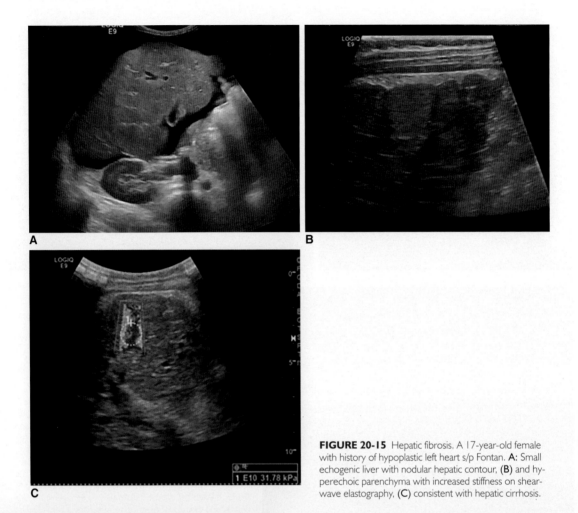

FIGURE 20-15 Hepatic fibrosis. A 17-year-old female with history of hypoplastic left heart s/p Fontan. **A:** Small echogenic liver with nodular hepatic contour, **(B)** and hyperechoic parenchyma with increased stiffness on shear-wave elastography, **(C)** consistent with hepatic cirrhosis.

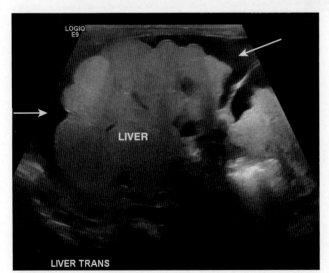

FIGURE 20-16 Hemochromatosis. Transverse image of the liver in a patient diagnosed with hemochromatosis demonstrating diffuse surface irregularities, increased parenchymal echogenicity, and free fluid (*arrows*). (Image courtesy of Primary Children's Hospital, Salt Lake City, UT.)

Hepatoblastoma is associated with Beckwith–Wiedemann syndrome (hemihypertrophy, macroglossia, hypoglycemia, organomegaly, and omphalocele), fetal alcohol syndrome, development of Wilms tumor, dysplastic kidney, and Meckel diverticulum.

A tumor should be considered resectable if it does not occupy more than one lobe, has no extrahepatic extension, and does not invade the portal vein. Although hepatoblastomas are often detected in advanced stages, unresectable tumors can be biopsied and converted to resectable tumors by chemotherapy. Chemotherapy is applied before surgery to shrink the tumor, resulting in improved operability.

Clinically, patients usually present with hepatomegaly or a painless, palpable abdominal mass in 90% of cases. In advanced cases, there can be accompanying fever, weight loss, pain, nausea, vomiting, jaundice, anemia, leukocytosis, adenopathy, and fractures due to bone metastases. Laboratory values include an elevation of AFP in 84% to 91% of cases, with a decrease after resection. There may also be a transaminase elevation, as well as anemia and thrombocytosis.

Sonographically, a hepatoblastoma appears as a solitary multinodular mass with a heterogeneous, hyperechoic pattern and indistinct borders (Fig. 20-17A–C).

Anechoic foci may also be present, representing necrosis or hemorrhage. Dense or coarse calcifications with posterior shadowing are also common. The differential diagnosis includes HCC, infantile hemangioendothelioma, and mesenchymal hamartoma.

Hepatocellular Carcinoma[10,11,25]

HCC, which is also known as hepatoma, affects children older than 3 years of age and has been associated with chronic

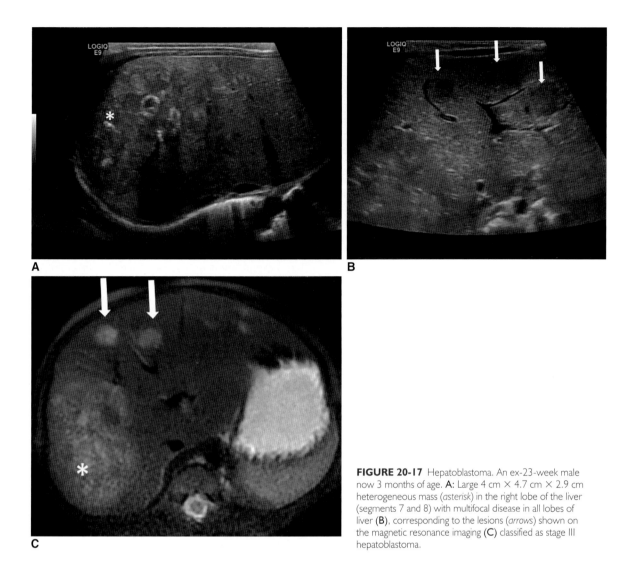

FIGURE 20-17 Hepatoblastoma. An ex-23-week male now 3 months of age. **A:** Large 4 cm × 4.7 cm × 2.9 cm heterogeneous mass (*asterisk*) in the right lobe of the liver (segments 7 and 8) with multifocal disease in all lobes of liver (**B**), corresponding to the lesions (*arrows*) shown on the magnetic resonance imaging (**C**) classified as stage III hepatoblastoma.

liver diseases, such as type I glycogen storage disease, Wilson disease, biliary atresia, and hepatitis. Pathologically, these lesions have characteristics that differentiate them from other hepatic lesions: daughter nodules, hepatic or portal tumor thrombosis, septa, and pseudocapsules. This tumor can be either well encapsulated or nonencapsulated and is commonly multicentric.

Clinically, the patient presents with sudden liver failure due to invasion of the tumor or thrombosis in the portal or hepatic veins, hepatomegaly, pain, GI bleeding, ascites, anorexia, hypoglycemia, anemia, weakness, and fever. Laboratory values include elevated AFP in 60% to 80% of cases.

Sonographically, the tumor may appear similar to a hepatoblastoma. It generally presents as a solid, hyperechoic mass and usually involves the entire liver. It can have well-defined or ill-defined borders. There may be anechoic areas within the mass representing necrosis or hemorrhage. An anechoic or hypoechoic halo or rim may also be seen. Tumor thrombi are frequently seen in the portal veins, hepatic veins, and IVC and should be documented if present.

The outcome for cirrhotic patients who develop HCC is poor. The differential diagnosis includes hepatoblastoma, abscess, focal nodular hyperplasia, adenoma, hemangiosarcoma, hemangioendothelioma, and biliary rhabdomyosarcoma.

Fibrolamellar Hepatocellular Carcinoma[10]

Fibrolamellar HCC is histologic subtype of HCC, which most commonly affects teenagers and young adults. Clinical findings include abdominal pain, mass, fever, weight loss, diarrhea, and vomiting. AFP levels are typically normal or mildly elevated. The tumor is usually solitary and well marginated with variable echogenicity. Some tumors demonstrate a central scar and/or focal calcifications. The sonographic appearance is so similar to other solid hepatic neoplasms that biopsy is needed to differentiate these tumors.

Mesenchymal Sarcoma[10,11]

Mesenchymal (embryonal) sarcoma is a rare malignant liver tumor that typically presents in patients aged 5 to 10 years, as a large fast-growing, round, singular mass with well-defined borders and a thick, fibrous pseudocapsule usually within the right lobe. It can contain multiple cystic spaces, hemorrhage, necrosis, and brown viscous material, as well as fibrous bands. It can easily spread to the abdominal cavity or to the diaphragm, with metastases to the lungs. Mesenchymal sarcoma is the fourth most common primary pediatric liver tumor following hepatoblastoma, infantile hemangioendothelioma, and HCC. Subtypes of mesenchymal sarcoma include embryonal sarcoma, rhabdomyosarcoma, angiosarcoma, and malignant mesenchymoma.

The clinical findings include abdominal pain and swelling, with a palpable mass. Jaundice is usually not present, and the AFP level is not increased.

Sonographically, mesenchymal sarcoma usually presents as a single hyperechoic mass containing anechoic areas, which represent the cystic spaces. It can also appear homogeneous and hyperechoic or as a complex lesion with anechoic areas as well as calcifications producing posterior shadowing.

Metastases[10]

The most common cause of metastatic hepatic neoplasms in children is neuroblastoma. Hepatic metastases are frequently associated with Wilms tumor, neuroblastoma, leukemia, and lymphoma. As in adults, the echogenicity and echotexture of metastases is variable: hypoechoic, isoechoic, hyperechoic and homogeneous, and heterogeneous or complex. Calcifications may be noted. Rarely are pediatric metastases diffuse, with diffuse disease most commonly associated with stage IV-S neuroblastoma.

Lymphoproliferative disorder can be a complication of solid organ transplant. Single or multiple hypoechoic masses in the liver may be noted sonographically; occasionally, diffusely infiltrating disease is found (Fig. 20-18A, B).

Lymphoma of the liver is more commonly secondary to non-Hodgkin lymphoma. Sonographically, discrete hypoechoic nodules are noted; hepatosplenomegaly may be present.

Hepatic Vascular Disorders

Vascular disorders of the liver include portal hypertension, Budd–Chiari syndrome, portal vein thrombosis, hepatic infarction, peliosis hepatis, and portal venous gas.

Portal Hypertension[19,27,28]

Portal hypertension is due to increased resistance to normal portal venous flow. The clinical presentation includes splenomegaly, ascites, caput medusa, and, in severe cases, hematemesis, hepatic encephalopathy, and hypersplenism. The obstruction to flow can be prehepatic (portal or splenic vein thrombosis), intrahepatic (secondary to cirrhosis and,

less commonly, hepatic vein obstruction), or posthepatic (secondary to congestive heart failure or constrictive pericarditis).

Sonographic findings include bidirectional or hepatofugal portal vein flow, development of varices, splenomegaly, a thicken lesser omentum, ascites, and evidence of cirrhosis. The portal vein may be dilated, but the size and number of varices or collaterals that develop as the disease progresses can reduce the diameter of the main portal vein. Respiratory variation in portal venous flow may be absent or reduced. Flow in the hepatic artery may increase to compensate for the decrease in blood to the liver via the main portal vein. The hepatic veins may demonstrate a loss of pulsatility and a monophasic flow pattern.

Portal Vein Thrombosis[19,27,28]

Portal vein thrombosis can be caused by thrombus or tumor invasion. Hepatoblastoma and HCC may involve tumor invasion of the portal vein. Nonmalignant thrombosis is associated with improper placement of UVC, dehydration, shock, sepsis, hypercoagulable states, and portal hypertension. Clinical presentation includes acute abdominal pain and, in some cases, splenomegaly. Portal vein thrombosis can be acute (enlarged, echogenic vein, absent flow with color Doppler or, in cases of tumor invasion, flow within the thrombus) or chronic (cavernous transformation of the portal vein, which is described as multiple tortuous vessels in the porta hepatis and nonvisualization of the portal vein).

Acute portal vein thrombosis may be anechoic and mimic a patent portal vein on grayscale imaging; however, color Doppler will confirm the finding of thrombosis. Additional sonographic findings in chronic portal vein thrombosis include the development of collaterals with the addition of pericholecystic collaterals in some cases (Fig. 20-19A–D).

Budd–Chiari Syndrome[19,27,28]

Budd–Chiari syndrome may be due to idiopathic occlusion or neoplastic invasion of the hepatic veins, usually secondary to hepatoblastoma, HCC, Wilms tumor, or thrombosis. Idiopathic causes of occlusion include hypercoagulable states, trauma, Gaucher disease, and cirrhosis. The primary sonographic findings include hepatomegaly, echogenic

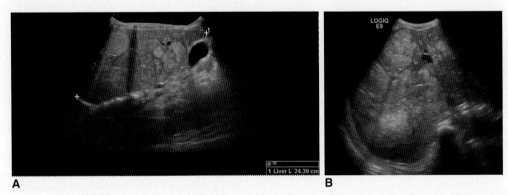

A   **B**

FIGURE 20-18 Liver metastasis. **A:** Longitudinal and transverse (**B**) images of the liver demonstrate multiple masses throughout the liver parenchyma. Findings compatible with extensive metastatic disease to the liver, particularly inferiorly and peripherally, with significant hepatomegaly.

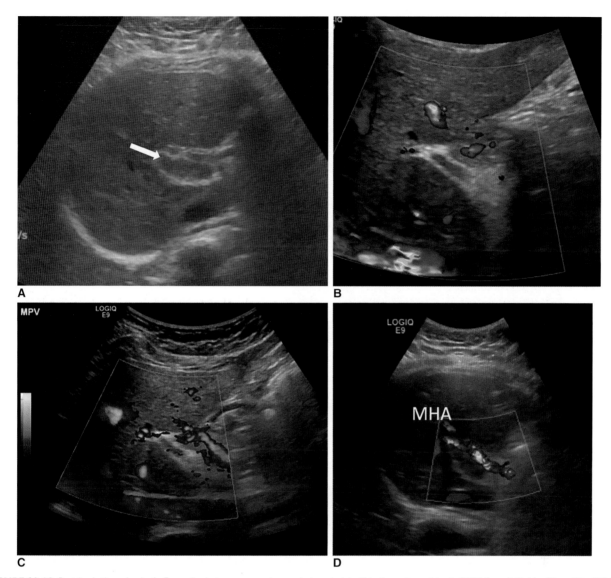

FIGURE 20-19 Portal vein thrombosis. **A:** Expansile, heterogeneous, hypoechoic material within the main portal vein (*MPV*) (*arrow*). **B:** Nonfilling of the MPV on power and color **(C)** Doppler, due to cavernous transformation. **D:** The main hepatic artery (*MHA*) is ectatic and hypertrophied, demonstrating turbulent blood flow on Doppler evaluation.

intraluminal clot, and the absence of hepatic vein flow using color and pulse-wave Doppler (Fig. 20-20A, B).

Secondary findings include ascites, pleural effusion, and gallbladder wall edema (Fig. 20-20C).

Nonvisualization of the hepatic veins is not specific evidence of hepatic vein occlusion because patent veins can be difficult to identify in the presence of hepatomegaly or cirrhosis. In the chronic stages, additional collateral pathways for hepatic vein flow can develop.

Occlusion of the vena cava may be due to a congenital membrane within the IVC (noted sonographically as a thin, hyperechoic band inside the IVC), neoplastic invasion, extrinsic tumor compression, enlarged caudate lobe, and thrombosis. Obstruction of the IVC can cause hepatic venous congestion and development of thrombus in the hepatic veins. Color and pulse-wave Doppler confirm the absence of flow in the obstructed portion of the IVC and abnormal flow in the hepatic veins. The IVC may be dilated inferior to the obstruction.

Portal Venous Gas

Air in the portal vein and its branches can be associated with umbilical venous catheterization, bowel surgery, and neonatal gastroenteritis. However, it is particularly important to recognize this entity in neonates because it can result from mesenteric ischemia due to small bowel obstruction or NEC, which occurs predominantly in premature and low birth weight infants with significant morbidity and mortality. Multiple echogenic foci can be seen moving within the vessels in the direction of blood flow, but acoustic shadowing and reverberation are not usually noted (Fig. 20-21A, B).

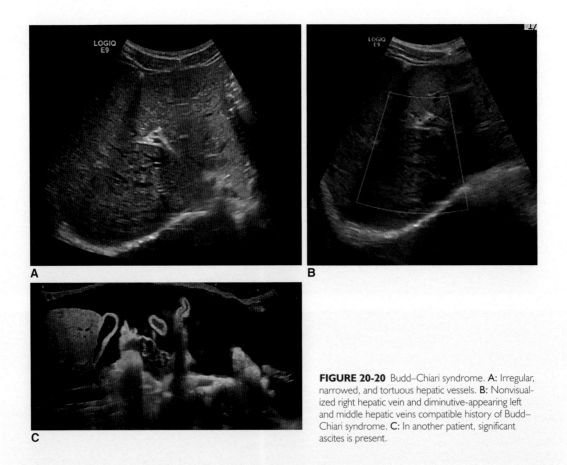

FIGURE 20-20 Budd–Chiari syndrome. **A:** Irregular, narrowed, and tortuous hepatic vessels. **B:** Nonvisualized right hepatic vein and diminutive-appearing left and middle hepatic veins compatible history of Budd–Chiari syndrome. **C:** In another patient, significant ascites is present.

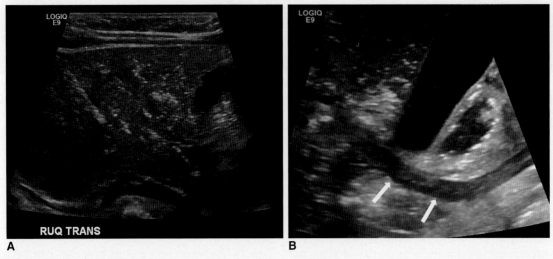

FIGURE 20-21 Portal venous gas. **A:** Transverse image of the liver demonstrates multiple echogenic foci without acoustic shadowing or reverberation associated with the portal venous branches. (Image courtesy of Primary Children's Hospital, Salt Lake City, UT.) **B:** Magnified view of the portal vein (*arrows*) showed real-time mobile foci compatible with portal venous gas.

GALLBLADDER AND BILIARY SYSTEM[29]

Although gallbladder disease is uncommon in children, it does occur. The normal sonographic appearance of the gallbladder is the same as in the adult patient: thin-walled, well-defined structure, with an anechoic lumen and echogenic walls.

Sonographic Examination Technique

Scan Technique

Patients are most commonly scanned in the supine and LPO positions. Additional patient positions, such as prone (especially in obese children), semi-erect, erect, and right posterior oblique (RPO), may be helpful.

The sonographer should acquire documentary images that clearly demonstrate the gallbladder and bile ducts in longitudinal and transverse planes. Evaluation, assessment, and documentation should include the gallbladder periphery; longitudinal and transverse sweeps extending past the medial, lateral, superior, and inferior borders of the gallbladder; and the total length of the bile duct should be evaluated. Normal maximal diameter of the common bile duct is calculated by age in children.

Congenital Anomalies[8,30,31]

Congenital anomalies of the biliary tract include biliary atresia, choledochal cyst, and, rarely, gallbladder ectopia, agenesis, or duplication (Fig. 20-22).

Biliary Atresia[16,19,30,32–35]

Elevated lab values of conjugated bilirubin (sometimes referred to as direct bilirubin) in the newborn have two major causes: diseases of the liver such as hepatitis and biliary tract abnormalities such as atresia. Signs and symptoms of neonatal cholestasis and neonatal hepatitis are similar to those of biliary atresia. In these conditions, patients present with jaundice at about 3 to 4 weeks of age. When infectious causes have been excluded, biliary atresia should be suspected.

It is extremely important to determine whether biliary atresia is present, because early identification significantly improves the clinical outcome of the patient. Biliary atresia requires surgical intervention, whereas neonatal hepatitis is treated medically. There are two surgical interventions for biliary atresia. Initially, the Kasai procedure is performed to develop a communication between the liver and the duodenum to promote drainage of bile and prevent liver failure. The success rate of this procedure is greatest when the intervention is performed before 8 weeks of age. The other treatment for biliary atresia is liver transplantation.

It is important to make sure that the patient is fasting appropriately to ensure visualization of the normally distended gallbladder. The manifestations of biliary atresia range from total absence of the biliary tree to a visibly patent gallbladder, cystic duct, and common bile duct. Sonographically,

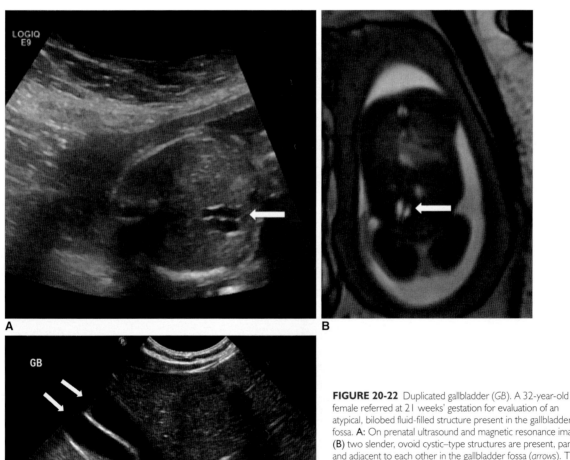

FIGURE 20-22 Duplicated gallbladder (*GB*). A 32-year-old female referred at 21 weeks' gestation for evaluation of an atypical, bilobed fluid-filled structure present in the gallbladder fossa. **A:** On prenatal ultrasound and magnetic resonance image (**B**) two slender, ovoid cystic–type structures are present, parallel and adjacent to each other in the gallbladder fossa (*arrows*). The most likely etiology for these findings is a duplicated GB. **C:** At 1-year follow-up: in the gallbladder fossa, there are two elongated tubular anechoic cavities that run parallel to each other and share a common wall, both cavities tapering as they approach the common bile duct at the porta. Maximum length measures up to 4 cm, diameter of each individual gallbladder cavity measures up to 9 mm wide. Gallbladder walls are regular throughout, measuring 1.5 mm in thickness. The common wall between the two GBs is thicker and measures 2 mm in thickness.

the gallbladder, cystic duct, common bile ducts, and intrahepatic bile ducts may or may not be seen, depending on the degree of atresia. Most commonly, the intrahepatic and extrahepatic bile ducts near the porta hepatis are absent. If a small, atretic gallbladder is seen, it can be reevaluated with extended fasting (up to 5 hours) to confidently demonstrate a lack of normal distention. If a rudimentary gallbladder is seen, a fasting measurement of less than 1.5 cm suggests atresia. It can also be checked postprandial to see if the size has changed. If it is not connected to the biliary system, there should be no change in its size.

The triangular cord sign is an important sonographic finding in biliary atresia and is seen as an echogenic tubular focus near the anterior branch of the right portal vein measuring greater than 4 mm in thickness. The liver is enlarged and diffusely hyperechoic. Microcyst in the porta hepatis may be noted. An increased hepatic artery diameter (>2 mm), splenomegaly (>6 mm), and polysplenia are also associated with biliary atresia (Fig. 20-23A–C). Ascites may be present. Shear-wave elastography shows promise as a method for differentiating biliary atresia from other hepatic pathologies.

Some patients with biliary atresia also have other congenital anomalies, such as anomalous origin of the hepatic artery, azygous continuation of the IVC, bilaterally bilobed lungs, preduodenal portal veins, abdominal malrotation, and visceral situs anomalies.

Care must be taken to ensure that a choledochal cyst is not mistaken for a normal gallbladder. The absence of the gallbladder may be the only sonographic sign of biliary atresia.

Choledochal Cyst[11,16,19,30,31,36]

Choledochal cyst is a congenital dilatation of the common bile duct that presents as abdominal pain, mass, and jaundice. Both sonography and hepatobiliary scintigraphy are used to establish the diagnosis of this disease, with CT and MRI providing additional information.

There are five main types of choledochal cyst. Type I is the fusiform dilatation of the common bile duct and is the most common form found in infants and children (Fig. 20-24A, B).

Type II presents as a diverticulum of the common bile duct and is the second most common (Fig. 20-25A).

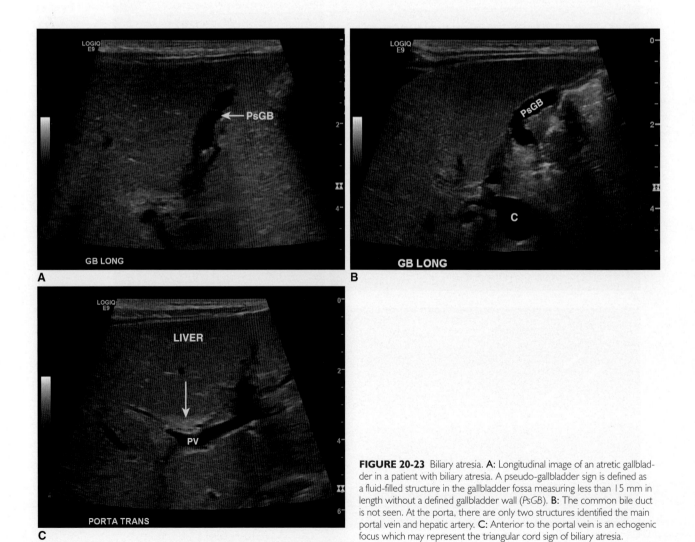

FIGURE 20-23 Biliary atresia. **A:** Longitudinal image of an atretic gallbladder in a patient with biliary atresia. A pseudo-gallbladder sign is defined as a fluid-filled structure in the gallbladder fossa measuring less than 15 mm in length without a defined gallbladder wall (*PsGB*). **B:** The common bile duct is not seen. At the porta, there are only two structures identified the main portal vein and hepatic artery. **C:** Anterior to the portal vein is an echogenic focus which may represent the triangular cord sign of biliary atresia.

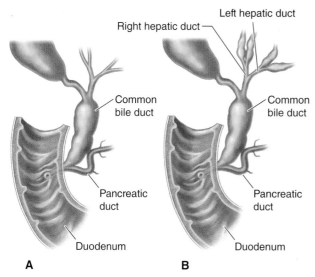

FIGURE 20-24 Choledochal cyst. **A:** Type I: concentric dilatation. **B:** Type IV: fusiform dilatation, concentric dilatation, with intrahepatic involvement.

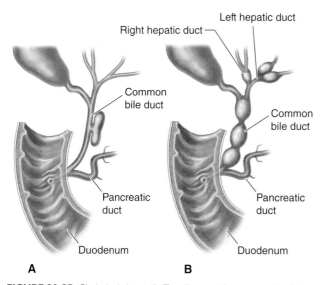

FIGURE 20-25 Choledochal cyst. **A:** Type II: eccentric common bile duct diverticulum. **B:** Type IV: rosary common bile duct diverticulum.

Type III is a congenital choledochocele, which is a cystic dilatation of the intraduodenal portion of the common bile duct. Type IV choledochal cysts are concentric dilatations of the common bile duct with intrahepatic ductal dilatation (Figs. 20-24B and 20-25B). Type V is Caroli disease in which the peripheral intrahepatic ducts are affected either diffusely or focally (Fig. 20-26).

Sonographically, a type I choledochal cyst appears as fluid-filled, well-defined mass in the porta hepatis adjacent to the gallbladder (Fig. 20-27A–C). The right, left, and common bile ducts may be seen entering the cyst, and the gallbladder is demonstrated as a separate cystic structure. If the cyst is large, it may contain sludge. A type II choledochal cyst demonstrates one or more diverticula or fluid-filled structures near or coming off the common bile duct. If there is intrahepatic ductal dilatation, type IV should be considered, and if peripheral ductal dilatation is identified,

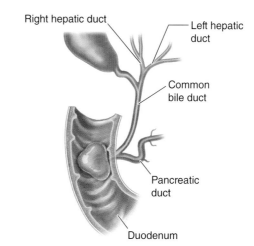

FIGURE 20-26 Choledochal cyst. Type III: congenital choledochocele.

Caroli disease (type V) cannot be ruled out. In types III and IV, intrahepatic ductal dilatation is noted.

Biliary atresia may be concurrent, in which case the choledochal cyst will be smaller and the intrahepatic ductal dilatation is absent.

Complications of untreated choledochal cyst include stone formation within the cyst, gallbladder or pancreatic duct, chronic biliary obstruction, chronic cholangitis, cirrhosis, biliary rupture with resulting biliary peritonitis, neoplasia (risk of adenocarcinoma increases with age), and pancreatitis.

Abnormal Gallbladder Size

If the patient is nonfasting, the gallbladder should be contracted (nondistended). In a fasting patient (4 to 6 hours), a small or nondistended gallbladder may indicate biliary atresia, congenital hypoplasia, acute viral hepatitis (AVH), cystic fibrosis, or chronic cholecystitis (uncommon in children). A large gallbladder may indicate prolonged fasting, hydrops, or obstruction of the cystic or common bile ducts. Administration of a fatty meal can be used in cases of gallbladder enlargement to determine whether the cystic duct is patent. The gallbladder is scanned before the fatty meal and should show emptying 45 minutes to 1 hour after the fatty meal if the cystic duct is patent.

Nonvisualization of the gallbladder is most commonly associated with biliary atresia or viral hepatitis. Less common etiologies include agenesis, ectopia, normal contraction after a meal, and the presence of sludge. A sludge-filled gallbladder can be isoechoic with the liver, making sonographic detection difficult.

Gallbladder Wall Thickening[16,18]

Diffuse gallbladder wall thickening is a nonspecific finding associated with numerous inflammatory and noninflammatory causes. In children, as in adults, a gallbladder wall thickness of 2 to 5 mm suggests disease, and thickness of 5 mm or more is considered indicative of disease. Inflammatory causes include acute and chronic cholecystitis. Noninflammatory causes include viral hepatitis, hepatic dysfunction, cirrhosis, hypoalbuminemia, pancreatitis, congestive heart

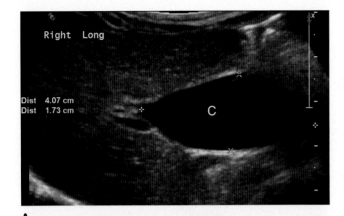

A

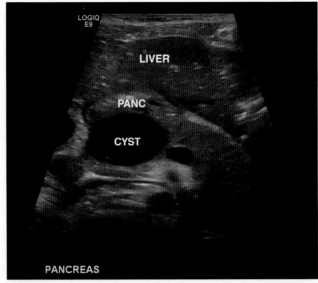

B

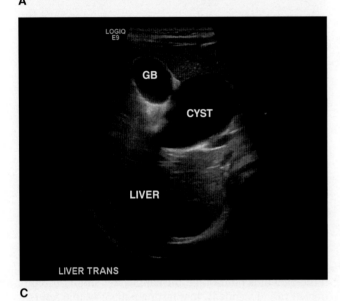

C

FIGURE 20-27 Choledochal cyst. **A:** A 3-day-old infant presents with jaundice and right upper quadrant cystic mass seen on a prenatal sonogram. A longitudinal scan of the right upper quadrant shows fusiform dilation of the common bile duct (between electronic calipers). This is compatible with a type I choledochal cyst. **B:** A choledochal cyst imaged posterior to the head of the pancreas in a transverse scanning plane. **C:** A choledochal cyst imaged posterior to the gallbladder (*GB*) during a transverse scan of the liver. (Image A: Courtesy of Rechelle Nguyen, Columbus, OH; Images **B** and **C**: Courtesy of Primary Children's Hospital, Salt Lake City, UT.)

failure, renal disease, bone marrow transplant, sepsis, and AIDS. Diffuse wall thickening may have several sonographic appearances, including uniformly echogenic, hypoechoic, or striated (hypoechoic and hyperechoic layers). In patients who are nonfasting, the gallbladder wall will demonstrate thickening because of the lack of distention of the gallbladder. Focal wall thickening is associated with cholecystitis or adenomyomatosis.

Cholelithiasis[16,19,37–39]

Cholelithiasis is the presence of one or more calculi (stones) in the gallbladder, cystic duct, or common bile duct. Biliary obstruction occurs if calculi are situated in the cystic or common bile ducts. Because bile salt secretion in infants is 50% of that in adults, it is assumed that any treatment that suppresses bile acid formation greatly increases the risk of gallstones. The incidence of gallstones is rising in children owing to the increase in childhood obesity, and pigmented stones are more common in children than cholesterol stones. Children with sickle cell disease have an increased incidence of cholelithiasis that is nearly double the general population.

Neonatal cholelithiasis is associated with congenital anomalies of the biliary system, total parenteral nutrition (TPN), dehydration, infection, hemolytic anemia,

extracorporeal membranous oxygenation (ECMO), and short-gut syndrome. Common causes of gallstones in older children and teenagers include cystic fibrosis, malabsorption, TPN, liver disease, Crohn disease, bowel resection, sickle cell disease, medication use by pediatric patients for congenital heart disease, and hemolytic anemia. Most children with gallstones are predisposed because of the presence of an underlying disease process; however, some gallstones are idiopathic.

The clinical presentation in younger children with gallstones includes nonspecific symptoms (jaundice, irritability), whereas older children and teens present with more classic symptoms of right upper quadrant pain, intolerance to fatty foods, nausea, and vomiting. The most common complication of gallstones in children is pancreatitis. Often, the gallstones resolve without treatment.

Gallstones and a sludge-filled gallbladder present sonographically as in older patients.

A neonate may be examined because gallstones were noted on a fetal sonogram; most resolve spontaneously within the first year of life. The formation of sludge within the gallbladder is associated with prolonged fasting, hyperalimentation, and extrahepatic bile duct obstruction. Patients with sickle cell disease and cystic fibrosis are predisposed to the formation of sludge.

Cystic duct stones are very difficult to demonstrate if the duct is not dilated. An impacted cystic duct stone can compress the adjacent common bile duct (Mirizzi syndrome), causing extrinsic bile duct dilatation and obstructive jaundice. Common bile duct stones can result in further complications, such as biliary obstruction, cholangitis, or pancreatitis.

Cholecystitis[39–41]

Acute or chronic cholecystitis in children has a number of causes: hypoalbuminemia, AVH, heart failure, renal failure, gallbladder carcinoma, ascites, multiple myeloma, congenital obstruction of the cystic duct or obstruction from an external source, biliary stasis, and portal node lymphatic obstruction.

Clinically, the patient can present with right upper quadrant pain, fever, vomiting, and a palpable right upper quadrant lump. The differential diagnosis includes cholecystitis, abdominal abscesses of the right upper quadrant, pancreatitis, appendicitis, peptic ulcer disease, and gallbladder torsion.

In a diseased state, the gallbladder wall presents sonographically as thickened, irregular, and highly reflective. A hypoechoic to anechoic halo seen surrounding the gallbladder wall is usually due to either infection of the wall itself or a disease process in the surrounding liver tissue (Fig. 20-28A, B). At times, sludge can be seen in the gallbladder owing to stasis.

Hydropic Gallbladder[42]

Hydropic gallbladder develops in acutely ill children who receive TPN or hyperalimentation therapy and in association with group B streptococcal sepsis, congestive heart failure, shock, chronic biliary tract obstruction, upper respiratory tract infection, gastroenteritis, and Epstein–Barr virus infection. Diseases such as Kawasaki (mucocutaneous lymph node) syndrome, leptospirosis, typhoid fever, ascariasis, *Salmonella*, or *Pseudomonas* may also present with gallbladder hydrops. Clinically, patients present with right upper quadrant pain, fever, dehydration, and abdominal distention. The reasons for hydropic gallbladder are unclear. Most of the time, a hydropic gallbladder resolves spontaneously.

Sonographically, the gallbladder is dramatically enlarged and completely anechoic with thin walls. Gallstones or sludge may be present. Such a gallbladder generally does not contract well, following a fatty meal (Fig. 20-29).

Biliary Obstruction[16,43,44]

Intrahepatic and extrahepatic bile duct obstruction may be due to the presence of neoplasm (rhabdomyosarcoma is the most common), enlarged lymph nodes in the porta hepatis compressing the bile duct, acute pancreatitis, biliary calculi, and biliary stricture (uncommon). Patients with biliary obstruction present with jaundice. Sonographically, the dilated intrahepatic bile ducts demonstrate as multiple anechoic irregularly branching structures, which are larger at the porta hepatis. The extrahepatic bile ducts demonstrate as round

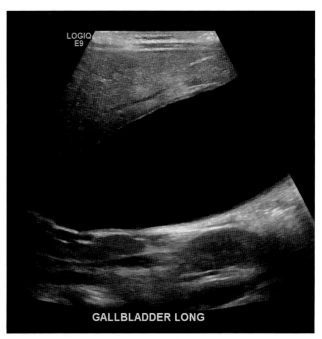

FIGURE 20-29 Hydropic gallbladder. A longitudinal scan of the gallbladder demonstrates a drastically enlarged gallbladder (measuring over 12 cm) with thin walls. Some echogenic foci are demonstrated anterior to the posterior gallbladder wall, possibly indicative of sludge. (Image courtesy of Primary Children's Hospital, Salt Lake City, UT.)

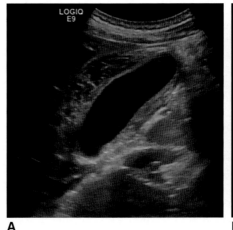 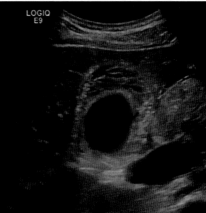

FIGURE 20-28 Cholecystitis. Longitudinal (**A**) and transverse (**B**) images of the gallbladder are on a 14-year-old patient with positive Murphy sign and acalculous cholecystitis. Note the markedly thickened irregular gallbladder wall.

A　　　　　**B**

or tubular anechoic structures near the porta hepatis and/or head of the pancreas. The sonographer should search for the point of obstruction and demonstrate the presence of a mass or calculus that is causing the obstruction. Pancreatitis usually causes the duct to taper significantly at the pancreatic head, whereas a mass, calculus, or stricture demonstrates as an abrupt change from a dilated to a narrowed or absent duct.

Dilated bile ducts may spontaneously rupture, causing neonatal jaundice and bile ascites or a biloma. The most common location for perforation is at the junction of the cystic and common bile ducts. Affected patients usually present in the first 3 months of life with ascites, mild jaundice, failure to thrive, and abdominal distention. Bilirubin values are elevated, but all of the other liver function tests are normal; this distinguishes biliary obstruction from neonatal hepatis syndrome and biliary atresia.

Bile plug syndrome (inspissated bile syndrome) can cause obstruction of the bile ducts. Liver abnormalities are not present in this syndrome, which primarily affects full-term infants. Risk factors include massive hemolysis, TPN, Hirschsprung disease, cystic fibrosis, and intestinal atresias. Echogenic material may be found within dilated ducts, and sludge may be noted in the gallbladder. Bleeding into the ducts from trauma, surgery, or biopsy can mimic the sonographic appearance of bile plug syndrome.

Sclerosing Cholangitis[16,19,30]

Sclerosing cholangitis is a chronic disease in which there is inflammatory fibrosis that obliterates the intrahepatic and extrahepatic bile ducts. This leads to the development of biliary cirrhosis, portal hypertension, and liver failure. Approximately 70% to 80% of children with sclerosing cholangitis have concurrent inflammatory bowel disease. The clinical presentation of sclerosing cholangitis is right upper quadrant pain and jaundice with abnormal liver function tests and elevated bilirubin.

Sonographic findings include thickening of the walls of the bile ducts, choledocholithiasis (intrahepatic and extrahepatic), cholelithiasis, and ductal strictures (Fig. 20-30A–E).

Biliary Neoplasm

Rhabdomyosarcoma[30,45,46]

Biliary rhabdomyosarcoma is a rare soft-tissue tumor occurring in children, usually between the ages of 1 and 5 years. It is the second most common cause of obstructive jaundice in older children after choledochal cyst and in neonates after biliary atresia.

Clinical signs are increasing abdominal girth, vomiting, pain, and weight loss. Usually, the diagnosis is delayed because these clinical symptoms are confused with those of infectious hepatitis. Laboratory values may include elevated total serum bilirubin, a marked increase in alkaline phosphatase, and normal or mildly elevated aspartate transaminase (AST). There may also be a moderate increase in the white blood cell count owing to subsequent cholangitis. Unlike hepatoblastoma or HCC, biliary rhabdomyosarcoma may not cause an increase in the AFP level. Biopsy and histologic examination are definitive for diagnosis.

Sonographically, rhabdomyosarcoma is predominantly solid, with hyperechoic formations and no posterior shadowing, as is commonly seen with stones. The tumor appears lobulated and is usually situated in the hilum of the liver. There may be cystic spaces representing intrahepatic radicles of the bile ducts. There may also be focal areas of necrosis and hemorrhage in the mass. Usually, dilated bile ducts surround the mass. Frequently, it is misdiagnosed as a choledochal cyst.

The favored method of treatment is surgery with adjuvant chemotherapy and radiation therapy.

PANCREAS

Sonography is currently the diagnostic procedure of choice for the examination of children with symptoms of pancreatic disease. Real-time sonography of the pancreas in infants and children is easily performed. Compared with adults, the pancreas is more easily seen in children because most are lean and have a large left hepatic lobe, which serves as an excellent window for visualizing the pancreas. The drawbacks of pancreatic sonography include technically unsatisfactory studies due to obesity or excessive bowel gas, and limited scanning surfaces when surgical dressings or ostomy sites are present.

Sonographic Examination Technique

Scan Technique

A standard examination of the pancreas includes transverse and longitudinal scans of the supine patient. The transverse scans may require some initial survey to determine the exact position of the gland because it generally lies oblique in the middle portion of the body, with the head lower than the body and tail. Longitudinal scans should be oriented to the true longitudinal axis of the pancreas, as determined by the transverse scans. It is common to examine the patient in different positions (i.e., upright, decubitus) to adequately visualize the pancreas. This is particularly important in the presence of disease because the scan must demonstrate the lesion's relationship to surrounding pancreatic structure and adjacent organs. Much of the pancreatic body and tail can be visualized with a coronal approach using the spleen as a sonographic window. Another helpful technique is to use the water-filled duodenum to outline the pancreas. The patient is given approximately 16 oz of water, and the progress of the water into the duodenum is checked periodically by the sonographer. When the duodenum is appropriately distended, the patient is repositioned until the water-filled duodenum outlines the area of the pancreas that is of interest. A fluid-filled stomach may also be helpful to outline the pancreatic tail. This technique, however, has several drawbacks: (1) many patients suffer severe nausea, and large amounts of water may induce vomiting; (2) fluid filling is contraindicated for fasting patients receiving intravenous fluid; and (3) the method can be time-consuming.

Technical Considerations

During pancreatic sonography, the gain control is usually at settings comparable to those used for scanning the liver. Determination of the normal pancreatic sonographic pattern

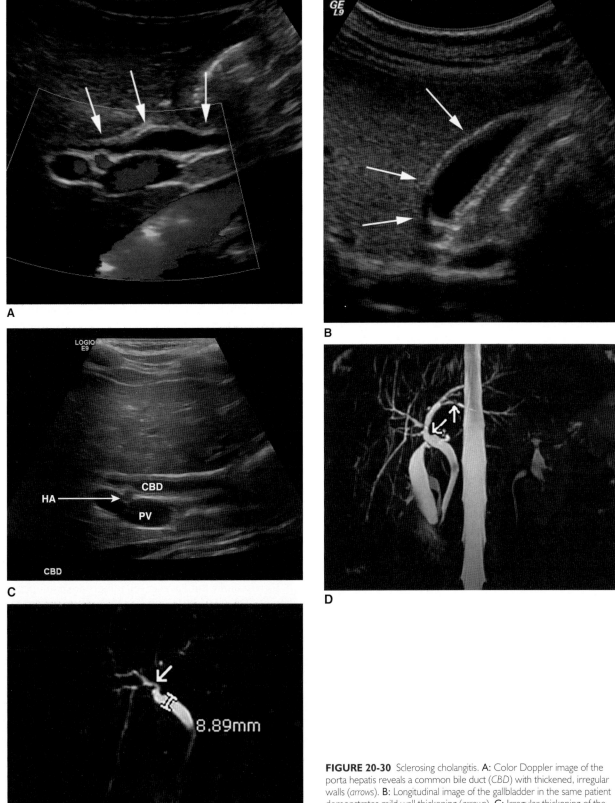

FIGURE 20-30 Sclerosing cholangitis. **A:** Color Doppler image of the porta hepatis reveals a common bile duct (*CBD*) with thickened, irregular walls (*arrows*). **B:** Longitudinal image of the gallbladder in the same patient demonstrates mild wall thickening (*arrows*). **C:** Irregular thickening of the wall keeping with known primary sclerosing cholangitis. **D & E:** Moderate irregularity noted within the biliary tree with several regions of apparent stenosis and somewhat beaded appearance (*arrows*).

is based on a comparison to the liver parenchymal pattern. In children, the normal pancreatic parenchyma is relatively homogeneous, with even, high-, and medium-level echo distribution. This is in contrast to the irregular echo texture, or "cobblestone" appearance, considered normal for adults. The normal pancreas is similar to or more echogenic than the liver parenchyma. Vascular structures abound in this area and should have a clearly echo-free pattern and not filled in by too high a gain setting. The transducer frequency selections should be made to obtain the highest resolution with adequate penetration.

Normal Anatomy

During a sonographic pancreatic study, the sonographer should pay particular attention to surrounding vascular landmarks, to the gland's shape and size, and to delineation of the pancreatic duct.

Attention to the surrounding vascular landmarks may be necessary to identify this rather small structure. Sonographic studies should also give specific attention to the size of the pancreas. The maximum anteroposterior (AP) diameters of the head, body, and tail are measured on transverse images obtained by angling the transducer to visualize more parenchyma. The entire gland can usually be seen in one image if it is oriented transversely across the abdomen, but often it lies oblique to some degree, with the tail more cephalad than the head and body, in which case it may be necessary to obtain several images to demonstrate the entire gland. The pancreatic duct is not always seen in normal patients. Usually appearing as a single echogenic line less than 1 mm, it can be located in the pancreatic body in a plane cephalad to the splenic vein.

Developmental and Congenital Anomalies

A very small pancreas (head only) is due to agenesis of the dorsal pancreas during the embryonic stage and is associated with polysplenia. Annular pancreas is the result of a bifid pancreatic head, which encases the duodenum. This anomaly is associated with duodenal atresia or stenosis.

Cystic Fibrosis[47–49]

Cystic fibrosis is a recessively inherited disease, with a prevalence of 1 in 3,500 in Caucasians and 1 in 17,000 in African Americans in the United States. Cystic fibrosis affects the exocrine glands in the lungs and GI tract, which produce abnormal highly viscous mucus. Those affected with cystic fibrosis have pancreatic exocrine dysfunction because of obstruction of the small ductules by mucoid secretions. The obstruction of the small ductules leads to subsequent tissue destruction and atrophy and eventual replacement of the pancreatic tissue with fibrosis and fat. Eventually, normal function is compromised, and pancreatic insufficiency results.

In cystic fibrosis patients, the pancreas is quite hyperechoic because of the replacement of normal pancreatic tissue by fibrosis and fatty tissue. Sonographically, apparent cysts may be found. Intraluminal calcifications can be found, but inflammatory changes are not common. Pancreatitis may occur but is not common, and notably, the sonographic appearance is not affected.

Other causes of a hyperechoic pancreas in childhood include steroid therapy, chronic pancreatitis, obstruction of the main pancreatic duct, and Cushing syndrome. Clinical and biochemical tests can distinguish these diseases from cystic fibrosis.

Congenital Cysts[48]

von Hippel–Lindau disease and autosomal polycystic disease are autosomal dominant disorders that can cause cysts in the pancreas as well as other organs (liver, kidney, adrenal glands, and spleen). Patients with von Hippel–Lindau disease also present with cerebellar, medullary, and spinal hemangioblastomas and pheochromocytomas.

Pancreatic Neoplasms[49–51]

Pancreatic neoplasms are uncommon in childhood, but their clinical appearance is similar to that in adults.

Pancreatic Carcinoma

Pancreatic carcinoma is a nonfunctioning tumor. Early diagnosis is difficult because of the variety and nonspecificity of early signs and symptoms. Because of this, the tumor is often large by the time it is discovered, and metastases to the liver, lymph nodes, and lung have already occurred.

Sonographically, pancreatic carcinoma usually appears as a localized, hypoechoic mass in comparison to the homogeneous texture of the normal pancreas. Focal enlargement is also an important sonographic clue. Lesions less than 2 cm are often difficult to detect, especially if they create only minor acoustic alterations.

Islet Cell Tumors

Approximately two-thirds of islet cell tumors are functional, producing a hormone that provokes the clinical suspicion of tumor early in the course of disease. Because of this, most islet cell tumors are small when first detected. The diagnosis is usually made by analyzing serum hormone levels. Therefore, in these cases, diagnostic imaging is used to localize rather than to diagnose.

The remaining third of islet cell tumors are nonfunctional. Owing to a lack of hormone secretion, they remain silent until they grow large enough to produce a palpable mass that obstructs the biliary system or the GI tract.

Sonographically, an islet cell tumor is a well-circumscribed, anechoic mass. It is important to search for metastatic disease, which may be the only reliable sign of malignancy. Sonography can be uniquely helpful in identifying the islet cell tumors in the operating room when all other modalities have failed. Direct pancreatic scanning can aid in tumor localization.

Insulinoma

Insulinoma, another tumor that occurs in childhood, is round, firm, and encapsulated, and 75% of the time is located in the body or tail of the pancreas. Clinically, patients present with hypoglycemia, which is often manifested in children by erratic behavior and seizures. Ectopic adenomas are rare, and most are benign.

Insulinomas sonographically appear as relatively small, hypoechoic, well-circumscribed masses. Insulinomas are sometimes difficult to accurately identify and isolate preoperatively. At surgery, palpation is used to aid in detection but is not always reliable. Intraoperative sonography is a more accurate method for detection. It provides better resolution, the field of view is such that access to the pancreas is improved, and the whole area of interest can be visualized and interrogated, unobscured by bowel gas and overlying structures.

Lymphoma

Lymphoma of the pancreas is a rare neoplasm. The involvement of the pancreas in a lymphatic process is usually secondary to primary lymph node disease. The neoplasm can be located anywhere in the pancreas, and symptoms depend on anatomic location.

The diagnosis of pancreatic lymphoma should be considered in several clinical situations: when a pancreatic mass develops in a patient known to have disseminated lymphoma, when fine-needle aspiration biopsy of a pancreatic mass reveals lymphocytes without evidence of carcinoma, and when a pancreatic mass is associated with chylous ascites.

Focal infiltration of the pancreas in lymphoma appears sonographically as a large, solitary, hypoechoic lesion. Differential diagnosis is facilitated by the presence of para-aortic lymphomas and the fact that the underlying disease is usually obvious at the time the pancreatic lesions are demonstrated.

Pancreatitis[8,47–49,52]

Pancreatitis is significantly less common in children than in adults but is not all that rare. Pediatric pancreatitis may have a variety of causes: (1) trauma (blunt abdominal trauma secondary to childhood accident, motor vehicle accidents, and child abuse); (2) infection (usually viral, such as mumps or mononucleosis); (3) toxicity (secondary to drugs such as prednisone and L-asparaginase); (4) heredity (an autosomal dominant disorder beginning in childhood); and (5) idiopathic. The most common of these is blunt abdominal trauma. To distinguish between the possible causes of pancreatitis, it is important to obtain a detailed patient history.

Acute Pancreatitis[19,48,49,52]

Acute pancreatic inflammation causes the escape of pancreatic enzymes from the acinar cells into surrounding tissues. Acute pancreatitis can usually be diagnosed with combined clinical and laboratory information without requiring pancreatic imaging. However, diagnostic imaging may be necessary when a wide variety of clinical symptoms, possible causes, and complications cause confusion. Nausea and vomiting are common and may precede or follow the onset of abdominal pain. Other frequent physical findings include fever, tachycardia, abdominal distention due to ileus, and abdominal tenderness. The use of sonography enables earlier diagnosis of acute pancreatitis in children with acute or chronic pain. Diagnostic imaging is also useful in defining the extent of the disease in the patient with suspected complications, such as necrotizing pancreatitis, hemorrhagic pancreatitis, pseudocyst formation, and superimposed infection.

The primary sonographic appearance in acute pancreatitis is of an enlarged, edematous gland that is less echogenic than the liver parenchyma (Fig. 20-31A). These characteristics are most obvious during the first hours after an acute attack. A dilated pancreatic duct is another indication of pancreatitis (Fig. 20-31B). A pancreatic ductal diameter of 1.5 mm should be considered abnormal. The pancreas' size and echo pattern usually return to normal as the disease resolves. The entire pancreas is usually involved, but sometimes, only portions are affected, particularly in pancreatitis by trauma. Follow-up examinations may help establish the diagnosis of pancreatitis by showing a decrease in the size of the pancreas. Sonography is also useful in the early detection of complications and the identification of associated biliary disease.

Complications of Acute Pancreatitis

After an episode of acute pancreatitis, a range of pathologic changes may develop in the gland and peripancreatic region.

Pseudocysts[11]

The best known complication of pancreatitis is pseudocyst formation. Pseudocysts can cause pain or bowel or

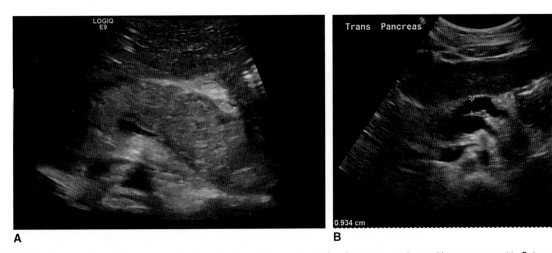

A **B**

FIGURE 20-31 Acute pancreatitis. **A:** The pancreas is enlarged in size and heterogeneous in echotexture, consistent with acute pancreatitis. **B:** In another patient, there is a markedly dilated pancreatic duct at 0.9 cm.

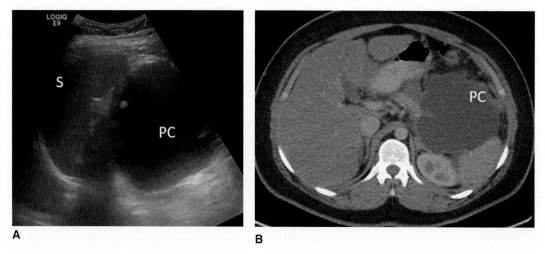

FIGURE 20-32 Pancreatic pseudocyst (*PC*). A 17-year-old male with type 2 diabetes mellitus, fatty liver, hyperlipidemia, and pancreatitis × 2 presents with 3 days of abdominal pain. **A:** Large left-sided pancreatic PC, medial to the spleen (*S*). **B:** A septated pancreatic PC replaces the distal body and tail of the pancreas, measuring approximately 11 cm × 8 cm × 10 cm on computed tomography.

biliary obstruction and can become infected. Pseudocysts are usually located in or adjacent to the pancreas but can occur anywhere in the abdomen or pelvis. Occasionally, pseudocysts may even extend into the mediastinum. Serial examinations are useful for monitoring enlargement and regression of pseudocysts. The majority of pseudocysts resolve spontaneously within 4 to 12 weeks, but those that develop mature, fibrous capsules are unlikely to be reabsorbed spontaneously. Recurrent abdominal pain, elevated serum amylase, and intermittent nausea and vomiting are common clinical symptoms consistent with this complication. When percutaneous drainage of the pseudocyst is indicated, sonographic guidance may be used.

Because children's pseudocysts often have a different pathogenesis, they may resolve more rapidly than the more common adult pancreatitis of biliary or alcoholic origin. Children's pseudocysts are less likely to recur following drainage.

Pseudocysts are usually anechoic masses, with a sharp back wall and increased through transmission. They may be single or multiple. Pseudocysts sometimes contain internal echoes emanating from pus and cellular debris (Fig. 20-32A, B).

Hemorrhage

Intrapancreatic hemorrhage with acute pancreatitis results from disruption of one or more pancreatic blood vessels. This is uncommon but is a potentially lethal complication that may produce a large pancreatic hematoma.

Sonographically, hemorrhagic pancreatitis appears as an inhomogeneous mass. Initially, acute hemorrhage into the pancreas may appear anechoic, but it becomes moderately echoic as organization occurs.

Phlegmon

A phlegmon is a solid inflammatory mass that may develop following acute pancreatitis. Composed of necrotic tissue mixed with inflammatory exudate and tissue edema, phlegmon may resolve spontaneously whenever the necrotic process is not progressive. With more severe episodes of

acute pancreatitis, a necrotizing process may predominate and provoke further complications (Fig. 20-33A–C). The patient is also at risk for developing a pancreatic abscess by bacterial seeding into necrotic tissue. A phlegmon appears as an anechoic mass in the pancreatic bed. Clinical history plus sonographic findings usually lead to the correct diagnosis.

Abscess

Abscess formation is more likely to occur in severe cases of pancreatitis with extensive necrosis. Marked by spiking fevers, chills, and a recurrence of abdominal pain 10 to 14 days after the initial episode, drainage is required in all cases because, untreated, mortality is usually 100%.

A pancreatic abscess can arise from different sources. A pancreatic phlegmon may develop into an abscess when the necrotic pancreatic and peripancreatic tissues are invaded by infection. An abscess can also occur in a pseudocyst in much the same way. Terminology can be confusing here because the infected pseudocyst is sometimes considered a different entity and not called an abscess.

Pancreatic abscess usually appears as a large anechoic mass in the pancreatic bed. The sonographic appearance varies with the amount of suppurative material and debris. Abscess walls are usually thick, irregular, and echogenic. When air bubbles are present, the pancreatic area appears highly echogenic with occasional shadowing. The air may obscure visualization on sonograms.

Chronic Pancreatitis[47–49]

Chronic pancreatitis, or chronic relapsing pancreatitis, is a clinical condition caused by repeated attacks of acute pancreatitis, which causes fibrosis and destruction of pancreatic cells.

A majority of the childhood cases of chronic relapsing pancreatitis have a definite familial clustering pattern and represent examples of the disease called hereditary pancreatitis. The likelihood that patients with "hereditary pancreatitis" will develop pancreatic carcinoma is increased, particularly for those with pancreatic calcifications.

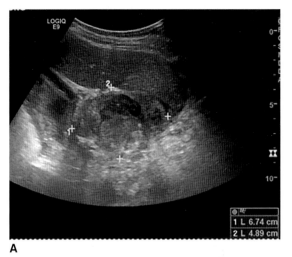

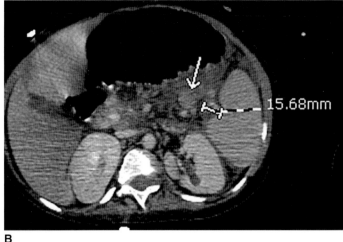

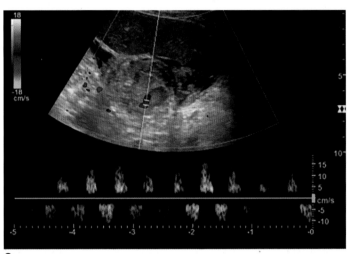

FIGURE 20-33 Pancreatic phlegmon with splenic artery aneurysm/pseudoaneurysm. **A:** Large phlegmon in the left upper quadrant extending to the splenic hilum consistent with necrotizing pancreatitis of the distal body and tail with surrounding phlegmon (*calipers*). **B:** There is a focal 1.4 cm × 1.7 cm dilatation of the splenic artery (*arrow*) at the superior aspect of the phlegmon with pulsatile swirling blood products (**C**).

Sonographically, in early stages of chronic pancreatitis, the pancreas is less echogenic than the normal liver parenchyma. This appearance is similar to that of acute pancreatitis. There may be dilatation of the main pancreatic duct or common bile duct caused by chronic pancreatitis. In advanced stages, the pancreas shrinks, develops irregular borders, and is more echogenic than usual. Calcifications and dilated ducts may also be present. The calcifications may be so pronounced and cause so much acoustic shadowing that pancreatic identification is difficult.

SPLEEN[53,54]

The normal sonographic appearance of the spleen and scan technique are the same in pediatric patients as in older patients. Much of the same pathologic processes occur in both populations. However, there are a few conditions unique to children. The most common indications for imaging the pediatric spleen are trauma and evaluating for congenital anomalies, such as polysplenia or asplenia. Spleen size is most often determined by measuring the length in a longitudinal, coronal plane from the dome to the inferior margin. Normal spleen size (based on length) has been established by age and weight. As a general guideline, the inferior margin of the spleen should not extend past the lower pole of the left kidney. In such cases, splenomegaly should be suspected (Table 20-1).

Developmental and Congenital Anomalies

Numerous syndromes and conditions are associated with asplenia and polysplenia. However, there are cases of isolated congenital asplenia in which an absent spleen is not affiliated with other developmental defects. It is important to differentiate between asplenia and polysplenia because they are associated with significant differences in anomalous systemic venous connections and tracheobronchial anomalies. For example, an abnormal renal vein confluence, although relatively rare, is frequently observed in asplenia. Also, congenital heart disease is typically more complex when associated with asplenia than polysplenia.

Asplenia

When evaluating for suspected asplenia, it is helpful to identify the vascular hilum of the spleen to differentiate it from the left lobe of the liver. Imaging the spleen adjacent to the left lobe of the liver in a transverse plane can increase diagnostic confidence in ruling out asplenia. It is important to

TABLE 20-1	Normal Splenic Length[54]
Age	**Length (Gender)**
0–3 months	4.4 (F) 4.6 (M)
3–6 months	5.2 (F) 5.8 (M)
6–12 months	6.3 (F) 6.4 (M)
1–2 years	6.3 (F) 6.8 (M)
2–4 years	7.5 (F) 7.6 (M)
4–6 years	8.0 (F) 8.1 (M)
6–8 years	8.2 (F) 9.0 (M)
8–10 years	8.7 (F) 9.0 (M)
10–12 years	9.1 (F) 9.8 (M)
12–14 years	9.8 (F) 10.2 (M)
14–17 years	10.3 (F) 10.7 (M)

F, female; M, male.

evaluate the entire abdomen for splenic tissue as "wandering spleen" may result in a nontraditionally located spleen. It is also worth noting that extralobar pulmonary sequestration below the diaphragm occurs more frequently on the left than the right. This entity can be similar in echogenicity and echotexture to the spleen and is associated with congenital anomalies.

Polysplenia

Polysplenia is defined as multiple splenules without a parent spleen typically located on the left side, although they may be bilateral. The most common anomaly affiliated with polysplenia is an interrupted IVC with azygous or hemiazygous continuation.

Splenomegaly

Splenomegaly refers to enlargement of the spleen. In pediatric patients, it is associated with sickle cell disease, portal hypertension, lymphoma, infectious mononucleosis, cardiac disease, infection, abscess, fungal microabscess, ECMO, and sepsis. Splenic cysts may be a cause of splenomegaly or palpable mass in the left upper quadrant of the abdomen and are the most common mass in the pediatric population. They have an appearance comparable to that of adults. Congenital cysts are considered "primary" and have an epithelial lining, whereas acquired or "secondary" cysts do not. Acquired cysts are also known as pseudocysts and, in children, are typically the result of prior trauma or affiliated with severe pancreatitis (Fig. 20-34A, B).

Infection

Splenic infection resulting in abscesses is associated with a variety of processes, including trauma, sickle cell disease, bacterial and fungal organisms, infarction, and pancreatitis. Splenic abscesses are much more common in immunocompromised children than those who are otherwise healthy. Fungal microabscesses should be suspected in children who are neutropenic with fever, abdominal pain, and an enlarged spleen. The most common type of fungal infection is *Candida* and may involve the liver and spleen. The appearance is typical of fungal infection in the adult population

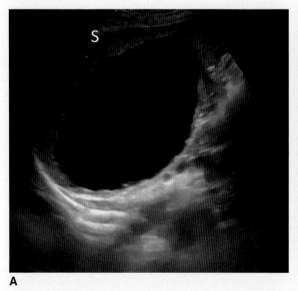

A

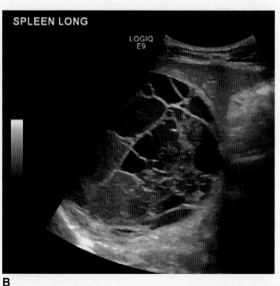

B

FIGURE 20-34 Splenic cyst. **A:** Large 18-cm cystic structure within the spleen (S) in a 14-year-old male. **B:** Rupture of preexisting very large splenic cystic lesion in the setting of blunt abdominal trauma in the same patient. Sonography now demonstrates a large multiloculated cyst within the S.

as multiple "bull's-eye" or "wheel-within-wheel" lesions. A high-frequency linear transducer should be utilized to visualize these microabscesses, which can be under 2 cm in diameter. In nonimmunocompromised children, cat-scratch disease should be considered. Infection with *Bartonella henselae* can result from being scratched by a cat or kitten. A small percentage of these patients can develop a systemic infection. These microabscesses are characterized as hypoechoic on ultrasound, may calcify, and often take months to resolve.

Splenic infarction, hematoma, and rupture in the pediatric population have the same etiology, pathologic progression (which may include infection), and sonographic appearance as in the general population.

Tumors

Lymphoma is the most common malignant mass of the spleen in childhood. On ultrasound, these masses tend to be hypoechoic, solitary, or multiple and may or may not have associated splenomegaly. Enlargement of retroperitoneal lymph nodes can help differentiate this disease from other conditions. Other than leukemia and lymphoma, tumors of the spleen are rare in children. Patients with leukemia may present with diffuse splenomegaly, but focal lesions are uncommon.

Hamartomas are the most common primary neoplasm of the spleen in children, although rare and benign. Sonographically, they are hypoechoic, avascular, and solid but may have a cystic component.

Hemangiomas of the spleen in children have a variable ultrasound appearance, as in the adult population. They may occur in as solitary lesions or in association with a syndrome, such as Beckwith–Wiedemann or Klippel–Trenaunay–Weber.

Lymphangioma, leiomyoma, and angiosarcoma are very uncommon in children and have a sonographic depiction similar to that of the adult population.

Metastatic involvement of the spleen, although rarely present in childhood, is most often related to neuroblastoma.

Sickle Cell Anemia

Young children with sickle cell disease or sickle cell trait may develop acute splenomegaly secondary to congestion of red pulp, causing intense pain. Acute splenic sequestration can be life-threatening because these patients may have a rapid drop in hematocrit and become hypotensive. Sonographically, the spleen is very large with hyperechoic and hypoechoic areas as a result of autoinfarction (Fig. 20-35A). In older children with sickle cell disease, the spleen becomes small and fibrotic from chronic autoinfarction and may calcify (Fig. 20-35B).

Gaucher Disease

Gaucher disease is the most common lysosomal storage disorder and predominantly affects those with Ashkenazi Jewish heritage. Hepatosplenomegaly and bone marrow involvement are hallmarks of the most common (non-neuropathic) form of this disease and contribute to anemia and thrombocytopenia. The spleen is markedly enlarged compared with the liver and is echogenic but may have small areas of hypoechogenicity or hyperechoic foci. The extent of splenic fibrosis and infarction is best depicted on MRI.

GASTROINTESTINAL TRACT[55,56]

Although sonography is not usually the modality of choice for evaluating the adult GI tract, sonography of the GI tract is readily performed in infants and children using a high-frequency linear transducer. Graded compression is utilized to displace bowel gas and permit visualization of

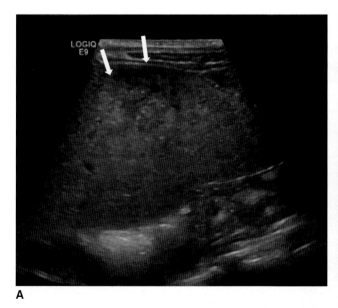
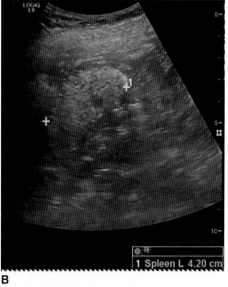

A   **B**

FIGURE 20-35 Sickle cell disease. **A:** Acute splenic sequestration. The spleen is moderately enlarged in size and demonstrates diffusely heterogeneous echotexture. The spleen measures 16.3 cm in maximum length and 7.6 cm in maximum width. Splenic parenchyma is diffusely heterogeneous with a mottled appearance characterized by innumerable tiny hypoechoic areas interspersed in the parenchyma. There is a relatively more hypoechoic and peripherally located area up to 4 cm × 3.5 cm × 3 cm size in the interpolar region, without any intrinsic vascularity (*arrows*). **B:** Atrophic echogenic spleen in a 14-year-old female with sickle cell disease.

the underlying structures. Hypertrophic pyloric stenosis (HPS), intussusception, and acute appendicitis are primarily evaluated using sonography.

Stomach

The normal gastric wall, including the mucosa and muscularis muscle layer, measures from 2.5 to 3.5 mm. The gastric wall's thickness can be assessed with the patient lying in the supine and RLO positions before and after ingestion of fluid. For such a study, the child should fast (Fig. 20-36A). With abnormalities associated with stomach wall thickening, the measurements and configuration remain unchanged when water is ingested. The stomach has an echogenic submucosa well seen with a fluid-filled stomach and an outer hypoechoic rim of muscle. A variety of abnormalities (e.g., eosinophilic gastritis, gastric ulcer, lymphoid hyperplasia, gastric hamartoma) have been reported to cause gastric wall thickening

of 5 to 15 mm. Ménétrier disease or transient protein losing gastropathy displays hypertrophy of the mucosa. The mucosa is thickened and echogenic, especially in the fundus and antrum. Lymphoma, Henoch–Schönlein purpura, and lymphangiectasia may look similar. In children with gastric ulcer disease, the thickening occurs in the antropyloric mucosa. Moderate or generalized thickening up to 5 mm was present with lymphoid hyperplasia, varioliform gastritis, and Crohn disease involving the stomach. The greatest amount of thickening (up to 10 mm) occurs in children with chronic granulomatous disease (Fig. 20-36B, C).

Pyloric Stenosis[55,57–63]

HPS most commonly affects first-born male infants between 2 and 10 weeks of age, with most patients presenting at 1 to 2 months of age. This idiopathic condition is caused by abnormal thickening of the antropyloric region of the stomach. Patients present with dehydration and frequent episodes of

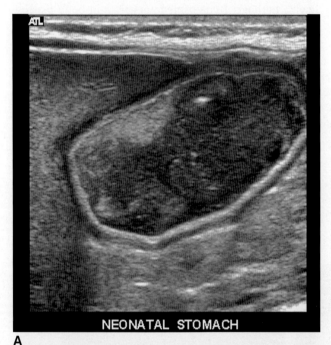

A

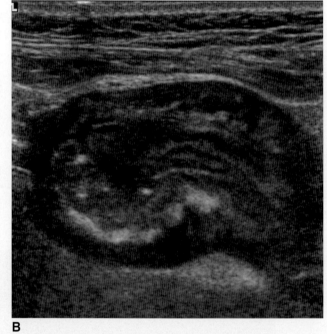

B

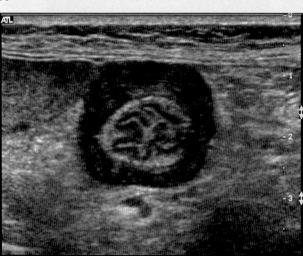

C

FIGURE 20-36 Stomach. **A:** In this image of a normal neonatal stomach filled with fluid, the hyperechoic submucosa can be clearly seen surrounded by the hypoechoic muscle layer. **B:** This image of the stomach demonstrates thickened submucosal and muscular layers. **C:** This transverse image of the stomach demonstrates a markedly thickened hypoechoic muscular layer. (Images courtesy of Phillip Medical Systems. Bothell, WA.)

projectile nonbilious vomiting; failure to thrive may also be noted. Sonography is highly sensitive and specific for the diagnosis of this condition, providing direct visualization of the pyloric muscle and passage of fluid through the pylorus (Fig. 20-37A, B). With pyloric stenosis, the stomach is often not empty, even if the patient has been fasting.

The patient should be examined in the supine and RPO positions; adjusting the position is particularly helpful when overlying bowel obscures the view. When possible, the patient should be fasting for 2 hours before the examination. The transverse plane demonstrates the long axis of the pylorus, and the longitudinal plane demonstrates its transverse axis. To identify the pylorus, scans should be made in the transverse plane, descending along the lesser curvature of the stomach through the left lobe of the liver, just to the right of the midline. The antrum of the stomach appears just medial to the gallbladder in the transverse plane, and the pylorus is continuous with the stomach. If the pylorus is not well visualized, the patient may be given water or nonmedicated liquid orally or through an enteric tube to better display the gastric lumen. The pylorus should be examined periodically while doing so, as an overly distended stomach can reposition the pylorus posteriorly, making it more difficult to evaluate. Images or video clips documenting fluid passing through the pyloric channel and into the duodenal bulb is an excellent way to rule out HPS.

The mass presents as a "doughnut" sign: an anechoic to hypoechoic muscle mass with a central lumen of increased echogenicity (Fig. 20-37C). Measurements should be made from the antrum of the stomach to the most distal portion of the identifiable channel (Fig. 20-37D). The diagnosis of pyloric stenosis can be made when the length from the antrum to the distal end of the channel exceeds 1.6 cm and the muscle thickness is 3 mm or larger (Fig. 20-37E, F). The numeric value of the elongated channel may be less important than the overall morphology of the pyloric canal and observations of gastric contents in real time. To differentiate from antritis, the stomach wall is always normal in patients with pyloric stenosis. The enlarged pyloric muscle is an abrupt change from the normal stomach wall.

Bezoar

Undigested material causing gastric or intestinal obstruction is known as a bezoar. Symptoms include early satiety, poor weight gain, vomiting, anorexia, and abdominal bloating. The most common type in infants is a lactobezoar, which consists of inspissated milk or infant formula. The phytobezoar is typically made up of poorly digestible plant or vegetable fibers and can be seen in patients with gastroparesis or other causes of poor gastric motility. Children with developmental delay or psychological disorders who chew on or eat hair or other material are at risk to develop a trichobezoar. Sonographically, a bezoar can appear as a solid or mottled mass in the stomach that may mimic the appearance of food. It may move to the dependent location in the stomach when the child is placed in a decubitus position. A bezoar form in the stomach and then become lodged in the small bowel, causing obstruction or perforation. Fluoroscopic upper GI or CT may help confirm or rule out this diagnosis.

Bowel Diseases of Infancy[8,52–59,64–66]

Abnormalities of the bowel typically diagnosed within the first year of life include small bowel obstruction, congenital anomalies such as midgut malrotation, bowel atresia, or meconium ileus.

Features of small bowel obstruction include hyperactive, dilated bowel loops with bowel wall thickening in some cases. Graded compression may be used in the sonographic evaluation of the small bowel. Sonography is useful when there is gasless abdominal distention. The normal small bowel wall thickness is 2 mm or less.

NEC is serious disease of preterm infants with a high mortality rate that requires urgent diagnosis and intervention. Preliminary research utilizing sonography shows promise for its use as an imaging modality that may have more prognostic value than abdominal x-ray. However, more studies are needed.

Atresias

Duodenal atresia, duodenal web, and duodenal stenosis are intrinsic causes of a dilated duodenum and stomach; the majority of obstructions at this level are intrinsic. (Extrinsic causes of an obstruction at this level include malrotation, duodenal duplication cyst, choledochal cyst, and annular pancreas.) Sonographically, the duodenum and stomach are seen as large anechoic structures; the esophagus may also be dilated. Duodenal atresia is common in patients with trisomy 21, 30% to 40% of patients with duodenal atresia have trisomy 21. A duodenal web may appear as an echogenic band in the proximal portion of the dilated duodenum.

Jejunal and ileal atresias are the most common causes of obstruction in the small bowel. Neonatal patients present with bilious vomiting, abdominal distention, and failure to pass meconium. Some of these patients will have associated abnormalities of midgut malrotation, gastroschisis, duodenal atresia, or tracheoesophageal fistula. The sonographic appearance is of multiple dilated loops of bowel in which active peristalsis can be seen.

Meconium Ileus

Meconium ileus is neonatal bowel obstruction due to abnormally thick meconium in the distal small bowel and is commonly associated with the presence of cystic fibrosis. The sonographic appearance includes echogenic bowel contents, dilated bowel loops, and decreased peristalsis.

A common complication of meconium ileus is antenatal meconium peritonitis and pseudocyst. It is also a complication of bowel atresia and in utero volvulus. Within 12 hours of perforation, calcifications can develop in the fetal abdomen, and echogenic ascites may be noted. These calcifications are easily identified in the fetal and neonatal abdomen. Meconium pseudocyst is a walled-off collection of meconium, which commonly contains calcifications (acoustic shadowing is noted) and may also contain air (shadowing or ring-down artifact may be noted).

Malrotation

Midgut malrotation of the small bowel mesentery is a result of arrested fetal gut development and is usually diagnosed within the first year of life. The mesentery may contain remnant peritoneal folds or shortened mesentery. Other anomalies

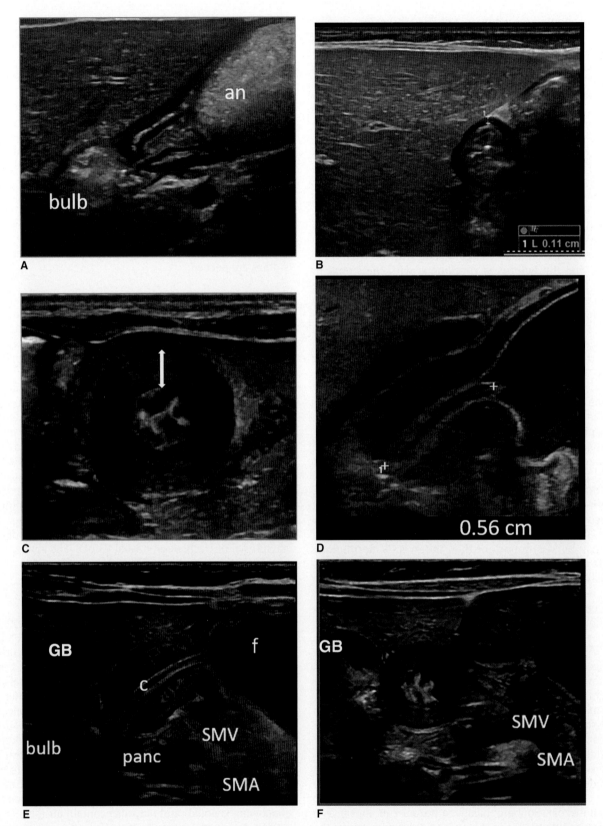

FIGURE 20-37 Hypertrophic pyloric stenosis (*HPS*). **A** and **B**: Longitudinal and transverse images demonstrate a normal pylorus. Gastric contents are seen in the antrum (*an*) and duodenal bulb (*bulb*). **C**: This transverse image of the pylorus demonstrates the doughnut sign with a thickened hypoechoic muscle layer. **D**: A longitudinal image of the pylorus demonstrates an elongated channel with a measurement from the antrum of the stomach to the distal end of the channel. A measurement of greater than 1.8 cm is considered abnormal. **E**: Long and transverse (**F**) axis images of the pylorus show a muscle thickness of 0.56 cm and an elongated pyloric channel (*C*) with a fluid-filled stomach in a 5-week-old boy with a history of 3 days of projectile vomiting and weight loss. The gallbladder (*GB*) is seen to the right of the pylorus and the pancreas (*panc*) posterior, with the superior mesenteric vein and artery medial (*SMV, SMA*). The triangular duodenal bulb just distal to the gastric antrum (*bulb*). Liquid is observed to pass readily from the antrum of the stomach into the duodenal bulb when the pyloric channel is normal. During this examination, fluid was not visualized passing through the elongated channel, consistent with HPS.

such as omphalocele, gastroschisis, diaphragmatic hernia, and duodenal atresia or web may coexist. Most patients present with bilious vomiting in the first month; abdominal sonography is useful to exclude other reasons for the vomiting.

The sonographer must demonstrate the relative positions of the SMV and superior mesenteric artery (SMA),

so careful scanning through the transverse axes of these vessels is crucial and should extend as inferiorly in the abdomen as possible. In patients with midgut malrotation, the normal positions of the SMV and SMA are reversed, with some cases presenting with the SMV directly anterior to the SMA (Fig. 20-38A). The SMA, which usually runs

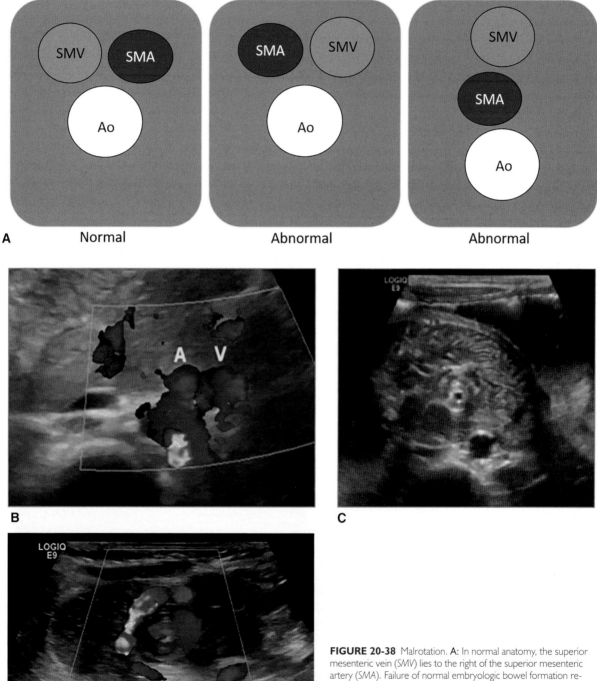

FIGURE 20-38 Malrotation. **A:** In normal anatomy, the superior mesenteric vein (*SMV*) lies to the right of the superior mesenteric artery (*SMA*). Failure of normal embryologic bowel formation reverses this relationship. Though reversal of this relationship may suggest malrotation, note that position of the vessels exists on a spectrum. Vessel position that deviates from the norm does not always imply malrotation is present. It is important to correlate sonographic findings with additional studies, including upper gastrointestinal. **B:** A 3-month-old male with vomiting demonstrates abnormal, clockwise swirling of mesenteric vessels in the midline abdomen along with a thickened loop of small bowel and its mesentery (**C**), forming the whirlpool sign (**D**). *Ao*, aorta.

inferior to the body of the pancreas, is pulled to the right side to lie anterior to the IVC or to the right of the aorta (Fig. 20-38B, C). Volvulus occurs when the bowel twists on itself and causes bowel obstruction. If volvulus is present, the whirlpool sign on grayscale and color Doppler has been shown to have 83% to 92% sensitivity and 100% specificity (Fig. 20-38D). The whirlpool appearance is a result of the mesentery and SMV wrapped around the SMA.

Hirschsprung Disease[55,67]

Hirschsprung disease (aganglionic megacolon) is a congenital disorder that is much more frequent in males than in females and is often associated with other anomalies, such as Down syndrome. It is usually manifested in early infancy and has been diagnosed in utero. Hirschsprung disease is caused by congenital absence of parasympathetic ganglion cells in the submucosal and intramuscular plexuses; the bowel becomes enormously dilated, and there is no peristaltic action in the aganglionic area. The aganglionic segment remains contracted without reciprocal relaxation and produces a functional obstruction. The area most frequently affected is the rectosigmoid.

The clinical manifestations depend on the length of aganglionosis or bowel distention. When the disease manifests in early infancy, the patient presents with abdominal distention, constipation, and vomiting and often appears malnourished and anemic. Hirschsprung disease can be suggested by sonography if the transition zone can be seen high in the sigmoid colon. The findings of distal colon obstruction are dilated distal small bowel and proximal colon, which may be quite echogenic from meconium. The findings of imperforate anus and atresia of the colon cannot be diagnosed by sonography, but by examining the patient from the perineal surface, the distance from the anus to the colon lumen can be measured.

Meckel Diverticulum

Meckel diverticulum is the most common congenital abnormality of the small intestine. It occurs when there is incomplete obliteration of the vitelline (omphalomesenteric) duct, and it can be a difficult diagnosis to make. It is a blind-ending outpouching of the ileum that can become infected (Fig. 20-39A–C). One of the complications is bowel obstruction. Most patients present before the age of 2 with painless rectal bleeding. Meckel diverticulum

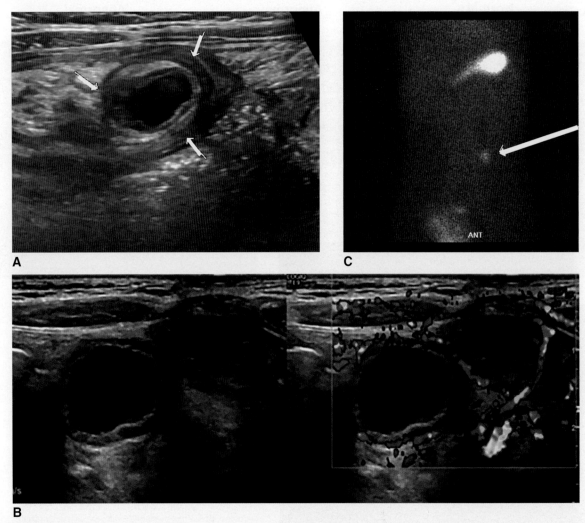

FIGURE 20-39 Meckel diverticulum. A 2-year-old male presents with emesis and recurrent colicky abdominal pain. **A:** Ultrasound reveals an acutely inflamed tubular fluid-filled pouch with gut signature in the left lower abdomen, with hyperemia (*arrows*) **(B)** suspicious for Meckel diverticulum. **C:** Nuclear medicine is useful in detecting the abnormally located mucosa of Meckel and confirmed the finding (*arrow*).

may also act as a lead point for intussusception. Most nonobstructive cases can be resolved by laparoscopic diverticulectomy.

Intussusception[8,11,52,58,62]

Intussusception is when the bowel telescopes on itself and is the most common obstructive bowel disorder of early childhood, found more frequently in males between the ages of 1 and 3 years. Intussusception occurs when a segment of bowel prolapses into a more distal segment (Fig. 20-40A–C). In the case of an ileocolic intussusception, ileum prolapses into the ascending colon. If the diagnosis is made early, the intussusception can easily be reduced by hydrostatic pressure before complications such as bowel obstruction, perforation, peritonitis, and vascular compromise (which, in turn, leads to edema of the bowel wall and gangrene) occur.

The most common type is ileocolic, followed by ileoileal and colocolic. Ninety percent of intussusceptions in children are ileocolic and typically occur between the ages of 3 months and 3 years. The child has a history of intermittent colicky abdominal pain, bloody stool, distention, and vomiting, and an abdominal mass may be palpable. Intussusception is rare in the first month of life. The majority of cases are idiopathic, but in children older than 3 years, there is greater likelihood of a lead point for the intussusception, such as a concurrent Meckel diverticulum, enteric duplication cyst, intestinal polyps, intramural hematoma, or a small bowel mass or tumor such as lymphoma. The incidence is higher for children who have undergone surgery and for those who have cystic fibrosis, appendicitis, or Henoch–Schönlein purpura.

Because sonography is now used as a screening procedure for patients with an abdominal mass as well as for children with vomiting and because the presentation of an intussusception is often not typical, there are sonographic patterns of intussusception that should be recognized. This is the so-called target pattern (multiple concentric anechoic rings surrounding a dense echogenic center) or the doughnut sign (an anechoic ring surrounding an echogenic center), or the pseudokidney appearance in the long axis (a reniform-shaped complex mass) (Fig. 20-40E–G). The intussuscipiens (the distal bowel into which the intussusceptum or proximal bowel herniates) does not usually suffer vascular compromise and so is not edematous but normally thin. As the intussusceptum becomes edematous, it compresses the bowel lumen, creating a hypoechoic ring with increased central echogenicity. Depending on the imaging plane, fluid may be present centrally in the obstructed bowel lumen. It is crucial to evaluate all quadrants of the abdomen and pelvis as an intussusception may extend all the way to the sigmoid colon.

In many pediatric hospitals, ileocolic intussusceptions are reduced with either hydrostatic pressure under sonographic or fluoroscopic guidance or retrograde flow of air or barium (Fig. 20-40H). Small bowel intussusception and unsuccessful reduction of an ileocolic intussusception may require surgical intervention. Incidence of intussusception is high within the first 24 hours following reduction, and these patients must be carefully monitored and reexamined if symptoms of intussusception recur.

Crohn Disease[50,58,68]

Crohn disease is the most common inflammatory disease of the small bowel. Approximately 25% of cases are diagnosed before adulthood, and its incidence is increasing in the pediatric population. The most common bowel segments affected are the terminal ileum and proximal colon. A child with Crohn disease typically present at age 10 years or older, and the most common clinical presentation is of abdominal pain, diarrhea, fever, and weight loss. Although contrast radiography examinations and endoscopy with biopsy have been the primary tools for diagnosis of this condition, technological advances in sonography are providing improved visualization of inflammatory bowel disease.

Sonographic evaluation of Crohn disease utilizes the graded-compression technique. The sonographic findings include concentric or eccentric thickened bowel walls, with the submucosal layer typically the thickest. A bowel wall measurement of 2.5 to 3 mm or more is abnormal. The bowel may be partially compressible or noncompressible with graded compression, and decreased peristalsis may be noted. Color Doppler imaging is used to demonstrate that the vascularity of the affected segment of bowel and actively inflamed bowel will show increased vascularity. However, this finding is nonspecific for Crohn disease because other bowel inflammations may have the same appearance. Increased flow in the SMA may be noted.

Areas of increased echogenicity (fibrofatty tissue proliferation in the mesentery) may appear to create a barrier around inflamed bowel loops, and enlarged lymph nodes may be seen. Reactive intraperitoneal free fluid may be present. The appendix may become thickened secondary to the spread of inflammation, with findings the same as acute appendicitis. Hypoechoic or complex masses in the right lower quadrant may be related to the presence of abscess or phlegmon. Sinus tracts or fistulas to other structures may be noted.

Other inflammatory conditions that cause small bowel wall thickening include cystic fibrosis, malabsorption syndromes, acute enteritis (which may mimic acute appendicitis), tuberculosis, histoplasmosis, *Campylobacter jejuni* infection, and *Salmonella typhosa* infection.

Duplication Cysts[52]

Enteric duplication cysts are benign and located along the mesenteric border of the bowel but do not communicate with the bowel. Most of these cysts are found in the ileum. Clinical findings include abdominal pain and distention, vomiting, and rectal bleeding. These cysts can be the lead point of intussusception and may cause pancreatitis if located near the ampulla of Vater.

Sonographically, enteric duplication cysts demonstrate as a well-defined, round, fluid-filled mass that is anechoic to hypoechoic with acoustic enhancement. Duplication cysts have a hypoechoic outer or muscular rim and a hyperechoic inner rim of mucosa. These layers allow differentiation from other cystic masses such as mesenteric or omental cyst, choledochal cyst, ovarian cyst, pancreatic pseudocyst, and abscess, which lack a mucosal wall (Fig. 20-41A–C). In some cases, the cyst may appear complex because of hemorrhage or debris.

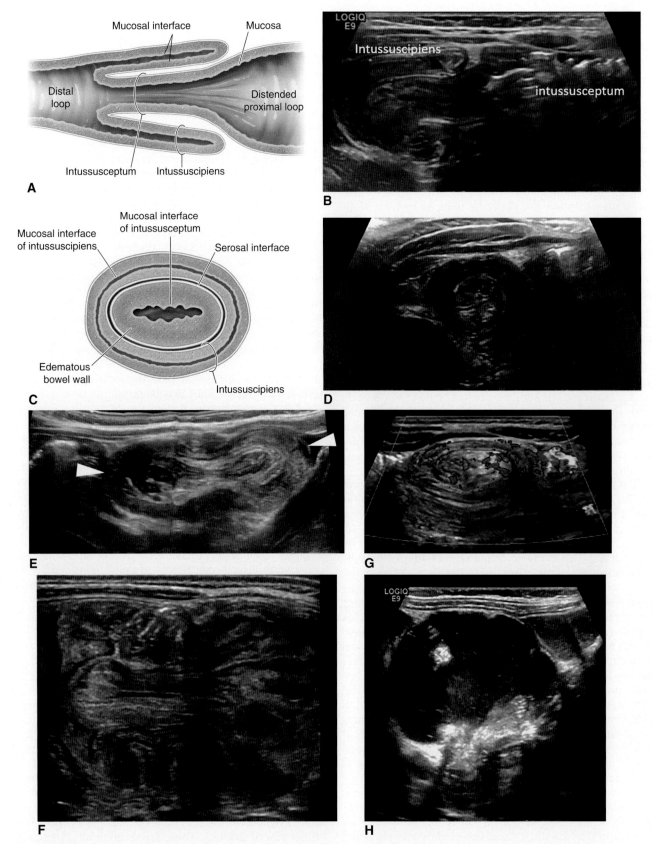

FIGURE 20-40 Intussusception. **A:** An illustration of intussusception caused by the proximal bowel loop telescoping into the lumen of the adjacent distal portion. **B:** Sonographic correlation of intussuscipiens and intussusceptum. **C:** A cross-sectional illustration of intussusception. **D:** Sonographic correlation of cross-sectional intussusception. A 20-month-old female presenting with bloody stool and vomiting. **E:** Grayscale panoramic image of the right upper quadrant showing a large structure (*arrowhead*) with concentric hypoechoic and hyperechoic rings. **F:** Longitudinal plane typical of intussusception. **G:** Robust flow seen on a color Doppler transverse image suggests viable bowel. **H:** Ultrasound-guided intussusception reduction. Under continuous sonographic guidance, a dilute solution of contrast was introduced into the colon via gravity until the intussusception was encountered. Further contrast filling resulted in successful reduction of the ileocolic intussusception, with observation of fluid filling distal small bowel loops.

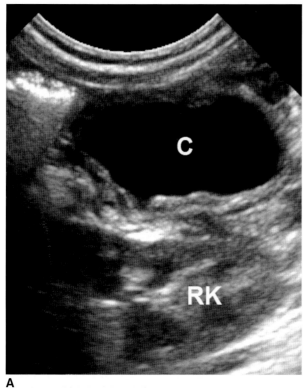

A

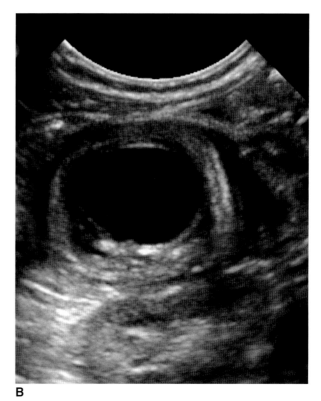

B

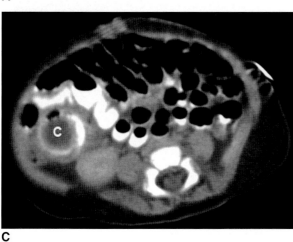

C

FIGURE 20-41 Duplication cyst. A 1-month-old patient presents with a history of a fever and bloody stool. The sonograms (**A, B**) of the right lower quadrant reveal a cystic structure with a thick wall. **C:** A computed tomography image on the same patient demonstrates the thick-walled cystic structure filled with simple fluid. A diagnosis of mesenteric duplication cyst was made with Meckel diverticulum as a differential diagnosis. *RK,* right kidney. (Images courtesy of Dr. Nakul Jerath, Falls Church, VA.)

Lymphoma[52]

The most common malignant mass of the small bowel is lymphoma. Most cases of bowel lymphoma are non-Hodgkin, presenting with palpable abdominal mass or with abdominal pain and vomiting (due to obstruction). The ileum is the most common site within the small bowel for lymphoma involvement, but multiple areas within the bowel may be affected. Sonographically, lymphoma of the small bowel demonstrates as hypoechoic bowel wall thickening or a focal hypoechoic or complex mass with areas of necrosis. The bowel lumen may be narrowed, and intussusception may occur. Other related findings can include splenomegaly and enlargement of the retroperitoneal and mesenteric lymph nodes.

Appendicitis[8,52,58,62,66]

The most common condition requiring emergency surgical intervention in children is acute appendicitis. The incidence

in the United States is 1 in 4,000 children under the age of 14. It is almost always associated with obstruction of the appendiceal lumen. The most common clinical presentation is periumbilical abdominal pain that migrates to the right lower quadrant, abdominal tenderness, fever, and leukocytosis, but the presentation may be variable, and other conditions, such as gynecologic disorders, can mimic appendicitis.

Sonography is the primary method of imaging for appendicitis in children because the abnormal appendix and surrounding tissues can be evaluated and other conditions, which may be mimicking appendicitis, can be found. The graded-compression technique is used to displace bowel gas and demonstrates the compressibility of the appendix (Fig. 20-42A). The examination is initiated by scanning transversely in the right midabdomen at about the level of the umbilicus, continuing caudad, with gradually increasing compression and then followed by reducing and then increasing the pressure of the transducer. This action allows

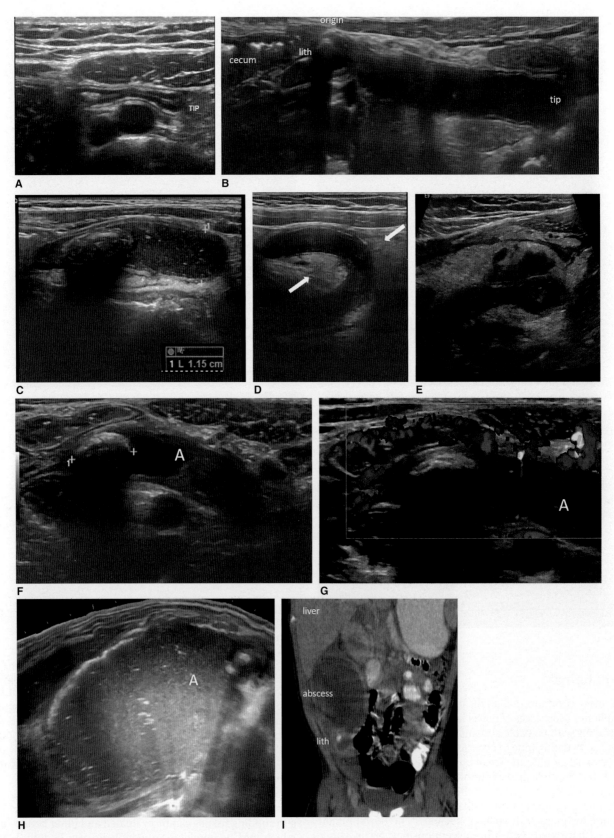

FIGURE 20-42 Appendicitis. **A:** The sonogram demonstrates the normal thin-walled appendix seen just anterior to the iliac vessels. **B:** Panoramic image of acute appendicitis. **C:** Longitudinal scan of right lower quadrant shows a dilated blind-ended tubular structure measuring 1.15 cm, representing an inflamed appendix. **D:** Longitudinal image of a dilated fluid-filled appendix is seen in the right lower quadrant, with mesenteric edema (*arrows*). **E:** Sonogram shows a dilated appendix with loss of normal wall structure, and adjacent irregular fluid pocket suggesting perforation and localized abscess. **F:** Echogenic appendicolith (*cursors*) is seen within the appendix (*A*). Note the acoustic shadowing from attenuation distal to the appendicolith. **G:** Hyperemia due to an inflamed appendix (*A*). **H:** A complex mass (*A*) seen in the right lower quadrant represents a large walled-off abscess in a patient with a ruptured appendix. **I:** A computed tomography was ordered and confirmed the findings of perforated appendicitis with appendicolith and large abscess, approximately 9.6 cm × 6.3 cm × 8.7 cm in the right hemiabdomen.

assessment of the compressibility of normal bowel. Normal cecum and terminal ileum are easily compressed with only moderate pressure. The inflamed appendix is most often visualized at the base of the cecal tip during maximum graded compression (Fig. 20-42B). Scanning at the point of maximum tenderness is useful. The abnormal appendix is a tubular, noncompressible, blind-ending structure and commonly has a target appearance of an outer hypoechoic muscular wall with an echogenic submucosa layer surrounding a fluid-filled center. The normal appendix should not exceed 6 mm in AP diameter (Fig. 20-42C, D).

An appendicolith (echogenic focus with acoustic shadowing) may be present in some cases of appendicitis (Fig. 20-42E, F). However, it is important to note that an appendicolith may be present in a normal appendix. Enlarged mesenteric lymph nodes, increased echogenicity of the pericecal area, and periappendiceal abscess may be noted as complications of perforation of the appendix (Fig. 20-42G).

Perforation, which occurs in 80% to 100% of children under the age of 3 years and 10% to 20% in ages 10 to 17 years, makes the diagnosis of appendicitis more difficult because the appendix may be no longer dilated or nonvisualized. Echogenic mucosa, increased echogenicity of periappendiceal mesentery, and a complex or fluid-filled focal collection (periappendiceal abscess) are the most common features of perforation. Major complications of perforation include abscess or phlegmon formation and peritonitis (Fig. 20-41H, I).

False-negative diagnosis of appendicitis may be due to focal appendicitis (infected tip and normal appendiceal origin and body) or nonvisualization of the appendix, which can occur with perforation or a retrocecal location. False-positive diagnoses are generally related to extension of inflammation from surrounding tissues, which may be seen in Crohn disease, tubo-ovarian abscess, or inflamed Meckel diverticulum.

RETROPERITONEUM[69–71]

The sonographic evaluation of the retroperitoneum is performed primarily to examine the kidneys, ureters, and urinary bladder and is discussed in the following chapter. The retroperitoneum also includes the muscles (psoas, quadratus lumborum), the crura of the diaphragm, and lymph nodes. Retroperitoneal hemorrhage, retroperitoneal fibrosis (rare in children), and presacral tumors can be evaluated with sonography.

Muscles

The retroperitoneal muscles may become involved in diseases that originate in the lymph nodes, kidneys, pancreas, duodenum, colon, and spinal column. Abscess can occur from bacteremia or adjacent inflammatory conditions; extension of lymphoma, Wilms tumor, Ewing sarcoma; and rhabdomyosarcoma originating in the muscle. The psoas muscle is a common location for abscess or changes related to neoplasm as well as hematoma in the hemophiliac patient. Correlation with clinical history is important.

Lymph Nodes

When multiple or large retroperitoneal lymph nodes are found during abdominal sonography of an infant or child, they are abnormal and are generally located near the aorta and IVC. Enlargement of lymph nodes in the retroperitoneum is most commonly associated with lymphoma, Wilms tumor, and neuroblastoma, but can be found in conjunction with other malignancies of the abdomen and pelvis. The sonographic appearance is of one or more hypoechoic homogeneous structures that may combine to appear as one large mass. The enlarged nodes can displace vessels and bowel anteriorly and displace the kidneys laterally (Fig. 20-43A, B).

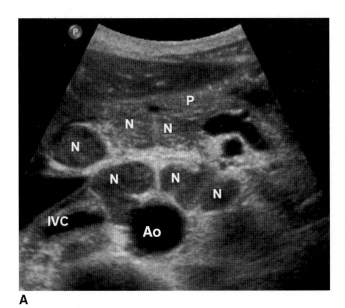

A

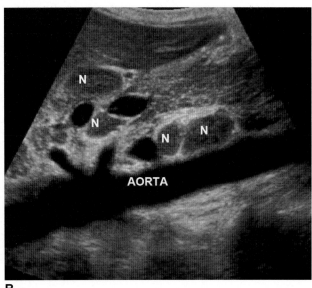

B

FIGURE 20-43 Lymphadenopathy. Transverse (**A**) and longitudinal (**B**) images demonstrate multiple hypoechoic lymph nodes (*N*) seen anterior to the aorta (*Ao*), adjacent to the pancreatic head (*P*) and porta hepatis. *IVC*, inferior vena cava. (Images courtesy of Philips Medical Systems, Bothell, WA.)

Neoplasms

Primary retroperitoneal tumors can arise from lymph channels, nerves, and connective tissues. Benign tumors include mature teratoma, hemangiomas, lipomatosis, lymphangioma, and neural tumors. Malignant tumors include rhabdomyosarcoma, fibrosarcoma, neuroblastoma, leiomyosarcoma, malignant germ cell tumor, malignant schwannoma, and Ewing sarcoma. Benign tumors are more likely to be hyperechoic with mature teratomas having a complex appearance due to fat, fluid, and bone contents (Fig. 20-44A–C). Malignant tumors are usually solid with variable echogenicity and a complex appearance due to hemorrhage or necrosis.

Presacral masses in children include sacrococcygeal teratoma (the most common), neuroblastoma, soft-tissue sarcomas, lymphoma, lipoma, anterior meningocele, sacral bone tumors, abscess, and rectal duplication.

There are four types of sacrococcygeal teratoma: type I that is predominately external, type II that is external with significant internal components, type III that is predominately internal, and type IV that is entirely presacral without external component or extension. These tumors occur most often in females, are predominately benign, and can be detected prenatally. The sonographic appearance of benign teratoma is of a predominately cystic structure with varied amounts of solid components (fat, calcification, bone, or teeth). Malignant teratomas are mostly solid but may contain cystic areas. Hydronephrosis or urine ascites from bladder rupture may be found. In most cases, CT and/or MRI are needed for a more accurate preoperative assessment.

Trauma

Retroperitoneal hemorrhage in children is associated with blunt abdominal trauma, although it can be a complication

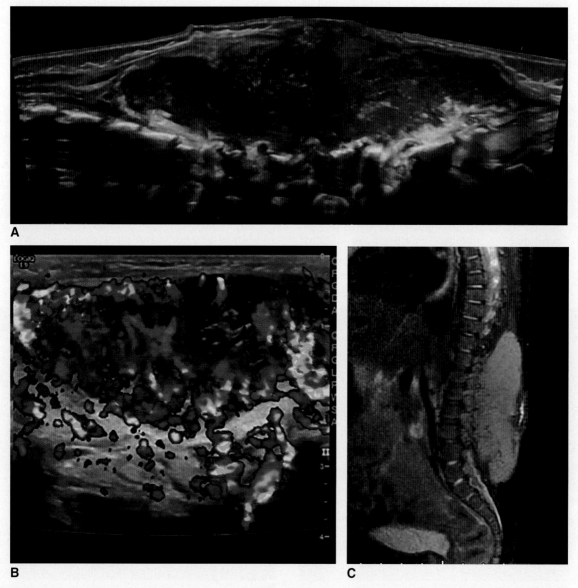

FIGURE 20-44 Retroperitoneal tumor in an ex-FT male born with large thoracolumbar mass. **A:** Ultrasound demonstrates a complex, hypervascular (**B**) structure to the right of midline. **C:** Large right-sided paraspinal soft-tissue tumor, invading the spinal canal from the lower T9 to S1, with severe cord compression. A diagnosis of fibrosarcoma was made by biopsy.

of renal biopsy or anticoagulant therapy. Hemorrhage associated with renal trauma first surrounds the kidney before extending into the retroperitoneal space. Sonography can detect the presence of fresh hemorrhage (anechoic) and follow the progress of the hemorrhage as it ages and changes in echogenicity.

Sonography has become one of the most important imaging modalities used for the evaluation of the pediatric urinary tract and adrenal glands. This is for several reasons. Unlike excretory urography and CT, sonography does not expose the child to ionizing radiation and does not carry the risk of a life-threatening anaphylactic contrast reaction.[72] Sonography can be performed portably, without sedation, and may be used for serial follow-up examinations. The examination cost is typically lower than the abovementioned modalities, and the ultrasound examinations are usually tolerated well by pediatric patients.

One of the most common ultrasound examinations ordered for the pediatric patient is the renal ultrasound. This is usually due to a suspected renal anomaly, which could be associated with abnormalities found in other body systems. Findings in prenatal sonography may also raise the question of renal anomalies.[11,73] For older infants and younger children, the most common reasons for ultrasound imaging referral are a workup for a urinary tract infection, enuresis, urgency, dysuria, and urinary reflux. Less common clinical indications of this examination include suspected mass palpation, unexplained hypertension, tuberous sclerosis, hemihyperplasia, prerenal or postrenal transplant evaluation, multicystic kidneys, polycystic kidneys, Prune belly syndrome, and the need for renal biopsy guidance.

KIDNEYS

Sonographic Technique

For evaluation of the kidneys, no preparation is necessary, although adequate hydration is preferred. Pediatric patients need not fast because the kidneys will be imaged from either the posterior surface (prone longitudinal or transverse scan planes) or the patient's side (coronal planes).

Most pediatric patients are evaluated in the prone position, but scanning children requires a certain amount of flexibility. When necessary, children may be scanned in the sitting position, decubitus positions, held in a parent's arms or lap, or across their parent's chest. Because children may be unable or unwilling to hold their breath or obey simple instructions, the sonographer must be prepared to scan from variable planes and positions to visualize all portions of the kidney. As part of the kidney examination, visualizing any portion of a dilated ureter is important. The bladder is also routinely examined as part of the urinary track sonographic evaluation.

For neonatal examinations, the higher frequency 10-MHz transducer affords exquisite resolution and detail of the kidney. Because the kidney is close to the posterior skin surface (0.5 to 3 cm) in young and premature infants, a 15-MHz transducer can provide excellent detail as long as penetration is adequate. A 7.5-MHz transducer is useful for scanning young children and older, thin children, providing excellent kidney detail. Either a curved-array or a linear-array transducer may be used.

Normal Sonographic Appearance

Sonographically, the renal pyramids or medulla of a normal newborn or infant can be identified as hypoechoic, triangular, or rectangular structures.[74] Sonographers unfamiliar with pediatric imaging have mistaken these structures for renal cysts (especially if a suboptimal transducer or transducer frequency is used). The renal pyramids show symmetric alignment within the kidneys cortical parenchyma. In 70% of kidneys, a compound renal pyramid or a normal hypoechoic medullary region occurs in the upper pole (50%), lower pole (30%), or middle region (20%). Compound calyces are a conglomerate of calyces that come to one infundibulum and are associated with compound pyramids. These fused medullary pyramids appear as an irregular, hypoechoic area. They are not associated with evidence of renal, pelvic, infundibular, or calyceal dilatation (Fig. 20-45A–D). If obstruction exists or other renal anomalies are present, the renal pyramids may be compressed and poorly visualized.

Renal lobulations are responsible for the irregular renal outlines seen in infants. The lobulations become less pronounced with age and disappear by about 6 years of age, although the normal junctional defects (triangular echogenic indentations in the cortex) on the anterior superior surface and the inferior posterior surface of the kidney may persist. The junctional parenchymal defect (also termed *interrenuncular defect*), an echogenic line from the renal cortex to the central sinus, separates the superior and inferior poles of the kidney and is a normal finding (Fig. 20-46).

The columns of Bertin are opposing infoldings of cortex, which are not separated by papillae. The cortex is thin compared with the medulla, and the renal sinus is less fat filled in infants and young children. The renal pelvis lies within the renal sinus during infancy. In childhood, half the renal pelvis is outside the renal sinus. The renal pelvis should measure less than 10 mm in the prone and supine positions.[74] The renal pelvic wall should not be visible. A wall may be thickened in cases of chronic infection, reflux, and chronic obstruction and is called urothelial thickening (Fig. 20-47). Urothelial thickening seen within the renal pelvis and in the ureters would be an abnormal sonographic finding.

Table 20-2 summarizes the normal infant and pediatric renal echo patterns. The cortical echogenicity in neonates and infants is greater than that in older children, especially in premature infants.[74–76] In older children, however, increased echogenicity in the cortex, although nonspecific, may indicate parenchymal disease. Causes of increased echogenicity are the same as for adults. Specific pediatric conditions include leukemia, progressive glomerulonephritis, nephrotic syndrome, renal artery stenosis, and chronic infection.[76]

Standard measurements of renal size have been published[77] and are related to the length of the kidney for age and also to the child's weight and body surface area.[78,79] These measurements are particularly useful for examining children who may have a diffuse process such as infection or leukemia.

Comparative measurements should be made to determine appropriate growth in children with chronic infection. Also, in children, the renal vein may be unusually prominent, including the intrahilar and sinus portions.

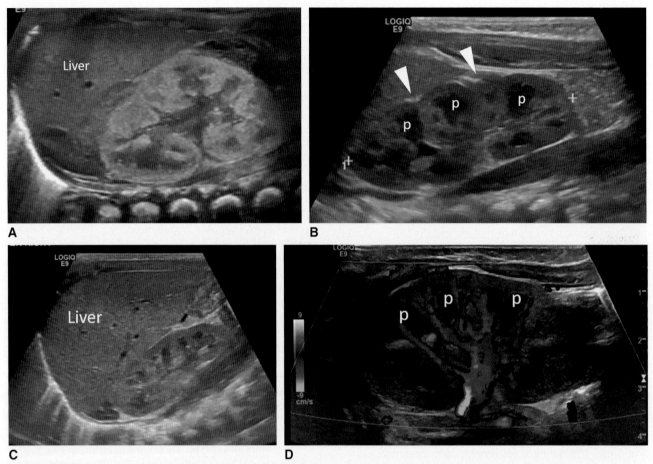

FIGURE 20-45 Normal kidneys. **A:** Longitudinal right kidney in a preterm neonate demonstrates the normal sonographic appearance. The pyramids are hypoechoic, and the echogenicity of the kidney cortex is greater than that of the adjacent liver. **B:** The normal neonatal kidney is seen in a longitudinal section with the hypoechoic to anechoic pyramids evenly spaced throughout the kidney. Note the normal mild fetal lobulation (*arrowheads*) and lack of renal sinus fat. **C:** Normal sonographic appearance of the right kidney in an infant. The cortex is isoechoic or slightly hypoechoic to the adjacent liver. **D:** Longitudinal view of the neonatal kidney demonstrates the normal renal vasculature with the interlobar vessels seen coursing between the renal pyramids (*p*). (Images **A** and **C**: Courtesy of Philips Medical Systems, Bothell, WA; Image **B**: Courtesy of GE Healthcare, Wauwatosa, WI; Image **D**: Courtesy of Jillian Platt, Falls Church, VA.)

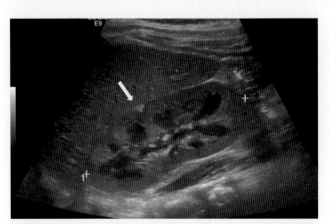

FIGURE 20-46 Junctional parenchymal defect (also termed *interrenuncular defect*). Longitudinal sonogram on a 9-year-old female with enuresis shows a normal kidney. Note the triangular defect in the upper pole (*arrow*).

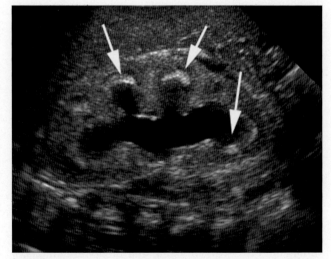

FIGURE 20-47 Thickened renal pelvic wall. This longitudinal sonogram of the kidney shows a dilated collecting system with a thick echogenic wall (*arrows*) in an infant with a history of posterior urethral valves and urinary tract infection. (Image courtesy of Dr. Nakul Jerath, Falls Church, VA.)

TABLE 20-2	**Normal Pediatric Renal Echo Pattern**	
Age	**Renal Structure**	**Echo Pattern**
Newborn	Cortex	More echoic than liver and spleen
	Sinus	Poorly defined because of paucity of fat in infants
6–8 weeks	Cortex	Isoechoic to liver and spleen
2–6 months	Cortex	Hypoechoic to liver and spleen
>6 months	Cortex	Hypoechoic to renal sinus

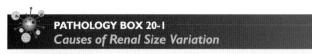

PATHOLOGY BOX 20-1
Causes of Renal Size Variation

Enlarged Kidney

Bilateral

Congenital: Duplication, cystic disease, storage disease, generalized visceromegaly, systemic infection

Acute: Pyelonephritis, glomerular nephritis

Neoplastic: Nephroblastomatosis, bilateral Wilms tumor, leukemia, lymphoma, tuberous sclerosis, or hamartoma

Vascular: Renal vein thrombosis, acute tubular necrosis, hemolytic uremia, sickle cell anemia

Obstructive: Congenital or acquired

Unilateral

Congenital: Duplication, cystic disease, cross-fused ectopia, horseshoe kidney

Infectious: Acute pyelonephritis, abscess

Neoplastic: Mesoblastic nephroma, Wilms tumor, angiomyolipoma or hamartoma, sarcoma, lymphoma

Vascular: Renal vein thrombosis, transplant complication (rejection or tubular necrosis)

Traumatic: Contusion, hematoma

Obstructive: Congenital, acquired

Small Kidneys

Bilateral

Congenital: Aplasia, hypoplasia

Acute: Pyelonephritis, glomerular nephritis

Infectious: Chronic pyelonephritis, reflux nephropathy with infarction

Vascular: Renal vein thrombosis, arterial occlusion (intrinsic or extrinsic)

Atrophic: Chronic obstruction, chronic recurrent infarction, chronic failure, dysplasia

Obstructive: Congenital or acquired

Unilateral

Congenital: Agenesis, hypoplasia

Infectious: Chronic, chronic reflux with infection

Vascular: Venous thrombosis, arterial obstruction (acquired or congenital)

Atrophic: Chronic obstruction, chronic infection and infarction, dysplasia

The renal vein can be distinguished from structures of the collecting system with color and/or pulsed Doppler. Fetal lobulations are present in most premature infants and in many newborns and infants.[75] By approximately 1 year of age, fetal lobulations should not be as evident, although, in some children, they persist as a normal variant. Fetal lobulation may be confused with scarring, but the pyelonephritic scar is usually opposite a clubbed calyx, whereas fetal lobulation is usually seen between the renal pyramids or calyces.

There is a great deal of variation in the size of pediatric kidneys. Large kidneys, by definition, are 2 standard deviations (SD) larger than the mean. Small kidneys are 2 SD smaller than the mean. An abnormality may be bilateral or unilateral, symmetric or asymmetric. There are a multitude of causes for an increase or decrease in the size of the kidneys (Pathology Box 20-1). Compensatory enlargement of a single functioning kidney usually occurs within 6 to 12 months following surgical removal of a kidney.

Duplex Doppler of the pediatric renal arteries demonstrates a sharp systolic peak with a continuous forward diastolic flow (Fig. 20-48A–D). With color-flow Doppler, it is easy to identify flow in the interlobar and arcuate arteries. The resistive indices (RIs) obtained in the interlobar and arcuate arteries should be less than 0.70.[80–82] In the normal neonate, the RI may exceed 0.70 but should be less than 0.70 by 6 weeks of age. The RIs are useful in helping to determine whether a dilated system is obstructed. The RI is increased in tubular interstitial disease and vascular disease, whereas frequently normal in glomerular disease.

Congenital Anomalies

Agenesis

Bilateral renal agenesis is associated with oligohydramnios, an unusually small amount of amniotic fluid. Renal agenesis is associated with Potter syndrome, features of which include abnormal facies with a small mandible and low-set ears. Affected infants also have pulmonary hypoplasia and frequently are stillborn or survive for only a very short time. They may live longer with hemodialysis, but eventually expire on account of renal failure. In cases of renal agenesis, the adrenal glands are usually well developed and may measure up to 3 cm in length (Fig. 20-49A, B).

It is important to use the highest resolution transducer available to achieve good definition of the adrenal glands and kidneys. With total renal agenesis, the bladder is also absent. Unilateral renal agenesis is more common and may be asymptomatic, in which case it may be detected only incidentally. Renal hypoplasia is probably due to renal infarction, possibly occurring in utero but more likely postpartum. Hypoplasia may result from unsuspected chronic atrophic pyelonephritis, unsuspected reflux nephritis, a hypoxic event, or decreased blood flow due to a vascular problem. Renal agenesis is a finding associated with

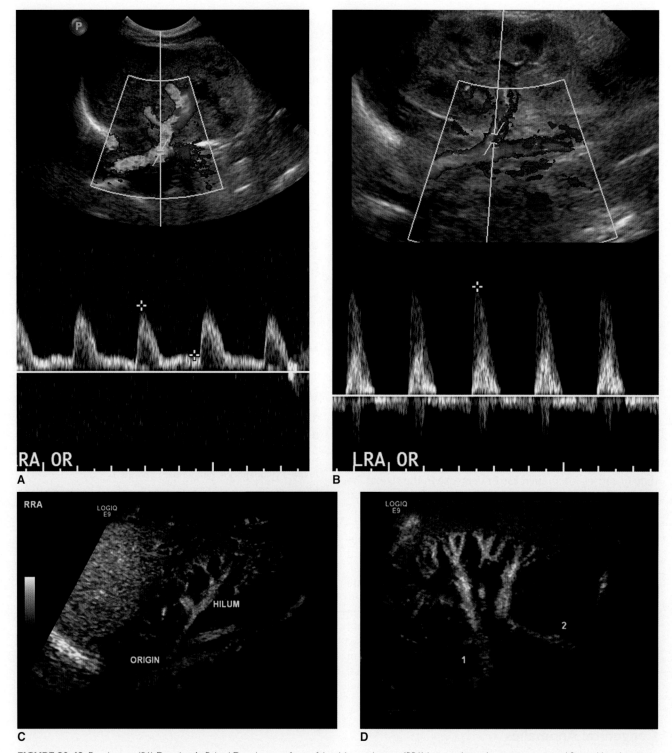

FIGURE 20-48 Renal artery (*RA*) Doppler. **A:** Pulsed Doppler waveform of the right renal artery (*RRA*) in a newborn demonstrates normal flow with a sharp systolic peak and continuous forward diastolic flow. **B:** Pulsed Doppler in a newborn with acute tubular necrosis demonstrates an abnormal waveform with reversed diastolic flow. **C:** B-flow image depicting the course of the RRA from origin to the hilum of the kidney. **D:** B-flow image demonstrating duplicated RAs in a 3-day-old female with hypertension. *LRA*, left renal artery.

numerous additional congenital and/or genetic anomalies (Pathology Box 20-2).

Hydronephrosis[11]

Hydronephrosis is a dilatation of the collecting system of the kidneys, specifically of the renal calyces, and renal pelvis.

Sonographically, hydroureters may be seen in conjunction with hydronephrosis (Fig. 20-50A–C). Congenital hydronephrosis results from mechanical or functional causes. If a dilated collecting system is identified, a voiding cystourethrogram (VCUG) is the examination of choice to determine whether reflux or outlet obstruction is responsible.[11,83] Dilatation does

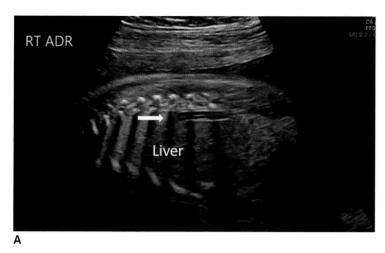

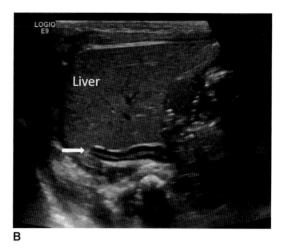

A **B**

FIGURE 20-49 Renal agenesis. A 32-year-old female referred for renal agenesis at 25 weeks' gestation. **A:** No right renal tissue is identified on prenatal ultrasound. The right adrenal gland is elongated consistent with absent right kidney (*arrow*). **B:** Postnatal examination performed at day of life 3 demonstrates empty right renal fossa, commensurate with prenatal diagnosis of right renal agenesis (*arrow*).

PATHOLOGY BOX 20-2
Associated Anomalies of Renal Agenesis and Hypoplasia

Cardiovascular	—
GI	Imperforate anus
	Esophageal atresia
Skeletal	Cervical and thoracic vertebral anomalies
	Klippel–Feil syndrome
	Duplicated uterus
	Duplicated vagina
Genital	Hypospadias
	Undescended testes
	Seminal vesicle cyst
	Absent vas deferens

not necessarily mean obstruction. Reflux accounts for up to 14% of cases of hydronephrosis. Reflux may occur with a variety of obstructive bladder lesions, such as Prune belly syndrome, posterior urethral valves, or neurogenic bladder with sphincter spasm.[1] Congenital hydronephrosis is the most common renal anomaly diagnosed among infants and children, frequently detected in utero.[75,84] Patients with congenital hydronephrosis may present with a palpable abdominal mass, flank pain, hematuria, and/or urinary tract infections.

Ureteropelvic Junction Obstruction

In infants, the most frequent site of obstruction is at the ureteropelvic junction (UPJ) (44%).[11,75,84–87] With hydronephrosis, there should be recognizable renal parenchyma surrounding the dilated collecting system. When hydronephrosis is more advanced, the fluid-filled calyces can be seen communicating with the dilated renal pelvis. In some cases, severe, progressive parenchymal thinning results in

the renal tissue being nonrecognizable, looking completely absent (Fig. 20-51A, B).

Distal Ureteral Obstructions

Distal ureteral obstructions are the next most prevalent cause of pediatric hydronephrosis (21%). Megaureter is an unusual condition being defined as a nonobstructed, nonrefluxing ureter caused by idiopathic dilatation. Usually, there is a distal stenosis or stricture, or the most distal ureter is unable to conduct a peristaltic wave.[11] In cases of bilateral hydronephrosis, the obstruction is going to be located distally, in the bladder or urethra. The bladder must be examined for obstructing masses such as dilated distal ureters that obstruct the bladder outlet as is common with ureterocele. A thick-walled small bladder with distention of the posterior urethra, such as that has been described in posterior urethral valves, can cause bladder outlet obstruction. A thick-walled bladder commonly indicates chronic distal obstruction. Children with distal urinary tract obstruction often present with recurrent urinary tract infections.

Duplicating Collecting Systems

The third most common cause of hydronephrosis is duplication of the collecting system (12%) (Fig. 20-52A–C). These lesions are recognized by dilatation of the upper pole calyx and a separate dilated ureter, which often can be followed to the level of the bladder. The upper pole may be dysplastic or hypoplastic. The upper pole ureter is dilated because of an abnormal ectopic insertion into the bladder with stenosis of the distal ureter.[11,88] It may also be due to an intravesicular obstruction of the distal ureter. When the ureter is obstructed in the area where it enters the bladder, the anterior wall of the ureter may balloon into the bladder lumen, forming an ureterocele (Fig. 20-52D, E). There may be dilatation, to a lesser degree, in the lower pole, either due to reflux or due to obstruction by the ectopic ureter. Unobstructed duplicated kidneys may be difficult to image in uncooperative children. The finding of infolding of cortical tissue into the medulla of the kidney and two renal sinuses, as well as a slight discrepancy in the length of the kidneys, should be clues to the existence of duplication. Kidney duplication is often bilateral.

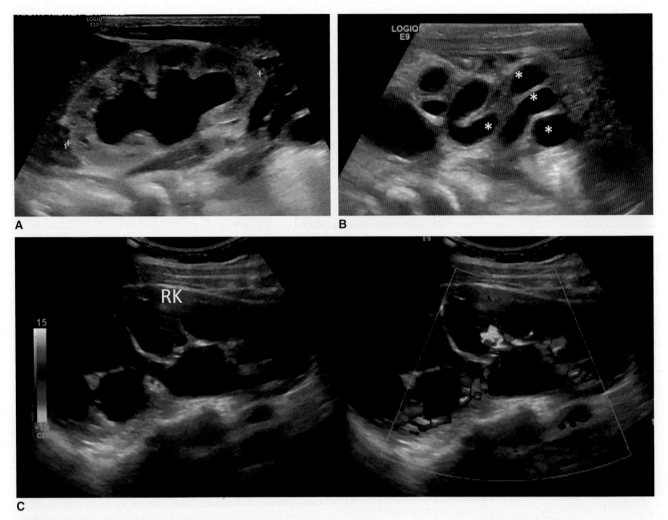

FIGURE 20-50 Hydronephrosis. **A** and **B**: Mild increased renal parenchymal echogenicity with preserved cortical medullary differentiation and moderate hydro-ureteronephrosis (*asterisk*) in a 1-day-old male with prenatal diagnosis of hydronephrosis. **C**: Dual-screen longitudinal grayscale and color Doppler image of the right kidney (*RK*) in an older pediatric child demonstrate dilatation of the calyces and renal pelvis.

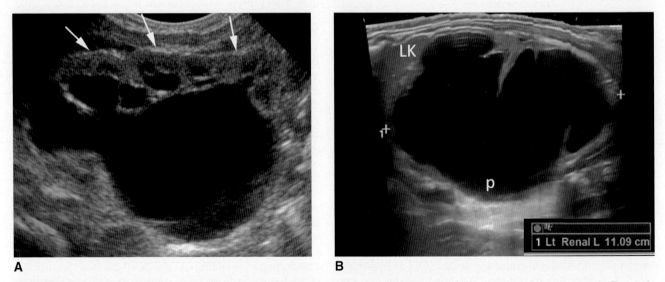

FIGURE 20-51 Ureteropelvic junction (*UPJ*) obstruction. **A**: Longitudinal sonogram of a neonatal kidney with an UPJ obstruction diagnosed prenatally. The renal pelvis and calyces are massively dilated. Renal parenchyma (*arrows*) is seen surrounding the dilated collecting system. **B**: Longitudinal image of a 2-month-old male with UPJ obstruction of the left kidney (*LK*). This image demonstrates the extended renal pelvis (*p*) and increased measurement of the kidney length.

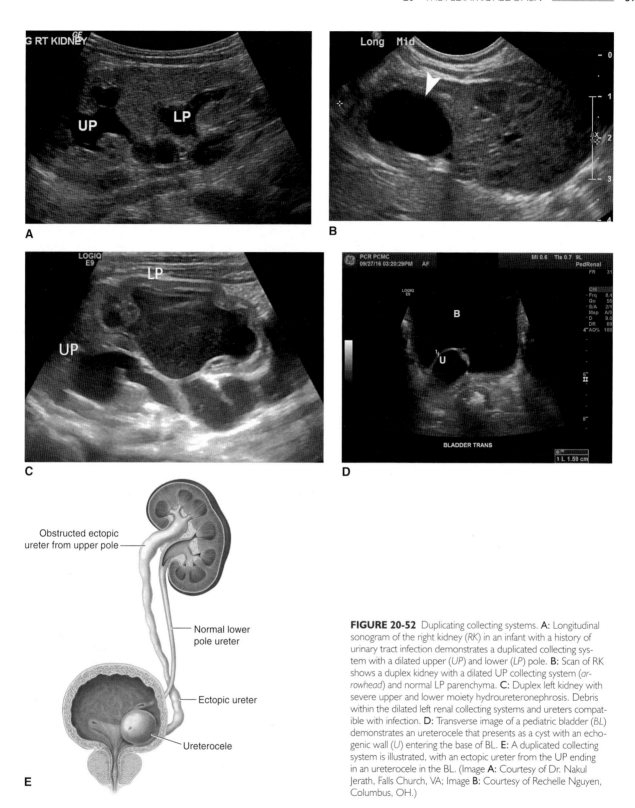

FIGURE 20-52 Duplicating collecting systems. **A:** Longitudinal sonogram of the right kidney (*RK*) in an infant with a history of urinary tract infection demonstrates a duplicated collecting system with a dilated upper (*UP*) and lower (*LP*) pole. **B:** Scan of RK shows a duplex kidney with a dilated UP collecting system (*arrowhead*) and normal LP parenchyma. **C:** Duplex left kidney with severe upper and lower moiety hydroureteronephrosis. Debris within the dilated left renal collecting systems and ureters compatible with infection. **D:** Transverse image of a pediatric bladder (*BL*) demonstrates an ureterocele that presents as a cyst with an echogenic wall (*U*) entering the base of BL. **E:** A duplicated collecting system is illustrated, with an ectopic ureter from the UP ending in an ureterocele in the BL. (Image **A:** Courtesy of Dr. Nakul Jerath, Falls Church, VA; Image **B:** Courtesy of Rechelle Nguyen, Columbus, OH.)

Posterior Urethral Valves

Posterior urethral valves account for 10% of cases of hydronephrosis and are the most common cause of urethral obstruction in boys, occurring in 1 in up to 8,000 boys.[11] A mucosal flap or folds or urethral tissue is responsible for the obstruction. These patients may be identified in utero with hydronephrosis or present with infection, voiding abnormalities, or retention.[89] Sonography demonstrates bilateral hydroureteronephrosis with parenchymal thinning (Fig. 20-53). The kidneys may be dysplastic with increased parenchymal echogenicity and cysts. They may be small and dysplastic. The ureters are dilated and tortuous. The bladder wall is thickened, and a dilated posterior urethra may be seen.[89]

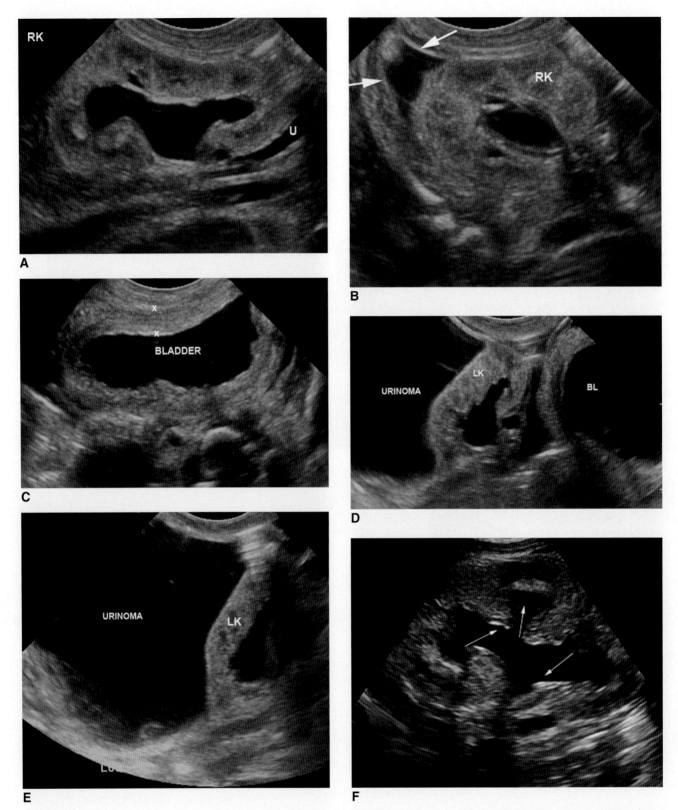

FIGURE 20-53 Posterior urethral valves. **A–E:** Sonographic examination of a male neonate with bilateral hydronephrosis diagnosed on a prenatal sonogram. The patient had urinary retention. A diagnosis of posterior urethral valves was made. **A:** Longitudinal image of the right kidney (*RK*) demonstrates hydronephrosis and echogenic renal parenchyma. The dilated ureter (*U*) is seen posterior to the kidney. **B:** Transverse image of the *RK* again demonstrates hydronephrosis and echogenic parenchyma. Free fluid is seen (*arrows*) and is consistent with an urinoma. **C:** The wall of the urinary bladder was markedly thickened (*between calipers*). **D:** Image of the left side demonstrates a large fluid collection displacing the left kidney (*LK*) inferiorly. The fluid collection is consistent with an urinoma resulting from a ruptured calyx. Hydronephrosis is also present in the LK, and the renal parenchyma is echogenic. The urinary bladder (*BL*) is seen inferior to the kidney and again demonstrates a thickened wall. **E:** In this longitudinal image, the urinoma is again seen in the left upper quadrant and is displacing the *LK*. **F–H:** Sonograms on a different male infant with a history of urinary tract infections. Longitudinal images of the RK (**F**) and LK

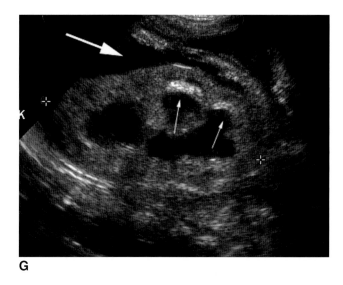

G

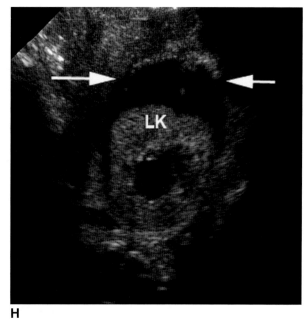

H

FIGURE 20-53 (*continued*) (**G**) demonstrate bilateral hydronephrosis. The walls of the collecting system are thickened and echogenic (*small arrows*) consistent with chronic obstruction or infection. A fluid collection is seen anterior to the *LK* (*large arrow*). **H:** Transverse image of the LK again demonstrates the fluid collection (*large arrows*) consistent with a small urinoma. The patient was diagnosed with posterior urethral valves. (Images courtesy of Dr. Nakul Jerath, Falls Church, VA.)

Ascites may be present, and perirenal or subcapsular fluid can be found.[90] The patient who develops a leak usually through an upper pole calyx has less dysplastic kidneys and better renal function due to decompression of the kidney.

Prune Belly (Eagle–Barrett) Syndrome

Prune belly syndrome presents with absent abdominal muscles, urinary tract abnormalities, and cryptorchidism.[73,91,92] It occurs in 1 in 50,000 live births and may rarely occur in females.[92] Many infants with Prune belly syndrome have small, cystic, dysplastic kidneys, but some have hydronephrotic kidneys. They may also have posterior urethral valves as well as abnormal musculature and lack of contractility of the bladder and ureteral walls. The flaccid, dilated bladder separates this condition from posterior urethral valves, as well as the clinical observation of the abnormal abdominal wall.

An obstructed kidney, from whatever cause, is an important indication for radionuclide scanning. Even with severely impaired function, radionuclide activity can be detected in an obstructed kidney. Notably, multicystic, dysplastic kidneys exhibit no function on radionuclide scanning, and this is a significant finding. Diuretic-augmented radionuclide scanning can, in some cases, differentiate significant obstruction from insignificant obstruction because of poorly functioning nonobstructed hydronephrotic systems.

Cystic Dysplastic Kidneys[93,94]

There are several classifications of cystic renal disease based on pathologic or radiographic findings. Sonographically, it may be difficult to differentiate many of the cystic diseases without a family history. Dysplastic kidneys may be small or large without cysts or have small cysts or very large ones. The cysts may involve only a portion of one kidney or both kidneys.

Multicystic Dysplastic Kidney[11,75]

Multicystic dysplastic kidney, probably the most common cystic dysplasia, is difficult to differentiate from hydronephrosis, but the distinction is important because multicystic dysplasia is a nonsurgical mass, whereas surgical correction of the obstruction may be done to salvage a hydronephrotic kidney. A multicystic kidney develops from a complete ureteral obstruction in utero. Terminal tubules become cysts, and as these cysts develop, they do not communicate and are eventually joined together by small connective tissue cords. There may be multiple cysts of varying sizes or a dominant or single cyst[21] (Fig. 20-54A–E). Multicystic kidneys may be bilateral, but this condition is inconsistent with life, and affected infants have a similar presentation to patients with renal aplasia, Potter syndrome, and respiratory difficulties.

A multicystic kidney may present as a very large mass at birth, as a progressive or decreasing cystic flank mass in utero, or as an unidentifiable kidney at a later age. Multicystic kidneys may enlarge after birth for up to 3 years. Sonography has been useful to document progressive decrease in the size and number of cysts. A distal ureter is present in multicystic disease, whereas, with agenesis, no ureter is present. The disorganized cysts do not communicate with the blind ureter, which is otherwise present. Reflux may occur into the blind ureter. Unilateral multicystic kidney disease may be associated with UPJ obstruction in the opposite kidney[11] (Table 20-3).

Hypoplasia and Dysplasia

Hypoplasia, a small but otherwise normal kidney, most often results from atrophy secondary to infection or from vascular occlusions with infarction. Dysplastic kidneys, however, may be large or small, and all are anatomically abnormal. Dysplasia is associated with urinary tract

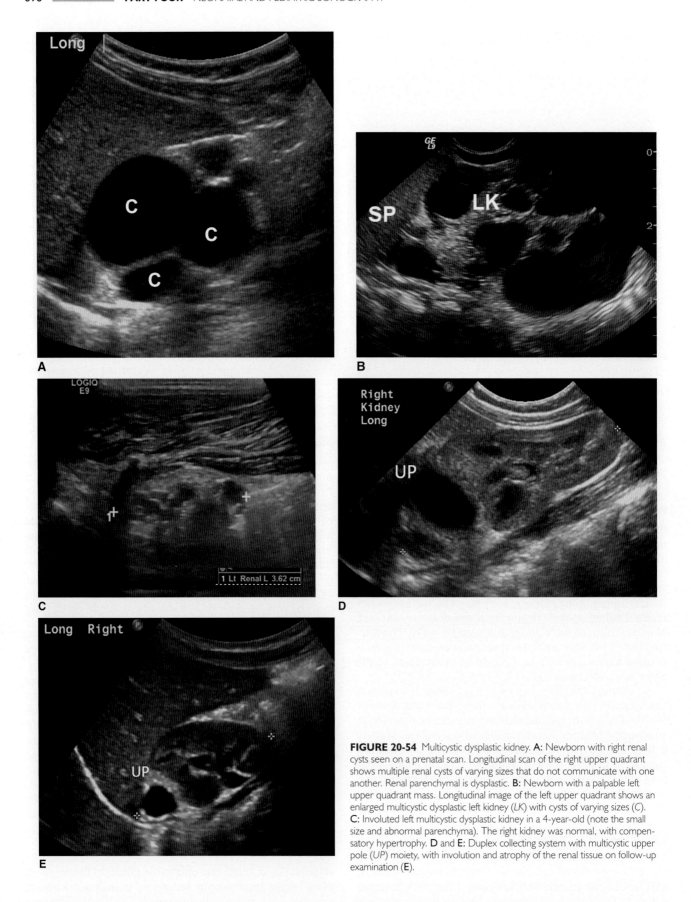

FIGURE 20-54 Multicystic dysplastic kidney. **A:** Newborn with right renal cysts seen on a prenatal scan. Longitudinal scan of the right upper quadrant shows multiple renal cysts of varying sizes that do not communicate with one another. Renal parenchymal is dysplastic. **B:** Newborn with a palpable left upper quadrant mass. Longitudinal image of the left upper quadrant shows an enlarged multicystic dysplastic left kidney (*LK*) with cysts of varying sizes (*C*). **C:** Involuted left multicystic dysplastic kidney in a 4-year-old (note the small size and abnormal parenchyma). The right kidney was normal, with compensatory hypertrophy. **D** and **E:** Duplex collecting system with multicystic upper pole (*UP*) moiety, with involution and atrophy of the renal tissue on follow-up examination (**E**).

TABLE 20-3 **Sonographic Differentiation of Hydronephrosis and Multicystic Disease**

Features	Multicystic Kidney	Hydronephrotic Feature Kidney
Reniform	2	4
Lobular	4	1
Parenchyma present	1	3
Continuity between cysts	1	1
Separated sinus	1	4
Interfaces	4	1
Largest cyst medial	1	4
Largest cyst peripheral	4	0
Single cyst	2	1

Reliability of findings ranges from 1 (least) to 4 (most).

malformations in 90% of the cases, usually obstruction. Dysplasia occurs with other malformations, such as an obstructed ureter, ureterocele with hydroureter, posterior urethral valves, and Prune belly syndrome. Ectopic kidneys are often dysplastic. The patient may have urinary ascites. The kidneys are often small and without the corticomedullary junction and pyramids seen in normal neonates. They may or may not have visible cysts. The renal pelvis may be small or dilated, and the ureter may be dilated for some distance. Caliectasis (dilatation of the renal calyx) is often not present. Congenital megacalyces and infundibular stenosis may be the same entity. Affected infants demonstrate asymptomatic hydrocaliectasis without obstruction, which is a radionuclide finding. The calyces are dilated, but the renal pelvis is of normal size, and the kidneys may appear small and hyperechoic.

Infantile Polycystic Kidney Disease

Infantile polycystic kidney disease or autosomal recessive polycystic kidney disease (ARPKD) is usually present at birth as symmetrically enlarged kidneys.[93] Although this condition is described as a cystic disease, the cysts result from tubular dilatation and are microscopic.[11,75] These cysts cause the pyramids or medulla of the kidney to reflect multiple bright echoes. At birth, the large kidneys are diffusely echogenic with poor differentiation of the renal sinus, medulla, and cortex.[75] Cortical echogenicity is increased, but with time, the thin cortex becomes anechoic. It is the medullary portion of the kidney that enlarges and causes stretching of the calyces and renal pelvis (Fig. 20-55A–F).

Congenital hepatic fibrosis is associated with ARPKD.[11,75] All patients who survive with recessive polycystic kidney disease eventually develop congenital hepatic fibrosis, although not all patients with congenital hepatic fibrosis have ARPKD[93,94] (Fig. 20-11D). Adult polycystic kidney disease and dysplastic kidneys are also associated with hepatic fibrosis. Children with less extensive renal involvement may present with liver disease or portal hypertension.[11] The liver cysts may be visualized without a microscope. Within

a given family, the presentation may vary, some members developed liver failure, and others developed renal failure.

Adult Polycystic Kidney Disease

Adult polycystic kidney disease or autosomal dominant polycystic kidney disease (ADPKD) may occur in the neonatal period.[94] ADPKD may affect one or both kidneys. Cysts described in the liver, pancreas, and lung in adults have not been described at this time in neonates. The cysts in neonates may range from 0.1 to 5 mm and can be difficult to visualize with sonography. The most common sonographic finding in the neonate is renal enlargement.[93] Of the cases described in the literature, only 50% had recognizable cysts at presentation. When visible, the cysts appear to be more cortical. Probably, the best way to separate ADPKD from ARPKD is by obtaining a family history or screening the rest of the family.[94] There is a 75% chance that other members of the family have the disease (Table 20-4).

Glomerular Cystic Disease

Glomerular cystic disease is a rare condition. It is hard to separate from ADPKD, ARPKD, and the hamartomas of tuberous sclerosis. At birth, the kidneys may be large and hyperechoic. With age, they become relatively smaller, and their echogenicity may decrease. Cortical cysts are present and are usually microscopic, but some may be macroscopic. Although the cortical echogenicity appears to resolve, there is persistent loss of the corticomedullary junction. Patients do not develop renal failure but may develop significant hepatic fibrosis and portal hypertension.

Medullary Cystic Disease

Medullary cystic disease usually presents as metabolic dysfunction in young adults.[95] There are two types.

Medullary sponge kidney or renal collecting tubular ectasia is usually diagnosed in people aged 10 to 30 years and on the basis of laboratory and radiologic findings. Neonatal cases of medullary sponge kidney are rarely seen.

Sonographically, medullary sponge kidney demonstrates a normal sonographic pattern, except for echogenic pyramids caused by calcium deposits. The findings are similar to renal tubular acidosis.[95]

Juvenile nephronophthisis or uremic medullary kidney disease is familial and may be autosomal dominant or recessive.[93] Patients present in adolescence. The kidneys may be normal or small, with increased parenchymal echogenicity and loss of the corticomedullary junction. There may be sonographically visible cysts at the corticomedullary junction (Fig. 20-56A, B).

Renal Cysts

Cystic disease may be associated with syndromes such as cerebral hepatorenal or Zellweger syndrome, tuberous sclerosis,[96] short rib polydactyly, orofacial digital syndrome, renal–retinal dysplasia, Conradi disease, Turner syndrome, von Hippel–Lindau disease, trisomy D or E, and Jeune asphyxiating thoracic dystrophy. Tuberous sclerosis can present initially with bilateral cystic kidneys. Acquired cysts have been described in patients on hemodialysis, especially after 3 years. Simple cysts are rare in children. Their frequency is less than 1%. Inflammatory cysts from tuberculosis or other abscesses do occur.

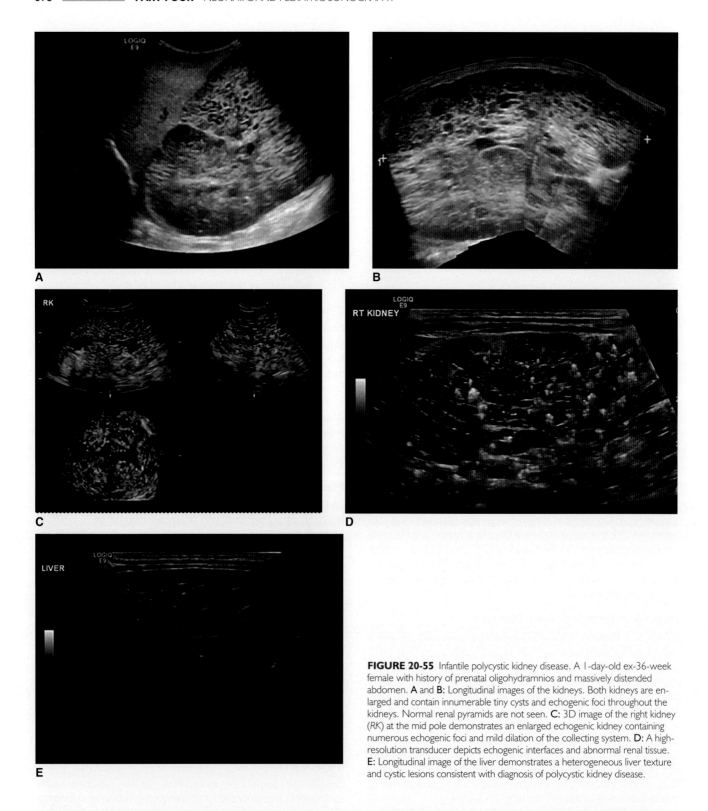

FIGURE 20-55 Infantile polycystic kidney disease. A 1-day-old ex-36-week female with history of prenatal oligohydramnios and massively distended abdomen. **A** and **B:** Longitudinal images of the kidneys. Both kidneys are enlarged and contain innumerable tiny cysts and echogenic foci throughout the kidneys. Normal renal pyramids are not seen. **C:** 3D image of the right kidney (*RK*) at the mid pole demonstrates an enlarged echogenic kidney containing numerous echogenic foci and mild dilation of the collecting system. **D:** A high-resolution transducer depicts echogenic interfaces and abnormal renal tissue. **E:** Longitudinal image of the liver demonstrates a heterogeneous liver texture and cystic lesions consistent with diagnosis of polycystic kidney disease.

TABLE 20-4	Sonographic Comparison of ARPKD, ADPKD, and GKD			
Disease	**Bilateral**	**Renal Size**	**Cysts**	**Inheritance**
ARPKD	+	Very large	Rare	Autosomal recessive
ADPKD	+	Variable	Rare	Autosomal dominant
GKD	+	Normal to huge	Variable	Sporadic

ADPKD, autosomal dominant polycystic kidney disease; ARPKD, autosomal recessive polycystic kidney disease; GKD, glomerulocystic kidney disease.

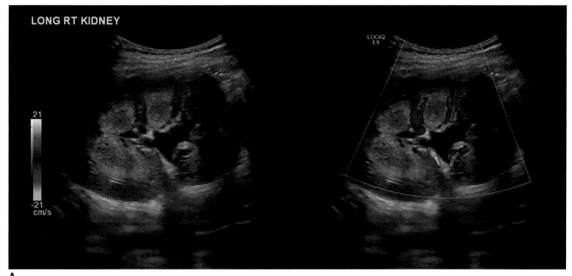

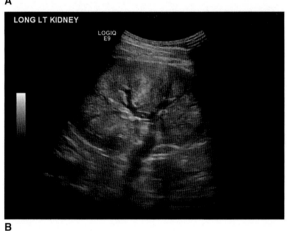

FIGURE 20-56 Longitudinal images of the right **(A)** and left **(B)** kidneys demonstrate abnormally medullary rays in a 3-year-old with medullary sponge kidneys.

Tumors[11]

When a sonographer examines any infant or child with an abdominal mass, there are three important things to determine.

1. The origin of the mass if possible. Can the mass be separated from the liver or kidney or other organ? Is the mass intraperitoneal or retroperitoneal? This may be difficult, but in children with little body fat, sonography can be more definitive than CT.
2. The extent of the mass. Does the mass extend beyond the organ of origin? Are there adjacent enlarged lymph nodes? Are the adjacent structures such as vessels (IVC or portal vein) displaced or invaded?
3. Metastases. Are there metastases to the liver? Of importance to renal tumors, is there involvement of the contralateral kidney?

Wilms Tumor

Wilms tumor is the most common malignant renal tumor in the pediatric population.[74] There are other malignant renal tumors that may occur, such as clear cell sarcoma and malignant rhabdoid tumor. Many of these tumors cannot be differentiated by any imaging study and are dependent on cytologic and/or histologic examination. The important thing is to determine whether the tumor is resectable or if there is bilateral involvement to preclude surgery.

Wilms tumor is the most common solid abdominal tumor in children, followed by neuroblastoma. It most often presents as a palpable mass but may cause nonspecific symptoms, such as pain, fever, malaise, and weight loss. The patient may also present with hematuria or hypertension. The peak age is 3 to 4 years, but adult and infant cases have been detected. Neonatal Wilms tumor has been described. This may be due to in utero malignant degeneration of nephrogenic rests.[97] Wilms tumor may involve the retroperitoneal nodes and frequently invades the renal vein and IVC and may extend into the heart.[74,98] Distant metastases may occur in the liver and lung. Therefore, these structures should be carefully examined as part of the evaluation of renal tumors. Wilms tumor may be bilateral.

There are congenital malformations associated with Wilms tumors, such as aniridia (absent iris), Beckwith–Wiedemann syndrome (omphalocele, macroglossia, and hypoglycemia), Drash syndrome (male pseudohermaphroditism, progressive nephritis, and Wilms tumor), and hemihypertrophy. Children at risk for Wilms tumor should have screening sonography at 3-month intervals up to at least 6 years of age.

Wilms tumors are large, well-circumscribed, smooth masses with a homogeneous echotexture slightly greater than the liver (Fig. 20-57A–C). The tumor has a pseudocapsule that separates it from normal renal parenchyma.[3] The mass may contain hypoechoic or cystic areas and may arise from the renal sinus, displacing and distorting the kidney. They may fill the pelvocaliceal system and obstruct the kidney. There is

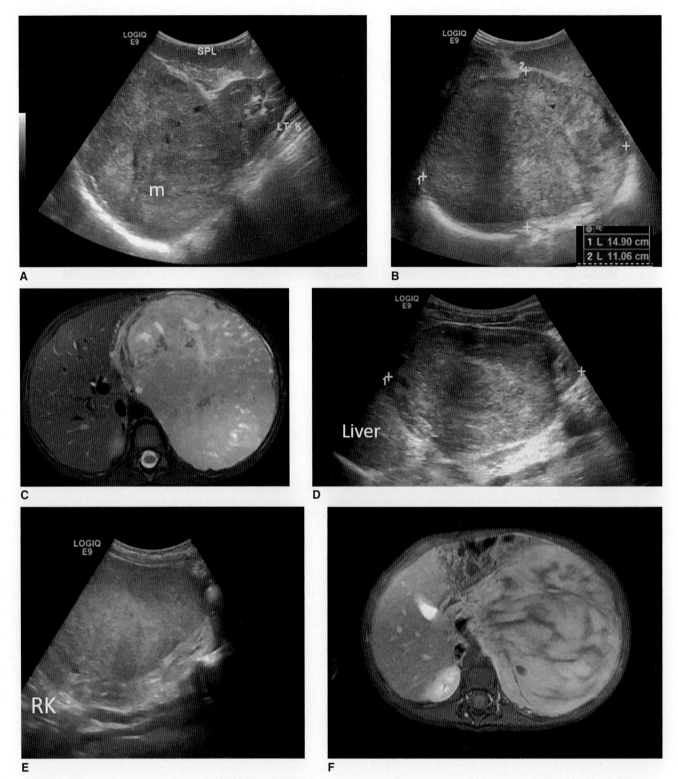

FIGURE 20-57 Malignant renal tumors. A 4-year-old male presented with a palpable abdominal mass. **A:** A transverse scan of the left upper quadrant demonstrates a large homogeneous solid mass (*m*) arising from the medial portion of the left kidney (*LT K*) diagnosed as a stage III Wilms tumor. **B:** The greatest dimension of the Wilms tumor (*M*) measured 14.9 cm. **C:** The mass demonstrates heterogeneous enhancement with multiple cystic/necrotic foci, as seen on magnetic resonance imaging. **D–F:** Longitudinal images of the right kidney (*RK*) in an infant with a clear cell carcinoma. A large solid well-defined mass with anechoic spaces is seen arising from the mid pole of the RK.

usually a portion of normal kidney that extends over the mass. The tumor may arise on a stalk from a single portion of the renal parenchyma. Anechoic or cystic spaces seen within the mass probably represent necrosis or hemorrhage but could be a remnant of a functioning calyx or infundibulum trapped in the mass. Rhabdoid tumors of the kidney are more likely to have calcification outlining lobulations (best imaged on CT) and subcapsular hematoma (Fig. 20-57D, E).

Nephroblastomatosis[75]

Nephroblastomatosis is a precursor of Wilms tumor and can be confused with it on histologic examination. Nephroblastomatosis has been found in 25% of patients with Wilms tumor and 100% of patients with bilateral Wilms tumors.[11]

It has also been found in cases of Beckwith–Wiedemann syndrome, aniridia, Denys–Drash syndrome, and hemihypertrophy. There are two patterns. The diffuse form is divided into the pancortical and superficial types. The former replaces the renal parenchyma, and the superficial has a subcapsular rind of primitive tissue surrounding normal cortex and medulla. This entity can be identified on sonography as a thick rim of hypoechoic or anechoic subcapsular tissue with irregular central contours and smooth outer margins (Fig. 20-58A–D). The kidneys are large. The sonographic and CT findings are very specific.

In multifocal nephroblastomatosis, there is persistence of primitive tissue along the columns of Bertin. The tissue ranges in size from microscopic rests to large masses in

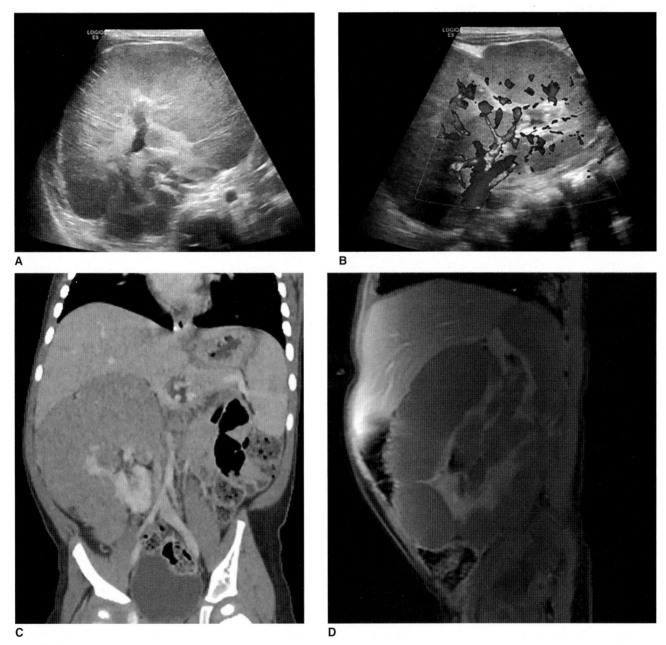

FIGURE 20-58 Nephroblastomatosis. **A:** Ultrasound demonstrates an ill-defined, massively enlarged kidney with numerous round lobular exophytic vascular masses (**B**) along the periphery of the right kidney in a 2-year-old male with nephroblastomatosis, also seen on coronal computed tomography (**C**) and sagittal magnetic resonance imaging (**D**).

the cortex.[11] The masses may be hypoechoic, anechoic, or isoechoic and only detectable when they alter renal contour or distort the collecting system.

Multilocular Cystic Nephroma

Also known as benign cystic nephroma, cystic hamartoma, cystic Wilms tumor, cystic lymphangioma, and multicystic nephroblastoma, a multilocular cystic nephroma presents as a mass with multiple thin-walled cysts or as septations within cysts. Normal renal parenchyma may be present elsewhere and is sharply demarcated from the mass. The presence of multiple cysts aids in the diagnosis of a multicystic nephroblastoma. These can occur at any age, and differentiation from a cystic Wilms tumor may be difficult without careful histologic review.

Mesoblastic Nephroma

Congenital mesoblastic nephroma is the most common abdominal neoplasm seen in the neonate and is sometimes diagnosed prenatally.[11,74,99,100] Solid renal tumors in infants younger than 3 months may represent congenital mesoblastic nephroma.[11,74] Mesoblastic nephroma is a unilateral or bilateral benign tumor composed of connective tissue, which can replace most of the renal parenchyma. Other names are fetal renal hamartoma, mesenchymal hamartoma of infancy, and benign Wilms tumor.[75,100] They present in neonates, whereas Wilms tumors are most common in children older than 2 years.[100] Although the tumor is considered benign, there is malignant potential; therefore, if the tumor is unilateral, it may be removed, as Wilms tumor would be; if bilateral, radiation and chemotherapy may be prescribed.[1] Sonographically, they resemble Wilms tumor presenting as a homogeneous mass with slightly increased echogenicity. They may be heterogeneous masses with necrosis or hemorrhage centrally (Fig. 20-59A–E).

Renal Cell Carcinoma

Renal cell carcinomas have rarely been reported in children.[74] These tumors have been found in association with tuberous sclerosis and von Hippel–Lindau disease. The tumors are isoechoic or slightly hypoechoic compared with the rest of the kidney. On CT, there is marked enhancement. Renal cell carcinoma is highly malignant in children.

Angiomyolipoma

Angiomyolipomas are hamartomatous masses frequently associated with tuberous sclerosis.[96] Patients with tuberous sclerosis present with seizures due to cortical hamartomas, red papular rash usually over the nose and cheeks, cardiac failure due to rhabdomyomas of the heart, and angiomyolipomas and cysts of the kidneys. Renal cysts and angiomyolipomas can help confirm the diagnosis of tuberous sclerosis. Angiomyolipomas are located within the renal cortex and are homogeneous, markedly hyperechoic, and, in cases of tuberous sclerosis, typically bilateral and multiple[74,96] (Fig. 20-60). There is an increased incidence of renal cell carcinoma associated with tuberous sclerosis.[96]

Acquired Pathology

Sonography may be used for evaluating pyelonephritis or infection of the upper urinary tract. Children under the age of 5 with a urinary tract infection typically undergo a sonographic examination of the urinary tract to evaluate for congenital anomalies.[88,101] The most common sonographic finding in the setting of pyelonephritis is enlargement of the kidneys. Areas of increased cortical echogenicity, and less often areas of decreased echogenicity, have been described in children with pyelonephritis (Fig. 20-61A–D). Additional sonographic indications include loss of corticomedullary differentiation and thickening of the walls of the renal pelvis or ureter (Fig. 20-62A, B).

Renal abscesses have been described on sonography as a hypoechoic mass with thick, irregular walls and distal acoustic enhancement. Often, the abscesses will include septations and mobile debris containing gas-forming organisms. Small abscesses may be treated with antibiotic therapy, whereas large abscesses may need to be drained and treated through percutaneous or surgical drainage. Mild scarring of a kidney due to chronic infection is a difficult sonographic diagnosis to make because the scars may be small and difficult to image and the calyces are not dilated. Sonography is not sensitive for the detection of acute inflammatory changes in the renal cortex.[101] Significant cortical scarring, especially if diffuse, may be easy to identify because of a decrease in overall renal size. Because acute pyelonephritis presents with renal enlargement, baseline measurements for following renal growth should be obtained at least 2 weeks after treatment.[102] In children with continuous lower urinary tract infections, renal measurements may be important to follow over a period of time, to ensure that the kidneys are growing properly. Sonography is also a useful screening tool to seek anatomic causes of infection, specifically obstruction.

Nephrocalcinosis

Nephrocalcinosis is the deposit of calcium in the kidney. It is associated with increased urine calcium from a variety of causes. Both kidneys are usually affected with focal echogenicity, with or without acoustic shadowing. Nephrocalcinosis may present with increased echogenicity of the renal pyramids (Fig. 20-63 A–C). Children may present with diffuse cortical nephrocalcinosis. In this situation, the kidneys are normal in size but very echogenic with a loss of the normal corticomedullary junction. Nephrocalcinosis can occur in children with renal tubular acidosis or a defect in tubular reabsorption, such as primary hyperoxaluria, cystinosis, and tyrosinemia.[95] Children with hypercalcemia—and particularly those infants receiving long-term furosemide for chronic lung or heart disease, hyperparathyroidism, medullary sponge, and Bartter syndrome—may present with hyperechoic medullary pyramids. Sonography in children at risk for nephrocalcinosis may identify hyperechoic pyramids. This could also represent sloughed papilla, blood clots, fungus balls, cellular debris, or proteinuria. Hyperechoic pyramids with normal urinary calcium have been seen in infancy and are associated with transient oliguria. Children at risk for urolithiasis due to urinary stasis or infection may have echogenic calculi in the ureter or bladder.

Renal Vascular Disease

Renal vascular problems in children are usually the result of trauma or other underlying conditions such as nephrotic syndrome, which predisposes the patient to renal vein thrombosis. Clot formation and emboli can occur in the renal arteries as a complication of umbilical artery catheterization and can

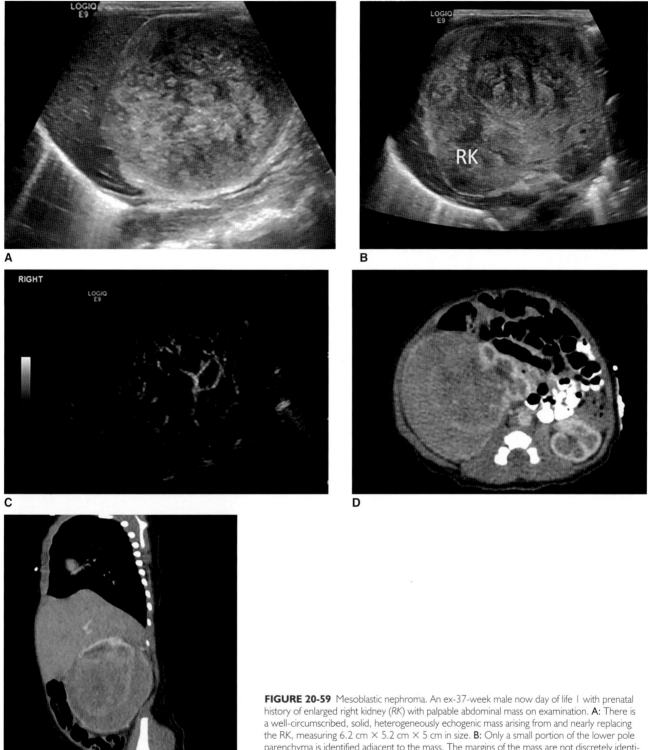

FIGURE 20-59 Mesoblastic nephroma. An ex-37-week male now day of life 1 with prenatal history of enlarged right kidney (*RK*) with palpable abdominal mass on examination. **A:** There is a well-circumscribed, solid, heterogeneously echogenic mass arising from and nearly replacing the RK, measuring 6.2 cm × 5.2 cm × 5 cm in size. **B:** Only a small portion of the lower pole parenchyma is identified adjacent to the mass. The margins of the mass are not discretely identified from the lower pole parenchyma. The mass also extends to the renal hilum. On grayscale ultrasound, there is a concentric pattern of hyperechoic and hypoechoic rings, giving it a whorled appearance. Corticomedullary differentiation is lost. **C:** B-flow demonstrates intrinsic neovascularity. **D** and **E:** Computed tomography correlation demonstrating a mass most compatible with congenital mesoblastic nephroma.

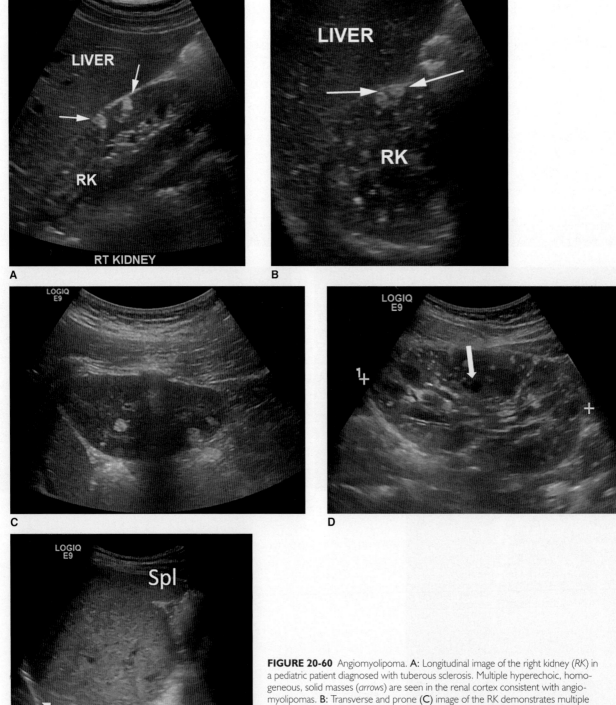

FIGURE 20-60 Angiomyolipoma. **A:** Longitudinal image of the right kidney (*RK*) in a pediatric patient diagnosed with tuberous sclerosis. Multiple hyperechoic, homogeneous, solid masses (*arrows*) are seen in the renal cortex consistent with angiomyolipomas. **B:** Transverse and prone (**C**) image of the RK demonstrates multiple echogenic foci seen throughout the renal cortex. The echogenic foci represent angiomyolipomas. A larger angiomyolipoma (*arrows*) is seen at the periphery of the cortex. **D:** In a different patient, a longitudinal image of the left kidney shows multiple echogenic foci throughout the cortex as well as a simple cyst (*arrow*) in the lower pole. **E:** In the spleen (*spl*), there is a large, well-circumscribed mass (*arrow*), consistent with splenic hamartoma in the setting of tuberous sclerosis. Splenic hamartomas, renal cysts, and angiomyolipomas are frequent abdominal manifestations seen in patients with tuberous sclerosis. Patients with tuberous sclerosis must be screened routinely because they are at a higher risk for renal cell carcinoma.

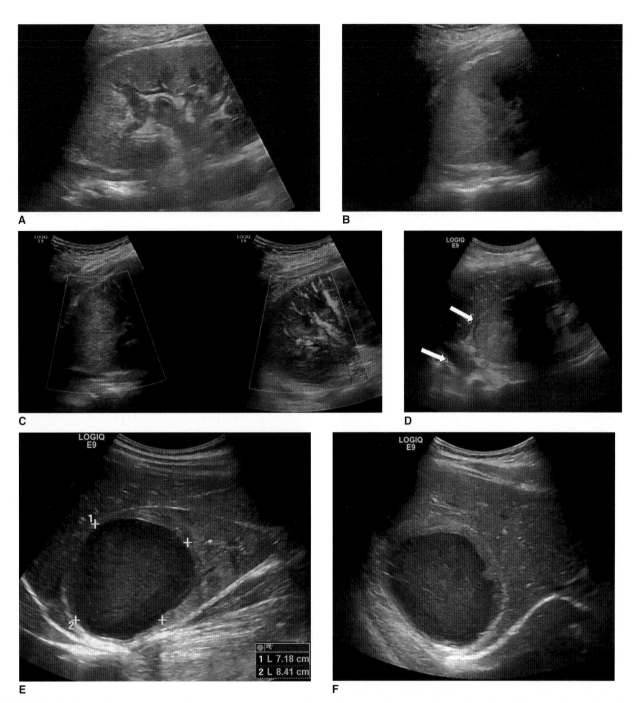

FIGURE 20-61 Pyelonephritis. An 11-year-old male presents with 5 days of fever, abdominal pain, and vomiting. **A:** There is an echogenic wedge-shaped segment in the upper pole of the right kidney with urothelial thickening of the collecting system. **B:** Magnified view showing the increased echotexture of the upper pole. **C:** Dual-screen image compares the upper pole of the right and left kidney with power Doppler and demonstrates hypovascularity on color and power Doppler. **D:** Perinephric fluid is present (*arrows*). **E:** Long and transverse (**F**) views of the right kidney with a well-circumscribed, thick-walled, hypoechoic lesion measuring up to 7.2 cm. Aspiration yielded 65 cm³ of pus.

result in hypoplasia of the kidneys. In small infants, it can be difficult to detect actual renal vein thrombosis because it often occurs in the small veins, but diffuse enlargement and increased echogenicity of the kidneys can be seen.

Trauma

Renal trauma is unusual in infants but may be related to a birth injury. The cause of a flank mass in a newborn is more often adrenal than renal parenchymal hemorrhage.

Sonographically, the appearance of hemorrhage changes over time and may be anechoic to complex. Hemorrhage may be subcapsular or perinephric. For imaging renal trauma in a child, CT is the modality of choice.

URINARY BLADDER

In infants, the bladder is an abdominal rather than a pelvic organ, and frequently, it is difficult to evaluate because the mere pressure of the transducer on the abdomen causes the

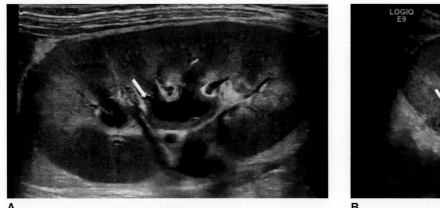

A

B

FIGURE 20-62 Urothelial thickening. A 7-year-old female with recent renal allograft presents with hematuria and increased creatinine. Longitudinal panoramic (**A**) and transverse (**B**) images demonstrate diffusely thickened walls (*arrows*) of the renal pelvis and ureter.

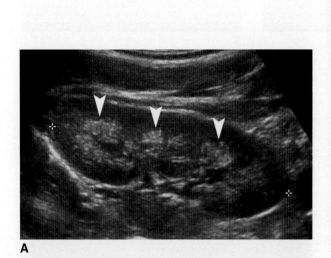

A

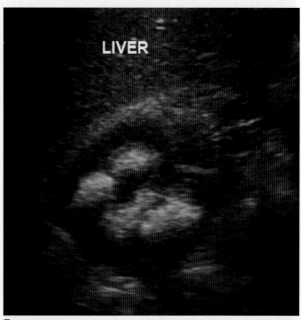

B

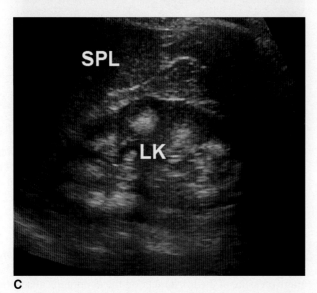

C

FIGURE 20-63 Nephrocalcinosis. A 3-year-old patient with a history of William syndrome and hypercalcemia. **A:** Longitudinal prone image of the right kidney shows increased echogenicity of the renal pyramids (*arrowheads*). (**B**) Transverse image of the right kidney demonstrates hyperechoic renal pyramids. **C:** Prone longitudinal image of the left kidney (*LK*) also demonstrates hyperechoic renal pyramids consistent with bilateral nephrocalcinosis. *SPL*, spleen.

bladder to evacuate. When it is necessary for an infant's bladder to be full, a Foley catheter can be used to fill it and the inflated balloon used to keep it full. It is unusual to see a very distended bladder in a normal neonate unless the mother received drugs during labor or delivery, which could affect the infant's nervous system for several hours, or the infant is receiving drugs that would inhibit voiding. Bladder distention may be caused by neurogenic disease or a pelvic mass. Cystic pelvic masses can be confused with the bladder, and care must be taken to clearly identify the bladder.

Congenital Anomalies

Urachal Abnormalities[83]

The urachus is a tubular structure continuous with the anterior dome of the bladder and extending outside the peritoneum to the umbilicus superiorly. Normally, during the fourth and fifth months of gestation, the urachus narrows to a small-caliber tube. The normal urachus is completely obliterated and fibrotic at or before birth, or it seals off in the neonatal period. Occasionally, the urachus persists. It may persist as a cord

from the umbilicus to the superior aspect of the bladder, producing an anterior superior vesical diverticulum, which is usually continuous with the bladder. It may remain as an open structure (patent urachus) between the umbilicus and the bladder, but usually only in cases of bladder outlet obstruction where the urachus decompresses the otherwise obstructed bladder. Such patients may exhibit an abdominal mass after the umbilical cord is clamped at birth. Sometimes, the urachus persists in continuity with the umbilicus, but not with the bladder; sometimes, it is continuous with the bladder, but not with the umbilicus. Urachal cysts may present as palpable midline abdominal masses, but more often, the patient presents with symptoms of an infection.

Sonography is useful for evaluating urachal cyst. The bladder is tethered anteriorly. Masses are continuous with the bladder, and the echo pattern is cystic or, if infected, complex (Fig. 20-64A–D).

The posterior urethral valve syndrome is another congenital urethral abnormality. The valve is a thin membrane positioned across the membranous portion of the penile urethra in boys. With secondary changes in the bladder,

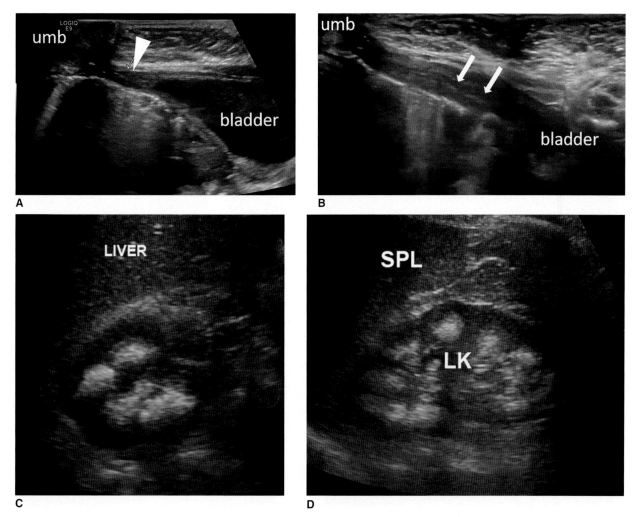

FIGURE 20-64 Urachal abnormalities. **A:** There is a tract extending from the dome of the bladder to the level of the umbilicus (*arrowhead*) with a small amount of fluid seen within (**B**) (*arrows*) consistent with patent urachus well demonstrated on the voiding cystourethrogram. **C** and **D:** Longitudinal scan of the pelvis demonstrates a hypoechoic tract (*arrows*) arising from the dome of the bladder to the umbilicus. **D:** A hypoechoic mass (*arrows*) is seen just posterior to the umbilicus, representing an infected patent urachus. The urachus was found to be patent at the bladder and closed to the umbilicus allowing a cyst to form. *LK*, left kidney; *SPL*, spleen. (Images **C** and **D**: Courtesy of Dr. Nakul Jerath, Falls Church, VA.)

ureters, or kidneys, it can obstruct voiding as previously described. Sonographically, the bladder wall may be thickened, and dilatation of the posterior urethra can be identified. The ureters are tortuous and dilated, and the kidneys have varying degrees of dysplasia. Children with Prune belly syndrome may have posterior urethral valves with hydroureteronephrosis and renal dysplasia, but the bladder is usually very large and flaccid.

Bladder Tumors

Rhabdomyosarcoma

Rhabdomyosarcomas often involve or arise from the bladder, prostate, uterus, or vagina of children. Depending on the point of origin, they may cause various changes in the urinary tract. With rhabdomyosarcoma of the bladder, patients present with hematuria, dysuria, retention, and urinary tract infection.[87] Sonographically, rhabdomyosarcomas are seen as a homogeneous polypoidal mass (Fig. 20-65A–D).[87] Masses within the bladder are often immovable blood clots that are adherent to the thick wall. The bladder may also be obstructed by sacrococcygeal teratoma.

Infection

Cystitis, the most common urinary tract infection in children, is 10 times more common in girls than in boys. In children with chronic cystitis, the bladder wall may be thickened, measuring greater than 0.3 cm with a full bladder and 0.5 cm with an empty bladder.[103] Usually, cystitis produces diffuse thickening of the bladder wall, which can be a nonspecific finding. Bladder wall changes may be asymmetrical with marked localized thickening of the wall, suggestive of a mass or pseudotumoral cystitis (Fig. 20-66A–F). If there

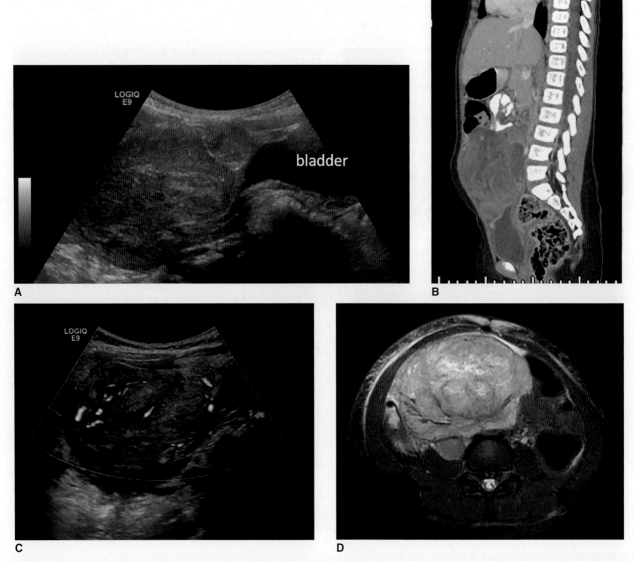

FIGURE 20-65 Rhabdomyosarcoma. A 3-year-old previously healthy female with new abdominal mass × 6 days. **A:** Sagittal ultrasound and computed tomography images demonstrate a large polypoidal mass. The urinary bladder is elongated with distortion of the bladder dome due to the mass (**B**). **C:** Color Doppler imaging verifies the presence of neovascularity within the mass. **D:** Magnetic resonance shows a well-circumscribed, solid heterogeneous mass measuring 11.7 cm × 9.3 cm × 7.5 cm.

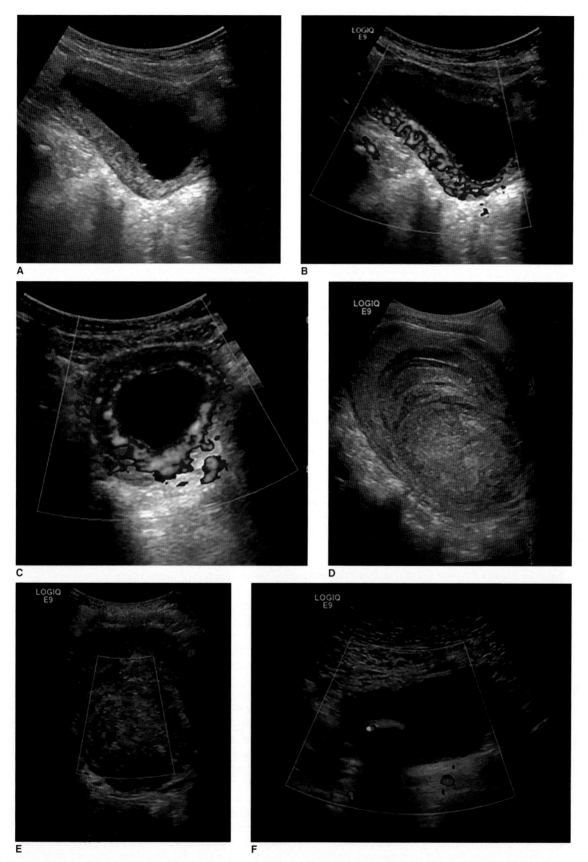

FIGURE 20-66 Bladder wall. **A:** Longitudinal image of a pediatric bladder demonstrates bladder wall thickening with asymmetric changes. **B:** Power Doppler confirms the presence of diffuse and increased blood flow within the thickened walls in long and transverse (**C**). A 15-year-old male with Ewing sarcoma presents with hematuria. **D:** The urinary bladder cavity is completely replaced by a large avascular lesion (**E**) with concentric alternating mid- and high-level echogenicity; reflecting a large intraluminal hematoma, consistent with hemorrhagic cystitis. A 7-year-old male with history of L4 to L5 myelomeningocele and neuropathic bladder. **E:** Large stone present in the bladder with twinkle artifact (**F**).

is evidence otherwise of acute infection, this should be treated conservatively and with follow-up sonography in a week to make sure that there is no progression of the mass to suggest tumor. Bladder calculi in children are extremely unusual unless there is urinary stasis in the bladder. Children with active urinary tract bleeding may show clots or blood in the bladder. Bladder perforation and trauma are best evaluated by cystography.

ADRENAL GLANDS

Diagnostic sonography is particularly useful in the examination of the neonatal adrenals. The right adrenal gland can be successfully imaged 97% of the time and the left adrenal gland 83% of the time. The ability to visualize the normal neonatal adrenal glands by sonography is due to several factors: (1) the neonatal adrenals are proportionally larger than adult glands (about one-third the size of the kidney at birth, as opposed to one-thirteenth in adults); (2) newborn infants' sparsity of perirenal fat affords better image resolution than the abundance of areolar fatty tissue surrounding the adult gland; and (3) the neonatal adrenal glands are closer to the skin surface, which permits the use of higher frequency transducers for sharper resolution of small structures.[104] In older infants and children, normal adrenal glands are sometimes difficult to identify, especially the left one. Adrenal sonography provides an opportunity to image from several directions, avoids the negative effects of ionizing radiation, is less expensive than CT, and can be performed at the bedside of a critically ill patient. The drawbacks of adrenal sonography include technically unsatisfactory studies resulting from the small size of the gland in older children, obesity, and overlying bowel gas.[104]

Sonographic Technique

Patient Preparation

Pediatric patients require no preparation for this examination but should be encouraged to be well hydrated. Adrenal visualization may be limited because the attenuation by bowel gas. Because air is a major culprit, it may be helpful to examine the patient after fasting using an approximate time line of 3 hours for patients younger than 1 year, 6 hours for patients aged 1 to 5 years, and 12 hours for older children.

Scan Technique

The accuracy of adrenal sonographic visualization varies greatly, depending on what technique is used and on the experience and skill of the operator. The age of the patient is also an important factor because the adrenal glands of neonates and young infants are larger and more easily identified.[105] It is not uncommon to examine the patient in different positions until the entire gland can be optimally visualized. The adrenal glands may be demonstrated by scanning from the flanks in longitudinal, coronal, and transverse planes. These planes are useful for avoiding overlying bowel.

The use of various decubitus and oblique positions may aid visualization.[104] A combination of transverse and longitudinal oblique scans has been reported to be accurate in identifying adrenal disease. When the patient lies in the decubitus position, the kidney falls forward, and the adrenal

gland may come into the scanning plane. However, because the gland is a complicated, folded piece of tissue, a single scan may demonstrate only part of it. For a complete adrenal evaluation, the sonographer should scan anterior as well as posterior to the gland until it is imaged in its entirety.

Another helpful technique in left adrenal gland visualization is the cava-suprarenal line position, in which the patient lies in a 45-degree LPO position while transverse scans are made from the right side to localize the left adrenal gland. The patient's position is then adjusted so that the acoustic beam lines up and passes through the IVC and aorta. The left adrenal gland is then visualized. Longitudinal planes are obtained by using the IVC and aorta as a double window for transmission.

The left adrenal gland is more difficult to visualize than the right one because of nearby stomach or bowel gas interference. This difficulty may be overcome by scanning through the intercostal spaces near the posterior axillary line. In difficult cases, it may be helpful to elevate the patient's left side, so that the adrenal area can be scanned through the spleen and kidney and behind the stomach gas bubble.

Technical Considerations

During adrenal scanning, the gain control setting should be comparable to that used for studying the liver. The normal adrenal glands have about the same echogenicity as the normal liver.

Normal Sonographic Appearance

The use of adjacent structural landmarks facilitates accurate localization of the adrenal glands. These paired retroperitoneal structures are located within the perirenal space. The right adrenal gland is pyramid shaped and lies over the kidney between the right crus of the diaphragm and the liver, posterior to the IVC. Any mass in the right adrenal area must be differentiated from a renal, hepatic, or retrocaval lymph node mass.

Imaging the left adrenal gland may be more difficult because of the numerous structures located in the left upper quadrant. The left adrenal is crescent shaped and lies anterior to the upper pole of the left kidney but lateral to the left crus of the diaphragm and posterior to the pancreatic tail. The esophagogastric junction is superior to the left gland and the fourth portion of the duodenum, inferior to it. It is important not to mistake the spleen, the splenic vessels, or the left renal vessels for the adrenal gland. These structures are usually distinguishable by their differing sonographic textures and contours, although masses originating in any of these structures can be mistaken for left adrenal masses or vice versa. A collapsed stomach or the duodenum can also be differentiated from the adrenal by the presence of "bright" central mucosal echoes and the real-time demonstration of peristalsis. The patient could drink clear liquids to aide in demonstrating the stomach if there is any question. Some splenic anatomic variations could also be mistaken for adrenal structures. The pediatric spleen varies in size and may have lobulations or additional splenules (accessory spleens). These findings can cause confusion and lead to misdiagnosis of an enlarged left adrenal gland or adrenal mass.[106]

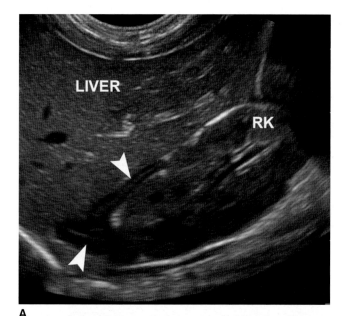

A

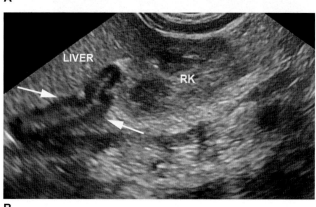

B

FIGURE 20-67 Normal neonatal adrenal gland. **A:** Longitudinal scan of right upper quadrant in a 35-week-old neonate shows the normal Y-shaped adrenal gland (*arrowheads*) superior to right kidney (*RK*). **B:** Longitudinal scan of the right upper quadrant in a term neonate shows the adrenal gland with the normal echogenic medulla surrounded by the hypoechoic cortex (*arrows*). (Image A: Courtesy of Monica Bacani, Columbus, OH; Image B: Courtesy of Jillian Platt, Falls Church, VA.)

The typical sonographic appearance of the adrenal gland is a Y- or V-shaped structure on longitudinal scans and a curvilinear structure on transverse scans[104] (Fig. 20-67A, B). The adrenal gland is made up of two parts: the medulla, which is sonographically visualized as a thin, echogenic central area, and the cortex, which appears as a thicker, anechoic zone surrounding the medulla. The newborn's adrenal cortex is relatively thick because it is composed of two layers: a thick fetal zone that occupies approximately 80% of the gland and a thin peripheral zone that will become the adult cortex. During the first year of life, the fetal zone undergoes involution, gradually shrinking, taking on a more typical adult appearance.[104]

Sonographic studies should note the size of the adrenal glands. The normal adrenal length ranges from 0.9 to 3.6 cm and the width between 0.2 and 0.5 cm. One study found no statistically significant difference in the size of right and left adrenals. It is important to note that with renal agenesis, the

adrenal gland is large and occupies the renal fossa. It may lose its typical Y or V shape but should not be mistaken for the kidney or another mass.[105]

Abnormal Findings

Tumors

Sonography can document the presence of adrenal masses, but it cannot differentiate tumor types.[106] Masses are usually more readily visualized than the normal gland. The sonographic appearance must be correlated with clinical and laboratory data to determine the type of lesion.[106] Adrenal masses usually appear as sonographically discrete lesions superior and medial to the upper pole of the kidney. A large mass may compress and deform the kidney, producing the appearance of tumor invasion. The most important feature for differentiating adrenal and renal masses is an interface or demarcation between the mass and the kidney. An adrenal mass shows such a demarcation, whereas a renal mass does not.

Neuroblastoma[11,107]

The most common adrenal tumors of childhood are the complex of neuroblastomas, which include ganglioneuromas, ganglioneuroblastomas, and neuroblastomas. All of the tumors are of neural crest origin, but the ganglioneuroma is considered less malignant and actually is a mature neuroblastoma.[105] Neuroblastoma is a tumor of infancy. Half the reported cases appear in the first year of life. Uncommon after age 8, neuroblastoma almost never occurs in adults.[108] It is important to note that these lesions can also arise from sympathetic ganglia in the lower abdomen, presacral region, chest, and even the neck and nasopharynx.[105] In the first year of life, almost all neuroblastomas involve the adrenal gland. The older the patient, the more likely the tumor is to arise outside the adrenal gland.[109] Children with abdominal neuroblastomas usually present with a palpable mass. It is less common for the presenting signs or symptoms to be caused by metastases. Pelvic tumors can cause urinary or GI symptoms. Clinically, systemic signs and symptoms, such as fever, weight loss, abdominal distention, irritability, hypertension, and anemia, are sometimes seen.[107,110] The prognosis for neuroblastoma is usually better in neonates and young infants than in older infants or children. Prognosis is also dependent on the site of origin of the tumor and the extent of disease at the time of diagnosis.[111] Early detection of the tumor is crucial to improve outcome.

Neuroblastoma is well known to have an unpredictable course.[108,112] Ordinarily, staging is based on the local extent of the lesion and the presence or absence of metastases. In most cases, patients with neuroblastoma present with advanced disease, having a large abdominal mass, or signs of metastases. Unlike Wilms tumor, most neuroblastomas are not "clean" lesions; usually, they spread rapidly beyond the confines of the adrenal glands, often crossing the midline in the abdomen and sometimes extending into the chest.[98] Calcification is a common finding in neuroblastoma, and calcifications are frequently irregular and visible in the primary tumor or its metastases.[105,109]

Sonographically, neuroblastoma is predominately echogenic, with poorly defined borders[107] (Fig. 20-68A–G). When

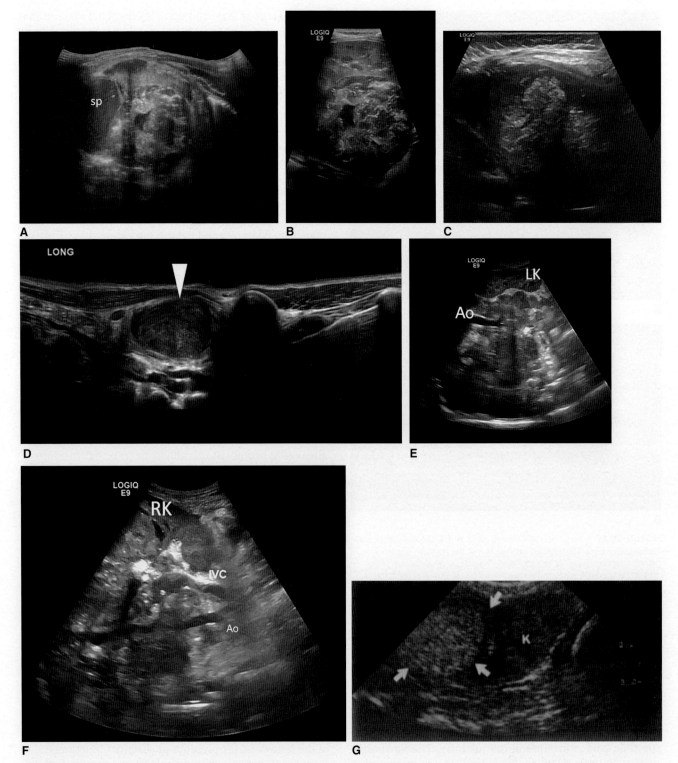

FIGURE 20-68 Neuroblastoma. An 11-year-old previously healthy male who presents with acute on chronic worsening back and abdominal pain found to have a large abdominal mass. **A–C:** There is an enhancing complex cystic and solid mass with coarse calcifications within the left abdomen measuring up to 15.1 cm in greatest dimension There is a predominantly cystic component within the superior aspect of this mass, which results in displacement of the spleen (*sp*). **D:** Left supraclavicular mass measuring up to 3.2 cm with additional regional prominent lymph nodes. Given the large retroperitoneal mass seen on abdominal ultrasound, the findings are consistent with neoplastic metastatic lymph node (*arrowhead*). **E:** A 6-year-old male with massive abdominal distention. **E:** Coronal image of a heterogeneous intra-abdominal mass. The inferior vena cava (*IVC*) and abdominal aorta and its major branches are encased circumferentially by the retroperitoneal mass (**F**). **G:** On this patient, the longitudinal sonogram of neuroblastoma (*arrows*) displaces the right kidney (*RK*) downward. Ao, aorta; *LK*, left kidney.

tumor calcification is present, focal echogenic areas can be seen producing acoustic shadowing. Hypoechoic areas within the neoplasm may result from necrosis. In the classic case of neuroblastoma arising from the adrenal gland, sonography clearly demonstrates the relationship of the tumor to the kidney, with its typical downward and outward displacement. Sonography is also useful for identifying urinary obstruction, vascular displacement and compression, nodal involvement, tumor extent, and liver involvement.[111] Extra-adrenal lesions exhibit a variety of configurations and relationships between the kidney and other organs.[105] Sonographic evaluation of neuroblastoma occurring in the chest and paraspinal area has obvious limitations. In these and other cases, CT more clearly demonstrates the extent and borders of the mass. Thus, even though sonography may originally make the diagnosis, CT is generally necessary to provide precise tumor mapping.[98] MRI also provides similar information important to both the initial diagnosis and post-treatment follow-up.[115]

The sonographer must attempt to differentiate the neuroblastoma from other abdominal masses, define the margins of the tumor, and identify any signs of metastatic disease. It may not be possible on the basis of the sonographic study alone to differentiate neuroblastoma from other solid tumors. Like Wilms tumor, neuroblastoma can metastasize to almost any organ.[112] In a neonate with a suprarenal mass, adrenal hemorrhage should be distinguished from necrotic neuroblastoma. An adrenal hemorrhage should show a characteristic pattern of resolution over a short time.

Adrenocortical Carcinoma

In children, adrenal gland tumors other than neuroblastomas are rare. The most common of these is the congenital adrenocortical carcinoma, which can produce virilizing symptoms or be linked with fetal alcohol syndrome or congenital hemihypertrophy and Beckwith–Wiedemann syndrome. Other clinical signs include abdominal mass, deepened voice, hypertension, seizures, and, rarely, weight loss. These lesions tend to be highly malignant and locally invasive[106] with frequent venous extension, regional lymph node involvement, and distant metastases to liver, lung, bone, and brain. Adrenocortical carcinoma is more common in adults than in children.[105]

Sonographically, adrenocortical carcinoma has a moderately echogenic complex pattern. The heterogeneous pattern probably represents areas of hemorrhage and necrosis dispersed throughout the tumor.[105] Calcification is seen in approximately one-fifth of the tumors. A thick, echogenic capsule-like rim may also be visualized in adrenocortical carcinoma.[111] Diagnostic imaging is an important tool for defining the extent of the primary tumor and determining the presence or absence of metastatic disease. Vascular extension is characteristic of adrenocortical carcinoma, and sonography can clearly demonstrate tumor extension into the IVC, hepatic veins, and right atrium. Metastasis in the retroperitoneum can also be visualized.

Pheochromocytoma

Pheochromocytomas are rare, functioning tumors that originate in chromaffin tissue. Fewer than 5% of all pheochromocytomas affect children, but most of those occur in the adrenal medulla. Pheochromocytomas may also be found in aberrant tissue along the sympathetic chain, the thorax, the para-aortic area, the aortic bifurcation, the retroperitoneum, and the bladder. Multiple pheochromocytomas are sometimes found in children, so it is important to search for a second and even a third lesion. In approximately 80% of pediatric cases, other family members are similarly affected, so careful examination of the child's immediate family is in order. Clinically, the diagnosis of pheochromocytoma is made by determination of urinary catecholamine excretion. Clinical symptoms include hypertension, headaches, palpitations, and diaphoresis.[108]

Sonographically, pheochromocytomas have a broad spectrum of appearance. A variety of internal echo patterns can be observed, including purely solid tumors, mixed solid and cystic masses, and cyst-like lesions. When lesions are large, they often contain areas of hemorrhage and necrosis, which result in a heterogeneous sonographic appearance (Fig. 20-69A–E).[106] Pheochromocytomas are almost always sharply encapsulated, producing a sharp, echogenic wall. Extra-adrenal masses are difficult to image sonographically and are often obscured by bowel gas.[106]

Metastases

Adrenal metastases often occur in a variety of adult malignancies but are rare in children.[110] Although metastases to the adrenal gland infrequently cause clinical symptoms, sonography is helpful for examining patients with known primary tumors for the progression of metastatic adrenal disease.[106] Such tumors are often bilateral and large.

Given the increased proportion of malignant lesions, adrenal masses in children and adolescents probably warrant resection unless they are seen in conjunction with a specific disorder, such as congenital adrenal hyperplasia (CAH).[113]

Sonographically, adrenal metastasis is nonspecific and may look identical to a primary adrenal tumor. Metastases appear solid, with varying degrees of echogenicity. Bilateral masses heighten the suspicion of adrenal origin.

Hemorrhage[114]

Adrenal hemorrhage in the newborn may result from prematurity, neonatal sepsis or hypoxia, or birth trauma inflicted on the rapidly involuting adrenal gland, particularly in large infants of diabetic mothers.[114,115] Often, more than one factor is responsible. Neonatal adrenal glands are susceptible to hemorrhage because of their large size and high vascularity.[114,115] Adrenal hemorrhage is most frequently identified between the second and seventh days of life. Clinically, there may be a palpable mass, anemia, hypotension, hyponatremia, jaundice, and scrotal discoloration in males.[114,115] Jaundice may occur because of the resorption of excessive hemoglobin from massive hemorrhage, but with massive hemorrhage, complete exsanguination of the infant can result.[115] Adrenal hemorrhage can also be identified after accidental blunt abdominal trauma[116] or child abuse in children. The hemorrhage is usually small, unilateral, in the right gland, and associated with ipsilateral intra-abdominal and intrathoracic injuries. Care should be taken not to incorrectly identify the hemorrhage as adrenal neoplasm, retroperitoneal blood, or hepatic or renal injury. An uncommon complication of adrenal hemorrhage is adrenal insufficiency.

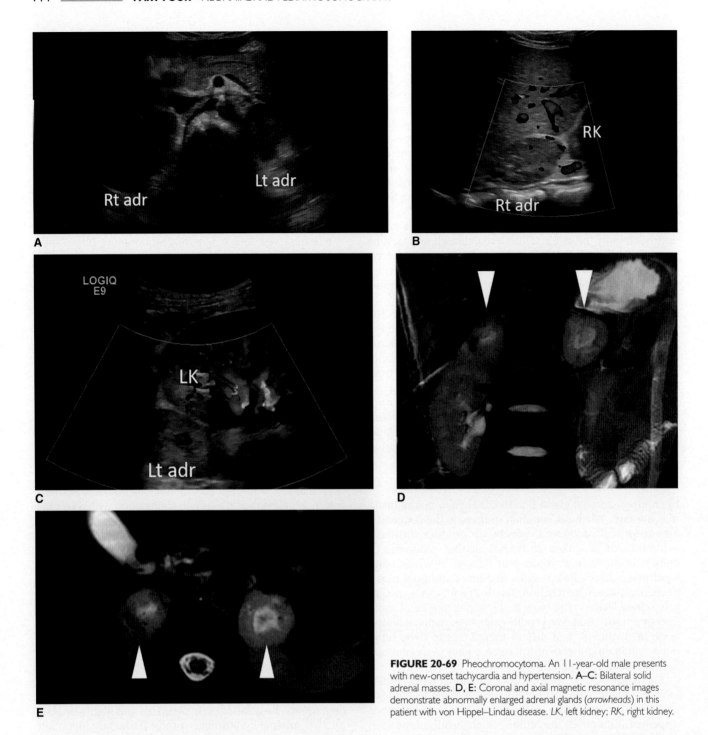

FIGURE 20-69 Pheochromocytoma. An 11-year-old male presents with new-onset tachycardia and hypertension. **A–C:** Bilateral solid adrenal masses. **D, E:** Coronal and axial magnetic resonance images demonstrate abnormally enlarged adrenal glands (*arrowheads*) in this patient with von Hippel–Lindau disease. *LK*, left kidney; *RK*, right kidney.

Sonographically, the appearance of adrenal hemorrhage depends on the age of the hemorrhage. Initially, hemorrhage appears as an echogenic mass in the suprarenal area. As it liquefies, the mass becomes progressively more anechoic so that, eventually, a suprarenal anechoic, cyst-like structure is visualized[105] (Fig. 20-70A–C). The diagnosis of adrenal hemorrhage may be established if sonography is repeated at 3- to 5-day intervals to observe the appearance of the mass as it changes from solid to cystic (Fig. 20-70D, E). Follow-up is appropriate at intervals of several weeks for 2 to 3 months because neuroblastoma may mimic the appearance of adrenal hemorrhage. Neuroblastoma will increase in size over time, whereas hemorrhage will resolve.[111] Elevated urinary catecholamines can also be indicative of neuroblastomas assisting with the differential diagnosis.

In most cases, the enlarged, hemorrhagic adrenal gland shrinks rapidly, and calcifications may become visible within a few weeks or months. Initially, the calcifications outline the enlarged anechoic adrenal gland in a rim-like manner. With time, as the adrenal becomes progressively smaller, the calcifications become more compact and eventually conform to the triangular configuration of the normal gland. Calcifications may be found incidentally on abdominal radiography or sonography. Documentation or adrenal hemorrhage is uncommon in these cases, but calcifications are assumed to be evidence of this. The calcified glands are echogenic.[115]

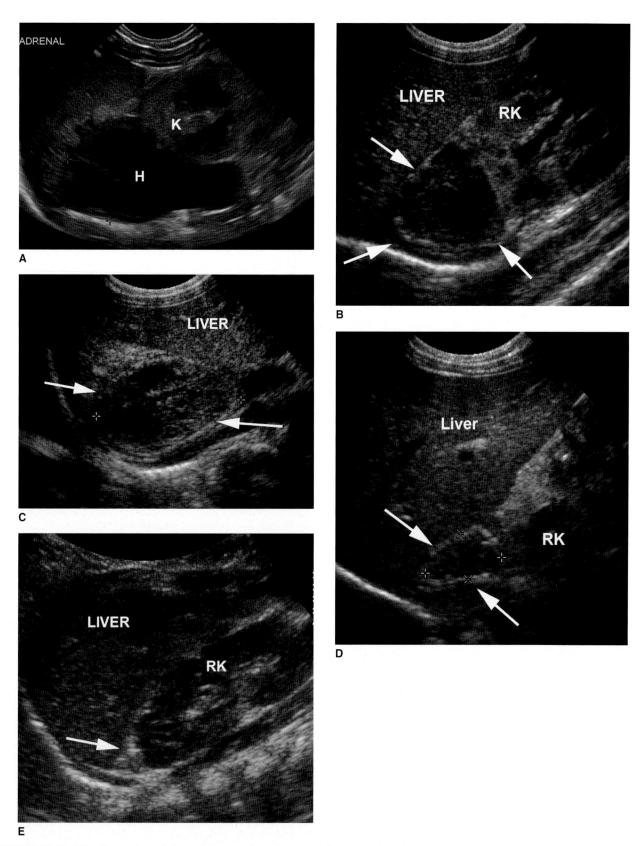

FIGURE 20-70 Adrenal hemorrhage. **A:** Prenatal sonogram showed a mass in left upper quadrant. Longitudinal scan of the left kidney (*K*) in the neonate shows a cystic mass (*H*) superior to kidney consistent with adrenal hemorrhage. **B–E:** Serial sonographic evaluations in a patient with adrenal hemorrhage following a traumatic delivery. Longitudinal (**B**) and transverse (**C**) images of the right upper quadrant 2 days after delivery demonstrate a heterogeneous mass (*arrows*) superior to the right kidney (*RK*). **D:** Follow-up examination 3 weeks later demonstrates a much smaller more echogenic mass (*arrows*) again seen superior to the RK. **E:** A second follow-up examination 6 weeks after delivery demonstrates complete resolution of the mass with only small residual calcifications (*arrow*, RK). Follow-up examination will help distinguish an adrenal hemorrhage from an adrenal tumor as an adrenal tumor should decrease in size over time. (Image **A:** Courtesy of Monica Bacani, Columbus, OH; Images **B–E:** Courtesy of Dr. Nakul Jerath, Falls Church, VA.)

Cysts

Adrenal cysts are rare.[106] They are usually unilateral, asymptomatic lesions that may be large and may cause hypertension. Adrenal cysts may occur secondary to hemorrhage or may be true cysts, such as retention cysts, cystic adenomas, or angiomatous cysts. Malignancies associated with adrenal cysts have not been reported.[106]

Sonographically, adrenal cysts usually appear as anechoic structures in the adrenal area that demonstrate well-defined walls and posterior acoustic enhancement. Typically, they displace the kidney inferiority and present a definite interface with the upper pole of the kidney. Some adrenal cysts contain debris and have irregular borders; for example, adrenal pseudocysts and hemorrhagic cysts. Adrenal cysts can simulate and must be distinguished from renal cysts, hydronephrosis, and splenic or pancreatic pseudocysts.[106]

Abscess

Adrenal abscesses are rare in children but have been documented in the neonatal period, probably the result of neonatal sepsis.[105] Bacterial seeding of adrenal hemorrhage is probably the cause of many adrenal abscesses.[110] The adrenals are relatively resistant to ordinary bacterial infection; although pyogenic abscesses can develop in the cortex with bacteremia, staphylococcal infections are the most common. The adrenal gland may also be involved by disseminated granulomatous disease. Adrenal abscesses are usually unilateral, but bilateral abscesses have been documented. Before 1946, adrenal tuberculosis accounted for nearly 90% of reported Addison disease cases in childhood. Since that time, histoplasmosis has become the most common childhood granulomatous disease of the adrenal gland. Infection of the adrenal gland by other fungi, particularly *Candida* (*Monilia*) or *Aspergillus*, may occur in terminal stages of leukemia or other hematopoietic diseases. Antibiotics alone are inadequate in treating a walled-off abscess, and percutaneous drainage is necessary.[111] Clinically, abscesses are characterized by fever, chills, and abdominal pain.

Sonographically, an adrenal abscess is identified as a relatively anechoic suprarenal mass, sometimes containing echogenic debris,[105] or a fluid–debris level with layering of debris altering with changes in position.[111] Abscesses are usually unilateral, although bilateral ones have been documented.[105] It can be difficult to sonographically distinguish between adrenal abscess and adrenal hemorrhage or neuroblastoma with central hemorrhage and necrosis. The failure of an adrenal hemorrhage to resolve or an increase in the size of a mass in an infant with fever should raise the suspicion of an abscess.[110] It is important to correlate the clinical history with the sonographic findings to make the correct diagnosis.[106]

Renal Agenesis

In patients with renal agenesis or severe renal hypoplasia (Potter syndrome) or ectopia of the kidney, the adrenal glands may become elongated and increase in thickness or may assume an unusual flattened or discoid shape.[110] Although this condition has been described as "hypertrophied," the adrenal gland is actually of normal weight and is normal in all other respects, except for shape.

In cases of renal agenesis, ectopia, or hypoplasia, it is important to recognize the characteristic sonographic appearance of the neonatal adrenals.[104] When normal renal tissue is absent, the adrenal gland preserves its typical echogenic medulla and hypoechoic cortex but enlarges, losing its characteristic Y or V shape and assuming a more elliptic, flattened shape. The distinctive appearance of the adrenal medulla and cortex should not be mistaken for the kidney.[104]

An enlarged adrenal gland without an adjacent kidney does not necessarily indicate renal agenesis because the kidney may merely be ectopic. Whenever enlarged adrenal glands are identified, a careful search should be made for renal tissue elsewhere in the abdomen or pelvis. Because renal agenesis is accompanied by Potter syndrome and pulmonary hypoplasia, it is important to identify affected fetuses and neonates because of direct therapeutic implications. The sonographic appearance of an elongated and thickened adrenal is probably the result of a lack of pressure from the kidney against the developing adrenal.

Congenital Adrenal Hyperplasia

CAH is an inborn error of the metabolism involving a deficiency of one of several enzymes necessary for normal steroid biosynthesis. It is transmitted as an autosomal recessive trait; the incidence is approximately 1 in 50 births in the United States.[112] The diagnosis of CAH depends on specific biochemical tests. The clinical signs include virilism in newborn females, premature masculinization in males, and advanced somatic development in both sexes.[110] Adrenocortical adenomas can develop in patients afflicted with CAH from hyperplastic tissue when the adrenal cortex undergoes increased hyperstimulation. Most cases of incidentally discovered adrenocortical adenomas (incidentalomas) have been reported in adults owing to increased CT and MRI scans being done for other diagnostic reasons. Lho et al reported a case of a 12-year-old girl with CAH, who developed an adrenocortical adenoma tumor despite being treated with steroids after birth.[117]

Sonographically, CAH is demonstrated by increased adrenal size. The adrenal glands become markedly enlarged, with preservation of the characteristic anechoic cortex and echogenic medulla. The enlargement involves the cortex predominantly, without obvious medullary enlargement, except in length. Sonographic adrenal measurements of 20 mm or more and a mean width of 4 mm or more are suggestive of the presence of adrenal hyperplasia. Sonography is used in CAH to measure the size of the adrenal glands to monitor the response to treatment and to reduce the likelihood of overtreatment and oversuppression and their effects on growth and maturation. Some neonates with biochemically proved CAH may have normal sonograms. Therefore, identification of sonographically normal-sized adrenal glands does not exclude CAH.

RELATED IMAGING PROCEDURES

Because no single procedure always provides all the necessary diagnostic information, the appropriate use of each modality requires an understanding of its strengths and weaknesses.

Radiographic Examinations

Intravenous pyelography (IVP) and the VCUG are used to evaluate the urinary tract in children and infants. Both examinations can provide information regarding congenital anomalies and the functionality of the urinary tract. VCUG is used to evaluate for reflux in cases of urinary tract infection. An IVP provides limited diagnostic information, and its importance has decreased with the introduction of sonography and CT. Both examinations have the disadvantage of using ionizing radiation and injected radiopaque contrast medium.

Computed Tomography

High-resolution CT can accurately image the normal kidneys and adrenal glands as well as tumors or masses, particularly in obese patients. It has been suggested that CT is the most important modality for assessment of primary and metastatic disease at the time of diagnosis and for follow-up. The advantages of CT are that it provides a more complete abdominal examination that is not limited by bowel gas, clearer definition of anatomic relationships, and very few unsatisfactory examinations. Disadvantages of CT include its ionizing radiation, opaque contrast material, relative expense, and limitation to imaging suite.

Magnetic Resonance Imaging

MRI demonstrates excellent soft-tissue contrast and is very helpful in differentiating among several diagnostic possibilities. MRI offers a combination of good anatomic information and tissue-specific information based on signal intensity. It is effective in diagnosing renal masses, adrenal hemorrhage, adrenal cortical carcinoma, metastases, pheochromocytoma (particularly ectopic lesions), and neuroblastoma, including staging (in children beyond the neonatal period). Magnetic resonance urography (MRU) has become more widely used and provides anatomic and functional information without the use of ionizing radiation.[86] MRU provides useful information in cases of complex congenital anomalies, urinary tract obstruction, and urinary tract infections.[86]

Nuclear Medicine Scintigraphy

Renal scintigraphy provides functional information about the urinary system and can provide valuable information in cases of congenital renal anomalies, obstruction, and reflux. Specifically, a metaiodobenzylguanidine (MIBG) scan can be used for detecting recurrent or metastatic adrenal tumors with fibrosis, distorted anatomy, or masses in an unusual location. Disadvantages include an increased dose of radiation, and the patient's thyroid gland must be blocked or protected during the scan.[118,119]

Positron Emission Tomography

Positron emission tomography can be utilized to target specific processes unique to certain types of tumors. Advantages are low radiation and no blocking of the thyroid needed (as in the MIBG scan). Disadvantages include an increased cost of the examinations.[118,119]

SUMMARY

- Sonography is the imaging modality of choice to evaluate the pediatric abdomen because it is portable, has no ionizing radiation, and provides excellent visualization of the abdominal organs and structures.
- Coarctation of the abdominal aorta is a rare congenital defect that causes severe hypertension, headaches, and fatigue in the pediatric population and a failure to thrive in the neonatal patient.
- Aortic thrombus is a complication of indwelling UACs in the neonate and presents clinically as absent femoral pulses, hematuria, cyanosis, hypertension, blanching of the lower extremities, and NEC.
- Thrombus in the IVC can be an extension of renal vein or iliac thrombosis.
- Tumor invasion into the IVC can occur from Wilms tumor, neuroblastoma, sarcoma, HCC, teratomas, and lymphoma.
- Benign neoplasms of the liver include hemangioendothelioma, cavernous hemangioma, and mesenchymal hamartoma.
- Liver cysts in the neonate and pediatric patient may be due to multicystic kidney disease, von Hippel–Lindau disease, hydatid disease, or trauma or may be simple congenital cysts.
- In patients with acute hepatitis, the liver may sonographically appear normal or may be enlarged and hypoechoic with prominent hyperechoic portal radicles.
- Liver abscesses may be amebic, pyogenic, or fungal.
- Fatty infiltration of the liver may be caused by malnutrition, malignancies, hyperalimentation, cystic fibrosis, Reye syndrome, glycogen storage disease, malabsorption syndrome, acute hepatitis, or obesity.
- With fatty infiltration, the liver appears echogenic with increased attenuation of the sound beam, causing decreased visualization of the posterior portions of the liver and the diaphragm.
- Cirrhosis of the liver in infants and children can be caused by biliary atresia, cystic fibrosis, chronic hepatitis, metabolic disorders, and medications.
- Malignant neoplasms of the liver that affect the pediatric population include hepatoblastoma, HCC, fibrolamellar HCC, and mesenchymal sarcoma.
- AFP is frequently elevated with hepatoblastoma and HCC but is typically normal with fibrolamellar HCC and mesenchymal sarcoma.
- Portal vein thrombosis can be caused by thrombosis or tumor invasion from hepatoblastoma or HCC.
- Conjugated hyperbilirubinemia in the newborn can be caused by neonatal hepatitis or biliary tract abnormalities such as biliary atresia.
- Biliary atresia can range from complete absence of the biliary tree to a rudimentary gallbladder and cystic duct or a visibly patent gallbladder, cystic duct, and common bile duct.

- A fasting gallbladder that measures less than 1.5 cm in the neonate with persistent jaundice is suggestive of biliary atresia.
- Choledochal cyst can present clinically with abdominal pain, palpable mass, and jaundice.
- There are five types of choledochal cysts; type I is the most common type diagnosed in the newborn and is a fusiform dilatation of the common bile duct.
- With sclerosing cholangitis, there is an inflammatory fibrosis that obliterates the intrahepatic and extrahepatic bile ducts, cirrhosis, portal hypertension, and liver failure and usually presents with concurrent inflammatory bowel disease.
- Rhabdomyosarcoma is a rare tumor of the biliary tract occurring between the ages of 1 and 5 that causes biliary obstruction and jaundice.
- In patients with cystic fibrosis, the pancreas is hyperechoic due to fibrosis and the replacement of normal pancreatic tissue with fatty tissue.
- Pancreatitis is less common in children than adults, but can be caused by blunt abdominal trauma, viral infection, drug toxicity, and hereditary disorders.
- Complications of pancreatitis include pseudocyst formation, phlegmon, hemorrhage, and abscess.
- HPS most commonly affects male infants between the ages of 2 and 10 weeks and presents with dehydration, projectile nonbilious vomiting, and possible failure to thrive.
- Pyloric stenosis can be diagnosed when the pyloric AP diameter exceeds 1.5 cm, the length of the channel exceeds 1.8 cm, and the muscle thickness exceeds 4 mm.
- Intussusception is found most frequently in males between the ages of 1 and 3 years and occurs when a segment of bowel prolapses into a more distal segment.
- Intussusception appears sonographically as a target pattern, multiple concentric anechoic rings surrounding an echogenic center, doughnut sign, anechoic ring surrounding an echogenic center, or pseudokidney sign, a reniform-shaped complex mass.
- Appendicitis is the most common surgical emergency in children and typically presents with periumbilical pain that radiates to the right lower quadrant, fever, and leukocytosis.
- The graded-compression technique is used to displace bowel gas and evaluate the right lower quadrant for appendicitis.
- The inflamed appendix is most often visualized at the base of the cecal tip as a tubular noncompressible structure with a target appearance in the transverse plane. The appendix should not exceed 6 mm in outer diameter.
- Sonography is widely used to evaluate the urinary tract and adrenal glands in the pediatric patient population because it can be performed portably; it does not employ ionizing radiation, contrast, or sedation; and it can be used for follow-up examinations.
- A 10-MHz transducer is used for neonatal examinations, whereas a 7.5-MHz transducer is more appropriate for older children.
- The medulla or renal pyramids are more prominent in infants and should not be mistaken for renal cysts.
- The renal pelvis should measure less than 10 mm in a normal kidney, and the wall should not be visible; a thickened wall may indicate chronic infection, reflux, or chronic obstruction.

- The cortex of the kidneys in newborns, especially premature infants, is more echogenic than the liver and spleen.
- Bilateral renal agenesis is incompatible with life and is associated with oligohydramnios and Potter syndrome; unilateral renal agenesis is more common and may be asymptomatic.
- In cases of renal agenesis, the adrenal gland may fill the renal fossa and should not be mistaken for the kidney.
- Congenital hydronephrosis is the most common renal mass in infants and children and most commonly results from an obstruction at the ureteropelvic junction.
- Duplication of the collecting system is a common cause of hydronephrosis because of the anomalous insertion of the ectopic ureter into the bladder; the upper pole collecting system is typically dilated.
- A ureterocele occurs when the ureter is narrowed at its distal insertion into the bladder; the anterior wall of the ureter projects into the bladder lumen, forming a ureterocele.
- Posterior urethral valves cause bilateral hydronephrosis, a thickened bladder wall, and dilated ureters.
- Multicystic dysplastic kidney may be hard to differentiate from hydronephrosis and is the result of a complete ureteral obstruction in utero.
- Hypoplastic kidney is a result of atrophy secondary to infection or vascular infarction.
- Infantile polycystic kidney disease presents at birth as symmetrically enlarged kidneys that are diffusely echogenic; the condition is associated with hepatic fibrosis.
- Simple renal cysts are rare in children and are usually associated with a syndrome such as tuberous sclerosis or von Hippel–Lindau disease.
- Wilms tumor is the most common malignant renal tumor in children and frequently presents before the age of 4 with pain, fever, malaise, weight loss, and a palpable abdominal mass.
- Wilms tumors are typically large, well-circumscribed, homogeneous masses that may contain cystic spaces within the mass representing necrosis or hemorrhage.
- Mesoblastic nephroma occur in infants younger than 3 months of age and may be unilateral or bilateral; sonographically, they resemble a Wilms tumor.
- Angiomyolipoma are echogenic, well-defined masses that are rare in children, except in cases of tuberous sclerosis, where they are typically bilateral and multiple.
- Cystitis is the most common urinary tract infection in children, occurs 10 times more often in females than in males, and may cause thickening of the bladder wall.
- The most common adrenal tumor of childhood is the neuroblastoma, which most commonly occurs in the first year of life.
- Sonographically, neuroblastomas are poorly defined, echogenic, solid masses that frequently have internal calcifications.
- Pheochromocytomas are rare, functioning adrenal gland medullary tumors that can occur in children and sonographically may appear solid, complex, or cystic.
- Adrenal hemorrhage may occur in the newborn as a result of prematurity, neonatal sepsis, birth trauma, or hypoxia; is most frequently identified between the second and seventh days of life; and may result in a palpable mass and anemia.
- Sonographically, the appearance of adrenal hemorrhage varies from echogenic to anechoic depending on the age of the hemorrhage.

REFERENCES

1. Redmon S. Pediatric sonography: funography for kids. *J Diag Med Sonogr*. 2007;23:110–112.
2. Fordham LA. Approach to the pediatric patient. *Ultrasound Clin*. 2009;4:439–443.
3. Baskin HJ. *Practical Pediatric Imaging*. Practical Imaging LLC; 2013.
4. Saif I, Seriki D, Moore R, et al. Midaortic syndrome in neurofibromatosis type 1 resulting in bilateral renal artery stenosis. *Am J Kidney Dis*. 2010;56:1197–1201.
5. Daghero F, Bueno N, Peirone A, et al. Coarctation of the abdominal aorta: an uncommon cause of arterial hypertension and stroke. *Circ Cardiovasc Imaging*. 2008:1:e4–e6.
6. Nagel K, Tuckuviene R, Paes B, et al. Neonatal aortic thrombosis: a comprehensive review. *Clin Padiatr*. 2010;222:134–139.
7. McAdams RM, Winter VT, McCurnin DC, et al. Complications of umbilical artery catheterization in a model of extreme prematurity. *J Perinatol*. 2009;29:685–692.
8. Miller CR. Ultrasound in the assessment of the acute abdomen in children: its advantages and its limitations. *Ultrasound Clin*. 2007;2:525–540.
9. Sigel MJ. Liver. In: Siegel MJ, ed. *Pediatric Sonography*. 4th ed. Lippincott Williams & Wilkins; 2011:214–274.
10. Varich L. Ultrasound of pediatric liver masses. *Ultrasound Clin*. 2010;5:137–152.
11. Milla SS, Lee EY, Buonomo C, et al. Ultrasound evaluation of pediatric abdominal masses. *Ultrasound Clin*. 2007;2:541–559.
12. Peddu P, Huang D, Kane PA, et al. Vanishing liver tumours. *Clin Radiol*. 2008;63:329–339.
13. Dubois J, Rypens F. Vascular anomalies. *Ultrasound Clin*. 2009;4:471–495.
14. Gow KW, Lee L, Pruthi S, et al. Mesenchymal hamartoma of the liver. *J Pediatr Surg*. 2009;44:468–470.
15. Feleppa C, D'Ambra L, Berti S, et al. Laparoscopic treatment of traumatic rupture of hydatid hepatic cyst—is it feasible?: a case report. *Surg Laparosc Endosc Percutan Tech*. 2009:19:e140–e142.
16. Siegel MJ. Jaundice in infants and children. *Ultrasound Clin*. 2006;1:431–441.
17. Mishra K, Basu S, Roychoudhury S, et al. Liver abscess in children: an overview. *World J Pediatr*. 2010;6:210–216.
18. Benedetti NJ, Desser TS, Jeffrey RB. Imaging of hepatic infections. *Ultrasound Q*. 2008;24:267–278.
19. Nievelstein RAJ, Robben SGF, Blickman JG. Hepatobiliary and pancreatic imaging in children—techniques and an overview of non-neoplastic disease entities. *Pediatr Radiol*. 2011;41:55–75.
20. Nanda K. Non-alcoholic steatohepatitis in children. *Pediatr Transplant*. 2004;8:613–618.
21. Alfire ME, Treem WR. Nonalcoholic fatty liver disease. *Pediatr Ann*. 2006;35:297–299.
22. Okka WH, Diego AA, Giovanna C, et al. Fatty liver: imaging patterns and pitfals. *Radiographics*. 2006;26(6):1637–1653.
23. Shorbagi A, Bayraktar Y. Experience of a single center with congenital hepatic fibrosis: a review of the literature. *World J Gastroenterol*. 2010;16:683–690.
24. Sirlin CB, Reeder SB. Magnetic resonance imaging quantification of liver iron. *Magn Reson Imaging Clin N Am*. 2010;18:359–381.
25. Tannuri AC, Tannuri U, Gibelli NE, et al. Surgical treatment of hepatic tumors in children: lessons learned from liver transplantation. *J Pediat Surg*. 2009;44:2083–2087.
26. Roebuck DJ, Olsen Ø, Pariente D. Radiological staging in children with hepatoblastoma. *Pediatr Radiol*. 2006;36:176–182.
27. Bittencourt PL, Couto CA, Ribeiro DD. Portal vein thrombosis and Budd-Chiari syndrome. *Clin Liver Dis*. 2009;13:127–144.
28. Harkanyi Z. Pediatric portal hypertension. *Ultrasound Clin*. 2006;1:443–455.
29. Siegel, MJ. Gallbladder and biliary tract. In: Siegel MJ, ed. *Pediatric Sonography*. 4th ed. Lippincott Williams & Wilkins; 2011:275–304.
30. Rozel C, Garel L, Rypens F, et al. Imaging of biliary disorders in children. *Pediatr Radiol*. 2011;41:208–220.
31. Mesleh M, Deziel DJ. Bile duct cysts. *Surg Clin North Am*. 2008;88:1369–1384.
32. Kanegawa K, Akasaka Y, Kitamura E, et al. Sonographic diagnosis of biliary atresia in pediatric patients using the "triangular cord" sign versus gallbladder length and contraction. *Am J Roentgenol*. 2003;181:1387–1390.
33. Humphrey TM, Stringer MD. Biliary atresia: US diagnosis. *Radiology*. 2007;244:845–851.
34. Lee MS, Kim MJ, Lee MJ, et al. Biliary atresia: color doppler US findings in neonates and infants. *Radiology*. 2009;252:282–289.
35. Aziz S, Wild Y, Rosenthal P, Goldstein RB. Pseudo gallbladder sign in biliary atresia: an imaging pitfall. *Pediatr Radiol*. 2011;41(5):620–626.
36. Souza LR, Pascoal G, Cappellari PF, et al. Giant choledochal cyst as a differential diagnosis for hepatic cyst. *J Diag Med Sonogr*. 2010;26:245–248.
37. Attalla BI. Abdominal sonographic findings in children with sickle cell anemia. *J Diag Med Sonogr*. 2010;26:281–285.
38. Walker TM, Hambleton IR, Serjeant GR. Gallstones in sickle cell disease: observations from the Jamaican cohort study. *J Pediatr*. 2000;136:80–85.
39. Punia RP, Garg S, Bisht B, et al. Clinico-pathological spectrum of gallbladder disease in children. *Acta Paediatr*. 2010;99:1561–1564.
40. Tsung JW, Raio CC, Ramirez-Schrempp D, et al. Point-of-care ultrasound diagnosis of pediatric cholecystitis in the ED. *Am J Emerg Med*. 2010;28:338–342.
41. Shukla RM, Roy D, Mukherjee PP, et al. Spontaneous gall bladder perforation: a rare condition in the differential diagnosis of acute abdomen in children. *J Pediatr Surg*. 2011;46:241–243.
42. Grisoni E, Fisher R, Izant R. Kawasaki syndrome: report of four cases with acute gallbladder hydrops. *J Pediatr Surg*. 1984;19:9–11.
43. Pryor JP, Volpe CM, Caty MG, et al. Noncalculous biliary obstruction in the child and adolescent. *J Am Coll Surg*. 2000;191:569–578.
44. Karrer FM, Bensard DD. Neonatal cholestasis. *Semin Pediatr Surg*. 2000;9:166–169.
45. Ali S, Russo MA, Margraf L. Biliary rhabdomyosarcoma mimicking choledochal cyst. *J Gastrointestin Liver Dis*. 2009;18:95–97.
46. Kitagawa N, Aida N. Biliary rhabdomyosarcoma. *Pediatr Radiol*. 2007;37:1059.
47. Nijs EL, Callahan MJ. Congenital and developmental pancreatic anomalies: ultrasound, computed tomography, and magnetic resonance imaging features. *Semin Ultrasound CT MR*. 2007;28:395–401.
48. Jackson WD. Pancreatitis: etiology, diagnosis, and management. *Curr Opin Pediatr*. 2001;13:447–451.
49. Vaughn DD, Jabra AA, Fishman EK. Pancreatic disease in children and young adults: evaluation with CT. *Radiographics*. 1998;18:1171–1187.
50. Chung E, Travis M, Conran R. Pancreatic tumors in children: radiologic–pathologic correlation. *Radiographics*. 2006;26:1211–1238.
51. Yu DC, Kozakewich HP, Perez-Atayde AR, et al. Childhood pancreatic tumors: a single institution experience. *J Pediatr Surg*. 2009;44:2267–2272.
52. Munden MM, Hill JG. Ultrasound of the acute abdomen in children. *Ultrasound Clin*. 2010;5:113–135.
53. Siegel MJ. Spleen and peritoneal cavity. In: Siegel MJ, ed. *Pediatric Sonography*. 4th ed. Lippincott Williams & Wilkins; 2011:305–338.
54. Hilmes MA, Strouse PJ. The pediatric spleen. *Semen Ultrasound CT MR*. 2007;28:3–11.
55. McCarten KM. Ultrasound of the gastrointestinal tract in the neonate and young infant with particular attention to problems in the neonatal intensive care unit. *Ultrasound Clin*. 2010;5:75–95.
56. Muradali D, Goldberg DR. US of gastrointestinal tract disease. *Radiographics*. 2015;35:50–68.
57. Hiorns MP. Gastrointestinal tract imaging in children: current techniques. *Pediatr Radiol*. 2011;41:42–54.
58. Sonanvane S, Siegel MJ. Sonography of the surgical abdomen in children. *Ultrasound Clin*. 2008;3:67–82.
59. Cohen HL, Greene EB, Boulden TP. The vomiting neonate or young infant. *Ultrasound Clin*. 2010;5:97–112.
60. Reed AA, Michael K. Hypertrophic pyloric stenosis. *J Diag Med Sonogr*. 2010;26:157–160.
61. Forster N, Haddad RL, Choroomi S, et al. Use of ultrasound in 187 infants with suspected infantile hypertrophic pyloric stenosis. *Australas Radiol*. 2007;51:560–563.
62. Junewick JJ. Decreasing radiation risks by increasing use of ultrasound in pediatric imaging. *Ultrasound Clin*. 2009;4:273–284.
63. Goldberg BB. *Atlas of Ultrasound Measurements*. Elsevier; 2006.
64. Applegate KE. Evidence-based diagnosis of malrotation and volvulus. *Pediatr Radiol*. 2009;39:S161–S163.
65. Patino MO, Munden MM. Utility of the sonographic whirlpool sign in diagnosing midgut volvulus in patients with atypical clinical presentations. *J Ultrasound Med*. 2004:23:S397–S401.

66. Rodriguez DP, Vargas S, Callahan MJ, et al. Appendicitis in young children: imaging experience and clinical outcomes. *Am J Roentgenol.* 2006;186:1158–1164.
67. Baltogiannis N, Mavridis G, Soutis M, et al. Currarino triad associated with Hirschsprung's disease. *J Pediatr Surg.* 2003;38:1086–1089.
68. Dillman JR, Smith EA, Sanchez RJ, et al. Pediatric small bowel Crohn disease: correlation of US and MR enterography. *Radiographics.* 2015;35(3):835–848.
69. Heflin D. The two extremes of sacrococcygeal teratomas. *J Diag Med Sonogr.* 2008;24:242–245.
70. Wu Y, Song B, Xu J, et al. Retroperitoneal neoplasms within the perirenal space in infants and children: differentiation of renal and non-renal origin in enhanced CT images. *Eur J Radiol.* 2010;75:279–286.
71. Rattan KN, Kadian YS, Nair VJ, et al. Primary retroperitoneal teratomas in children: a single institution experience. *Afr J Paediatr Surg.* 2010;7:5–8.
72. Sidhu M, Coley BD, Goske MJ, et al. Image gently, step lightly: increasing radiation dose awareness in pediatric interventional radiology. *Pediatr Radiol.* 2009;39:1135–1138.
73. Becker AM. Postnatal evaluation of infants with an abnormal antenatal renal sonogram. *Curr Opin Pediatr.* 2009;21:207–213.
74. Paltiel HJ. Sonography of pediatric renal tumors. *Ultrasound Clin.* 2007;2:89–104.
75. Lawande A. Ultrasonography in pediatric renal masses. *Ultrasound Clin.* 2010;5:433–441.
76. Kasap B, Soylu A, Türkmen M, et al. Relationship of increased renal cortical echogenicity with clinical and laboratory findings in pediatric renal disease. *J Clin Ultrasound.* 2006;34:339–342.
77. Michel SC, Forster I, Seifert B, et al. Renal dimensions measured by ultrasonography in children: variations as a function of the imaging plane and patient position. *Eur Radiol.* 2004;14:1508–1512.
78. Creel SA, Anderson J, Michael K, et al. Evaluation of pediatric renal size by sonography. *J Diag Med Sonogr.* 1999;15:1–6.
79. Pantoja Zuzuárregui JR, Mallios R, Murphy J. The effect of obesity on kidney length in a healthy pediatric population. *Pediatr Nephrol.* 2009;24:2023–2027.
80. Ozçelik G, Polat TB, Aktas S, et al. Resistive index in febrile urinary tract infections: predictive value of renal outcome. *Pediatr Nephrol.* 2004;19:148–152.
81. Okada T, Yoshida H, Iwai J, et al. Pulsed Doppler sonography of the hilar renal artery: differentiation of obstructive from nonobstructive hydronephrosis in children. *J Pediatr Surg.* 2001;36:416–420.
82. Yildirim H, Gungor S, Cihangiroglu MM, et al. Doppler studies in normal kidneys of preterm and term neonates: changes in relation to gestational age and birth weight. *J Ultrasound Med.* 2005;24:623–627.
83. Zamir G, Sakran W, Horowitz Y, et al. Urinary tract infection: is there a need for routine renal ultrasonography? *Arch Dis Child.* 2004;89:466–468.
84. Sivit CJ. Sonography of pediatric urinary tract emergencies. *Ultrasound Clin.* 2006;1:67–75.
85. Al Aaraj MS, Badreldin AM. *Ureteropelvic Junction Obstruction.* StatPearls Publishing; 2022. https://pubmed.ncbi.nlm.nih.gov/32809575/
86. Singh H, Ganpule A, Malhotra V, et al. Transperitoneal laparoscopic pyeloplasty in children. *J Endourol.* 2007;21:1461–1466.
87. Renjen P, Bellah R, Hellinger JC, et al. Pediatric urologic advanced imaging: techniques and applications. *Urol Clin North Am.* 2010;37:307–318.
88. Sidhu R, Bhatt S, Dogra VS. Ultrasonography of the urinary bladder. *Ultrasound Clin.* 2010;5:457–474.
89. Bernardes LS, Aksnes G, Saada J, et al. Keyhole sign: how specific is it for the diagnosis of posterior urethral valves? *Ultrasound Obstet Gynecol.* 2009;34:419–423.
90. Heikkilä J, Taskinen S, Rintala R. Urinomas associated with posterior urethral valves. *J Urol.* 2008;180:1476–1478.
91. Metwalley KA, Farghalley HS, Abd-Elsayed AA. Prune belly syndrome in an Egyptian infant with Down syndrome: a case report. *J Med Case Rep.* 2008;2:322.

92. Lin CC, Tsai JD, Sheu JC, et al. Segmental multicystic dysplastic kidney in children: clinical presentation, imaging finding, management, and outcome. *J Pediatr Surg.* 2010;45:1856–1862.
93. Garel L. Renal cystic disease. *Ultrasound Clin.* 2010;5:15–59.
94. Sweeney WE Jr, Avner ED. Diagnosis and management of childhood polycystic kidney disease. *Pediatr Nephrol.* 2011;26:675–692.
95. El-Sawi M, Shahein AR. Medullary sponge kidney presenting in a neonate with distal renal tubular acidosis and failure to thrive: a case report. *J Med Case Rep.* 2009;3:6656.
96. Letourneau K, Harrington C, Reed M, et al. Tuberous sclerosis complex: typical and atypical sonographic findings. *J Diag Med Sonogr.* 2005;21:491–496.
97. Ritchey ML, Azizkhan RG, Beckwith JB, et al. Neonatal Wilms tumor. *J Pediatr Surg.* 1995;30:856–859.
98. Mehta SV, Lim-Dunham JE. Ultrasonographic appearance of pediatric abdominal neuroblastoma with inferior vena cava extension. *J Ultrasound Med.* 2003;22:1091–1095.
99. Celik H, Kefeli M, Tosun M, et al. Congenital mesoblastic nephroma: prenatal diagnosis by sonography. *J Diag Med Sonogr.* 2009;25:112–115.
100. Fuchs IB, Henrich W, Brauer M, et al. Prenatal diagnosis of congenital mesoblastic nephroma in 2 siblings. *J Ultrasound Med.* 2003;22:823–827.
101. Bauer R, Kogan BA. New developments in the diagnosis and management of pediatric UTIs. *Urol Clin North Am.* 2008;35:47–58.
102. Pickworth FE, Carlin JB, Ditchfield MR, et al. Sonographic measurement of renal enlargement in children with acute pyelonephritis and time needed for resolution: implications for renal growth assessment. *Am J Roentgenol.* 1995;165:405–408.
103. Bellah RD, Epelman MS, Darge K. Sonography in the evaluation of pediatric urinary tract infection. *Ultrasound Clin.* 2010;5:1–13.
104. Oppenheimer DA, Carroll BA, Yousem S. Sonography of the normal neonatal adrenal gland. *Radiology.* 1983;146:157–160.
105. Hayden KC Jr, Swischuk LE. *Pediatric Ultrasonography.* Lippincott Williams & Wilkins; 1987.
106. Worthen NJ. Adrenal sonography. In: Sarti D, ed. *Diagnostic Ultrasound: Text and Cases.* 2nd ed. Year Book Medical Publishers; 1987.
107. Perry CL. Sonographic evaluation of neuroblastoma. *J Diag Med Sonogr.* 2009;25:101–107.
108. Dunnick NR, Korobkin M. Imaging of adrenal incidentalomas: current status. *Am J Roentgenol.* 2002;179:559–568.
109. Arce GJ, Arce TY, Angerri FO, et al. Retroperitoneal ganglioneuroma in the infancy. *Actas Urol Esp.* 2008;32:567–570.
110. Shackelford GD. Adrenal glands, pancreas and other retroperitoneal structures. In: Siegel MJ, ed. *Pediatric Sonography.* 2nd ed. Raven Press; 1995.
111. Silverman FN, Kuhn JP. *Caffey's Pediatric X-Ray Diagnosis: An Integrated Imaging Approach.* Vol 2. CV Mosby; 1993.
112. Filiatrault D, Hoyoux C, Benoit P, et al. Renal metastases from neuroblastoma. Report of two cases. *Pediatr Radiol.* 1987;17:137–138.
113. Pescovitz OH, Eugster EA. *Pediatric Endocrinology: Mechanisms, Manifestations, and Management.* Lippincott Williams & Wilkins; 2004.
114. Valdespino RS. The importance of sonography in the evaluation of neonatal adrenal hemorrhage. *J Diag Med Sonogr.* 2009;25:221–225.
115. Abdu AT, Kriss VM, Bada HS, et al. Adrenal hemorrhage in a newborn. *Am J Perinatol.* 2009;26:553–557.
116. Soundappan SV, Lam AH, Cass DT. Traumatic adrenal haemorrhage in children. *ANZ J Surg.* 2006;76:729–731.
117. Lho SR, Park SH, Jung MH, et al. A case of adrenocortical adenoma following long-term treatment in a patient with congenital adrenal hyperplasia. *Korean J Pediatr.* 2007;50:302–305.
118. Willatt JM, Francis IR. Radiologic evaluation of incidentally discovered adrenal masses. *Am Fam Physician.* 2010;81:1361–1366.
119. Sahdev A, Willatt J, Francis IR, et al. The indeterminate lesion. *Cancer Imaging.* 2010;10:102–113.

CHAPTER 21

The Neonatal Head

TARA K. CIELMA AND ANJUM N. BANDARKAR

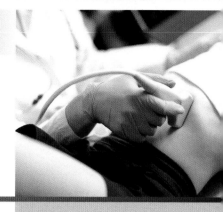

OBJECTIVES

- Review developmental anatomy of the brain and intracranial vascular structures.
- Identify the sonographic appearance of the normal brain in neonates and infants.
- Describe the systematic evaluation of the neonatal brain.
- Discuss Doppler evaluation of intracranial vessels.
- Describe the physiologic and maturation differences in the sonographic appearance of the preterm and term neonatal brain.
- Illustrate ischemic injury of the preterm and term infant.
- Identify the risk factors for the development of an intracranial hemorrhage (ICH) and illustrate the sonographic appearance of ICH.
- Describe the mechanism, etiologies, and sonographic appearance of hydrocephalus.
- Identify types of traumatic hemorrhage including birth trauma and non-accidental injury.
- Identify ultrasound findings in the setting of congenital infections.
- List common pathologies including congenital malformations of the brain that can be visualized sonographically.
- Describe the evaluation of cranial sutures to assess for craniosynostosis.

GLOSSARY

cerebellum posterior portion of the brain composed of two hemispheres; lies below the tentorium

cerebral spinal fluid (CSF) surrounds the brain and the spinal cord to protect the brain and spinal cord from injury

cerebrum largest section of the brain; divided into two hemispheres joined by the corpus callosum

choroid plexus echogenic cluster of cells located within the lateral ventricles responsible for the production of CSF

corpus callosum largest white matter structure in the brain; contains nerve tracts that allow communication between the right and left hemispheres of the brain

falx cerebri fold of dura mater that divides the two hemispheres of the brain

fontanelle soft spot between the cranial bones; anterior, posterior, and mastoid fontanelles are used as acoustic windows during sonographic examination of the neonatal brain

gyri various infolds of the cerebral cortex, surrounded by sulci

hypoxia lack of oxygen

infant human baby 1 month to 1 year of age

KEY TERMS

agenesis of the corpus callosum

anterior cerebral artery

cerebellar hemorrhage

Chiari malformation

coarctation of the lateral ventricle

cytomegalovirus

Dandy–Walker complex

germinal matrix hemorrhage

holoprosencephaly

hydrocephalus

hypoxic–ischemic encephalopathy

increased intracranial pressure

intracranial hemorrhage

macrocephaly

middle cerebral artery

periventricular leukomalacia

porencephaly

prominent periventricular blush

resistive index

subarachnoid space

TORCH complex

vein of Galen malformation

(continued)

meninges membranous coverings of the brain and spine

neonate human baby less than 1 month of age

porencephaly cyst or cavity in the brain usually as a result of a destructive lesion

sulci linear structures that separate gyri

suture fibrous, immovable joints that connect the skull bones

thalamus paired ovoid structures in the central brain responsible for relaying nerve impulses and carrying sensory information into the cerebral cortex

Cranial sonography has evolved into a vital clinical tool and is the primary modality for screening, monitoring, and follow-up of intracranial hemorrhage (ICH), hydrocephalus, ischemic lesions, and congenital malformations of the neonatal and infant brain. Its widespread utilization is the result of its proven diagnostic value, improved sensitivity and specificity, bedside availability, nonionizing nature, and its cost-effectiveness compared with other imaging modalities.

The overall aim of this chapter is to provide an introduction to cranial sonography for sonographers of all experience levels. The chapter discusses exam indications, scanning protocols, sonographic anatomy, normal variants, and common intracranial pathology and anomalies. For a more comprehensive study of intracranial anomalies, there are several texts the reader should reference.[1,2]

TECHNIQUE

The anterior fontanelle is the primary acoustic window to image the brain. The closure of the anterior fontanelle begins at about 9 months of age and is usually complete by approximately 15 months of age. However, the fontanelle may remain patent in patients with extreme prematurity and in conditions like osteogenesis imperfecta, and hypophosphatasia. Routine images are obtained in coronal and sagittal planes. The posterior fontanelle (PF), mastoid (posterolateral) fontanelle (MF), and sphenoid fontanelle have shown considerable diagnostic value as adjuvant imaging approaches to the routine anterior fontanelle approach. The squamosal portion of the temporal bone allows interrogation of the circle of Willis. The foramen magnum provides visualization of the upper spinal canal in patients with Chiari malformation. An illustration of their clinical utility will be discussed further in this chapter.

A small-footprint, high-frequency, 7-to-10-MHz phased-curved array or sector transducer is typically used to image the neonatal brain. A lower-frequency (5 to 7 MHz) transducer may be needed for older infants with closing fontanelles or infants with a large amount of hair. Some infants may require a lower frequency, such as 4 MHz, to penetrate the temporal bone for transaxial Doppler imaging. A small-footprint, high-frequency linear transducer (9 to 18 MHz) is useful for imaging superficial structures, such as the superior sagittal sinus (SSS), superficial cortex, or the extracranial space around the convexity of the brain.[3] Coupling gel and standoff pads may be used to achieve optimal skin-to-transducer contact to characterize structures in the near field. Color and spectral Doppler are utilized to assess intracranial hemodynamics.

Preterm infants (defined as delivery prior to 36 weeks of gestation) in the intensive care nurseries are at high risk for infections because of their immature immune systems. Transducers and cables must be cleaned thoroughly between each patient. Proper hand-washing technique, adherence to isolation protocols, and the use of single-use gel packets will help minimize the spread of infection. Before proceeding with the scan, the examiner needs to communicate with the nurse in charge of the infant to discuss any potential complications that may arise during scanning and to solicit help with ventilator tubes or other equipment that may need to be rearranged in order to access the fontanelles. There are also some procedural precautions that need to be observed in order to prevent additional stress on the preterm infant. These precautions include limiting head and neck movement to minimize the risk of dislodging critical airway support; minimizing pressure to the anterior fontanelle to avoid bradycardia; and maintaining thermal regulation to prevent heat loss. Opening the isolette doors should be avoided when possible. Scanning through the portholes of the isolette and the use of prewarmed gel can help the infant maintain thermal stability during the sonography examination.

NORMAL BRAIN ANATOMY

The brain and spinal cord comprise the central nervous system (CNS). Three protective membranes, called meninges, cover and protect the brain and spinal cord from injury, to allow the passage of CSF and to support vascular structures. They consist of the dura mater, arachnoid mater, and pia mater. The dura mater is the outer layer and the most resilient of the three. It attaches to the inside of the cranial vault and partitions the intracranial space through folds into separate compartments. The arachnoid space forms the middle layer, forming a bridge around the cortical sulci. The pia mater surrounds the innermost surface of the cerebral cortex, and closely follows the contours of the gyri and sulci.

Cerebrospinal Fluid

The CSF surrounds the brain and the spinal cord. Largely produced by choroid plexus (CP), this fluid acts like a buffer to help cushion the brain and spinal cord from injury, removes waste products, and serves to regulate intracranial pressure. The brain maintains a balance between the amount of CSF that is generated and the amount that is absorbed.

Fontanelles

The anterior fontanelle (also known as bregma) is formed at the junction of the coronal, sagittal, and frontal sutures. Closure occurs at approximately 9 to 15 months of age. The PF is formed by the junction of the lambdoid and sagittal sutures and may be palpated above the level of the occipital protuberance. Closure occurs at approximately 2 to 6 months of age. The mastoid fontanelle (MF) (also known as posterolateral) is located at the junction of the squamosal, lambdoidal, and occipital sutures. Closure occurs at approximately 6 to 18 months of age. The sphenoid fontanelle (also known as anterolateral) is located at the intersection of the sphenoid, parietal, temporal, and frontal bones. Closure occurs at approximately 6 months of age (Fig. 21-1).

Divisions of the Brain

The brain can be divided into the cerebrum, the cerebellum, and the brainstem. The cerebrum is the largest section and is divided into right and left cerebral hemispheres and is separated by a fissure or groove called the interhemispheric (longitudinal) fissure. The falx cerebri is a section of dura that lies within this fissure. The cerebrum is composed of both gray and white matter. The outer portion, called the cortex, is composed of gray matter, whereas the white matter is found deeper within the cerebrum.

The cortex is divided into four lobes: frontal, parietal, occipital, and temporal. The brainstem is a stalk-like structure connecting the cerebral hemispheres with the spinal cord. It consists of three parts: the midbrain, pons, and medulla oblongata. The cerebellum is located at the back of the brain beneath the occipital lobes and is separated from the

cerebrum by the tentorium (a fold of dura). The cerebellum is composed of two hemispheres with a median structure called the vermis that connects the two hemispheres. The cavity containing the cerebellum, fourth ventricle, brain stem, and cranial nerves is called the posterior fossa.[3]

Ventricles

The purpose of the ventricular system is to provide a pathway for the circulation of CSF. The ventricular system is composed of four ventricles: the paired lateral ventricles and the midline third and fourth ventricles. The paired lateral ventricles are the largest of the ventricles and are located on either side within the cerebrum of the brain. They are divided into four segments: the frontal (anterior) horn, body, temporal, and occipital (posterior) horn. The trigone (atrium) of the lateral ventricle is the region where the anterior, occipital, and temporal horns converge.

The paired lateral ventricles drain into the third ventricle through the foramen of Monro and the third ventricle drains into the fourth through the aqueduct of Sylvius. The fourth ventricle drains into the subarachnoid space through the foramina of Luschka and Magendie and then into the basal cistern. CSF flows upward around the brain to the vertex, where it is resorbed by the arachnoid granulations into the superior sinuses. CSF also flows around and down the spinal subarachnoid space.[3]

Choroid Plexus

The CP is responsible for the production and regulation of CSF. The largest part of the CP, which is known as the glomus, is seen as an echogenic structure within the lateral ventricles at the level of the trigone. It tapers as it courses anteriorly and ends at the caudothalamic groove. The CP never extends anterior to the foramen of Monro into the frontal horns or posteriorly into the occipital horns. CP is also present in the roof of the third and fourth ventricles.

Corpus Callosum

The two sides of the cerebrum are joined by the corpus callosum. The corpus callosum is the largest white matter structure in the brain and contains nerve tracts that allow communication between the right and left hemispheres of the brain. It is divided into the rostrum, genu, body, and splenium (posterior part) and forms the roof of the lateral and third ventricle.

Caudate Nucleus

Located in each hemisphere of the brain, the caudate nucleus is the most medial of the four basal ganglia. It is an elongated, curved mass of gray matter, and it consists of head, body, and tail. The head and body form part of the floor of the anterior horn of the lateral ventricle, and the tail curves back toward the anterior, forming the roof of the inferior horn of the lateral ventricle.

Thalamus

The thalami are paired structures of gray matter situated between the cerebral cortex and the midbrain. They are

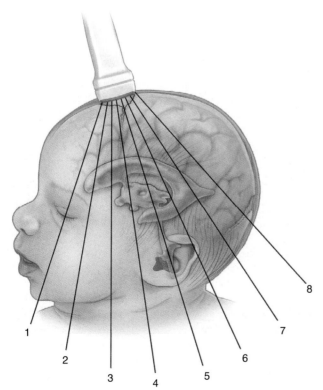

FIGURE 21-1 Coronal scan planes (*1 to 8*). Coronal imaging planes via the anterior fontanelle approach.

located in the center of the brain, one beneath each cerebral hemisphere, next to the third ventricle. The thalami can be thought of as relay stations for nerve impulses carrying sensory information into the cerebral cortex.

Fissures

There are five major fissures that divide the cerebral hemispheres: interhemispheric fissure, Sylvian fissure, parieto-occipital fissure, transverse fissure, and central fissure. The interhemispheric fissure (also known as the falx or longitudinal fissure) divides the cerebrum into right and left hemispheres. The Sylvian fissure (also known as lateral fissure) divides the frontal and parietal lobes from the temporal lobe. The parieto-occipital fissure separates the occipital lobe from the parietal lobe. The transverse fissure separates the cerebrum from the cerebellum. The central fissure (also known as fissure of Rolando) separates the frontal and parietal lobes.

Cisterna Magna

The cisterna magna (CM) is a fluid-filled structure that communicates with the fourth ventricle. It lies between the cerebellum and the dorsal surface of the medulla.

SCANNING PROTOCOL

Neurosonography should be performed in a standardized manner with a specific sequence of images and key anatomical structures identified on each scan. Most premature infants will have serial scans over the course of their hospital stay, and a standard approach will ensure that consistency be maintained from examiner to examiner. The examiner should also know the approximate gestational age of the infant. This will aid in differentiating age-related features from pathology.

Coronal Scanning Protocol

Scanning in the coronal plane via the anterior fontanelle should minimally include six to eight images. Magnified image planes should be incorporated to draw attention to suspicious areas or to enhance the visualization of abnormal areas. Maintaining side-to-side symmetry while scanning in the coronal plane is a technique that will require some practice; however, doing so is essential to obtaining a good study. Representative coronal sections are obtained by systematically angling the transducer from the frontal lobe of the infant brain to the occipital cortex, anterior to the orbital ridge, past the occipital lobes. The scanning planes are depicted in Figure 21-1. In the coronal plane, by convention, image labeling should have the right side of the brain projected on the left side of the image.

The most anterior coronal image is obtained through the frontal lobes of the cerebral cortex at the level of the orbital ridge and the interhemispheric fissure (Fig. 21-2). This scan is anterior to the frontal horns. The next scan should include the triangular-shaped, fluid-filled frontal horns and the head of the caudate nuclei adjacent to the lateral walls of the ventricles. The fluid-filled cavum septi pellucidi can be seen between the frontal horns of the lateral ventricles.

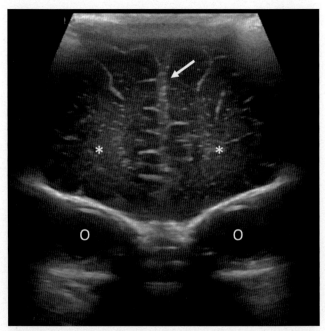

FIGURE 21-2 Frontal lobes. Coronal image at the level of the frontal lobes shows the interhemispheric fissure *(arrow)*, normal echogenicity of the frontal lobes *(asterisks)*, and orbital ridges *(O)*. This image is anterior to the frontal horns and lateral ventricles.

Anterior to the cavum is the corpus callosum (Fig. 21-3). The next scan is slightly more posterior and is obtained at the level of the foramen of Monro. This is where the lateral ventricles and the third ventricle communicate. The normal slit-like third ventricle is often difficult to visualize owing to volume averaging; its transverse diameter often falls within the beam width. Slight off-axis angulation will offset the

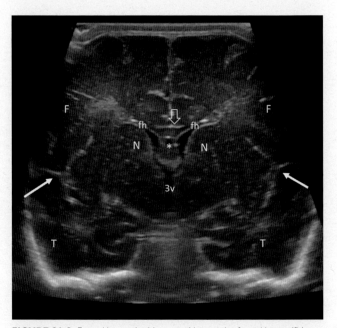

FIGURE 21-3 Frontal horns. In this coronal image, the frontal horns *(fh)* appear as triangular-shaped, fluid-filled spaces separated by the cavum septi pellucidi *(asterisk)*. The head of the caudate nuclei *(N)* lie adjacent to the lateral walls of the ventricles. The hypoechoic corpus callosum *(cc)* forms the roof of the cavum. The third ventricle *(3v)* can also be seen. The echogenic Y-shaped Sylvian fissures *(arrows)* are seen laterally. *F*, frontal lobe; *T*, temporal lobe.

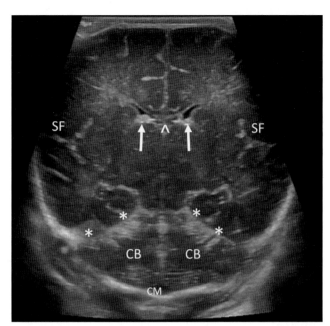

FIGURE 21-4 Coronal view posterior to the third ventricle. The echogenic CP is seen in the floor of the lateral ventricle *(arrows)* and the roof of the third ventricle *(caret)*. The Y-shaped Sylvian fissures *(SF)* are seen laterally. Also visible are the echogenic tentorium *(asterisks)*, the cerebellar hemispheres *(CB)*, and the cisterna magna *(CM)*.

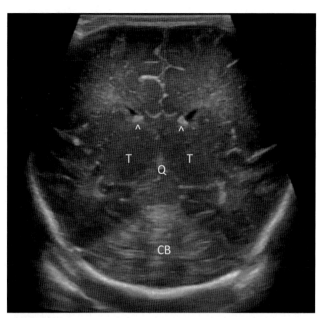

FIGURE 21-5 Quadrigeminal cistern. Coronal image taken at the level of the quadrigeminal cistern. The star-shaped echogenic quadrigeminal cistern *(Q)* is seen inferior to the thalami *(T)*. The cerebellum *(CB)* and the echogenic choroid plexus *(CP, carets)* in the floor of the lateral ventricles are also visualized.

beam thickness effect and will often allow visualization of the normal third ventricle. When dilated, it can be imaged quite easily. Continuing with further posterior angulation, the echogenic CP can be seen in the floor of the lateral ventricle and in the roof of the third ventricle. This scan is slightly posterior to the third ventricle. The echogenic V-shaped tentorium can be seen in this scan anterior to the cerebellum. Posterior to the vermis of the cerebellum is the CM. The Y-shaped Sylvian fissure can also be seen in this plane (Fig. 21-4). With more posterior angulation, the next scan demonstrates the echogenic star-shaped quadrigeminal cistern posterior to the thalami. Posterior to the tentorium is the posterior fossa containing the echogenic cerebellum (Fig. 21-5).

Angling slightly more posterior, the trigones of the lateral ventricles dominate this section. The glomi of the CP fill most of the lateral ventricles at this level. The periventricular parenchyma lateral to the ventricles should be evaluated carefully. These areas represent the periventricular white matter, and the echogenicity of this area should not be brighter than the CP (see the section on Prominent Periventricular Blush). A benefit of the coronal plane is that it allows contralateral comparison of the echogenicity between the CP and the periventricular parenchyma. Increased echogenicity of this area should arouse suspicion for hemorrhage/infarction and requires follow-up evaluation (Fig. 21-6). The final and most posterior scan predominantly visualizes the gyri and sulci of the occipital lobe, the periventricular white matter, and the posterior interhemispheric fissure (Fig. 21-7).[3]

Sagittal/Parasagittal Scanning Protocol

The transducer is rotated 90 degrees from the coronal plane and, starting at the midline, is angled medial to lateral sequentially through each cerebral hemisphere via the anterior fontanelle. The scanning planes are depicted in Figure 21-8. Image labeling, by convention, places the anterior aspect of the brain on the left side of the image. The midline, right side, and left side need to be annotated, respectively. In the midline, the crescentic hypoechoic corpus callosum is visualized just above the cavum septum pellucidum and vergae (seen in premature infants only). Superiorly, the corpus callosum is surrounded by the hyperechoic pericallosal

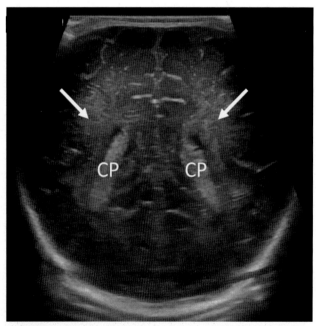

FIGURE 21-6 Choroid plexus *(CP)*. Coronal scan at the level of the trigones of the lateral ventricles. The largest part of the CP can be seen occupying most of the lateral ventricles. The periventricular white matter (also known as the optic radiation) is located lateral to the ventricles *(arrows)*.

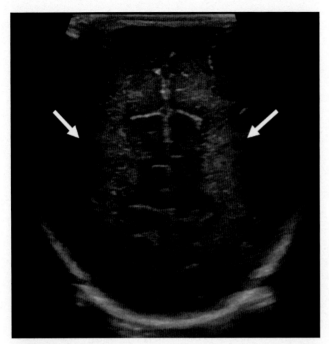

FIGURE 21-7 Occipital lobes. Coronal image taken posterior to the occipital horns of lateral ventricles shows the normal echogenic periventricular white matter *(arrows)* and the occipital cortex.

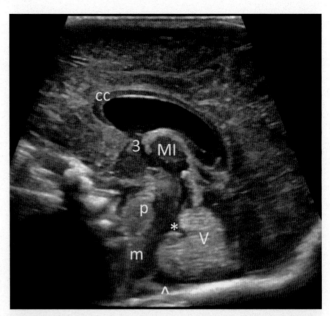

FIGURE 21-9 Sagittal midline. Normal midline sagittal image on a term infant. The hypoechoic corpus callosum *(CC)* is seen anterior to the cavum septum pellucidum. The third *(3)* and fourth *(*)* ventricles are visible in this plane. Posterior to the fourth ventricle is the echogenic vermis of the cerebellum *(V)* and the cisterna magna *(CM, caret)*. Anterior to the fourth ventricle is the pons *(p)* and medulla *(m)*. *MI,* massa intermedia.

sulci, which contains the pericallosal artery. The vascular pulsations from these vessels can be appreciated on real-time imaging. Inferior to the corpus callosum is the third ventricle. Anterior to the echogenic vermis of the cerebellum is the triangular-shaped fourth ventricle. The moderately echogenic midbrain is anterior to the fourth ventricle, and

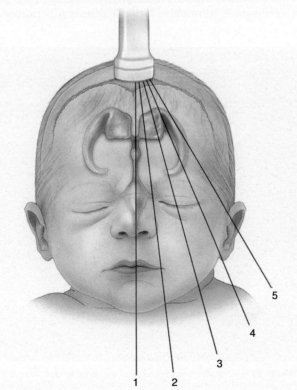

FIGURE 21-8 Sagittal scan planes. Sagittal/parasagittal imaging planes via the anterior fontanelle approach.

the echogenic cerebellar vermis is posterior to the fourth ventricle (Fig. 21-9). The CM is seen inferior to the vermis and should always be visualized. Absence of the CM is indicative of pathology. Parasagittal images are obtained by angling the transducer from the midline through the right and left cerebral hemispheres from medial to lateral (or lateral to medial). The main anatomic landmark in the next image is the caudothalamic groove. The anterior extent of the CP tapers to a point into this groove, which is formed by the head of the caudate nucleus anteriorly and the thalamus posteriorly. The head of the caudate nucleus is slightly more echogenic than the thalamus. In the premature neonate, the fragile germinal matrix (GM) is located in these areas and is a common site for hemorrhage (see further discussion under the section on Intracranial Hemorrhage). This is an area where a magnified image plane is recommended (Fig. 21-10). With continued angulation laterally, the next image is through the lateral ventricle. The frontal horn of the lateral ventricle is more medial than the occipital horn; thus, to visualize the entire ventricle, the anterior part of the transducer needs to be angled obliquely with the front end of the transducer angled medially and the posterior part angled slightly more lateral. This parasagittal section will visualize a good portion of the frontal horn and body of the lateral ventricle. The thalamus is seen inferior to the head of the caudate nucleus, and the CP should taper into the caudothalamic groove (Fig. 21-11). Angling more laterally, the highly echogenic glomus of the CP is seen filling the trigone of the lateral ventricle and has a comma-shaped configuration because it courses posterior toward the temporal horn (Fig. 21-12). There should be no CP extending anterior to the third ventricle or into the occipital horn. Several images may be needed to image the complete ventricular system. The temporal horn or occipital horn will need to be imaged separately because it is not always possible to

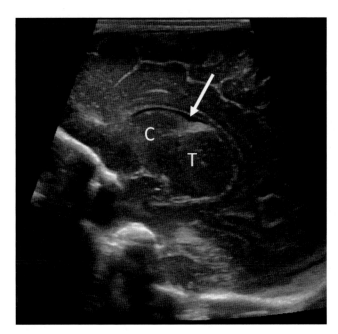

FIGURE 21-10 Caudothalamic groove. Parasagittal scan at the level of the caudothalamic groove. Head of the caudate nucleus *(C)* is seen anterior to the thalamus *(T)*. Between these two structures is the caudothalamic groove or notch *(arrow)*, which contains the anterior extent of the choroid plexus *(CP)*.

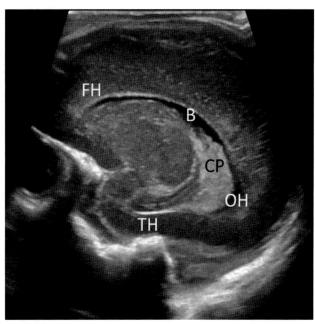

FIGURE 21-12 Parasagittal choroid plexus. Parasagittal scan through the body *(B)* of the lateral ventricle. The echogenic choroid plexus *(CP)* is seen within the trigone of the ventricle. *FH*, frontal horn; *OH*, occipital horn; *TH*, temporal horn.

line up the entire ventricular system in one plane. In a nondilated ventricular system, the temporal and occipital horn may be difficult to visualize. As on the coronal section, the periventricular white matter lateral and posterior to the trigones of the lateral ventricles requires careful evaluation. This area should not be brighter than the CP. Angling more lateral to the ventricle, the next scan demonstrates the far lateral periventricular white matter tracts and the echogenic Sylvian fissure. On real-time scanning, the middle cerebral artery (MCA) branches can be seen pulsating within this fissure (Fig. 21-13).[3]

Supplemental Views

Supplemental windows exist to augment the diagnostic accuracy of the neurosonogram. These alternative acoustic windows allow improved access to visualize and detect pathologic

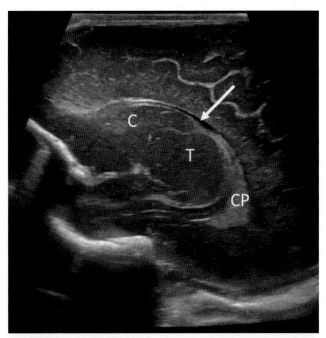

FIGURE 21-11 Lateral ventricle. Parasagittal through the lateral ventricle. The highly echogenic choroid plexus *(CP)* is seen within the body of the lateral ventricle and tapers at the caudothalamic groove *(arrow)*. The caudate nucleus *(C)*, anterior to the thalamus *(T)* is again noted. This is the location of the germinal matrix *(GM)* in premature infants.

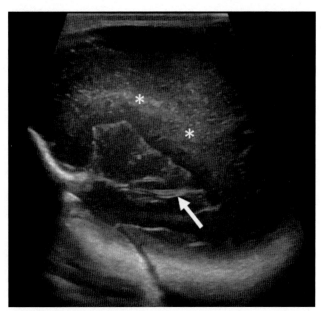

FIGURE 21-13 Sylvian fissure (lateral fissure). Parasagittal scan lateral to the ventricle. The Sylvian fissure *(arrow)* is seen in this image. Pulsations from branches of the middle cerebral artery *(MCA)* can be seen on real-time scanning. Normal periventricular white matter *(asterisks)* lateral to the ventricle.

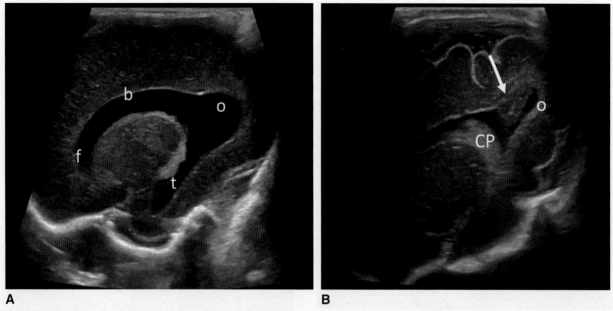

A   **B**

FIGURE 21-14 Posterior fontanelle *(PF)*. **A:** Image taken from the *PF* demonstrates the ventricular system. Frontal horn *(f)*, body *(b)*, temporal horn *(t)*, and occipital horn *(o)*. Compare the occipital horn in images **(A)** and **(B)**. **B:** Note the presence of hypoechoic tissue with a central echogenic sulcus projecting into the medial wall of the occipital horn. This is the calcar avis *(arrow)*. Doppler imaging is useful to differentiate between normal anatomy and hemorrhage. *CP*, choroid plexus.

conditions and structural malformations in the brainstem, cerebellum, and subarachnoid cisterns. The PF provides an enhanced view of the glomus of the CP, its extension into the body and temporal horn of the ventricle. It allows better visualization of the occipital horn, facilitating the detection of intraventricular blood clot from normal structures, like the calcar avis (Fig. 21-14). The MF depicts a superior view of the cerebral peduncles, thalamus, quadrigeminal cistern, cerebellar hemispheres, vermis, and the CM by avoiding the echogenic tentorium (Fig 21-15).

Spectral and Color Doppler Imaging of the Brain

Valuable cerebrovascular hemodynamic information can be gained by adding color, B-flow, power, and spectral Doppler imaging to the exam. Duplex imaging allows the assessment of intracranial anatomy (Fig. 21-16), the patency of arterial and venous structures (Fig. 21-17), blood flow dynamics, and velocity measurements.[4] This is critical when establishing a diagnosis such as increased

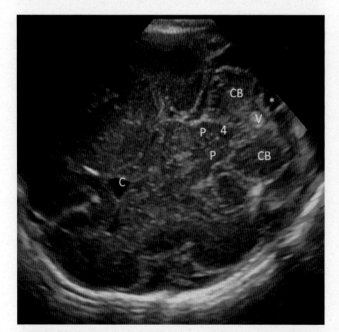

FIGURE 21-15 Posterior fossa. Normal posterior fossa structures obtained via the mastoid fontanelle *(MF)*, depicting a normal fourth ventricle *(4)*, cerebellar hemispheres *(CBs)*, midline vermis *(v)*, cisterna magna *(CM, *)*, cavum *(C)*, cerebral peduncles *(P)*.

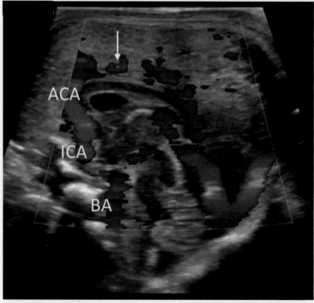

FIGURE 21-16 Color Doppler. Normal sagittal color flow midline image depicting the anterior cerebral artery *(ACA)*, internal carotid artery *(ICA)*, basilar artery *(BA)*, and pericallosal artery *(arrow)* as it courses over the corpus callosum.

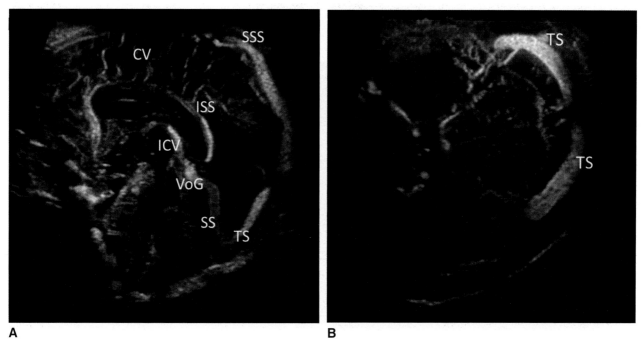

A **B**

FIGURE 21-17 A: B-flow image of veins and (**B**) dural venous sinuses. The dural sinuses drain venous blood via the internal jugular vein. The superior sagittal sinus *(SSS)* also assists with the production of cerebrospinal fluid *(CSF)*. CVs, cortical veins; *EDV*, end diastolic velocity; *ICV*, internal cerebral vein; *ISS*, inferior sagittal sinus; *PSV*, peak systolic velocity; *SS*, straight sinus; *TS*, transverse sinus; *VoG*, vein of Galen.

intracranial pressure, asphyxia, brain injury, and brain death. Doppler may be performed through the anterior fontanelle or transtemporal, through the sphenoid fontanelle (Fig. 21-18). Placing probe 1 cm anterior and superior to the tragus of the ear enables access to the circle of Willis, a ring of vessels that sit at the base of the brain. It is formed anteriorly by the internal cerebral artery (ICA) as it terminates into the MCA, anterior cerebral artery (ACA), and posterior communicating artery (Fig. 21-19) and joins with the vertebrobasilar system, composed of the vertebral and basilar arteries. The role of the circle of Willis is to supply collateral circulation and decrease blood pressure, through pressure equilibrium, in the brain. The MCA provides approximately 80% of blood to the cerebral

hemispheres. The ACA and pericallosal artery are well seen through the anterior fontanelle, whereas the MCA is best evaluated from the transtemporal acoustic window (owing to the parallel angle of insonation). The resistive index (RI) (defined as PSV − EDV / PSV) is influenced by several factors, including peripheral vascular resistance, blood volume, and flow velocity. An increase in diastole will result in a decreased RI, whereas a decrease in diastole will result in an increased RI. Resistive indices decrease from full-term to preterm neonates owing to the maturation of cerebrovascular autoregulation (Table 21-1). Larger cerebral arterial vessels typically yield values between 0.71 and 0.80 in most neonates; resistive indices may also be influenced by a variety of conditions related to hemodynamics (Table 21-2).[2]

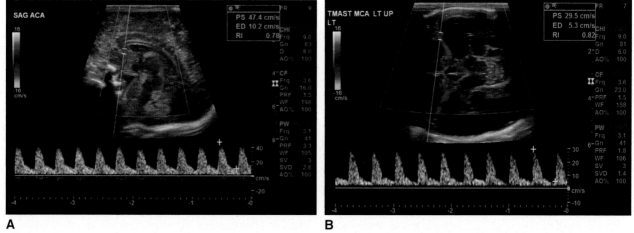

A **B**

FIGURE 21-18 Normal arterial spectral Doppler flow pattern of the anterior cerebral artery *(ACA)* (**A**) and middle cerebral artery *(MCA)* (**B**).

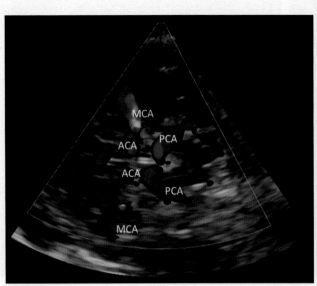
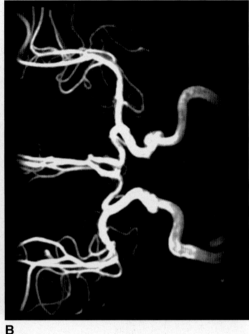

A   **B**

FIGURE 21-19 Transtemporal view of the circle of Willis. **A:** Anterior cerebral artery (*ACA—A1 segment*), middle cerebral artery (*MCA—M1 segment*), posterior cerebral artery (*PCA*). **B:** MR (Magnetic Resonance) angiogram depicting the circle of Willis.

TABLE 21-1	**Normal Arterial Doppler Hemodynamics in the Newborn (ACA)**
Preterm infant	RI 0.5–1.0 (mean 0.78)
Term infant	RI 0.6–0.8 (mean 0.71)
1–24 months	RI 0.6
>24 months	RI 0.43–0.58

ACA, anterior cerebral artery; RI, resistive index.

TABLE 21-2	**Conditions that Influence the Resistive Index**
Increased RI	**Decreased RI**
Hydrocephalus	Luxury perfusion owing to birth asphyxia
Edema	Term infant
Subdural hematoma	
Patent ductus arteriosus	
Congenital heart disease	

RI, resistive index.

Venous drainage of the brain can be assessed by imaging the veins and dural venous sinuses. Superficial veins empty into the SSS and lie on the surface of the cerebral hemispheres. Deep veins, including the internal cerebral vein and vein of Galen (VoG), drain into the straight sinus. Optimization of the Doppler technique is key in obtaining diagnostic information.

Three-Dimensional Sonography

Three-dimensional (3D) sonography has gained acceptance as a component of clinical imaging. Although the early applications of 3D sonography focused on obstetrical, gynecologic, and cardiac applications, this technique is showing promise as an emerging technique in imaging the brain.[5,28] Recent advances in computer technology and improvements in reconstruction software and transducer technology have driven the expansion. 3D imaging capabilities are available on most sonography systems.

Some of the advantages of 3D over two-dimensional (2D) scanning are a decrease in the examination time, less variability among operators, and the capability of viewing anatomy and pathology in an infinite number of scanning planes unattainable through 2D scanning. 3D sonography also provides additional benefits for education and training because the data can be virtually rescanned and manipulated at a workstation long after the exam is completed. A typical 2D neonatal head scan takes approximately 10 to 15 minutes to perform. The time needed for 3D image acquisition is only a few minutes. Rapid acquisition of data reduces the duration of stimulation to the infant and may have the potential of reducing some musculoskeletal injuries suffered by sonographers. The digital data sets are saved and recalled for reconstruction and interpretation at an offline computer. Recent advances in volumetric sonography have enabled the volumetric data to be viewed in tomographic slices (Fig. 21-20) and in multiplanar mode (Fig. 21-21), in which the reconstructed axial plane is comparable to other modalities like computed tomography (CT) and magnetic resonance imaging (MRI). With this technique, a volumetric transducer sweeps through the brain acquiring a volume of images. After capturing the volume data set, the images are sliced into axial, coronal, and sagittal planes.[4]

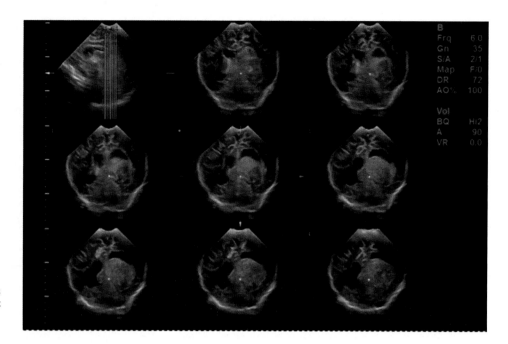

FIGURE 21-20 Tomographic ultrasound imaging *(TUI)*. TUI demonstrates large parenchymal hemorrhage in an ex 24-week infant with *ventriculoperitoneal (VP)* shunt failure.

NORMAL VARIANTS

Sonographic Features of the Mature versus Immature Brain

Sonographically, certain features are markers of prematurity and should not be misinterpreted as abnormal. The premature brain changes significantly in appearance from 26 weeks until term, including development of sulci. Knowing the approximate gestational age of the infant will aid in differentiating age-related features from pathology.

Cavum Septi Pellucidi, Cavum Vergae, and Cavum Veli Interpositi

The cavum septi pellucidi is a CSF-filled space lying between the frontal horns of the lateral ventricles. In very premature infants, a posterior extension of the cavum septi pellucidum, called the cavum vergae, is often seen. On the coronal scan, it can be seen lying between the bodies of the lateral ventricles, and on the midline sagittal scan, it can be seen posterior to the corpus callosum (Fig. 21-22). Closure of this space starts at approximately 6 months of gestation and progresses from the posterior to the anterior. The cavum veli interpositi (Fig. 21-23) is another subcallosal CSF-filled cavity that must be differentiated from a VoG aneurysm. In late-gestation infants, only the anterior cavum septum pellucidum may be appreciated. This fetal structure typically closes by 3 to 6 months after birth, but it may remain open into adulthood in approximately 15% of patients.

Brain Parenchyma

In the very premature infant, the sulci and gyri are not fully developed, and the brain appears quite smooth and featureless (Fig. 21-24). Sulci development begins to appear during the fifth month of gestation. Generally, the sulci are not seen sonographically until about 26 weeks of gestation. Before the age of 24 to 26 weeks of gestation, the area of

the insula is exposed, and the Sylvian fissure is wide open. The sonographic appearance of widely separated Sylvian fissures on the coronal/parasagittal section is a marker of extreme prematurity. As the brain continues to mature, specific sulci become visible. The sulci branch and bend further in the eighth and ninth months with the development of secondary and tertiary sulci.[4] A smooth cortical surface of the brain, with absence of sulcation, may be caused by a malformation of neuronal migration, termed lissencephaly.

Prominent Periventricular Blush

Nearly all premature and some term infants show an increased echogenicity in the parenchymal region around the peritrigonal area of the ventricles. This appearance has been termed the "peritrigonal blush"[7] or the "periventricular halo."[8] When scanning through the anterior fontanelle, the orientation of the normal fiber tracts superior and posterior

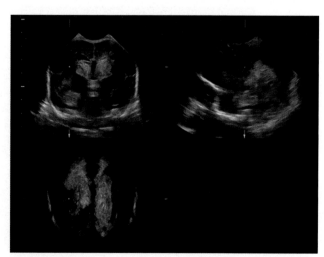

FIGURE 21-21 Multiplane imaging depicts extensive areas of grade IV periventricular hemorrhagic infarction involving bilateral temporal and posterior parietal regions.

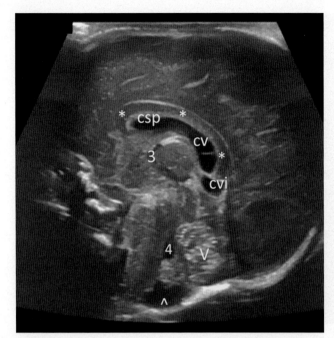

FIGURE 21-22 Cavum vergae and interpositi. Sagittal midline scan of a neonate (ex 23 weeks gestation). The midline cystic cavum septi pellucidi (*csp*), cavum vergae (*cv*), and cavum veli interpositi (*cvi*) are prominent in this preterm infant. Superior to the cavum is the hypoechoic corpus callosum (*asterisk*). The third (*3*) and fourth (*4*) ventricles are seen in this plane with the fourth ventricle seen as a triangular lucency indenting the vermis (*V*). The cisterna magna (*CM, caret*) is visible posterior to the vermis and the midbrain is seen anterior to the fourth ventricle.

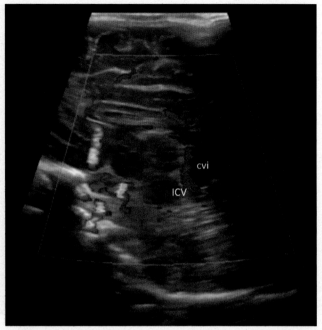

FIGURE 21-23 Cavum veli interpositi (*cvi*). The internal cerebral veins (*ICVs*) are seen coursing inferior to this structure, thereby differentiating it from other cystic lesions such as pineal cyst.

to the peritrigonal area is perpendicular to the interrogating sound beam, thus producing this increased echogenicity. Scanning through the PF (Fig. 21-25) places these fiber tracts more parallel to the beam, and in most cases, the blush disappears (Fig. 21-26). The change in echogenicity of this area from the anterior fontanelle approach to the PF approach is because of the anisotropic effect of scanning. Anisotropy refers to the difference in echogenicity of an organ based on its orientation to the sound beam. This normal finding must be differentiated from the abnormal

increased echogenicity caused by periventricular leukomalacia (PVL). If the increased peritrigonal echogenicity persists on the PF section, follow-up scans are needed to check for the evolution of PVL.

Ventricular Size

Ventricular size also varies with maturity. The ventricles of the preterm infant appear relatively larger than those of a term infant. Narrow slit-like ventricles, particularly in the frontal horn, can be seen in most normal, full-term infants. Slit-like ventricles can also be seen in infants with cerebral edema; however, there are often other associated findings. Some degree of ventricular asymmetry can be seen in 20%

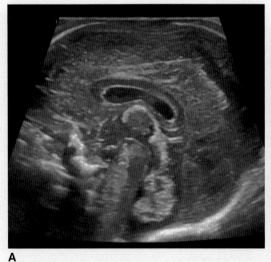

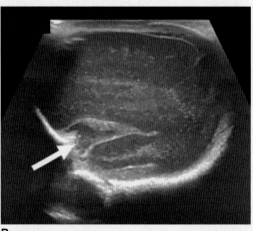

FIGURE 21-24 Maturation patterns. Sagittal (**A**) and parasagittal (**B**) scans of an ex 23-week premature infant. The brain parenchyma is smooth owing to underdeveloped gyri and sulci. Coronal scan behind the foramen of Monro at insular level

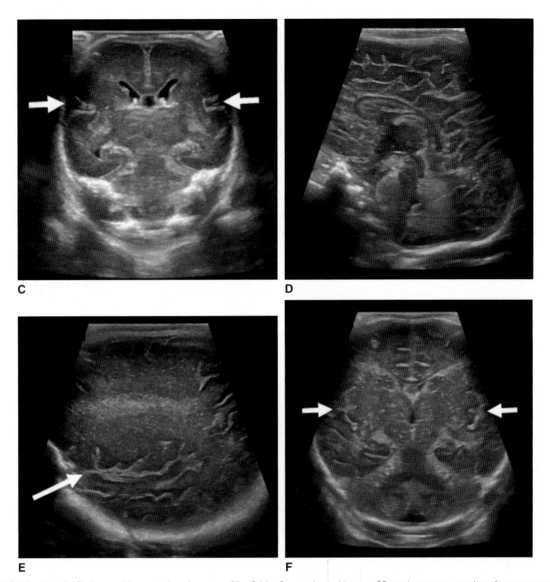

FIGURE 21-24 *(continued)* **(C)** shows wide-open triangular space of the Sylvian fissures *(arrows)* in an ex 22-week neonate, a marker of extreme prematurity (continued). Sagittal **(D)** image of a full-term infant. Note the formation and branching of the gyri and sulci. Parasagittal plane **(E)** and coronal plane **(F)** depict closure of the triangular area of the Sylvian fissure and insula.

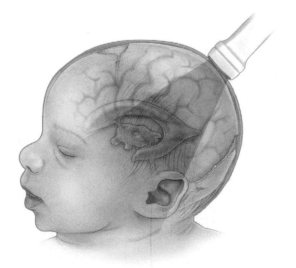

FIGURE 21-25 Posterior approach. Sagittal imaging plane through the posterior fontanelle *(PF)*. Coronal plane is obtained by rotating the transducer 90 degrees.

to 40% of infants with the left ventricle often larger than the right[9] (Fig. 21-27).

Coarctation of the Lateral Ventricle (Connatal Cyst)

Cranial sonograms will occasionally demonstrate cystic areas adjacent to the superolateral angles of the lateral ventricles. Coarctation of the lateral ventricle is an unusual variant that consists of a focal approximation of the ventricle wall at the external angle of the lateral ventricle at the level of the foramen of Monro. These are also known as connatal cysts. Unilateral or bilateral cystic areas located adjacent to the superolateral margins at the external angle of the lateral ventricle are a normal variant and should not be confused with hemorrhage or ischemia (Fig. 21-28). Position of these cystic areas as related to the external angle of the frontal horn of the lateral ventricle is the key in differentiating them from other cystic lesions. Lesions, such as cystic PVL, are located above the external angle, and GM cysts are located below.[9]

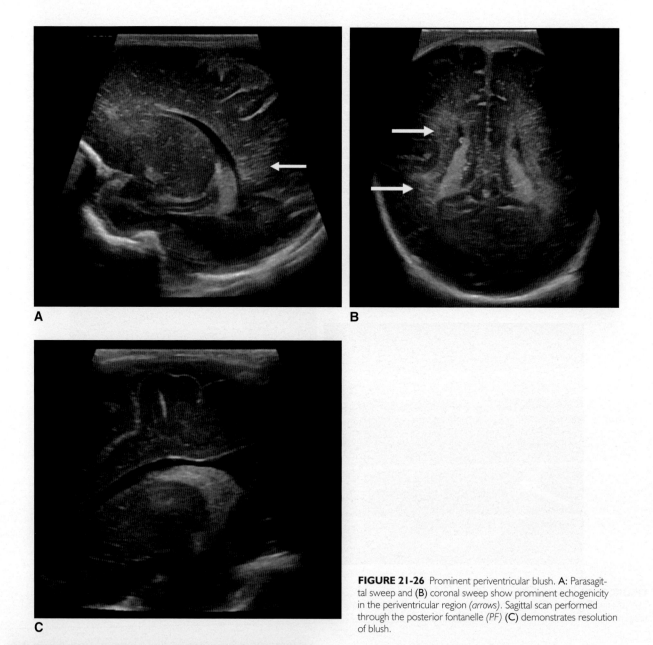

FIGURE 21-26 Prominent periventricular blush. **A:** Parasagittal sweep and **(B)** coronal sweep show prominent echogenicity in the periventricular region *(arrows)*. Sagittal scan performed through the posterior fontanelle *(PF)* **(C)** demonstrates resolution of blush.

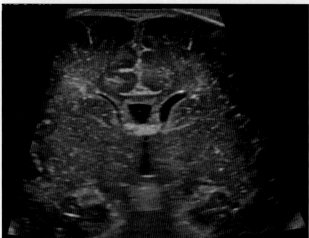

FIGURE 21-27 Ventricular asymmetry (a 2-mm difference is present at the diagonals of the right and left frontal horns at the level of the foramen of Monro). Coronal scan shows the left lateral ventricle larger than the right. This is considered a normal variant.

INTRACRANIAL PATHOLOGIES

Intracranial Hemorrhage

One of the main indications for cranial sonography is to evaluate the premature neonate for ICH. ICH is a major cause of neonatal morbidity and mortality in premature infants. Prognosis varies with the extent and severity of the hemorrhage.

Germinal Matrix Hemorrhage

GM hemorrhage is a complication occurring in the first weeks of life of premature infants. The majority of ICH usually occurs within the first 3 days of life, with about 50% occurring on day 1, 25% on day 2, and 15% on days 3 to 4. By 72 to 96 hours, 80% to 90% of ICH has occurred.[2,10]

Preterm neonates with a birth weight less than 1,500 g and a gestational age of less than 32 weeks have the greatest risk for developing cerebral events, such as ICH. Screening and serial cranial sonography are necessary in this group because ICH can occur without clinical signs. Most bleeds originate in the GM, which is a fetal structure located in

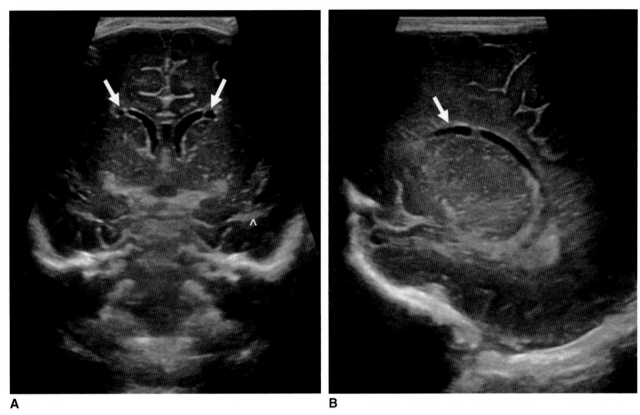

A **B**

FIGURE 21-28 Coarctation of lateral ventricles (connatal cyst). **A:** Coronal. **B:** Sagittal scan shows bilateral cysts *(arrows)* at the external angle of the frontal horns of the lateral ventricles.

the subependymal region of the lateral ventricles. The most prominent portion lies between the head of the caudate nucleus and the thalamus at the caudothalamic groove. The GM is not seen sonographically as a discrete structure; however, it is important to understand its location, development, and the effects of certain physiologic stressors that make it predisposed to hemorrhage.

The GM is a metabolically active, highly vascular network composed of immature fragile blood vessels with poor supporting connective tissues. Between 8 and 28 weeks of gestation, the GM produces neurons and glial cells, which migrate to populate the cerebral cortex during embryologic development. The GM reaches its greatest size at approximately 23 to 24 weeks of gestation. It continues to regress, and involution is usually complete by the 36th week of gestation; therefore, the incidence of GM is low in term infants. Hypoxia (decreased oxygen) predisposes premature infants to the loss of autoregulation of cerebral circulation. Loss of autoregulation allows fluctuations in blood pressure to be transmitted to the cerebral circulation, which leads to hypotension and vascular dilatation. These factors along with the structurally fragile nature of the GM vasculature predispose it to hemorrhage.[3,10]

Classification of Intracranial Hemorrhage

The most widely used classification to grade the severity of ICH is that of Papile and colleagues.[12] ICH is divided into four grades (see Pathology Box 21-1).

Grade I Hemorrhage

The area of the caudothalamic groove is the primary site for hemorrhage in preterm infants. On the parasagittal scan, the

---

PATHOLOGY BOX 21-1
Intracranial Hemorrhage[11]

Grade I	GM (subependymal hemorrhage)
Grade II	Intraventricular hemorrhage without ventricular dilatation
Grade III	Intraventricular hemorrhage with ventricular dilatation
Grade IV	IPH with or without ventricular dilatation

GM, germinal matrix; IPH, intraparenchymal hemorrhage.

CP should taper to a point at the caudothalamic groove. The CP does not extend anterior to the third ventricle into the frontal horns of the lateral ventricles. GM hemorrhage, subependymal hemorrhage (SEH), or grade I hemorrhage appears as a bulbous focal area of increased echogenicity at the inferolateral area of the floor of the frontal horn on the coronal section and anterior to the caudothalamic grove on the parasagittal section. The hemorrhage can be unilateral or bilateral. Over time, the clot evolves and liquefies, creating a cystic center (Fig. 21-29). This grade of hemorrhage is the mildest form of ICH and carries no long-term neurologic sequelae.[3,13]

Grade II Hemorrhage

When GM hemorrhage ruptures through the ependymal lining and enters the ventricular cavity, it is classified as a grade II ICH. Ventricular dilatation is not present in a grade II hemorrhage. Distinguishing hemorrhage from the normal echogenic CP can be quite difficult in a nondilated ventricle. Clot can adhere to the normal choroid, causing it to appear irregular and

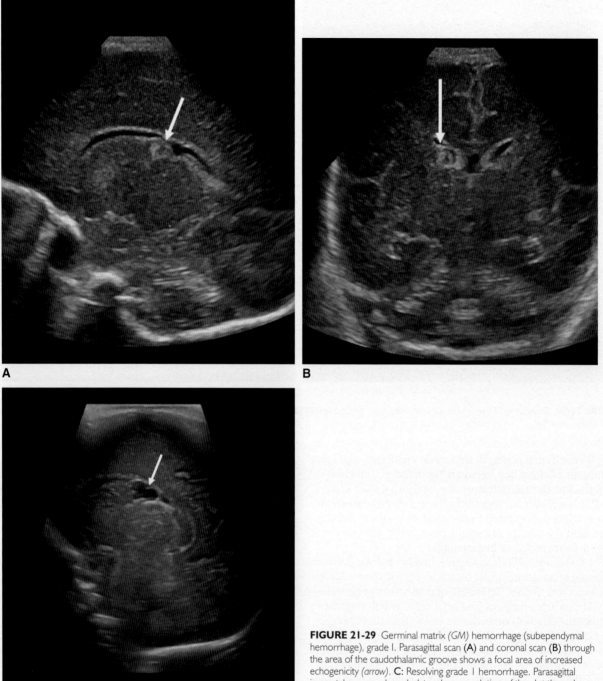

FIGURE 21-29 Germinal matrix *(GM)* hemorrhage (subependymal hemorrhage), grade I. Parasagittal scan **(A)** and coronal scan **(B)** through the area of the caudothalamic groove shows a focal area of increased echogenicity *(arrow)*. **C:** Resolving grade I hemorrhage. Parasagittal image taken several weeks later shows evolution of the clot through liquefaction *(arrow)*.

thickened. Doppler imaging may help in differentiating blood flow in the normal CP from nonvascular clot. Most often, the blood accumulates and migrates to the most dependent part of the ventricle, the occipital horn. Intraventricular echogenicity anterior to the foramen of Monro or in the occipital horn may be the only sign of a grade II hemorrhage. Scanning through the PF can aid in determining the presence or absence of blood in the occipital horns.[14,15] Echogenic material in the occipital horn utilizing the PF section should be suspicious for a grade II hemorrhage (Fig. 21-30).[3,12]

Grade III Hemorrhage

Grade III ICH consists of intraventricular hemorrhage with ventricular dilatation. Initially, hemorrhage may completely fill the lateral ventricular cavity, forming a cast of the ventricle with the contour of the ventricles becoming rounded (Fig. 21-31). Over a period of weeks, the clot begins to resolve and becomes less echogenic owing to internal liquefaction. The clot gradually retracts, and fragmentation may occur, resulting in small segments of clot moving freely within the ventricle. With real-time scanning, the movement of these low-level echoes can be appreciated.

When the third ventricle is dilated, a structure called the massa intermedia (MI) can be seen. It connects the two thalami and crosses the third ventricle and should not be mistaken for a clot (bleed). Often, the lining of the ventricles becomes thickened and echogenic after a bleed because of

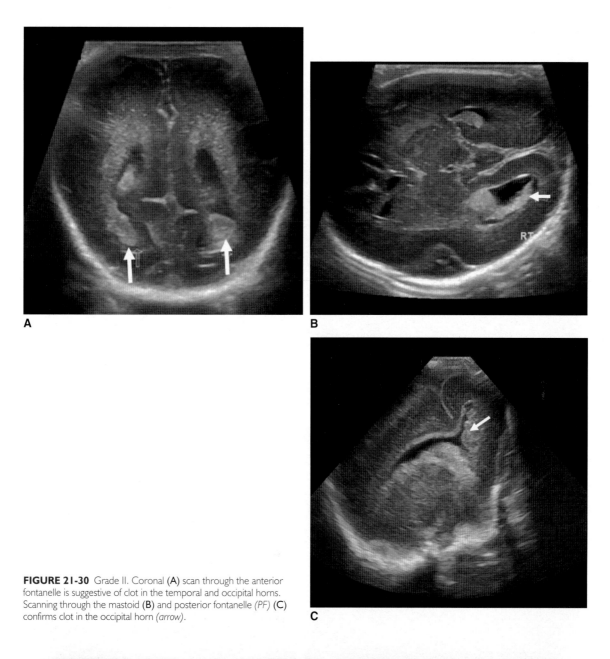

FIGURE 21-30 Grade II. Coronal (**A**) scan through the anterior fontanelle is suggestive of clot in the temporal and occipital horns. Scanning through the mastoid (**B**) and posterior fontanelle *(PF)* (**C**) confirms clot in the occipital horn *(arrow)*.

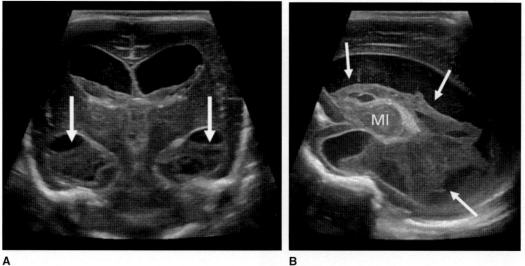

FIGURE 21-31 Grade III. Coronal scan (**A**) shows clot in both lateral ventricles with hydrocephalus *(arrow)*. Parasagittal scan (**B**) demonstrates blood-filled lateral ventricle with clot filling the entire ventricle and forming an echogenic cast of the ventricle *(arrow)*. *MI*, massa intermedia.

irritation from the breakdown of blood products. Posthemorrhagic hydrocephalus (PHH) is often a complication.[3,13] (See the section on Hydrocephalus.)

Grade IV Hemorrhage

Grade IV ICH is characterized by parenchymal involvement with or without ventricular dilatation. Traditionally, this was considered to be because of an extension from a ventricular bleed; however, it is now considered to be the result of a venous infarction secondary to the obstruction of the terminal veins by GM hemorrhage.[9,16] When the draining veins become obstructed, the area they drain becomes congested, and this leads to venous infarction and subsequent hemorrhagic necrosis of the periventricular white matter. Intraparenchymal hemorrhage (IPH) is most common in the frontal and parietal lobes (Fig. 21-32).

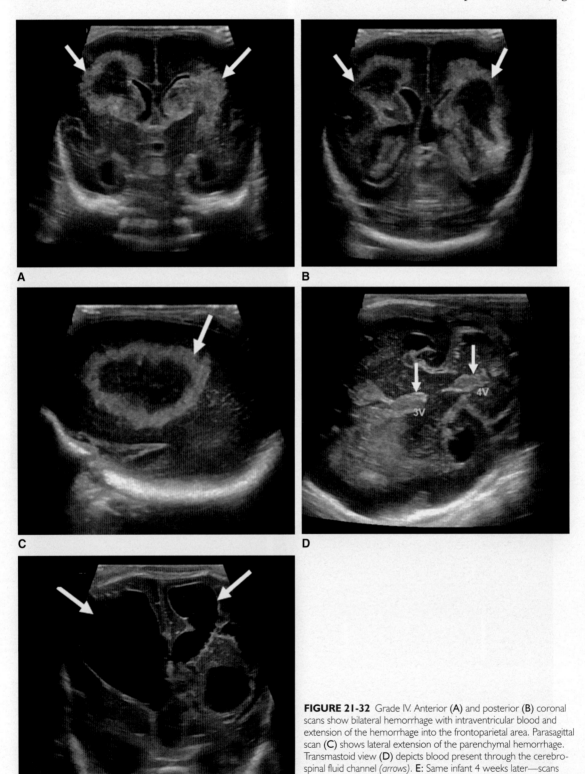

FIGURE 21-32 Grade IV. Anterior (**A**) and posterior (**B**) coronal scans show bilateral hemorrhage with intraventricular blood and extension of the hemorrhage into the frontoparietal area. Parasagittal scan (**C**) shows lateral extension of the parenchymal hemorrhage. Transmastoid view (**D**) depicts blood present through the cerebrospinal fluid channel *(arrows)*. **E:** Same infant 4 weeks later—scans show a large area of porencephaly in the area of the brain involved by the hemorrhagic infarction *(arrows)*. This cystic cavity communicates with the adjacent ventricles.

Over time, the clot demonstrates characteristic evolution with retraction from the surrounding brain parenchyma. An area of porencephaly can develop, which represents resorption of the infarcted area of brain parenchyma. Porencephaly is defined as fluid-filled spaces that have replaced normal brain parenchyma owing to the result of a destructive process. These areas may or may not communicate with the ventricular system. These cysts rarely resolve. Long-term neurologic sequelae include deficits, such as cerebral palsy, developmental delays, and seizures.[3,13]

Hydrocephalus

Hydrocephalus is a progressive dilatation of the ventricular system that is a result of impairment of CSF dynamics or brain parenchymal loss. PHH is a common complication of intraventricular hemorrhage (IVH) and may initially result from an acute increase in ventricular size because of hemorrhage, later by the obstruction of the outflow tracts of the ventricles or by the occlusion of the arachnoid granulations with blood. When these membranes swell, the normally small channels (e.g., foramina of Monro and aqueduct of Sylvius) become blocked.[3]

If the obstruction occurs within the ventricular system, it is referred to as noncommunicating hydrocephalus, whereas if it occurs outside the ventricular system (extraventricular), the term communicating hydrocephalus is applied.[17] The trigones and the occipital horns of the lateral ventricles are initially the first parts of the ventricular system to dilate. A chemical ventriculitis resulting from blood products within the CSF causes thickening and increased echogenicity of the ependymal lining of the ventricular system (Fig. 21-33).

The classic clinical signs of hydrocephalus; increasing head size; bulging of the anterior fontanelle; and separation of the cranial sutures, bradycardia, apnea, and increased intracranial pressure (ICP) often lag behind the onset of ventricular dilatation by days or weeks. For this reason, serial sonograms are often required to monitor the progression of hydrocephalus.

Infants with progressive hydrocephalus and elevated ICP may require the placement of a shunt or ventricular reservoir. Hemodynamic changes in response to fontanelle compression during Doppler sonography can be a useful technique in identifying infants with elevated ICP and in determining optimal timing for shunt placement. This method involves the compression of the anterior fontanelle with the transducer while obtaining a spectral Doppler tracing from the pericallosal branches of the ACA, easily located in the midline sagittal section. The Doppler gate is positioned in the artery, and a spectral tracing is obtained without any fontanelle compression. The fontanelle is then gently compressed with the transducer while another spectral Doppler tracing is obtained. The duration of the pressure should not exceed 3 to 5 seconds. Prolonged or continuous compression should be avoided, and pressure should be discontinued if the infant's heart rate decreases. An RI is obtained from both spectral Doppler tracings. An increase in RI of greater than 0.1 above a baseline measurement or reversal of flow in diastole is an indication of elevated ICP (Fig. 21-34). If reversal of flow is present without compression, this is suggestive of an increase in ICP, and fontanelle compression is not recommended.[18]

Shunt tubes are highly echogenic on the sonogram and can be seen as bright parallel lines if imaged perpendicularly to their long axis (Fig. 21-35). Otherwise, they will appear as echogenic foci with distal shadowing. Sonography is useful in monitoring ventricular size after shunt placement.

Cerebellar Hemorrhage

Detection of hemorrhage within the cerebellum is difficult to visualize from the traditional anterior fontanelle approach. This is primarily because of the poor delineation of the posterior fossa structures from the anterior fontanelle approach. Recent utilization of the MF, as an alternate acoustic window, has improved the visualization of the infratentorial structures of the posterior fossa—especially the cerebellum—and should routinely be incorporated as part of the protocol when performing sonography of the neonatal brain. From the anterior fontanelle approach, the posterior fossa structures lie in the far field of the transducer beam, and many of these structures lie parallel

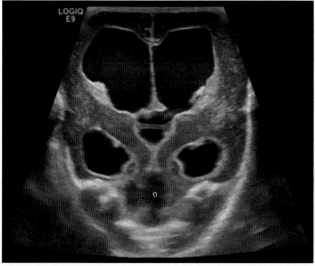
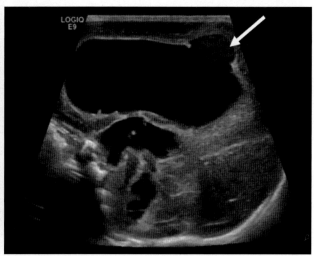

A **B**

FIGURE 21-33 Post-hemorrhagic hydrocephalus. Coronal (**A**) and sagittal (**B**) scans show hemorrhage, hydrocephalus, and an area of porencephaly *(arrow)* with residual clot in the lateral ventricles. The ependymal lining is increased in echogenicity, consistent with ependymitis (chemical ventriculitis).

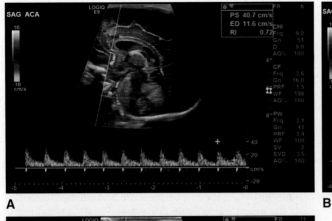

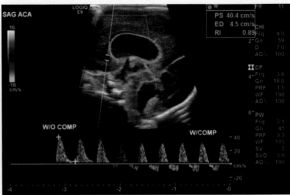

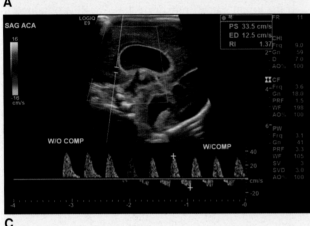

FIGURE 21-34 Spectral Doppler with brief compression of anterior fontanelle. Sagittal midline (**A**) of a normal spectral Doppler signal from a branch of the pericallosal artery demonstrating a normal resistive index (*RI*). Sagittal midline in a neonate with post-hemorrhagic hydrocephalus (**B**) *without* compression shows elevated RI, but with preserved diastole. With brief fontanelle compression (**C**), the waveform demonstrates reversal of flow in diastole, of greater than 17%, indicating elevated intracranial pressure.

to the sound beam. Utilizing the MF places these structures in a more optimal focal zone of the transducer and at a more perpendicular orientation to the sound beam. Also, by utilizing the MF approach, the highly echogenic tentorium can be avoided, thus improving visualization of the cerebellum.[14,19,20]

Mastoid scanning is best performed with the infant's head on the side. The most accessible side should be used, with care taken to indicate on the images which side of the brain is nearest the transducer. Axial and coronal scanning can be performed depending on the desired anatomical information. For the coronal section, the transducer is placed over the MF just behind the pinna of the ear and rotated until the desired structures of the posterior fossa are seen. Orientation of the transducer places the notch toward the top of skull for a coronal section (Fig. 21-36). Four to five images are obtained in this plane, angling from superior to inferior. Images are obtained from the

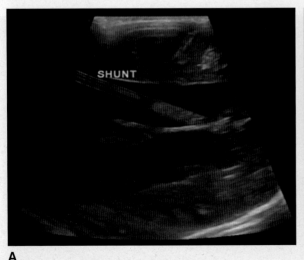

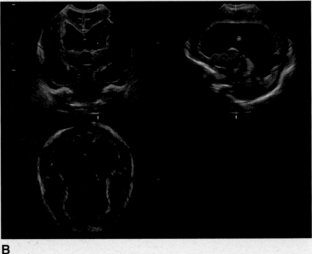

FIGURE 21-35 Transmastoid scan (**A**) shows bright parallel lines from a shunt (*arrow*) in a dilated ventricle. Three-dimensional multiplanar view (**B**) depicts shunt location.

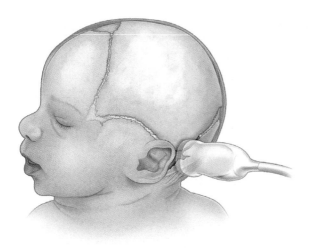

FIGURE 21-36 Mastoid fontanelle *(MF)*. Image shows the placement of transducer over MF.

tentorium cerebelli superiorly through the fourth ventricle, the cerebellar hemispheres, vermis, and CM inferiorly. For an axial section, the transducer is positioned above the tragus of the ear with the notch of the transducer toward the infant's face.

Cerebellar hemorrhage may be clinically silent in presentation and only discovered on a routine cranial sonogram. Cerebellar hemorrhages may or may not be associated with supratentorial hemorrhage (Fig. 21-37). Posterior fossa hemorrhages have also been associated with traumatic delivery and infants on extracorporeal membrane oxygenation (ECMO).[21,22] The MF approach permits a more comprehensive evaluation of the third and fourth ventricles in the presence of hydrocephalus.

Hypoxic–Ischemic Encephalopathy

Hypoxia is the lack of adequate oxygen and ischemia is the lack of adequate blood flow to a region. Hypoxic injury encephalopathy occurs mainly in full-term infants during the neonatal period owing to lack of oxygen supply to the brain. It is one of the most common causes of brain injury and neurologic dysfunction in newborns, posing significant risk for morbidity and mortality. The damage is correlated to the duration of injury, extent of hypoxia, and age of the neonate. Doppler sonography is a critical component to assess brain perfusion. Mild hypoxic–ischemic encephalopathy (HIE) produces decreased RI owing to significant diastolic hyperemia, whereas severe HIE increases cerebral resistivity, effectively decreasing the RI.[24]

Periventricular Leukomalacia

PVL is the most common hypoxic–ischemic brain injury in premature infants. The white matter most affected is the parenchyma adjacent to the region of the peritrigonal area of the posterior lateral ventricles and the frontal cerebral white matter just anterolateral to the frontal horns. In premature infants, the blood flow watershed area is located in the periventricular area and is a zone of end arteries that lack collateral circulation. When blood supply to this area is decreased, ischemia occurs and leukomalacia (softening of white matter) results.[13,17]

Sonographically, acute PVL initially appears as an increase in echogenicity in these areas. PVL is almost always bilateral and symmetric. The echogenicity of these regions should not be greater than that of the CP (Fig. 21-38). Sonography has limited sensitivity in detecting acute PVL because of the difficulty in differentiating it from the normal periventricular blush that is seen in most premature infants. (See the section on Normal Variants.) The later changes of PVL are the formation of cysts in the periventricular area. These findings may only become apparent over a period of weeks after the initial insult. The cystic spaces represent areas of necrosis and cavitation (Fig. 21-39). Neurologic sequelae associated with PVL include cerebral palsy, developmental abnormalities, intellectual impairment, and visual disturbances.

Traumatic Brain Injury, Brain Death

Although the diagnosis of brain death is clinical, Doppler sonography can provide an ancillary component to measure

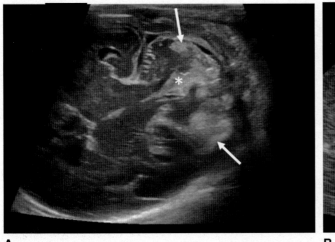
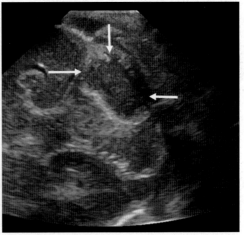

A   **B**

FIGURE 21-37 Cerebellar hemorrhage. **A:** Coronal image shows large echogenic acute hemorrhage within each cerebellar hemisphere *(arrows)* and clot *(asterisk)* in dilated fourth ventricle. **B:** Magnified view of unilateral evolving subacute cerebellar hemorrhage in a preterm neonate *(arrows)*.

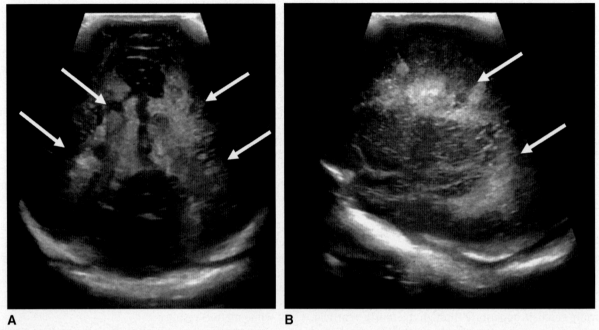

FIGURE 21-38 Periventricular leukomalacia *(PVL)* in a premature infant. **A:** Posterior coronal scan shows symmetrically increased echogenicity *(arrows)* in the periventricular areas bilaterally. **B:** Parasagittal scan shows increased echogenicity at the lateral angles of the ventricle *(arrows)*.

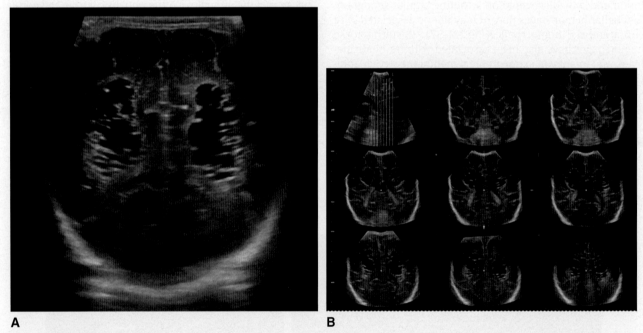

FIGURE 21-39 Periventricular leukomalacia *(PVL)*. Coronal **(A)** and three-dimensional tomographic ultrasound imaging *(TUI)* **(B)** image depicts extensive cystic changes in the parieto-occipital periventricular and subcortical white matter compatible with evolving PVL.

the systolic, diastolic, and mean flow velocities, as well as calculating the pulsatility and RI of the cerebrovascular system. Transcranial Doppler is used to assess intracranial autoregulation and identify vasospasm and is helpful to evaluate neurovascular response to therapy and predict neurologic outcomes in patients with traumatic brain injury (Figs. 21-40 to 21-43).

Intracranial Extra-Axial Collections

Extra-axial fluid collections are a relatively common finding on cranial sonograms and are easily demonstrated as anechoic areas on gray scale imaging. This fluid is usually seen within the interhemispheric fissure and over the convexities of the brain.

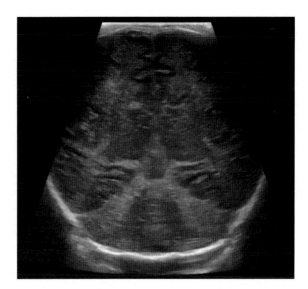

FIGURE 21-40 Full-term female with meconium aspiration. Diffusely heterogeneous patchy appearance of the brain parenchyma with increased echogenicity in the subcortical white and periventricular matter, relatively dark hypoechoic appearance of parasagittal gray matter and increased gray–white differentiation, all findings favor hypoxic–ischemic encephalopathy *(HIE)*.

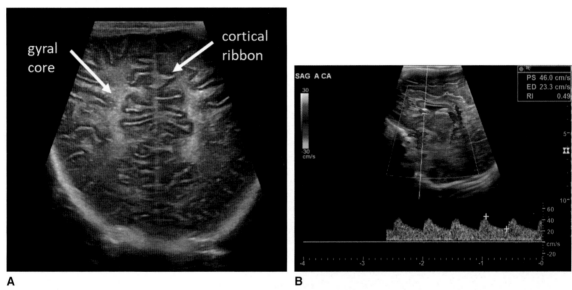

A   **B**

FIGURE 21-41 Coronal image (**A**) of a 42-week-born via stat C-section after failed home birth with slit-like appearance of the lateral ventricles, obliteration of extra-axial spaces, and diffuse increased echogenicity within the periventricular parenchyma and visualized sulci consistent with cerebral edema. Spectral Doppler demonstrates decreased resistive indices related to arterial vasodilation (**B**) in this patient with prolonged asphyxia.

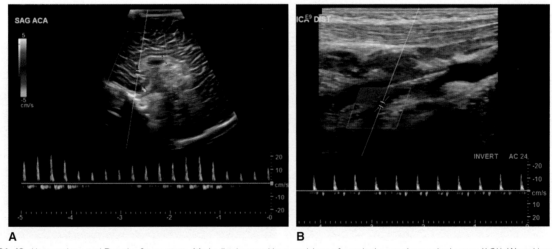

A   **B**

FIGURE 21-42 Abnormal spectral Doppler flow pattern. Markedly abnormal intracranial waveforms in the anterior cerebral artery *(ACA)* (**A**) and internal cerebral artery (**B**) with damped arterial peaks, absent/reverse flow signal in diastole. Findings compatible with brain parenchymal resistance to flow in an infant with traumatic brain injury s/p motor vehicle collision.

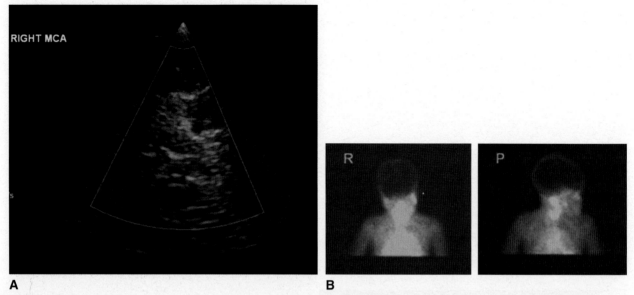

A　**B**

FIGURE 21-43 Anoxic brain injury. Absence of intracranial flow in the middle cerebral artery *(MCA)* **(A)** on ultrasound. Nuclear medicine **(B)** demonstrates unchanged and irreversible cessation of function of the brain and brainstem, consistent with brain death.

Color flow or power Doppler and a high-frequency linear array transducer are used to differentiate subarachnoid from subdural fluid collections. Fluid in the subarachnoid space produces a cortical vein (CV) sign, whereas subdural fluid does not. Superficial cortical blood vessels lie between the pia and arachnoid. Fluid in the subarachnoid space displaces cortical vessels away from the brain surface toward the cranial vault. The CVs can be seen bridging the fluid collection (Fig. 21-44). Fluid in the subdural space displaces cortical vessels toward the brain surface and contains no crossing vessels.[22]

Subarachnoid fluid is commonly seen with benign macrocrania of infancy (Fig. 21-45) and in former premature infants (Fig. 21-46). Measurement should be taken in a coronal plane at the foramen of Monro through the anterior fontanelle.[25] Using a high-frequency transducer, measure the craniocortical, sinocortical, and interhemispheric widths (Table 21-3). The craniocortical width is the distance between the cerebral

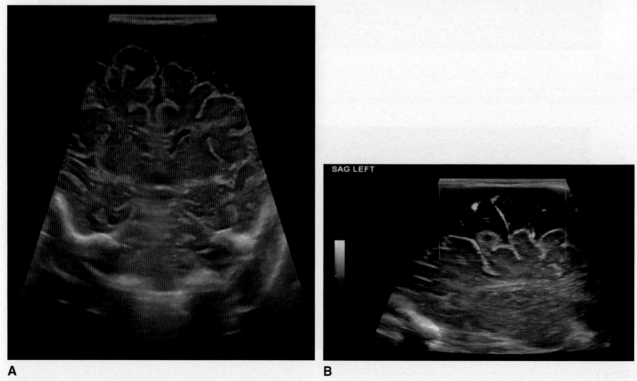

A　**B**

FIGURE 21-44 Moderate to large–volume extra-axial fluid overlying the bilateral cerebral hemispheres with mass effect on the left frontal convexity **(A)**. Traversing vessels are consistent with subarachnoid space location **(B)**.

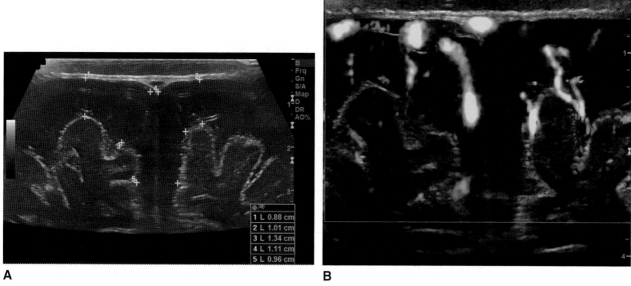

FIGURE 21-45 Enlarged bifrontal extra-axial spaces (**A** and **B**), most suggestive of benign enlargement of the subarachnoid spaces of infancy *(BESSI)*.

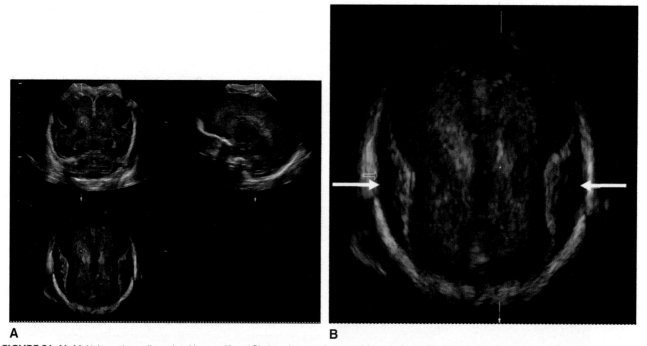

FIGURE 21-46 Multiplanar three-dimensional images (**A** and **B**) show increased extra-axial spaces *(arrows)* in this extreme prematurity neonate.

cortex and calvarium. The sinocortical width is the diagonal distance between the cerebral cortex and the lateral wall of the SSS. The interhemispheric width is measured at the widest distance between the hemispheres. Subdural fluid is usually blood; is related to infection, traumatic delivery (Fig. 21-47); and should be considered in cases of child abuse in the appropriate setting (Fig. 21-48).

TABLE 21-3 Measurements of the Extra-Axial Space[26]	
Craniocortical width	0.3–6.3 mm
Sinocortical width	0.4–3.3. mm
Interhemispheric width	0.5–8.2 mm

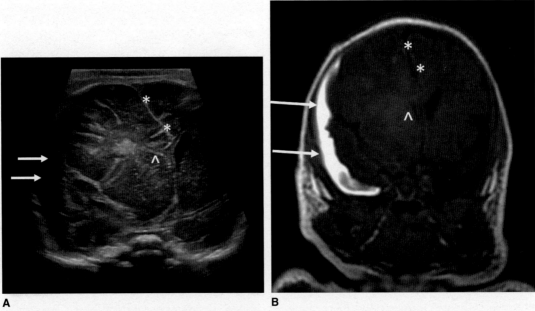

FIGURE 21-47 Subdural hemorrhage on ultrasound *(US)* **(A)** and magnetic resource imaging *(MRI)* **(B)**. Large hypoechoic extra-axial fluid collection consistent with subdural hemorrhage involving the right hemisphere *(arrows)* with significant midline shift *(asterisks)*, effacement of the lateral ventricular system on the right *(caret)*, and mild enlargement of the ventricular system on the left.

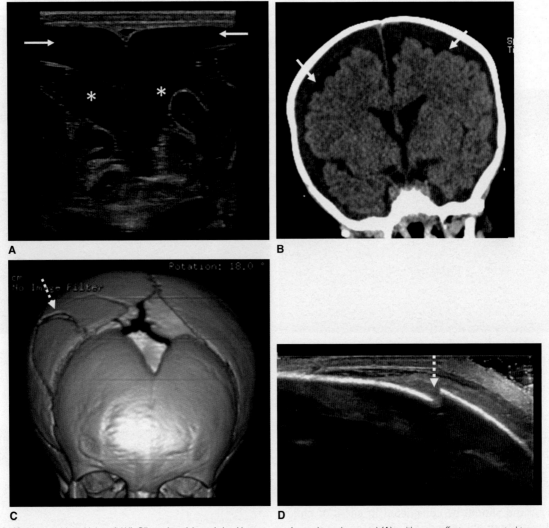

FIGURE 21-48 Non-accidental injury *(NAI)*. Bilateral evolving subdural hematomas *(arrows)* on ultrasound **(A)**, with mass effect on computed tomography *(CT)* **(B)**, and right parietal skull fracture depicted on the three-dimensional CT reformat **(C)** and ultrasound **(D)**. Increased subarachnoid space indicated by *asterisks*.

Extracranial Extra-Axial Fluid Collections (Birth Trauma)

Birth trauma can have several etiologies, ranging from small maternal pelvis, an infant large for gestational age, prolonged labor, abnormal fetal presentation, or instrument-assisted delivery. The main injuries include cephalohematoma, caput succedaneum, and subgaleal hematoma. Cephalohematomas are subperiosteal collections and occur gradually, presenting hours or days after birth. They are limited by the boundaries of the bone, and do not cross suture lines (Fig. 21-49). Cephalohematomas begin to calcify peripherally within the first month and generally resolve by 2 to 3 months of age. Caput succedaneum is a subcutaneous collection of serosanguinous fluid and resolves spontaneously. Subgaleal hemorrhage is an accumulation of blood in the subaponeurotic space—which lies between the epicranial aponeurosis and the periosteum—and is not limited to suture lines (Fig. 21-50). If progressive, these fluctuant masses can cause severe complications such as hypovolemic shock and death.

Agenesis of the Corpus Callosum

The corpus callosum forms during the third and fourth months of fetal life. Complete or partial agenesis is possible and depends on the stage of callosal development when the intrauterine insult occurs. Complete agenesis usually occurs before 12 weeks of gestation. The direction of embryonic

TABLE 21-4 Features of Agenesis of the Corpus Callosum
Widely separated lateral ventricles
Widened interhemispheric fissure
Colpocephaly
Dilated and elevated third ventricle
"Sunburst" sign of sulci and gyri perpendicular to the third ventricle
Dorsal interhemispheric cyst (may or may not be present)

development is from anterior to posterior; therefore, in partial agenesis, the posterior portion is absent. Agenesis of the corpus callosum can occur as an isolated condition or in combination with other cerebral abnormalities, including Chiari II malformation, Dandy–Walker syndrome, holoprosencephaly, and septo-optic dysplasia (also known as de Morsier syndrome)[2] (Table 21-4).

Sonographically, agenesis of the corpus callosum presents as the complete or partial absence of the hypoechoic band usually seen in the midline superior to the third ventricle. The third ventricle may be displaced upward between the separated frontal horns. On the coronal scan, the frontal horns of the lateral ventricles are widely separated and sharply angled laterally, and the occipital horns have a parallel orientation and a teardrop shape. There is relative enlargement of the posterior horns (colpocephaly). Best seen on the midline sagittal image is the radial arrangement of the medial sulci and gyri above the third ventricle, also known as the "sunburst sign" rather than the normal parallel orientation when the corpus callosum is present (Fig. 21-51).

Dandy–Walker Complex

The Dandy–Walker complex is a term used to indicate a spectrum of anomalies of the posterior fossa that include the Dandy–Walker malformation and Dandy–Walker variant. The classic Dandy–Walker malformation is characterized by cystic dilatation of the fourth ventricle, superior elevation of the tentorium, partial or complete absence of the vermis, and small cerebellar hemispheres (Fig. 21-52). Hydrocephalus is present in 80% of cases.[2,27,28]

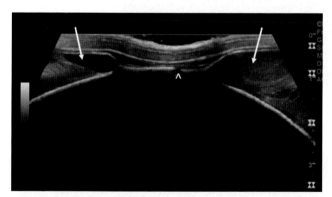

FIGURE 21-49 Cephalohematoma. Large bilateral occipital cephalohematomas *(arrows)*, do not cross suture line *(caret)*, with internal heterogeneity indicative of resorbing blood products

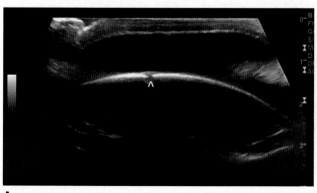

A

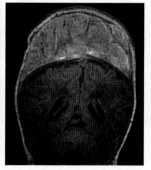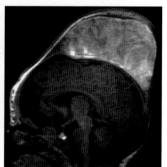

B

FIGURE 21-50 Subgaleal hematoma. Biparietal hypodense subgaleal fluid collection on **(A)** ultrasound and **(B)** magnetic resource imaging *(MRI)*. Note the fluid overlapping and crossing across the suture *(caret)*.

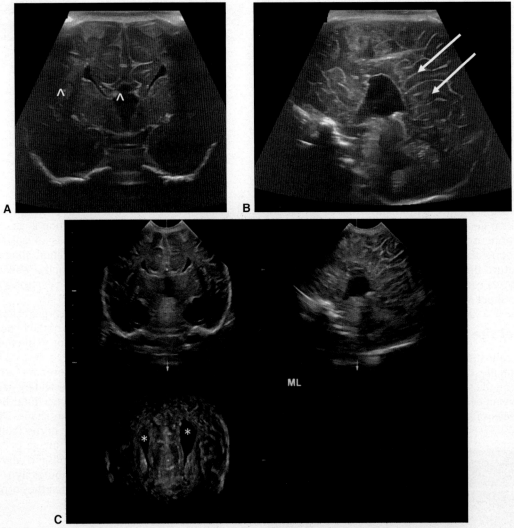

FIGURE 21-51 Agenesis of corpus callosum. Coronal (**A**), sagittal (**B**), and three-dimensional (**C**) imaging depict the absence of the corpus callosum with widely separated frontal horns (*caret*), sunburst sign (*arrows*), associated diffuse ventriculomegaly and colpocephaly (*asterisk*).

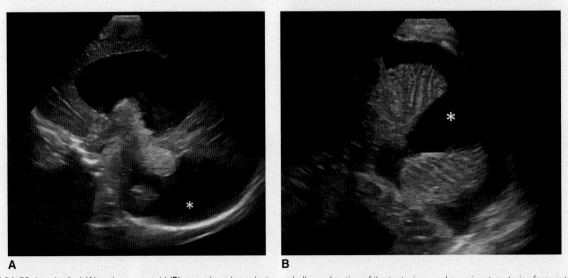

FIGURE 21-52 Longitudinal (**A**) and transmastoid (**B**) scans show hypoplastic cerebellum, elevation of the tentorium, and prominent posterior fossa extra-axial spaces (*asterisk*) consistent with Dandy–Walker malformation.

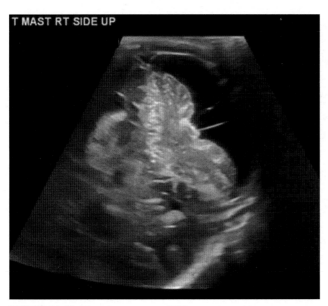

FIGURE 21-53 Mega cisterna magna *(CM)* seen as a prominent retrocerebellar cerebrospinal fluid *(CSF)* containing space with a normal fourth ventricle and normal cerebellum.

Dandy–Walker malformation is frequently associated with other intracranial anomalies. These include partial or complete agenesis of the corpus callosum, holoprosencephaly, and occipital encephalocele. Extracranial anomalies include cystic renal disease as well as chromosomal and cardiac abnormalities. Dandy–Walker variant refers to a milder form of the Dandy–Walker malformation. The fourth ventricle is slightly to moderately enlarged, the cerebellar hemispheres are normal, and there is variable hypoplasia of the cerebellar vermis. Hydrocephalus is usually not present.[2]

A mega CM, arachnoid cyst, and Blake pouch cyst can be confused with a Dandy–Walker cyst. Arachnoid cysts do not communicate with the fourth ventricle. A mega CM (Fig. 21-53) is a normal variant typically seen as prominent retrocerebellar CSF space with a normal vermis, a normal fourth ventricle, and a normal cerebellar hemispheres. Blake pouch cyst is a benign cystic malformation of the posterior fossa characterized by a midline outpouching of the superior medullary velum into the CM that results from failure of the rudimental fourth ventricular tela choroidea to regress during embryogenesis (Table 21-5).

TABLE 21-5 Features of Dandy-Walker Malformation

Enlarged posterior fossa

Dilated fourth ventricle

Elevated tentorium

Small cerebellar hemispheres

Vermian dysgenesis

Chiari Malformation

The Chiari malformation is a complex congenital malformation of the brain involving the hindbrain and has been classified into three main types. Type I is a downward displacement of the cerebellar tonsils without displacement of the fourth ventricle. Chiari II malformation is the most common type seen in infants and neonates and is nearly always associated with myelomeningocele. It is characterized by a relatively small posterior fossa; downward displacement of the cerebellum, medulla, and fourth ventricle into the upper spinal canal; and elongation of the pons and fourth ventricle. Hydrocephalus is present in varying degrees and tends to worsen after repair of the myelomeningocele because CSF can no longer decompress into the spinal defect. These patients are treated with the placement of a ventriculoperitoneal shunt in which the proximal end is placed in the lateral ventricles and the distal end is placed in the peritoneal cavity. Chiari III malformation is rare and is characterized by a high cervical encephalomeningocele containing the medulla, fourth ventricle, and cerebellum.[1,2,29]

Sonographic findings in Chiari II malformation include hydrocephalus with a prominent MI; inferior pointing of the frontal horns of the lateral ventricles referred to as the "bat-wing" appearance; and downward displacement and elongation of the cerebellum and fourth ventricle with loss of visualization of the CM. The posterior fossa is small, and the tentorium appears low and dysplastic (Fig. 21-54). The occipital horns of the lateral ventricles are larger than the frontal horns (colpocephaly), and there is usually a partial or complete absence of the corpus callosum.

Vascular Malformation

The vein of Galen malformation (VGM) is the most common intracranial vascular anomaly presenting in the neonatal period. The VGM is a midline cerebral arteriovenous malformation, which causes dilatation of the VoG. Large arteries from the anterior and posterior cerebral artery (PCA) circulation feed the malformation. These abnormal feeding vessels drain into the VoG, causing it to become markedly enlarged. Most VGMs present during the neonatal period.

Neonates classically present with congestive heart failure and a cranial bruit. Because of shunting of blood into the lower resistive VoG, perfusion of blood to the periphery of the brain can be decreased, causing brain atrophy and calcifications.

Sonographic features include a well-circumscribed anechoic or hypoechoic mass in the midline posterior to the third ventricle. Hydrocephalus may be present. Color Doppler identifies feeding and draining vessels and is helpful in demonstrating turbulent flow within the VoG. Spectral Doppler shows elevated systolic and diastolic flow velocities and damped plasticity (Fig. 21-55).

Although sonography can identify vascular malformations, MRI is required to identify the feeding arteries and draining veins (Fig. 21-56). Angiography remains the definitive examination to identify vascular anatomy more accurately prior to embolization therapy.

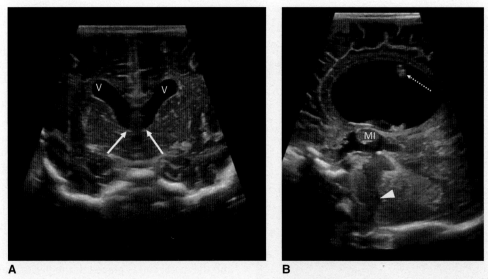

FIGURE 21-54 Chiari malformation. **A:** Coronal sonogram through the anterior fontanelle shows "bat-wing" appearance of the frontal horns of the lateral ventricles *(V)* and inferior pointing of the frontal horns *(arrows)*. **B:** Sagittal scan shows prominent massa intermedia *(MI)*; the posterior fossa is small and low lying, and the cisterna magna *(CM)* is obliterated. The fourth ventricle is flattened and displaced caudally *(arrowhead)*. A ventricular shunt catheter is also present *(dotted arrow)*.

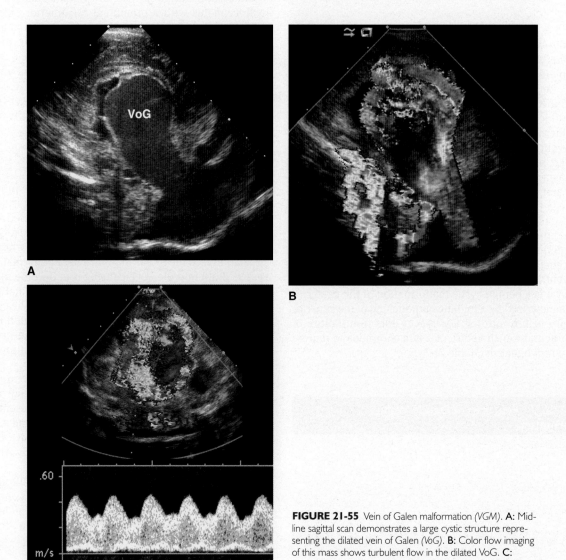

FIGURE 21-55 Vein of Galen malformation *(VGM)*. **A:** Midline sagittal scan demonstrates a large cystic structure representing the dilated vein of Galen *(VoG)*. **B:** Color flow imaging of this mass shows turbulent flow in the dilated VoG. **C:** Coronal scan with spectral Doppler demonstrates increased systolic and diastolic flow velocities.

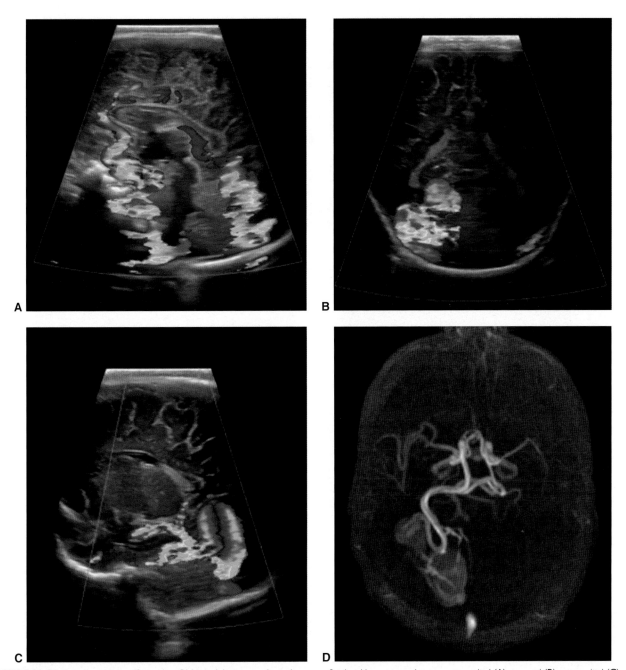

FIGURE 21-56 Arteriovenous malformation. Right occipitotemporal arteriovenous fistula with venous varices seen on sagittal (**A**), coronal (**B**), parasagittal (**C**) ultrasound, and coronal MR venogram (**D**).

Sinus pericranii is an uncommon vascular anomaly in which intracranial dural sinuses communicate with epicranial venous structures through transosseous venous channels (Fig. 21-57).

Holoprosencephaly

Holoprosencephaly represents a spectrum of congenital malformations that result from a disorder of diverticulation in which the primitive forebrain (prosencephalon) fails to divide into two separate cerebral hemispheres. There are three distinct forms of holoprosencephaly depending on the degree of diverticulation: alobar, semilobar, and lobar.

A wide variety of midline craniofacial anomalies is associated with these malformations.[30]

Alobar holoprosencephaly is the most severe form. There is a thin pancake-like primitive cerebrum covering a horseshoe-shaped midline monoventricle. The corpus callosum, third ventricle, and interhemispheric fissures are absent, and the thalami are fused (Fig. 21-58). The optic tracts and olfactory bulbs are also absent. Infants born with this form are usually stillborn or die shortly after birth. Facial anomalies are severe and can include close-set eyes (hypotelorism), cleft lip and/or palate, single central eye (cyclopia), a nose located on the forehead (proboscis), or missing facial features.[2]

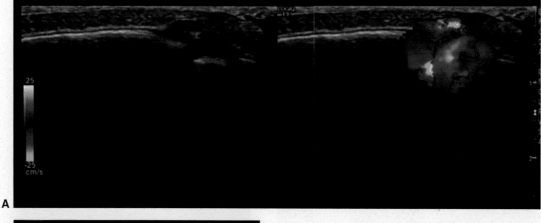

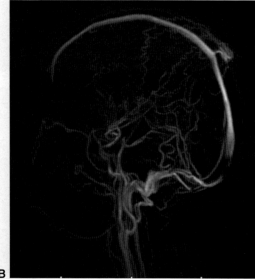

FIGURE 21-57 Pulsatile soft tissue mass in the posterior midline scalp contains extracranial vessels communicating with the intracranial superior sagittal sinus *(SSS)* across the cranial defect, compatible with sinus pericranii, as seen on ultrasound **(A)** and magnetic resource imaging *(MRI)* **(B)**.

Semilobar holoprosencephaly or incomplete forebrain division results in partial separation of the cerebral hemispheres posteriorly; however, a single ventricle persists (Fig. 21-59). The occipital and temporal horns may be formed. A small portion of the falx may be present, along with variable degrees of fusion of the thalami. The third ventricle is small or absent.

The least severe form is lobar holoprosencephaly. Facial anomalies are much milder, and there is nearly complete separation of the hemispheres with the formation of the falx, interhemispheric fissure, third ventricle, and normal posterior fossa (Table 21-6).

Intracranial Infection

The most common neonatal congenital infections are those referred to as the TORCH complex (toxoplasmosis, others, rubella, cytomegalovirus [CMV], and herpes simplex). CMV is the most common, with toxoplasmosis as the second most common. The transmission of congenital infections occurs via the placenta except for herpes simplex virus, which is usually transmitted at the time of birth as a result of contact with lesions in the vagina.

The diagnosis of CNS infections is made clinically, and the role of sonography is to diagnose complications resulting from infections. Parenchymal calcifications and lenticulostriate vasculopathy are sonographic findings that can be seen with neonatal infections. Parenchymal calcifications are the classic sonographic finding and can be seen with or without distal acoustic shadowing and can vary in number and location (Fig. 21-60). Other complications include abscess (Fig. 21-61), infarction, encephalomalacia, and hydrocephalus.[3]

Lenticulostriate vasculopathy is characterized by linear branching of echogenic foci within the basal ganglia and thalamus. These echogenic foci may be unilateral or bilateral and follow the distribution of the lenticulostriate vessels (Fig. 21-62). This finding, however, is not specific for the TORCH infections and can be seen in a wide range of nonspecific clinical conditions: fetal alcohol syndrome, intrauterine cocaine exposure, hypoxic/ischemic conditions, cardiac disease, and chromosomal abnormalities.[24,31]

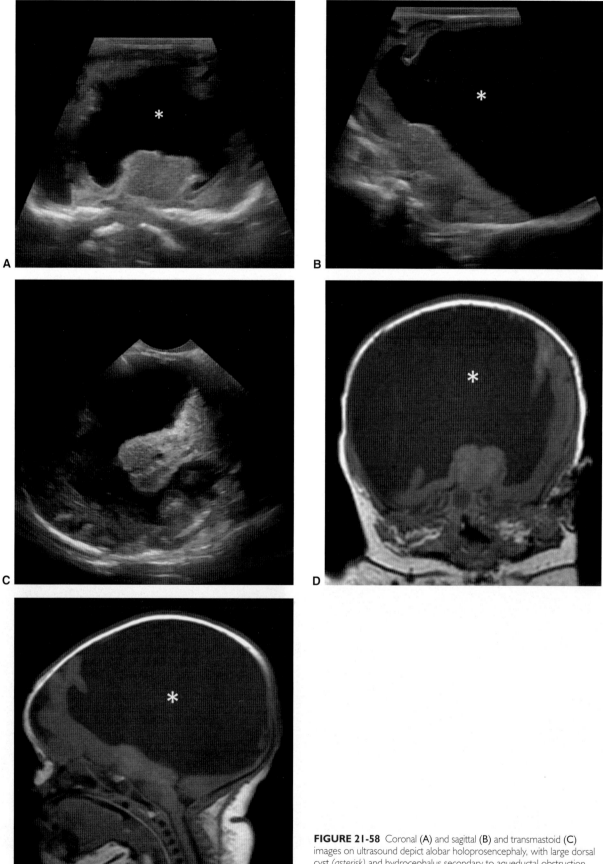

FIGURE 21-58 Coronal (**A**) and sagittal (**B**) and transmastoid (**C**) images on ultrasound depict alobar holoprosencephaly, with large dorsal cyst *(asterisk)* and hydrocephalus secondary to aqueductal obstruction. Coronal (**D**) and sagittal (**E**) MR included for correlation.

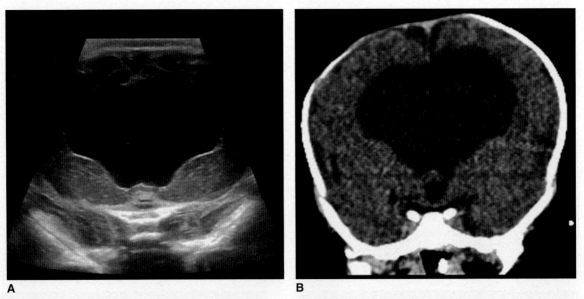

FIGURE 21-59 Semilobar holoprosencephaly. Severe lateral ventriculomegaly with absence of septum pellucidum and corpus callosum on coronal ultrasound (A) and computed tomography (CT) (B), with fusion of the frontal lobes, reflecting semilobar holoprosencephaly.

TABLE 21-6	**Characteristics of Holoprosencephaly**[31]		
Finding	**Alobar (Complete)**	**Semilobar**	**Lobar (Incomplete)**
Ventricles	Holosphere	Frontal segmentation	Frontal horn fusion
Corpus Callosum	Absent	Absent genu	Partial
Cavum Septi Pellucidi	Absent	Absent	Absent
Falx	Absent	Partial	Formed
Thalami	Fused	Partial separation	Separated
Craniofacial anomaly	Severe	Variable	Absent or mild

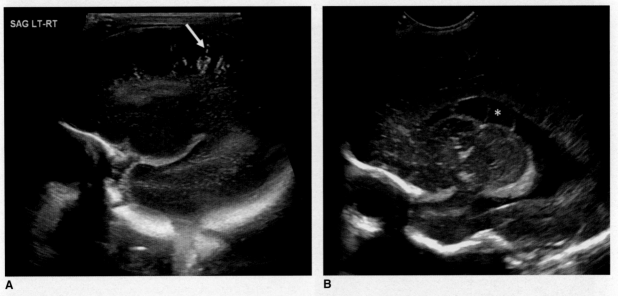

FIGURE 21-60 TORCH. Parasagittal (A) image depicts linear hyperechoic foci (arrow) of vasculopathy along the parietal and occipital lobes. Prominent germino-lytic cysts (asterisk) in the caudothalamic groove (B) with a mixture of cystic somponents and layering blood products with fluid–fluid levels. Findings consistent with provided history of elevated cytomegalovirus (CMV)-specific antibodies.

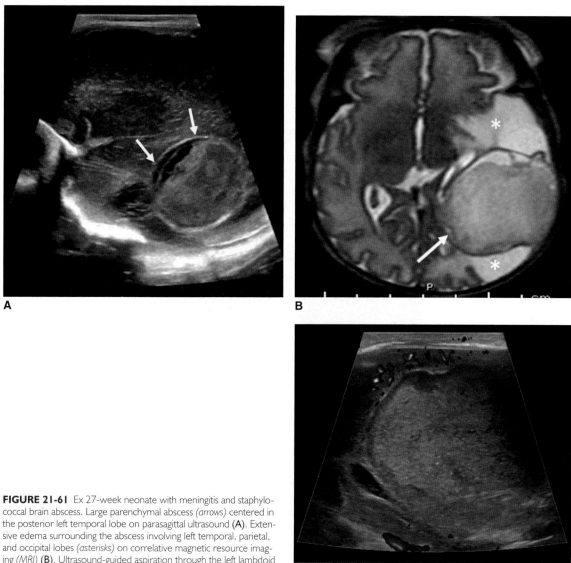

FIGURE 21-61 Ex 27-week neonate with meningitis and staphylococcal brain abscess. Large parenchymal abscess *(arrows)* centered in the posterior left temporal lobe on parasagittal ultrasound (**A**). Extensive edema surrounding the abscess involving left temporal, parietal, and occipital lobes *(asterisks)* on correlative magnetic resource imaging *(MRI)* (**B**). Ultrasound-guided aspiration through the left lambdoid suture (**C**) drained 20 cc of purulent fluid.

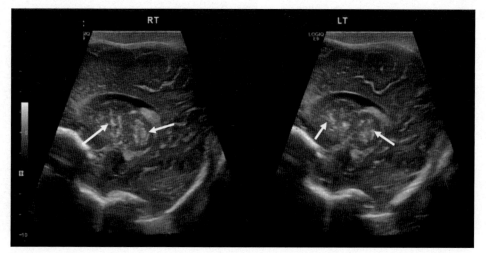

FIGURE 21-62 Lenticulostriate vasculopathy. Parasagittal section shows bilateral branching of echogenic foci in the basal ganglia representing mineralized deposits along the lenticulostriate vessels *(arrows)*.

Neoplasms

The majority of perinatal brain tumors arise in the supratentorial compartment. The most common neoplasm is teratoma, followed by glioma, astrocytoma, and CP papilloma (Fig. 21-63). Although rare, atypical teratoid rhabdoid tumor can also be encountered in patients with genetic syndromes (Fig. 21-64). Infants may present with increased head circumference, seizure, local deficits, and tense or bulging fontanelle. Ultrasound serves an excellent

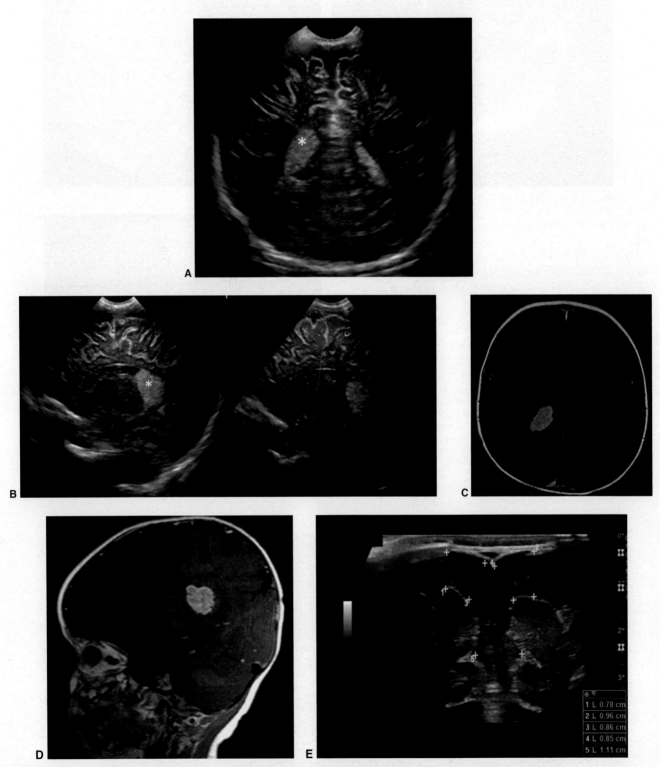

FIGURE 21-63 A 6-month-old infant with macrocephaly. Choroid plexus neoplasm *(asterisk)* centered within the atrium of the right lateral ventricle on coronal **(A)** and sagittal **(B)** ultrasound, and axial **(C)** and sagittal **(D)** magnetic resource imaging *(MRI)*. Prominent extra-axial spaces **(E)**. Pathology confirmed choroid plexus papilloma.

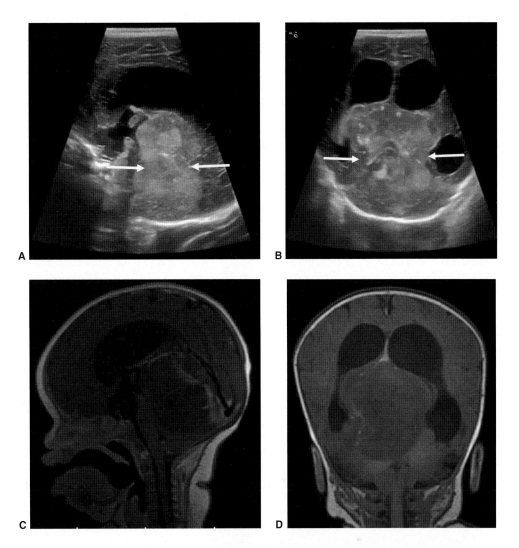

FIGURE 21-64 Sagittal (**A**) and coronal (**B**) screening scan for a 2-month-old infant with macrocephaly. Ultrasound *(US)* reveals hydrocephalus and a large complex mass within the posterior fossa. Sagittal (**C**) and coronal (**D**) MR correlation. Pathology confirms atypical teratoid rhabdoid tumor (WHO grade IV).

first-line tool in screening infants with macrocephaly or tense fontanelle.

Craniosynostosis

Sutures are immovable fibrous bands of tissue that connect the skull bones. When these joints fuse prematurely, normal brain and skull development is altered and pathologic changes occur. Cranial deformation depends on which suture prematurely closed. Sagittal synostosis results in a long and narrow head, termed scaphocephaly. Metopic synostosis, known as trigonocephaly, results in a triangular-shaped forehead and hypotelorism. Bicoronal synostosis is known as brachycephaly and causes a wide and flat head. Lambdoid synostosis, termed posterior plagiocephaly, results in a flattened occiput. Fontanelles serve as landmarks for the study. The probe is placed vertically on the suture line between the adjacent fontanelle and scanned for evidence of ridging (Fig. 21-65). Sonography is a reliable screening tool to assess suture patency in patients with abnormal head shape.

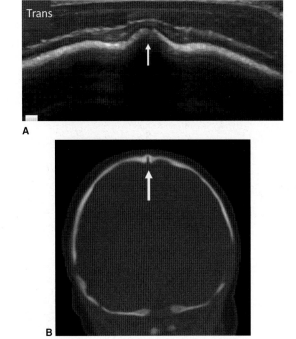

FIGURE 21-65 Craniosynostosis. Sagittal suture demonstrates ridging *(arrow)* on ultrasound (**A**) and computed tomography *(CT)* (**B**).

SUMMARY

- Fluid in the subarachnoid space will displace cortical vessels away from the brain surface toward the cranial vault, and the cortical veins will be seen bridging the fluid collection.
- Fluid in the subdural space displaces cortical vessels toward the brain surface and contains crossing vessels which are not seen.
- Agenesis of the corpus callosum presents sonographically as an absence of the hypoechoic band seen in the midline superior to the third ventricle, which may be displaced upward between the separated frontal horns.
- With agenesis of the corpus callosum, a radial arrangement of the medial sulci and gyri above the third ventricle is seen and referred to as the "sunburst sign."
- The Dandy–Walker complex is a term used to indicate a spectrum of anomalies of the posterior fossa that include the Dandy–Walker malformation and the less severe Dandy–Walker variant.
- The Chiari malformation is a complex congenital malformation of the brain involving the hindbrain.
- The VGM is a midline cerebral arteriovenous malformation, which causes dilatation of the vein of Galen.
- Holoprosencephaly represents a spectrum of congenital malformations in which the primitive forebrain (prosencephalon) fails to divide into two separate cerebral hemispheres.
- Depending on the degree of diverticulation, holoprosencephaly is divided into alobar, semilobar, and lobar varieties.
- TORCH complex (toxoplasmosis, others, rubella, CMV, and herpes simplex) are the most common neonatal congenital infections and present sonographically as parenchymal calcifications.
- Three-dimensional sonography continues to evolve and has the potential to decrease the examination time, improve consistency among sonographers, and provide an infinite number of scan planes from one volume data set.
- With the increasing survival rate of very low–birth weight neonates, sonography will continue to play a major role in the diagnosis, follow-up, and management of intracranial problems in sick neonates.
- The anterior fontanelle is the primary acoustic window used to image the neonatal brain; the PF and MF can also be utilized.
- Closure of the anterior fontanelle begins at about 9 months, making imaging after this time difficult.
- A small-footprint, high-frequency 7- to 10-MHz phased curved array or sector transducer is used to image the neonatal brain; a linear transducer may be used to image the subarachnoid and subdural spaces.
- The brain is divided into the cerebrum, cerebellum, and brain stem.
- The ventricular system provides a pathway for the circulation of CSF and is made up of the paired lateral ventricles and the midline third and fourth ventricles.
- The corpus callosum lies in the midline and contains nerve tracts that allow communication between the right and left hemispheres of the brain.
- A standardized protocol, including coronal and sagittal images, should be used when evaluating the neonatal brain.
- Coronal evaluation should include images from the frontal lobe of the brain to the occipital cortex with the right side of the brain displayed on the left side of the image.
- Sagittal evaluation should include images from the right and left hemispheres and the midline with the anterior aspect of the brain on the left side of the image.
- The sonographic appearance of the premature brain differs from that of the mature brain, and these differences should not be mistaken for pathology.
- Sulci are not seen sonographically until 26 weeks of gestation; therefore, the very premature brain appears smooth.
- An increased area of echogenicity, termed peritrigonal blush, is seen in the parenchymal region around the peritrigonal area of the ventricles in most premature infants.
- Scanning through the PF should cause the blush to disappear; however, if it persists, follow-up scans are needed to check for the evolution of PVL.
- ICHs are classified as grades I to IV based on their severity.
- GM ICH typically occurs within the first 3 days of a premature infant's life, and neonates with a birth weight less than 1,500 g and a gestational age of less than 32 weeks are at the greatest risk.
- Grade I ICHs include GM or SEH.
- Grade II ICHs are intraventricular hemorrhages that occur without ventricular dilatation.
- Grade III ICHs are intraventricular hemorrhages with ventricular dilation.
- Grade IV are the most severe and consist of IPH with or without ventricular dilatation.
- Hydrocephalus is a dilatation of the ventricular system and can be classified as communicating or noncommunicating.
- PVL is the most common hypoxic–ischemic brain injury in premature infants and affects the parenchyma adjacent to the region of the peritrigonal area of the posterior lateral ventricles and the frontal cerebral white matter just anterolateral to the frontal horns.
- Initially, PVL appears sonographically as an increased area of echogenicity; over time, cystic spaces form as a result of necrosis.

REFERENCES

1. Rumack CM, Drose JA. Neonatal and infant imaging. In: Rumack CM, Wilson SR, Charboneau JW, Levine D, eds. *Diagnostic Ultrasound*. Vol 2. 4th ed. Elsevier Mosby; 2011:1558–1636.
2. Siegel MJ, ed. Brain. In: *Pediatric Sonography*. 4th ed. Lippincott Williams & Wilkins; 2011:43–117.
3. Fox TB. Sonography of the neonatal brain. *J Diagn Med Sonogr*. 2009;25:331–348.
4. Riccabona M. Neonatal neurosonography. *Eur J Radiol*. 2014;83(9):1495–1506.
5. Malhoul IR, Eisenstein I, Sujov P, et al. Neonatal lenticulostriate vasculopathy: further characterization. *Arch Dis Child Fetal Neonatal Ed*. 2003;88:F410–F414.
6. Riccabona M, Nelson TR, Weitzer C, Resch B, Pretorius DP. Potential of three-dimensional ultrasound in neonatal and paediatric sonography. *Eur Radiol*. 2003;13:2082–2093.
7. Worthen NJ, Gilbertson V, Lau C. Cortical sulcal development seen on sonography: relationship to gestational parameters. *Ultrasound Med*. 1986;5:153–156.
8. DiPietro MA, Brody BA, Teele RL. Peritrigonal echogenic "blush" on cranial sonography: pathologic correlates. *Am J Roentgenol*. 1986;146:1067–1072.
9. Grant EG, Schellinger D, Richardson JD, Coffey ML, Smirniotopoulous JG. Echogenic preventricular halo: normal sonographic or neonatal cerebral hemorrhage. *Am J Roentgenol*. 1983;140:793–796.
10. Rosenfeld DL, Schonfeld SM, Underberg-Davis S. Coarctation of lateral ventricles: an alternative explanation for subependymal pseudocyst. *Pediatr Radiol*. 1997;27:859–897.
11. Hobar JD, Leahy KA, Lucey JF. Ultrasound identification of lateral ventricular asymmetry in premature infants. *Clin Radiol*. 1983;35:29–31.
12. Bassen H. Intracranial hemorrhage in the preterm infant: understanding it, preventing it. *Clin Perinatol*. 2009;36:737–762.
13. Papile LA, Burstein J, Burstein R, Koffler H. Incidence and evolution of subependymal and intraventricular hemorrhage: a study of infants with birth weights less than 1,500 gm. *J Pediatr*. 1978;92:529–534.
14. Ishak GE. Germinal matrix hemorrhage (GMH). In: Thappa M, Weinberger E, eds. *Pediatric Imaging: A Teaching File*. Lippincott Williams & Wilkins; 2013:166–167.
15. DiSalvo DN. A new view of the neonatal brain: clinical utility of supplemental neurologic US imaging windows. *Radiographics*. 2001;21:943–955.
16. Flavia C, Goya E, Rosselló J, et al. Posterior fontanelle sonography: an acoustic window into the neonatal brain. *Am J Neuroradiol*. 2004;25:1274–1282.
17. Ghazi-Birry HS, Brown WR, Moody DM, Challa VR, Block SM, Reboussin DM. Human germinal matrix: venous origin of hemorrhage and vascular characteristics. *Am J Neuroradiol*. 1997;18:219–229.
18. Benson JE, Bishop MR, Cohen HL. Intracranial neonatal neurosonography: an update. *Ultrasound Q*. 2002;178:89–114.
19. Taylor GA, Madsen JR. Neonatal hydrocephalus: hemodynamic response to fontanelle compression: correlation with intracranial pressure and need for shunt placement. *Pediatr Radiol*. 1996;201:685–689.
20. Enriquez G, Correa F, Enriquez G, et al. Mastoid fontanelle approach for sonographic imaging of the neonatal brain. *Pediatr Radiol*. 2006;36:532–540.
21. Luna JA, Goldstein RB. Sonographic visualization of the neonatal posterior fossa abnormalities through the posteriolateral fontanelle. *Am J Roentgenol*. 2000;174:561–567.
22. Bulas DI, Taylor GA, Fitz CR, Revenis ME, Glass P, Ingram JD. Posterior fossa intracranial hemorrhage in infants treated with extracorporeal membrane oxygenation: sonographic findings. *Am J Roentgenol*. 1991;156:571–575.
23. Merrill JD, Piecuch RE, Fell SC, Barkovich AJ, Goldstein RB. A new pattern of cerebellar hemorrhages in preterm infants. *Pediatrics*. 1998;102:62–66.
24. Coley BD, Rusin JR, Boune DR. Importance of hypoxic/ischemic conditions in the development of cerebral lenticulostriate vasculopathy. *Pediatr Radiol*. 2000;30:846–855.
25. Libicher M, Tröger J. US measurement of the subarachnoid space in infants: normal values. *Radiology*. 1992;184(3):749–751. doi:10.1148/radiology.184.3.1509061
26. Govaert P, de Vries LS. *An Atlas of Neonatal Brain Sonography*. Vol 2. Mac Keith Press; 2010.
27. Chen CY, Chou TY, Zimmerman RA, Lee CC, Chen FH, Faro SH. Pericerebral fluid collection: differentiation of enlarged subarachnoid spaces from subdural collections with color Doppler US. *Radiology*. 1996;201:389–392.
28. Epelman M, Daneman A, Blaser SI, et al. Differential diagnosis of intracranial cystic lesions at head US: correlation with CT and MR imaging. *Radiographics*. 2006;26:173–196.
29. Nixon J, Weinberger E. Dandy Walker malformation (DWM). In: Thappa M, Weinberger E, eds. *Pediatric Imaging: A Teaching File*. Lippincott Williams & Wilkins; 2013:164–165.
30. Ishak GE. Chiari II malformation with lumbosacral myelomeningocele. In: Thappa M, Weinberger E, eds. *Pediatric Imaging: A Teaching File*. Lippincott Williams & Wilkins; 2013:132–133.
31. Ishak GE. Holoprosencephaly. In: Thappa M, Weinberger E, eds. *Pediatric Imaging: A Teaching File*. Lippincott Williams & Wilkins; 2013:136–167.

CHAPTER 22

The Infant Spine

TARA K. CIELMA AND ANJUM N. BANDARKAR

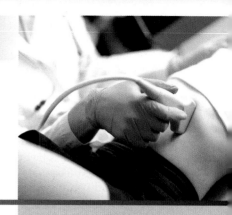

OBJECTIVES

- Describe the embryological development of the spine.
- Define the process for sonographic evaluation of the spine.
- List the clinical indications for sonographic evaluation of the spine.
- Depict the normal sonographic appearance of the neonatal spinal canal and cord.
- Illustrate normal variants that may simulate pathology.
- Describe open and closed spinal dysraphism.
- Identify the sonographic appearance of congenital anomalies of the spine.

GLOSSARY

cauda equina a collection of nerve roots at the end of the spinal column; includes lower lumbar and sacral nerve roots; Latin for horse's tail because of its appearance

central echo complex the echogenic interface of the spinal cord

conus medullaris the most caudal (terminal) portion of the spinal cord

dura outermost layer of the covering of the spinal cord

epidural space space between the outermost layer of the spinal cord, the dura, and the spinal column

filum terminale tapering end of the spinal cord, caudal to the conus medullaris

hydromyelia dilatation of the central canal of the spinal cord

low-lying cord conus ending below the L2 to L3 disk space

myelomalacia softening of the spinal cord frequently caused by a lack of blood supply

simple sacral dimple cutaneous indentation located in the midline, close to the gluteal cleft, without additional stigmata

syrinx fluid-filled cavity in the spinal cord

ventriculus terminalis cerebrospinal fluid-filled, ependyma-lined cavity within the conus medullaris

KEY TERMS

conus medullaris

diastematomyelia

dorsal dermal sinus

filar cyst

lipomyelocele

lipomyelomeningocele

myelocele

myelomeningocele

pilonidal sinus

sacral dimple

spinal lipoma

terminal myelocystocele

tethered cord

ventriculus terminalis

Sonography is a useful first-line imaging tool when evaluating the spinal canal and cord in infants with suspected spinal anomalies. It is expedient and cost-effective, with no known side effects or harmful exposure to radiation. However, owing to the obvious bony nature of the spine, the utility of sonography is generally limited to infants under the age of 6 months. Other potential uses include guidance during interoperative procedures, interventional radiology, and settings in which there is an acoustic window in an older child.

Sonography is possible in infants because the posterior spinous processes are not yet ossified, thus providing an acoustic window. Sonography of the spine becomes increasingly difficult as these bones begin to ossify. Its diagnostic value decreases at 3 months, and it is nearly nondiagnostic after 6 months unless there is delayed ossification or a posterior defect of the vertebral bodies.[1] Sonography can be utilized in the surgical setting through a surgically created acoustic window. Known spinal defects where the posterior spinal elements are missing can also be used as an acoustic window to image the spinal canal.

Clinical indications for spinal sonography include evaluation of spinal dysraphism and any associated mass, including meningoceles, myelomeningoceles (MMCs), lipomyelomeningoceles, and lipomas.[2] Patients with lumbosacral cutaneous stigmata, including pigmented spots, hairy nevus, dermal sinuses, dimples, and hemangiomas, may be evaluated for an associated tethered spinal cord.[3-5] Sonographic evaluation readily detects spinal tumors, masses, cysts, and syrinx. Acquired lesions, such as cord birth trauma, subarachnoid and epidural hemorrhage, and epidural abscess, can also be detected in the infant.[6] Intraoperative use of spinal sonography is helpful to localize intramedullary lesions, including tumors, cysts, hydrosyrinx, and vascular malformations, which may otherwise be difficult to locate by direct visualization of the cord.

SONOGRAPHIC TECHNIQUE

High-frequency linear transducers provide detailed evaluation of the spinal cord and the nerve roots. Linear or sector transducers with frequencies ranging from 8 to 15 MHz are used routinely.[1,7] High-resolution hockey stick probes may be used to evaluate dimples. Sector transducers may be useful in older patients, where the acoustic window is smaller owing to progressive ossification. Dual screen images can extend the field of view to image longer sections of the spine. Panoramic views, which are now readily available on many machines, provide an extended field of view to encompass the length of the spine.[7] Panoramic imaging is especially helpful when determining the level of the conus (Fig. 22-1) and its relationship to the lumbosacral junction.

To evaluate the spine, the patient should be placed in a position such that the acoustic window is optimized. The infant patient may be placed prone over a towel or pillow. This will round out the back, creating a slight kyphosis.[7] A decubitus position can also be helpful because the legs can be tucked up in front of the body, increasing the splaying of the spinous processes.[7] A warm blanket, bottle, or pacifier

can be helpful during this examination because it will help keep the patient still.

The examination should include longitudinal and axial images from the craniocervical junction to the coccyx. The rounded surface of a curvilinear transducer will optimize imaging of the craniocervical junction.[7] For the remainder of the examination, a linear transducer is placed midline, directly over the spine. An exception is made for the older child, where a parasagittal approach may diminish shadowing from the ossified spinous process.[7] The level of the conus medullaris, as well as the position of the spinal cord in the spinal canal, is documented. During the examination, cord and nerve root motion should be detected and noted. Any cutaneous lesion should be documented and evaluated for associated tracts or masses.

NORMAL ANATOMY

The spinal canal and cord can be observed from the base of the skull to the tip of the coccyx. Scanning from a posterior approach, in the sagittal plane, the canal will be anechoic. The echogenic vertebral bodies and hypoechoic intervertebral disks border the length of the spinal canal anteriorly.[7] Posteriorly, the canal is bordered by the hypoechoic spinous processes and the narrow echogenic epidural space. An intense linear echo, representing the arachnoid-dural layer, is seen lining the canal both anteriorly and posteriorly. Between the echogenic dura, the hypoechoic spinal cord is situated centrally to slightly anterior and is surrounded by anechoic cerebrospinal fluid (CSF) of the subarachnoid space[8] (Fig. 22-2A, B). The subarachnoid space or thecal sac extends into the sacral region.

In the sagittal plane, the cord is a hypoechoic, tubular structure bordered by two echogenic, nearly parallel lines anteriorly and posteriorly and by a linear echogenic central canal[8] (Fig. 22-3A). Between 1 and 3 months of age, the cervical, thoracic, and lumbar segments of the spine are 5.3 ± 0.29, 4.4 ± 0.42, and 5.8 ± 0.66, respectively.[8] The spine is larger in the cervical and lumbar regions because of the number of nerves in these areas. The spinal cord tapers to a point and terminates at the conus medullaris between L1 and L2. The conus gives way to the filum terminale, which is surrounded by the echogenic strands of the cauda equina[8] (Fig. 22-3B). The filum terminale can be slightly more echogenic and thicker (≤2 mm) than the surrounding nerve roots.[8,9] The roots of the cauda equina form a collection of less echogenic linear strands that move freely with changes in patient positioning and with crying. The filum terminale and nerve roots extend into the distal portion of the thecal

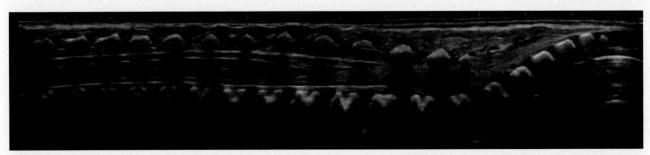

FIGURE 22-1 Extended field-of-view image. This feature enables the sonographer to display the full length of the spine in one image. This image displays the thoracic spine to the sacrum.

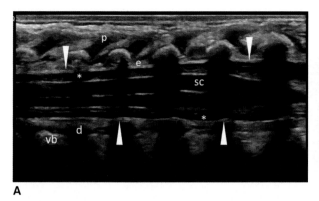
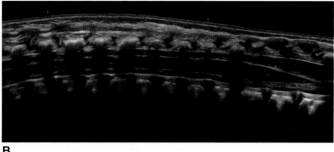

A   B

FIGURE 22-2 Spinal canal. **A:** This image is annotated. The canal is bordered anteriorly by the echogenic vertebral bodies (*vb*) with hypoechoic intervertebral disks (*d*) and posteriorly by the hypoechoic spinous processes (*p*). The canal is surrounded by a thin, brightly echogenic layer that represents the arachnoid/dural layer (*arrowheads*). Just posterior to the arachnoid/dural layer and anterior to the spinous process is the epidural space (*e*). Anechoic cerebrospinal fluid (*asterisk*) encompasses the hypoechoic spinal cord (*sc*) and occupies the subarachnoid space. **B:** Compare this image with the annotated image.

sac. Inferior to the thecal sac, the echogenic vertebral bodies are noted coursing posteriorly toward the skin surface (Fig. 22-3C). Caudal to the sacrum are two to three hypoechoic coccygeal segments. The coccyx is hypoechoic because of its cartilaginous nature (Fig. 22-3D).

In the axial plane, the spinal cord appears as an oval to round hypoechoic structure located within the spinal canal, with an echogenic circumferential border and echogenic dot centrally. The cord is surrounded by CSF, which is contained by the echogenic dura surrounding the canal (Fig. 22-4A). Posteriorly, the spinous process is noted centrally as a small hypoechoic circle. The echogenic vertebral arches are seen posterior and lateral on both sides of the canal. The cord diameter is larger in the cervical region, narrows through the thoracic segment, and then enlarges again near

the conus. As the spinal cord tapers to the conus, the cord diameter diminishes to a small hypoechoic circle. The filum terminale appears as a slightly thicker, round, echogenic, centrally located nerve arising from the tip of the conus (Fig. 22-4B). The nerves of the cauda equina appear as smaller echogenic dots surrounding the conus and filum (Fig. 22-4C). Because of these surrounding nerves, it can be difficult to differentiate the filum from the cauda equina.[8] As the thecal sac tapers distally, the sacral vertebral bodies appear as echogenic round structures in the far field, which gives way to the hypoechoic round cartilaginous bones of the coccyx just below the skin surface.

Ascertaining the exact level of the vertebral column allows determination of normal or abnormal levels of the position of the conus medullaris and exact localization of

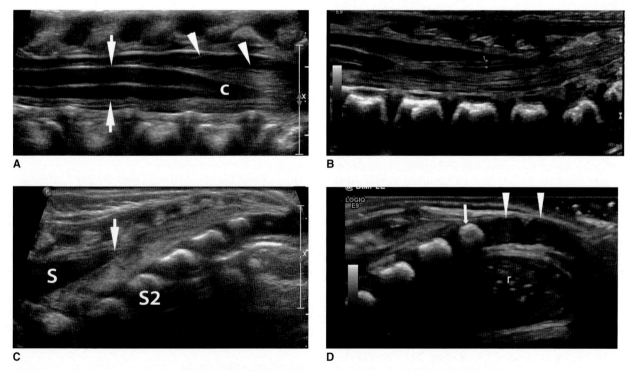

A   B

C   D

FIGURE 22-3 Normal longitudinal spinal cord. **A:** The hypoechoic cord is defined by two parallel echogenic lines anteriorly and posteriorly (*arrows*) with an echogenic central canal. The cord tapers to the conus medullaris (*c*) and echogenic nerve roots are observed extending distally (*arrowheads*). **B:** The echogenic filum terminale (*calipers*) extends from the conus and floats among the echogenic nerve roots in the anechoic cerebrospinal fluid. **C:** The hypoechoic thecal sac (*S*) comes to a point (*arrow*) and terminates at S2. The echogenic sacral vertebral bodies are coursing posterior toward the skin. **D:** The hypoechoic coccyx contains two to three cartilaginous segments, one of which is partially calcified (*arrow*). The air-filled rectum (*R*) is seen anterior to the coccyx.

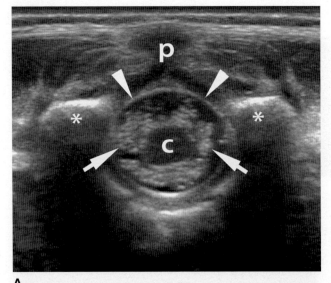

A

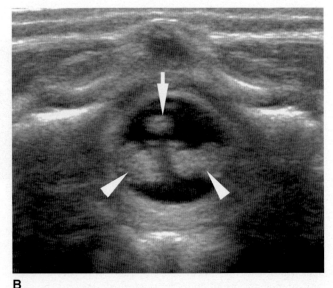

B

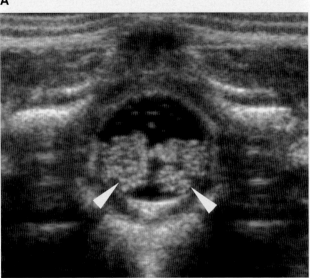

C

FIGURE 22-4 Normal transverse spinal cord. **A:** The hypoechoic spinal cord (c) is surrounded by the echogenic nerve roots of the cauda equina (*arrows*). Cerebrospinal fluid surrounds the cord that is contained by the echogenic dura (*arrowheads*) encompassing the canal. Echogenic vertebral arches (*asterisk*) are noted posterior and laterally joining with the hypoechoic spinous process (*p*) posteriorly. **B:** A slightly more prominent echogenic round filum terminale (*arrow*) floats among echogenic nerve roots (*arrowheads*). **C:** Nerve roots can appear as small echogenic dots (*arrowheads*) or clump together, sometimes obscuring the filum terminale.

intraspinal abnormalities. As stated previously, the spinal cord should terminate between L1 and L2. Determination, however, can be difficult.[10] In the earlier reports of sonography use in the spine, methods used to determine the exact level in the spinal cord included palpation of the end of the lower ribs (said to indicate the level of L2). Another method involves determining the supracristal line by connecting the top of the palpated iliac crest (supposed to transect the L3 to L4 space). A more objective method of determining the level of the conus is to count vertebrae up from the sacrum or down from the thoracolumbar junction. Generally, there are five sacral vertebrae and five lumbar vertebrae. Starting at S5 (the last echogenic structure in the sacrum), count cephalad five vertebrae to the lumbosacral junction (LSJ) (S1/L5) and then five more vertebrae to the thoracolumbar junction (T12/L1) (Fig. 22-5). The count could be confirmed by locating T12 by following the last rib to the junction with the spine and counting lumbar vertebrae caudally. Another way to confirm the level of the conus is to visually identify the LSJ and count upward.[7] The LSJ is identified by the transition from the relatively straight line of the lumbar vertebral bodies to the gentle kyphosis of the sacrum.[10] Because there can be variants in the bony anatomy, if the level of the conus is uncertain, an X-ray may be needed to confirm the level. Using sonographic guidance, a radiopaque marker can be placed on the skin, over the tip of the conus, and an X-ray of the spine obtained.[11] The X-ray will confirm any variant in the bony anatomy and the level of the conus.

Normal Variants

There are a few normal variants that can be discovered during sonography of the spine. These variants are incidental findings and have no significant clinical implications. They should be identified and documented to prevent further unnecessary testing.[11]

Ventriculus Terminalis

The *ventriculus terminalis* is a slight widening of the distal central canal. The dilated area is linear to slightly irregular and is anechoic. The widening is thought to be caused by the

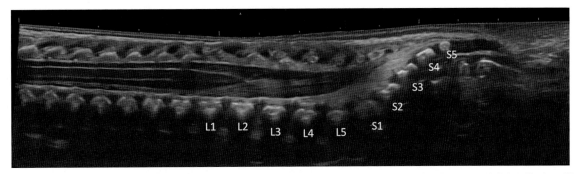

FIGURE 22-5 Counting vertebrae. Utilizing an extended field-of-view image, starting with the fifth sacral vertebral body, count cephalad and backward five vertebrae ending at the first sacral vertebra. Continue counting five more lumbar vertebrae ending at the first lumbar vertebra. Note the gentle curve of the sacral vertebral bodies as it meets the more straight lumbar vertebrae at the lumbosacral junction.

incomplete resolution of the embryonic terminal ventricle and is sometimes referred to as *the fifth ventricle.*[11,12] Typically, it disappears after the first few months of life[7] (Fig. 22-6).

Filar Cyst

A *filar cyst* is an ovoid midline anechoic structure just inferior to the tip of the conus medullaris. It is thought to be an ependyma-lined cyst that develops during embryogenesis. Some consider this the ventriculus terminalis, whereas others define it as the fifth ventricle. This structure is 8 to

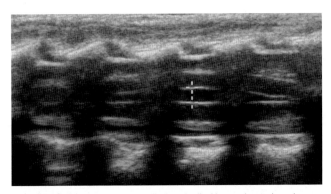

FIGURE 22-6 Ventriculus terminalis. Longitudinal image shows the echogenic walls of the central canal are slightly separated by anechoic fluid near the conus (*cursors*). Note that the central canal widening is confined to the distal cord and does not extend cranially into the thoracic spinal cord.

10 mm long and 2 to 4 mm in the transverse diameter[7,8,11] (Fig. 22-7).

CONGENITAL ANOMALIES

Spinal dysraphism refers to an array of spinal abnormalities caused by inadequate or improper fusion of the neural tube (NT) early in fetal life.[13] The incidence of spinal dysraphism is 0.5 to 0.8 per case per 1,000 births.[13] Most commonly, the defect occurs in the lower spine, although any part of the spine may be affected. The spectrum of spinal dysraphism can be categorized into two major groups. An *Open spinal dysraphism* (OSD) is characterized by neural tissue exposed without skin covering. A *closed spinal dysraphism* (CSD) is a skin-covered spinal abnormality. Owing to the obvious defect, open dysraphisms, like myeloceles and MMCs, are easily classified.

The second group, closed dysraphisms, can present with a skin-covered subcutaneous mass or various cutaneous markers. CSDs presenting with a subcutaneous mass include lipomyelocele/lipomyelomeningocele and myelocystocele. Closed dysraphisms without a subcutaneous mass-like tethered cord, spinal lipoma, diastematomyelia, or a dorsal dermal sinus (DDS) can present with various cutaneous markers that can indicate an underlying abnormality. These cutaneous markers are typically located in the midline lumbosacral region and include hair tufts, sacral dimples or pits,

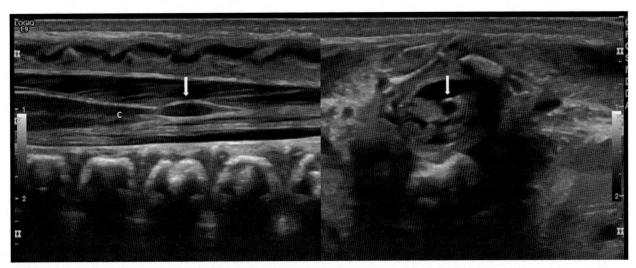

FIGURE 22-7 Filar cyst. A longitudinal view of the conus and nerve roots demonstrates a small anechoic fluid collection (*arrow*) among the nerve roots just inferior to the conus medullaris (*c*).

pigment changes, hemangiomas, and skin tags.[14–17] Nearly all of the previously mentioned anomalies are associated with a tethered cord (Fig. 22-8A–C).

Embryology

A brief summary of embryogenesis can provide some understanding as to why these anomalies occur. Development of the NT begins early in fetal life and is completed around the eighth week of gestation.[1,7] The NT (which becomes the spinal cord) starts as a flat plate comprised of a single layer of ectodermal cells.[7,18] Skin and nerve tissue will differentiate from the single ectodermal layer.[18] The neural plate begins to fold in the center, creating two opposing ridges. As the fold deepens, the ridges come together and fuse, forming a tube starting in the middle and extending superiorly and inferiorly.[7] During the fusion, the ectoderm separates from the NT. Mesenchymal cells separate from the ectoderm to become the bony spine, meninges, and muscle.[1] Because the fusion of the NT and separation of the ectodermal and mesenchymal layers occur simultaneously, any disruption in the process can lead to spinal abnormalities.[7]

Open Spinal Dysraphism

Myelocele/Myelomeningocele

Myeloceles and MMCs represent two forms of spinal dysraphism in which there is a failure of the spinal cord to fold into an NT with a herniation of the leptomeninges through a defect in the dura matter. The NT persists as a flat plate. This occurs in 2 out of every 1,000 births.[8] A myelocele presents as a flat plate of neural tissue flush with the skin surface (Fig. 22-9A). The neural plate, of the more common MMC, is elevated above the skin surface owing to an enlarged underlying subarachnoid space[16] (Fig. 22-9B). The developmental process stopped in the area of the defect because the NT did not fuse.[8] The ectoderm failed to separate from the NT and the mesenchymal cells did not migrate to form the bones. The skin, paraspinal musculature, and bony vertebral arches overlying the defect are attached and splayed lateral to the defect. The spinal cord is tethered at the level of the abnormality. Because the pathology is visible

and the risk of infection is high, preoperative evaluation is not necessary.[16] Some of the problems these patients will encounter are decreased lower limb function to paralysis, bladder and bowel dysfunction, and hydrocephalus.[16]

In patients with MMC and myelocele, sonography displays absent spinous processes in the midline, the laminae are everted anteriorly, and the paraspinal musculature rotates anteriorly with the laminae.[19] The *myelocele* or *MMC* is a fluid-containing anechoic mass that is continuous with the spinal canal through the defect in the spine (Fig. 22-9C). The spinal cord is low in position and may extend over the entire length of the canal, never tapering into the conus, and terminate into the dorsal plate of neural tissue. The fluid-filled sac may contain fibrous septa that may be difficult to distinguish from nerve roots. Real-time evaluation will be helpful in that nerve roots demonstrate arterial-like pulsations, provided that the tension from the tethered cord is not so great as to completely dampen these pulsations. Postoperatively, a sac-like enlargement of the subarachnoid space is often seen (Fig. 22-9D). Owing to the bony defect, sonographic evaluation may be useful to diagnose any associated abnormality such as lipoma, hydromyelia, and retethering. Associated lipomas will appear as echogenic masses that may be situated between the cord and the posterior defect or into which the cord may insert. Concurrent hydromyelia will be manifested by a centrally positioned anechoic collection within the spinal cord that will displace the cord peripherally. The hydromyelia may be focal, or it may extend over the entire length of the cord.

Closed Spinal Dysraphism

Tethered Cord

A *tethered cord* is a low-lying cord with a thickened filum terminale. It is almost always associated with dysraphic spinal anomalies. Physically, a tethered cord as well as dysraphic states can present with a wide range of symptoms. OSDs and CSDs can cause decreased lower limb, bowel, and urinary function.[20,21] Tethered cord symptoms are similar but may present later as a child grows and the spinal cord is pulled tight, causing neurological symptoms.[8,20] For this

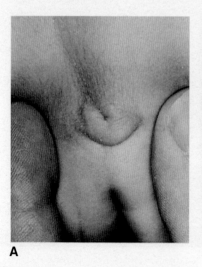
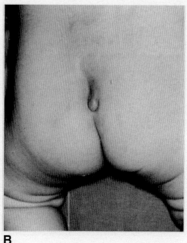
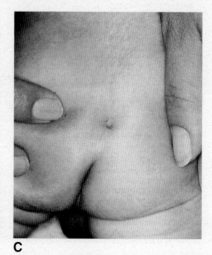

A   **B**   **C**

FIGURE 22-8 Closed spinal dysraphisms present with various cutaneous markers. **A:** Clinical appearance of a skin-covered subcutaneous mass. **B:** Depicts a midline pit over the lumbar spine and a skin tag. **C:** Depicts a deep sacral pit.

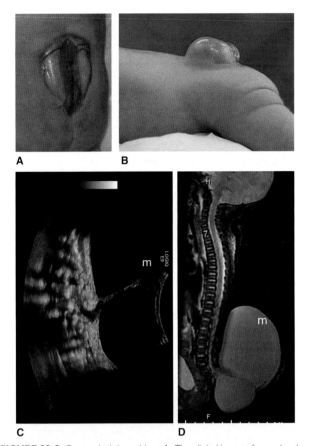

FIGURE 22-9 Open spinal dysraphism. **A:** The clinical image of a myelocele demonstrates the midline open, flat neural plate and tissues flush with the skin. **B:** The clinical image of a myelomeningocele demonstrates the neural plate elevated above the skin surface owing to an enlarged underlying subarachnoid space. **C:** Large multilobulated cystic mass with thick septation and communication with the central canal consistent with myelomeningocele (*m*). **D:** Large myelomeningocele (*m*) at the S2 level. Spinal cord terminates in a neural placode along the dorsal surface of the MMC.

reason, early detection can decrease nerve damage because the cord is surgically released before it is pulled tight and damaged. Clinically, aside from obvious lumbar masses, any abnormal markings over the midline spine should be investigated for possible spinal anomalies. As mentioned previously, hair tufts, vascular malformations, deep dimples, skin tags, and deep clefts, especially in the lumbar region or higher, are highly suspicious for a spinal abnormality. Also, patients with anal or urogenital malformations or VACTERL (vertebral defects, anal or duodenal atresia, cardiac defects, tracheoesophageal fistula, renal anomalies, and limb malformations) syndrome have a high association with tethered cord.[17,20,21]

Sonographically, the spinal cord is low in position (Fig. 22-10A). The conus is considered abnormally low at or below the L3 vertebral level.[5,11] The spinal cord will be pulled dorsally. The conus will be abnormally elongated and may lack the normal tapering (Fig. 22-10B).[1,11] The cord and nerve roots will also have decreased motion. Instead of floating freely in the CSF, the nerve roots will be floating more dorsally and lack normal movement. The filum terminale, if not associated with a dysraphic mass, may be abnormally thick (>2 mm) or fatty[5] (Fig. 22-10C). A fatty filum can also be an incidental finding and is known as *tight filum terminale syndrome.* The abnormally thick filum gets tethered in the distal canal, which may or may not cause symptoms.[9]

Diastomyelia

Diastomyelia is the separation of the spinal cord into two hemicords.[4,16] The split cord can be separated by a bony or fibrous septum, which can make imaging difficult.[16] This defect most commonly occurs in the thoracolumbar region and is usually associated with a cutaneous marker in the region of the defect.[4,9] The two hemicords reunite to form a single distal cord in the majority of cases. It is associated

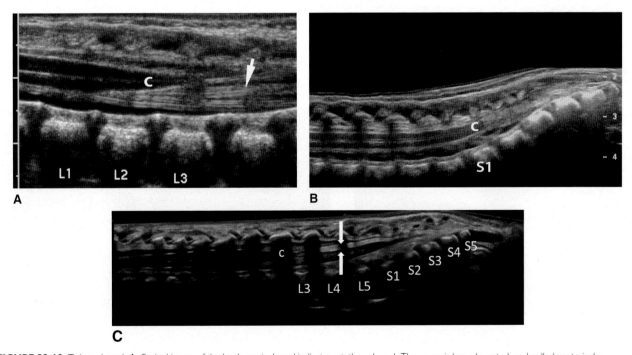

FIGURE 22-10 Tethered cord. **A:** Sagittal image of the lumbar spinal cord indicates a tethered cord. The conus is low, elongated, and pulled posteriorly. The nerve roots are also pulled more posteriorly (*arrow*). **B:** The extended field-of-view image of the lumbosacral spine demonstrates an extremely low conus and dorsally displaced spinal cord. The conus (*c*) ends at S1. **C:** Longitudinal image of a fatty filum (*arrows*) with a conus ending at L2–L3.

with tethered cord, scoliosis, clubfoot, vertebral anomalies, and dilatation of the central canal (hydromelia).[4,8,9]

Sonographic diagnosis is made in the axial plane with demonstration of two hemicords, each with its own central echo complex[4,8] (Fig. 22-11A–D). Evaluation in the sagittal plane will fail to detect its presence because the hemicords will not be visible simultaneously. The septum separating the hemicords may cause an acoustic barrier, making diagnosis difficult. Associated severe scoliosis can also limit the sonographic window.

Dorsal Dermal Sinus

The DDS is a thin, epithelial-lined tract that passes from the skin toward the spinal canal.[16,19,22] Dermal sinuses represent a very focal disruption in the development or fusion of the spinal canal. They are most common in the lumbosacral region; however, they can occur in any region of the spine. Clinically, they manifest as deep midline dimples or pits. They should not be confused with a sacral dimple located in the gluteal fold.[16] Patients are at risk of developing meningitis because of the open tract to the spinal canal.[14,23]

Sonographically, a dermal sinus appears as a midline opening/defect that leads to the deep tract of the sinus. Appearance may vary depending on the width of the lumen.

The sinus tract may appear as a single echogenic band if the lumen is very narrow or as a triple tract with two parallel lines of echogenicity with a central hypoechoic space if the lumen is large enough to be visualized (Fig. 22-12A, B). It is frequently difficult, if not impossible, to trace the sinus into the canal itself. If the spinal cord is low in position, tethering from an intraspinal extension of the sinus can be suspected. In addition, an abnormal focus of echogenicity within the canal suggests an associated dermoid.

Sacral Dimple/Pilonidal Sinus

The *sacral dimple* or *pit* is the most common reason an infant is referred for spinal sonography. This skin anomaly, which quite possibly is a normal variant, is located within the gluteal fold less than 2.5 mm from the anus.[5,7,14] The dimple can be blind ending or associated with a pilonidal sinus/tract that extends to the coccyx. Sonographically, sacral dimples appear as an indentation or a pit in the skin that leads to a hyperechoic or hypoechoic tract (Fig. 22-13). If there is an associated pilonidal cyst, the sinus will widen deeply into a fluid collection. Again, the pilonidal sinus should not be confused with a DDS because it has no connection to the normal spine. Pilonidal sinus tracts communicate with the exterior and often contain fluid and hair particles. Hairs

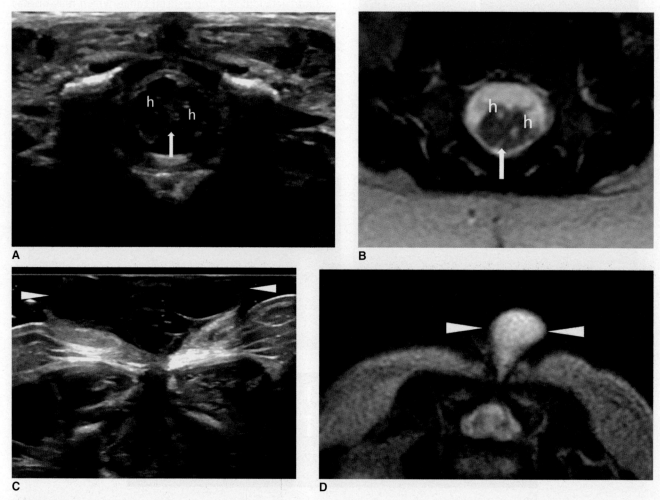

FIGURE 22-11 Diastematomyelia. **A:** The transverse spinal cord image on ultrasound and magnetic resonance imaging (*MRI*) (**B**) demonstrates two hemicords (*h*), each with its own central echo complex, separated by a fibrous septum (*arrow*). **C:** One hemicord terminates in a meningocele (*arrowheads*) on the sonogram and MRI image (**D**).

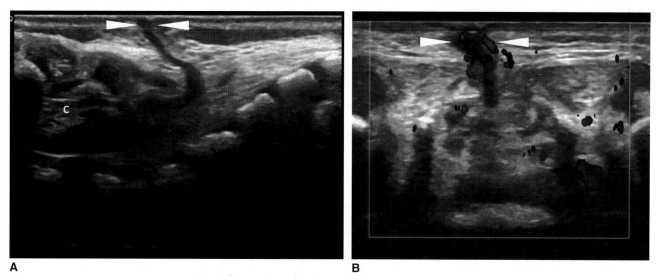

A **B**

FIGURE 22-12 Dorsal dermal sinus. **A:** The longitudinal extended field-of-view image displays a hypoechoic tract (*arrowheads*) extending from the skin to the spinal canal and terminating in diffusely echogenic tissue surrounding a low conus (*c*). **B:** In the axial plane, a hypoechoic tract (*arrowheads*) with an echogenic component representing a dermoid is noted in the thoracic spine.

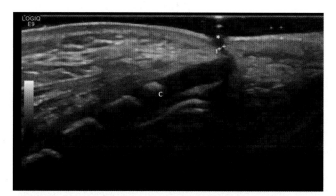

FIGURE 22-13 Pilonidal sinus. The patient presented with a simple sacral dimple. Longitudinal image over the dimple (*asterisk*) shows a hypoechoic tract (*arrowhead*) coursing toward the coccyx (*c*) in this longitudinal image.

forming around the gluteal cleft may break off and serve as foreign bodies. Penetration into the skin can cause a cyst or abscess around the natal cleft.

Spinal Lipoma

Spinal lipomas are collections of fat and connective tissue that appear at least partially encapsulated and have a definite connection with the spinal cord.[19] There are three major types: (1) lipomyeloceles/lipomyelomeningoceles (most common), (2) intradural lipomas, and (3) lipomas of the filum terminale. These defects make up 20% to 50% of closed spinal defects[9] (Fig. 22-14). Lipomas are caused when mesenchymal cells separate and migrate too early and end up in the not-yet-closed NT. The cells develop into fat, thus causing the fatty masses.[8] They will appear hyperechoic or mixed in echogenicity.

The most common of the three, lipomyelocele/lipomyelomeningocele, presents with a skin-covered back mass typically located in the lumbar region.[8] Both abnormalities are associated with a midline bony defect and an echogenic fatty mass that distorts and tethers the spinal cord.[22] The difference between the lipomyelocele and lipomyelomeningocele is similar to the difference between a myelocele

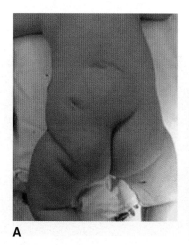

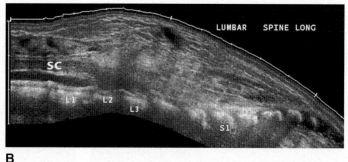

A **B**

FIGURE 22-14 Lipomyelomeningocele. **A:** The clinical marker on this patient shows the dimple left of midline and the *red markings* are slightly higher and are midline. **B:** This infant presented with a skin-covered lumbar mass. In this longitudinal image, the spinal cord (*sc*) is low and tethered by a diffuse echogenic mass. The distal cord is displaced anteriorly and disappears into the echogenic mass.

and an MMC. The lipomyelocele stays within the spinal canal, whereas the lipomyelomeningocele has an enlarged subarachnoid space and the fatty mass extends through the posterior bony defect[16] (Fig. 22-14B).

The last two spinal lipomas, intradural lipoma and lipoma of the filum terminale, are different from the lipomyelocele/lipomyelomeningocele because they are not associated with a subcutaneous mass. They also differ in that they may or may not be associated with a tethered cord.[19] An intradural lipoma lies within the spinal cord and is completely confined by the dura. The echogenic mass can be located in the lumbosacral region and sometimes higher in the cervicothoracic area.[16] Lipomas of the filum terminale can present as a thickened filum (>2 mm) or a small echogenic fatty mass associated with the filum (Fig. 22-15A, B). A fatty filum can be an incidental finding (Fig. 22-16A, B).

Terminal Myelocystocele

A *terminal myelocystocele* is a skin-covered, fluid-filled lumbar mass protruding through a dysraphic defect.[9] The fluid-filled cyst is an abnormal dilatation of the terminal ventricle that communicates with the central spinal cord

canal. The cyst does not communicate with the subarachnoid space.[16] Although the etiology is unclear, it is suggested that an abnormal circulation of CSF results in a massively dilated terminal ventricle.[8]

Sonographically, a large skin-covered, fluid-filled mass is identified in the lumbar region. The central canal widens and directly communicates with the fluid-filled sac. The large sac herniates through the dysraphic defect, creating a large lumbar mass[9] (Fig. 22-17). Hydromelia (dilated central canal) can be seen extending superiorly in some cases.

Myelocystocele is associated with omphalocele, bladder exstrophy, and imperforate anus. As with other spinal dysraphisms, patients suffer from decreased lower extremity and poor bladder/bowel function.[16]

Miscellaneous Spinal Abnormalities

Vertebral Anomalies

Locating the position of the conus medullaris may be difficult in patients with vertebral body anomalies. Butterfly vertebrae, block vertebrae, and hemivertebrae may be encountered

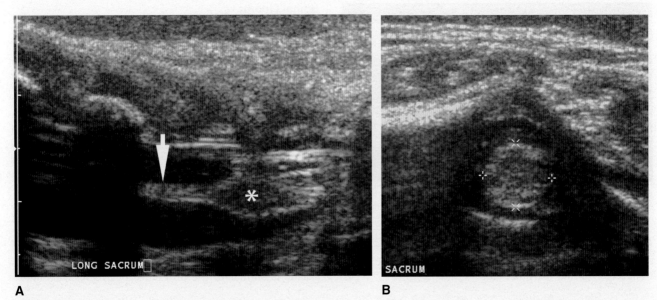

A **B**

FIGURE 22-15 Filum lipoma. **A:** The longitudinal image shows the filum terminale (*arrow*) expanded by a focal echogenic mass (*asterisk*). The lipoma is confined to the filum. **B:** Transversely, the echogenic lipoma is obvious (*cursors*), surrounded by cerebrospinal fluid, and located posterior to the echogenic nerve roots.

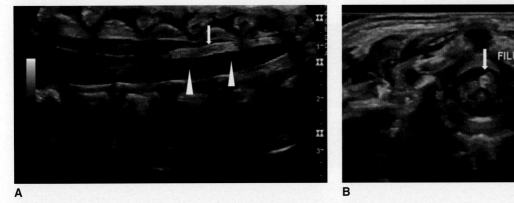

A **B**

FIGURE 22-16 Fatty filum. **A:** The transverse image of the lumbar spine documents an incidental prominent fatty filum in an otherwise normal examination. **B:** The prominent filum (*arrow*) floats posterior to the more anterior group of nerve roots (*arrowheads*).

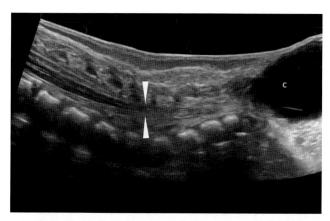

FIGURE 22-17 Myelocystocele. The longitudinal image of the spinal cord shows the spinal cord splitting (*arrowheads*) and the central canal ballooning into the large lumbar cystic (c) mass.

during a routine spinal sonography examination. Butterfly vertebrae is a cleft of the vertebra, or failure of fusion, owing to persistent notochord tissue between the lateral halves of the vertebrae body. Block vertebrae occurs with two adjacent vertebral bodies fail to separate (Fig. 22-18). Hemivertebrae is a congenital disruption of vertebral body development. In cases with variable ossification, using a radiopaque BB and marking the suspected location can assist in determining the corresponding location.

Sacrococcygeal Teratoma

Sacrococcygeal teratoma is the most common type of germ cell tumor, occurring in the neonatal or newborn period.[24,25] The majority of these lesions are benign; risk of malignancy increases with age. Altman proposed a classification of four main types, which helps to characterize components and describe their location prior to surgical intervention. Postnatal detection may occur during soft tissue and spinal evaluation in infants with gluteal fluctuation or sacral mass (Fig. 22-19A–H).

Spinal Cord Injuries

Sonography can be useful in the evaluation of birth trauma to the spinal cord, especially because it is portable. Although the majority of cases are evaluated by magnetic resonance imaging (MRI), sonography may be used because of sedation issues as well as portability. Sonography can also be utilized after failed lumbar puncture (LP) to evaluate for epidural hematoma.

Typically, spinal cord injury resulting from birth trauma occurs during a difficult breech delivery. Severe spinal cord injury is infrequent, but it may manifest sonographically as cord edema, hematomyelia, and hemorrhage outside the cord. Subacute or serial follow-up evaluation may help identify a focal area of cord narrowing from myelomalacia, which will appear as focal increased echogenicity of the cord with obliteration of the central echo complex. Extramedullary, hematomas resulting from trauma displace and compress the spinal cord. They can appear echogenic or anechoic depending on their chronicity. The older the hematoma, the more anechoic it becomes. Acute hemorrhage is more echogenic.

LPs are performed routinely for infants with sepsis to obtain CSF for culture.[26] Unfortunately, approximately 50% of LPs in neonates are unsuccessful.[26] Because there is a network of vessels in the epidural space and the thecal sac, a significant hematoma can occur after a failed or traumatic LP.[27] Sonography is utilized after a failed LP to confirm the presence of CSF to avoid another failed attempt.[26]

Following a failed LP, the lumbar region of the epidural space and the thecal sac should be evaluated for blood products. Sonographically, as mentioned previously, hematomas vary in echogenicity depending on age. Acutely, the epidural space will be enlarged and filled with echogenic blood compressing the thecal sac. As the thecal sac is compressed, the CSF is displaced cephalad[27] (Fig. 22-20A, B). As the hematoma resolves, it will become more anechoic (Fig. 22-20C). The compression will become less severe, and the CSF will return slowly. Blood in the thecal sac appears as debris-filled CSF. Once reaccumulation of CSF is confirmed, a sonography-guided LP can be performed to assure a successful outcome.[28]

Tumor/Intraoperative Sonography

The use of sonography in the evaluation of spinal cord tumors is not routine in the initial evaluation and diagnosis, but it is used in the operating room and following therapy or treatment. Evaluation can be performed through the laminectomy defect to localize the tumor, to follow postoperative complications (syrinx or cyst formation, recurrent disease, or myelomalacia), or to evaluate response to therapy (Figs. 22-21 and 22-22).

Sonographic characteristics of intramedullary tumors include expansion of the spinal cord with the tumor itself usually demonstrating homogeneous or heterogeneous increased echogenicity. Some tumors, however, may have

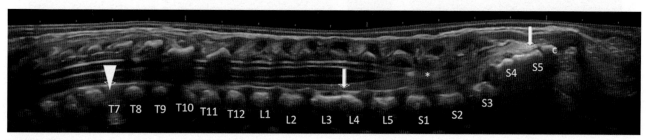

FIGURE 22-18 Vertebral segmentation anomalies. In this extended field-of-view image, a hemivertebra is demonstrated at T5, whereas L1 to L2 and S4 to S5 depict block vertebrae. In addition, there is a low-lying cord terminating at L3 and a fatty and thickened filum terminale.

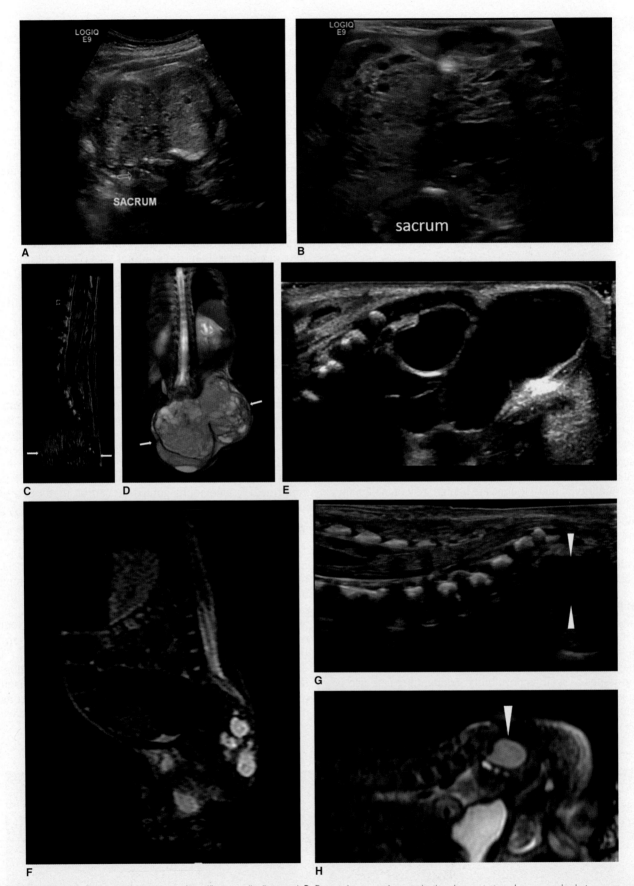

FIGURE 22-19 **A:** Sacrococcygeal teratoma (type II), prenatally diagnosed. **B:** Postnatal sonography examination demonstrates a large, complex heterogeneous mixed hypo-/hyperechoic mass, situated just above the sacrum. **C:** Magnetic resonance imaging (MRI) depicts intrapelvic and intraspinal components, consistent with sacrococcygeal teratoma (*arrows*). **D:** Sacrococcygeal teratoma type III. Multicystic mass (*arrows*) with presacral component seen on ultrasound (**E**) and MRI (**F**) (*arrowhead*). **G** and **H:** Sacrococcygeal teratoma, type IV, in a 1-week-old female with anal stenosis. Low-lying cord, vertebral anomalies, and presacral mass seen anterior to the coccyx (*arrowhead*), resembling the rectum. MRI (**H**) demonstrates multiple cystic components, not appreciated on the sonogram.

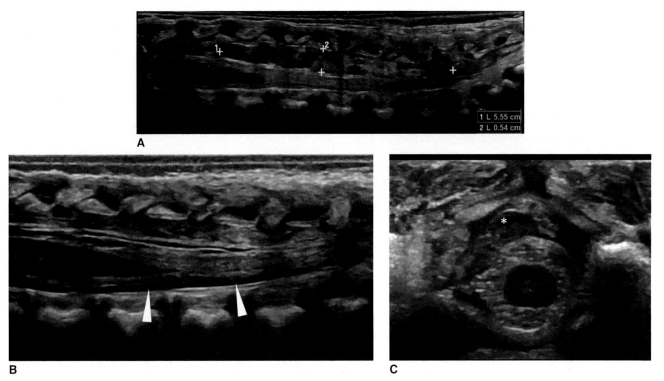

FIGURE 22-20 Bleeding after lumbar puncture. **A:** Longitudinal and axial (**B**) images of the lumbar spine after a failed lumbar puncture demonstrate mixed echogenicity blood in the epidural space. The enlarged epidural space is compressing the thecal sac (*arrowheads*). The echogenic nerve roots are compressed together. No cerebrospinal fluid is identified. **C:** The hematoma begins to resolve (*asterisk*), becoming less echogenic, with less compressed nerve roots and visible cerebrospinal fluid.

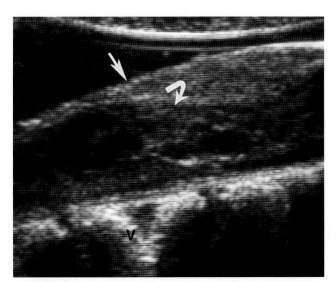

FIGURE 22-21 Intraoperative sonography. Intraoperative sonogram in the longitudinal section through a laminectomy defect in a 9-year-old boy, who had resection of brain tumor 3 years earlier. The spinal cord (*arrow*) is expanded by a heterogeneously echogenic mass (*curved arrow*), which was a metastatic pilocytic astrocytoma of the cord at pathology (*v*, vertebrae).

an echo texture that is indistinguishable from the normal cord and are apparent only because of the change in the caliber or margins of the cord itself. The central echo complex is either partially or totally obliterated by the tumor. There may or may not be associated cystic structures present. Extramedullary tumors are most frequently echogenic with respect to the spinal cord and displace the spinal cord. Whereas the central echo complex is at least partially obliterated by intramedullary tumors, it is usually preserved when extramedullary tumors are present.

Intraoperative sonography during neurosurgical procedures allows for localization of intramedullary tumor,[29,30] differentiates cystic from solid components,[29,31] identifies and localizes spinal arteriovenous malformations, and provides guidance for placement of shunts in the treatment of syrinx.

The technique used for intraoperative sonography evaluation involves scanning, with the patient in a prone position, through the laminectomy defect. Before the dura is opened, sterile saline is used to fill the defect. Gel should be applied to a high-frequency transducer and enclosed in a sterile probe cover. The neurosurgeon or radiologist will perform the scanning while the technologist operates the machine.

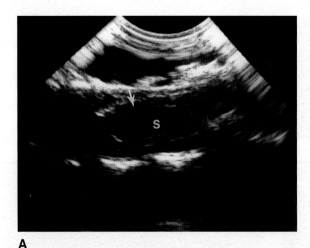

A

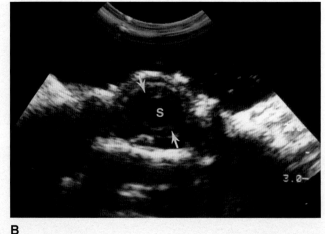

B

FIGURE 22-22 Sonography-guided drainage. Intraoperative sonography was performed for guidance in drainage of a syrinx in the cervical spinal cord in a 7-year-old boy. Both a longitudinal section (**A**) and an axial section (**B**) were obtained via a laminectomy defect. The spinal cord (*arrow*) is displaced peripherally by an anechoic fluid collection, which is the syrinx (*s*) in the center of the spinal cord.

SUMMARY

- Sonographic evaluation of the spine can be performed in infants up to 6 months of age as well as in patients with congenital or postsurgical defect in the posterior arch of the vertebrae.
- A low-lying cord with a thickened filum terminale is almost always associated with dysraphic spinal anomalies.
- The conus is considered abnormally low at or below the L3 vertebral level.
- With a tethered cord, the cord and nerve roots will have decreased motion.
- Diastematomyelia is the separation of the spinal cord into two hemicords.
- The DDS is a thin, epithelial-lined tract that passes from the skin toward the spinal canal as a result of a very focal disruption in the fusion of the spinal canal.
- DDSs manifest as deep midline dimples or pits, but they should not be confused with a sacral dimple located in the gluteal fold.
- The sacral dimple or pit is the most common reason an infant is referred for spinal sonography.
- The sacral dimple can be a blind ending or associated with a pilonidal cyst that extends to the coccyx; however, the pilonidal sinus has no connection to the normal spine.
- Spinal lipomas, which make up 20% to 50% of closed spinal defects, are collections of fat and connective tissue that appear at least partially encapsulated and have definite connection with the spinal cord.
- Trauma to the spinal cord during birth can present sonographically as cord edema, hematomyelia, and hemorrhage outside the cord.
- The most frequent use will be in the infant with a sacral dimple or other midline cutaneous abnormalities, in which, evaluation of the cord and the level of the conus medullaris is desired to exclude the presence of a tethered cord.
- Intraoperative use in cooperation with the neurosurgeon for the localization of tumors, cysts, and other lesions as well as in the setting of trauma has become widely accepted.

- Clinical indications for sonographic evaluation of the neonatal spine include patients with lumbosacral skin anomalies such as pigmented spots, hairy nevus, dermal sinuses, dimples, and hemangiomas.
- A high-frequency (8 to 15 MHz) linear transducer is routinely used to evaluate the neonatal spine.
- The infant should be placed prone on a towel or pillow to provide an optimal acoustic window.
- The level of the conus medullaris, as well as the position of the spinal cord in the spinal canal, is documented along with visualization of normal cord and nerve root motion.
- Between the echogenic dura, the hypoechoic spinal cord is situated centrally to slightly anterior and is surrounded by anechoic CSF.
- The spinal cord tapers to a point and terminates with the conus medullaris between L1 and L2.
- The conus gives way to the filum terminale, which is surrounded by the echogenic strands of the cauda equina.
- The roots of the cauda equina form a collection of less echogenic linear strands that move freely with changes in patient positioning and with crying.
- Spinal dysraphism refers to an array of spinal abnormalities caused by inadequate or improper fusion of the NT early in fetal life.
- Most defects occur in the lower spine, although any part of the spine may be affected.
- Spinal dysraphisms are classified as open or closed depending on whether the lesions are covered by skin.
- Myelocele and the more common MMC are two forms of spinal dysraphism in which there is a herniation of the leptomeninges through a defect in the dura matter.
- With myelocele and MMC, the skin, paraspinal musculature, and bony vertebral arches overlying the defect are attached and splayed lateral to the defect, and the spinal cord is tethered at the level of the abnormality.
- The myelocele or MMC is a fluid-containing anechoic mass that is continuous with the spinal canal through the defect in the spine.

REFERENCES

1. Dick EA, Patel K, Owens CM, et al. Spinal ultrasound in infants. *Br J Radiol.* 2002;75:384–392.
2. Coley BD, Siegel MJ. Spinal ultrasonography. In: Siegel MJ, ed. *Pediatric Sonography.* 4th ed. Lippincott Williams & Wilkins; 2011:647–673.
3. Bates D, Ruggieri P. Imaging modalities for evaluation of spine. *Radiol Clin North Am.* 1991;29:675–690.
4. Hung PC, Wang HS, Lui TN, et al. Sonographic findings in a neonate with diastematomyelia and a tethered spinal cord. *J Ultrasound Med.* 2010;29:1357–1360.
5. Ben-Sira L, Ponger P, Miller E, et al. Low-risk lumbar skin stigmata in infants: the role of ultrasound screening. *J Pediatr.* 2009;155:864–869.
6. Gudinchet F, Chapuis L, Berger D. Diagnosis of anterior cervical spinal epidural abscess by US and MRI in a newborn. *Pediatr Radiol.* 1991;21:515–517.
7. Deeg KH, Lode HM, Gassner I. Spinal sonography in newborns and infants—Part I: method, normal anatomy and indications. *Ultraschall Med.* 2007;28:507–517.
8. Unsinn KM, Geley T, Freund MC, et al. US of the spinal cord in newborns: spectrum of normal findings, variants, congenital anomalies, and acquired diseases. *Radiographics.* 2000;20:923–938.
9. Dick EA, de Bruyn R. Ultrasound of the spinal cord in children: its role. *Eur Radiol.* 2003;13:552–562.
10. Beek FJ, van Leeuwen MS, Bax NM, et al. A method for sonographic counting of the lower vertebral bodies in newborns and infants. *Am J Neuroradiol.* 1994;15:445–449.
11. Lowe LH, Johanek AJ, Moore CW. Sonography of the neonatal spine: part I, normal anatomy, imaging pitfalls, and variations that may simulate disorders. *Am J Roentgenol.* 2007;188:733–738.
12. Kriss VM, Kriss TC, Coleman RC. Sonographic appearance of the ventriculus terminalis cyst in the neonatal spinal cord. *J Ultrasound Med.* 2000;19:207–209.
13. Drolet BA, Chamlin SL, Garzon MC, et al. Prospective study of spinal anomalies in children with infantile hemangiomas of the lumbosacral skin. *J Pediatr.* 2010;157:789–794.
14. Schenk JP, Herweh C, Günther P, et al. Imaging of congenital anomalies and variations of the caudal spine and back in neonates and small infants. *Eur J Radiol.* 2006;58:3–14.
15. Robinson AJ, Russell S, Rimmer S. The value of ultrasonic examination of the lumbar spine in infants with specific reference to cutaneous markers of occult spinal dysraphism. *Clin Radiol.* 2005;60:72–77.
16. Rossi A, Biancheri R, Cama A, et al. Imaging in spine and spinal cord malformations. *Eur J Radiol.* 2004;50:177–200.
17. Cornette L, Verpoorten C, Lagae L, et al. Closed spinal dysraphism: a review on diagnosis and treatment in infancy. *Eur J Paediatr Neurol.* 1998;2:179–185.
18. Sneineh AK, Gabos PG, Keller MS, et al. Ultrasonography of the spine in neonates and young infants with a sacral skin dimple. *J Pediatr Orthop.* 2002;22:761–762.
19. Naidich TP, Radkowski MA, Britton J. Real-time sonographic display of caudal spinal anomalies. *Neuroradiology.* 1986;28:512–527.
20. O'Neill BR, Yu AK, Tyler-Kabara EC. Prevalence of tethered spinal cord in infants with VACTERL. *J Neurosurg Pediatr.* 2010;6:177–182.
21. Kim SM, Chang HK, Lee MJ, et al. Spinal dysraphism with anorectal malformation: lumbosacral magnetic resonance imaging evaluation of 120 patients. *J Pediatr Surg.* 2010;45:769–776.
22. Sorantin E, Robl T, Lindbichler F, et al. MRI of the neonatal and paediatric spine and spinal canal. *Eur J Radiol.* 2008;68:227–234.
23. Lin KL, Wang HS, Chou ML, et al. Sonography for detection of spinal dermal sinus tracts. *J Ultrasound Med.* 2002;21:903–907.
24. Barnewolt CE. The pediatric spinal canal. In Rumack CM, Wilson SR, Charboneau, JW, et al., eds. *Diagnostic Ultrasound.* Vol 2. 3rd ed. Elsevier Mosby; 2005:1793–1828.
25. Siegel MJ. *Pediatric Sonography.* 4th ed. Lippincott Williams & Wilkins; 2011:647–674.
26. Baxter AL, Fisher RG, Burke BL, et al. Local anesthetic and stylet styles: factors associated with resident lumbar puncture success. *Pediatrics.* 2006;117:876–881.
27. Coley BD, Shiels WE II, Hogan MJ. Diagnostic and interventional ultrasonography in neonatal and infant lumbar puncture. *Pediatr Radiol.* 2001;31:399–402.
28. Molina A, Fons J. Factors associated with lumbar puncture success. *Pediatrics.* 2006;118:842–844.
29. Brunberg JA, DiPietro MA, Venes JL, et al. Intramedullary lesions of the pediatric spinal cord: correlation of findings from MR imaging, intraoperative sonography, surgery and histologic study. *Radiology.* 1991;181:573–579.
30. Kawakami N, Mimatsu K, Kato F. Intraoperative sonography of intramedullary spinal cord tumours. *Neuroradiology.* 1992;34:436–439.
31. Kochan JP, Quencer RM. Imaging of cystic and cavitary lesions of the spinal cord and canal. The value of MR and intraoperative sonography. *Radiol Clin North Am.* 1991;29:867–911.

CHAPTER 23

The Infant Hip Joints

CHARLOTTE HENNINGSEN

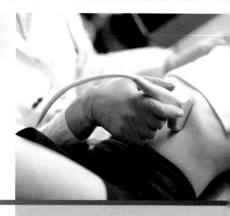

OBJECTIVES

- Describe the embryologic development of the hip joint.
- Illustrate the bones and joints of the hip.
- List the risk factors associated with the developmental dysplasia of the hip.
- Define the process for sonographic evaluation of the hip.
- Describe the etiologies of hip effusion.
- Identify the sonographic appearance of hip effusion.
- Define proximal femoral focal deficiency.

KEY TERMS

developmental dysplasia of the hip

hip effusion

proximal femoral focal deficiency

septic arthritis

transient synovitis

GLOSSARY

abduct to move away from the midline

adduct to move toward the midline

arthrocentesis to remove fluid from a joint through a needle

arthroplasty joint replacement

erythrocyte sedimentation rate a nonspecific indicator for inflammation; a measurement of the time it takes for red blood cells to settle in a tube of unclotted blood

mesoderm the middle germ cell layer that contributes to the embryologic development of connective tissue, bone, blood, muscle, vessels, and lymphatics

osteomyelitis infection of the bone marrow and bone

torticollis a head that is held sideways owing to a muscle contraction

Developmental dysplasia of the hip (DDH) describes a range of dysplasia that includes instability, subluxation, and frank dislocation. DDH was previously known as *congenital dysplasia of the hip*, but most dislocations occur after birth. The overall frequency of DDH is 20:1,000 live births, with dislocations occurring in 1 to 2 out of 1,000 births, and many of the milder manifestations resolve spontaneously shortly after birth.[1] Early diagnosis and treatment are important to avoid significant and permanent disability. Clinical assessment and sonography are the two most common methods utilized in the detection of DDH.[2] This chapter provides an overview of the development and anatomy of the hip and explores the risk factors associated with DDH. Sonographic evaluation for DDH is explained in addition to other diseases that can affect the hip, including hip effusion and focal femoral deficiency.

EMBRYOLOGY

There are three germ layers from which all body systems form: the ectoderm, the mesoderm, and the endoderm. The bones, connective tissues, and muscles are derived from the mesoderm. The initial development of the mesoderm occurs in the latter part of the third week postconception, which marks the beginning of bone formation. From the mesoderm, mesenchymal cells arise that are concentrated in the cephalic end of the body and, along with cells derived from the neural crest, contribute to the development of the face and head. The ossification of the bones of the arms and legs begins at the end of the third week, which marks the end of the embryonic period, although the development of bones continues into adult life. Initially, the limbs arise as buds with the distal ends developing into paddle-like structures from which the bones continue to develop and fingers and toes arise. Myoblasts differentiate to develop into the muscles of the long bones. The joints of the body begin to develop during the sixth week, and during the seventh week of development, the upper and lower limbs will rotate on their longitudinal axes.[3]

ANATOMY

The bones of the hip joint are composed of the pelvic girdle and the femur. The hip bone or coxal bone is composed of the ilium, ischium, and pubis (Fig. 23-1). The acetabulum is located at the lateral aspect of these bones and is joined by a growth plate, the triradiate cartilage. This creates an articulation point for the femur. The proximal aspect of the femur, the femoral head, is rounded and sits in the acetabulum. At the rim of the acetabulum sits a lip of cartilage called the *acetabular labrum* (Fig. 23-2). The femoral head is contiguous with the neck, which is contiguous with the diaphysis or shaft of the femur. The femoral head is cartilaginous at birth and the acetabulum is composed of cartilage and bone. The femoral head begins to ossify from the center outward at 2 to 8 months of age (Fig. 23-3).[4]

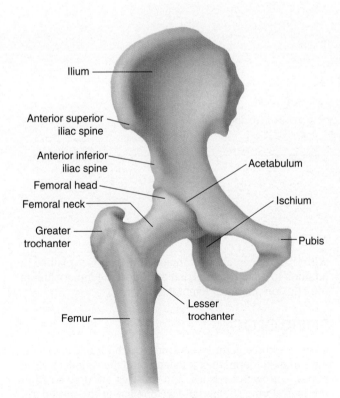

FIGURE 23-1 Hip joint anatomy. The illustration of the anterior hip joint shows the ilium, ischium, and pubis forming the hip bone. The acetabulum is located at the lateral aspects and has the triradiate cartilage (growth plate), which creates an articulation point for the femoral head.

The cartilaginous characteristics allow for sonographic evaluation of the hip in infants. It is also because of the large cartilaginous component of the hip that it is subject to molding with normal development dependent on the femur being in good contact with the acetabulum. Additionally, during fetal development, maternal hormonal influences contribute to the laxity of fetal ligaments, which may in turn create a vulnerable atmosphere for the hip to become subluxable or dislocatable.

DEVELOPMENTAL DYSPLASIA OF THE HIP

DDH occurs most frequently at birth but may also appear throughout infancy. The cause may be mechanical as a result of positional influences in utero and after birth, or the cause may be physiologic—resulting from a response to maternal hormones in utero or physical makeup after birth.

Risk Factors

Several risk factors have been identified for DDH, including breech birth and positive family history, especially if a parent or sibling is affected.[5] High birth weight, multiple gestations, knee dislocations, limited abduction, and increased gestational weeks at birth are also risk factors. Torticollis and clubfoot have also been identified. Tight swaddling of infants with legs extended and adducted has also be implicated as a causative factor.[6] The left hip has been identified as being more commonly affected than the right.[7] Conversely, there are protective factors that guard against DDH including decreased birthweight and premature delivery.[6] Education in appropriate swaddling techniques has also greatly reduced the risk of DDH in those populations.

Clinical Assessment

A routine neonatal screening typically includes clinical assessment of both hips. The assessment should be completed by experienced hands and when the infant is relaxed. Even in experienced hands, sonographic evaluation may detect instabilities that are undetected by clinical examination; however, research has shown that many of these dysplasias will become normal without treatment.[2] More significant dysplasias can lead to osteoarthritis, low back pain, disability, and diminished quality of life and require surgical treatment, including hip arthroplasty in adult life.[1] A proper diagnosis, which results in the best treatment plan, is dependent on the expertise of the individual examining the infant.

Barlow and Ortolani Maneuvers

The Barlow and Ortolani tests are two maneuvers for assessing hip stability. With the Barlow maneuver, the examiner attempts to push the femoral head posteriorly out of the socket, and with the Ortolani maneuver, the examiner attempts to reduce a recently dislocated hip.

The Barlow provocative maneuver test is performed on a supine infant with legs flexed at 90 degrees. The examiner grasps the symphysis pubis and sacrum with one hand while the other hand is placed over the knee area and adducts the leg. Slight outward pressure is then exerted over the

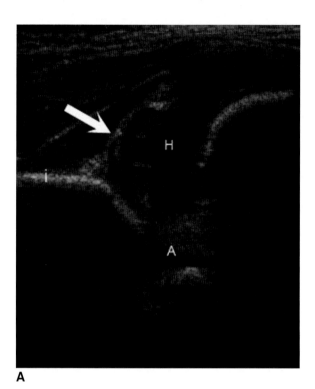

A

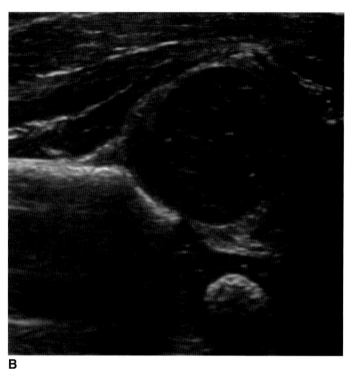

B

FIGURE 23-2 Coronal sections. **A:** A coronal section of the hip with the leg in the neutral position shows the femoral head *(H)*, the iliac line superiorly *(i)*, the labrum *(arrow)*, and the acetabulum *(A)*. **B:** This coronal section in a flexed position demonstrates a similar anatomy; however, the femoral neck is not seen.

knee and distal thigh area in an effort to dislocate the hip. A palpable sensation of movement called a *clunk* is felt as the femoral head exits the acetabulum posteriorly.[5,8,9]

The Ortolani maneuver is performed on a supine infant and the index and middle fingers of the examiner are placed along the greater trochanter with the thumb placed along the inner thigh. The hip is flexed to 90 degrees and held in

a neutral position as the hip is gently abducted, simultaneously lifting the leg anteriorly. A palpable physical movement called a clunk is felt as the dislocated femoral head reduces into the acetabulum.[8,9]

Palpable and, at times, audible clunks are strong positive Barlow and Ortolani signs.[5,8,9]

Visual Assessment

Other features that arouse suspicion include asymmetry of thigh folds, a positive Allis or Galeazzi sign, and discrepancy of leg lengths. These physical findings alert the examiner that abnormal relationships of the femoral head to the acetabulum (dislocation and subluxation) may be present.

A visual assessment should be performed for signs that would raise suspicion of DDH. Dislocation can be observed using the Allis or Galeazzi sign of the relative shortness of the femur by noting that when the knees are flexed, one knee will appear lower than the other. For unilateral hip dysplasia, the Allis or Galeazzi sign can be assessed with the patient in the supine position with the knees flexed, noting limb-length discrepancy. Other visual signs include a shortening of the thigh, redundant and asymmetric skin folds on the thigh of the affected leg, and asymmetry of gluteal folds.[2,8,9] A female profile with an increased pelvic width and the appearance of a waist may also be noted. A positive clinical examination may prompt a follow-up sonographic examination. To reduce the likelihood of a false-positive examination owing to laxity of the muscles in response to maternal hormones, sonographic examination of the hip should be performed between 4 and 6 weeks of age.[10] In a toddler, DDH may present as an abnormal gait.[2]

FIGURE 23-3 Ossification. The femoral head ossification is seen on a 5-month-old female.

Sonographic Evaluation

Preparation

The literature describes a variety of techniques to examine infants for DDH with sonography. Most authors agree that to obtain the best results, it is important for the infant to be relaxed and cooperative. The best time to examine the infant will be immediately following or during feeding. Additionally, it may be helpful to have distractions such as toys available during the examination. It is beneficial to position bolsters of foam or rolled bedding on both sides of the body to aid in stabilizing the infant when scanning in a decubitus position; scanning in the supine position is also acceptable. Parents can be valuable during the examination by helping to hold the infant and by calming the infant with soothing conversation.

Preparation for the examination includes removing clothing below the waist that might impede making contact with the infant's hip. Clothing above the waist should not be removed and care must be taken to maintain the infant's warmth. It is recommended that the diaper be left in place, exposing each side as it is being examined. A warm room and warm gel are a must to maintain as much cooperation as possible.

A linear transducer is preferred over a sector transducer owing to the larger footprint and better near-field resolution. The highest frequency that allows adequate penetration should always be utilized to achieve the best resolution possible.[5] Sonography of the hip is best performed up to 6 months of age, whereas between 6 months and 1 year of age, radiography is more reliable owing to the increasing bony ossification that will eventually preclude adequate sonographic imaging caused by shadowing.

Technique

In the 1980s, sonography of the hip was introduced by Graf, an Austrian orthopedic surgeon. Graf used static images with a coronal approach, measuring the acetabular depth. A dynamic technique was then developed by Harcke and others, which evaluated femoral head coverage.[11] The current guidelines recommend imaging with and without stress, utilizing either the measurement technique or assessing for femoral head coverage. Imaging planes include the coronal plane without stress and the transverse plane with and without stress maneuvers. To assess for asymmetry, both hips must be included in the protocol.[5] The infant can be imaged in the supine or decubitus position. It is easiest to assess if the sonographer holds the transducer in one hand and the infant's leg in the other hand.

Reproducibility and accuracy are important aspects of the sonographic examination. There is a learning curve for the sonographer, during which time, experience with normal and abnormal hips should be obtained.

Coronal Scan Plane

The coronal scanning plane may be obtained with the hip in a neutral or flexed position and the infant may be either in a decubitus or a supine position (Fig. 23-2). The transducer is placed at the lateral aspect of the hip, providing a longitudinal image of the hip from the coronal plane.[4,5] In this scan plane, the femoral head can be identified sitting in the acetabulum. The iliac line will be identified superiorly, and the bony shaft of the femoral neck will be identified inferiorly. The iliac line should appear as a straight line, which is important in making an accurate assessment. If the iliac appears concave, the transducer should be positioned slightly more anteriorly, and if the iliac line appears to incline laterally, then the transducer should be positioned slightly more posteriorly. In the coronal/neutral scan plane, the leg can either be extended or remain in a neutral position. Care should be taken to guard against forcing the leg beyond what would be a natural extension. In an infant, the physiologically neutral state maintains an approximate 15 to 20 degrees of flexion.

Both the alpha and beta angles can be obtained using the coronal scan plane; however, the alpha angle is the measurement most commonly obtained. To obtain the angles, a sonography hip applications package may be used or lines may be drawn on the image. The first line is aligned with the ilium and extends through the head of the femur. The second line extends from the ilium along the labrum. The third line extends from the bony edge of the acetabulum at the triradiate cartilage to the lowest point of the ilium. The alpha angle is the angle formed between the first and second lines (Fig. 23-4). The beta angle is the angle formed between the first and third lines. The alpha angle is defined as the bony or osseous roof of the acetabulum and the beta angle is defined as the cartilaginous roof of the acetabulum. The angles can be used to measure the depth of the acetabulum and the position of the acetabular labrum. The alpha angle has been used as the primary measure for hip dysplasia. When the alpha angle is at least 60 degrees, it is considered normal.[5] Furthermore, utilizing the Graf classification,[12] the hip can be classified using the criteria presented in (Table 23-1).

It should be noted that both premature and newborn infants may present with type II hips and may only require follow-up to determine if treatment is necessary, because many of these hips may appear normal at 4 to 6 weeks of age without medical intervention.

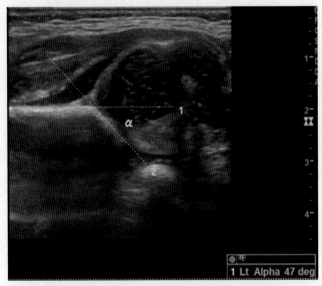

FIGURE 23-4 Alpha angle. On the longitudinal image obtained with a coronal scan plane, there is an alpha angle of 47 degrees in a 2-week-old female scanned owing to increased risk factors of positive family history and breech delivery.

TABLE 23-1	Graf Classification
Classification	**Criteria**
Type I hip	Normal, alpha angle >60 degrees
Type II hip	Normal if newborn, up to 3 mo of age; indicates slowed development, alpha angle 44–60 degrees
Type III hip	Dislocated hip, alpha angle <43 degrees
Type IV hip	Gross dislocation, alpha angle not measurable

The coronal scan plane also allows for an assessment of femoral head coverage with respect to how well it is contained in the acetabulum and whether or not the femoral head is in contact with the acetabular floor. At least 50% of the femoral head will normally sit in the acetabulum (Fig. 23-5A).[4] A dislocated hip will sit completely out of the acetabulum. Although indexes and application software have been developed to quantify the percentage of coverage, a qualitative assessment is commonly thought to be sufficient and can be classified as shallow, intermediate, or deep (Fig. 23-5B).

A coronal/flexion image is made in the coronal scan plane with the hip held at a 90-degree angle. The transducer should be positioned at the lateral aspect of the hip and in a coronal plane with respect to the acetabulum similar to the coronal/neutral scan/position. When viewing a coronal/flexion sonogram, the normal hip will demonstrate the femoral head nestled against the acetabulum and a straight, echogenic iliac line. When the hip is subluxable, posterior, superior, and lateral displacement of the femoral head will be identified. With hip dislocation, the femoral head will appear completely out of the acetabulum (Fig. 23-6).

In the flexed position, the infant's hip can be stressed when scanning by exerting downward pressure and simultaneously adducting and abducting the hip slightly. A stress

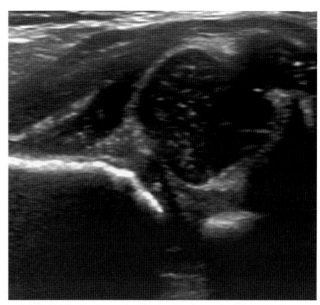

FIGURE 23-6 Hip dislocation. The femoral head is completely out of the acetabulum, which is consistent with dislocation in this 10-week-old girl.

maneuver utilizing a push–pull method can also be used to test for instability. Additionally, utilizing an abduction maneuver, similar to the Ortolani maneuver, can demonstrate whether or not a subluxed or dislocated hip is reducible.[4,5] Images are then obtained noting any movement of the femoral head (Fig. 23-7). The sonogram should be labeled with the scan plane, the flexed position, and whether the hip is stressed or unstressed.

Transverse Scan Plane

In the transverse scan plane, the transducer is rotated 90 degrees from the coronal orientation. The transverse image may also be obtained in a neutral or flexed position; however, current guidelines suggest that the flexion position

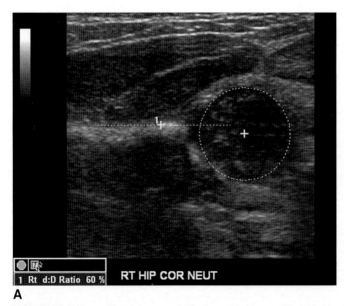

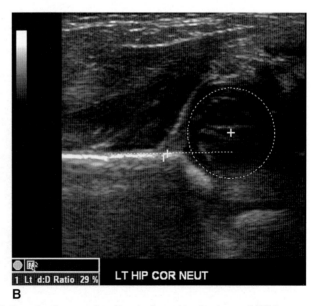

A   **B**

FIGURE 23-5 Femoral head coverage. **A:** On the coronal image of the right hip with the patient in a neutral position, the femoral head coverage of 60% is consistent with a normal examination. **B:** On the coronal image of the left hip, the femoral head coverage of 29% is seen in a 2-month-old in a neutral position with a positive clunk on physical examination. The interpretation report stated the presence of shallow coverage of the femoral head.

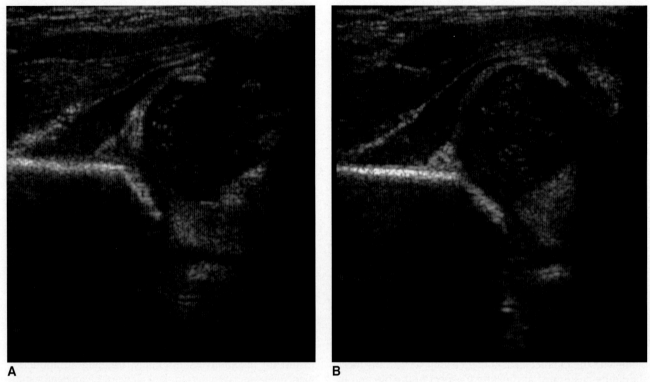

FIGURE 23-7 Subluxation. Stress maneuvers demonstrate subluxation in this 3-month-old with bilateral developmental dysplasia of the hip *(DDH)*. Compare the image made **(A)** without stress with the image made **(B)** with stress and note the movement of the femoral head.

is adequate.[5] In the transverse/flexion, the image is made from a transverse scan plane with the femur flexed to 90 degrees. The transducer may need to be shifted slightly posterolaterally on the infant's hip to obtain the image plane of the femoral shaft and the ischium as they form a U- or V-configuration around the femoral head (Fig. 23-8A).[4]

The relationship of the femoral head to the acetabulum should then be observed by performing stress maneuvers, which may include a piston maneuver and/or abduction and adduction. If the hip is abnormal, the femoral head will be positioned away from the ischium and soft tissue echoes will be identified in-between. If the hip is dislocated,

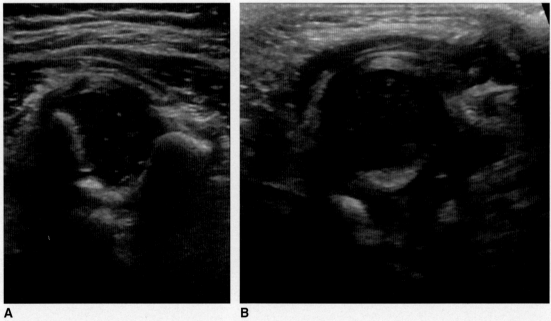

FIGURE 23-8 Transverse image/flexion position. **A:** On a transverse image made with the patient in the femur flexed to 90 degrees, U-configuration formed by the femoral shaft and the ischium can be identified with the femoral head nestled deeply in the center in this normal image. **B:** In a different patient, the femoral head can be identified elevated out of the acetabulum.

the U-configuration will not be identified (Fig. 23-8B). Additionally, the sonographer may be able to observe reduction of the dislocation by abducting the hip. Images should be made of each scan plane with the proper annotation of each stress maneuver. Measurements are not taken in this imaging plane.

HIP EFFUSION

When young children present with hip pain, the diagnosis can be variable with a the extent of severity ranging from innocuous to a true emergency. Clinically, patients can present with localized pain, limping or refusal to bear weight, limited movement, irritable behavior, and fever.[13] Sonography can evaluate for the presence of a hip effusion, and the evaluation of the aspirate of that effusion can differentiate between transient synovitis versus septic arthritis. In geographically endemic areas, Lyme arthritis may also be considered, albeit rare. Though Lyme arthritis usually affects the knee, it can also affect the hip and has a similar clinical presentation.[14]

Transient synovitis is a common cause of a painful hip in children between 3 and 8 years of age.[13] It is a self-limiting disease that can be treated with anti-inflammatory medication and rest.[15] Though symptoms may be similar to patients with septic arthritis, they may present at the milder end of the spectrum. Patients may present with a history of a recent upper respiratory infection, or gastrointestinal or urinary tract infection, although most patients will be afebrile at the time of the onset of hip pain.[13] Once symptoms abate, there are no long-term effects.

Septic arthritis is a serious bacterial infection that can present with more severe clinical symptoms than transient synovitis, but clinical differentiation may be difficult, although children will usually present with a fever. In addition, the patient may show elevated erythrocyte sedimentation rate, C-reactive protein level, and serum white blood cell count.[13] Septic arthritis is considered a medical emergency requiring rapid treatment in order to avoid long-term sequelae, including avascular necrosis of the femoral head, osteomyelitis, systemic sepsis, limb-length discrepancy, and osteoarthritis of the hip joint.[16] Sonography-guided arthrocentesis is utilized to aspirate the fluid for laboratory evaluation. When septic arthritis is confirmed, it usually leads to hospitalization for intravenous antibiotics; however, surgical intervention may also be required in more severe cases. The arthrocentesis can also have the added benefit of providing some pain relief to the child.

Sonographic Technique

Patients presenting for sonography-guided arthrocentesis may be placed under general anesthesia or given local anesthesia with sedation. The patient is placed in the supine position with the legs placed in a neutral position. A linear transducer should be utilized and the highest frequency possible. Imaging is performed from the anterior aspect of the leg with the transducer oriented oblique, parallel to the long axis of the femoral neck. A normal hip capsule will usually have a concave appearance and with the presence of an effusion, it bulges outward (Fig. 23-9). The hip capsule is usually 2 to 5 mm in thickness and should be

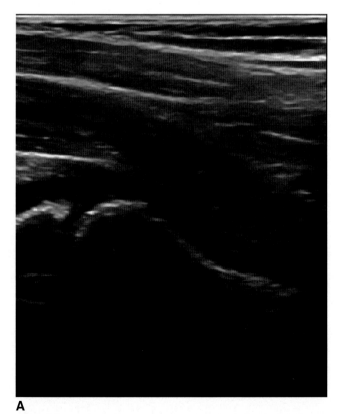
A

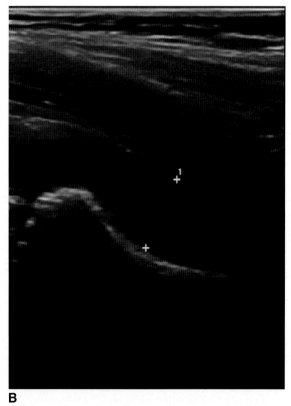
B

FIGURE 23-9 Hip joint capsule. **A:** A longitudinal image demonstrates a normal hip capsule. **B:** This longitudinal image on an afebrile 4-year-old boy with right-sided hip pain shows the right joint capsule with an effusion measuring 10.1 mm in diameter. The patient's left hip capsule was normal.

symmetric, so both hips should be imaged for comparison. An abnormal appearance is defined as a capsular thickness of greater than 5 mm or a 2-mm difference between both hips, assuming it is not a bilateral process.[17] Once an effusion is identified, sonographic guidance for aspiration may be performed.

FEMORAL FOCAL DEFICIENCY

Proximal femoral focal deficiency (PFFD) is a rare congenital anomaly involving the proximal femur and the acetabulum. The range of severity of PFFD greatly varies from decreased ossification to absence of the hip joint with significant shortening or absence of the femur. PFFD has been attributed to an in utero vascular event and has also been associated with numerous syndromes.[12,18] Other in utero factors that may be associated to PFFD include diabetes, drugs, viral infections, radiation, and trauma.[18] Clinically, these infants may present with a short lower extremity. Radiographic imaging, sonography, and magnetic resonance imaging (MRI) may be utilized in the evaluation of PFFD.[19] Sonographic evaluation is not definitive but may be able to identify the presence or absence of the femoral head or a lack of connection between the femoral head and shaft.[12]

DIAGNOSIS AND TREATMENT

Screening

Sonography has become an excellent screening modality for the identification of hip dysplasias and other hip joint pathology in infants. There is, however, controversy as to when infants should be screened and which infants should be screened. Clinical screening is available to most newborns, but it does not identify all abnormalities. A sonography screening program appears to identify a number of the abnormalities that may be missed by clinical assessment; however, the cost-effectiveness of a sonography screening program is questioned. The current recommendation is to screen all newborns with physical examination and utilize sonographic assessment for those infants with an abnormal clinical examination and those with a compelling risk factor that would place the infant at increased risk for the development of hip abnormalities.[1] If the sonography examination is scheduled when the infant is 6 weeks of age, the time lapse provides an opportunity for physiologic laxity to resolve, which diminishes the need for follow-up treatment; however, if the newborn is screened earlier owing to an abnormal physical examination, follow-up may be required before determining if treatment is necessary.[5]

Follow-Up

Once an infant has been diagnosed with a hip abnormality of mild instability, subluxation, a dislocatable hip, or frank dislocation, various treatment methods may be utilized depending on the severity of the abnormality. Sonography of the hip may be utilized to follow a borderline hip that will typically become normal within a few weeks without treatment. Treatment plans may include placing the infant in a Pavlik harness, bracing the lower extremities, casting, or surgical reduction. The Pavlik harness is considered the gold standard for treatment of DDH, with a reported success rate of up to 95%. The Pavlik harness is designed to brace the hip in abduction and flexions; so, the acetabulum will remodel as the femoral head is placed to rest, centered in the acetabular socket. Other advantages of the harness include affordability, the ability to adequately monitor the hip sonographically, and the ability to change diapers without removal of the harness. Sonographic evaluation of the treatment progress can be performed with the infant in the harness; it can assist in determining when the harness can be removed and as follow-up, once harness use has been discontinued. The harness is typically removed after 6 weeks, if evaluation of the hip demonstrates proper position of the femoral head.[1,2] It is important to remember that stress maneuvers should not be performed while the infant is in the Pavlik harness, nor should it be removed unless requested by the orthopedic surgeon.[5]

When treatment of the Pavlik harness fails or an older child presents late with DDH, splinting, bracing, or casting may be performed. Closed or open reductions of dislocations may also be necessary under anesthesia. Sonographic follow-up may be inadequate and this point, and a radiograph, MRI, and/or computed tomography (CT) may be used in monitoring the position of the femoral head.[1]

OTHER IMAGING MODALITIES

In the past, radiographic imaging of the infant hip was widely used. Because the newborn hip is primarily composed of cartilage, the radiograph may fail to identify marginal abnormalities. Radiographic examination is less costly to perform and may be more effective at 6 months and older, when the ossification centers are more likely to be evident. Using CT for infant hip imaging is primarily indicated for follow-up rather than screening. It is especially useful, as previously noted, when imaging casted patients and when sonographic evaluation is suboptimal. The advantages of using MRI for screening and follow-up include the fact that it is an excellent modality for identifying musculoskeletal abnormalities and, like sonography, does not use ionizing radiation. The major disadvantages of MRI for screening are that it is expensive and the long examination time requires sedation.

SUMMARY

- The bones of the hip joint are composed of the pelvic girdle (ilium, ischium, and pubis), the acetabulum, the triradiate cartilage (growth plate), and the femoral head.
- DDH, previously known as congenital dysplasia of the hip, describes a range of dysplasia that includes instability, subluxation, and frank dislocation.
- The risk factors of DDH include breech position, positive family history, and being swaddled with legs adducted and fixed in position.
- There is a higher incidence of DDH in the first born, females, infants with high birth weights, and in multiple gestations.
- The Barlow test, Ortolani test, and visual assessment are used to screen for DDH.
- The sonography procedure should include an evaluation of both hips in coronal and transverse scan planes with neutral and flexed patient positions.
- The alpha angle can be obtained in the coronal scan plane.
- There are four types of hip joint classifications using criteria developed by Graf.
- Sonography assessment of the hip is best performed up to 6 months of age after which time radiography is more reliable owing to increasing bony ossification.
- Evaluation of both hips is included in the protocol.
- The reproducibility and accuracy of the sonography examination rely on the skill, knowledge, and experience of the sonographer who has performed multiple examinations on both normal and abnormal hips.
- The Pavlik harness is considered the gold standard for treatment of DDH.

ACKNOWLEDGMENT

The author would like to acknowledge Tara Cielma, BS, RDMS, RDCS, RVT, RT(S), Children's National Hospital, Washington, DC, for her valuable assistance in gathering images for this chapter.

REFERENCES

1. Clarke NMP, Taylor CC, Judd J. Diagnosis and management of developmental hip dysplasia. *Paediatr Child Health*. 2016;26:252–256.
2. Alsaleem M, Set KK, Saadeh L. Developmental dysplasia of hip: a review. *Clin Pediatr*. 2015;54:921–928.
3. Moore KL, Persaud TVN. *Before We Are Born: Essentials of Embryology and Birth Defects*. 6th ed. Saunders; 2003.
4. Henningsen C, Kuntz K, Youngs, D. *Clinical Guide to Sonography, Exercises for Critical Thinking*. Mosby; 2014.
5. American Institute of Ultrasound in Medicine. AIUM-ACR-SPR-SRU practice parameter for the performance of an ultrasound examination for detection and assessment of developmental dysplasia of the hip. *J Ultrasound Med*. 2018;9999:1–5.
6. Onay T, Gumustas SA, Cagirmaz T, Aydemir AN, Orak MM. Do the risk factors for developmental dysplasia of the hip differ according to gender? A look from another perspective. *J Paediatr Child Health*. 2019;55:168–174.
7. Zimri FUK, Shah SSA, Saaiq M, Qayyum F, Ayaz M. Presentation and management of neglected developmental dysplasia of hip (DDH): 8-years' experience with single stage triple procedure. *Pak J Med Sci*. 2018;34:682–686.
8. Krader CG. Developmental dysplasia of the hip. June 1, 2017. https://www.contemporarypediatrics.com/view/developmental-dysplasia-hip
9. Committee on Quality Improvement and Subcommittee on Developmental Dysplasia of the Hip. Clinical practice guideline: early detection of developmental dysplasia of the hip. *Pediatrics*. 2000;105:896–905.
10. Kolarsky P, Haber R, Bialik V, Eidelman M. Developmental dysplasia of the hip: what has changed in the last 20 years? *World J Orthop*. 2015;6:886–901.
11. Harcke HT, Grissom LE. Infant hip sonography: current concepts. *Semin Ultrasound*. 1994;15:256–263.
12. Siegel MJ, ed. Musculoskeletal system and vascular imaging. In: *Pediatric Sonography*. 4th ed. Lippincott Williams & Wilkins; 2011:602–646.
13. Neville DNW, Zuckerbraun N. Pediatric nontraumatic hip pathology. *Clin Emerg Med*. 2016;17:13–28.
14. Cruz AI, Anari JB, Ramirez JM, Sankar WN, Baldwin KD. Distinguishing pediatric Lyme arthritis of the hip from transient synovitis and acute bacterial septic arthritis: a systematic review and meta-analysis. *Cureus*. 2018;10(1):e2112. doi:10.7759/cureus.2112
15. Ohtsuru T, Murata Y, Morita Y, Munakata Y, Kato Y. A case of Legg-Calve-Perthes disease due to transient synovitis of the hip. *Case Rep Orthop*. 2016;2016:7426410. doi:10.1155/2016/7426410
16. Bachur RG, Adams CM, Monuteaux MC. Evaluating the child with acute hip pain ("irritable hip") in a Lyme endemic region. *J Pediatr*. 2015;166:407–411.
17. Cruz CI, Vieira RL, Mannix RC, Monuteaux MC, Levy JA. Pint-of-care hip ultrasound in a pediatric emergency department. *Am J Emerg Med*. 2018;36:1174–1177.
18. Mailath-Pokorny M, Timor-Tritsch IE, Monteagudo A, Mittal K, Konno F, Santos R. Prenatal diagnosis of unilateral proximal femoral focal deficiency at 19 weeks' gestation: case report and review of the literature. *Ultrasound Obstet Gynecol*. 2011;38:594–597.
19. Subbaran K. Proximal femoral focal deficiency (PFFD) imaging spectrum. *J Med Sci Res*. 2015;3:90–93.

PART FIVE

SPECIAL STUDY SONOGRAPHY

CHAPTER 24

Organ Transplantation

KEVIN D. EVANS

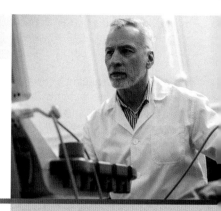

OBJECTIVES

- Describe each part of the comprehensive patient history including laboratory values and medications and its importance in evaluating the patient with an organ transplantation.

- Describe the clinical presentations, pathologies, and sequelae leading to the need for an organ transplantation.

- Differentiate between organ donations from a living donor and one harvested from a cadaver.

- Illustrate the most common surgical placements for the renal, pancreas, and liver allografts with a rationale for each location.

- Correlate the sonography evaluation of a transplant patient to include the grayscale parenchymal echogenicity, Doppler data, and medical complications associated with pathology or rejection.

- Demonstrate completing a diagnostic sonography examination on patients with a renal, pancreas, and/or liver transplant.

- Discuss other procedures used to evaluate patients with organ transplants.

KEY TERMS

allograft

Doppler

heterotopically

histocompatibility

perfusion

GLOSSARY

allograft graft transplanted between genetically nonidentical individuals of the same species

histocompatibility the state of a donor and recipient sharing a sufficient number of histocompatibility antigens so an allograft is accepted and remains functional

immunosuppressive medication pharmaceutical agents prescribed to prevent or decrease the immune response

Sonographic evaluation of transplanted organs is a routine exam completed in most general sonography departments. However, a true understanding of the sonographic information and its diagnostic value continues to evolve. As with many sonography examinations, a holistic approach is needed to ensure that the data acquired are placed in context with the many other pieces of diagnostic information obtained on these patients.

COMPREHENSIVE PATIENT HISTORY

Prior to conducting a sonographic examination on a patient with a transplanted organ, it is of utmost importance to obtain a comprehensive patient history. Accomplishing this task will require access to the patient's electronic medical record so that a thorough search can be conducted to gather information, such as the origin of the native organ disease, site of transplantation, preexisting malignancy or infections, and any other medical issue that could impact the activity of the organ.[1] This information is gathered each time a transplant patient returns to the hospital with a change in their health following a transplant procedure or hospital discharge. Typically, these patients provide an extensive oral history, which needs to be checked against their medical record for accuracy.

An additional piece needed in making the diagnosis is a review of the patient's current clinical laboratory values with a focus on the typically most sensitive tests[2] (Table 24-1). It is also advised to consult the record for information on the patient's immune status and any pathology report that might be available. Screening patients for the presence of an infectious disease is also paramount.

As with conducting any sonography examination, it is imperative to spend time evaluating the previous imaging studies in order to form a diagnostic baseline for the current study to be performed. Often, Doppler information and the grayscale dimensions of the transplanted organ can provide important formative information while new information is being gathered. The interpreting physician's reports, the postoperative notes, and the transplant surgeon's diagrams cumulatively provide the background material that can prove to be invaluable during the sonographic examination because they will expedite the time spent in examination.

Patients are usually good at self-reporting their medications, and—although valuable to the interpreting physician, this information needs to be verified against their medical record. Most patients will be taking some amount of immunosuppressive medication, with the most common being cyclosporine A (CsA), sirolimus (Rapamycin), or tacrolimus (Prograf), and patients often take some accompanying levels of steroids.[2] These drugs must be closely monitored to ensure that they are providing the proper protection because lower levels lead to rejection and higher levels can contribute to toxicity. High-pressure liquid chromatography is considered to be the current gold standard for obtaining quantitative information about drug levels.[2] Certainly, these values can be important to the referring physician who has to assemble all the diagnostic information to adjust the patient's treatment plan.

A comprehensive patient history can assist the sonographer in obtaining and in evaluating the images and Doppler data. Sonography of the transplanted organ is a key part of the diagnostic workup and is a vital part of a holistic plan of action in determining the proper medical course of action.

TABLE 24-1	**Sensitive Clinical Laboratory Tests[2]**
Entity	**Laboratory Test**
Kidney	Creatinine
Liver	Gamma-glutamyl transferase
	Alanine aminotransferase
	Aspartate aminotransferase
Pancreas	Amylase
	Lipase
	Blood glucose
Inflammation	Cytokines
	Chemokines

CLINICAL PRESENTATION

A patient diagnosed with chronic renal failure likely undergoes some form of dialysis to reduce nitrogen-containing wastes that have accumulated in the blood stream. A failure to clear nitrogen-containing wastes from the body results in increased blood urea and creatinine. This condition is referred to as uremia. Uremia has a toxic effect on different body systems, such as the gastrointestinal and nervous systems, causes the skin to take on a yellow color, and also causes itching. These physical manifestations are a combination of uremia and developing anemia in the patient. The inability to synthesize erythropoietin, which governs the production of red blood cells, results in the development of anemia.[3] Either hemodialysis three times a week or peritoneal dialysis, which is often done at home at night, should assist the patient in reducing uremia and anemia. However, the process is very hard on the cardiovascular system.[4]

Cirrhosis of a patient, and its poor prognosis, is one condition that leads to liver transplantation.[5] A patient is deemed a candidate for liver transplantation when the patient's underlying disease becomes so threatening that the risk of surgery is less than the continued life expectancy with the native liver. The 1-year survival rate for a liver transplant patient is 87% and the 1-year graft survival rate is 80.3%.[1] The causes for liver failure and ultimate transplantation are hepatitis C, alcoholic liver disease, and cryptogenic cirrhosis.[1] Those patients with metastatic cancer, active substance abuse, sepsis, and compromised cardiac function are not typical candidates for liver allograft.[1] Patients with portal vein thrombosis are considered high risk because it complicates the surgical procedure and results in lower survival rates.

Uncontrolled diabetes manifests in a variety of pathologies, and many type I diabetics are more likely to seek pancreatic allografts. Since diabetics are at risk for chronic renal failure, there is a tendency to advocate for a dual transplant of a kidney and pancreas. A simultaneous pancreas and kidney transplant (SPK) is reportedly 85% successful, whereas a pancreas following a renal transplant (PAK) is only 78% effective and a pancreas transplant alone (PTA) is only 77% effective.[2]

Successful transplantation of solid organs has dramatically improved in the short term, with first-year rejection rates dropping; however, the long-term survival rates of transplants have remained unchanged—so, more data are needed on long-term survival of transplanted organs. The least amount of data on survival exists for PTA.[6]

SURGICAL PLACEMENT

The orientation of the transplanted organ anatomy or allograft is very often dictated by the medical condition of the patient at the time of surgical implantation. The term allograft is defined as graft transplanted between genetically nonidentical individuals of the same species.[7] The medical condition of the allograft recipient can vary according to the severity of the recipient's underlying disease.

There are two types of organ donations: donation from a living donor or one harvested from a cadaver. The benefits of matching the donor and recipient are that both the cellular and humoral rejection pathways can be suppressed. The use of immunosuppressive drugs is necessary to avoid these cellular pathways; however, they do not protect the recipient from fungal, viral, and other infections.[2] The postsurgical risks for infection are coupled with the challenge to regulate the immunosuppressive drugs to achieve an optimal balance for the patient.

Renal Allograft

Renal allografts are surgically implanted in a superficial placement in either the right or left lower abdomen.[4] Although the renal allograft can be placed transperitoneal or intraperitoneal, the surgical preference is an extraperitoneal placement, which is usually in the right iliac fossa.[8] Compared with the left iliac fossa, the right iliac fossa is nearer to major vessels and the urinary bladder. If the transplanted kidney is placed heterotopically, the right kidney is transplanted in the left iliac fossa or the left kidney is transplanted in the right iliac fossa.[8]

En block is a type of harvesting that preserves cadaveric ureters, main renal arteries and veins, segments of the suprarenal and infrarenal arteries and veins, as well as segments of the aorta, and inferior vena cava (IVC).[1] In the case of a cadaveric transplant with a donor renal artery and a portion of the aorta, multiple donor arteries are anastomosed end-to-side to the external iliac artery using a Carrel patch.[1,8,9] In the case of a living donor transplant harvested with only the main renal artery, the artery is anastomosed either end-to-end to the internal iliac artery or end-to-side to the recipient external iliac artery[8] (Fig. 24-1). Hilar fat and adventitia surrounding the ureter are harvested to maximize the blood supply to these areas.[1] The ureter is implanted directly into the superolateral wall of the bladder, via ureteroneocystostomy.[1] The ureter can also be joined to the native ipsilateral ureter, otherwise known as an ureteroureterostomy.[9] Although the health of the recipient is of primary concern, it is also important to be aware of any intrinsic pathology that might be passed on from the donor and donated tissue.

Pancreatic Allograft

The pancreatic allograft is implanted as a whole organ and placed either in the pelvis or the upper abdomen. In the pelvis, the pancreatic allograft is oriented vertically and the arterial anastomosis is made with the iliac artery. The donor's portal vein is sewn into the external iliac vein and a stump of the donor's duodenum is inserted so that it empties into the recipient's urinary bladder.[1] In the upper abdomen, the pancreatic allograft is oriented diagonally and this placement attaches the donor's portal vein to the recipient's superior mesenteric vein (SMV). The donor's duodenal stump is sutured into the recipient's jejunum, which is much like a Roux-en-Y gastric bypass procedure.[1]

An alternative procedure that is growing in popularity is a pancreatic islet allotransplantation. This alternative procedure is based on the harvesting of pancreatic islets, also called islets of Langerhans. These tiny clusters of cells are scattered throughout the pancreas and the transplantation procedure begins with taking the islets from the pancreas of a deceased organ donor and then purifying, processing, and transferring them into the living donor. The transplantation procedure requires that a physician (typical interventional radiologist) inserts a catheter into the recipient's portal vein to inject the pancreatic islet cells. The cells are infused, or pushed, slowly into the liver through the catheter. Usually, the patient receives a local anesthetic and a sedative. In some cases, a surgeon performs the transplant using general anesthesia. The purpose is to seed the native pancreas with cells that will spur the organ into proper function and relieve the patient from insulin injections.[10]

Liver Allograft

The surgery for a liver allograft is quite complex because it requires that four vascular connections as well as a biliary anastomosis be made for proper perfusion and drainage. The hepatic artery is typically anastomosed by either suturing in the donor's celiac artery to the recipient's split right and left hepatic or at the branch point of the gastroduodenal and proper hepatic arteries.[1] In some cases, an interposition graft must be used to hook the donated celiac axis directly into the recipient's aorta.

The donated portal vein is end-to-end anastomosed to the recipient's portal vein. In the situation of a portal vein thrombosis, a jump graft may be needed in order to unite the vessels around the area of thrombosis.

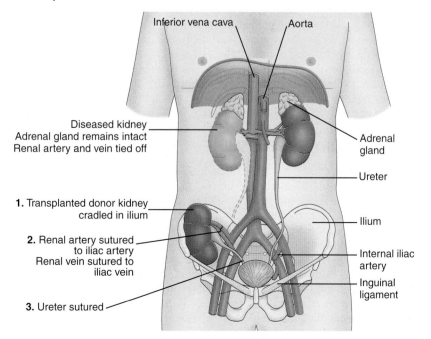

FIGURE 24-1 Renal transplantation. The illustration shows the diseased kidney, which may be removed with the renal artery and vein tied off. The transplanted kidney is placed in the iliac fossa. The donor renal artery is sutured to the iliac artery, the donor renal vein is sutured to the iliac vein, and the donor ureter is sutured to the superolateral urinary bladder wall of the recipient.

The IVC is transected above and below the donated liver so that these vascular connections can be made with an end-to-end anastomosis with the native IVC. Additional surgical techniques, such as a side-to-side or an end-to-side connection between the donor IVC and the recipient's IVC, are connections that are likely made between the donor's IVC and the stump of the recipient's hepatic veins.

The donor's bile duct can be united with the recipient's biliary system by an end-to-end anastomosis after the gallbladder has been removed. A T-tube can be left in place for those patients that have a diseased biliary tree. Those with advanced biliary disease may need a choledochojejunostomy.

This type of allograft is typically provided as a result of a cadaver donation; however, living donations are sometimes made. These partial donations involve a right hepatectomy for segments V, VI, VII, and VIII along with the right hepatic vein.[1] But, regardless of the donation source, the anastomotic connections must be carefully interrogated to ensure that the vascular connections are not stenotic and provide adequate perfusion to the allograft.

ALLOGRAFT PHYSIOLOGY

The renal allograft has an average life span of 7 to 10 years; however, this is increased for those who receive a living donor organ to a life span expectancy between 15 and 20 years of function.[1,9] Upon transplantation, the renal allograft experiences a margin of hypertrophy of up to 15% in size within the first 2 weeks postsurgically. It is also expected to increase in volume by 40% and maintain its final size and shape about 6 months postoperatively.[1]

Pancreatic allografts have a reported survival rate of 95% at 1 year and have decreasing rates of acute rejection (AR). As many as 80% of pancreatic transplant recipients are freed from insulin injections after 1 year postoperatively.[1] Postoperative monitoring of active rejection is necessary along with increased immunosuppressive therapy to avert ischemia of the allograft.[11]

Liver allografts should begin functioning immediately and the normal flow anticipated in the hepatic artery is a rapid acceleration of less than 100 ms. The flow should be continuous throughout the diastole with a resistive index (RI) between 0.5 and 0.7.[12] The portal vein will have hepatopetal flow into the liver and may appear turbulent. Additionally, the hepatic veins should demonstrate their expected phasic flow that crosses the Doppler baseline owing to changes in the cardiac cycle. Assessing perfusion and determining the patency of the IVC are important factors in predicting the success of the liver transplant procedure.

LABORATORY TEST RESULTS

Renal allografts can be monitored in conjunction with imaging by analyzing biomarkers. The two most frequently monitored during AR are increased levels of blood urea nitrogen (BUN) and creatinine. Alongside these lab tests, the electrolytes for the patient need to be closely monitored for changes. If the rejection episode progresses, the laboratory values for BUN and creatinine will also continue to escalate.[13] An estimated glomerular filtration rate (eGFR) can be derived for a kidney transplant, and careful evaluation is needed when the values drop below 10 rnl/rnin.[12] A successful renal allograft should have a mean eGFR value of between 50 and 60 mL/hour.[14] One of the most popular equations for deriving eGFR in kidney transplant recipients is the Modification of Diet in Renal Disease (MDRD). This formula takes in several factors for calculating the mean GFR (mGFR).[15] Research has suggested that a 30% drop in eGFR during the first and third years posttransplantation is associated with a negative outcome for transplant survival.[16]

The pancreatic allograft provides exocrine secretions of amylase, lipase, and anodal trypsinogen into the bladder, which help to provide biomarkers of acute acinar cellular injury. Elevated levels of amylase and lipase are indicative of inflammation.[13] An increase in parenchymal water content is associated with rejection and is thought to be related to a swelling in overall allograft size.[17] Blood glucose also provides a measure of endocrine function.

The liver allograft should be monitored for function with biomarkers that are typically used for a native liver. The allograft is expected to function at an optimal level and any decrease in function may be an indicator of tissue ischemia. Sonographic evaluation of the vascular patency of the liver allograft is indicated owing to abnormal liver function biomarkers.

SONOGRAPHIC ANATOMY

Renal Allograft

The renal allograft must be evaluated sonographically for its size and overall echogenicity. The grayscale images that are chosen for inclusion in the patient's record should demonstrate the echogenicity of the cortex as well as the renal sinus. The normal sonographic appearance of the renal cortex is hypoechoic with prominent medullary pyramids that are anechoic. The thickness and the qualitative assessment of the renal allograft cortex will be highly relevant for gauging the potential for rejection and possible ischemia of the tissue. Because the cortex is the primary site for urine production, close attention needs to be paid to this area of the allograft. The renal allograft sinus is normally hyperechoic and contains the hilum for vascular insertion as well as the pelvis for urine excretion. Depending on the stage of transplantation, small amounts of fluid can be visualized within the renal pelvis, especially immediately after the postoperative period. If there is confusion in identifying vessels versus the ureteropelvic junction, power Doppler is a good diagnostic tool to clarify the anatomic difference. Color and power Doppler are the primary diagnostic tools for the evaluation of renal transplants and facilitate a rapid assessment of global renal artery perfusion and venous patency.[12] The current technology allows for definitive visualization of the main, anterior, and posterior divisions of the renal artery and vein. Additionally, within the renal sinus and cortex, Doppler allows for the assessment of the segmental, interlobar, and arcuate arteries with the corresponding veins (Fig. 24-2).

The normal renal allograft has a low-resistance vascular bed, which is characterized by streamlined systolic flow and continuous forward flow during diastole. The normal main renal artery has a velocity that ranges between 80 and 118 cm/second.[12] As mentioned earlier, the renal allograft will be expected to increase in size during the postsurgical period. Resolution of any fluid collections adjacent to the renal allograft should be carefully documented because these have the potential to compress vital arterial flow to the allograft or venous drainage from the allograft.

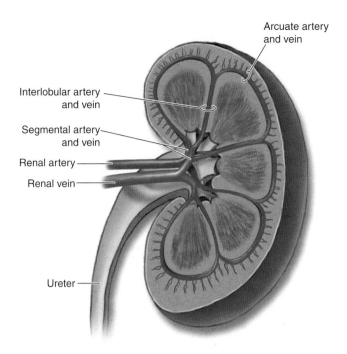

FIGURE 24-2 Vascular assessment. Doppler evaluation of the renal allograft includes the renal sinus and renal cortex as well as the segmental, interlobar, and arcuate arteries with the corresponding veins.

Pancreatic Allograft

The sonographic appearance of a pancreatic allograft is very similar in echogenicity to that of native pancreas (Fig. 24-3A). The transplant is surgically placed either vertically in the right lower quadrant or diagonally in the upper abdomen for enteric drainage into the portal vein. Regardless of its placement, patency of the vasculature associated with the transplanted pancreas is important to assure proper perfusion of the tissue (Fig. 24-3B). The arterial and venous flow should be carefully documented to determine the potential for resistance. Spectral Doppler should document monophasic venous flow and low-resistant arterial waveforms (Fig. 24-3C, D). The pancreatic duct should also be visualized to ensure that pancreatic digestive enzymes and juices are being generated and are flowing out of the allograft. Extra pancreatic fluid collections should be carefully monitored. Again, the documentation of fluid collections adjacent to the pancreatic allograft has the potential to compress the vascular flow directed into and out of the organ. Bowel gas in the abdomen or pelvis limits the evaluation of the area around the pancreatic allograft.

Liver Allograft

The transplanted liver is in many ways similar in echogenicity to the normal healthy liver (Fig. 24-4A, B). The portal triad of the portal vein, hepatic artery, and bile duct must be

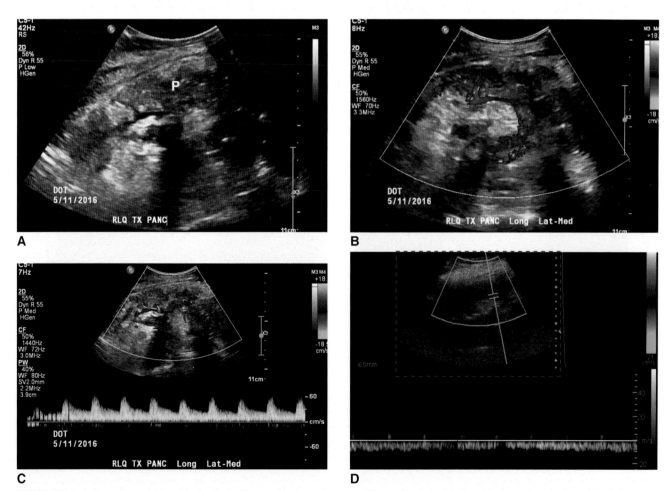

FIGURE 24-3 **A:** Grayscale evaluation. The longitudinal image of the normal pancreas *(P)* transplant located in the pelvis shows normal echogenicity similar to a native pancreas. **B:** Color Doppler evaluation. The longitudinal section of the pancreas demonstrates vascular patency and perfusion of the allograft. **C, D:** Spectral Doppler evaluation. The images of the transplanted pancreas sonograms document both **(C)** the presence of arterial flow and **(D)** venous patency.

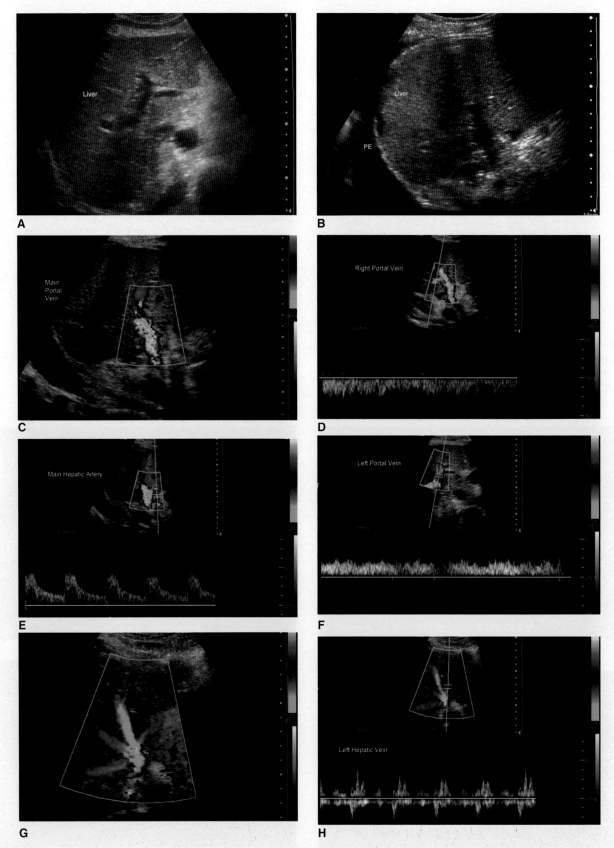

FIGURE 24-4 A, B: Grayscale liver allograft. The echogenicity of the transplanted liver is similar to the native liver. **A:** The longitudinal image is obtained on a liver allograft transplanted 8 days previously. **B:** The transverse image of the liver allograft demonstrates normal echogenicity on a patient with an associated right pleural effusion *(PE)*. **C–F:** Evaluation of portal triad vessels. **C:** Color Doppler images of turbulent main portal vein of a liver allograft. **D:** Spectral Doppler tracing of the forward flow into the right branch of the portal vein. **E:** Spectral Doppler tracing of the main hepatic artery perfusing the liver allograft. **F:** Spectral Doppler tracing of the left portal vein with forward flow into the left lobe of the allograft. Evaluation of hepatic veins. **G:** Color Doppler evaluation of the hepatic veins within the liver allograft. **H:** Spectral tracing of the turbulent flow within the left hepatic vein in the liver allograft.

carefully documented to ensure that the surgical anastomosis between the allograft and the native vasculature is patent (Fig. 24-4C–F). Additionally, the hepatic veins must also be evaluated to ensure that they are patent and flowing in the correct direction and draining into the IVC (Fig. 24-4G, H). Doppler waveforms within the hepatic artery, portal vein, and hepatic veins should be recorded to ensure that proper perfusion of the allograft is accomplished. Angle correction of the Doppler cursor to at most 60 degrees is necessary in order to capture accurate and reproducible spectral waveforms of the flow in the segments of vessels interrogated. The sonographic evaluation of the liver allograft is highly dependent on the documentation of flow in the intrahepatic and extrahepatic vessels. Often, if patency and correct direction of flow are not demonstrated, the patient will have more invasive vascular studies and/or will return to the surgical suite. Since narrowing or occlusions within the vasculature are a risk, careful interrogation at points both inside and outside of the liver allograft needs to be made. The portal vein should be sampled in the main, right, and left branches to ensure hepatopetal flow. Owing to the importance of these measurements, careful use of the sonographic equipment is required to provide quick and accurate results.

SONOGRAPHIC TECHNIQUE AND ASSESSMENT

Since the placement of the renal/pancreatic allograft is in the iliac fossa of the lower abdominal quadrant, a 3- to 6-MHz curvilinear transducer with an adjustable bandwidth frequency will provide high-resolution images. The liver transplant is much more difficult to investigate in patients who have a fresh transplant, postoperatively. These patients are heavily bandaged, and many times, the only area for contact scanning with a transducer is below the rib cage. On occasion, bandages can be adjusted to provide an intercostal space for sonographic investigation of the liver and associate vessels.

All three primary transplanted organs (renal, pancreas, and liver) will require the use of Doppler to generate both quantitative and qualitative information on the perfusion of the allograft. Again, a 3- to 6-MHz transducer that can provide duplex imaging will facilitate the interrogation of vessels at specific locations throughout the transplanted tissue. All Doppler interrogations need to be angle corrected to at most 60 degrees so that the quantitative values can be compared and reproduced. Attention to detail for each grayscale image and Doppler waveforms is required, so image optimization needs to be a primary concern. At the end of imaging, most sonographic equipment allows the sonographer to complete post-processing of images, which can ensure a quality image or volume clip was acquired. Often, spectral waveforms are set up to be autocalculated, and this needs to be carefully scrutinized to ensure that proper waveforms have been selected by the software for analysis. It is advisable to consider manual calculation for those waveforms that appear to have been neglected or disregarded by the software during autocalculation. The precision demanded by these studies requires that the sonographer and sonologist carefully review all images and data generated for each and every patient in the laboratory.

Each selected sonographic image needs to be carefully labeled for the anatomy and vessel being imaged and the orientation of the transducer. The use of Doppler measurements taken at varied segments of the vasculature will require proper annotation such that the sonologist and subsequent sonographers can be assured that the data were taken from discrete locations within the allograft and the supporting vessels. Again, a key component to these studies is accuracy and reproducibility, and this includes proper annotation of the images selected by the sonographer. Ultimately, these images and Doppler waveforms will be used as a guide for subsequent follow-up examinations throughout the life of the allograft.

Renal Allograft

Grayscale Sonographic Imaging

Evaluation of the renal allograft is highly dependent on the representative images presented to the sonologist for interpretation. High-quality images that have been carefully optimized for sonographic technique are required. It is advisable that the sonographer utilize the width of the frequency bandwidth to ensure proper penetration of the allograft and the surrounding pelvic anatomy. Since the renal allograft has a more superficial position in the lower abdomen/pelvis, it has a more reflective quality than what is normally encountered with the native kidney. This may require post-processing of the image to achieve a suitable presentation. Allografts tend to have an appearance much like a pediatric renal study with the noted prominence of the renal pyramids within the cortex. This can give an erroneous, false-positive appearance of a dilated collecting system (Fig. 24-5A, B). Sonographic documented abnormalities in the renal allograft are associated diagnostically with three root causes: parenchymal pathology, prerenal pathology, and postrenal complications.[1,9]

It is difficult to detect the early stages of parenchymal pathology, within the cortex of the allograft because both acute accelerated rejection (AAR) and acute tubular necrosis (ATN) appear the same sonographically. Both AAR and ATN cause subtle changes in the dimensions of the allograft. Color Doppler is also not very helpful in the early stages of these two pathologies.[1] What can be noticed at an early stage in the parenchyma are focal regions of cortical hypoechoic spaces that are indicative of edema and possible necrosis of the tissue.[12] The pyramids can appear to be prominent, but this is rather nonspecific and some swelling of the cortex adds to its thickness. An important sonographic sign of disease is the loss in differentiation between the cortex and the medullary sinus. This blending of the echogenicity of these tissues has also been seen as a result of nephrotoxicity from CsA. Chronic rejection is associated with a loss of renal allograft function after 3 months. The kidney begins to atrophy, and interstitial fibrosis becomes noticeable sonographically. This atrophy of the tissue is believed to be a result of recurrent episodes of AR. The allograft can be measured from the sonogram and compared to previous studies; however, a biopsy is needed to confirm the diagnosis.[9]

Prerenal pathologies are most often fluid collections or other entities that cause compression of the vascular flow to the renal allograft. In the early stages following transplant surgery, lymph collections, hematomas, or even urinomas

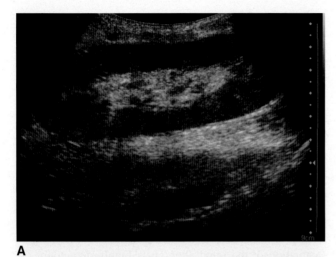

A

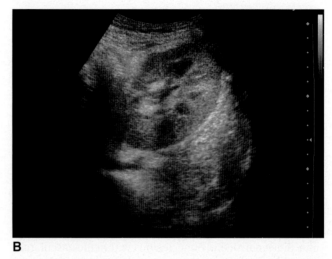

B

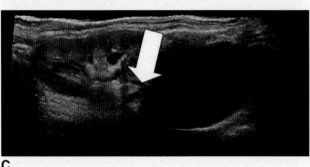

C

FIGURE 24-5 Grayscale evaluation. The sonographic evaluation of a renal allograft uses (**A**) a transverse transducer orientation to obtain a longitudinal image and (**B**) a longitudinal transducer orientation to obtain a transverse image. The superficial surgical placement of the renal allograft allows for visualizing prominent renal pyramids within the cortex. **C**: Lymphocele. A large lymphocele poses an obstruction to the vasculature and ureter of the renal allograft. The *white arrow* indicates the "mass effect" compressing the renal artery, vein, and ureter. (Image courtesy of General Electric HealthCare, Inc., Milwaukee, WI.)

can create a mass effect that occludes blood flow to and from the organ. Fluid collections can either naturally resolve or be drained to relieve the pressure and help to restore vascular perfusion (Fig. 24-5C). More information on these entities is presented in the section on Allograft Pathology and Rejection in this chapter.

Postrenal complications are intrinsic or extrinsic lesions that result in the obstruction of the ureter and prevent urine drainage from the allograft. Some of the previously presented fluid collections can also cause compression of the ureter and can cause hydronephrosis within the transplant. Again, the mass effect needs to be removed in order to restore normal urine flow to the bladder.

Doppler

Color and power Doppler are very helpful in identifying arteries and veins within the renal allograft as well as global perfusion within the cortex[18] (Fig. 24-6A). Likewise, color or power Doppler are extremely helpful in detecting areas that lack perfusion and could indicate areas of early ischemia.[1]

Spectral interrogation of the renal allograft has been an evolving diagnostic tool, and benchmarking for spectral data points is strengthened by continued published research. Spectral tracings of the interlobar arteries should be obtained from the upper, middle, and lower portion of the allograft with a low-filter setting, maximum gain, and a small velocity scale to profile the spectral peak. An RI of at most 0.8 and/ or a pulsatility index (PI) of at most 1.5 have been suggested as normal parameter for diagnostic purposes[12] (Fig. 24-6B, C). Published research has posed morphologic indicators for spectral Doppler to document a rejection episode[12] (Pathology

Box 24-1, Fig. 24-6D, E). Quantitatively, spectral Doppler information can be compared to published clinical guidelines that can help suggest that the allograft is undergoing a rejection episode. RI values of at least 0.9 and/or PI values of at least 1.8 are regarded as abnormal findings.[10,19]

The American College of Radiology (ACR) publishes criteria for guidance as to the most effective imaging examinations for specific conditions. These criteria are based on systematic reviews of the published evidence as to the diagnostic sensitivity for the imaging examinations recommended (ACR Appropriateness). When considering a patient for renal transplant dysfunction, the ACR Appropriateness Criteria recommend sonography of the kidney transplant with a rating of 9. The rating corresponds to "usually appropriate" and makes it the highest-ranked choice for making this diagnostic evaluation.[19] These criteria are updated on a regular basis and this particular recommendation is based on research available prior to 2012. Interestingly, these criteria also mention that contrast-enhanced ultrasound (CEUS) has demonstrated diagnostic information relative to the diagnosis of chronic allograft nephropathy.[19] Any contrast imaging of the native or transplant organ needs to be carefully planned and implemented to ensure that the patient and allograph are properly protected. The ACR also has an important guide and criteria, which should be consulted before attempting contrast imaging in adults or children.[20]

Recent research conducted in Europe with pulse inversion imaging (PII) and contrast imaging was done to assess the function of the cortical perfusion of an allograft suspected of AR.[21,22] These studies adjusted the overall power to low diagnostic levels, and then after bolus injection, assessed

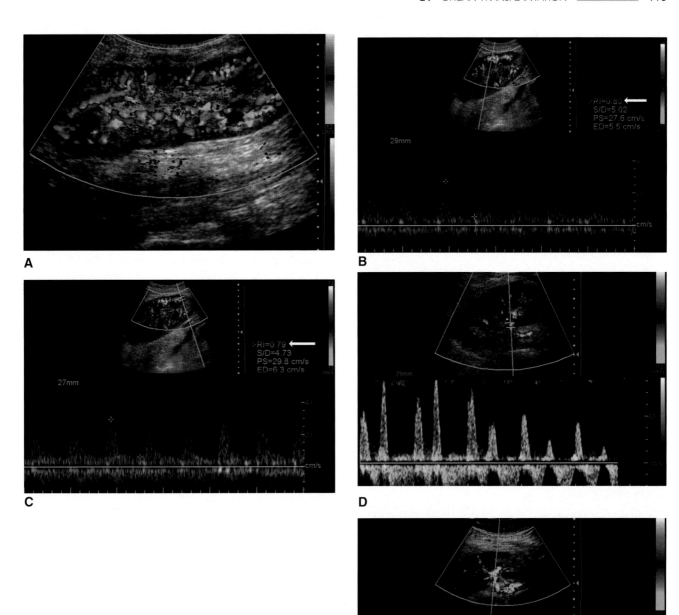

FIGURE 24-6 A–C: Color Doppler assessment. **A:** The sonogram shows the normal vasculature and cortical perfusion within the renal allograft. **B:** A spectral tracing is seen of the midportion of a lobular artery in a renal allograft with a resistive index *(RI)* value of at most 0.80 *(arrow)*. **C:** A spectral tracing on this patient in the lower portion of a lobular artery in a renal allograft with an *RI* value of at most 0.80 *(arrow)*. **D, E:** Quantitative documentation of rejection. **D:** The spectral Doppler tracing documents a highly resistant renal artery in the hilum of the allograft. **E:** On this patient, the spectral Doppler tracing displays a steep spectral peak and spectral broadening.

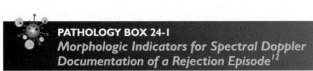

PATHOLOGY BOX 24-1
Morphologic Indicators for Spectral Doppler Documentation of a Rejection Episode[12]

1. High-resistance waveforms
2. Sharp, narrow spectral peaks
3. The second spectral peak is higher than the first spectral peak.
4. Minimal or absent diastolic flow
5. Reversal of flow in diastole

the cortex with increased overall power and the shattering of microbubbles in the contrast. This revealed detailed information about the cellular activity of the allograft. The dynamic ability to determine the rate at which contrast clearance was obtained gave functional information about the transplanted organ. The levels of evidence provided by these studies point to the progression of using sonography to document pathology at the level of the glomerulus. It is hoped that these techniques could someday be approved for use in the United States.

Pancreatic Allograft

The pancreas are difficult to evaluate owing to their placement in the body and the amount of bowel gas encountered while scanning. Color and power Doppler can be very helpful in identifying the vasculature and obtaining spectral tracings. As with any transplanted organ, it is important to determine whether there is reversal of flow and if all the tissue is adequately perfused. Sonographic information should be paired with medical laboratory testing to present a complete picture of the health of the allograft. An RI of 0.7 has been published as a clinical guide to suggest possible acute pancreatic allograft rejection.[12] Interestingly, a study conducted by Wong et al.[11] used biopsy specimens to confirm that AR in selected pancreatic allografts was best suggested by using grayscale images that demonstrated a heterogeneous echotexture and an overall increase in graft size.[11] Although rigorous, the research is limited by the number of patients studied; so, biopsy results on a larger number of pancreatic allografts would assist in establishing these sonographic features as a clinical benchmark.

The American Institute of Ultrasound in Medicine (AIUM) provides guidelines on the use of sonography to evaluate the transplanted pancreas. These guidelines promote the use of sonography to screen the transplant pancreas and to establish a baseline after surgery. It is also advocated as a follow-up to abnormal findings from a prior transplant sonogram. It is also considered very beneficial for assessing graft dysfunction in patients with abnormal laboratory values or clinical findings.[23]

Liver Allograft

The liver allograft should have a native liver sonographic appearance with minimal fluid collections surrounding the organ. These fluid collections should resolve within 7 to 10 days postoperatively. The biliary system should have a normal appearance with the measurements following those guidelines established for a postcholecystectomy patient. The anastomosis of the common bile duct should be carefully scrutinized in order to ensure that a stricture has not developed and biliary obstruction will not ensue. Grayscale evaluation of the caliber of the common bile duct and wall thickness can be important diagnostic indicators.

The American Association for the Study of Liver Diseases and the American Society of Transplantation jointly published clinical guidelines for liver allograft testing, and strongly recommended magnetic resonance imaging (MRI), computed tomography (CT), endoscopic retrograde cholangiopancreatography (ERCP), and sonography as appropriate modalities.[24] They also state that rejection can only be reliably diagnosed on the basis of the histology from a liver biopsy.[24]

ALLOGRAFT PATHOLOGY AND REJECTION

Human lymphocytic antigens (HLAs) are classified into three classes, each located on chromosome 6, which must be matched between the donor and recipient in order to prolong allograft survival.[1] This process leads to measuring histocompatibility. The timing for surgery is also important because it allows the donated tissue to be warm and functional,

ideally 24 to 48 hours after harvest. Cold-transplanted renal tissue will often require dialysis to encourage function of the newly implanted allograft.[12]

Renal Allograft

Parenchymal Pathology

Acute accelerated, acute, and chronic rejection are general terms and should be considered imprecise because these terms are not well suited to categorize patients for diagnosis and treatment. These terms are best used to represent a continuum of assaults that affect the parenchyma and longevity of a renal allograft.

The condition known as AAR, or hyperacute, should not occur if proper steps have been made to ensure major histocompatibility (MHC) between the donor and the recipient.[25] Circulating antibodies prior to transplantation are available and can cause an immediate rejection at the vascular level. Graft rejection during surgery in the presensitized patient causes a series of vascular reactions, which are widespread. AAR begins with acute arteritis and arteriolitis and leads to massive vessel thrombosis and ischemic necrosis owing to the binding of humoral antibodies. All arteries and arterioles exhibit acute necrosis as a result of binding to humoral antibodies. To minimize the potential for AAR, it is vital to adhere to rigorous preadmission testing, crossmatch, and typing of HLA, thereby avoiding antibodies that can develop against the donor's lymphocytes. AAR has become less of a concern owing to the histocompatibility testing, and as a result it, occurs in less than 0.4% of transplants.[1,5] Heart and liver transplants become available on a very emergent basis affording little advanced notice to the patient or the healthcare team. Therefore, the same level of histocompatibility testing cannot be accomplished, which results in a higher percentage of HLA rejection in these emergent types of transplants.

The early necrosis of the cortical filtration system, referred to as acute tubular necrosis, is most often detected within the first few days after transplantation of the allograft. ATN can be reduced by allowing the patient to undergo dialysis to assist the allograft to achieve maximal function. ATN has been noted in 10% to 30% of transplanted patients and is often attributed to the transplantation of cold preserved tissue.[14] The process "delayed graft function," which includes ATN, describes diminished activity and a variety of clinical problems.[25] Distinguishing between an AR episode and ATN is difficult clinically because the symptoms and signs of AR are rare, whereas ATN has been commonly noted in cadaveric grafts[1] (Fig. 24-7A–C).

The next phase of concern has been labeled acute rejection and it typically occurs in 40% of patients from the first to third week posttransplantation (Fig. 24-7D–F). AR is believed to be manifest owing to activity from cellular and humoral/antibody pathways.[1,14] The cellular pathway of AR encompasses rejection that is attributed to tubule-interstitial rejection, transplant endarteritis, and transplant glomerulitis. The humoral/antibody pathway of AR is believed to cause fibrinoid arterial wall necrosis and rare forms of AAR.[25] A transplant biopsy is indicated in order to histologically classify the cause of a suspected rejection episode. The treatment to reverse AR is accomplished by utilizing high doses of steroids or antibody therapy. Flu-like symptoms, fever, and malaise, along with graft tenderness, are some of

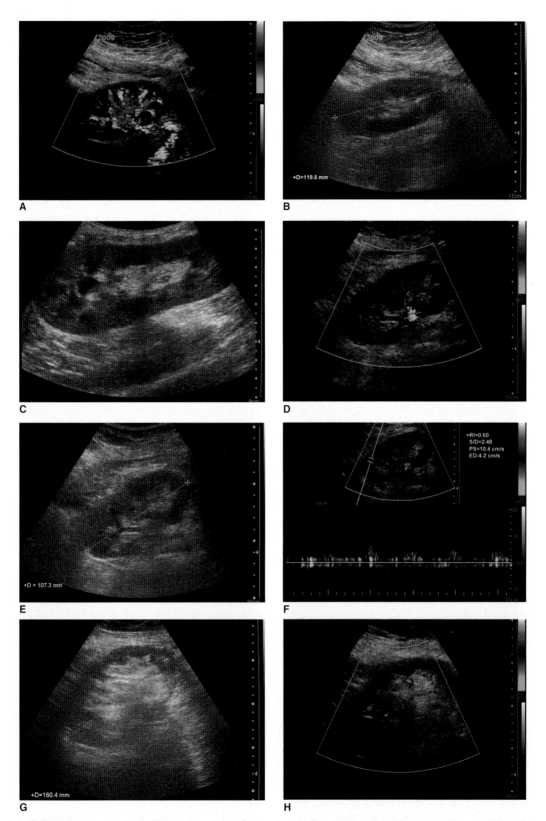

FIGURE 24-7 **A–C:** Third day postoperative. **A:** The longitudinal, lateral-to-medial color Doppler image is used to evaluate the allograft for perfusion. **B:** Grayscale imaging is used to obtain the baseline measurements. This sonogram demonstrates a longitudinal image of the right kidney measuring 119.5 mm in length. **C:** The longitudinal sonogram shows prominent pyramids within the parenchyma of the superficially located renal allograft. **D–F:** Acute rejection *(AR)*. The second-day postoperative sonographic evaluation provides evidence to suspect *AR* of the right renal allograft. The three images are of the renal allograft surgically paced in the right lower quadrant. **D:** The color Doppler sonogram documents lack of perfusion in the allograft parenchyma. **E:** The grayscale sonogram documents swelling of the parenchyma. **F:** The spectral Doppler sonogram documents diminished flow in the lobular arteries in the upper pole of the renal allograft. **G, H:** Chronic rejection. **G:** The grayscale image of the right renal allograft is seen in a longitudinal section using a lateral-to-medial transducer orientation. The sonogram shows the documentation of a chronic rejection episode with a noticeable thin cortex compared to the sinus. **H:** The color Doppler sonogram made through the hilum of the right kidney shows documentation of a chronic rejection episode in a renal allograft with diminished cortical flow.

the reported symptoms by patients who are undergoing an AR episode.[1] In these cases, the patient's symptoms are not specific enough to indicate AR as a potential for renal disease and can be manifest owing to an allograft's "previous life."

These two pathways that contribute to AR are not sharply divided and work together to reject the donation of the transplanted organ. The cellular pathway is based on the activity that occurs within a period of 10 to 14 days. During this time, mononuclear cells infiltrate and invade, causing edema and parenchymal damage. Further damage is created at the cellular level by these mononuclear cells, which further permeate into the glomerulus and peritubular capillaries, which begins to cause focal tubular necrosis. The antibody pathway is also actively engaged and contributes to rejection more than was previously believed. Humoral antibodies react and cause narrowing of the arterioles, which results in infarction or renal cortical atrophy. These resulting lesions resemble arteriosclerotic thickening.[1,2] Specific antibodies are identified as the instigators of tissue rejection. CD4 and CD8 are two specific antibodies that work in tandem to activate separate processes that result in a rejection of the allograft.[2] The immune complex is activated by requiring T-cell activation and that is caused by both CD4 and CD8. A direct recognition of foreign tissue is made by CD8, which unites with T cells to lysis the allograft cells through the vascular membrane. This allows direct attack on the renal parenchyma and is considered an antigen class I process.[2] An indirect recognition of the donated tissue is made by CD4, which unites with B lymphocytes to attack the allograft with an aggressive macrophage. This process increases vascular permeability and allows more mononuclear cells to collect and results in cellular death. This indirect attack through the permeability of mononuclear cells is classified as an antigen class II process.[2]

The life of an allograft is jeopardized by episodes of rejection, and these bouts are conceptualized as a continuum of infiltration that moves from AR to a more chronic condition that results in sclerosed renal cortical tissue. The sclerosing renal cortical tissue ends in a diagnosis of chronic allograft rejection (CR). CR is theorized to culminate in the loss of function in the renal parenchyma owing to the aforementioned mononuclear infiltration (Fig. 24-7G, H). This loss of function within the allograft is completed by long-standing arteritis and is termed interstitial fibrosis. This fibrotic renal tissue is likely caused by the healing and scarring that occurred from earlier inflammatory episodes. CR is diagnostically inferred with sonography owing to the reduction in size of the transplanted organ. A change in the echogenicity of the allograft as well as a change in vascular perfusion can be noted. An interesting point to consider is that CsA nephrotoxicity can have a similar sonographic appearance much like rejection.[12,26]

A critical assault on the parenchyma of the renal allograft is a stenosis of the anastomosed renal artery.[14] Renal artery stenosis (RAS) quickly curtails the arterial flow into the allograft and compromises its parenchymal function. RAS occurs at a rate of 10% and occurs within 1 to 3 years after surgical implantation.[14] The grayscale evaluation of this pathology would cause a decrease in the size of the allograft and, in the long term, would demonstrate ischemic tissue. Spectral Doppler has been used to document proper arterial flow through the united renal artery. Stenotic areas within the transplant renal artery display a peak systolic velocity greater than 200 cm/second with distant turbulence.[12] Interrogation of vessels within the allograft would demonstrate diminished flow and dampened waveforms.

A thrombosis within the allograft vein or artery is considered to be rare.[12,14] A venous thrombosis in the allograft would demonstrate a reversal of flow in diastole prior to the clot and an absence of venous flow beyond the obstruction. An arterial thrombosis, although rare, would occur in the first month and often is hard to distinguish from AAR or AR.

Prerenal Pathology

Infection can occur postoperatively, and this can negatively influence the function of the newly transplanted kidney. One of the most difficult infections to treat is polyoma-BK virus nephropathy (PVN), which has been blamed for up to 10% of allograft failures.[25] Unfortunately, there are no potent drugs to treat PVN.[25] Infections can be localized and arise from otherwise sterile fluid collections. An abscess is hallmarked by a patient that presents with fever, leukocytosis, and pain.

Much like the disease of the native kidney, pyelonephritis can attack at the cellular level and is believed to be the result of bacteria that has ascended from the bladder. This infection of the renal parenchyma can be caused by obstruction, stasis, reflux, or the spread of *Escherichia coli*.[13] A renal allograft that has survived an episode of hydronephrosis can be susceptible to attack by bacteria that has communicated upward and contaminated the cortex. Recurrent urinary tract infections (UTIs) are another contributor to the spread of *E. coli* to the allograft.[13] The sonographic appearance is an echogenic cortex, loss of corticomedullary junction, and inflammatory changes surrounding the allograft. An alternative form of this infection is emphysematous pyelonephritis, which results in air developing in the collecting system. The sonographic appearance comprises of bright echogenic foci with distal dirty shadowing.

An abscess can occur weeks to months after the transplant surgery and sonographically presents as a well-defined collection of contents that vary from anechoic to echogenic in appearance. These infectious collections can cause the compression of the vasculature as a prerenal pathology.

A prerenal pathology that can result in compression of the vascular structures of an allograft is perinephric fluid collections.[14] A common fluid collection that can be noted in association with a renal transplant is a localized hematoma. A hematoma presents asymptomatically and is often found sonographically immediately after surgery. A hematoma can be anechoic at an early stage and progress to a more mixed echogenicity. Hematomas are generally absorbed and should decrease in size over time.

Another asymptomatic fluid collection associated with a renal allograft is a lymphocele. The patient with a lymphocele presents asymptomatically and again can have an obstructed ureter owing to this postrenal complication (Fig. 24-5C). A lymphocele is typically found postsurgically between the first and second months. It is believed to be caused by an interruption of lymphatics that occurred at the time of surgery. Sonographically, these fluid collections can be multilocular with thin septa and anechoic fluid. Commonly, they are located between the lower pole of the transplant and the urinary bladder.

A urine leak or urinoma is another prerenal pathology that can be discovered sonographically. Urinomas are well defined; appear anechoic; and on rare occasions, can also cause compression of the ureter. A urinoma has been reported in association with 6% of renal allografts and is usually discovered in the first month after surgery.[1]

The detection of an arteriovenous malformation (AVM) can be made with color or power Doppler, and these are often created as a result of biopsy trauma.[12,14]

Postrenal Complication

Hydronephrosis is the most common postrenal complication; however, some slight dilation of the collecting system is common postoperatively.[12] Compression of the ureter or stricture at the site of anastomosis of the ureter to the urinary bladder could result in pressure in the collecting system. Careful surveillance of the renal allograft to detect dilatation of the collecting system is paramount (Fig. 24-8).

Pancreatic Allograft

The pancreatic allograft is susceptible to many of the same risks for early rejection as a renal allograft. Combining immunosuppressive drugs and histocompatibility testing helps to reduce the incidence of AR in these patients. AR is commonly suspected when there is an incidence of a 50% drop in timed urine amylase output.[1] This indicates diminished allograft function, which is likely caused by humoral/cellular attack and injury to the tissue. The pancreatic tail is usually fixed when implanted in the left lower quadrant because the descending colon can physically hold it in place.[1] The pancreatic tail develops an attachment to the lateral parietal peritoneum. The placement in the lower quadrant makes the pancreatic allograft tail an ideal location for biopsies to determine a true rejection episode.

The second contributor to the loss of a pancreatic allograft is vascular thrombosis, which has a 2% to 19% incidence.[1] Thrombosis can cause AR of the allograft prior to the first month postoperatively and chronically afterward. This occurs because of the slower rate of perfusion in the pancreatic allograft. The rate of flow is much lower compared with the renal transplant. Thrombosis can cause pancreatic ischemia and pulmonary embolus, as well as pancreatitis. An arterial malformation is considered to be rare and therefore not commonly considered as a cause for rejection.

Liver Allograft

The most significant liver allograft pathology are biliary strictures, which can develop and can result in complications in as many as 25% of patients.[27] The onset of a biliary

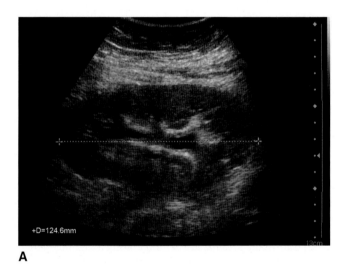

A

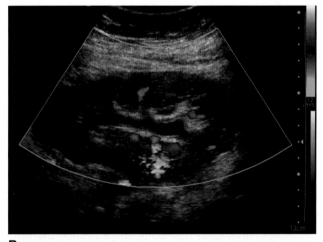

B

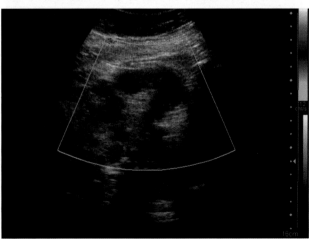

C

FIGURE 24-8 Hydronephrosis. **A:** The grayscale longitudinal sonogram shows documentation of a hydronephrotic renal allograft and a baseline measurement. **B:** The color Doppler longitudinal sonogram shows documentation of a hydronephrotic renal allograft and continued perfusion of the tissue. **C:** The grayscale and color Doppler sonogram shows documentation of a hydroureter, which confirms a postrenal complication.

stricture is complicated by the fact that the nerve supply to the liver allograft is minimal, and patients have no sense of impending obstruction. Often, they present with painless jaundice and abnormal liver function tests. This requires a careful investigation to determine the location of the stricture, which could be either intrahepatic or extrahepatic. The process of transplantation can be the cause of postsurgical scarring, which results in a narrowing of the biliary system. A sonogram can demonstrate a focal area of dilation proximal to the area of stricture. A stricture needs to be surgically corrected to avoid biliary obstruction and subsequent bacteria that can develop owing to stasis. Ascending cholangitis develops owing to an overgrowth of bacteria that moves through the biliary tree.[1] These pathologic conditions are commonly reviewed and managed with ERCP.

Recurrent sclerosing cholangitis can occur after 350 days posttransplant and sonographically can present much like acute sclerosing cholangitis.[1] This condition permits bacteria such as enteric flora, cytomegalovirus, and cryptosporidium to invade the liver allograft. Sonographically, this can be noted as thickening of the ducts and diverticulum-appearing outpouchings of the common bile duct.[1]

An additional concern is the development of sludge in the biliary tree, which has been seen in up to 29% of liver allograft patients as late as 8.5 years postoperatively.[1] The development of sludge is not clearly understood; however, it has been linked to bacterial infection, rejection, biliary obstruction, and biliary leaks. Since the presence of sludge in the biliary tree has the ability to promote sclerosing cholangitis, it is important to document the sonographic pathology and amend medical treatment to avert ischemia of the allograft. It is important to also ensure that bile is not leaking from the site of biliary anastomosis.

The sphincter of Oddi must also be closely evaluated to make sure that it is not dysfunctional and the source of biliary stasis. Although this is a more infrequent pathology associated with the liver transplant patient, an ERCP is an appropriate procedure to evaluate the insertion of the common bile duct to the ampulla of Vater. An ERCP can help to decompress the biliary system and ensure that digestive juices are freely flowing into the duodenum.[1]

The potential of hepatic artery thrombosis is a major clinical concern and must be closely monitored because the biliary system is highly dependent on the hepatic artery for its arterial blood supply as well as for overall organ perfusion. Capturing a spectral Doppler tracing that documents forward flow in the hepatic artery is often difficult but can save the patient from additional imaging studies, such as angiography. The use of Doppler to detect hepatic artery thrombosis is reported to be as high as 92%.[28] As collateral vessels begin to form throughout the liver, diminished flow can be expected as these new vascular connections are forming.

Stenosis of the hepatic artery is also a secondary concern owing to narrowing that can occur at the anastomotic site. The incidence of stenosis of the hepatic artery can be caused by the surgical technique, catheters used during surgery, or a rejection episode. The patient will present with abnormal liver function tests and biliary ischemia.[1] Duplex sonography can be used to directly investigate the course of the hepatic artery and detect areas of high flow or turbulence. Spectral waveforms can also be helpful, and a tardus parvus

signal, suggests a stenosis proximally.[1] Since the hepatic artery is difficult to directly investigate throughout its entire course, angiography may be the best imaging choice if a stenosis is suspected. Evaluation of the portal vein must also be completed to ensure that hepatopetal flow has been restored and maintained. If recanalizations of varices are noted, then a portal vein thrombosis or stenosis should be suspected. Grayscale images of the portal vein will be helpful in confirming if a portal vein thrombosis has developed; however, an acute thrombosis can be anechoic and easily missed. This makes the use of duplex necessary to record a spectral tracing and to document the direction of flow at several points within the liver.

SARS-CoV-2 Implications

As patients survive one of the most deadly pandemics in modern history, unknown sequelae may impact their overall health. Patients in need of organ transplantation or having received an allograph are likely highly susceptible to contracting the severe acute respiratory syndrome coronavirus 2 (SARS-CoV-2) virus. Those that survived the acute phase of the infection are now reporting long-term consequences of the coronavirus disease (COVID-19). These patients likely have experienced latent effects of the virus moving through the vascular system and attacking the liver, kidneys, pancreas, or their corresponding allographs. The evolution of care for COVID-19 survivors is in its infancy; however, the World Health Organization (WHO) provides a variety of tools for the assessment, management, and ongoing care of these patients.[29] WHO has already provided global advice that patients who have contracted either severe and/ or critical SARS-CoV-2 may develop post-intensive care syndrome (PICS).[30] These patients can present with a variety of deficits such as physical deconditioning, respiratory, swallow, cognitive, and mental health symptoms.[30] The use of sonography is an important diagnostic tool for providing surveillance of these patients with PICS as well as those who have recuperated at home. Those transplant patients that survived COVID-19 with a mild case of infection can still report with some form of these symptoms and possible organ dysfunction. At the time of this writing, scientific evidence is still being gathered; however, cohort studies of renal transplant patients are demonstrating a high incidence of mortality, and the status of being immunosuppressed likely is a contributing factor.[31] It is understandable that patients with poor allograph function, over 60 years of age, and with cardiac pathology were the least able to survive the acute SARA-CoV-2 infection.[32]

Those patients who have survived COVID-19 have been referred to as "COVID long-haulers" and this denotes their ongoing battle with many of the deficits outlined previously. Transplant patients need even closer diagnostic scrutiny owing to their susceptibility and potential for organ failure. Grayscale and duplex sonography provide a low-cost, highly portable, and nonionizing technique to assess the function of the allograph in COVID long-haulers. As the scientific evidence is gathered, these patients need to be imaged using a protocol that would be used to determine a rejection episode. At this early point of assessing COVID transplant survivors, one pathology that is important to note is a prevalence of arterial stenosis seen in renal transplants.

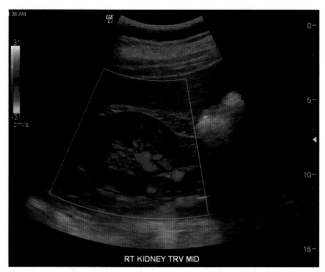

FIGURE 24-9 Right renal sonogram of a 35-year-old COVID-19 male survivor who had borderline cortical thickness, as part of the imaging assessment. This transverse color Doppler sonogram illustrates high-quality vascular flow in the renal artery and native kidney perfusion. This same methodology of vascular assessment can be applied to the COVID-19 transplant survivor.

In a study of pediatric transplanted kidneys, the use of sonography was key in detecting stenosis likely caused by the inflammatory residual of the SARS-CoV-19 virus.[33] See Figure 24-9.

OTHER PROCEDURES

Renal Allograft Biopsies

The gold standard for diagnosis is the evaluation of core tissue from the allograft. Biopsies are more accurate when the procedure is sonographically guided. It has been reported that using sonography to guide a biopsy procedure increases the probability of obtaining renal cortex in 75% to 90% of patients.[34] The percentage increases when the core samples can be immediately evaluated with an electron microscope and accuracy approaches 100%.

TABLE 24-2   **Renal Allograft Biopsy Criteria**[22]
1. Obtain at least two biopsy cores for standard light microscopic evaluation.
2. A biopsy sample needs to contain greater than 12 glomeruli (located in the deep cortex).
3. A biopsy sample needs to contain greater than two large interlobular arteries/branches of arcuate arteries (with at least two to three layers of medial smooth muscle cells).
4. The sample should contain a portion of the medulla.

Besides defining the diagnosis of rejection, a biopsy has a significant impact on the treatment of the patient. Biopsy results have helped modify the treatment of 27% to 46% of patient cases, have revised therapies in 42% to 83% of patient cases, and have helped to avoid the use of additional immunosuppressive therapy in 19% to 30% of patient cases.[25] In order to ensure that the pathologist can provide these important diagnostic results, a proper sample of the allograft is needed. Histology can pinpoint the cause of rejection from a broad spectrum of diseases that can be superimposed on the rejection episode.[25] It is also important to obtain tissue from the allograft during the rejection episode so that a morphologic episode can be diagnosed. Waiting until an episode has concluded will make the diagnosis less definitive and only document sclerosis.[25] A biopsy gun is an important tool, and utilizing sonographic guidance is recommended; so, criteria can be followed to obtain sufficient tissue and to ensure that a diagnostic sample is obtained from the renal allograft[25] (Table 24-2).

The research conducted by Bartlett et al.[17] documents the usefulness of taking a biopsy sample of both the renal and pancreatic allograft to determine the extent of a rejection episode.[17] Securing biopsies of both allografts helps ensure that the appropriate medical therapy is used and the overall dosages are regulated. Sonography guidance is vital and helps with the appropriate diagnosis to tailor treatment for patients with compromised health owing to rejection (Fig. 24-10).

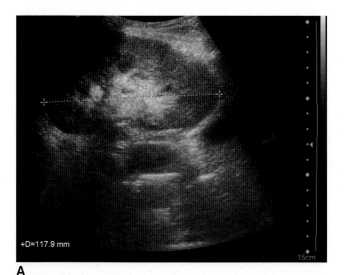

A

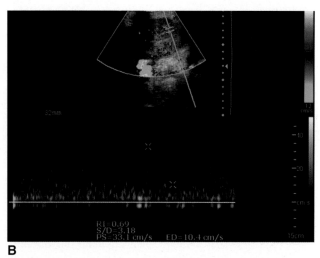

B

FIGURE 24-10 A 17-year-old renal allograft. **A:** The grayscale longitudinal sonogram of the renal allograft documents parenchymal echogenicity, which aids in tailoring treatment for patients with compromised health owing to rejection. **B:** The color and spectral Doppler evaluation shows perfusion within the cortex of the renal allograft.

Computed Tomography

CT has been described as a central imaging modality, and other imaging options are utilized when a CT is deemed inconclusive. Owing to the use of ionizing radiation and patient dose, CT is not a primary imaging tool for transplant patients because these patients are generally followed through their clinical course for changes in their medical status postoperatively. CT is very helpful as part of the workup of potential donors when screening for compatibility.[35] Three-dimensional (3D) CT and CT angiography (CTA) studies provide preoperative assessment of renal donors and give the surgeon important information about the ureters, number of vessels, and the location of renal arteries.[36] This allows for preplanning of the living allograft surgical procedure and the associated complications that might be encountered.

CT examination can play a role in the evaluation of the pancreatic allograft because it is usually surgically placed in the lower pelvis and is often partially obscured by bowel gas and other pelvic organs. A CT evaluation can help to define all the margins of the pancreatic allograft and also detect the associated fluid collections. CT can also provide added information for those liver allograft patients with extrahepatic biliary duct strictures. A study of 38 patients demonstrated that helical CT provided a volumetric image that predicted the donated right liver lobe volume with 92% of actual graft volume.[37] Detailed CT sectional images of the duodenum and ampulla of Vater would allow the site of obstruction to be located and perhaps avoid the need to undergo an ERCP.

Nuclear Medicine

A nuclear medicine allograft study requires the injection of a radioisotope into the transplant recipient's venous system. This allows the radionuclide to circulate back through the arterial system and traces perfusion of the allograft suspected of rejection. Using a camera to collect the radiation emitted by the patient over the site of the allograft provides information regarding the function of the organ. A lack of vascular perfusion within the allograft would suggest that the arterial supply is being rejected and is under a state of vasodilatation even though the volume of flow is inadequate. A function study of the allograft is very helpful to determine whether acute or chronic ischemia has occurred. Positron emission tomography (PET) studies coupled with CT have been shown to be helpful in monitoring perfusion in posttransplant patients and also could aid in regulating medical therapy.[38]

SUMMARY

- Sonography of patients with organ transplantations requires a holistic approach to ensure the data acquired are placed in contexts with all diagnostic information.
- A comprehensive patient history includes a thorough check of the patient's electronic medical record with the evaluation of current clinical laboratory values, immunosuppressive drugs, other medications, surgical placement of the organ, immune status, pathology reports, and imaging examinations.
- Patients with clinical presentations including chronic renal failure, hepatitis C, alcoholic liver disease, cryptogenic cirrhosis, and/or type I diabetics are the most likely candidates for organ transplantation.
- The two types of organ donations are from a living donor and one harvested from a cadaver.
- Renal allografts can be placed transperitoneal or intraperitoneal, but the surgical preference is an extraperitoneal placement, usually in the right iliac fossa.
- The pancreatic allograft is oriented vertically in the pelvis or diagonally in the upper abdomen.
- The liver allograft is surgically placed in the right upper quadrant and involves complex anastomosis of vasculature and biliary ducts.
- The renal allograft has an average life span of 7 to 10 years for a harvested organ from a cadaver and 15 to 20 years for an organ from a living donor organ.
- One year following transplantation, successful pancreatic allografts free 80% of the recipients from insulin injection.
- With a liver allograft, flow should be continuous throughout diastole with a RI between 0.5 and 0.7.
- Postoperatively, the renal, pancreas, and liver transplants should be evaluated with both grayscale for the parenchymal echogenicity and with Doppler to generate both quantitative and qualitative information on the perfusion of the allograft.
- Acute accelerated renal allograft rejection can be greatly diminished with rigorous preadmission testing, crossmatch, and typing of HLA to help avoid antibodies against the donor's lymphocytes.
- Renal allograft pathologies, which increase the incidence of rejection, are classified as parenchymal pathology, prerenal pathology, and postrenal complications.
- The primary contributors to the loss of a pancreatic allograft include diminished function likely caused by humoral/cellular attach and injury to the tissue or vascular thrombosis.
- Biliary strictures are the most significant liver allograft pathology, and vascular thrombosis, stenosis, and flow direction are also of major clinical concern.
- Patients surviving CoV-19 need to be carefully evaluated for signs of chronic disease and concomitant organ transplant compromise.
- Other procedures to evaluate the health of an allograft include biopsy, CT, and nuclear medicine.
- Follow-up examination accuracy and reproducibility are possible when each study includes proper annotation of the images, which includes labeling the anatomy, vessels, and the orientation of the transducer.

DEDICATION

Dedicated to my sister who was the recipient of my kidney donation more than 35 years ago.

REFERENCES

1. Muradali D, Chawla T. Organ transplantation. In: Rumack CM, Wilson SR, Charbonneau JW, eds. *Diagnostic Ultrasound*. 4th ed. Vol 1. Elsevier Mosby; 2011:639–707.
2. Mitchell RN, Kumar V. Diseases of immunity. In: Kumar V, Cotran RS, Robbins SL, eds. *Basic Pathology*. 7th ed. Elsevier Saunders; 2003:103–164.
3. Eisenberg RL, Johnson NM. Urinary system. In: Eisenberg RL, Johnson NM, eds. *Comprehensive Radiographic Pathology*. 6th ed. Elsevier Mosby; 2016:216–247.
4. Brown ED, Chen MYM, Wolfman NT, Ott DJ, Watson NE Jr. Complications of renal transplantation: evaluation with US and radionuclide imaging. *Radiographics*. 2000;20:607–622.
5. Kowalczyk N, Mace JD. Hepatobiliary system. In: Kowalczyk N, Mace JD, eds. *Radiographic Pathology for Technologists*. 5th ed. Elsevier Mosby; 2009:140–160.
6. Fiorina P, Venturini M, Folli F, et al. Natural history of kidney graft survival, hypertrophy, and vascular function in end-stage renal disease type 1 diabetic kidney-transplanted patients: beneficial impact of pancreas and successful islet cotransplantation. *Diabetes Care*. 2005;28(6):1303–1310.
7. Stedman TL, Dirckx JH. *Stedman's Concise Medical Dictionary for the Health Professions*. Lippincott Williams & Wilkins; 2001:50.
8. Kobayashi K, Censullo ML, Rossman LL, Kyriakides PN, Kahan BD, Cohen AM. Interventional radiologic management of renal transplant dysfunction: indications, limitations, and technical consideration. *Radiographics*. 2007;27:1109–1130.
9. Wise A, Cox LA, Long BW. Renal transplant: a review. *J Diagn Med Sonogr*. 1998;14:60–66.
10. National Institute of Diabetes and Digestive and Kidney Diseases. Pancreatic islet transplantation. Accessed August 30, 2021. https://www.niddk.nih.gov/health-information/diabetes/overview/insulin-medicines-treatments/pancreatic-islet-transplantation
11. Wong JJ, Krebs TL, Klassen DK, et al. Sonographic evaluation of acute pancreatic transplant rejection: morphology-Doppler analysis versus guided percutaneous biopsy. *AJR Am J Roentgenol*. 1996;166:803–807.
12. Pellrtito JS, Zwiebel WJ. Ultrasound assessment of native renal vessels and renal allografts. In: Zwiebel WJ, Pellerito JS, eds. *Introduction to Vascular Ultrasonography*. 5th ed. Elsevier Saunders; 2005:611–636.
13. Hall R. *The Ultrasound Handbook*. 3rd ed. Lippincott Williams & Wilkins; 1999.
14. Baxter GM. Ultrasound of renal transplantation. *Clin Radiol*. 2001;56:802–818.
15. Salvador CL, Hartmann A, Åsberg A, Bergan S, Rowe AD, Mørkrid L. Estimating glomerular filtration rate in kidney transplant recipients: comparing a novel equation with commonly used equations in this population. *Transplant Direct*. 2017;3(12):e332.
16. Clayton PA, Lim WH, Wong G, Chadban SJ. Relationship between eGFR decline and hard outcomes after kidney transplants. *J Am Soc Nephrol*. 2016;27(11):3440–3446.
17. Bartlett ST, Schweitzer EJ, Johnson LB, et al. Equivalent success of simultaneous pancreas kidney and solitary pancreas transplantation: a prospective trial of tacrolimus immunosuppression with percutaneous biopsy. *Ann Surg*. 1996;224:440–452.
18. Schwenger V, Korosoglou G, Hinkel UP, et al. Real-time contrast-enhanced sonography of renal transplant recipients predicts chronic allograft nephropathy. *Am J Transplant*. 2006;6:609–615.
19. American College of Radiology Appropriateness Guidelines. Clinical condition: renal transplant dysfunction. Revised 2016. https://acsearch.acr.org/docs/71096/Narrative/
20. American College of Radiology. *ACR Manual on Contrast Media*. American College of Radiology; 2020. https://www.acr.org/-/media/ACR/files/clinical-resources/contrast_media.pdf
21. Lefevre F, Correas JM, Briancon S, Hélénon O, Kessler M, Claudon M. Contrast-enhanced sonography of the renal transplant using triggered pulse-inversion imaging: preliminary results. *Ultrasound Med Biol*. 2002;28:303–314.
22. Lockhart ME, Wells CG, Morgan DE, et al. Reversed diastolic flow in the renal transplant: perioperative implications versus transplants older than 1 month. *AJR Am J Roentgenol*. 2008;190:650–655.
23. American Institute of Ultrasound in Medicine. AIUM practice parameter guidelines for the performance of an ultrasound examination of solid-organ transplants. 2020. http://www.aium.org/resources/guidelines/solidorgantransplants.pdf
24. Lucey MR, Terrault N, Ojo L, et al. Long-term management of the successful adult liver transplant: 2012 practice guideline by the American Association for the Study of Liver Diseases and the American Society of Transplantation. *Liver Transpl*. 2013;19(1):3–26.
25. Nickeleit V. The pathology of kidney transplantation. In: Ruiz P, ed. *Transplantation Pathology*. Cambridge University Press; 2009:45–110.
26. Weinberg K, Telegrafi S. The urinary system. In: Hagen-Ansert SL, ed. *Textbook of Diagnostic Ultrasonography*. 7th ed. Vol 1. Elsevier Mosby; 2012:355–421.
27. Demetris AJ, Minervini M, Nalesnik M, Randhawa PS, Sasatomi E, Demetris AJ. Histopathology of liver transplantation. In: Ruiz P, ed. *Transplantation Pathology*. Cambridge University Press; 2009:111–184.
28. Flint EW, Sumkin JH, Zajko AB, et al. Duplex sonography of hepatic artery thrombosis after liver transplant. *AJR Am J Roentgenol*. 1988;151:481–483.
29. World Health Organization. Coronavirus disease (COVID-19) technical guidance: patient management. https://www.who.int/emergencies/diseases/novel-coronavirus-2019/technical-guidance/patient-management
30. World Health Organization. Clinical management of COVID-19 patients: living guidance. https://app.magicapp.org/#/guideline/j1WBYn/section/L0bkdE
31. Elias M, Pievani D, Randoux C, et al. COVID-19 infection in kidney transplant recipients: disease incidence and clinical outcomes. *J Am Soc Nephrol*. 2020;31(10):2413–2423.
32. Oto OA, Ozturk S, Turgutalp K, et al. Predicting the outcome of COVID-19 infection in kidney transplant recipients. *BMC Nephrol*. 2021;22(1):1–6.
33. Berteloot L, Berthaud R, Temmam S, et al. Arterial abnormalities identified in kidneys transplanted into children during the COVID-19 pandemic. *Am J Transplant*. 2021;21(5):1937–1943.
34. Damjanov I, Perry AM, Perry, KD. *Pathology for the Health Professional*. 6th ed. Elsevier Mosby; 2022:263-280.
35. Kamell R, Kruskal JB, Pomfret EA, Keogan MT, Warmbrand G, Raptopoulos V. Impact of multidetector CT on donor selection and surgical planning before living adult right lobe liver transplantation. *AJR Am J Roentgenol*. 2001;176:193–200.
36. Flak B. Computed tomography of the body. In: Seeram E, ed. *Computed Tomography: Physical Principles, Clinical Applications, and Quality Control*. 4th ed. Elsevier; 2016:383–408.
37. Pomfret A, Pomposelli JJ, Lewis WD, et al. Live donor adult liver transplantation using right lobe grafts: donor evaluation and surgical outcome. *Arch Surg*. 2001;136:425–433.
38. McCormack L, Hany T, Hubner M, et al. How useful is PET/CT imaging in the management of post-transplant lymphoproliferative disease after liver transplantation? *Am J Transplant*. 2006;6:1731–1736.

CHAPTER 25

Point-of-Care

JAVIER ROSARIO

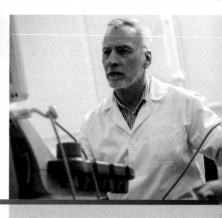

OBJECTIVES

- Define what point-of-care sonography (POCUS) encompasses and how it is being utilized.
- List some of the primary applications for POCUS.
- Explain the common acoustic windows, probe placement, and anatomy seen in certain types of examinations.
- Discuss the importance of evaluating certain anatomical perspectives for possible pathologies.
- Demonstrate the clinical application and sonographic differentiation for certain types of limited examinations.

GLOSSARY

cardiac tamponade mechanical compression of the heart resulting from large amounts of fluid collecting in the pericardial space and limiting the heart's normal range of motion

coaptation refers to normal vein walls touching with compression

deep vein thrombosis (DVT) the formation or presence of a thrombus within a vein

diagnostic peritoneal lavage (DPL) a surgical procedure used to insert a catheter through the abdominal wall and fascia; a syringe is attached to the catheter to aspirate fluid; bleeding is confirmed when gross blood is aspirated; saline solution is injected into the catheter, then it is drained and analyzed

hemothorax accumulation of blood in the pleural cavity (the space between the lungs and the walls of the chest)

hollow viscous injury blunt force injury specific to the gastrointestinal tract system occasionally resulting in perforation and leakage of enteric contents

laparotomy incision made into the abdomen to insert a camera (laparoscope) into the abdomen to visualize and examine the abdomen and pelvic structures and spaces

lumen inside space of a tubular or cellular structure

parietal pleura pleura that lines the inner chest walls and covers the diaphragm

pericardial effusion presence of fluid within the pericardium

pneumothorax the abnormal presence of air between the lung and the wall of the chest (pleural cavity), resulting in collapse of the lung

sonologist clinician who has the ability to both perform and interpret bedside ultrasonography

subcutaneous emphysema presence of abnormal quantities of air within subcutaneous tissue

visceral pleura pleura that covers the lungs

KEY TERMS

bedside sonography

extended focused assessment with sonography in trauma (eFAST)

emergency sonography

focused assessment with sonography in trauma (FAST)

point-of-care ultrasonography (POCUS)

Point-of-care (POC) sonography—or, more commonly, point-of-care ultrasonography (POCUS)—can be characterized into five fundamental clinical categories: diagnostic, monitoring, procedural guidance, resuscitation, and symptom- or sign-based. Using POCUS for *diagnostic imaging* allows the clinician to focus on distinctive organ pathologies based on the patient's presenting signs and symptoms. Having the ability to quickly distinguish between normal and abnormal anatomical findings allows for tapering of differential diagnoses and determining the best management strategies, while still at the bedside or in the immediate clinical setting. Focused ultrasonographic examinations can be performed on any organ or cavity that full diagnostic sonography currently excels at. *Monitoring* of certain conditions via POCUS allows for specific serial sonographic assessments of a patient's known condition or to observe the effects of an ongoing intervention. The use of ultrasound for *procedural guidance* has long been proven to reduce complications and enhance success rates because of its ability to dynamically and in real time visualize and track the procedural process. The adoption of POCUS in the trauma setting specifically during *resuscitation* and evaluation of traumatic injuries during cardiac arrest has been widely accepted and is already a well-established application within the guidelines of traumatic evaluation. The ability to immediately assess and direct emergent interventions by swiftly diagnosing tension pneumothorax, cardiac tamponade, and massive intraperitoneal fluid is well appreciated within the literature.[1-3] Skilled clinicians may be able to determine cardiac standstill, clotting within ventricular and atrial chambers, or visualization of subtle contractions or fibrillation during cardiac arrest and appropriately guide care. A *symptom- or sign-based evaluation* carries many advantages because of its ability to rapidly assess patients with their given signs and symptoms and may help further improve the diagnostic accuracy of the differential diagnosis while also offering the avoidance of ionizing radiation. Today, many subspecialties are using POCUS as a principal tool to their daily practices. The term sonologist may be interchanged or used when clinicians performing these studies are making direct clinical determinations based on their findings.

Throughout the last decade, ultrasound imaging and information systems have continued decreasing in size, while at the same time becoming more sophisticated and increasing their usability. These advances have increased the versatility, mobility, and integration of a broad spectrum of clinical applications in which they can be used. For this reason, sonography is far from being limited to the traditional radiology or cardiology settings. Sonography continues to

establish itself as an indispensable tool in the evaluation of acute patients in many realms within the prehospital, hospital, and in the field/office setting. The technological advancements in instrumentation allow for a less complicated user interface, which increases the ease of operating the equipment and allows for its application in multiple health care settings.

POCUS has been described as sonographic imaging used to enhance and advance patient care during a specific encounter or procedure. Today, POCUS covers a broad spectrum of medical specialties in a variety of settings because it has been shown to improve the safety and effectiveness of patient care.[4-6] Most clinical applications involve answering a specific question, or set of questions, through a focused and directed sonographic examination to better assess if a condition or pathology is present or the cause of the patient's symptoms.

For several decades, the use of ultrasound evaluations for patient care has become an integral part of specialties like emergency medicine (EM) and acute and critical care. Recently, there has been increasing interest on the utility of POCUS for patient care in almost every medical and surgical specialty.[7] Now, POCUS is used to evaluate most body systems and virtually every disease process with great effectiveness (Table 25-1).

This chapter focuses on some of the primary indications for sonographic examination in the POC setting and discusses how sonography is more readily utilized on both acute and stable patients in diverse areas of clinical practice.

PERFORMANCE STANDARDS

Sonography is a well-established, reliable, and noninvasive diagnostic tool. This concept of quick and limited sonographic imaging began spreading in Japan and Europe in the 1970s.[2] However, it was not until the 1980s and 1990s that physicians in the United States began publishing studies focused on the depiction of free fluid or blood within the peritoneal and pericardial spaces to aid with critical trauma settings. Since that time, the use of targeted sonographic assessments has evolved and has been utilized in multiple specialties within medicine. As the medical profession continues to gain experience with sonography and as the technology continues to ascend, its varied use in more clinical applications and in a broader spectrum of disciplines is continually growing as well.[8-10]

The growth in the applications of these sonographic assessments has led to an evolving standard of care developed from what began as best practice for emergency department trauma care to now being included in inpatient units and

TABLE 25-1 **Medical Specialties Currently Using Point-of-Care Ultrasonography Applications[11]**		
Anesthesia	Obstetrics and Maternal–Fetal Medicine	Pulmonary Medicine
Cardiology	Neonatology	Radiology and Interventional Radiology
Critical Care Medicine	Nephrology	Rheumatology
Dermatology	Neurology	Trauma Surgery
Emergency Medicine	Ophthalmology	Urology
Endocrinology and Endocrine Surgery	Orthopedic Surgery	Vascular Surgery
General Surgery	Otolaryngology	
Gynecology	Pediatrics	

TABLE 25-2 Summary of Practice Guidelines for Emergency Sonography[13–15]

1. Typically, emergency sonography is a goal-directed focused examination that answers brief and important clinical questions in an organ system or for a clinical symptom or sign involving multiple organ systems.
2. Emergency sonography is complementary to the physical examination but should be considered a separate entity that adds anatomic, functional, and physiologic information to the care of the emergent patient.
3. Emergency sonography is performed, interpreted, and integrated in an immediate and rapid manner dictated by the clinical scenario. It can be applied to any emergency medical condition in any setting with the limitations of time, patient condition, operator ability, and technology limitations.
4. The information gained from the emergency sonography examination is the basis for immediate decisions about further evaluation, clinical management, and therapeutic interventions.
5. Emergency sonography requires emergency physicians to be knowledgeable in the indications for sonography applications, competent in image acquisition and interpretation, and able to integrate the findings appropriately in the clinical management for each patient.

outpatient settings.[11,12] As with any growth, there are continued challenges to ensure whether its full potential and diagnostic abilities are being reached. These include but are not limited to adequate training, proper documentation and image archiving for all to adhere to, meeting standard competencies, and proper governance or oversight. Once these important criteria have been established and fulfilled, proper continuing education requirements should be met, and the necessary skill sets should continually be developed. Another important factor to successful POCUS adaptation is the utilization of proper equipment. The lack of proper equipment may limit the type of applications available for patient care and the thoroughness of its adoption.

Professional associations have developed recognized guidelines, recommendations, and standardizations for bedside sonographic examinations because POCUS has branched to become an extra set of skills that can enhance the traditional clinical examination. Two well-known associations that have shown strong support to the use of POCUS with websites containing valuable clinical information include the American College of Emergency Physicians and the American Institute of Ultrasound in Medicine.[13,14] A brief summary of the practice guidelines for emergency sonography published by these organizations is given in Table 25-2. Each publication includes standards for personnel, education, protocols, risk management, quality control, quality improvement, and scanning equipment and maintenance.

CLINICAL APPLICATIONS

Emergency Medicine

For several decades, the specialty of EM has established itself as a leader in the education and advancement of POCUS in the clinical setting. Emergency physicians receive training in POCUS since their early training in residency and have established robust guidelines for its use in the clinical setting (Table 25-3).[13] For advanced and expanded applications, there are over 120 EM-focused fellowship programs providing advanced clinical ultrasound training under standardized curricula and guidelines.[15] Whereas most of these guidelines are EM-specific, other medical professionals have taken interest in POCUS applications and use these to formulate their own individual and specialty-specific guidelines. The following sections will further break down these POCUS core applications. However, to obtain more expanded evaluations of specific organ systems, other chapters of this book may be recommended.

TABLE 25-3 Outline of the 12 Emergency Medicine Core Applications

Trauma	Urinary tract
Pregnancy	Deep vein thrombosis
Cardiac/hemodynamic assessment	Soft tissue/musculoskeletal
Abdominal aorta	Ocular
Airway/thoracic	Bowel
Biliary	Procedural guidance

Trauma and Extended Focused Assessment with Sonography in Trauma Examination

The focused assessment with sonography in trauma (FAST) examination originated in the United States in the early 1990s and was likely the original POC rapid sonographic examination.[16,17] The FAST examination and the extended FAST (eFAST) examination are two protocols used to detect sequelae of trauma in emergency sonography. Implementing the eFAST for emergency sonography provides a rapid evaluation tool for the everyday practice of trauma and/or acute patient care, which can significantly improve patient care and triage and balance the differences between medical and surgical emergencies. Following the advanced trauma life support (ATLS) guidelines, it can be utilized in both stable and unstable patients, in conjunction with the physical examinations, resuscitation, and stabilization. The concept behind the FAST examination is based on the fact that many life-threatening injuries cause bleeding in the pericardium, thorax, abdomen, and pelvic regions. The primary purpose of the FAST examination is the methodical search for anechoic free fluid (i.e., blood in the appropriate setting) in the dependent regions of the pericardium, pleural spaces, intraperitoneal spaces, and the retroperitoneum. The primary purpose of the eFAST examination is to extend the search for a pneumothorax in this same scenario.

The eFAST examination can be up to 96% specific for detecting any amount of intraperitoneal free fluid[18] and nearly perfect for the detection of intraperitoneal bleeding significant enough to cause shock and an emergent laparotomy.[19–23] The use of the eFAST examination has made the use of diagnostic peritoneal lavage (DPL) obsolete in the acute evaluation of traumatic injuries. It is important to understand that the eFAST examination does not provide a comprehensive examination of the underlying pathology. However, there are major benefits to performing this noninvasive bedside examination, which can be performed on pregnant women and children, without the risk of exposure to ionizing radiation or nephrotoxic contrast agents.

Patients who benefit from the eFAST examination include those with traumatic injuries who are hemodynamically stable or unstable, patients with worsening clinical status from initial presentation, and those with penetrating trauma with multiple wounds or unclear trajectory. The limitations of this examination include the inability to differentiate blood from other fluids (ascites, urine), difficulty in identifying injured abdominal organ(s), views that may be limited in patients with subcutaneous emphysema or patients with hollow viscous injury (free air in the abdomen), and difficulty examining obese patients.

Learning to perform and interpret the eFAST examination involves understanding how to best visualize the dependent portions of the abdomen and pelvic structures to include the diaphragm on each side, liver, lungs, spleen, kidneys, and urinary bladder. The examination, like all other sonographic examinations, is operator dependent. The following sections will describe these protocols in more depth.

Trauma: Preparation

The eFAST examination protocol is performed with the patient in a supine position. Though not routinely used, patients may also be evaluated in the Trendelenburg position to help free abdominal fluid movement to the most dependent portions.[22] Typically, a 3.0-to-5.0-MHz frequency curvilinear transducer is used to optimally resolve and evaluate the entire organ system for this examination. Alternatively, a similar frequency phased array probe can be used. Normal sonographic findings for this area include the absence of intraperitoneal fluid along with the normal echogenicity typically demonstrated in the abdomen and pelvis. The abdomen and pelvic anatomic regions, common acoustic windows, and scanning planes for the FAST examination and overall emergency assessments are presented below. The basic questions answered by this POCUS examination are highlighted here.

Basic questions to answer in the eFAST examination:

1. Is there free fluid in the *abdomen*?
2. Is there free fluid in the *thorax*?
3. Is there increased fluid in the *pericardium*?
4. Is there evidence of a *pneumothorax*?
5. Is this causing patient symptoms?

eFAST Evaluation Recommended Order (Fig. 25-1)

1. *Right upper quadrant view* (RUQ)
2. *Left upper quadrant view* (LUQ)
3. *Pelvic/bladder view*
4. *Cardiac view* (parasternal long axis or subxiphoid)
5. *Lungs* (right and left)

Trauma: Right Upper Quadrant

The probe is placed in the midaxillary line between the 8th and 12th rib spaces. For this view, liver is used as an acoustic window to avoid the adjacent air-filled bowel. Sagittal oblique and a coronal scanning planes are used with the notch of the probe (also known as the probe marker) placed toward the patient's head. This is an excellent scanning plane for visualizing the hepatorenal space located between the liver capsule and the fatty fascia of the right kidney. When fluid

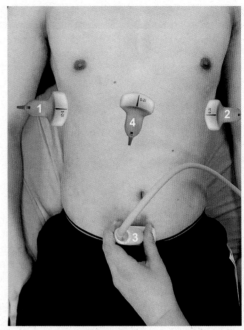

FIGURE 25-1 Coronal placement on the probe in the right upper quadrant between the 8th and 12th intercostal spaces with the patient in supine position.

filled, this potential space is also known as Morison pouch (Fig. 25-2A). Small superior probe sliding or angulations allow for evaluation of the right pleural space. With inferior probe sliding or angulations, the inferior pole of the right kidney and the right paracolic gutter can be surveyed. Both longitudinal oblique and coronal planes can be obtained to view the interface between the liver and right kidney. It is important to follow the lower edge of the liver caudally, until a sufficient view of the hepatic tip is obtained (Fig. 25-2B) because this may be an area of early fluid accumulation in trauma[24] (Fig. 25-2C).

Trauma: Left Upper Quadrant

The scanning orientation for this view is the same as for the right upper quadrant with the probe placed on the left side at the midaxillary line, but now between the 7th and 10th rib space owing to the smaller-sized spleen. This can be a challenging view because of the smaller size of the spleen and often requires the probe to be placed closer to the posterior axillary line for proper visualization. This image plane will demonstrate the relationship of the spleen and left kidney (Fig. 25-3). Both longitudinal oblique and coronal planes should be obtained to view the interface between the spleen and left kidney. With superior probe angulations, the left pleural space can be visualized. The probe should be rotated and angled to follow the renal anatomic plane to visualize fluid, if present, above the left kidney or in the left paracolic gutter.

Trauma: Pelvic Cavity

When the patient is in a supine position, the pelvis is the most dependent part of the peritoneal cavity. A fluid-filled urinary bladder typically provides a proper acoustic window to investigate for fluid anterior to the bladder, the rectouterine space in females, and behind the bladder, the rectovesical

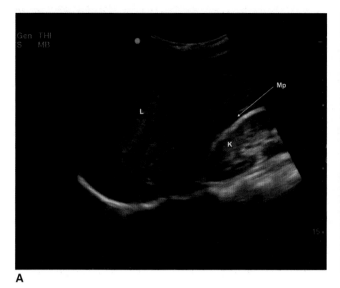

A

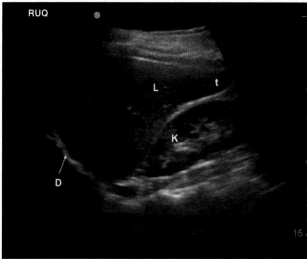

B

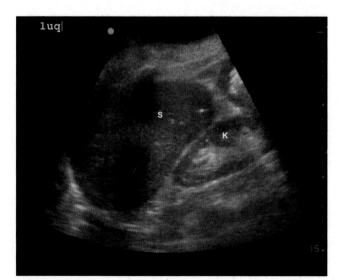

C

FIGURE 25-2 **A:** Coronal plane of right upper quadrant *(RUQ)*. The sonogram demonstrates anechoic free fluid in the Morison pouch *(Mp)*. The liver *(L)* is noted anterior to the right kidney *(K)*. **B:** Longitudinal image of right upper quadrant. The full extent of the liver is displayed. The hepatic tip *(t)* annotates the inferior aspect of the liver. **C:** Coronal plane of the right upper quadrant showing evidence of free fluid in the hepatic tip.

FIGURE 25-3 Coronal image of the left upper quadrant. The sonogram demonstrates the relationship of the spleen *(S)* and the left kidney *(K)*. There is no anechoic blood or fluid identified.

pouch in males or rectouterine pouch in females (Fig. 25-4A). A Trendelenburg position may be used if satisfactory images are not obtained with the patient in a supine position. Evaluation of the pelvic cavity using both longitudinal and transverse planes should be performed.

If free fluid is present, it is most often located superior and posterior to the urinary bladder and the uterus.[22] Be aware of the possibility of a distended or overly distended urinary bladder being mistaken for free fluid in the pelvis (Fig. 25-4B).

Trauma: Pericardial Effusion

Sonography of the pericardial space to evaluate for fluid collections is a well-documented practice performed in a variety of clinical settings, especially in trauma.[25-28] For this examination, the clinician can continue with the curvilinear probe. If needed, a phased array (commonly known as cardiac probe) can be used. In the absence of fluid collections, the parietal and visceral pericardia are typically indistinguishable from each other, visualized as a combined hyperechoic line. The subxiphoid window is the most commonly used

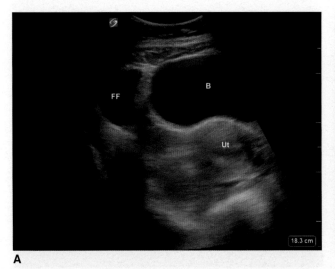
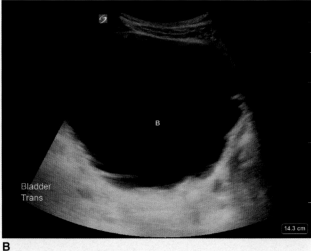

FIGURE 25-4 **A:** Transverse plane, midline pelvis. There is a collection of anechoic free fluid *(FF)* noted lateral to the bladder *(B)* and superior to the uterus *(Ut)*. **B:** Transverse plane, midline pelvis. The urinary bladder *(B)* is distended. Care should be taken not to mistake the anatomy as a large free fluid collection.

and convenient method to sonographically visualize cardiac structures, including the pericardial sac. With the transducer oriented transversely and angled superiorly in the subxiphoid region/window, the four-chamber cardiac image can be recognized. The liver serves as an acoustic window, and often, a small segment of the liver can be visualized in the near field. The base of the heart, including both atria, should be located to the patient's right and is slightly posterior. The apex of the heart is located more to the patient's left and is situated more anteriorly and inferiorly. If any of the four chambers are not fully visualized within this acoustic window, an attempt should be made to adjust the transducer orientation, so that it is almost parallel to the skin of the anterior torso. In certain patients, especially those with abdominal distention or pain, the subxiphoid window may not be optimal; therefore, familiarity and mastery of all cardiac scanning planes, discussed below, will help to rule out any pericardial or cardiac pathology.[29]

The pattern of two hypoechoic ribs interrupted by a central hyperechoic pleural line is referred to as the bat sign (two ribs forming the wings superiorly and the pleural line forming the body inferiorly) (Fig. 25-5A). A sonographic finding that is often noted, which can be seen with cardiac imaging, is the presence of up to 10 mL of normal serous physiologic fluid and sometimes a small amount of pericardial fat.[30]

The detection of pericardial fluid is evident by its hypoechoic presence surrounding the heart (located within the pericardial sac) (Fig. 25-5B, C). Small effusions are smaller than 1 cm in size, moderate effusions between 1 and 2 cm in size, and large effusions are greater than 2 cm in size.[31] In the acute traumatic setting, the hypoechoic echogenicity can be consistent with blood such as what is found within the cardiac chambers. When present, blood collections will most often be noted in the subxiphoid window between the liver and right side of the heart. In the parasternal window, blood will most often be noted superior to the right ventricle, or even posteriorly as it outlines the free wall of the left atria and ventricle (Fig. 25-5D). The descending aorta may be used as a landmark for the posterior aspect of the pericardial sac and is often another site for pericardial fluid collections. Hemorrhage has the ability to quickly collect between the

visceral and parietal space, which causes hypotension owing to the cascade of increasing intrapericardial pressure, which in turn causes a decrease in right heart filling, which then causes decreased LV stroke volume. Even small pericardial effusions can set this cascade in motion, causing tamponade (see the section on Cardiac Examination below). In the event of a pericardial effusion, it is imperative that patients receive immediate treatment to avoid the life-threatening clinical course with the onset of tamponade physiology.

Trauma: Pneumothorax

Sonography is more sensitive than chest radiography or physical examination for the evaluation of a pneumothorax.[32-36] The eFAST examination is easily mastered by proper identification of the normal anatomy and its appearance during normal respiration. The curvilinear probe can be used for this examination by decreasing the depth of penetration to allow for better resolution. Alternatively, a high-frequency linear probe can be used for even better visualization of the pleura and ribs (Fig. 25-6A). The parietal pleura can be visualized in the near field, distal to the echogenic ribs with distal shadowing, which serves as a sonographic landmark. Air has a high acoustic impedance; therefore, the air-filled lung covered by visceral pleura is a potent reflector of the ultrasound beam, blocking sound penetration deeper into the chest and producing a bright linear interface that moves with respiration.

With the transducer oriented toward the patient's head at the intercostal space, one or two ribs will be identified, and subcutaneous tissue and muscle can be visualized between the rib shadows. Finally, the pleura itself is located within 1 cm of depth from the rib space, with the parietal pleura immediately distal to the chest muscle. The pleura is identified by its pronounced superficial echogenic line.

There are two techniques that can be used for the eFAST examination of the parietal and visceral pleura to rule out a pneumothorax. The first is to identify the normal back-and-forth movement of the pleural layers, corresponding to the patient's respirations. This is known as the "sliding sign." The second is to identify comet tail artifacts at the pleural interface.[32,34] The sliding should be readily appreciated

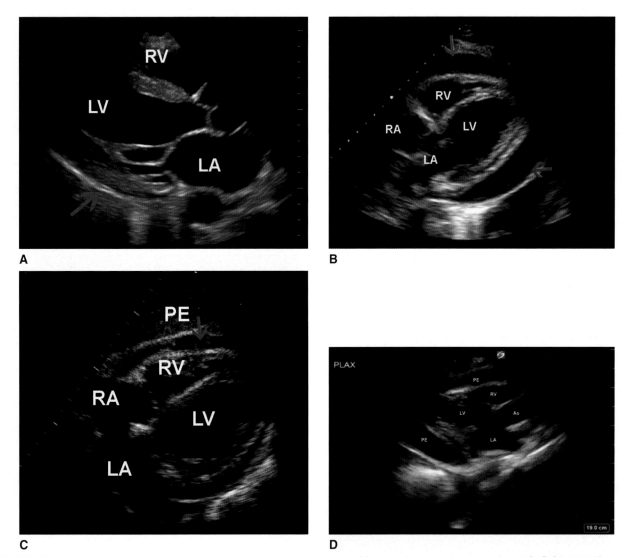

FIGURE 25-5 **A:** Parasternal long axis. The sonogram demonstrates the close proximity of the parietal and visceral pericardia *(arrow)*. **B, C:** Subxiphoid four chambers. The sonograms demonstrate a pericardial effusion *(arrow)*. **D:** Parasternal long axis *(PLAX)* showing pericardial effusion *(PE)*. *Ao,* aortic root; *LA,* left atrium; *LV,* left ventricle; *PE,* pericardial effusion; *RA,* right atrium; *RV, right ventricle.* (**A:** Courtesy of Zonare Medical Systems, Mountain View, CA.)

once the echogenic reflectors (parietal pleura and visceral pleura) just distal to the ribs are seen in real time with the visceral pleura sliding back and forth under the parietal pleura with patient respiration (Fig. 25-6B). The sliding sign and moving comet tail artifacts are synchronized with respiratory movement. Absence of the sliding sign indicates that there is a possible pneumothorax. Finding a sliding sign can immediately rule out a pneumothorax at this particular location; however, multiple areas should be evaluated, especially in the absence of the sliding sign. Although this imaging finding can be present along any and all acoustic windows in the upper thorax, with the patient in the supine position, the more superior location is the common site for a pneumothorax.

A second sonographic technique used to identify a pneumothorax is with the application of M-mode (motion mode), which is used to detect motion along a select line of interrogation (line of site). In this technique, motion creates waves or curves, and stillness creates straight horizontal lines. A tracing is displayed by placing the M-mode cursor on the pleura between the ribs. The M-mode will reveal parallel lines above the pleural line corresponding to the motionless parietal tissue of the chest wall. In the presence of sliding, a homogeneous granular (sandy) pattern is seen below the pleural line because of the corresponding constant motion of the underlying lung. This normal lung sliding motion has the appearance of a sandy beach intersecting with rolling waves and is known as the "seashore sign" (Fig. 25-6C, D).[33,34] In the case of pneumothorax with absent normal sliding, the M-mode reveals a series of parallel horizontal lines, suggesting complete lack of movement both over and under the pleural line. This pattern is known as the "barcode sign" or "stratosphere sign."[33-35] Although absent lung sliding suggests pneumothorax, it can occur in the presence of many other conditions, such as main stem intubation, acute respiratory distress syndrome, or pleural adhesions.[37]

If a pneumothorax is suspected, one should attempt to document the size or extent of the pneumothorax by localizing the point on the chest wall, where the normal lung pattern can be seen. The "lung point" sign determines where the visceral pleura begins to separate from the chest wall at the margin of the pneumothorax. At this point, both absent

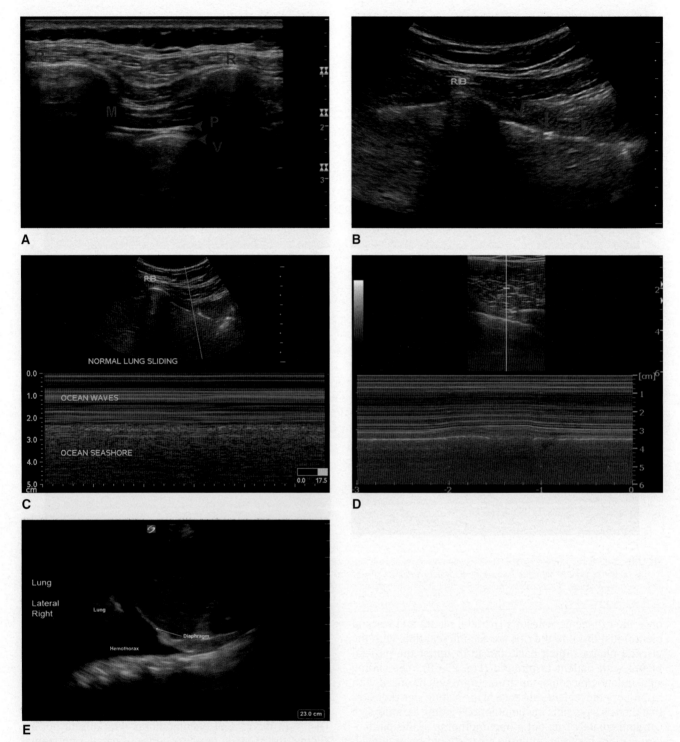

FIGURE 25-6 A: Transverse plane of the upper thorax. The echogenic ribs *(R)* can be seen with normal distal shadowing. The intercostal muscles *(M)* are seen between the ribs. Distal to the ribs, the parietal pleura *(P)* lining the chest wall is seen, and distal to this is the visceral pleura *(V)*. The parietal pleura and visceral pleura should be visualized sliding over each other with respiration *(arrowheads)*. **B:** Longitudinal plane of the upper thorax. The echogenic rib *(RIB)* can be seen with its normal distal shadowing. The parietal and visceral pleura are noted in close proximity *(red arrows)*. On normal individuals, a sliding motion caused by the movement of the mobile visceral pleural during respiration along the static parietal pleura to slide over one another with patient respirations can be observed in real time. **C** and **D:** M-mode (motion mode) tracing of the upper thorax. The grayscale image corresponds anatomically with the M-mode tracing. The nonmobile superficial structures of the chest, ribs, and muscle above the pleural line correspond to the "ocean waves" on the M-mode display. The moving parietal and visceral pleura are noted in the "ocean seashore" area, with normal air in the lungs corresponding to the inhomogeneous M-mode tracing below. **E:** Coronal plane. The sonogram shows a hemothorax in the costophrenic angle and within the pleural cavity as the diaphragm is located inferiorly. (**B–D:** Courtesy of Zonare Medical Systems, Mountain View, CA. **D:** Courtesy of Mathew Ahern, Salt Lake City, UT.)

and normal lung sliding can be demonstrated between the pneumothorax and the normal lung.[27] At the lung point position during expiration, no sliding is seen; but, with inspiration, the lung inflates and the visceral pleura moves up in apposition with the parietal pleura beneath the probe and sliding is again seen.[35] The ability to demonstrate the alternating lung sliding and absence of lung sliding within the same field is diagnostic of pneumothorax with a sensitivity of 66% and specificity of 100%.[26–28]

The incidence of a hemothorax after blunt or penetrating chest injury can be noted sonographically as an anechoic or hypoechoic fluid collection localized to the costophrenic angle.[36,37] Visualizing an intact diaphragm inferiorly will allow for the certainty that the fluid collection rests within the pleural cavity (Fig. 25-6E). If there is a pleural cavity fluid collection, the lung may sometimes be identified as a triangular structure superior to the diaphragm and should display rhythmic movement corresponding to the patient's respirations.

Thorax

Lung sonography is effective in deciphering between the differential diagnosis of acute pulmonary edema and acute respiratory failure. Sonographic examinations help practitioners differentiate between pneumonia, hemothorax, lung contusions, and pneumothorax, and better identify the best location for tube thoracostomy or thoracentesis guidance. During the COVID-19 pandemic, lung sonography has proven useful in the diagnosis and management of patients from the point of triage to intensive care.

Biliary Examination

Basic Questions to Answer for the Biliary Examination

1. Is there evidence of gallstones?
2. Is there biliary wall thickening?
3. Is there fluid surrounding the biliary wall/pericholecystic fluid?
4. Is there a sonographic Murphy sign?

POCUS is a reliable and valuable tool in identifying biliary tree disease in the acute patient.[40] Using sonography avoids ionizing radiation, allows for a rapid assessment, and is highly sensitive and specific for gallbladder disease.[40] The evaluation of the entire biliary tree allows for the assessment of cholelithiasis, the presence of biliary sludge within the gallbladder lumen, gallbladder wall thickening, pericholecystic fluid, a more accurate sonographic Murphy sign, and/or bile duct dilatation.

The absence or presence of gallbladder stones is often the primary purpose of utilizing POCUS to evaluate the biliary tree for acute cholecystitis. However, acalculous cholecystitis should be considered with the appropriate clinical presentation, including sonographic findings of gallbladder wall thickening, pericholecystic fluid, and a sonographic Murphy sign. The gallbladder should be evaluated in both the longitudinal and transverse planes by sweeping from the neck inferiorly to the fundus superiorly. The gallbladder wall should be measured, and the gallbladder fossa must be examined for fluid collections and edema.

Biliary Examination Preparation

As is the case with most abdominal examinations, a 3.0-to-5.0-MHz frequency curvilinear transducer is used to optimally evaluate the entire organ. Alternatively, a similar frequency phased array probe can be used. Ideally, the patient should be fasting 6 to 8 hours prior to sonographic assessment because typically this avoids the gallbladder from contracting. However, in the POC setting, this may not always be an option because it would make the gallbladder appear contracted and harder to find.

Because the gallbladder is not fixed to body walls like other gastrointestinal organs, it can have a variety of positions in the right upper quadrant, and the patient can be repositioned from a supine into a left lateral decubitus position, to allow for better visualization of the gallbladder by moving it more to the midline. This repositioning can also aid in visualizing mobile stones or sludge as they shift location with patient movement (Fig. 25-7A). If possible, the patient can be asked to hold the right arm above the

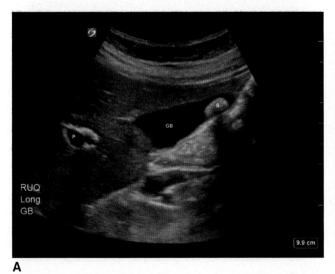

A

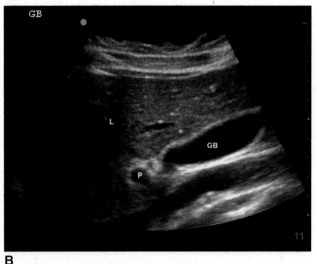

B

FIGURE 25-7 A: Longitudinal plane of the gallbladder *(GB)* demonstrating a gallbladder stone *(S)* within. **B:** Longitudinal plane of the *GB* demonstrating its relationship to the liver *(L)* and portal vein *(P)*.

head to widen the intercostal spaces. If the ribs are still blocking the view, the patient can be asked to hold a deep breath to further widen the intercostal spaces. Additionally, the probe can be rotated slightly obliquely to align with the intercostal spaces.

Biliary Imaging

To identify the location of the gallbladder, the probe can be positioned on the patient's right in the anterior–axillary line at the level of the 10th to 11th intercostal spaces or around the mid-epigastric region, with the indicator facing the patient's head. The gallbladder neck is attached to the main lobar fissure (MLF), thus this structure can be used as a landmark to find the gallbladder. Once the MLF is identified, you can tilt (or fan) the tail of your probe in either direction slowly to find the gallbladder (Fig. 25-7B).

Identifying the common bile duct (CBD) and intrahepatic ducts can be challenging, often requiring significant practice and training in POCUS. As seen in Figure 25-8, when the gallbladder is found, the portal vein would be seen in the leading edge of the screen, often referred to as the "exclamation sign." The portal triad (CBD, hepatic artery, and portal vein) can be seen in the short axis. This view is also known as the "Mickey Mouse Sign," with the CBD and hepatic artery, as the "ears," and the portal vein, as the "head," making up the structure (Fig. 25-8).

The CBD is located anterior to the main portal vein in the porta hepatis. The inside diameter of the CBD should be measured and assessed for choledocholithiasis or any masses. Color Doppler should be used to decipher the difference between any similarly appearing vascular structure and the CBD. Additional information about the performance of biliary ultrasound, images, and its findings can be found in Chapter 8.

Renal Examination

Patients presenting with undifferentiated flank pain can be rapidly assessed using POCUS with good accuracy and without the exposure to radiation or contrast injection.[40–42] Focused renal sonography is often utilized to detect and grade hydronephrosis and can be used to assess for renal calculi with or without obstruction of flow.

> **Basic Questions to Answer for the Renal Examination**
> 1. Is there evidence of hydronephrosis?
> 2. Is there evidence of intrarenal stones?
> 3. Is there evidence of obstruction by ureteral bladder jets?

Renal Examination Preparation

For this examination, the patient can initially be in the supine position. However, there may be the need to roll the patient on the left or right side to position the probe directly over the kidneys. As is the case with other peritoneal and retroperitoneal examinations, a 3.0-to-5.0-MHz frequency curvilinear or similar frequency phased array transducer should be used to optimally evaluate the renal system. Occasionally, the patient may need to be asked to maintain a certain breathing pattern (breath holds or exhalation to allow better visualization of the kidneys). Figure 25-9 shows several important structures that need to be identified when performing ultrasound of the kidneys.

Renal Imaging

The examination is started with the patient in supine position and the probe indicator toward the patient's head at the right midaxillary line around the 10th to 11th intercostal space and swept from a lateral-to-medial perspective. Occasionally, the transducer may need to be rotated 10 to 20 degrees counterclockwise to get in-between the rib spaces and optimize the view. Once the longitudinal view is complete, the kidney should be centered on the screen, and the transducer should be rotated 90 degrees counterclockwise, with the probe indicator pointing posteriorly and swept from the superior to inferior poles to obtain the short-axis

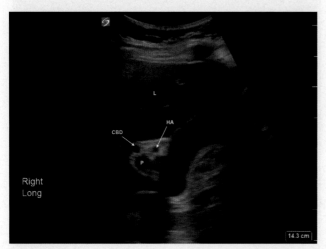

FIGURE 25-8 Short-axis evaluation of the portal triad, which includes the common bile duct (CBD), the hepatic artery (HA), and the portal vein (P). L, liver.

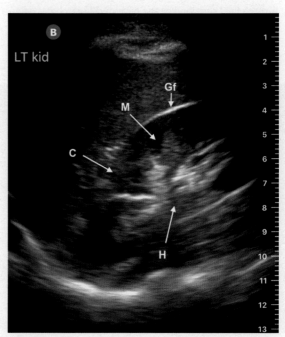

FIGURE 25-9 Longitudinal plane of the left kidney indicating the location of important anatomic structures. C, cortex; Gf, Gerota fascia; H, renal hilum; M, medullary pyramids.

views. In the majority of cases, the liver can be used as an acoustic window in the right upper quadrant with the occasional need to turn patients on a left lateral decubitus position to image through the right flank.

The technique for scanning the left kidney is very similar to that of the right kidney. However, the left kidney is positioned slightly superior and posterior in comparison to the right kidney owing to the smaller-sized spleen. The probe is similarly placed with the probe indicator toward the patient's head between the 8th and 10th intercostal spaces of the left posterior axillary line. The same techniques of counterclockwise rotation and probe tilting may be needed to visualize in-between the rib spaces. Later, with the kidney centered, the probe is rotated 90 degrees counterclockwise to achieve the short-axis views. As with the right side where the liver is used as an acoustic window, on the left side, the spleen is often used as a sonographic window.

It should be noted that the right kidney is often slightly larger and more inferior and anteriorly placed when compared with the left kidney. Gerota fascia and perinephric fat appear hyperechoic, whereas the normal renal cortex should appear homogenous and hypoechoic in comparison with both the hepatic and splenic parenchyma. The renal sinus normally appears hyperechoic because of its fat consistency. The proximal ureter located in the renal hilum is typically not well seen sonographically unless it is distended.

An enlarged fluid-filled or anechoic area within the renal sinus is indicative of hydronephrosis and can be seen progressing up and into the renal calyces. Hydronephrosis is categorized into mild, moderate, and severe (Fig. 25-10A–C). Renal calculi can be seen with sonography; however, its sensitivity for detection can sometimes be challenging. Renal stones are typically hyperechoic and should display posterior acoustic shadowing because of their high densities.

Urinary Bladder

As is the case with the rest of the renal evaluation, a 3.0-to-5.0-MHz frequency curvilinear transducer is used to evaluate the bladder. Typically, focused bladder studies are performed to assess for total bladder or postvoid volume; calculi; urinary catheter placement; and, in the setting of suspected obstructive uropathy, for the presence or absence of ureteral jets. If a suspected kidney stone is lodged within the ureter or ureterovesical junction, there may be an absence of ureteral jets on the obstructed side when scanning the bladder. The right and left ureters enter the urinary bladder in the inferior and posterior aspects at the level of the trigone. When the bladder is distended and filled with anechoic fluid, its contents act as an excellent window for a detailed survey of the bladder's intraluminal contents.

The bladder can be visualized from the suprapubic window approach in a sagittal plane. Beginning at midline,

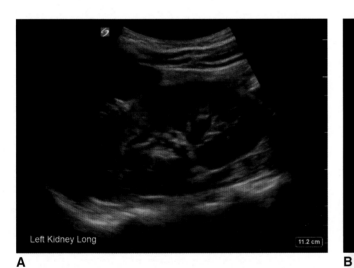

A

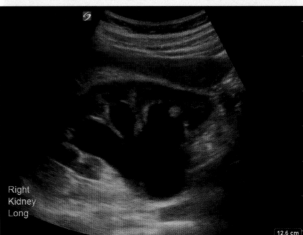

B

C

FIGURE 25-10 Longitudinal planes of kidneys showing different grading of hydronephrosis **A:** Mild hydronephrosis. **B:** Moderate hydronephrosis. **C:** Severe hydronephrosis.

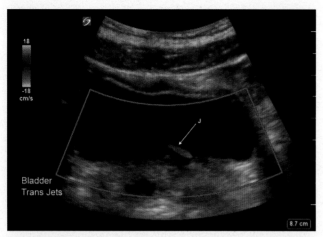

FIGURE 25-11 Transverse plane of the urinary bladder showing evidence of a left ureteral jet (*J*) indicating no obstruction.

the transducer can be swept toward the patient's right and toward the patient's left to demonstrate both midline and parasagittal aspects of the bladder. With the patient in the same supine position, the transducer can be rotated 90 degrees counterclockwise to obtain the transverse plane at the superior edge of the pubic symphysis and the ultrasound beam can be directed posteriorly and sweep up superiorly.

To evaluate for ureteral jets properly, the probe should be in the transverse plane of the bladder and the color Doppler scale set to about 10 to 20 cm/second. Alternatively, the power Doppler function can be used. Urine is not continuously released into the bladder, and the release actually occurs at regular intervals. Therefore, it may take up to 5 to 10 minutes to see if there are any ureteral jets (Fig. 25-11).

A bladder volume can easily be acquired by measuring the distance from wall to wall in three orthogonal planes. Bladder volume = (0.75 × width × length × height). Occasionally, urinary catheter placement can be observed while the bladder is distended as the more echogenic intraluminal echoes of the bladder are seen within the anechoic fluid in the bladder, thus aiding in confirmation of proper catheter placement (Fig. 25-12). Additional information on renal ultrasonography can be found in Chapter 12.

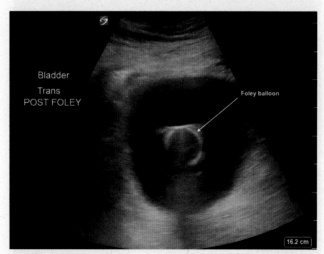

FIGURE 25-12 Transverse plane of the urinary bladder confirming placement of the foley catheter.

Cardiac Examination

> **Basic Questions to Answer for the Cardiac Examination**
> 1. Is there evidence of abnormal ejection fraction?
> 2. Is there evidence of pericardial fluid/tamponade?
> 3. Is there evidence of fluid overload?
> 4. Is there evidence of chamber size abnormalities?
> 5. Is there evidence of aortic root enlargement? (optional)

Bedside POCUS echocardiography in the emergency or acute care setting is a rapid and dynamic method of evaluating patients suspected of having some form of life-threatening impaired cardiac disease prompted by the patient's presentation. Its primary applications are directed toward the detection of at least five direct observations or abnormalities. These include the ability for detecting pericardial effusions, obtaining a qualitative left ventricular ejection fraction, ventricular size equality, aortic root diameter examination, and inferior vena cava (IVC) diameter with breathing variation.[37] In addition, they also include the detection of cardiac motion in patients with pulseless electrical activity or ventricular dysrhythmias during cardiac arrest.[30,43–46] In the trauma setting, cardiac sonography is a defined component of the FAST examination.

Cardiac Examination Preparation

Bedside echocardiography is usually completed using a low-frequency phased array probe, also known as a cardiac probe. The patient can typically be positioned in a supine or left lateral recumbent for better visualization of each cardiac portion during the examination. The subxiphoid, parasternal, and apical regions provide the three common acoustic windows used in emergency echocardiography (Table 25-4).

Cardiac Imaging

There are five main views obtained in POCUS echocardiography: a parasternal long-axis (PLAX), a parasternal short-axis (PSAX), an apical four-chamber (A4C), a subcostal long-axis (SCLA or IVC view), and a subcostal four-chamber (SC4C or subxiphoid) view. As with most conventional sonography, pertinent findings should optimally be confirmed in at least two planes. However, time constraints, patient acuity, patient mobility, and patient habitus may limit certain views.[37,47] In the case of images obtained in emergency POCUS echocardiography, there may be variation in the use of the probe indicator. Some POCUS experts will use an EM convention for cardiac imaging with the probe marker oriented to the patient's right, which keeps the anatomic right on the screen-left, as is the convention for other ultrasound (US) imaging.[48] This is in contrast to the image and probe orientation utilized in traditional cardiology-performed ultrasonography but has been recognized as an accepted modification and may be conceptually easier, particularly when performing these cardiac assessments as part of an integrated examination such as FAST or the rapid US for shock and hypotension (RUSH).[49] For simplicity, the views shown in this section will maintain cardiology ultrasound orientation.

Cardiac Effusion and Tamponade

Pericardial tamponade is an established finding often presenting in certain medical or traumatic conditions and

TABLE 25-4 Common Acoustic Windows in Emergency Echocardiography

Acoustic Window	Probe Position	Probe Placement	Anatomy	Sonographic Image
Subxiphoid	Just inferior to the xiphoid tip of the sternum; transducer angled superiorly toward left shoulder			
Parasternal long axis	Third to fifth intercostal space, left side of sternum, directly over heart		Right ventricle / Right atrium / Left ventricle / Left atrium	Right ventricle / Aorta / Left atrium / Left ventricle
Parasternal short axis	Same position as parasternal long axis; rotate transducer 180 degrees clockwise	Right ventricle / Left ventricle	Right ventricle / Left ventricle / Left atrium / Right atrium	
Apical	Patient in left lateral decubitus position; transducer placed at point of maximum impulse on the lateral chest wall (often just below the nipple)			

can be rapidly recognized sonographically. It is classically demonstrated by visualizing an anechoic space surrounding the heart (pericardial effusion) with the collapse of the right ventricle (RV) or during diastole. Findings of an effusion should prompt the clinician to look for tamponade physiology. As pressures inside the pericardium elevate, bedside imaging will show a progression of findings beginning with collapse of the right atrium (RA) in systole, collapse of the RV in diastole, and finally left ventricle (LV) collapse.[50] In slightly more advanced imaging, tamponade physiology can also be demonstrated on echocardiography by exaggerated respiratory variation of ventricular in-flow velocities. Another sign of tamponade is the loss of respiratory variation in the IVC. This is sonographically noted by the loss of collapse in the anteroposterior plane of the IVC with forceful inhalation or a "sniff" test performed by the patient (Fig. 25-13).

Cardiac Ejection Fraction

Emergency physicians and properly trained practitioners on POCUS echocardiography can accurately make a qualitative assessment of the global left ventricular ejection fraction (LVEF), usually categorized as "hyperdynamic" (LVEF > 65%), "normal" (LVEF 50% to 65%), "moderately depressed" (LVEF 30% to 50%), or "severely depressed" (LVEF < 30%).[51,52] Sonography is clearly superior in assessing normal versus reduced LV function when compared with chest radiography, physical examination, electrocardiogram, and blood chemistries.[43] For example, in a patients presenting with dyspnea, poor LV function often coupled with a dilated or plethoric IVC and B-lines on thoracic images may indicate a fluid overload and congestive heart failure.

The POCUS evaluation and visual determination of LVEF can be obtained using the PLAX as an initial window.

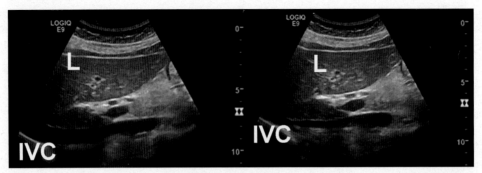

FIGURE 25-13 Longitudinal plane of upper abdomen. Normal respiratory variation is seen when comparing the two longitudinal sonograms of the upper abdomen. The left image displays the inferior vena cava (*IVC*) with expiration and the right image demonstrates the normal 50% collapse of the *IVC* with inspiration. *L*, liver.

This view includes a good portion of the LV, including the septum, apex, and posterior LV wall, and provides good visualization of the anterior leaflet of the mitral valve (MV), allowing for the assessment of E-point septal separation (EPSS), which can be used to determine the ejection fraction (EF). The anterior movement of the MV toward the septum can be used for visual estimation or measured quantitatively using M-mode to measure the smallest distance from valve tip to the septal wall during diastole filling (Fig. 25-14). This is a surrogate measurement of EF. This is a measure of filling of the ventricle, which if intact will push the leaflet toward the septal wall. Generally, measurements above 7 mm correlate with a depressed EF and measurements above 10 mm indicate severely depressed EF. One can assess the overall cardiac contractility by qualitatively observing the relative percentage of change in the movement of ventricular endocardial walls from relaxation during diastole to contraction during systole. A uniformly and circumferentially contracting endocardium is indicative of good function. Additional views may be obtained for further global EF assessment.

Cardiac Activity

Additional primary applications of emergent cardiac sonography include the evaluation of gross cardiac activity in the setting of cardiopulmonary resuscitation. Although the SC4C view is commonly used during cardiac arrest, almost any

of the described views can be used in the determination of cardiac activity. It is recommended that clinicians choose a view or position that will not interrupt the ongoing resuscitation efforts.[53] Occasionally, the use of echocardiography during cardiac arrest may help with adequate positioning of compressor hands during chest compressions to avoid obstructing the outflow tract and compressing the ventricles. Most recently, some emergency departments are including the use of transesophageal echocardiography (TEE) for the evaluation of cardiac arrest. TEE can be an option to the properly trained and credentialed physician to investigate multiple aspects of cardiopulmonary resuscitation.

In the setting of a pulseless patient, the lack of cardiac activity carries a grave prognosis. Multiple possibilities relating to low flow states can contribute to the presence of electrical activity without a palpable pulse. The sonographic evaluation of cardiac structures can allow for the rapid dynamic visualization of heart wall contractions because they may occur undetected. Some studies have indicated that ultrasound may aid in the identification of occult ventricular fibrillation (Vfib), also known as fine Vfib, in apparent cases of asystole cardiac arrest. Having this immediate diagnostic tool allows for the prompt correction of decision-making, which may be a potential life-saving event.[54]

Inferior Vena Cava and Volume Status

Recently, there exists some controversy over the correlation of IVC measurements to other quantitative measures of RA pressure; however, the qualitative assessment of the IVC may be clinically helpful, especially when it is plethoric or completely collapsed.[55] Assessment of the IVC can be important to the management of patients in shock and is now a routine part of cardiac assessments. IVC examination with sonography offers a quick noninvasive estimation and can help direct the assessment of volume status and possibly volume responsiveness.

Using the subxiphoid window, the IVC in a longitudinal view can be used to correlate the right atrial pressure and elevated central venous pressure based on distention and collapsibility with each respiration.[56,57] Using the liver as an acoustic window, this view is ideal to evaluate the hepatic veins emptying into the IVC and the IVC emptying into the right atrium. When a low intravascular volume is present, the percentage of collapse of the vessel will be proportionally higher than in intravascular volume-overload states. This phenomenon can be measured quantitatively with the caval index formula (Fig. 25-15). The closer the caval index percentage is to 100, the closer the IVC is to complete collapse, indicative

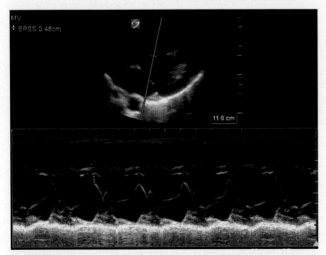

FIGURE 25-14 The parasternal long-axis plane is used to measure the excursion of the mitral valve toward the septal wall. This is known as the E-point septal separation (*EPSS*).

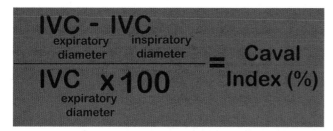

Volume Overload = Increased intravascular volume, minimal collapse

Volume Depletion = Diameter of IVC will decrease >50%

FIGURE 25-15 Inferior vena cava (*IVC*) formula used to calculate volume overload.

of volume depletion. With the same thought process, the closer the caval index is to 0, the lesser is the collapse with inspiration, suggestive of volume overload. When cardiac tamponade is suspected, this interrogation will allow for a sensitive assessment of whether intrapericardial pressure exceeds the right atrial and central venous pressure. With minimal to no inspiratory collapse after deep inspiration, cardiac tamponade should be considered.

The patient should be in a supine position with the transducer in a subxiphoid acoustic window and the probe marker pointing toward the patient's head; this will allow for a longitudinal plane of section of the IVC as it enters into the right atrium. In this view, the proper calculations can be made 2 cm from where the IVC enters the right atrium. This measurement can also be obtained using the motion mode or M-mode during inspiration and expiration. The ability to dynamically determine patient clinical status and when to intensify, stop, or continue diuretic therapy is paramount.[58-60]

Cardiac Chambers

In healthy patients, the RV is a low-pressure chamber with a thin wall and will be relatively smaller than the LV. As pressures increase in the pulmonary arteries owing to acute or chronic obstructions, the RV may begin to increase in size because of its high compliance. If the ratio approaches 1:1 when compared with the LV, a diagnosis of RV dilation can be made (Fig. 25-16). In patients presenting with

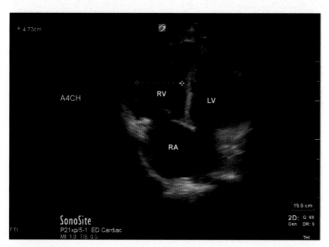

FIGURE 25-16 Apical four-chamber view of the heart showing evidence of right ventricle (*RV*) enlargement in comparison to the left ventricle (*LV*). RA, right atrium.

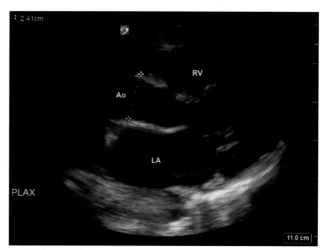

FIGURE 25-17 The parasternal long-axis plane is used to measure the diameter of the aortic root (*Ao*) from outer wall to inner wall. *LA*, left atrium; *RV*, right ventricle.

undifferentiated chest pain, shortness of breath, hypotension, or syncope, the presence of any RV dilatation should raise the diagnostic suspicion of an acute pulmonary embolism (PE).[56] This evaluation is typically done in the A4C view, which allows for direct comparison of both ventricular chambers.

Another structure in which the chamber size is commonly evaluated is the aortic outflow tract or aortic root. This structure is best visualized in the PLAX view. Aneurysmal disease of the thoracic aorta predisposes to aortic dissection.[56] The aortic root should be measured from the outside wall to inside wall at the widest visible point during diastole (Fig. 25-17). A thoracic aortic root of over 4.5 cm is considered aneurysmal and one less than 4.0 cm is considered normal.

Aortic Examination

Located medially, the abdominal aorta is a retroperitoneal vascular structure with an anechoic lumen. When clinically suspected, POCUS can be utilized to assess for abdominal aortic aneurysm (AAA) or dissection. There are several aortic catastrophic pathologies that should be recognized such as aneurysms, thrombosis, rupture of the vessel, or even dissection of the intimal layer.[61] The aorta can be evaluated with POCUS from the root, arch, and descending portions in the cardiac views through to the xiphoid process to the umbilicus in abdominal views. The abdominal aorta commonly contains small intraluminal calcifications, has a pulsatile flow, is surrounded by retroperitoneal fat, and is located medial to the IVC in the abdomen. It is paramount to recognize the difference between the abdominal aorta and the IVC with assurance (Fig. 25-18).

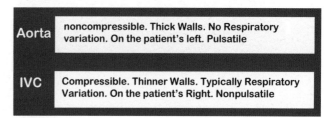

Aorta	noncompressible. Thick Walls. No Respiratory variation. On the patient's left. Pulsatile
IVC	Compressible. Thinner Walls. Typically Respiratory Variation. On the patient's Right. Nonpulsatile

FIGURE 25-18 A comparison of aorta and inferior vena cava (*IVC*) characteristics.

Aorta Preparation

With a low-frequency curvilinear probe in hand, the patient can start the examination in a supine position. To begin this examination, one must determine whether the thoracic or abdominal portion of the aorta is of concern. In certain circumstances, it is recommended to evaluate the entirety of the aorta, such as the case with dissection.

Aortic Imaging

For evaluation of the abdominal aorta, the patient should be in a supine position with the transducer in the subxiphoid acoustic window (midline) and the probe marker pointing toward the patient's right. To identify the abdominal aorta, the vertebral spine can be used as an initial anatomic landmark. The aorta lies anterior and to the patient's left in relation to the vertebral spine with the IVC found on the anatomic right. In this transverse plane, the aorta can be followed from the proximal aspect superiorly in the abdomen down to the bifurcation of the iliac arteries, more inferiorly. The maximal diameter should be obtained in at least three positions in the abdomen (proximal, mid, distal) to identify AAAs. A great landmark for the proximal portion of the aorta is the celiac axis. However, this can be a technically difficult view to obtain, and some clinicians choose the highest point at which the aorta can be measured in the epigastric abdomen. The middle, or midportion, of the aorta is usually right below the renal arteries, the most common area for AAAs to happen. Finally, the distal aorta can be observed at the level of the inferior mesenteric artery (IMA) (Fig. 25-19A–C). An additional view that needs to be obtained is the bifurcation of the distal aorta to the iliac arteries. Then, additional investigation can be made by rotation of the probe by 90 degrees with the indicator toward the patient's head. In this view, the aorta can be visualized as a single tubular structure as the probe slides inferiorly (Fig. 25-19D). Typically, an aortic aneurysm is diagnosed when the diameter from outer wall to outer wall is greater than 3.0 cm. The dilatation of all three layers of the aorta (intima, media, and adventitia) by definition describes a true aneurysm[62] (Fig. 25-20). The presence of any fluid collection proximal to this structure should also be noted.

If the thoracic aorta is of concern, investigation can begin by obtaining a measurement of the aortic root as seen in the cardiac PLAX view (Fig. 25-17). An additional, more advanced, view is the suprasternal view where the probe is placed at the superior sternal notch. This view allows visualization of the aortic arch (Fig. 25-21). This may require hyperextension and lateral rotation of the patient's neck to allow for probe manipulation and optimal visualization.

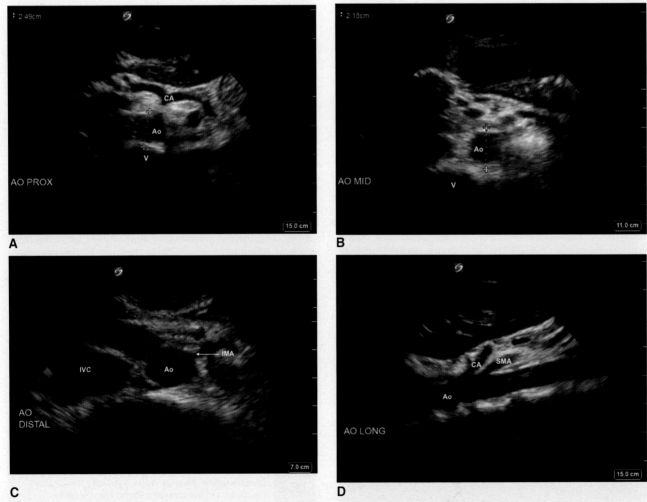

A

B

C

D

FIGURE 25-19 **A:** Transverse plane of proximal aorta *(Ao)* showing its relationship to the celiac artery *(CA)* with the vertebral spine *(V)* as the anatomical landmark. **B:** Transverse plane of the mid-aorta *(Ao)* with the vertebral spine *(V)* shown as the anatomical landmark. **C:** View of the distal aorta *(Ao)* with its vertebral shadow *(V)* and the anatomical location of the inferior mesenteric artery *(IMA)*. Notice the difference in location, size, and shape of the inferior vena cava *(IVC)*. **D:** Longitudinal plane of the aorta *(Ao)* with the adjacent proximal arteries, celiac artery *(CA)* and superior mesenteric artery *(SMA)*.

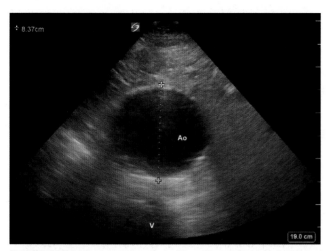

FIGURE 25-20 Transverse plane view of the mid-aorta *(Ao)* with evidence of a large (8.37 cm) abdominal aortic aneurysm. *V,* vertebral body.

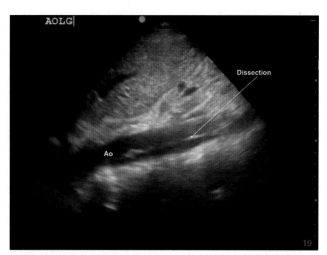

FIGURE 25-22 Longitudinal plane view of the proximal and mid-aorta *(Ao)* showing a bright echogenic line within the vessel, indicative of a classic "dissection flap" or intimal tear.

When dissection is suspected, the aorta can be examined in its entirety for determination of an intimal flap. This flap can be seen as an additional, pulsatile, hyperechoic line within the anechoic lumen of the aorta. Visualization of this intimal flap can sometimes be seen more clearly in the longitudinal plane (Fig. 25-22).

Vascular Access

Sonography is an effective tool to help guide the insertion and placement of vascular catheters into both arterial and venous structures. Tracking of the needle in real time helps reduce mechanical complications inherent to catheter placement leading to complications, such as pneumothorax or arterial puncture. High-frequency linear transducers aid in providing excellent resolution of vascular anatomy and differentiation of proximal structures. The safety profile of ultrasound utilization for venous access over anatomical access has been well established in the literature.[63–66] Arteries and veins have well-defined sonographic characteristics, which distinguish them from other anatomical structures and between themselves. For instance, arteries are less collapsible with pressure, pulsatile, and round, whereas veins are not as round, are easily compressible with pressure, and can vary in dimension with inspiration and expiration (Fig. 25-23A, B).

Vascular Access Preparation

Prior to insertion of the needle, the area should be scanned first to identify the most proximal and superficial insertion sites and to identify vital structures surrounding the vascular structure of interest. Vascular access can be further divided into three modalities: peripheral, central, or arterial. The determination of which modality is needed will be dependent on the patient's needs. When there are multiple failed attempts by palpation by appropriately trained personnel, ultrasound-guided peripheral insertion is typically pursued. There are multiple indications for central access, but it is typically suited for critically ill patients who require frequent blood draws, vasoactive agents (e.g., vasopressors or vasodilators), medication drips, or when central venous pressures need to be accurately monitored. Arterial lines are usually suited for constant monitoring of systemic blood pressure, interventional catheter insertion and/or arterial blood gas analysis.

Vascular Procedures and Imaging

For peripheral veins and upper-extremity arterial access, the patient can be positioned in a supine or sitting position with the desired arm externally rotated. Commonly, the distal upper arm and proximal forearm are used for ultrasound evaluation and vein selection is based on the size of the vessel, surrounding structures, and depth.

Although the best detail will be obtained in the longitudinal plane to track the needle's course, the transverse plane is often used, so as to prevent the probe from sliding away from the desired vessel and into an undesired neighboring one (e.g., puncturing an artery instead of a vein). The vessel of interest should be centered in the transverse view on the screen to allow for depth perception and identification of adjacent structures. The lowest depth setting that allows for good visualization of the vessel should be used. The depth of the vessel selected should also take into account the length of the needle being used. Once identified, the needle can be inserted at a 45-to-60-degree angle and the needle tip should be identified on the screen by slowly sweeping and subtly tilting the transducer. The needle should be advanced only a few millimeters at a time, while continually

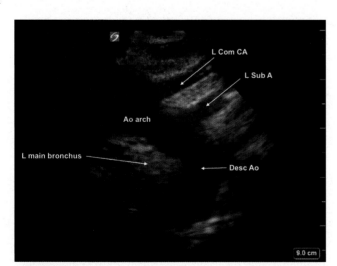

FIGURE 25-21 Transverse plane suprasternal view or the aortic *(Ao)* arch and associated vessels. *Desc Ao,* descending aorta; *L Com CA,* left common carotid; *L main bronchus,* left main bronchus; *L Sub A,* left subclavian artery.

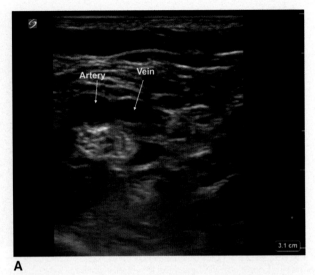

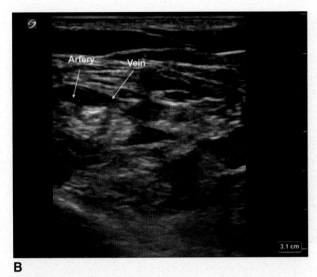

A   **B**

FIGURE 25-23 A: Transverse plane of forearm vessels. Notice the different appearance of the walls between the artery and the vein. **B:** Transverse plane of same forearm vessels with application of mild compression. Notice the collapsibility of the vein in comparison to the artery.

and sweeping the transducer proximally to the patient while always visualizing the needle tip. When the needle tip encounters the vessel of interest, the more anterior aspect of the vessel will be seen to "tent" or displace the anterior wall inferiorly toward the lumen, followed by the vessel being punctured and the needle being placed within the lumen. At this time, the angle of insertion can be decreased to allow for further placement of the needle within the lumen. Proper placement should be evidenced by both a "flash" of blood within the catheter and by a smooth insertion of the catheter (Fig. 25-24). Any resistance of passage should be concerning for inappropriate or incomplete placement.

Central venous access follows similar preparation and probe manipulations. However, this procedure is considered sterile, and proper safety measures should be undertaken prior to this procedure being attempted. The three most common locations for access are the internal jugular vein, subclavian vein, and femoral vein.

Deep Vein Thrombosis

The clinical diagnosis of lower-extremity deep vein thrombosis (DVT) is often hindered by its variable and unpredictable presentation, as well as the reality that many nonthrombotic conditions produce signs and symptoms suggestive of DVT.[67,68] However, the relatively superficial location and the lack of overlying skeletal structures or bowel gas allow for the seemingly simplistic sonographic evaluation of peripheral veins.[69,70] The limited venous graded compression emergency protocol pursues areas in which turbulence poses the greatest risk for developing thrombosis. This graded compression evaluation includes the sonographic imaging of the common femoral vein, the saphenous junction, the proximal deep and superficial femoral vein, and the popliteal vein. Of importance, the superficial femoral vein is part of the deep venous system, but to avoid confusion, it should simply be referred to as the *femoral vein*.

Deep Vein Thrombosis Preparation

To begin the examination, place the lower extremities in a dependent position. This can be done with the patient in a supine position and elevating the head of the bed approximately 15 to 40 degrees (reverse Trendelenburg). The leg

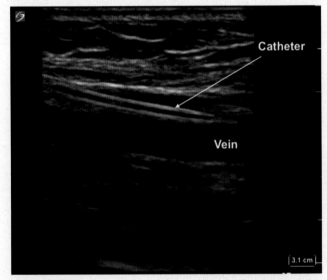

FIGURE 25-24 Longitudinal evaluation of a vessel after successful catheter placement. This view can be used to confirm adequate insertion into the vascular system.

in question should be abducted and rotated externally with slight flexion of the knee, also known as frog leg position. A high-resolution linear array transducer with a frequency ranging between 5.0 and 9.0 MHz should be utilized.

Deep Vein Thrombosis Examination

The targeted evaluation of the deep venous system has two components: a primary and a secondary. The primary component uses grayscale imaging and a transverse plane to visualize the vein and to use the transducer to apply systematic, intermittent compression. Very little pressure is needed to collapse veins because their walls are thin and venous pressure is low. Venous patency is confirmed with the release of pressure, and in the presence of a clot, coaptation does not occur because the vein will typically not collapse.

The secondary component is the integration of Doppler techniques into the exam, assessing for flow characteristics and confirming venous patency in the setting of a suspected clot. In normal veins, color flow should fill the vessel lumen from wall to wall (Fig. 25-25A). In the presence of

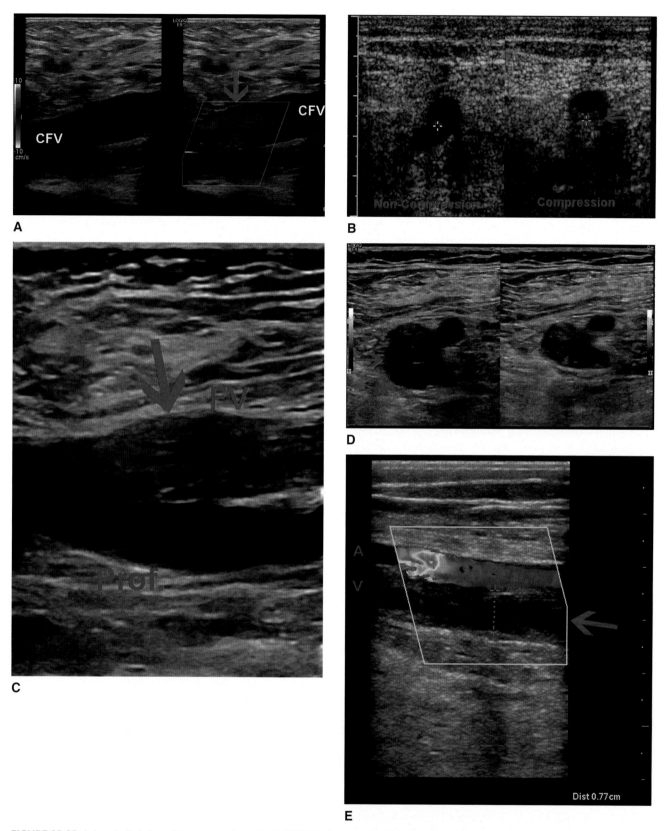

FIGURE 25-25 A: Longitudinal plane of the common femoral vein *(CFV)*. The image on the left demonstrates the grayscale image. The image on the right displays normal intraluminal filling of the vein, with color Doppler *(arrow)*. **B:** Transverse superior femoral artery *(A)* and vein *(v)*. The image on the left shows the vessels without compression. The image on the right displays the position of the superior femoral vessels but with compression, and there is a change in shape and the vein completely collapses *(arrow)*. **C:** Longitudinal plane of the superior femoral vein *(FV)* and the profunda vein *(Prof)*. The sonogram shows an echogenic intraluminal clot *(arrow)* seen in the femoral vein. **D:** Transverse mid-femoral vein. The image on the left corresponds to a noncompressed vein with an echogenic clot in its lumen *(arrow)*. The image on the right demonstrates the inability of the lumen walls to coapt with compression *(arrow)*. **E:** Color Doppler imaging through the superior femoral vein *(V)* and artery *(A)*. The artery displays good vascular flow *(blue color pixels)*. In the femoral vein, there is no Doppler shift; thereby, it lacks color flow *(arrow)*.

clot, areas of flow disturbances within the venous lumen can be seen as blood flows around the obstruction, which does not allow the lumen of the vein to fill with color.[71,72]

With the transducer perpendicular to the skin surface, at a level just inferior to the inguinal canal, the common femoral vein and femoral artery should be noted in a transverse plane. With mild pressure applied to the transducer, on the surface of the leg, the normal venous lumen should completely collapse with immediate coaptation of its walls (Fig. 25-25B). The degree of pressure required varies and will depend on the depth and location of the vein. The artery often becomes misshaped but should not readily collapse.

Once the common femoral vein and artery are identified, transverse, systematic, and intermittent compression should be performed every 1 to 2 cm through the level of the superior femoral vein, past the junction of the common femoral, deep femoral, and superficial femoral vessels.[73] Transverse compression should then continue into the popliteal fossa, at the level of the popliteal vein, and through the popliteal trifurcation.

In the presence of clot, an intraluminal hyperechogenicity is often seen, which leads one to suspect thrombus (Fig. 25-25C). Because an acute clot is often anechoic or hypoechoic and an older or chronic clot is more echogenic, the true hallmark diagnosis for DVT rests in the inability to completely compress the lumen of the vein (Fig. 25-25D).[69,70] In the longitudinal plane, color Doppler should be applied to any venous segment in question of a successful compression or one containing internal echoes. If an obstructive process is located in the vein, color will not persistently fill the entire lumen (Fig. 25-25E).

Obstetrics

First Trimester Evaluation

Female patients often present to the emergency department with pain and bleeding. Vaginal bleeding within the first trimester occurs in approximately 25% of all pregnancies.[74-76] It is in this setting that POCUS has become of value in assessing the first trimester pregnancy. The main utility of POCUS in this setting is to effectively rule-in a viable intrauterine pregnancy (IUP). Panebianco et al. found that when an endovaginal (EV) or transvaginal (TV) approach was taken with patients presenting to the emergency department with early first trimester pregnancy complications, emergency room length of stay was significantly shortened. When the examination was indeterminate in the emergency department and patients were then seen in the radiology setting, the patients' length of stay was no longer than if they had foregone the TV examination in the emergency department and waited for their study to be completed in radiology.[77] This section will describe some of the basics of the first trimester POCUS examination, but more in-depth reading and practice are recommended for adequate diagnostics and evaluation.

First Trimester Preparation

Using POCUS in this trimester with the serum beta-human chorionic gonadotropin (β-hCG) helps to distinguish among many differential diagnoses of first trimester pathology, as outlined in Table 25-5.[78] Imaging can be performed with a transabdominal (TA) or TV sonography, to improve resolution. For earlier first trimester imaging, a TV probe is used with the patient in a lithotomy position. There are some limitations for the use of TV probes in certain settings that

TABLE 25-5	**Terminology Used in the First Trimester of Pregnancy**
Viable pregnancy	Findings consistent with the potential to result in liveborn baby.
Nonviable pregnancy	Findings do not support the result of a liveborn baby, including ectopic and failed IUP.
Intrauterine pregnancy of uncertain viability	Findings show an intrauterine gestational sac without a heartbeat or definitive signs of pregnancy failure.
Pregnancy of unknown location	Findings of a positive pregnancy test with no definitive findings of IUP or ectopic pregnancy via transvaginal ultrasound.

IUP, intrauterine pregnancy.

are dependent on national recommendations on probe cleaning and disinfection. It is understood that the resolution and details obtained with TV probes can be superior to TA probes in the early stages of pregnancy. It is important to recognize that despite the benefits of POCUS in identifying some of these key abnormalities, the misinterpretation of these studies can lead to interventions that damage pregnancies that might have had normal outcomes.[79] This section aims to describe some of the basic findings but should not be used as a comprehensive guide on how to manage first trimester pregnancy presentations.

First Trimester Imaging

The transducer should be covered with a sheath prior to its use and inserted into the vaginal canal until the longitudinal plane of the uterus is noted in the midline. Movement of the transducer from the midline plane into the right lateral and left lateral aspects of the pelvic cavity will allow for visualization of the entire uterus and the adnexal structures. Angling the transducer posteriorly and more inferiorly allows for visualization of the cervical canal and the pouch of Douglas. These structures should be well examined for the possibility of a cervical ectopic pregnancy, missed abortion, or spontaneous abortion and for free fluid in the posterior cul-de-sac. By rotating the transducer counterclockwise in a 90-degree plane, the uterus and adnexa can be examined in the orthogonal transverse plane, from their inferior to superior aspects, with high resolution.

Thickening of the endometrium in the midline of the uterus in the first stage of pregnancy can typically be noted in the fourth gestational week. However, a thickened endometrium (>17 mm) does not assure an intrauterine pregnancy or rule out any pregnancy-related pathologies that may be present.[77-80] At about 5 weeks gestational age, the gestational scan shows a small cyst-like fluid collection with well-rounded edges and no visible contents inside located within the central echogenic portion of the uterus.[78] The yolk sac, a circular structure seen within the gestational sac measuring 3 to 5 mm in diameter, typically appears at about 5½ weeks of gestation (Fig. 25-26). The fetal pole embryo is first seen adjacent to the yolk sac at about 6 weeks, at which time the heartbeat is present as a flickering motion.[78] At this stage in pregnancy, the cardiac activity should be noted between 110 and 175 beats/minute.

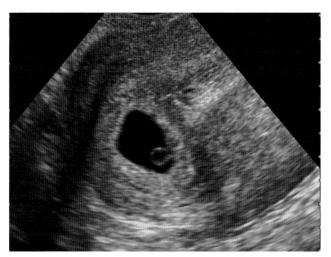

FIGURE 25-26 The yolk sac within an early gestational sac. This is actually the secondary yolk sac (secondary umbilical vesicle). (Image and legend courtesy of Paula Woletz in Stephenson MA. *Diagnostic Medical Sonography Obstetrics and Gynecology.* 3rd ed. Lippincott; 2012.)

There is considerable overlap between β-hCG levels in viable intrauterine pregnancies, nonviable intrauterine pregnancies, and ectopic pregnancies; hence, a single β-hCG measurement does not distinguish reliably among them.[81] Given all these limitations, a hemodynamically stable woman with presumptive diagnosis of ectopic pregnancy should probably not be treated with abortive medications or surgical management with such limited amount of data and known variation.[78]

In symptomatic patients presenting to the emergency department, ectopic pregnancy is a true concern to be ruled "out" or ruled "in." During the fifth week of gestation in the setting of a positive β-hCG and no sonographic evidence of an intrauterine pregnancy, ectopic pregnancy should be considered.[82] Visualizing a fluid-filled structure in the endometrial canal does not rule out an ectopic pregnancy because these can also be signs of an intrauterine pseudo-sac, which is often noted with ectopic pregnancies. It is necessary to only make the diagnosis of an intrauterine pregnancy when a yolk sac is noted within this fluid collection presumed to be the gestational sac. Even with the assurance of a gestational sac containing a yolk sac, the presence of a heterotopic pregnancy is possible.[83,84] A gestational mean sac diameter of 25 mm or greater without an embryo is abnormal, representing pregnancy failure. A visible heartbeat could be seen by about 6 weeks and is usually clearly depictable by 7 weeks. If this is observed, the probability of a continued pregnancy is better than 95%.[85] If a previously noted gestational sac has been documented and the patient presents with bleeding after 8 to 9 weeks and no fetal cardiac activity can be visualized, this becomes concerning for an missed abortion (Fig. 25-27A, B). A missed abortion or blighted ovum

A

B

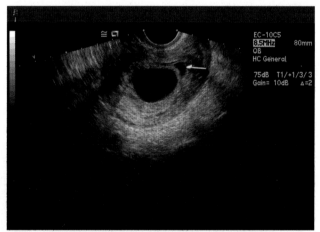

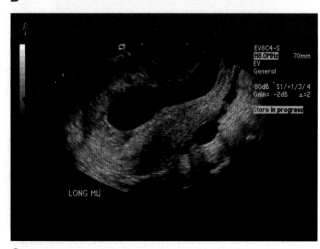

FIGURE 25-27 A: Transabdominal image of a blighted ovum. **B:** Endovaginal image of the same empty sac. Note the beginning of sac separation from the uterine wall. **C:** Impending abortion. The low position of the gestational sac and the open cervix indicate imminent expulsion of the uterine contents. (Image and legend courtesy of Paula Woletz in Stephenson MA. *Diagnostic Medical Sonography Obstetrics and Gynecology.* 3rd ed. Lippincott; 2012.)

C

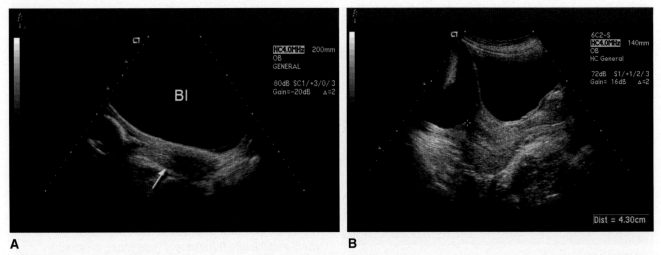

FIGURE 25-28 Impending abortion. **A:** The position of the gestational sac, lower uterine segment, and open cervix *(arrow)* can indicate an imminent expulsion of the uterine contents or the cervix and lower uterine segment is compressed with an overfull bladder. *Bl*, bladder. **B:** An appropriately filled bladder. The calipers indicate the cervical length measurement between internal and external os. The gestational sac is imaged superior to the internal os and the cervix demonstrates a slight opening. (Image and legend courtesy of Malka Stromer in Stephenson MA. *Diagnostic Medical Sonography Obstetrics and Gynecology.* 3rd ed. Lippincott; 2012.)

will typically present sonographically with a misshaped gestational sac with absence of a fetal pole or cardiac activity (Fig. 25-27C).

POCUS can also evaluate for other pathology that may explain the patient's symptoms, such as ovarian torsion or cysts, gestational trophoblastic disease, or early placental disorders.

Third Trimester Evaluation

Third trimester evaluations and emergencies can be time-critical presentations. A prompt evaluation of both the fetal and maternal safety often includes the rapid

assessment of fetal viability, fetal heart rate, fetal lie, placental parameters, and amniotic fluid, specifically in the setting of trauma. POCUS allows for the rapid evaluation of all of these parameters with no invasiveness to the fetus or radiation exposure. By placing the transducer in a longitudinal plane slightly superior to the symphysis pubis, the lower uterine segment should be visualized in the midline demonstrating the cervical canal (Fig. 25-28), which should measure greater than 3 cm in length.[81,86,87] The cervical canal should be evaluated for competency insofar as the absence of funneling of the internal os as well as its length (Fig. 25-29).

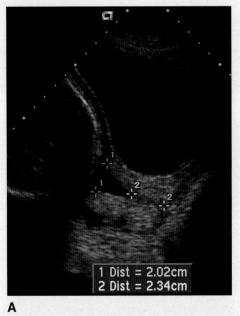

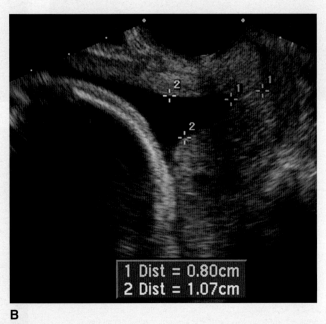

FIGURE 25-29 Short funneled cervix. **A:** Transabdominal view demonstrates a dilated cervix measuring 20.2 mm (+1 calipers) at the internal os. The length of the residual closed cervix is 23.4 mm (+2 calipers). **B:** Endovaginal view of the cervix (in another case) demonstrates a dilated cervix measuring 10.7 mm dilated (+2 calipers) at the internal os. Residual closed cervix measures 8.0 mm (+1 calipers). (Image and legend courtesy of Malka Stromer in Stephenson MA. *Diagnostic Medical Sonography Obstetrics and Gynecology.* 3rd ed. Lippincott; 2012.)

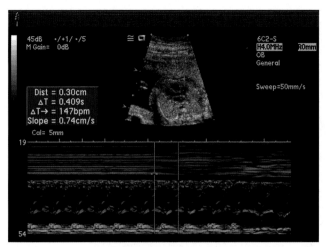

FIGURE 25-30 A normal M-mode tracing obtained through the aortic root. (Image and legend courtesy of Marium Holland and Joan M. Mastrobattista in Stephenson MA. *Diagnostic Medical Sonography Obstetrics and Gynecology*. 3rd ed. Lippincott; 2012.)

The fetal lie can be confirmed by locating the fetal head and following the spine down to the fetal pelvis. By locating the fetal thorax, cardiac activity can be quickly ascertained by its persistent contractions ranging between 120 and 160 beats/minute. By utilizing the M-mode technique (sonography displays echo amplitude and shows the position of moving reflectors), an accurate heart rate can be found on placing the cursor through the chest and cardiac structures and counting the beats per minute (Fig. 25-30).

Amniotic fluid should be noted in all four quadrants of the uterus, with pockets deeper than 2 cm when measured in the anterior to posterior plane. The placenta should be identified and evaluated for any sonographic sign of separation or retroplacental clot, or intraplacental anechoic areas representing possible subchorionic hematoma (Fig. 25-31).[88]

Superficial and Soft Tissues

The skin and many soft-tissue structures are relatively superficial, making them an ideal candidates for sonographic evaluation.[89,90] Foreign body–related injuries may be difficult to visualize with other imaging modalities depending on their compositions. The echo patterns or sonographic characteristics of foreign bodies will depend on the size, nature, area of implant, and importantly the length of time within the body, which allows for different inflammatory aspects to develop and sonographic artifacts to appear. Cellulitis is commonly clinically seen because it is the most commonly encountered type of soft-tissue infection and has a well-known sonographic appearance.[91,92] The hyperemic pattern of the inflamed subcutaneous fat surrounded by the anechoic fluid along the connective tissue planes is distinctive for inflamed tissue. Given the clinical presentation, cellulitis often exhibits along with the sonographic characteristics of cellulitis, POCUS can be further utilized to rule out abscess formation in these areas. Sonography can also provide for the dynamic evacuation and drainage of an abscess or aid in the dynamic guidance of foreign body removal.

A linear array transducer is typically used for superficial imaging because of its greater resolution at shallower depths. If an open wound is being examined, it should be covered prior to the application of gel or the transducer. Because most superficial structures are imaged in the near field, it may be helpful to use a copious amount of gel or a standoff pad to allow for the area of interest to be imaged in the most optimally focused zone of the transducer.

Soft-Tissue Imaging

Because sonography is able to provide a three-dimensional description of the size, shape, and location of subcutaneous lesions, it has become an integral tool in the bedside evaluation of skin and subcutaneous lesions. Using a high-frequency and high-resolution transducer, the sonographic characteristics about a lesion's quality (solid, cystic, complex) and inner structure (inhomogeneous, calcific, fluid filled, necrotic, hypoechoic, hyperechoic, homogenous) can quickly be obtained (Fig. 25-32). Color and power Doppler imaging are routinely emphasized for their ability to evaluate inflammation levels, angiogenesis that is often related to benign versus malignant lesions, and to

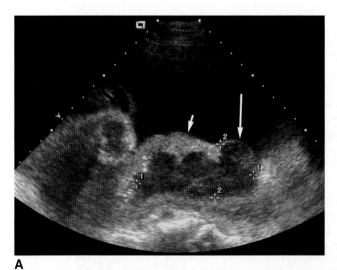

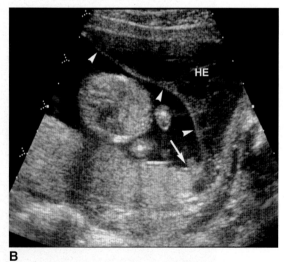

A **B**

FIGURE 25-31 Placental abruption. **A:** There is a hypoechoic, retroplacental hematoma *(long arrow and calipers)* lifting the edge of the placenta *(short arrow)*. **B:** The hypoechoic hematoma *(HE)* lifts the edge of the placenta *(arrow)* under the chorionic membrane *(arrowheads)*. (Image and legend courtesy of Malka Stromer in Stephenson MA. *Diagnostic Medical Sonography Obstetrics and Gynecology*. 3rd ed. Lippincott; 2012.)

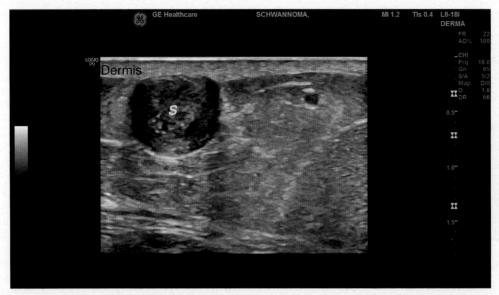

FIGURE 25-32 Transverse view of a superficial lesion just posterior to the dermis in the left lateral neck. Upon gross specimen dissection, this mass was found to be a schwannoma *(S)*.

distinguish between cystic and solid lesions.[93,94] To sum up the main dermatologic clinical applications, they include but are not limited to benign tumors, skin cancer, vascular anomalies, cosmetic field, nail disorders, and inflammatory diseases (Fig. 25-33).[95] The reader is recommended to refer to Chapter 27 for more information and image examples.

Lymph Node Imaging

Sonography can assess the size, shape, echogenicity, borders, and vascularity both within and proximal to many lymph node chains and within the lymph nodes themselves. Normal lymph nodes are distributed along the course of lymphatic vessels and can be divided into the medulla and cortex, within a think fibrous capsule. The central medulla is hyperechoic because of lymphatic cords and sinuses, whereas the outer cortex is hypoechoic because of lymphoid follicles. Vascular supply is obtained via the central fatty area known as the hilum, which can readily be appreciated in the normal lymph node with both color and power Doppler imaging.

A high-frequency transducer should be utilized for the best resolution of the superficial structures, unless the lymph node of interest is located too deeply, in which case a curved array transducer may be more advantageous. POCUS not only allows for a thorough lymphatic assessment but is also readily utilized for the guidance of fine-needle aspiration or core-needle biopsy.[91] The reader is recommended to refer to Chapter 27 for more information and image examples.

Regional Anesthesia

As with other subspecialties in medicine, anesthesiologists began seeing the potential of POCUS decades ago. The ability

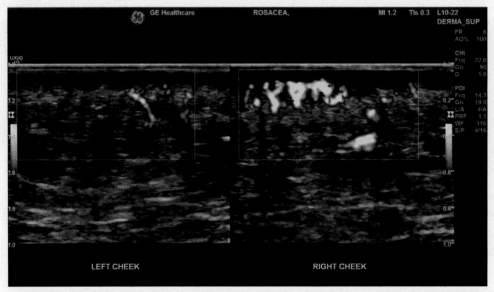

FIGURE 25-33 Rosacea. Images of the left and right cheeks demonstrate this chronic skin condition. Rosacea is characterized by superficial dilated blood vessels highlighted using power Doppler imaging.

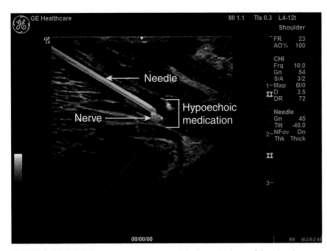

FIGURE 25-34 Pain management nerve block procedure of the shoulder. Guidance for the injection of nerve numbing medication is a common point-of-care sonography application.

to evaluate complex and varied anatomy as well as to dynamically evaluate an injection site significantly improved patient care in this field.[96] Today, POCUS is being used by anesthesiologists to offer guidance for difficult venous access, epidural space identification, especially in cases of difficult anatomy, to better delineate nerve plexuses for regional anesthesia and for cardiac cases using transesophageal echocardiography. The ability to dynamically visualize in a cross-sectional aspect the anatomical structures of interest during invasive procedures can enhance the process with both normal and variant anatomy. Nerve block failure can also be decreased by utilizing dynamic imaging while placing local anesthesia. By actually observing the contact of local anesthetic with the nerve, there is more of an assurance the correct nerve is being anesthetized and avoidance of inadvertent vessels being punctured. The scope of regional nerve blocks has also been adopted in acute care settings, such as the emergency department, where a nerve block may potentially benefit and improve patient care when there is no immediate access to anesthesiology for this procedure (Fig. 25-34).

Pain Management

Pain management providers have been convinced of the benefits related to sonography-guided anesthesia to manage chronic pain. The application of ultrasound in pain management has increased at an incredible rate both on the therapeutic and on the diagnostic level with uses for intraoperative analgesia and postoperative pain control.[97] Although magnetic resonance imaging (MRI), computerized tomography (CT), and fluoroscopy all have their places in advanced pain management practices, POCUS has been recognized for its ability to enhance performance with its dynamic guidance, adding to the therapeutic effectiveness. Furthermore, sonographic technologies and procedures continue to evolve and improve strengthening the diagnostic capabilities of POCUS within pain management. Given that musculoskeletal disorders are a common finding for pain physicians, a clinical diagnosis based on patient physical examination, history, signs, and symptoms can be more accurately obtained with the use of sonography. Bedside sonographic imaging allows for

transient conditions to be realized with manipulation and adjustments that static imaging does not allow for.[98] As sonography continues to develop new techniques and becomes more accessible and easier to use, it opens up many more treatment and diagnostic opportunities for pain management.

Musculoskeletal

Rheumatology and Sports Medicine

Goal-directed musculoskeletal sonography is increasingly being used as a bedside tool in aiding to diagnose pathologies in musculoskeletal structures, such as injuries of the muscles, tendon, ligament, bursa, bony structures, cartilage, joints, and subcutaneous tissue. Another large benefit to utilizing sonography with musculoskeletal symptomatic patients is the real-time guidance of procedures that can be greatly enhanced by ultrasound's dynamic ability.[98]

Sonography can add both a different and complimentary dimension to imaging when compared with the traditional modalities of plain radiography, CT, and MRI. Advantageously, POCUS does not require radiation, is financially feasible, often readily available, and an option for patients with a contraindication to MRI, including those with a pacemaker or other surgical hardware. For instance, some neuromas can be visualized and confirmed in the clinical setting using sonography with the same efficacy as MRI offers.[99]

One of the most appealing advantages to utilizing sonography over other imaging modalities in musculoskeletal issues is its ability to dynamically evaluate structures at will (see Fig. 18-15). This can readily improve pathologic interpretation when combined with clinical relevance in answering targeted patient-care questions while manipulating the structure under question. Dynamic joint assessment can also allow for a more thorough depiction of joint and tendon movements and stability and structural abnormalities, ligamentous injury, and mechanical impingement.

Swollen and tender joints are a common clinical symptom in the musculoskeletal practice. In recent years, musculoskeletal POCUS has played a pivotal role in the detection, diagnosis, and monitoring of commonly occurring rheumatic diseases in terms of early detection, grading, and treatment of synovitis. Many studies have validated its superiority over the traditional physical examination for conditions such as synovitis of the knee joint, synovial hypertrophy, effusion and related pathologies (Fig. 25-35).[100-102] In the case of synovitis, this is largely because of the fact that sonography can visualize minimally thickened synovium, which is not yet perceivable by clinical palpation, as well as depict an array of different types of arthritis and injuries around and within joints.

Utilizing power Doppler imaging in rheumatologic POCUS for the evaluation of arthritis allows for examination of structures and inflammation at a microvascular level. Most musculoskeletal examinations are fairly superficial, allowing a linear array transducer to provide good resolution. However, some studies, such as hip examinations, may require not only a wider field of view but also a lower frequency to penetrate the deeper structures such that a curvilinear transducer will provide.

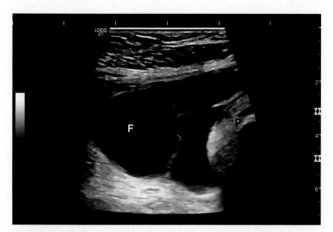

FIGURE 25-35 Longitudinal midline image of the knee. A large fluid collection with internal septations (F) is noted anterior to the patella (P).

The area of interest should be scanned similar to other parts of the human body with the transducer oriented in the longitudinal aspect of the structure being the "longitudinal plane" and 90 degrees to this being the orthogonal "transverse plane." Many pieces of sonography equipment are capable of imaging in a panoramic view, elongating the displayed field of view on the monitor. This is often used to image structures that have a longer dimension, allowing for the full visualization of the area of interest. For instance, an elongated muscle may be more appreciated if seen in its entirety, especially when pathology can be evaluated for its relational perspectives.

Musculoskeletal sonography also has some limitations, which must be recognized and appreciated by those relying on it. Artifacts, such as anisotropy, and a high operator dependence on both a solid knowledge base and a strong background in sonographic imaging techniques are a requirement for complete and accurate results, devoid of artifacts. When imaging any part of the human body, it is important to have the correct type of equipment to gather the most information, and this becomes very important when imaging dynamic and superficial structures as well.

CONCLUSIONS

POCUS continues to offer the ability to make timely critical decisions and to guide many procedures. There is solid evidence showing how POCUS can improve traditional techniques in the diagnosis and management of the acutely unwell medical patient. There is no doubt that POCUS has been a practice-changing technology for the care of patients in the acutely ill and emergent settings. The practice of POCUS has transcended beyond the space of radiology and EM with many other specialties finding ways to apply in their practice. As sonography remains less harmful, noninvasive, and inexpensive in comparison with other imaging modalities, there is no question that the adaptation of POCUS will continue growing over the decades.

It is the ability to look inside the human body dynamically and in real time that helps clinicians narrow the differential diagnoses early on in a patient's evaluation and helps guide decisions regarding further testing or treatment, thereby, improving patient care with rapid answers, treatments, and guided care.

SUMMARY

- POCUS in the emergency department has expanded beyond the traumatic patient workup.
- Emergency POCUS includes the ability to rapidly and accurately perform targeted emergent studies and examination protocols that can aid in identifying disease and guiding its treatment.
- The use of ultrasound in EM allows for a more thorough and expedient care of critical patients and holds the potential of unveiling immediate data to manage emergent situations.
- Emergency sonography is an excellent imaging modality to evaluate for life-threatening injury and to utilize clinical expertise over time for evaluating patients or immediate surgical consultation.
- Owing to its multiple benefits, POCUS is transcending beyond the practice of radiology and EM into other specialties.
- The use of POCUS in any setting should be standardized by training pathways and further supported by specialty-specific guidelines.

REFERENCES

1. Kortbeek JB, Al Turki SA, Ali J, et al. Advanced trauma life support, 8th edition, the evidence for change. *J Trauma.* 2008;64:1638–1650.
2. Hoffenberg S. The history and philosophy of emergency ultrasound. In: Cosby K, Kendall J, eds. *Practical Guide to Emergency Ultrasound.* Lippincott Williams & Wilkins; 2006:1–3.
3. Heller M, Melanson SW. Applications for ultrasonography in the emergency department. *Emerg Med Clin North Am.* 1997;15:735–744.
4. Mjolstad O, Dalen H, Graven T, Kleinau JO, Salvesen O, Haugen BO. Routinely adding ultrasound examinations by pocket-sized ultrasound devices improves inpatient diagnostics in a medical department. *Eur J Intern Med.* 2012;23(2):185–191. doi:10.1016/j.ejim.2011.10.009
5. Gulič TG, Makuc J, Prosen G, Dinevski D. Pocket-size imaging device as a screening tool for aortic stenosis. *Wien Klin Wochenschr.* 2016;128(9/10):348–353. doi:10.1007/s00508-015-0904-6
6. Solomon SD, Saldana F. Point-of-care ultrasound in medical education-stop listening and look. *N Engl J Med.* 2014;370(12):1083–1085.
7. Adhikari S, Amini R, Stolz LA, Blaivas M. Impact of point-of-care ultrasound on quality of care in clinical practice. *Rep Med Imaging.* 2014;2014(7):81–93.
8. American College of Emergency Physicians. Use of ultrasound by emergency physicians. *Ann Emerg Med.* 2001;38:469–470.
9. Rubin M. Cardiac ultrasonography. *Emerg Med Clin North Am.* 1997;15:745–762.
10. Nelson BP, Melnick ER, Li J. Portable ultrasound for remote environments. Part II: current indications. *J Emerg Med.* 2011;40(3):313–321.
11. Moore CL, Copel JA. Current concepts: point-of-care ultrasonography. *N Engl J Med.* 2011;364(8):749–757. doi:10.1056/NEJMra0909487
12. Ault MJ, Rosen BT. Portable ultrasound: the next generation arrives. *Crit Ultrasound J.* 2010;2(1):39–42.

13. Ultrasound guidelines: emergency, point-of-care and clinical ultrasound guidelines in medicine. *Ann Emerg Med.* 2017;69(5):e27–e54. doi:10.1016/j.annemergmed.2016.08.457

14. American Institute of Ultrasound in Medicine. AIUM practice guideline for the performance of the focused assessment with sonography for trauma (FAST) examination. Accessed June 6, 2017. http://www.aium.org/publications/guidelines/fast.pdf

15. Lewiss RE, Tayal VS, Hoffmann B, et al. The core content of clinical ultrasonography fellowship training. *Acad Emerg Med.* 2014;21(4):456–461. doi:10.1111/acem.12349

16. Rugolotto M, Chang C, Hu B, Schnittger I, Liang DH. Clinical use of cardiac ultrasound performed with a hand-carried device in patients admitted for acute cardiac care. *Am J Cardiol.* 2002;90:1040–1042.

17. Hendrickson RG, Dean AJ, Costantino TG. A novel use of ultrasound in pulseless electrical activity: the diagnosis of an acute abdominal aortic aneurysm rupture. *J Emerg Med.* 2001;21: 141–144.

18. Wherrett LJ, Boulanger BR, McLellan BA, et al. Hypotension after blunt abdominal trauma: the role of emergent abdominal sonography in surgical triage. *J Trauma.* 1996;41:815–820.

19. Jehle D, Guarino J, Karamanoukian H. Emergency department ultrasound in the evaluation of blunt abdominal trauma. *Am J Emerg Med.* 1993;11(4):342–346.

20. Reardon R, Moscati R. Beyond the FAST exam: additional applications of sonography in trauma. In: Jehle D, Heller M, eds. *Ultrasonography in Trauma: The FAST Exam.* American College of Emergency Physicians; 2003:107–126.

21. Moscati R, Reardon R. Clinical application of the FAST exam. In: Jehle D, Heller M, eds. *Ultrasonography in Trauma: The FAST Exam.* American College of Emergency Physicians; 2003:39–60.

22. Abrams BJ, Sukumvanich P, Seibel R, Moscati R, Jehle D. Ultrasound for the detection of intraperitoneal fluid: the role of Trendelenburg positioning. *Am J Emerg Med.* 1999;17:117–120.

23. Nishijima DK, Simel DL, Wisner DH, Holmes JF. Does this adult patient have a blunt intra-abdominal injury? *JAMA.* 2012;307(14):1517–1527. doi:10.1001/jama.2012.422

24. Lobo V, Hunter-Behrend M, Cullnan E, et al. Caudal edge of the liver in the right upper quadrant (RUQ) view is the most sensitive area for free fluid on the fast exam. *West J Emerg Med.* 2017;18(2):270–280. doi:10.5811/westjem.2016.11.30435

25. Mandavia D, Joseph A. Bedside echocardiography in chest trauma. *Emerg Med Clin North Am.* 2004;22:601–619.

26. Dulchavsky SA, Schwarz KL, Kirkpatrick AW, et al. Prospective evaluation of thoracic ultrasound in the detection of pneumothorax. *J Trauma.* 2001;50:201–205.

27. Lichtenstein D, Meziere G, Biderman P, Gepner A. The "lung point": an ultrasound sign specific to pneumothorax. *Intensive Care Med.* 2000;26:1434–1440.

28. Tayal VS, Kline JA. Emergency echocardiography to detect pericardial effusion in patients in PEA and near-PEA states. *Resuscitation.* 2003;59:315–318.

29. Smith-Bindman R, Aubin C, Bailitz J, et al. Ultrasonography versus computed tomography for suspected nephrolithiasis. *N Engl J Med.* 2014;371(12):1100–1110. doi:10.1056/NEJMoa1404446

30. Chan D. Echocardiography in thoracic trauma. *Emerg Med Clin North Am.* 1998;16:191–207.

31. Imazio M, Mayosi BM, Brucato A, Adler Y. Pericardial effusion triage. *Int J Cardiol.* 2010;145(2):403–404. doi:10.1016/j.ijcard.2010.04.031

32. Zhang M, Liu ZH, Yang JX, et al. Rapid detection of pneumothorax by ultrasonography in patients with multiple trauma. *Crit Care.* 2006;10(4):R112.

33. Kirkpatrick AW, Sirois M, Laupland KB, et al. Hand-held thoracic sonography for detecting post-traumatic pneumothoraces: the extended focused assessment with sonography for trauma (EFAST). *J Trauma.* 2004;57:288–295.

34. Stone MB. Ultrasound diagnosis of traumatic pneumothorax. *J Emerg Trauma Shock.* 2008;1:19–20.

35. Lichtenstein D, Meziere G, Lascols N, et al. Ultrasound diagnosis of occult pneumothorax. *Crit Care Med.* 2005;33:1231–1238.

36. Alrajhi K, Woo MY, Vaillancourt C. Test characteristics of ultrasonography for the detection of pneumothorax: a systematic review and meta-analysis. *Chest.* 2012;141(3):703–708. doi:10.1378/chest.11-0131

37. Via G, Hussain A, Wells M, et al. International evidence-based recommendations for focused cardiac ultrasound. *J Am Soc Echocardiogr.* 2014;27(7):683.e1–683.e33. doi:10.1016/j.echo.2014.05.001

38. Woo KC, Schneider JI. High-risk chief complaints I: chest pain—the big three. *Emerg Med Clin North Am.* 2009;27:685–712.

39. Abboud PC, Kendall J. Emergency department ultrasound for hemothorax after blunt traumatic injury. *J Emerg Med.* 2003;25:181–184.

40. Jain A, Mehta N, Secko M, et al. History, physical examination, laboratory testing, and emergency department ultrasonography for the diagnosis of acute cholecystitis. *Acad Emerg Med.* 2017;24(3):281–297. doi:10.1111/acem.13132

41. Wong C, Teitge B, Ross M, Young P, Robertson HL, Lang E. The accuracy and prognostic value of point-of-care ultrasound for nephrolithiasis in the emergency department: a systematic review and meta-analysis. *Acad Emerg Med.* 2018;25(6):684–698. doi:10.1111/acem.13388

42. Pathan SA, Mitra B, Mirza S, et al. Emergency physician interpretation of point-of-care ultrasound for identifying and grading of hydronephrosis in renal colic compared with consensus interpretation by emergency radiologists. *Acad Emerg Med.* 2018;25(10):1129–1137. doi:10.1111/acem.13432

43. Perera P, Mailhot T, Riley D, Mandavia D. The RUSH exam: rapid ultrasound in shock in the evaluation of the critically ill. *Emerg Med Clin North Am.* 2010;28:29–56.

44. Plummer D. Principles of emergency ultrasound and echocardiography. *Ann Emerg Med.* 1989;18(12):1291–1297.

45. Tang A, Euerle B. Emergency department ultrasound and echocardiography. *Emerg Med Clin North Am.* 2005;23:1179–1194.

46. Volpicelli G. Usefulness of emergency ultrasound in nontraumatic cardiac arrest. *Am J Emerg Med.* 2011;29(2):216–223.

47. Chisholm CB, Dodge WR, Balise RR, Williams SR, Gharahbaghian L, Beraud AS. Focused cardiac ultrasound training: how much is enough? *J Emerg Med.* 2013;44(4):818–822. doi:10.1016/j.jemermed.2012.07.092

48. Moore C. Current issues with emergency cardiac ultrasound probe and image conventions. *Acad Emerg Med.* 2008;15(3):278–284. doi:10.1111/j.1553-2712.2008.00052.x

49. Seif D, Perera P, Mailhot T, Riley D, Mandavia D. Bedside ultrasound in resuscitation and the rapid ultrasound in shock protocol. *Crit Care Res Pract.* 2012;2012:503254. doi:10.1155/2012/503254

50. Nagdev A, Stone MB. Point-of-care ultrasound evaluation of pericardial effusions: does this patient have cardiac tamponade? *Resuscitation.* 2011;82(6):671–673. doi:10.1016/j.resuscitation.2011.02.004

51. Moore CL, Rose GA, Tayal VS, Sullivan DM, Arrowood JA, Kline JA. Determination of left ventricular function by emergency physician echocardiography of hypotensive patients [published correction appears in *Acad Emerg Med.* 2002;9(6):642]. *Acad Emerg Med.* 2002;9(3):186–193. doi:10.1111/j.1553-2712.2002.tb00242.x

52. Randazzo MR, Snoey ER, Levitt MA, Binder K. Accuracy of emergency physician assessment of left ventricular ejection fraction and central venous pressure using echocardiography. *Acad Emerg Med.* 2003;10(9):973–977. doi:10.1111/j.1553-2712.2003.tb00654.x

53. Gilman LM, Ball CG, Panebianco N, Al-Kadi A, Kirkpatrick AW. Clinical performed resuscitative ultrasonography for the initial evaluation and resuscitation of trauma. *Scand J Trauma Resusc Emerg Med.* 2009;17:34.

54. Rabiei H, Rahimi-Movaghar V. Application of ultrasound in pulseless electrical activity (PEA) cardiac arrest. *Med J Islam Repub Iran.* 2016;30:372.

55. Blehar DJ, Dickman E, Gaspari R. Identification of congestive heart failure via respiratory variation of inferior vena cava diameter. *Am J Emerg Med.* 2009;27:71–75.

56. Kennedy Hall M, Coffey EC, Herbst M, et al. The "5Es" of emergency physician-performed focused cardiac ultrasound: a protocol for rapid identification of effusion, ejection, equality, exit, and entrance. *Acad Emerg Med.* 2015;22(5):583–593. doi:10.1111/acem.12652

57. Killu K, Coba V, Huang Y, Andrezejewski T, Dulchavsky S. Internal jugular vein collapsibility index associated with hypovolemia in the intensive care unit patients. *Crit Ultrasound J.* 2010;2(1):13–17. doi:10.1007/s13089-010-0034-3

58. Goonewardena SN, Gemignani A, Ronan A, et al. Comparison of hand-carried ultrasound assessment of the inferior vena cava and N-terminal pro-brain natriuretic peptide for predicting readmission after hospitalization for acute decompensated heart failure. *JACC Cardiovasc Imaging.* 2008;1:595–601.

59. Stawicki S. Braslow BM, Panebianco NL, et al. Intensivist use of hand-carried ultrasonography to measure IVC collapsibility in estimating intravascular volume status: correlations with CVP. *J Am Coll Surg.* 2009;209(1):55–61.

60. Kent A, Bahner DP, Boulger CT, et al. Sonographic evaluation of intravascular volume status in the surgical intensive care unit: a prospective comparison of subclavian vein and inferior vena cava collapsibility index. *J Surg Res.* 2013;184(1):561–566.

61. Ruff AL, Teng K, Hu B, Rothberg MB. Screening for abdominal aortic aneurysms in outpatient primary care clinics. *Am J Med.* 2015;128(3):283–288.
62. Bhatt S, Dogra VS. Catastrophes of abdominal aorta: sonographic evaluation. *Ultrasound Clin.* 2008;3(1):83–91.
63. Lamperti M, Bodenham AR, Pittiruti M, et al. International evidence-based recommendations on ultrasound guided vascular access. *Intensive Care Med.* 2012;38:1105–1117.
64. Espinet A, Dunning J. Does ultrasound-guided central line insertion reduce complications and time to placement in elective patients undergoing cardiac surgery. *Interact Cardiovasc Thorac Surg.* 2004;3(3):523–527.
65. Leung J, Duffy M, Finckh A. Real-time ultrasonographically-guided internal jugular vein catheterization in the emergency department increases success rates and reduces complications: a randomized, prospective study. *Ann Emerg Med.* 2006;48(5):540–547.
66. Brass P, Hellmich M, Kolodziej L, Schick G, Smith AF. Ultrasound guidance versus anatomical landmarks for internal jugular vein catheterization. *Cochrane Database Syst Rev.* 2015;1(1):CD006962. doi:10.1002/14651858.CD006962.pub2
67. ACEP Clinical Policies Committee. Clinical policy: critical issues in the evaluation and management of adult patients presenting with suspected lower-extremity deep venous thrombosis. *Ann Emerg Med.* 2003;42:124–135.
68. Blaivas M, Lambert MJ, Harwood RA, Wood JP, Konicki J. Lower-extremity Doppler for deep vein thrombosis—can emergency physicians be accurate and fast? *Acad Emerg Med.* 2000;7:120–126.
69. Jang T, Docherty M, Aubin C, Polites G. Resident-performed compression ultrasonography for the detection of proximal deep vein thrombosis: fast and accurate. *Acad Emerg Med.* 2004;11:319–322.
70. Jacoby J, Cesta M, Axelband J, Melanson S, Heller M, Reed J. Can emergency medicine residents detect acute deep venous thrombosis with a limited, two-site ultrasound examination? *J Emerg Med.* 2007;32:197–200.
71. Fox J. Lower extremity venous studies. In: Cosby K, ed. *Practical Guide to Emergency Ultrasound.* Lippincott Williams & Wilkins; 2006:255–266.
72. Kline JA, O'Malley PM, Tayal VS, Snead GR, Mitchell AM. Emergency-clinician performed compression ultrasonography for deep venous thrombosis of the lower extremity. *Ann Emerg Med.* 2008;52:437–445.
73. Theodoro D, Blaivas M, Duggal S, Snyder G, Lucas M. Real-time B-mode ultrasound in the ED saves time in the diagnosis of deep vein thrombosis (DVT). *Am J Emerg Med.* 2004;22:197–200.
74. Snell BJ. Assessment and management of bleeding in the first trimester of pregnancy. *J Midwifery Womens Health.* 2009;54(6):483–491. doi:10.1016/j.jmwh.2009.08.007
75. Wendt K. An outcomes evaluation of an emergency department early pregnancy assessment service and early pregnancy assessment protocol. *Emerg Med J.* 2014;31(e1):e50–e54. doi:10.1136/emermed-2013-202887
76. McRae A, Murray H, Edmonds M. Diagnostic accuracy and clinical utility of emergency department targeted ultrasonography in the evaluation of first-trimester pelvic pain and bleeding: a systematic review. *CJEM.* 2009;11(4):355–364.
77. Panebianco NL, Shofer F, Fields JM, et al. The utility of transvaginal ultrasound in the ED evaluation of complications of first trimester pregnancy. *Am J Emerg Med.* 2015;33(6):743–774.
78. Doubilet PM, Benson CB, Bourne T, Blaivas M; Society of Radiologists in Ultrasound Multispecialty Panel on Early First Trimester Diagnosis of Miscarriage and Exclusion of a Viable Intrauterine Pregnancy. Diagnostic criteria for nonviable pregnancy early in the first trimester. *N Engl J Med.* 2013;369(15):1443–1451. doi:10.1056/NEJMra1302417
79. Doubilet PM, Benson CB. First, do no harm... To early pregnancies. *J Ultrasound Med.* 2010;29(5):685–689. doi:10.7863/jum.2010.29.5.685
80. Stein JC, Wang R, Adler N, et al. Emergency physician ultrasonography for evaluating patients at risk for ectopic pregnancy: a meta-analysis. *Ann Emerg Med.* 2010;56(6):674–683.

81. Condous G, Kirk E, Lu C, et al. Diagnostic accuracy of varying discriminatory zones for the prediction of ectopic pregnancy in women with a pregnancy of unknown location. *Ultrasound Obstet Gynecol.* 2005;26:770–775.
82. Crochet JR, Bastian LA, Chireau MV. Does this woman have an ectopic pregnancy? The rational clinical examination systematic review. *JAMA.* 2013;309(16):1722–1729.
83. Chadee A, Rezai S, Kirby C, et al. Spontaneous heterotopic pregnancy: dual case report and review of literature. *Case Rep Obstet Gynecol.* 2016;2016:2145937. doi:10.1155/2016/2145937
84. Arsala L, Danso D. Spontaneous heterotopic triplet pregnancy with tubal rupture: a case report and literature review. *J Investig Med High Impact Case Rep.* 2014;2(2):2334. doi:10.1177/2324709614531556
85. Wendt K, Crilly J, May C, et al. A collaborative framework for managing pregnancy loss in the emergency department. *J Obstet Gynecol Neonatal Nurs.* 2009;38:730–738.
86. Berghella V, Roman A, Daskalakis C, Ness A, Baxter JK. Gestational age at cervical length measurement and incidence of preterm birth. *Obstet Gynecol.* 2007;110:311–317.
87. Mella MT, Berghella V. Prediction of preterm birth: cervical sonography. *Semin Perinatol.* 2009;33(5):317–324.
88. Di Salvo DN. Sonographic imaging of maternal complications of pregnancy. *J Ultrasound Med.* 2003;22(1):69–89.
89. Marin JR, Dean AJ, Bilker WB, Panebianco NL, Brown NJ, Alpern ER. Emergency ultrasound-assisted examination of skin and soft tissue infections in the pediatric emergency department. *Acad Emerg Med.* 2013; 20(6):545–553.
90. Adhikari S, Blaivas M. Sonography first for subcutaneous abscess and cellulitis evaluation. *J Ultrasound Med.* 2012; 31(10): 1509–1512.
91. Adams CM, Neuman MI, Levy JA. Point-of-care ultrasonography for the diagnosis of pediatric soft tissue infection. *J Pediatr.* 2016;169:122–127. doi:10.1016/j.jpeds.2015.10.026
92. Chen KC, Lin AC, Chong CF, Wang TL. An overview of point-of-care ultrasound for soft tissue and musculoskeletal applications in the emergency department. *J Intensive Care.* 2016;4:55. doi:10.1186/s40560-016-0173-0
93. Schmid-Wendtner MH, Dill-Müller D. Ultrasound technology in dermatology. *Semin Cutan Med Surg.* 2008;27(1):44–51.
94. Moehrle M, Blum A, Rassner G, Juenger M. Lymph node metastases of cutaneous melanoma: diagnosis by B-scan and color Doppler sonography. *J Am Acad Dermatol.* 1999;41(5):703–709.
95. Wortsman X, Alfageme F, Roustan G, et al. Guidelines for performing dermatologic ultrasound examinations by the DERMUS group. *J Ultrasound Med.* 2016;35(3):577–580. doi:10.7863/ultra.15.06046
96. Gupta PK, Gupta K, Prashant K, Dwivedi AN, Jain M. Potential role of ultrasound in anesthesia and intensive care. *Anesth Essays Res.* 2011;5(1):11–19.
97. Neal JM, Brull R, Chan VW, et al. The ASRA evidence-based medicine assessment of ultrasound-guided regional anesthesia and pain medicine: executive summary. *Reg Anesth Pain Med.* 2010;35(2):S1–S9. doi: 10.1097/AAP.0b013e3181d22fe0.
98. Jacobson JA. Shoulder US: anatomy, technique, and scanning pitfalls. *Radiology.* 2011;260:6–16.
99. Xu Z, Duan X, Yu X, Wang H, Dong X, Xiang Z. The accuracy of ultrasonography and Magnetic Resonance imaging for the diagnosis of Morton's neuroma: a systematic review. *Clin Radiol.* 2015;70(4):351–358.
100. Grassi W, Tittarelli E, Pirani O, Avaltroni D, Cervini C. Ultrasound examination of metacarpophalangeal joints in rheumatoid arthritis. *Scand J Rheumatol.* 1993;22:243–247.
101. Kane D, Balint P. Sturrock R. Ultrasonography is superior to clinical examination in the detection and localization of knee joint effusion in rheumatoid arthritis. *J Rheumatol.* 2003;30: 966–971.
102. Balsa A, de Miguel E, Castillo C, Peiteado D, Martín-Mola E. Superiority of SDAI over DAS-28 in assessment of remission in rheumatoid arthritis patients using power Doppler ultrasonography as a gold standard. *Rheumatology.* 2010;49(4):683–690.

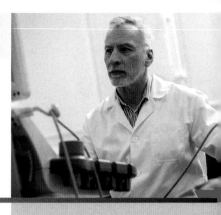

CHAPTER 26

Interventional Procedures

AUBREY J. RYBYINSKI

OBJECTIVES

- Describe the benefits of sonography-guided interventional procedures.
- Discuss the indications and contraindications for sonography-guided interventional procedures.
- Explain the role of the sonographer during sonography-guided interventional procedures.
- Discuss the difference between a fine-needle aspiration and a core biopsy and the benefits of each procedure.
- List common sonography-guided interventional procedures and the potential complications involved in each.

GLOSSARY

coagulopathy a defect in the body's mechanism for blood clotting

core biopsy a procedure that utilizes a hollow core biopsy needle to remove a sample of tissue frequently with a biopsy gun

fine-needle aspiration a procedure that utilizes a small needle attached to a syringe, in which a vacuum is created and sample cells are aspirated for evaluation

fresh frozen plasma a form of blood plasma that contains all of the clotting factors except platelets that is used to treat patients with a coagulopathy prior to interventional procedures

international normalized ratio (INR) a value used to standardize prothrombin time results between institutions because it adjusts for variations in processing; it is expressed as a number

partial thromboplastin time (PTT) laboratory test used to evaluate for blood clotting abnormalities

pneumothorax a collection of air or gas in the pleural cavity of the chest between the lung and the chest wall that creates pressure on the lung

prostate-specific antigen (PSA) a laboratory examination that measures the level of PSA, a protein produced by the prostate gland, in the blood; an elevated level can indicate the presence of prostate conditions such as prostate cancer, benign prostatic hypertrophy, and prostatitis

prothrombin time (PT) laboratory test used to evaluate for blood clotting abnormalities; the time it takes the blood to clot after thromboplastin and calcium are added to the sample is recorded

pseudoaneurysm a complication that can occur after cardiac catheterization or angioplasty in which a hematoma is formed by a leakage of blood from a small hole in the femoral artery

KEY TERMS

abscess drainage

adrenal biopsy

breast biopsy

liver biopsy

lung biopsy

lymph node biopsy

musculoskeletal biopsy

pancreatic biopsy

paracentesis

prostate biopsy

pseudoaneurysm repair

renal biopsy

sonography-guided procedure

thoracentesis

thyroid biopsy

The use of sonographic guidance has proven to be an invaluable asset to clinicians and patients for diagnostic and therapeutic procedures. Sonographic guidance techniques are continuing to improve with advances in transducer and equipment technology as well as increased operator experience. Sonographic guidance is frequently used for localizing organs, masses, and fluid collections in the abdomen, chest, neck, pelvis, and retroperitoneum. The most successful sonography-guided procedures have all the personnel involved work together as a team, and this includes the sonographer, physician, nurse, cytologist, and patient. This chapter focuses on those guidance procedures performed within the sonography department.

SONOGRAPHY-GUIDED BIOPSY

Percutaneous biopsy has become the widely accepted technique for confirmation of suspected malignant masses and characterization of many benign lesions in various locations throughout the body. Many of these masses are in locations that once required computed tomography (CT) guidance or open surgery, but now equipment and procedures allow for successful sonography-guided biopsy. The popularity of sonography guidance has increased steadily because it is minimally invasive, accurate, and relatively safe. Minimally invasive procedures are cost effective because patients may not require complex surgical interventions, long hospital stays, or excessive recovery times. In many cases, patients leave the same day after the procedure and quickly return to their normal activities. The ability to accurately characterize a disease lowers the number of additional examinations to confirm diagnosis, potentially decreasing the amount of radiation exposure.

Unlike other imaging modalities, sonography is readily available, inexpensive, and reproducible and can provide guidance in multiple imaging planes, allowing for multiple patient positions and approaches to be considered. The greatest advantage, however, is that it permits the real-time visualization of the needle tip because it passes through tissue planes into the target area. This allows for precise needle placement and avoidance of important structures. Studies have shown that an accurate diagnosis can be made in 95% of cases regardless of the sample size. In addition, color flow Doppler imaging can help prevent complications by identifying and helping the clinician to avoid vascular structures that may be in the needle's path.

Traditionally, the use of sonography for guided biopsy was for large, superficial, or cystic masses. With improvements in technology and biopsy techniques, small, deeply located, and solid masses can also undergo successful and accurate biopsy. Biopsy of deep masses and masses in obese patients can be difficult with sonography because of the difficulty in lesion visualization resulting from sound attenuation in the soft tissues. Similarly, not all lesions can be visualized by sonography because they may be isoechoic to the surrounding tissues. Lesions located within or behind bone or gas-filled bowel cannot be visualized because of nearly complete reflection of sound from the bone or air interface. Frequently, biopsies of the breast, liver, kidney, prostate, thyroid, parathyroid, and cervical nodes are easily performed. However, other sites within the body can undergo biopsy if the lesion is adequately visualized. A good rule of thumb is that any mass that is well visualized on ultrasound should be amendable to a sonography-guided biopsy. A major factor in the success of sonography-guided biopsy lies in the experience and comfort level of the sonographer and radiologist.[1]

Indications and Contraindications

A biopsy is performed to definitively diagnose the nature of a lesion. The major indication for biopsy is the suspicion of either primary malignancy or metastatic disease. As a diagnostic tool evaluating potentially malignant conditions, biopsy is indicated for initial evaluation before both surgical and nonsurgical interventions such as the administration of chemotherapy or radiation. For example, a biopsy could be performed to differentiate a metastatic mass from a second primary malignancy in a patient with a known primary malignancy. Frequently, biopsies are performed to evaluate the nature of an indeterminate lesion, such as a solitary solid hepatic mass in a patient with no history of malignancy. Infrequently, a biopsy is performed for the confirmation of a mass that is suspected of being benign.[2,3]

The three contraindications to needle biopsy include uncorrectable coagulopathy, unsafe biopsy route, and an uncooperative patient. Although there are studies stating that compromised coagulopathy is not a contraindication for fluid aspiration and superficial or low-risk biopsies, it is presented to provide general knowledge.[4] If the patient's coagulopathy is unavailable within the patient's medical record, the patient should get routine lab tests, known as a coagulation study. The three tests—prothrombin time (PT), partial thromboplastin time (PTT), and international normalized ratio (INR)—measure the time it takes for the blood to form a clot. These tests are simple, and results are usually available within 2 to 3 hours. Owing to the variability of the PT and PTT values between institutions, the World Health Organization implemented the INR. This value standardizes results between institutions because it adjusts for variations in processing and is expressed as a number.

Mild coagulopathies may occur secondary to the use of blood thinners, such as Plavix, aspirin, and warfarin, and some antibiotics.[5] If a coagulopathy is present, the procedure may be delayed and the causative drug discontinued until the laboratory values return to normal. Patients who cannot wait for values to normalize can be administered fresh frozen plasma or vitamin K. An important consideration is given to patients in whom the need for biopsy outweighs any risk.

The choice of biopsy route is crucial to success, and a safe route must be chosen. A biopsy path going through major vessels or highly vascular structures increases the risk of hemorrhage. Bowel, the trachea, and other adjacent organs must also be avoided. An uncooperative patient also contraindicates needle biopsy. Patient cooperation is necessary for success because uncontrolled motion during the biopsy increases the potential for laceration and hemorrhage. It may be necessary to administer a form of sedation to a potentially uncooperative pediatric, senile demented, or mentally challenged patient.[6]

Types of Sonography-Guided Procedures

Sonography can be used for biopsies, core biopsies, needle placement for fluid drainage or mass localization (including fiducial marker or post-biopsy clip placement), insertion of a nephrostomy tube in an obstructed kidney, and collecting fluid from an abscess. Most often, the biopsies are used to confirm if a lesion is benign, malignant, or infected to help determine an appropriate treatment plan. These methods are less invasive than open and closed surgical procedures because the incisions of the latter are much larger and require some level of local or general anesthesia.

Fine-Needle Aspiration

Fine-needle aspiration (FNA) with sonographic guidance is a widely accepted technique for the confirmation of suspected malignant masses and characterization of many benign lesions in various locations. Even with a palpable, discrete lesion, ultrasound allows controlled sampling of different regions within the lesion. For this type of biopsy, a "fine" or "thin" needle, most often 20G to 27G, is utilized and attached to a syringe (Fig. 26-1). These needles allow for multiple passes and are considered low risk because of the needle's relative thickness. As the name indicates, this technique uses aspiration to sample cells or fluid from a mass and is optimal for lesions lying superficially or at a moderate depth.[2] Specimens may also be obtained using a capillary action technique involving an up-and-down motion of the needle within the mass. This technique reduces trauma to the cells, which in turn decreases the amount of background blood on cytologic evaluation. FNA is a reliable and safe method of obtaining tissue samples, allowing cellular evaluation for cytologic examination. FNA success is measured in terms of aspirating enough cells and maintaining patient comfort. The overall accuracy increases when a cytopathologist evaluates the specimens during the procedure to determine if additional tissue aspiration is required for diagnosis.[7] With FNA, the cells are disorganized and no longer maintain the spatial arrangement they originally had in the lesion. In order to preserve the spatial arrangement of the cells, a core biopsy sample must be taken.[8] FNA is performed predominately on thyroid nodules, parathyroids, and lymph nodes. It is important to make sure that the appropriate transducer is selected. The transducer should offer the highest frequency while maintaining visualization of the area to be sampled.

Core Biopsy

A core needle biopsy is a procedure that involves removing small samples of tissue using an automated hollow core

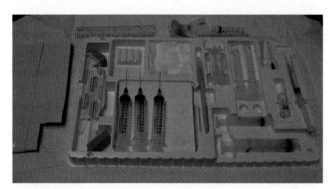

FIGURE 26-1 Procedure tray. Commercially available prepackaged procedure trays contain antiseptic solution and needles attached to syringes. This procedure tray is set up for a thyroid fine-needle aspiration.

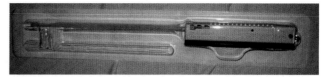

FIGURE 26-2 Biopsy gun. Core samples throughout the body can be obtained using a commercially available biopsy gun. The sterile, prepackaged devices are available in a variety of gauges with different shaft and sample lengths.

needle commonly referred to as a "biopsy gun" (Fig. 26-2). The biopsy gun makes a loud noise when activated. It is important to make the patient aware of the noise to minimize patient alarm and patient motion during the procedure. As the name implies, the core biopsy needle facilitates the removal of a core sample of tissue and is a larger gauge than the needle used for FNA. Core biopsy needles are most often 14G to 19G, offer various throw lengths, and have a tissue-cutting tip. The device is cocked and then inserted within the mass. A button is then pushed lunging the needle forward, which takes and stores a sample within a slot on the inner needle. In a core biopsy, the larger needle allows for a "core" tissue sample for analysis. The larger sample can be recut into smaller samples, which can be used for further analysis, offering a more definitive histologic evaluation.[9] The larger sample can aid in the diagnosis of parenchymal disease, involving the breast, kidney, liver, prostate gland, and transplanted organs.

Needle Selection

Each biopsy technique has its advantages and disadvantages, as does each needle type. There are a wide variety of needles commercially available, which vary in gauge, length, and tip configuration. An important consideration when choosing the appropriate needle is the amount of tissue required for accurate pathologic diagnosis.[10] The bore size of the needle is inversely related to its gauge. For example, a 16G needle will offer a larger specimen than a 27G needle. The choice of needle should be made with respect to the area being sampled and the risks that may be increased due to complications associated with larger bore needle.

Although real-time visualization of the needle is one of the greatest strengths of sonography, it is often the most technically challenging. The sonographic appearance of a needle is either a hyperechoic line or dot depending on which imaging plane is used (Figs. 26-2 and 26-3). Larger-caliber needles with a larger reflectivity surface are more readily visualized than the smaller-gauge needles. If the needle is not visualized at first because of misalignment, usually, maneuvering the transducer should allow for visualization. The needle and transducer should be in the same plane to produce the best visualization. The ability to see the needle tip will improve the more perpendicular the needle is to the transducer. Needles that are made specifically for sonography-guided procedures are commercially available and are designed to aid in visualization, although any needle used for biopsy should be able to be visualized sonographically if aligned correctly. Experience results in improving both needle alignment and needle visualization.

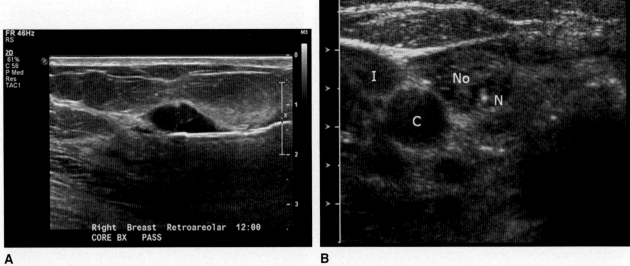

A　　　　　　　　　　　　　　　　　　　　**B**

FIGURE 26-3 Needle visualization. **A:** An image of the needle coursing through a breast mass perpendicular to the transducer. In this plane, the needle tip and shaft are visualized as an echogenic line. **B:** Only the needle tip, represented as an echogenic dot is appreciated within a thyroid nodule when the needle tip crosses the sound beam. *C,* carotid artery, *I,* internal jugular vein; *M,* mass; *N,* needle; *No,* nodule.

PROCEDURE

Role of the Sonographer

The sonographer plays an important role in interventional procedures. It is important to be able to locate the pathology of interest and offer a recommendation for the best and safest approach. Interventional sonographers must not only possess basic sonographic knowledge but also be able to optimize images for the detection of subtle masses and utilize features such as color Doppler to find a biopsy path that does not course through a blood vessel. The sonographer must also be familiar with instrumentation technologies to include harmonics and compound imaging and consider transducer selection based on the area of interest, location, footprint size, and transmit frequency. During the procedure, the sonographer makes use of different patient positioning techniques that aid in the best approach and is aware of how breathing affects the movement of the mass. The sonographer is one of the first people the patient interacts with and can reassure the patient with a simple smile and an introduction to the procedure. Building a positive rapport from the beginning is invaluable. The sonographer can coach and support the patient during the procedure to put them at ease and to make the procedure easier for all involved.

Preprocedure

After the patient's medical record is evaluated for appropriate history, lab values, and other imaging studies, informed consent must be obtained. Written informed consent has a detailed explanation of the major complications and should be discussed in the patient's native language. The patient should be apprised of the indications and alternatives and be able to understand and cooperate with instructions before and during the procedure.[11] After informed consent is obtained, everyone in the procedure room must pause for

a time out. A time out allows the staff to verify the correct patient is present and confirm the procedure and procedure site. The sonographer may document the time out on an image (Fig. 26-4). Before, during, and after the procedure, a radiology nurse monitors vital signs by electrocardiogram (ECG) and pulse oximetry.

One of the pitfalls of biopsy involves performing the procedure on the incorrect mass. The best way to avoid this is having the images from the prior exam in the procedure room for immediate and direct comparison. A limited sonography examination must be performed to confirm the results of the prior examination and to determine the best biopsy approach. Depending on the department, the designated interventional ultrasound equipment may be the oldest piece of equipment. If you are not able to reproduce the area of interest on preprocedure imaging, try to use a newer piece of equipment as that should have improved resolution.

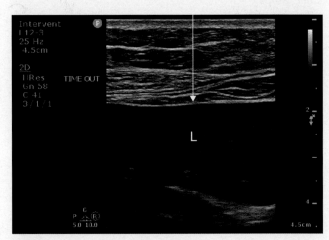

FIGURE 26-4 Time out. The procedure type, location, and time are documented when a "time out" is taken during the procedure. The *arrow* demonstrates the depth to the liver (*L*) capsule as a likely path for biopsy.

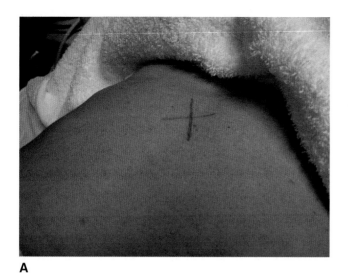

A

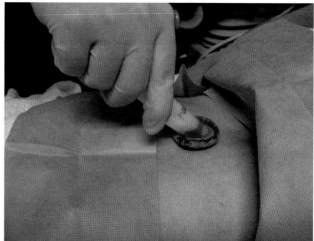

B

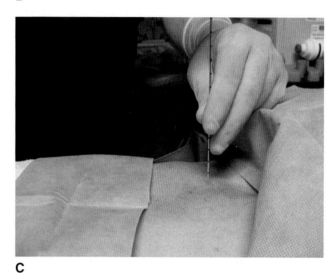

C

FIGURE 26-5 Preprocedure. These images were obtained during the pre-procedure setup for a left lobe liver biopsy. **A:** An "X" is placed over the best location for sampling. **B:** The area is then cleaned with an antiseptic solution and covered with sterile drapes. **C:** The biopsy gun is being lined up before being inserted for sampling.

Possible approaches will be discussed with the performing physician and an "X" should be placed on the area where the needle will break the skin line (Fig. 26-5). Measuring the distance from the skin to the area of interest will help determine the length of the procedure needle needed (Fig. 26-6). During the procedure, it is preferable for the sonographer to stand on the opposite side of the stretcher than the physician but on the same side as the imaging equipment for ease of use. In the case requiring the sonographer to be positioned on the side opposite the sonography equipment or behind the physician, support staff can be directed to adjust instrumentation controls. It is always important to use optimal scanning ergonomics.

Most sonography-guided biopsies are performed on an outpatient basis, and the patient can leave after completion or after a few hours of observation. There are generally no dietary restrictions before a biopsy; however, some institutions recommend nothing by mouth (NPO) or only having a light breakfast prior to a liver biopsy to contract the gallbladder. Patients may experience some level of anxiousness before the procedure and medication is prescribed and administered on a case-by-case basis. Many biopsies are performed using only 1% lidocaine as a local anesthetic to relieve pain. The

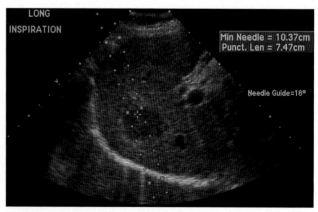

FIGURE 26-6 Needle guide. By using the needle guide mode on the sonography equipment, the sonographer can determine the minimum needle and puncture lengths to the area of interest. Note the parallel white dots that offer a guide as to where the needle will travel during the probe-guided biopsy.

injection of lidocaine can be described to the patient as a "bee sting." Increasing the pH of 1% lidocaine by adding 1 part of 1 mEq/mL of sodium bicarbonate to 9 or 10 parts of lidocaine can reduce the discomfort and enhance anesthetic tissue dispersion. For deeper or painful lesions, conscious sedation with intravenous Versed (midazolam) or Valium (diazepam) and pain control with Dilaudid (hydromorphone hydrochloride) or Sublimaze (fentanyl) is used.[10] The level of sedation should be carefully monitored, so that patients can still cooperate with inspiration and expiration requests. Intravenous access can be established to administer medications during or after the procedure.

During Procedure

All patients are vulnerable to infection; therefore, aseptic or sterile technique must be maintained during the procedure. A sterile technique prevents contamination to the patient and to the specimen obtained by eliminating microorganisms. Those involved directly in the procedure will wear sterile gloves, and the ultrasound transducer may be covered with a sterile plastic sheath (Fig. 26-7). The biopsy site will be cleaned with an antiseptic solution and draped. The transducer cover may degrade the quality of the ultrasound image, and in such cases, a povidone-iodine (Betadine) solution or sterile acoustic gel can preserve sterility and act as an acoustic medium.

Because one of the greatest benefits is real-time visualization, most sonography-guided interventional examinations use the procedure. Biopsies are performed probe-guided or free hand. The probe-guided technique uses a needle guide fixed to the ultrasound transducer. The main advantage of this technique is that it keeps the needle within the plane of the sonographic image as it is advanced toward the biopsy target. The disadvantage is, however, the fixed relationship between the needle and probe reduces operator freedom in choosing the needle path.[12] When the transducer guide attachment is utilized, the needle guide mode on the sonography equipment can display the path the needle will travel (Fig. 26-8). For physicians who prefer a "freehand" approach during biopsy, the needle is freely inserted into the patient without the use of a needle guide. The freehand technique requires the operator to manipulate the sonography probe with one hand and the biopsy needle with the other (Fig. 26-9). The chief advantage is its versatility. The probe and needle can be positioned independently to achieve the best image of the lesion and a needle path free of intervening structures. To monitor the needle tip on its course to the target, the operator must maintain the needle within the plane of the ultrasound beam.[12]

Postprocedure

Regardless of the method used for biopsy, representative images must be made during and after the procedure. There is no standardized postprocedure care for biopsy or FNA. Postprocedural images evaluate for complications such as hematomas. After a superficial biopsy, the patient may be given an ice pack to hold over the incision site. Cold ice causes the capillaries to constrict and facilitates clotting. The patient is typically monitored for 2 to 4 hours post–liver biopsy. Vital signs will be taken after the procedure and before the patient is discharged.

Complications and Risks

The complications of a sonography-guided biopsy are rare, but those involved in the procedure as well as the patient undergoing the biopsy should be aware of them. Most of these procedures are simple, safe, and performed as an outpatient procedure. Performing a minimally invasive biopsy can prevent the patient from undergoing unnecessary surgery. Localized pain, vasovagal reaction, and hematoma formation are the most encountered complications, but the complications could become as serious as death. The

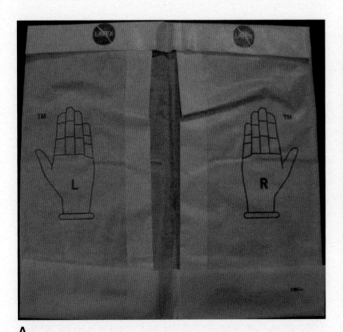

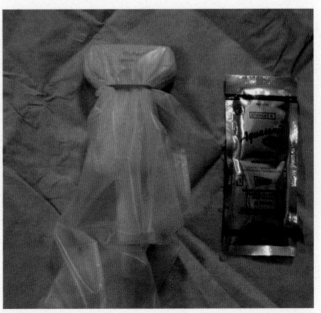

A   **B**

FIGURE 26-7 Sterile technique. **A:** Sterile gloves and (**B**) a transducer covered by a sterile sheath help maintain an aseptic environment. The sterile gel is usually located within the transducer cover. The commercially available prepackaged sterile gloves and transducer covers help maintain a sterile technique and reduce the risk of infection.

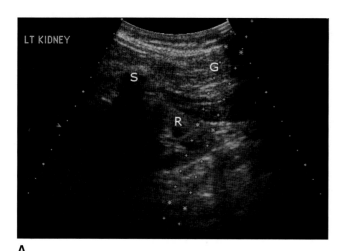

A

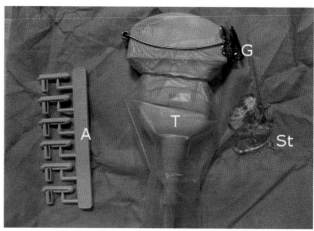

B

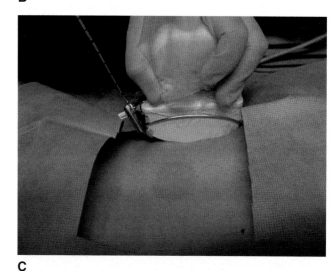

C

FIGURE 26-8 Probe-guided procedure. **A:** The biopsy guide offers a representative pathway the needle will travel during the procedure. The image was right–left inverted for this renal biopsy. Inverting the image and transducer facilitates many biopsy procedures. *R,* kidney; *S,* rib shadow. **B:** The transducer (*T*) is prepared for the procedure. The reusable sterile biopsy bracket (*G*) is placed on the transducer over the sterile cover. The disposable sterile needle guides (*A*) are available in a variety of gauges and clip onto the biopsy bracket. Sterile gel (*St*) is placed on the sterile drape for use during the procedure. **C:** The needle is being inserted through the needle guide.

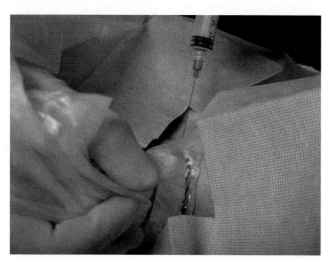

FIGURE 26-9 Freehand technique. This left thyroid fine-needle aspiration is performed using the freehand technique. The needle is freely inserted into the patient without the use of a transducer guide using real-time visualization to guide positioning the needle.

incidence of hematoma is related to the number of passes and needle gauge necessary to obtain an adequate sample. Pain may be more common with lesions or masses that are situated deeply. Other complications include swelling, pancreatitis, biliary leakage, peritonitis, and pneumothorax. Anytime the skin is punctured, there is a risk of bleeding and infection, which diminishes by maintaining a sterile technique. Infrequently, the needle may pass through an unintended target such as a vessel, loop of bowel, or an adjacent structure (Fig. 26-10). The frequency of complications is often related to organ vascularity and location as well as the needle gauge selected for the procedure.

COMMON PROCEDURES

Percutaneous Drainage

Indications for percutaneous drainage are broad, but the purpose is to remove infected fluid, such as pus, from the body. An abscess can form after surgery or an infection such

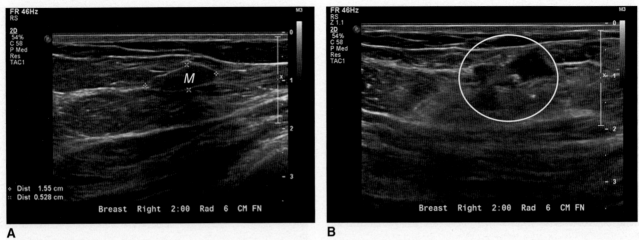

A   **B**

FIGURE 26-10 Post-biopsy hematoma. **A:** Image of a solid breast mass (*M*) obtained during preprocedure scanning. Retrospective imagine review did not show an image was obtained with color Doppler imaging to demonstrate any vessel in the biopsy path. **B:** Post-biopsy image showing a hematoma (*arrow*). (Image courtesy of Jeanine Rybyinski RDMS, RVT, Inspira Health Network, Vineland NJ.)

as appendicitis. Abscess drainages are usually performed if a patient has been on antibiotics with no change in symptoms. The aspirated fluid undergoes laboratory testing to determine what, if any, antibiotics could successfully treat the condition. An abscess can form anywhere in the body, and the drainage may include the insertion of a tube or aspirating the fluid into a syringe (Fig. 26-11).

Adrenal Biopsy

The adrenal glands biopsy on the organs located superior to each kidney may be performed if there is either a unilateral or a bilateral adrenal gland mass. Owing to anatomic location, the right adrenal gland is more amendable to a sonography-guided biopsy through a transhepatic approach.

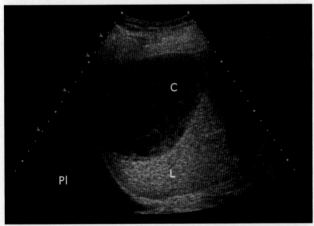

A

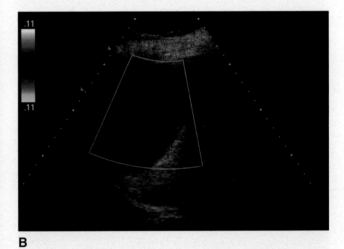

B

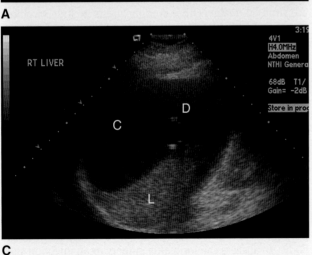

C

FIGURE 26-11 Fluid drainage. The patient presents for a sonography-guided drainage procedure of the right liver. **A:** Longitudinal imaging of the right liver lobe shows a complex area in the liver and the patient also has a pleural effusion. **B:** The color Doppler image demonstrates no flow within the complex area. **C:** The echogenic circle is the end of the drainage catheter. *C*, complex area; *D*, drainage catheter; *L*, liver; *Pl*, pleural effusion.

Accurate patient positioning is crucial for success. The procedure may require an oblique, decubitus, or even a prone position.

Paracentesis

A paracentesis procedure is used to remove ascites. The paracentesis can be performed for diagnostic or therapeutic reasons. Diagnostic indications include a new onset of ascites and ascites of unknown etiology. The collected fluid can be sent for laboratory examination to diagnose its cause and determine if it is infected. The most common causes of ascites are cirrhosis and malignancy. Other causes include heart failure, tuberculosis, dialysis, and pancreatic disease. Therapeutic paracentesis is performed when the cause is already known, and the fluid is removed for patient comfort. The entire abdomen is evaluated before paracentesis to locate the largest or deepest pocket (Fig. 26-12). A left lower quadrant site is generally the best because the abdominal wall is relatively thinner and the depth of fluid is typically greater.[13] When evaluating the abdomen for the largest pocket of fluid, it is important not to apply excess probe pressure because it distorts and diminishes the actual volume of fluid (Fig. 26-13).

Breast Biopsy

Patients presenting with suspicious breast findings are referred for core biopsy, FNA biopsy, or needle localization of a mass. The use of sonography is only advised if the suspected mass is well visualized. For palpable lesions, FNA is able to rapidly provide a diagnosis. A thin needle is used with FNA biopsy to obtain cells for cytologic evaluation. The main disadvantages of FNA breast biopsy are (1) the inability to distinguish between in situ and invasive cancer and (2) the significant rate of nondiagnostic samples and false-negative results primarily attributed to inexperience of the individual obtaining the biopsy.[14] A core needle biopsy offers a more definitive histologic diagnosis, avoids inadequate samples, and may permit the distinction between invasive versus in situ cancer (Fig. 26-14). For nonpalpable abnormalities, core biopsy is replacing wire localization and excision.[14] A clip is placed in the area of a core sample to identify the region on follow-up examinations or subsequent wire localization and excision (Fig. 26-15). Wire localization performed using ultrasound guidance is faster and better tolerated than the comparable mammographic localization. In women with nonpalpable microcalcifications, the use of wire localization and excision is tailored to each case after collaboration

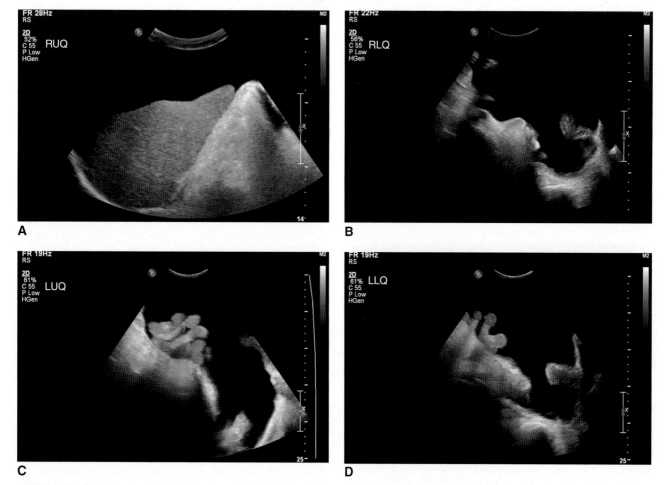

A

B

C

D

FIGURE 26-12 Paracentesis planning. Prior to a paracentesis, images are made from all four abdominal quadrants. **A–D:** When comparing these longitudinal sections from the four anatomic locations in the same patient, ascites is demonstrated throughout the abdomen. For this patient, the best area for catheter placement is the left lower quadrant (*LLQ*), which contains the most fluid.

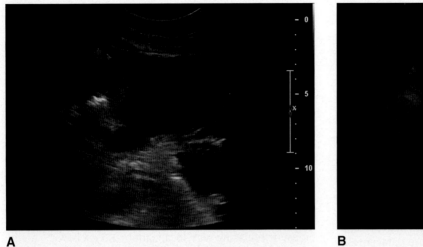

FIGURE 26-13 Probe pressure. The two sonograms of the right upper quadrant show how probe pressure affects the amount of ascites visualized. **A:** Image made with light probe pressure. **B:** Image made with a moderate amount of probe pressure, which makes the amount of ascites appear less than in (**A**).

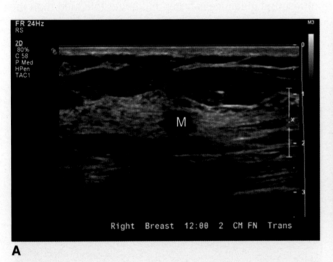
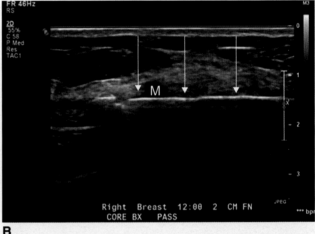

FIGURE 26-14 Core biopsy. **A:** The sonogram made prior to the biopsy procedure demonstrates the location of a solid breast mass (*M*). **B:** During the core biopsy, the sonogram demonstrates both the solid breast mass (*M*) and the echogenic line of the needle (*arrows*) within the mass. (Images courtesy of Jeanine Rybyinski, RDMS, RVT, Inspira Health Network Vineland, NJ.)

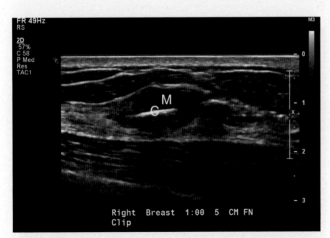

FIGURE 26-15 Clip Placement. The sonogram shows the echogenic line representing a clip (*C*), which was inserted into the suspicious breast lesion that was sampled (*M*). The clip placement shows which area or lesion was previously sampled. (Images courtesy of Jeanine Rybyinski, RDMS, RVT, Inspira Health Network Vineland, NJ.)

between the radiologist and surgeon. Wire localization is becoming less popular owing to the use of nonradioactive surgical guidance technology. This technology uses a clip placed in soft tissue, lymph node, or breast masses. The area of interest is then found using a radar system in the operating room and the area is excised by the surgeon. Symptomatic cysts may undergo a sonography-guided aspiration (Fig. 26-16).

Liver Biopsy

A liver biopsy is performed after a thorough clinical evaluation in patients with abnormal biochemical tests or liver lesions. Sonography-guided liver biopsy can be performed with either an FNA or by obtaining a core sample. Indications include the diagnosis, grading, and staging of parenchymal liver diseases, abnormal liver tests with unknown etiology, fever of unknown origin, diagnosis of a mass, and developing treatment plans based on histologic analysis.[15] Proper

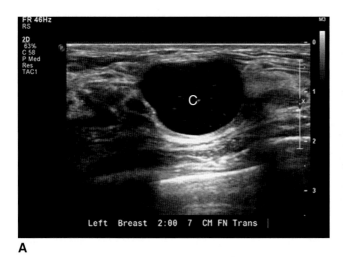

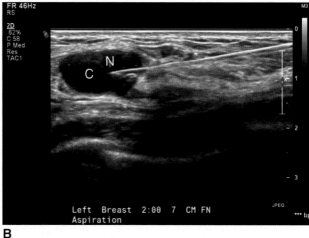

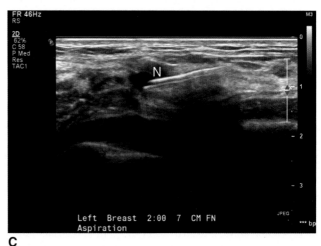

FIGURE 26-16 Breast cyst aspiration. **A:** Prior to the aspiration procedure, a sonogram shows a complex cyst (*C*). **B:** During the procedure, the needle (*N*) tip can be seen within the cyst (*C*). **C:** As the procedure progresses, the sonogram shows the cyst was nearly aspirated and the needle (*N*) is still seen in place. (Images courtesy of Jeanine Rybyinski, RDMS, RVT, Inspira Health Network Vineland, NJ.)

patient preparation is essential because it can reduce complications. Coagulation studies are obtained because some liver disorders elevate bleeding times. Patients are asked to remain NPO or have a light fatty meal to force gallbladder contraction, so it is less likely to be injured. The success of sonography-guided focal liver lesions is highly dependent on obtaining enough tissue for analysis, and although studies have proven ultrasound-guided technique is effective in lesions as small as 1.3 cm, it is recommended for superficial masses with a diameter greater than 3 cm.[15] A liver FNA is used to sample suspected masses, whereas a core sample allows for parenchymal disease to be assessed (Fig. 26-17). The left lobe is easily biopsied using a subxiphoid approach. This approach is generally better tolerated by patients and is more accurate than a blind right lobe biopsy.[16] Complications include bile leak, pneumothorax, and hematoma formation. After the biopsy samples are completed, postprocedural images should be obtained to evaluate for potential complications.

Lung Biopsy

Sonography is becoming more widely accepted and offers a safer alternative to CT for biopsy of the pleural space, lung, and mediastinal masses. Indications include evaluation of

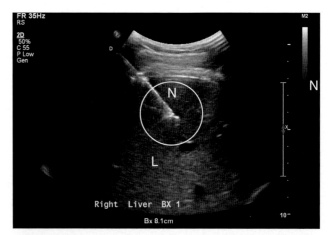

FIGURE 26-17 Liver biopsy. The transverse sonogram made during a core biopsy of a hypoechoic liver mass (*circle*) shows the needle (*N*) within the liver (*L*). (Image courtesy of. Briana Reis RDMS, RVT, Navix Diagnostix, Taunton, MA.)

a previously found abnormality, mass, or pleural effusion. Sonography-guided lung biopsies are commonly performed on masses close to a rib or the diaphragm. Owing to the variation of lung location during respiration, the procedure should be performed in a single breath to minimize complications. Depending on the location of the mass, different patient positions may be necessary to determine the safest approach. Complications include pneumothorax, bleeding in the lung, and infection.

Lymph Node Biopsy

Lymph nodes are part of the immune system and are found in the neck, behind the ears, in the axilla, and in the chest, abdomen, inguinal area, and groin. Normal lymph nodes are usually hard to feel and difficult to visualize sonographically. Lymph nodes can enlarge and become tender usually because of some type of infection. The swelling can also be caused by a cut, scratch, insect bite, tattoo, drug reaction, or malignancy. Most lymph nodes are superficial and amendable to a sonography-guided biopsy. The sonographer can use the curved or linear transducer and apply moderate pressure to reduce the distance the needle must travel and to move adjacent bowel out of the way. Color Doppler imaging is used to avoid any blood vessel that courses within the needle path. Lymph nodes can be sampled by FNA or core biopsy.

Musculoskeletal Biopsy

Sonography is used to localize masses found throughout the body for biopsy. Sonographic guidance can be used to efficiently acquire specimens from a variety of soft-tissue tumors and disease processes. If biopsy of a soft-tissue malignancy is performed, consultation with the surgeon is necessary to ensure that the biopsy tract is removed during the surgical procedure. Both fine-needle and core needle biopsy specimens can be obtained. Sonography can also be used to localize affected muscle groups and biopsy bone lesions when cortical destruction is present and to facilitate the passage of a needle into the medullary cavity.[10] Complications include bone fracture of the biopsy site, neurologic injury secondary to anesthetizing major motor nerves that may create paresis or paralysis, and bleeding or infection.

Pancreatic Biopsy

Pancreatic biopsy is indicated whenever there is a pancreatic mass or pancreatitis of unknown etiology. Sonographically, the pancreas can be difficult to visualize because of

its anatomic location, and during biopsy, bowel gas may obscure the image. During the procedure, moderate probe pressure can move and keep bowel loops away as well as shorten the needle path. Color Doppler imaging is used to search for blood vessels and determine the safest biopsy route (Fig. 26-18). Despite its location and relational anatomy, complications during pancreatic biopsy are rare.

Thoracentesis

Thoracentesis is the removal of pleural fluid, and the procedure can be performed for diagnostic or therapeutic purposes. Diagnostic indications include a unilateral effusion, bilateral effusions of different sizes, pleurisy, fever, an ECG and laboratory values inconsistent with heart failure, and an effusion that does not resolve with heart failure therapy. A sonogram to evaluate pleural fluid should be performed with the patient in the same position as during the thoracentesis, preferably upright leaning over a table. Sonography is used to localize fluid collections, especially loculated effusions[17] (Fig. 26-19). The puncture site should be one to two rib spaces below the level at which breath sounds decrease or disappear on auscultation, above the ninth rib to avoid subdiaphragmatic puncture, and midway between the spine and posterior axillary line where the ribs are easily palpated. Therapeutic paracentesis is performed when the cause is already known, and the fluid is removed for patient comfort. Complications include pain, bleeding, pneumothorax, infection, spleen or liver puncture, and vasovagal events.

Prostate Biopsy

The prostate is biopsied to confirm malignancy. Indications for biopsy include elevated prostate-specific antigen (PSA), abnormal digital rectal examination, or palpable nodules. Before the procedure, the patient receives enema to clear the feces in the rectum that could obscure imaging. The patient is most commonly positioned in left lateral decubitus position. A high-frequency endocavitary transducer is inserted into the rectum to evaluate the prostate. The prostate should be surveyed in sagittal and coronal planes, and a volume measurement should be recorded.

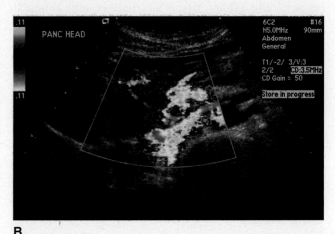

A   **B**

FIGURE 26-18 Pancreatic mass. **A:** The grayscale transverse image of the pancreas (*P*) demonstrates a mass (*M*) in the pancreatic head. The gallbladder (*G*) is seen lateral to the pancreatic head. The inferior vena cava (*I*) is seen posterior to the pancreas. **B:** A color Doppler image demonstrates the surrounding vascularity. (Images courtesy of Patricia Perez, RDMS, RVT, Inspira Health Network Vineland, NJ.)

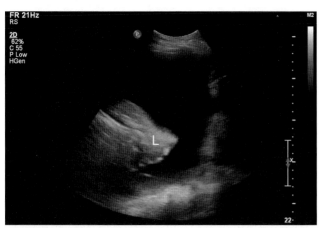

FIGURE 26-19 Pleural effusion. The sonogram of the right pleural space prior to thoracentesis. Ultrasound is useful at determining the best incision site and to confirm that the lung (*L*) is not near the incision site. (Image courtesy or Briana Reis RDMS, RVT, Navix Diagnostix, Taunton MA.)

Prostate cancer occurs most frequently in the peripheral zone; therefore, adequate sampling must be obtained from this region. Many techniques have been established, but the most common technique uses the coronal plane, and two representative samples are taken from the apex, base, and mid-segments, from the right and left as well as a sample from the central zone. Additional samples should be obtained from suspicious or hypoechoic areas[18] (Fig. 26-20). When obtaining biopsy samples on the left side, puncturing the urethra is a complication that can be avoided by inverting the transducer right to left while rotating the transducer 180 degrees. Other complications include vasovagal episodes, rectal bleeding, and hematuria.

Pseudoaneurysm Repair

A pseudoaneurysm forms when an arterial puncture site fails to seal, which allows arterial blood to spread into the surrounding tissues and form a pulsatile hematoma. They typically occur in the femoral artery and are iatrogenic. The number of pseudoaneurysms has increased significantly because of the exponential growth of interventional cardiology (Fig. 26-21). Several therapeutic strategies have been developed to treat this complication. They include sonography-guided compression repair, surgical repair, and minimally invasive percutaneous treatments such as thrombin injection. It is important to note that sonography-guided compression repair has considerable drawbacks, including long procedure time, patient discomfort, and a relatively high recurrence rate in patients receiving anti-coagulant therapy. Compression repair has been shown to be less successful in patients with pseudoaneurysms larger than 3 to 4 cm in diameter and those who cannot tolerate the associated discomfort. Complications include acute pseudoaneurysmal enlargement, rupture, vasovagal reactions, deep vein thrombosis, atrial fibrillation, and angina. Moreover, sonography-guided compression repair requires the availability of an ultrasound device and the presence of skilled personnel during the procedure. The technique involves applying compression on the pseudoaneurysm neck with the ultrasound transducer until the flow within the neck is obliterated. Pressure is applied for a period of 1 minute, with the procedure repeated 10 times. At the end of each period, compression is released briefly to assess pseudoaneurysm patency and to reposition the transducer. Care must be taken to avoid compromising flow within the underlying femoral artery. After successful thrombosis, patients should be kept supine for a few hours, with the affected leg in the stretched position.

Percutaneous thrombin injection has gained popularity despite complications associated with the initial use of high-dose thrombin (average dose of 1,100 IU). The technique was refined when low-dose thrombin injections were studied and proven to have the same efficacy and consistently high success rates. Compared with surgical repair, the treatment of pseudoaneurysms with thrombin injection offers many advantages. The success rate of thrombin injection is 97%, even with patients treated with therapeutic levels of anti-coagulants.[19] Treatment can usually be completed within several minutes. Common complications of thrombin injection include distal migration of the thrombin. It is also possible that if the thrombin is injected in a diluted concentration, it may not remain in the cavity long enough to form a clot.

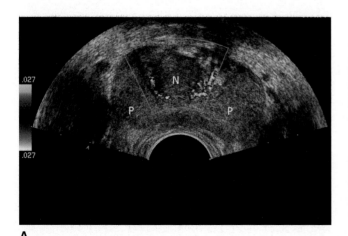

A

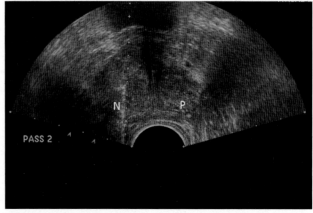

B

FIGURE 26-20 Prostate biopsy. **A:** Before the biopsy, the prostate gland (*P*) is evaluated for nodules. This color flow image demonstrates a nodule (*N*) that will be sampled. **B:** During the biopsy, the prostate gland sonogram demonstrates the needle as an echogenic line (*N*) along the needle guide (*dotted line*).

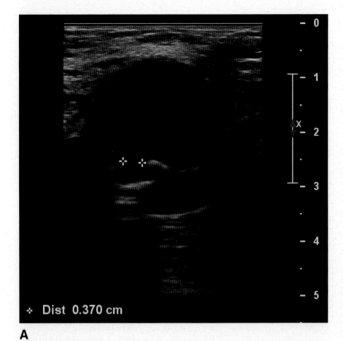

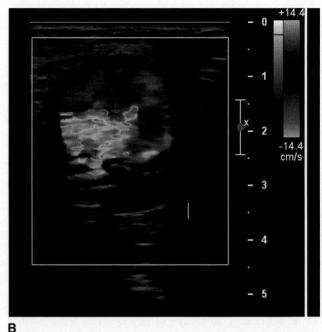

A **B**

FIGURE 26-21 Pseudoaneurysm. **A:** A transverse sonogram on a patient following postcardiac catheterizations demonstrates pseudoaneurysm in the common femoral artery. The neck is marked by calipers and is small enough for a thrombin injection intervention. **B:** The color Doppler sonogram demonstrates turbulent flow within the pseudoaneurysm.

Renal Biopsy

Renal biopsies are typically performed based on clinical history or laboratory values. Indications include isolated glomerular hematuria, isolated non-nephrotic proteinuria, nephritic syndrome, acute nephritic syndrome, suspected renal lymphoma, focal renal lesion, deteriorating renal function, and unexplained acute renal failure. Generally, these procedures are performed to obtain a core tissue sample to evaluate parenchymal and glomeruli disease rather than sample a mass, and as such, the kidney with the least associated risk is biopsied.[20] Biopsy of a renal transplant can also be performed to evaluate for graft rejection. A lower pole biopsy site is optimal owing to a decreased risk of major vessel puncture. Renal biopsies are performed probe-guided, not free hand, to minimize risk and improve success. The kidney is sampled in the sagittal plane with the patient in the prone position. Inverting the image right to left and turning the transducer so that the notch points toward the patient's feet can aid in biopsy access (Fig. 26-22). Common complications include pain, infection, hematoma formation, and rarely, puncture of the adjacent organs. The risk of complication is higher in patients with advanced renal insufficiency as well as hypertension and amyloidosis.[4,21]

Thyroid and Neck Biopsy

Thyroid, parathyroid, and other neck masses can be safely sampled by FNA. The success of FNA depends on the size of the lesion and the extent of cystic involvement.[22] Recent literature discourages FNA on nodules less than 10 mm because these microcarcinomas infrequently metastasize and carry a small risk of recurrence and mortality after surgical removal. Sonography offers real-time visualization; however, accurately aspirating cells from nodules smaller than 10 mm

is difficult and may lead to false-negative results. The Society of Radiologists in Ultrasound guidelines recommends FNA of nodules 10 mm or greater only when microcalcifications are present, 15 mm or greater if completely or predominantly solid or if coarse calcifications are present, and 20 mm or greater if predominantly cystic nodules are with a solid component are present[23,24] (Fig. 26-23). Cystic nodules offer a cytologic diagnostic challenge because negative findings are not reliable but a finding of malignancy is reliable. For nodules that are complex, the cystic competent can be aspirated followed by sampling of the residual solid component.[25] If a large cystic mass is causing pain or discomfort, the cyst

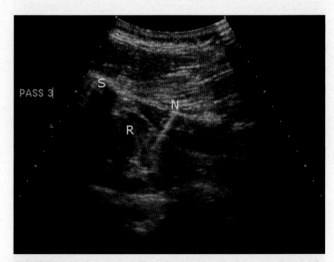

FIGURE 26-22 Renal biopsy. The left kidney sonogram is inverted right–left, which facilitates both transducer and biopsy needle placement. The echogenic line represents the needle (*N*) as it obtains the sample. *R*, left renal tissue; *S*, rib shadow.

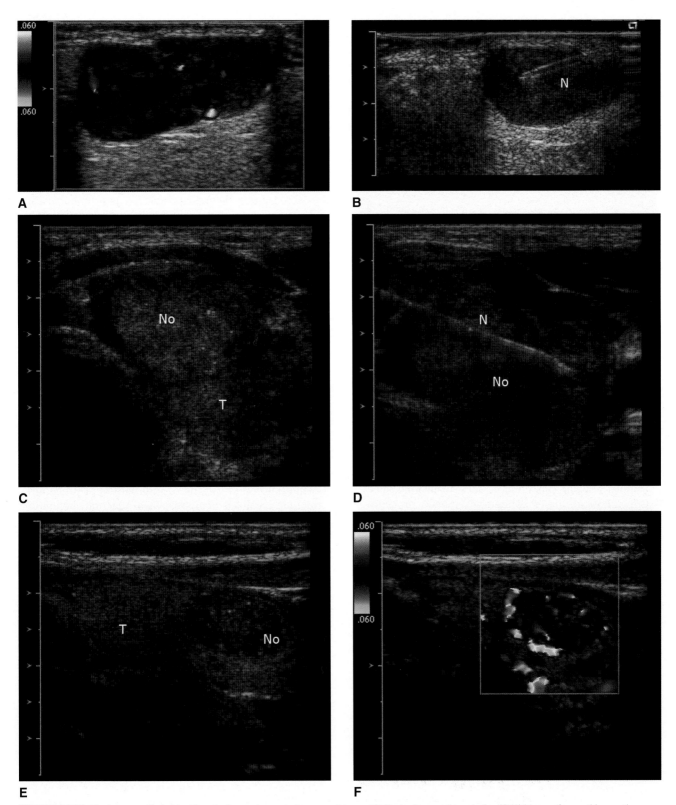

FIGURE 26-23 Neck masses. **A:** A color Doppler image demonstrates a parotid mass. **B:** During fine-needle aspiration (*FNA*) biopsy of a parotid mass, the needle is clearly visible within the mass (*N*). This mass was diagnosed as an early malignancy. **C, D:** The sonograms show a large thyroid nodule (*No*) that underwent successful FNA. The needle (*N*) can be seen within the nodule. *T*, thyroid. **E, F:** The longitudinal sonograms of the thyroid gland (*T*) demonstrate vascular flow to a heterogeneous nodule (*No*) with microcalcifications in the lower pole of the gland. Microcalcifications increase the risk of malignancy.

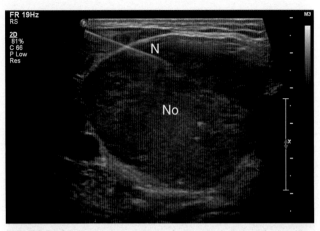

FIGURE 26-24 Thyroid lesions. During fine-needle aspiration of a thyroid nodule (*N*), this sonogram was made and demonstrates the needle tip (*arrow*) within the nodule.

can be aspirated to alleviate symptoms (Fig. 26-24). Doppler ultrasound is used to evaluate any vessel that may lie in the needle path. Another technique used for obtaining cells is the fine-needle capillary (FNC) technique. Advantages of FNC include minimal trauma, tissue pressure, and capillary action. This method removes the syringe plunger and only uses the to-and-fro motion of the needle to obtain cells. The technique aspirates a smaller but more concentrated sample. FNC does not obtain as many cells as FNA, and having a cytopathologist evaluate the specimens during the procedure drastically increases the overall accuracy because they can determine if additional tissues are required for diagnosis. For these procedures, the patient is placed in a supine position and has both arms to the side. A rolled towel can be placed under the nape of the neck. This eases stress and makes the anterior neck more accessible. Common complications include pain, bleeding, infection, and puncture of adjacent vessels such as the internal jugular vein or carotid artery.

SUMMARY

- Sonography-guided interventional procedures include fluid drainages, tube placements, biopsies, FNAs, and core biopsies.
- Benefits of sonography-guided interventional procedures include the following: no ionizing radiation, less invasive than surgery, less expensive than alternative procedures, can be performed with the patient in different positions, allow for real-time visualization of procedure, and color Doppler imaging can aid in vessel visualization.
- Contraindications to sonography-guided procedures include coagulopathy, unsafe biopsy route, and an uncooperative patient.
- FNA is performed with a thin needle, 20G to 27G, attached to a syringe to remove cells for evaluation.
- Core biopsy is performed with a larger-gauge, 14G to 19G, biopsy gun and is used to remove a larger sample of tissue.
- The size and type of needle chosen depend on the type of procedure, area of interest, amount of tissue needed for evaluation, and the risk involved. Needle gauge is inversely proportional to the diameter of the needle.
- A needle guide keeps the needle in plane with the transducer for easier visualization but limits the path the needle can take; freehand procedures allow for more versatility because the needle and transducer can be maneuvered independently, but needle visualization can be a challenge. The needle is best seen when the needle is in the same plane as the ultrasound beam and is more perpendicular to the transducer.
- Potential complications of interventional procedures include localized pain, vasovagal reaction, hematoma formation, and infection.
- Common sonography-guided interventional procedures include abscess drainage, adrenal biopsy, diagnostic and therapeutic paracentesis, breast biopsy, liver biopsy, lung biopsy, lymph node biopsy, musculoskeletal biopsy, pancreatic biopsy, diagnostic and therapeutic thoracentesis, prostate biopsy, pseudoaneurysm repair, renal biopsy, and thyroid biopsy.

REFERENCES

1. DeJong R. Ultrasound-guided interventional techniques. In: Hagan-Ansert S, ed. *Textbook of Diagnostic Ultrasonography.* Vol 1. 8th ed. Elsevier Mosby; 2011:467–498.
2. Rumack CM, Wilson SR, Charboneau JW. Ultrasound-guided biopsy and drainage of the chest, abdomen and pelvis. In: Rumack CM, Wilson SR, Charboneau JW, eds. *Diagnostic Ultrasound.* Vol 1. 5th ed. Elsevier Mosby; 2011:597–622.
3. American Institute of Ultrasound in Medicine. AIUM practice guidelines for the performance of selected ultrasound guided procedures. 2014. Accessed March 30, 2021. http://www.aium.org/resources/guidelines/usGuidedProcedures.pdf
4. Walker TG. *Interventional Procedure.* Lippincott Williams & Wilkins; 2012
5. Humes D. *Kelley's Textbook of Internal Medicine.* 3rd ed. Lippincott Williams & Wilkins; 2000.
6. Shin HJ, Amaral JG, Armstrong D, et al. Image-guided percutaneous biopsy of musculoskeletal lesions in children. *Pediatr Radiol.* 2007;37:362–369.
7. Afify AM, Al-Khafaji BM, Kim B, et al. Endoscopic ultrasound-guided fine needle aspiration of the pancreas: diagnostic utility and accuracy. *Acta Cytol.* 2003;47:341–348.
8. Domanski H. *Atlas of Fine Needle Aspiration Cytology.* 2nd ed. Springer; 2018.
9. Shah VI, Raju U, Chitale D, et al. False-negative core needle biopsies of the breast: an analysis of clinical, radiologic, and pathologic findings in 27 consecutive cases of missed breast cancer. *Cancer.* 2003;97:1824–1831.
10. Hallet R. Musculoskeletal biopsy: percutaneous needle technique. Musculoskeletal procedures. *eMedicine: Medscape.* 2009. Accessed May 24, 2010. http://emedicine.medscape.com/article/399094-overview
11. Rockey DC, Caldwell SH, Goodman ZD, et al. Liver biopsy. *Hepatology.* 2009;49:1017–1044.
12. Pramit P, Brooks D, Wolfe R. Sonographically guided biopsy of focal lesions: a comparison of freehand and probe-guided techniques using a phantom. *Am J Roentgenol.* 2005;184:1652–1656.
13. Thompson TW, Shaffer RW, White B, et al. Paracentesis. *N Engl J Med.* 2007;355:19–23.

14. Verkooijen HM. Diagnostic accuracy of stereotactic large-core needle biopsy for nonpalpable breast disease: results of a multicenter prospective study with 95% surgical confirmation. *Int J Cancer.* 2002;99:853–859.

15. Chhieng DC. Fine needle aspiration biopsy of liver: an update. *World J Surg Oncol.* 2004;2:1186–1194.

16. Plecha DM, Goodwin DW, Rowland DY, et al. Liver biopsy: effects of biopsy needle caliber on bleeding and tissue recovery. *Radiology.* 1997;204:101–104.

17. Koh DM, Burke S, Davies N, et al. Transthoracic ultrasound of the chest: clinical uses and applications. *Radiographics.* 2002;22:15–23.

18. Yang X. *Interpretation of Prostate Biopsy. An Illustrated Guide.* Springer; 2020.

19. Stolt M, Braun-Dullaeus R, Herold J. Do not underestimate the femoral pseudoaneurysm. *Vasa.* 2018;47(3):177–185. doi:10.1024/0301-1526/a000691

20. Stock KF, Slotta-Huspenina J, Kübler H, Autenrieth M. Innovative Ultraschalldiagnostik bei Nierentumoren [Innovative ultrasound-based diagnosis of renal tumors]. *Urologe A.* 2019;58(12):1418–1428. doi:10.1007/s00120-019-01066-y

21. Whittier WL, Korbet SM. Timing of complications in percutaneous renal biopsy. *J Am Soc Nephrol.* 2004;15(1):142–147.

22. Feldkamp J, Führer D, Luster M, Musholt TJ, Spitzweg C, Schott M. Fine needle aspiration in the investigation of thyroid nodules. *Dtsch Arztebl Int.* 2016;113(20):353–359. doi:10.3238/arztebl.2016.0353

23. McCartney CR, Stukenborg GJ. Decision analysis of discordant thyroid nodule biopsy guideline criteria. *J Clin Endocrinol Metab.* 2008;93:3037–3044.

24. Durante C, Grani G, Lamartina L, Filetti S, Mandel SJ, Cooper DS. The diagnosis and management of thyroid nodules: a review [published correction appears in *JAMA.* 2018 Apr 17;319(15):1622]. *JAMA.* 2018;319(9):914–924. doi:10.1001/jama.2018.0898

25. Suen K. Fine-needle aspiration biopsy of the thyroid. *CMAJ.* 2002;167(5):491–495.

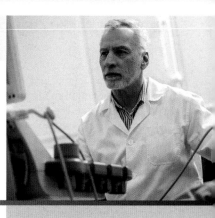

CHAPTER 27

Foreign Bodies

TIM S. GIBBS

OBJECTIVES

- Identify and give examples of different types of soft-tissue foreign bodies (STFBs) based on composition.
- Explain sensitivity and specificity.
- List the important information the sonographer should obtain from the patient interview and patient chart prior to providing a comprehensive sonography evaluation.
- Differentiate the different sonographic appearances of STFBs based on composition, location, age, and artifacts.
- Describe the role of the sonographer prior to, during, and following sonography-guided foreign body (FB) removal.
- Explain the limitations of sonography and the advantages of other imaging modalities used to image STFBs.

GLOSSARY

granuloma a tumor-like mass formation that usually contains macrophages and fibroblasts and forms as a result of chronic inflammation and isolation of the infected area

hyperemia an increase in the quantity of blood flow to a body part; increased blood flow as in the inflammatory response

in vitro when referring to a biologic process, it is made to occur in a laboratory vessel or in a controlled experimental environment but does not occur within a living organism or in a natural setting

in vivo when referring to a biologic process, it occurs or is made to occur within a living organism or natural setting

occult in reference to foreign bodies (FBs), the term refers to something hidden from view

radiolucent a tissue or material that allows transmission of X-rays and appears more dense (dark) on a radiograph; also known as nonradiopaque; for a FB, the material will often blend in and cannot be differentiated from the surrounding soft tissue

radiopaque a tissue, contrast, or material that attenuates or blocks radiation; the tissue, contrast, or material will appear bright on the radiograph

KEY TERMS

foreign bodies

granuloma

hypoechoic halo

inorganic

organic reverberation

rim

sensitivity

shadowing

soft tissue

specificity

Conventional radiography, fluoroscopy, computed tomography (CT), magnetic resonance imaging (MRI), nuclear medicine, and sonography have been used to demonstrate the presence of foreign bodies (FBs). The purpose of this chapter is to present the sonographic scanning technique to recognize, locate, and assist in the removal of various types of soft-tissue foreign bodies (STFBs) in superficial structures. Increasing sonographer and clinician awareness and confidence to choose sonography for STFB detection, localization, and removal may result in increased diagnostic accuracy and decreased diagnostic expense.

COMPOSITION OF FOREIGN BODIES

FBs can be separated into three distinct categories based on their composition (Table 27-1). *Organic material* refers to biologic plant material and animal products. *Inorganic materials* are usually man-made products composed of minerals or made from minerals but are not animal or vegetable in origin. *Metallic materials* are those products with a metal alloy.

Sensitivity and Specificity

Radiographic imaging for FBs has been used for many years with some degree of success. Because radiography relies on the density of the FB, it has varied sensitivities for imaging the different types of FBs. Radiography detects 98% of radiopaque objects such as gravel, most glass, and metal[1]; however, radiography detects only 15% or less of radiolucent FBs such as wood, plastic, some glass, and cactus spine.[2] Despite the poor sensitivity of radiography to demonstrate many organic objects and some inorganic objects, conventional radiography remains the most commonly used imaging study for the evaluation of FBs in the emergency department.[3] Consequently, many FBs are missed on initial evaluation. In fact, missed FBs are the second

leading cause of malpractice lawsuits against emergency medicine physicians.[4,5] Wound care litigation constitutes 5% to 20% of lawsuit claims against emergency medicine physicians and results in 3% to 11% of monetary rewards.[6,7]

Sonography performs well in demonstrating the FBs traditionally considered the most difficult to image on radiographic studies. In a retrospective study where radiography failed to demonstrate a STFB, sonography had a sensitivity of 95% and a specificity of 89%.[8,9] In a prospective study using cadaver feet and wooden FBs, Jacobson et al.[10] reported that sonography can reveal wooden FBs as small as 2.5 mm in length with 86.7% sensitivity and 96.7% specificity. At the time of this study, the resolution of the sonography equipment either makes visualizing FBs smaller than 2.5 mm more difficult or limits adequate visualization. The equipment used today are capable of resolving objects within ±1 mm. Most recently, Mecado and Hayre[11] compared direct digital radiography (DDR) with sonography and concluded that sonography remains superior in identifying and detecting smaller FBs.

Sonography Equipment

Whenever possible, a 7-to-18-MHz high-resolution, linear array transducer should be used to obtain the images.[12] A large-footprint transducer is generally preferable for initial FB imaging and localization, but a small-footprint transducer may be used when indicated. Maximizing image size by using a large, high-resolution monitor also facilitates FB identification. It may be difficult to identify small FBs on smaller monitors seen on some portable equipment. The visualization of superficial FBs may be facilitated by use of a water bath (Fig. 27-1). When it is necessary to increase the near field length for better visualization of the skin

TABLE 27-1	Composition of Foreign Bodies
Organic	Plant material (thorn, wood, etc.) Animal products (bee stinger, barb, etc.)
Inorganic	Glass, gravel, plastic (acrylic), pencil lead, graphite, and so forth
Metallic	Wire, needle, fish hook, and so forth

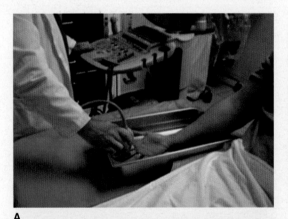

A

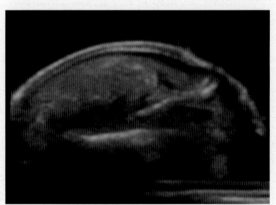

B

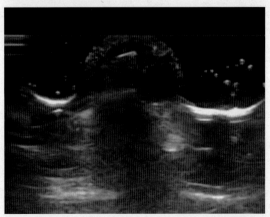

C

FIGURE 27-1 Water bath. **A:** The photograph demonstrates using a water bath to scan the finger. **B:** The sonogram demonstrates a hyperechoic foreign body that was a broken toothpick located in the finger. **C:** Represents the broken tip of a toothpick within a finger along with the original path while immersed in the water bath. (Photo and image **A** and **B:** Courtesy and permission of Robert Tillotson DO, RDMS, FACEP, FAAEM, Stevens Point, WI.)

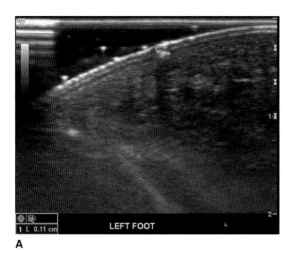

A

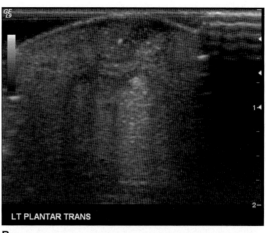

B

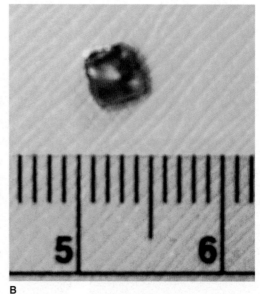

C

FIGURE 27-2 Increase in the near field length can be achieved by using a standoff gel pad or thicker layer of scanning gel, which can help to demonstrate superficial foreign bodies. **A:** On a sonogram of the foot, the punctate, hyperechoic material was diagnosed as gravel. **B:** The transverse sonogram of the left plantar image demonstrates glass as hyperechoic echoes in this foot of a 1-year-old infant. **C:** The transducer-to-skin surface distance of a standoff gel pad is seen on this transverse image, which demonstrates the hyperechoic glass located in the right forehead.

surface and to place a superficial FB in the focal zone, the sonographer can use a standoff gel pad[13-15] or something as simple as a thicker layer of scanning gel[10] (Fig. 27-2).

Imaging Technology

Shadowing and reverberation artifacts are helpful in both identifying and locating an FB. Newer technology does not provide any apparent improvement when imaging FBs and actually may make detection more difficult. Two of these instrumentation selections are tissue harmonics imaging (THI) and instrumentation that uses transmit beam-steering to create multiple imaging angles and then combines these microimages from different viewing angles into a single compounded image. The use of multiple imaging angles reduces shadow artifact, which is an important secondary sign in the detection of FBs (Fig. 27-3).

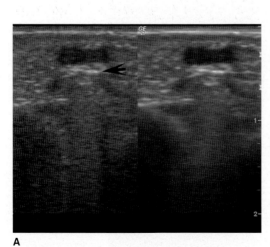

A

B

FIGURE 27-3 **A:** Compare the edge shadowing (*arrow*) and resolution of the glass foreign body of the image on the left made with normal instrumentation and the sonogram on the right made with crossbeam instrumentation. **B:** After removing the glass fragment, the foreign body is seen on the centimeter ruler.

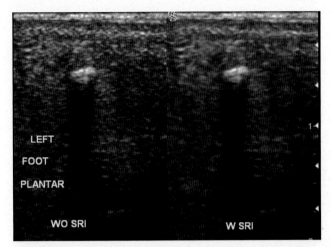

FIGURE 27-4 A toothpick in the plantar surface of the foot is seen on these two images. Compare the foreign body image without speckle reduction (*WO SRI*) to the image with speckle reduction (*W SRI*).

The same is true for THI, where shadowing is diminished or eliminated completely. Only the speckle reduction imaging (SRI) feature has helped improve image quality over normal imaging parameters (Fig. 27-4).

Color and power Doppler imaging may further increase sensitivity because the normal inflammatory reaction materializes in a hypoechoic ring around the FB as a result of hyperemic flow.[16] Color Doppler parameters should be set to visualize slow flow (low velocity) to help determine if reactive hyperemia is present.[16] Varying the transducer angle in relation to the FB will ensure the best color flow image is obtained with the highest Doppler shift.

EVALUATING COMPOSITION, LOCATION, AGE, AND APPEARANCE

Before beginning the imaging examination, the patient interview should be conducted and the patient's chart reviewed. If a radiographic procedure has already been performed, the radiographs should be reviewed. The information that is helpful prior to scanning includes ascertaining the type of material, the mechanism of injury to include the point of entry, and the duration of symptoms.

Composition

The organic FB is the most difficult to locate and is rarely demonstrated on radiography; however, organic FBs are easier to locate and demonstrate on sonography. The echogenic pattern of an organic FB varies with its indwelling age. Some inorganic FBs can be difficult to image using radiography but present little challenge for sonography. Metallic FBs can be seen on radiography and sonography. Metals and most glass are radiopaque (with metals being more radiopaque than glass) and relatively easily seen with radiography (Fig. 27-5).

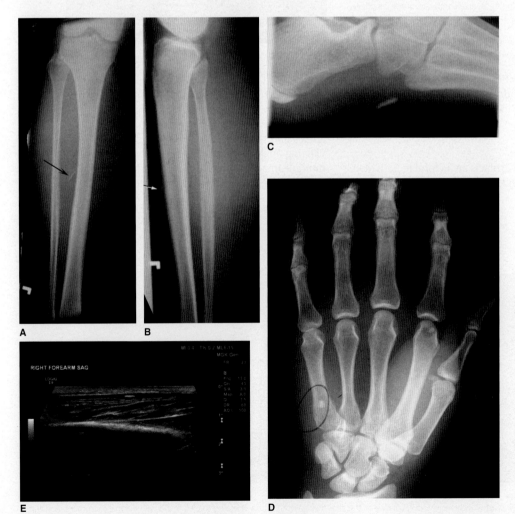

FIGURE 27-5 Metal and most types of glass are radiopaque foreign bodies that can be demonstrated and located on radiographs whereas others are invisible. A metal sewing needle (*arrows*) can be seen in the lower leg on this (**A**) anterior-to-posterior projection and (**B**) the lateral projection of the tibia and fibula. **C:** A glass foreign body is seen on a lateral projection of the plantar surface of the foot. **D:** On a posterior-to-anterior projection of the hand, a glass foreign body (*circle*) is seen near the proximal end of the fifth metacarpal (*circle*). **E:** Ultrasound of a silicone fragment from a broken fish tank injury.

Location

When locating an FB, radiographs should be use if available to provide further information regarding the location, depth, and composition of the FB. When used, radiographs should be obtained in two perpendicular projections (imaging planes) in order to triangulate the location. The FB will only be radiographically visualized if its density is greater than the surrounding soft tissue.

Radiographs may assist in targeting the location for initial insonation. This is especially helpful when external signs such as swelling or redness are not present. A working knowledge of the normal soft-tissue structures can assist in separating normal structures from that of the FB (Fig. 27-6A). By documenting these anatomic structures and their relationship to the FB (veins, arteries, tendons, etc.), the physician can plan the best approach for its removal to diminish postoperative complications[14] (Fig. 27-6B).

The smaller the FB, the more difficult it is to visualize.[17] The depth of an FB will determine the optimal frequency of the transducer. Ideally, the highest frequency possible that allows adequate depth of penetration should be utilized. Every attempt should be made to visualize the FB perpendicular to the transducer to minimize the potential errors in location and position within the soft tissue[14] (Fig. 27-7). When the FB is visualized, its location should be marked on the overlying skin for the physician to use during sonography-guided FB removal.

Age

Based on the duration of symptoms before imaging, the FB may be described in one of three age categories: acute, intermediate, or chronic[18] (Table 27-2). The sonographic appearance of a STFB will correlates with the type and age of the retained material.

In the acute phase, the FB will present as a bright echogenic structure with shadowing, owing to the strong reflection of air in an organic FB, the material composition of an inorganic FB, or the alloy in a metallic FB. The term dirty shadowing is used when the reflection is caused by the refracting properties of small gas bubbles and the high

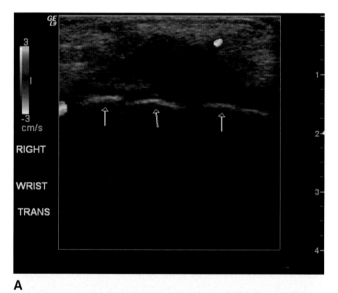

A

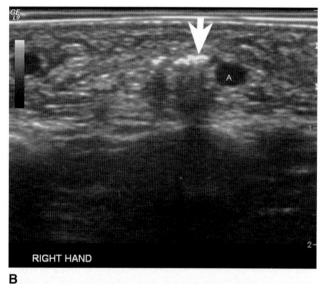

B

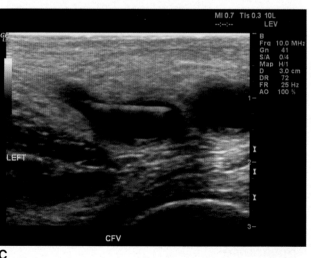

C

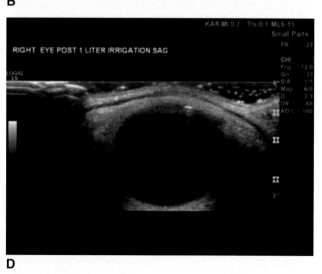

D

FIGURE 27-6 Knowledge soft-tissue structures and anatomic relationships is important to enable differentiating anatomy from a foreign body and to identify the foreign body location. **A:** A transverse sonogram demonstrates three linear echogenic structures (*arrows*). The structures are three right carpal bones but were mistaken for foreign bodies. **B:** A sonogram of the right hand shows the relationship of the foreign body (*arrows*) to an artery (*A*). **C:** Broken needle with the tip still within the vein. **D:** Glass fragment still present under the upper eyelid after copious irrigation.

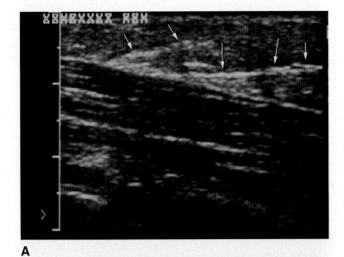

A

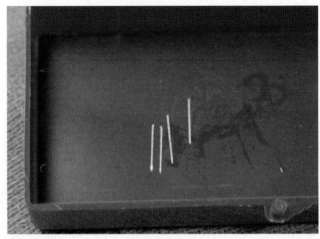

B

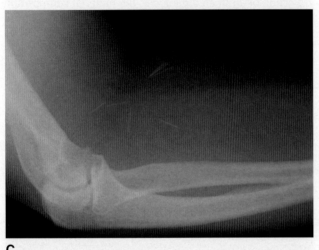

C

FIGURE 27-7 This patient with 26-G hypodermic needles imbedded in her upper forearm presented a difficult challenge. **A:** Imaging perpendicular to the proximal forearm best demonstrated the needles (*arrows*). **B:** The four superficial needles were easily demonstrated and removed. **C:** The lateral view of the right elbows made with fluoroscopy during removal demonstrates six radiopaque needles that were not seen sonographically.

impedance of a gas.[3] The term clean shadowing is used when it is caused by attenuating properties (Fig. 27-8). A potential pitfall usually occurs with a projectile FB when there is air within the wound, which can obscure the visualization of the FB. This may be diminished or avoided by using multiple imaging angles after evaluating the FB with perpendicular beam. After 24 hours from the beginning of the acute phase, a hypoechoic ring develops around the FB, representing an inflammatory reaction to the FB.[19,20] The hypoechoic halo helps locate an FB because it highlights its location[16] (Fig. 27-9).

In the intermediate injury phase with an organic FB, air is slowly replaced with fluid. The sound penetrates through the FB without the shadowing artifact from the air that was present in the acute phase. At this point, the inflammatory response to the FB will appear with a more pronounced hypoechoic halo seen surrounding each type of FB. The

hypoechoic ring can be used to improve both the sensitivity and specificity of the sonography examination.[17] Toward the end of this phase, the inflammatory response increases and the hypoechoic halo surrounding the FB becomes even more pronounced (Fig. 27-10). This inflammatory response may demonstrate an increased vascular perfusion on color or power Doppler.[16]

In the chronic phase, the appearance of the organic FB is similar to the acute phase in that air is replaced by bodily fluid (Fig. 27-11). As the chronic stage progresses, a dense granular material develops encapsulating all three types of FBs. This is the body's response to wall off the foreign material.[20] The inflammatory response can result in a clean shadow similar to that of bone (Fig. 27-12). If the granular material attenuates sound, the FB in this stage may be easier to locate and demonstrate with sonography. When located superficially, the FB and associated granuloma may easily be palpated, aiding in documenting its location.

Appearance

The changing sonographic appearance of retained FBs can assist in their detection and can be used to draw attention to the actual FB itself (Table 27-3). Most FBs are echogenic.

TABLE 27-2	Age of the Foreign Body
Acute phase	Injury less than 3 d
Intermediate phase	Injury within 3–10 d
Chronic phase	Injury more than 10 d

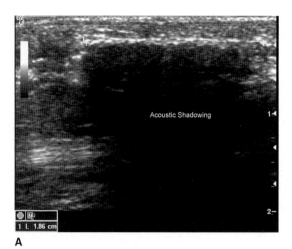

A

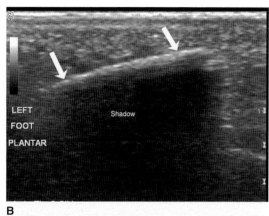

B

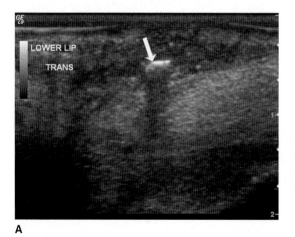

C

FIGURE 27-8 Shadowing. **A:** The linear echogenic foreign body is seen with distal acoustic shadowing. **B:** The sonogram of an acute injury to the plantar surface demonstrates a linear echogenic toothpick (*arrows*) with distal shadowing. **C:** The sonogram of a slanted echogenic foreign body (*arrows*) shows distal clean shadowing (*AS*).

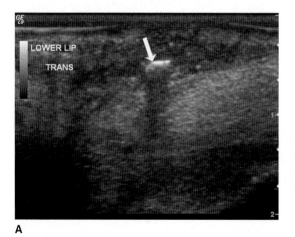

A

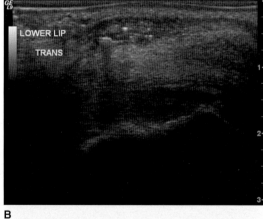

B

C

FIGURE 27-9 Hypoechoic rim. **A:** The transverse sonogram shows a large broken tooth fragment imbedded in the lower lip with surrounding exudation. There is acoustic shadowing distal to the linear echogenic tooth fragment (*arrow*). **B:** On the same patient, a transverse sonogram shows multiple small tooth fragments, which appear echogenic and are located in the lower lip with a surrounding inflammatory process. **C:** On this patient, a transverse sonogram shows the glass foreign body in the forehead with the early formation of a hypoechoic rim.

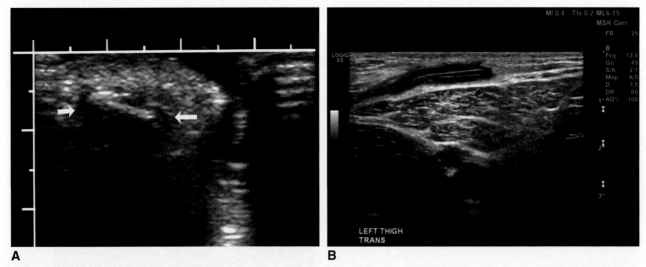

FIGURE 27-10 A: This sonogram demonstrates a linear echogenic wood splinter in the finger with some distal acoustic shadowing. A hypoechoic halo (*arrows*) representing an inflammatory reaction to the foreign body is forming around the wooden foreign body. **B:** Tip of a Spanish bayonet plant with hypoechoic halo.

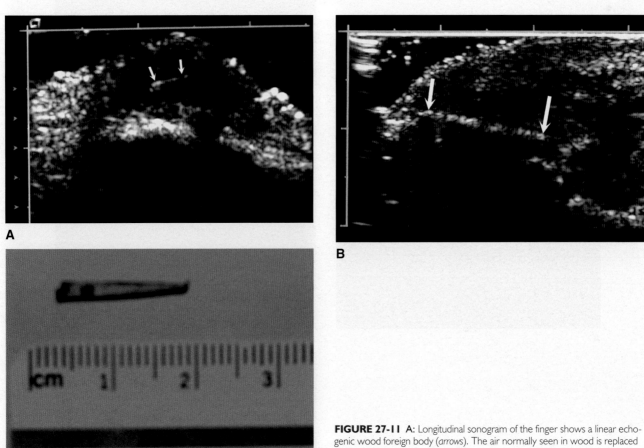

FIGURE 27-11 A: Longitudinal sonogram of the finger shows a linear echogenic wood foreign body (*arrows*). The air normally seen in wood is replaced by fluid, which results in the loss of an acoustical shadow. **B:** On this patient, the sonogram was made on a wooden splinter (*arrows*) in the late intermediate early chronic stage. The splinter loses the acoustic shadow as air owing to fluid replacement. **C:** The 2-cm splinter is seen after removal.

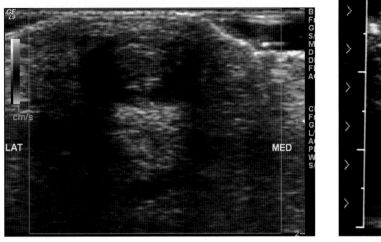

A

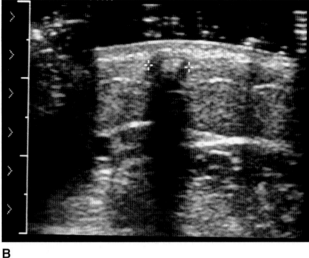

B

FIGURE 27-12 A: The transverse sonogram on the plantar surface shows the formation of a granuloma from a 3-month-old glass foreign body. **B:** This transverse sonogram shows a 5.6-mm granuloma from a retained bee stinger. In this patient, the attenuation by the granular material creates a clean shadow distal to the granuloma and foreign body.

TABLE 27-3	**Appearance of Retained Foreign Bodies**

- Echogenic with clean shadowing
- Echogenic with dirty shadowing
- Echogenic with distal ring down
- Echogenic with hypoechoic ring surrounding it

Artifacts created by FBs may help identify their location. Comet tail artifacts can be seen with both metallic and glass FBs[9,21] (Fig. 27-13). Clean or dirty posterior shadowing may also be seen with an FB or with fragments from an FB of varying thicknesses and shapes. A potential pitfall of relying on shadowing is that air within the soft tissue can mimic the appearance of an FB (Fig. 27-14).

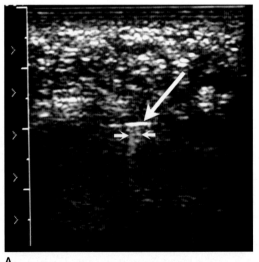

A

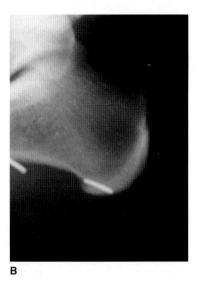

B

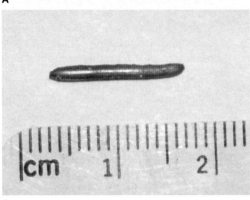

C

FIGURE 27-13 This patient presented with a history of being injured with a wire. **A:** The sonogram shows the wire (*arrow*) located 2-cm deep, posterior, and lateral to the calcaneus. Distal to the wire, the *short arrows* mark the comet tail artifact that is caused by closely spaced reverberation echoes. **B:** The radiopaque wire can be seen on a lateral radiograph of the calcaneus. **C:** The 1.5-cm wire is measured after its removal.

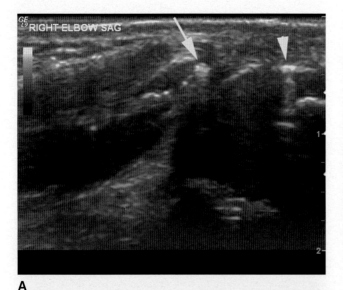

A

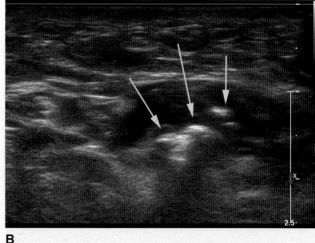

B

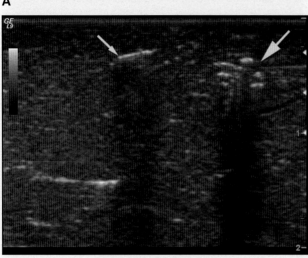

C

FIGURE 27-14 A: The longitudinal sonogram of the right elbow demonstrates glass (*arrow*) embedded in soft tissue near air (*arrowhead*), which can mimic a foreign body. **B:** The air (*arrows*) seen on this sonogram through soft tissue can mimic foreign bodies. **C:** On this sonogram, one can see shadowing from the foreign body (*small arrow*) and from the air (*large arrow*), which was introduced with a lidocaine injection.

SONOGRAPHY-GUIDED FOREIGN BODY REMOVAL

Once located, the depth, size, shape, and orientation or position of the FB should be determined and sonographically documented. A three-dimensional localization should be made by scanning the area of interest in both the longitudinal and transverse orientations, with attention to detecting an FB and imaging any associated posterior acoustic shadowing or reverberation echoes.[13,19,20] It is important to mark the surface of the skin with an indelible marker directly over the FB. To facilitate this, a paper clip may be inserted between the patient and the transducer to create a shadow on the FB. The transducer is then removed and a mark is placed at the skin surface. If the FB is a small square or round BB-sized object, a dot is sufficient to mark its location. If the FB is a linear object like a needle or toothpick, both ends of the FB should be marked and connected by a dotted line. This provides the physician with information regarding which direction to pull out the material (Fig. 27-15).

The location and distance of the FB from an acute entry wound can help the physician determine if removing the FB through the original track is feasible or whether a more direct approach is required. Trauma to the surrounding soft tissue is reduced whenever the FB can be removed through the original injury track. The physician may only need to enlarge the track slightly to provide access for the forceps. Using sonographic guidance for FB removal can result in reducing the size of incision with a less traumatic dissection to find and remove the material.[14] When using direct sonographic imaging to guide the forceps, it may be necessary to use a small-footprint sector transducer in place of a linear transducer (Fig. 27-16).

When an open wound is present, the physician needs to determine if the FB may be removed through the tract it entered. In order to determine the best approach and minimize postoperative complications, the tract's angle and characteristics as well as the surrounding structures and their relationship to the FB should be ascertained. To further assist in the removal of small FBs, a needle or guide wire may be inserted with the tip placed at the FB. This provides a path of dissection through which the FB may be removed[14] (Fig. 27-17). The region adjacent to the FB is anesthetized, a small forceps is placed to the extraction site, and the FB is removed. Some physicians use hydraulic dissection prior to extracting the FB to minimize tissue

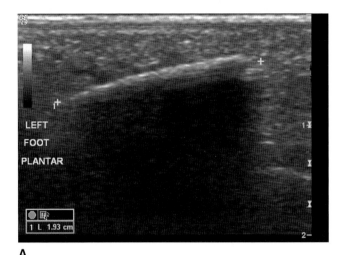

A

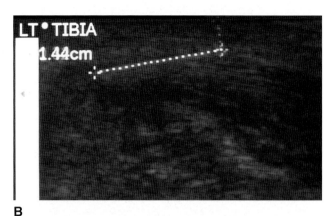

B

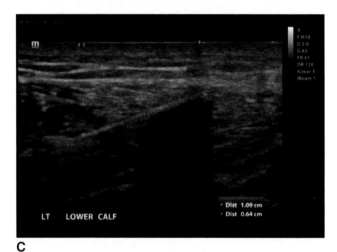

C

FIGURE 27-15 Documenting foreign body location. **A:** The sonographer should annotate the image so the physician can see related anatomy and the angle of the foreign body in relationship to the skin surface. **B:** The annotation should include the length of the foreign body. **C:** The depth of the foreign body in the soft tissue and the skin surface marked.

damage. This is accomplished by injecting fluid along the removal path as well as the location of FB itself. This technique separates the material from soft tissue, allowing the physician to grasp and remove the material with minimal damage to the soft tissue (Pathology Box 27-1).

If the site is old and the original track has closed, determining the FB position can result in a smaller incision

and decreased dissection for its removal. This results in decreased risk of complications as well as a faster recovery period. Untreated or retained FBs can result in inflammation, infection, tendon or nerve injury, and allergic reaction[15,19,22] (Fig. 27-18). Infection is the most common complication with nerve injury a distant second.[2,19] If a patient presents with a history of recurrent localized infections, the patient

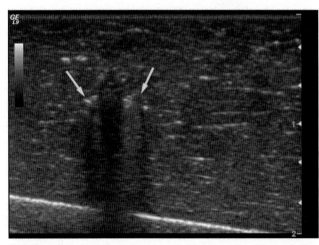

FIGURE 27-16 During sonography-assisted removal, this sonogram shows the forceps (*arrows*) holding a glass fragment prior to removal.

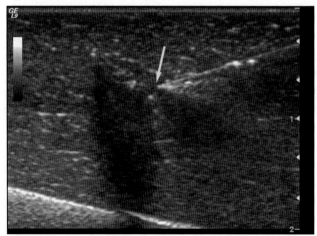

FIGURE 27-17 The sonogram shows the placement of the needle tip (*arrow*) adjacent to a glass fragment.

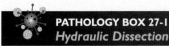

PATHOLOGY BOX 27-1
Hydraulic Dissection

While anesthetizing the extraction site under ultrasound guidance, the physician will inject lidocaine into the soft tissue along the extraction path. This results in less traumatic tissue separation prior to forceps removal of the FB. Another advantage is less air infiltrating the tract, allowing for unobscured ultrasound visualization during its removal.

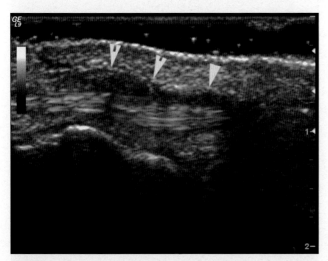

FIGURE 27-18 The longitudinal sonograms show hypoechoic inflammation (*arrows*), surrounding the tendon.

should be asked about recent or remote trauma that may lead to a necessary search for a retained FB.[6]

Once the initial learning curve is overcome, sonographic guidance results in reduced time for FB localization and removal, smaller incisions, and less traumatic dissections.[14] A physician spent 20 minutes in a failed attempt to remove a glass FB seen on the radiograph in Figure 27-5D. On the same patient, the FB was removed in less than 1 minute using the sonography image seen in Figure 27-3A to reveal the FB location and the appropriate path of dissection.

After removal, the site should be reimaged to evaluate if the removal was a complete success. A postremoval sonography evaluation precaution will help prevent retained FBs, which can result in inflammation, infection, tissue injury, and allergic reaction[15,19,22] (Fig. 27-19).

LIMITATIONS OF SONOGRAPHY

Although sonography is effective in localizing FBs, there are limitations to its successful use. The major limitation is that the examination relies on the skill, knowledge, experience, and accuracy of the sonographer. Although sonography has demonstrated superficial FBs less than 2 mm in size, it can be challenging for imaging objects that are smaller and/or not superficially located. FBs may also be obscured by bony structures and air within the wound. Varying the imaging angles can decrease obscuration from bone. Imaging prior to wound exploration or irrigation may decrease the introduction of air bubbles into the field of view. Air within the open cavity or removal site creates difficulty for sonographic imaging because it can mimic the appearance of an FB or obscure an FB. Air is introduced with the injection of a numbing anesthetic such as lidocaine and can result in almost total obliteration of an FB on the sonography image (Fig. 27-20).

False-positive findings can occur as a result of calcifications, scar tissue, fresh hematoma, or air trapped in the soft tissues.[19] Air within the tract created by an FB is seldom a problem for sonography if imaging is performed before any surgical intervention. Small glass fragments can mimic the appearance of air when the wound is still open. With a good understanding of normal anatomic structures, this potential risk with an open wound can

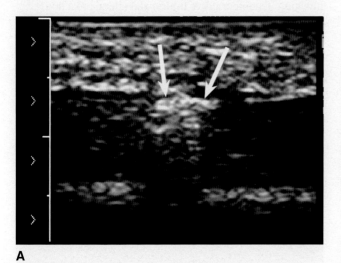

A

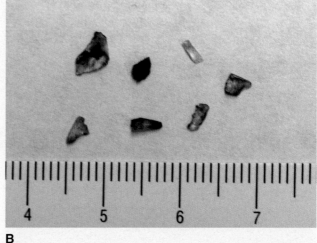

B

FIGURE 27-19 Removing glass from the forearm. **A:** After sonography-guided removal of three small glass shards, the rescanning of the area showed that foreign bodies (*arrows*) were still present. **B:** Seven more glass shards were eventually removed.

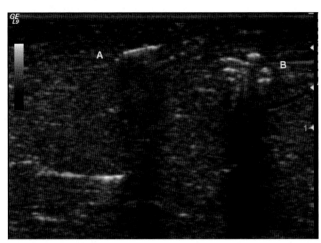

FIGURE 27-20 The sonogram on the left (*A*) shows a glass foreign body as a linear echogenic structure in the tissue with some distal attenuation. Following injection with lidocaine, the sonogram on the right (*B*) shows air bubbles interfering with visualizing the glass foreign body. Note the distal acoustic shadowing.

be minimized (Fig. 27-20). Prior unsuccessful attempts at removing an FB can result in scar tissue that can distort the normal anatomic structures, making a definitive identification problematic.

COMPARING IMAGING MODALITIES

Conventional radiography is capable of visualizing metal, glass, and stone in bone, muscle, and air but is limited to demonstrating graphite only in muscle.[23] Most organic and inorganic FBs are radiolucent and cannot be visualized on radiography in bone, muscle, or air.

On a CT image, wood is poorly seen and difficult to image in muscle, but it may be seen in the presence of air[23] (Fig. 27-21A, B). CT imaging does detect metal, glass, stone, and graphite in bone and muscle. The greatest advantage of CT over conventional radiography or sonography is its capability of demonstrating FBs in air.[23] CT scanning is a more expensive imaging procedure, uses ionizing radiation, and may require sedation when used with pediatric patients.[19]

MRI is of limited use in the early detection of an FBs because the modality is more expensive and its availability is more limited. For safety reasons, MRI should not be used for metallic FBs and other unknown types of FBs. The usefulness of MRI in FB evaluation is in providing detailed information regarding tissue inflammatory reactions, osteoblastic or osteolytic changes, and secondary tissue reactions that can aid in determining the presence and location of an otherwise occult FB.[24]

Sonography has been proven more effective and less expensive than CT imaging, eliminating the problem of radiation exposure.[9] The widespread availability and low cost of sonography make it the best choice for determining the presence of FBs. Sonographic imaging may not be utilized because of a lack of knowledge, experience, and confidence with sonographic findings, which prompt physicians to order imaging procedures.[18] The American College of Emergency Physicians published guidelines recognizing FB detection and removal as a unique and evolving application of emergency sonography.[25] Sonography should become the main imaging tool used for the detection and localization of STFBs because of its sensitivity compared with the lack of sensitivity of other imaging modalities, because it is noninvasive compared with ionizing radiation or magnet safety seen in other modalities, and because it provides a high-resolution, real-time evaluation.[10,14,26]

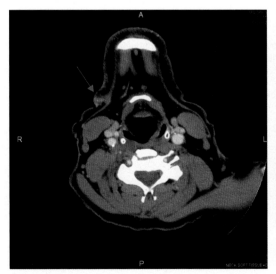

A

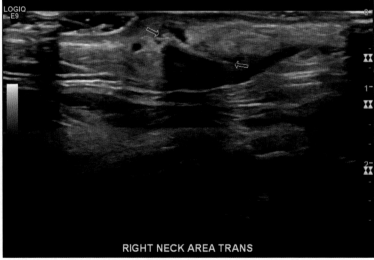

B

FIGURE 27-21 Comparison of computed tomography (CT) and sonography demonstrating the same wood tree splinter in the neck of a professional tree trimmer. **A:** CT scan of the splinter (*arrow*) located in the patient's neck inferior to the right mandibular ramus. **B:** Sonogram of the same splinter.

SUMMARY

- Sonographer and clinician awareness to use sonography for STFB recognition, localization, and removal may result in decreased diagnostic expense and increased diagnostic accuracy.
- When using high-frequency transducers to obtain high-resolution imaging, sonography is sensitive and specific for the detection of STFBs, which has been demonstrated in vivo[11,12] and in vitro.[5,24]
- Sonography examinations rely on the skill, knowledge, and accuracy of the sonographer who pays attention to the composition, location, age, and artifacts associated with FBs.
- The experienced sonographer has an important role prior to, during, and following sonography-guided FB removal.
- Recognizing FB detection and removal is a unique and evolving application of emergency sonography.
- Sonography should become the main imaging tool used for the detection and localization of STFBs because of its sensitivity, because it is noninvasive, and because it provides a high-resolution, real-time evaluation.

REFERENCES

1. Manthey DE, Storrow AB, Milbourn JM, et al. Ultrasound versus radiography in the detection of soft-tissue foreign bodies. *Ann Emerg Med.* 1996;28:7–9.
2. Anderson MA, Newmeyer WL, Kilgore ES Jr. Diagnosis and treatment of retained foreign bodies in the hand. *Am J Surg.* 1982;144:63–67.
3. Lyon M, Brannam L, Johnson D, et al. Detection of soft tissue foreign bodies in the presence of soft tissue gas. *J Ultrasound Med.* 2004;23:677–681.
4. Dunn JD. Risk management in emergency medicine. *Emerg Med Clin North Am.* 1987;5:51–69.
5. Schlager D, Sanders AB, Wiggins D, et al. Ultrasound for the detection of foreign bodies. *Ann Emerg Med.* 1991;20:189–191.
6. Bass AM, Levis JT. wound foreign body removal. *Medscape: eMedicine.* January 2010. Accessed August 8, 2010. http://emedicine.medscape.com/article/1508207-overview
7. Pfaff JA, Moore GP. Reducing risk in emergency department wound management. *Emerg Med Clin North Am.* 2007;25:189–201.
8. Bray PW, Mahoney JL, Campbell JP. Sensitivity and specificity of ultrasound in the diagnosis of foreign bodies in the hand. *J Hand Surg Am.* 1995;20:661–666.
9. Gilbert FJ, Campbell RS, Bayliss AP. The role of ultrasound in the detection of non-radiopaque foreign bodies. *Clin Radiol.* 1990;41:109–112.
10. Jacobson JA, Powell A, Craig JG, et al. Wooden foreign bodies in soft tissue: detection at US. *Radiology.* 1998;206:45–48.
11. Mecado LNS, Hayre CM. The detection of wooden foreign bodies: an experimental study comparing direct digital radiography (DDR) and ultrasonography. *Radiography.* 2018;24(4):340–344.
12. Rooks VJ, Sheils WE, Murakami JW. Soft tissue foreign bodies: a training manual for sonographic diagnosis and guided removal. *J Clin Ultrasound.* 2020;48(6):330–336.
13. Fornage BD, Schernberg FL. Sonographic diagnosis of foreign bodies of the distal extremities. *Am J Roentgenol.* 1986;147:567–569.
14. Shiels WE II, Babcock DS, Wilson JL, et al. Localization and guided removal of soft-tissue foreign bodies with sonography. *Am J Roentgenol.* 1990;155:1277–1281.
15. Soudack M, Nachtigal A, Gaitini D. Clinically unsuspected foreign bodies: the importance of sonography. *J Ultrasound Med.* 2003;22:1381–1385.
16. Davae KC, Sofka CM, DiCarlo E, et al. Value of power Doppler imaging and hypoechoic halo in the sonographic detection of foreign bodies: correlation with histopathologic findings. *J Ultrasound Med.* 2003;22:1309–1313.
17. Jarraya M, Hayashi D, de Villiers RV, Roemer FW, Murakami AM, Cossi A, Guermazi A. Multimodality imaging of foreign bodies of the musculoskeletal system. *Am J Roentgenol.* 2014;203(1):92–102.
18. Gibbs TS. The use of sonography in the identification and removal of soft tissue foreign bodies. *J Diagn Med Sonogr.* 2006;22:5–21.
19. Boyse TD, Fessell DP, Jacobson JA, et al. US of soft-tissue foreign bodies and associated complication with surgical correlation. *Radiographics.* 2001;21:1251–1256.
20. Saboo SS, Saboo SH, Soni SS, et al. High-resolution sonography is effective in detection of soft tissue foreign bodies: experience from a rural Indian center. *J Ultrasound Med.* 2009;28:1245–1249.
21. Ziskin MC, Thickman DI, Goldenberg NJ, et al. The comet tail artifact. *J Ultrasound Med.* 1982;1:1–7.
22. De La Torre C, Toribio J. Sea-urchin granuloma: histologic profile. A pathologic study of 50 biopsies. *J Cutan Pathol.* 2001;28:223–228.
23. Aras MH, Miloglu O, Barutcugil C, et al. Comparison of the sensitivity for detecting foreign bodies among conventional plain radiography, computed tomography, and ultrasonography. *Dentomaxillofac Radiol.* 2010;39:72–78.
24. Voss JO, Maier C, Wüster J, et al. Imaging foreign bodies in head and neck trauma: a pictorial review. *Insights Imaging.* 2021;12(1):20.
25. American College of Emergency Physicians. Emergency ultrasound guidelines. *Ann Emerg Med.* 2009;53:550–570.
26. Gooding GA, Hardiman T, Sumers M, et al. Sonography of the hand and foot in foreign body detection. *J Ultrasound Med.* 1987;6:441–447.

Note: Page numbers followed by "*b*," "*f*," and "*t*" denotes boxes, figures, and tables respectively.